UVEITIS

Commissioning Editor: *Russell Gabbedy*
Development Editor: *Sharon Nash*
Editorial Assistant: *Poppy Garraway*
Project Manager: *Gopika Sasidharan*
Design: *Stewart Larking*
Illustration Manager: *Bruce Hogarth*
Illustrator: *Martin Woodward*
Multimedia Producer: *Fraser Johnston*
Marketing Manager(s) (UK/USA): *Richard Jones/Helena Mutak*

UVEITIS

FUNDAMENTALS AND CLINICAL PRACTICE

Fourth Edition

Robert B. Nussenblatt, MD, MPH
Chief, Laboratory of Immunology, National Eye Institute
Acting Scientific Director, National Center
for Complimentary and Alternative Medicine
Centre for Human Immunology, Clinical Centre
National Institutes of Health
Bethesda, Maryland

Scott M. Whitcup, MD
Executive Vice President
Head, Research and Development
Chief Scientific Officer
Allergan, Inc.
Irvine, California

Department of Ophthalmology
Jules Stein Eye Institute
David Geffen School of Medicine at the University of
California, Los Angeles
Los Angeles, California

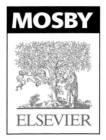

MOSBY

ELSEVIER

is an imprint of Elsevier Inc.

First edition 1989
Second edition 1996
Third edition 2004

Notices
Knowledge and best practice in this field are constantly changing. As new research and experience broaden our understanding, changes in research methods, professional practices, or medical treatment may become necessary. Practitioners and researchers must always rely on their own experience and knowledge in evaluating and using any information, methods, compounds, or experiments described herein. In using such information or methods they should be mindful of their own safety and the safety of others, including parties for whom they have a professional responsibility.

With respect to any drug or pharmaceutical products identified, readers are advised to check the most current information provided (i) on procedures featured or (ii) by the manufacturer of each product to be administered, to verify the recommended dose or formula, the method and duration of administration, and contraindications. It is the responsibility of practitioners, relying on their own experience and knowledge of their patients, to make diagnoses, to determine dosages and the best treatment for each individual patient, and to take all appropriate safety precautions.

To the fullest extent of the law, neither the Publisher nor the authors, contributors, or editors, assume any liability for any injury and/or damage to persons or property as a matter of products liability, negligence or otherwise, or from any use or operation of any methods, products, instructions, or ideas contained in the material herein.

ISBN: 978-1-4377-0677-3
British Library Cataloguing in Publication Data

Nussenblatt, Robert B.
   Uveitis : fundamentals and clinical practice. – 4th ed. – (Expert consult. Online and print)
   1. Uveitis.
   I. Title   II. Series   III. Whitcup, Scott M.
   617.7'2 – dc22

   ISBN-13: 9781437706673

Library of Congress Cataloging in Publication Data
A catalog record for this book is available from the Library of Congress

your source for books,
journals and multimedia
in the health sciences

www.elsevierhealth.com

Working together to grow
libraries in developing countries

www.elsevier.com | www.bookaid.org | www.sabre.org

ELSEVIER   BOOK AID International   Sabre Foundation

The
publisher's
policy is to use
**paper manufactured
from sustainable forests**

Printed in China
Last digit is the print number: 9 8 7 6 5 4 3 2 1

Contents

PART 5: UVEITIC CONDITIONS NOT CAUSED BY ACTIVE INFECTION

Foreword

Since the last edition of this book in 2004, there again has been tremendous progress in understanding the basis for intraocular inflammation, and a number of novel immunotherapies for autoimmune diseases has become available for physicians. Advances in immunology, molecular biology, cell biology, imaging, and other aspects of the biomedical sciences continue to foster new approaches to the study of inflammatory diseases, both in the eye and in the rest of the body. Nevertheless, the diagnosis and treatment of uveitis remains a significant challenge for ophthalmologists and other health care practitioners.

Fortunately, scientific advances have led to improvements in our ability to study the disease and optimize the way we approach the patient with uveitis. Genetic studies have identified new pathogenic mechanisms of ocular inflammation. Since the last edition of this book, these studies have implicated the complement pathway in the pathogenesis of age-related macular degeneration. New diagnostic and analytical tools, including advances in ocular coherence tomography have improved the way we diagnose patients and assess their response to therapy.

I have had the opportunity to work closely with Dr. Whitcup and Dr. Nussenblatt for more than two decades. Both are widely recognized as leading authorities in the field of uveitis. The fourth edition of Uveitis: Fundamentals and Clinical Practice remains the authoritative text and will be of great use to ophthalmologists and other doctors who see and manage patients with ocular inflammatory disease. The book remains unique—it is not only a thorough review of the basic and clinical science of uveitis but also a practical guide to the diagnosis and management of patients with inflammatory eye disease.

In Part 1, the authors start with a thorough discussion of the fundamentals of inflammation and review the immunology of uveitis. In Part 2, they provide an organized description of the diagnostic approach to the patient with ocular inflammation. The ophthalmic history and examination, diagnostic testing, and guides to developing a differential diagnosis are reviewed. This section also provides an insight into the evaluation of the uveitis literature. In Part 3, the authors offer the reader a thorough approach to the medical and surgical therapy of uveitis, followed by a section on infectious uveitic conditions in Part 4, and 13 chapters related to diseases and syndromes of uveitis in Part 5.

The chapters are definitive yet practical reviews on their individual topics and they are well integrated to cover the entire field with few omissions and little duplication. Chapters are well-illustrated and this edition has been newly formatted with color figures and photographs throughout the text. For example, the chapter on acquired immunodeficiency syndrome (AIDS) remains comprehensive, up to date, yet readable. Results from important clinical trials are succinctly summarized. There is an excellent presentation of cases and photographs that emphasize both the disorder and the treatment of patients with ocular complications of AIDS.

There have been a number of important additions and updates to this new edition. In addition to the chapter on AIDS, the chapter on medical therapy has been extensively updated and reviews a number of new therapeutic approaches to patients with inflammatory disease, including biologic agents that block tumor necrosis factor. Dr. Whitcup has expanded the discussion of bacterial and fungal causes of uveitis, and this is now divided into two chapters, Chapters 9 and 10, and has added a discussion of evidence-based medicine in the section on diagnosis. Dr. Nussenblatt has written a new chapter discussing the role of inflammation in other retinal diseases including age-related macular degeneration and diabetic retinopathy. In addition to new color illustrations throughout the book, key concepts have been added to each chapter to focus the reader on the key take-home messages.

The authors have divided this edition of the book into 31 chapters and brought each of their individual strengths into this partnership. They worked together for almost a decade at the National Eye Institute, and their cohesive approach to uveitis benefits the reader. The scholarship and experience of the authors provide a unified textbook that can be read cover to cover, or used as a reference guide that is at the forefront of clinical medicine. Each chapter is authoritatively presented, well-illustrated, and practical. The authors have again given us an excellent textbook on uveitis, which ophthalmologists and other practitioners will find useful in taking care of their patients. This is a book which will be frequently used by clinicians and will improve the care of the challenging patient with uveitis.

Stephen J. Ryan, MD
President
Doheny Eye Institute
Grace and Emory Beardsley Professor of Ophthalmology
Keck School of Medicine of the University of
Southern California (USC)

Preface

The 21st century may be remembered as the true golden age of medicine. Advances in molecular biology, immunology, pharmacology, and drug discovery that began and matured over the last 50 years will lead to substantive changes in the way we diagnose and treat our patients with uveitis in the decades to come. Prior to 1950, treatment for uveitis was severely limited. Many physicians treated patients with uveitis by inducing hyperpyrexia. Patients were placed into steam baths where their temperatures were raised to 40 to 41 degrees centigrade for four to six hours. Although occasionally successful, Sir Stewart Duke-Elder did note that the treatment was poorly tolerated and often dangerous for the patient. In 1949 Philip Hench and colleagues reported the successful use of corticosteroids for the treatment of rheumatoid arthritis. Ophthalmologists were quick to use corticosteroids for the treatment of ocular inflammatory disease, and interestingly, despite profound improvements in immunotherapy, steroids remain the mainstay of therapy even today.

However, many patients remain resistant or become intolerant to corticosteroid therapy. Spawned by the need for better immunosuppression for transplant surgery, a number of new and effective immunosuppressive agents have been developed. More recently, a number of novel immunologic therapies have aided physicians in the treatment of autoimmune disease. Drugs that specifically target cytokines and cytokine receptors are now commonly used in the treatment of diseases such as rheumatoid arthritis and increasingly employed in the treatment of severe uveitis. Intravitreal injections and sustained-release intravitreal implants have allowed physicians to deliver high amounts of drugs to target tissues in the eye while avoiding systemic side effects. Nevertheless, the cause of many forms of uveitis remains unknown, and vision loss is still an all too common occurrence in our patients.

Even since the publication of the third edition of our book, there have been a number of significant advances in basic science, technology, and clinical medicine that impact our approach to uveitis. First, the field of immunology continues to move forward. New cytokines and inflammatory pathways have led to a better understanding of disease pathogenesis and novel therapeutic targets. The roles of IL-23 and Th17 cells in autoimmune disease and uveitis have been described and new therapies are being developed that target this pathway. Second, new technologies are changing the way we diagnose and follow our patients. Ocular coherence tomography is now commonly used to evaluate macular edema and assess the response to therapy. PCR is more frequently used to diagnose infectious etiologies for uveitis and allow specific antimicrobial therapy for patients who were previously misdiagnosed. Third, we have new therapies in our armamentaria, including novel immunosuppressive agents and biologics that target key inflammatory cytokines, cell adhesion molecules, inflammatory cells, or other critical components of the inflammatory response. Fourth, advances in drug delivery allow us to administer high amounts of drugs directly to the diseased tissues and minimize systemic exposure and treatment-limiting side effects.

The goal of this fourth edition of Uveitis: Fundamentals and Clinical Practice remains the same as that of the first three – to provide a comprehensive text presenting a practical approach to the diagnosis and treatment of various forms of the disease. The book includes a review of the fundamentals of ocular immunology but focuses on the clinical aspects of the disease. We believe that our book will be of value not only to ophthalmologists, optometrists, and other eye care providers, but also to internists, rheumatologists, and other physicians who see patients with diseases associated with uveitis.

Again, the text is divided into five parts. Part 1 includes a single chapter on the immunology of uveitis. Part 2 on diagnosis includes detailed discussion of the medical history, clinical examination, and diagnostic testing in the patient with uveitis. Part 3 includes two chapters covering the medical and surgical therapy of uveitis. In Part 4, uveitic syndromes with known infectious etiologies are reviewed. In Part 5, a number of other uveitic diseases and syndromes are included – some which may have an infectious etiology that has not been elucidated. With improvements in our diagnostic testing, we are identfying specific infections as the cause for more forms of uveitis. We now know that *Tropheryma whipllei* causes Whipple's disease, and the section on uveitis associated with this disease has now been moved from the chapter on anterior uveitis to the chapter on bacterial and fungal diseases. Finally, we have added a chapter on the role of inflammation in diseases other than uveitis, including macular degeneration.

We have based this book, to a large extent, on our clinical experience, both at the National Eye Institute where both of us spent time seeing patients together, and at the Jules Stein Eye Institute. We owe a great deal of thanks to Alan Palestine who helped make the first edition of the book a reality and continue to express our gratitude to Chi-Chao Chan, Igal Gery, and Rachel Caspi for their knowledge and friendship and to our fellows for their inquisitiveness and comradeship. We must also thank the photographers of the National Eye Institute and a number of our colleagues for obtaining the artful clinical photographs. Importantly, we must thank our patients who value the opportunity to contribute to the understanding of their disease in an attempt to help others.

Finally, we thank our families and friends for their support and tolerance in allowing us to work on yet another edition of the book.

Scott & Bob

Dedication

To Rosine, Veronique, Valerie, and Eric.
Bob

I would like to dedicate this book to my father whose love, support, humor, and inquisitiveness will always be a part of me; and to my family and friends.
Scott

For our colleagues and patients.

Acknowledgments

We would like to thank the photographers and ophthalmic technicians of the National Eye Institute for their assistance in obtaining photographs, angiograms, and other materials for the book. We also want to thank our colleagues who supplied outstanding images that help to bring our text to life.

Elements of the Immune System and Concepts of Intraocular Inflammatory Disease Pathogenesis

Robert B. Nussenblatt

Key concepts

- T cells play an important role in the pathogenesis of uveitis.
- The eye is very active immunologically, with ocular resident cells interacting with the immune system.
- Uveitogenic antigens are found in the eye, and immunization of animals with these antigens induces experimental uveitis, often resembling the human condition.
- Similar immune responses can be seen in the experimental models of uveitis as in the human condition.

In an ever-changing field, a review of the immune system is the subject of numerous books, courses, and scientific articles. However, certain principles have been established that, in the main, have survived the test of time and rigorous scrutiny. The aim of this chapter is to provide the reader with the essentials needed to follow a discussion on mechanisms proposed for intraocular inflammatory disease; therefore, topics relevant to the understanding of that subject are addressed. In addition, selected themes thought to be important in understanding the unique ocular immune environment and pathogenesis are covered. It is clear to any observer of immunology that a detailed description of immune events would be far beyond the scope of this book, and it would hubris to think otherwise. For those well versed in this field, parts of this chapter may be somewhat superfluous.

The development of the immune system is an extraordinary product of evolution. Its goal is to recognize that which is different from self, so its initial role is to respond to foreign antigens with an innate immune response that is geared to rapidly clear the body of the foreign invader. 'Innate immunity' is restricted to the non-antigen-specific immune response involving phagocytic cells that engulf and destroy invaders, humoral factors such as the complement system and receptors on antigen-presenting cells such as phagocytes called 'toll-like receptors' that interact with the invaders' molecules. This activates the antigen-presenting cell to initiate the 'adaptive' immune response. Clearly the invader may return, and so the adaptive immune response is in place to respond. The adaptive immune response is antigen specific and deals with the invaders that escaped the innate immune mechanism or have returned. The adaptive immune response consists of both B and T cells, and portions of these populations acquire the properties of memory cells of the secondary immune response. This adaptive immune response connotes an immune memory, hence the development of a complex way in which high-affinity molecules and cell-surface markers can distinguish between the invader and self. A given of this concept is that self antigens are not attacked: that is, an immune tolerance exists. Part of our story deals with the immune system's appropriate response to outside invaders (such as *Toxoplasma*) and the other part deals with understanding (and trying to explain) the response to autoantigens. The dynamic is not as simple as outlined; in fact, it starts as an appropriate response to a foreign antigen and then changes to an abnormal response against the eye. Many mechanisms, such as molecular mimicry, have been proposed.

To achieve this complex but highly specific immune response requires multiple players. Some of these are reviewed in the first part of this chapter. In the second part findings and theories of disease mechanisms relevant to the ocular diseases discussed in later chapters are introduced.

Elements of the immune system

The immune system is the result of several cell types, including lymphocytes (T and B cells), macrophages, and polymorphonuclear cells. However, additional cells, such as dendritic cells in the skin and spleen and ocular resident cells in the eye, also should be included. These components add up to a complex immune circuitry or 'ballet,' which in the vast number of individuals responds in a way that is beneficial to the organism.

Macrophages/monocytes

Phagocytic cells originate in the bone marrow. The concept that phagocytosis is important for the immunologic defense of the organism was proposed by Metchnikoff at the end of the nineteenth century. The macrophage, which is relatively large (15 µm), has an abundant smooth and rough endoplasmic reticulum. Lysosomal granules and a well-developed Golgi apparatus are also found. Several functional, histochemical, and morphologic characteristics of these cells can be noted (**Table 1-1**). In addition to the phagocytic

*The author thanks Drs William Paul and Igal Gery for reviewing this chapter. The helpful parts of the chapter are due to their good and wise counsel. The parts that are less so are due to my own shortcomings. RBN

Table 1-1 Macrophage characteristics

Histochemical	Surface Antigens	Receptors	Functions
5′-Nucleotidase	OKM1	Fc	Phagocytosis
Esterase	Class II antigens	IgM	Pinocytosis
Alkaline phosphodiesterase		Lymphokine	Immune activation
Aminopeptidase		Lactoferrin	Secretory
Insulin			Microbicidal
		Cb3	Tumoricidal
		Fibrinogen	
		Lipoprotein	

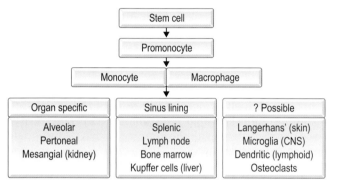

Figure 1-1. Macrophage differentiation.

characteristics already alluded to, these cells contain esterases and peroxidases, and bear membrane markers that are typical of their cell line (i.e., OKM1 antigen and F4/80). Other cell-surface markers are also present, such as class II antigens, Fc receptors (for antibody), and receptors for complement. These enzymes and cell markers help to identify this class of cells as well as their state of activation. The presence of esterase is a useful marker to distinguish macrophages from granulocytes and lymphocytes. Monocytes will leave the bloodstream because of either a predetermined maturational process or induced migration into an area as a result of chemotactic substances, often produced during inflammatory events. Once having taken up residence in various tissues, they become macrophages, which are frequently known by other names (**Fig. 1-1**). Dendritic cells, such as Langerhans' cells, are found in the skin and cornea, and play an important role in activating naive lymphocytes.

Macrophages play at least three major roles within the immune system. The first is to directly destroy foreign pathogens as well as clearing dying or diseased tissue. Killing of invading microbes is in part mediated by a burst of hydrogen peroxide (H_2O_2) activity by the activated macrophage. An example with ocular importance is the engulfment of the toxoplasmosis organism, with the macrophage often being a repository for this parasite if killing is inadequate. The second is to activate the immune system. Macrophages or other cells with similar characteristics are mandatory for antigen-specific activation of T lymphocytes. Internalizing and processing of the antigen by the macrophage are thought

to be integral parts of this mechanism, and the macrophage (or dendritic cell) is often described as an antigen-presenting cell (APC). Other cells, such as B cells, can also serve this function. The macrophage and lymphocyte usually need to be in close contact with one another for this transfer to occur. Another requirement is for the cells to have in common a significant portion of their major histocompatibility complex (MHC), genes that express various cell-surface membranes essential for cellular communication and function. Thus this MHC stimulation leads to the initiation of an immune response, ultimately with both T and B cells potentially participating. Other cell-surface markers are needed for activation. This 'two-signal' theory has centered on other cell-surface antigens, such as the B7–CD28 complex. The engagement of B7 (on the macrophage side) with CD28 enhances the transcription of cytokine genes. Third, the macrophage is a potent secretory cell. Proteases can be released in abundance, which can degrade vessel surfaces and perivascular areas. Degradation products that result from these reactions are chemotactic and further enhance an immune response. Interleukin (IL)-1, a monokine with a molecular weight of 15 000 Da, is produced by the macrophage (as well as other cells) after interaction with exogenous pathogens or internal stimuli, such as immune complexes or T cells. IL-1 release directly affects T-cell growth and aids this cell in releasing its own secretory products. IL-1 is noted to act directly on the central nervous system, with a by-product being the induction of fever. Still other macrophage products stimulate fibroblast migration and division, all of which have potentially important consequences in the eye.

Macrophages produce IL-12 and IL-18 (once called interferon (IFN)-γ-inducing factor), IL-10, and transforming growth factor (TGF)-β. In a feedback mechanism, IFN-γ can activate macrophages, and the production of IL-12 by the macrophage plays an important role in T-cell activation. The role of macrophages in the eye still needs to be fully explored. One concept (in a disease not usually thought of as being immune driven) is that chronically activated macrophages congregate at the level of the retinal pigment epithelium (RPE), inducing the initial changes that lead to age-related macular degeneration.

Dendritic cells

Although macrophages play an important role, it is conjectured that dendritic cells are important macrophage-like cells in tissue. They are a subset of cells, perhaps of different lineage from macrophages, from which they can be distinguished by a lack of persistent adherence and by the bearing of an antigen, 33D1, on their surface, features that macrophages do not possess. The major role of dendritic cells is to serve as initiators of T-cell responses, for both CD4+ and CD8+ cells. Like macrophages, dendritic cells produce IL-12, an important activator of T-cell responsiveness. They are rich in MHC II intracellular compartments, an important factor in antigen presentation. The MHC class II compartments will move to the surface of the cell when the dendritic cell matures, stimulated by IFN-α and the CD40 ligand. Dendritic cells are special in that they inhabit tissues where foreign antigens may enter. Experiments with painting of the skin brought seminal observations. Antigens painted on the skin are 'brought' to the draining lymph nodes by the dendritic cells of the skin (Langerhans' cells) where T-cell activation can occur. What is interesting is the migratory nature of these cells: they constantly carry important information to peripheral centers of the immune response. Whether dendritic APCs can activate T cells efficiently in the tissues themselves is an open question and is important to our understanding of immune responses in the eye. Dendritic cells are thought to be the APCs (or one of the major players) in corneal graft rejection. Thus the concept of removing dendritic cells from a graft has been proposed and used in experimental models. However, there is an opposing concept that peripheral immune tolerance, induced by antigens that foster programmed cell death (apoptosis), may depend on presentation of antigen bydendritic cells in the tissue.

T cells

T cells are found in large numbers in the systemic circulation. Lymphocytes are broadly divided into two major categories, T cells and B cells (discussed later). These appellations are based on initial observations in chickens, in which a subgroup of lymphocytes homed to the thymus, where they underwent a maturational process leading to the heterogeneous population now recognized as 'thymus-dependent' or T cells. The thymus, the first lymphoid organ to develop, has essentially two compartments, the cortex and the medulla. Within the thymus are found epithelial cells, thymocytes (immature lymphocytes), occasional macrophages, and more mature lymphocytes. The highly cellular cortex is the center of mitoses, with large numbers of immature thymocytes and epithelial cells adhering to each other. As the thymocytes mature to T cells they migrate to the medulla and are ultimately released into the systemic circulation. Major alterations occur to the thymocyte during this maturational process. There is the activation of specific genes needed for only this portion of the lifecycle of the cells. In addition, lifelong characteristics are acquired. These include the development of specific receptors that recognize particular antigens, the acquisition of MHC restriction needed for proper immune interactions, and the acquisition of various T-cell functions, such as 'killing' and 'helping' other cells. These cells are activated by a complex of structures on their surface. The T-cell receptor (specific to the antigen that is being presented to the cell), the CD3 complex, and the antigen cradled in either an MHC class I or II cassette are needed. Other cofactors are also needed for very robust activation.

Some important qualities possessed by these cells are their immunologic recall or anamnestic capacity; this increases the number of specific cells as well as changing them into a 'memory' phenotype. They also have the capacity to produce cellular products called cytokines (**Table 1-2**). A T cell previously sensitized to a particular antigen can retain this immunologic memory (see below) essentially for its lifetime. With a repeat encounter, this memory response leads to an immune response that is more rapid and more pronounced than the first. Such an example is the positive skin response seen after purified protein derivative (PPD) testing.

The central role of the T cell in the immune system cannot be overemphasized. T cells function as pivotal modulators of the immune response, particularly by helping B-cell production of antibody and augmenting cell-mediated reactions through further recruitment of immunoreactive cells. T cells also may downregulate or prevent immune reactions through active suppression. In addition to these 'managerial' types of roles, some T-cell subsets are known to be cytotoxic and are recognized as belonging to the predominant cells in transplantation rejection crises. The accumulated evidence supports the importance of T cells in many aspects of the intraocular inflammatory process – from the propagation of disease to its subsequent downregulation.

Major subsets of T cells

The functions that have been briefly described are now thought to be carried out by at least three major subsets of T cells, with these cells identified either through functional studies or through monoclonal antibodies directed against antigens present on their surface. It was observed early on that T cells (as well as other cells) manifest myriad different molecules on their surface membranes, some of which are expressed uniquely at certain periods of cell activation or function. It was noted that certain monoclonal antibodies directed against these unique proteins bind to specific subsets of cells, thereby permitting a way to identify them (**Table 1-3**). The antibodies to the CD3 antigen (e.g., OKT3) are directed against an antigen found on all mature human T cells in the circulation; approximately 70–80% of lymphocytes in the systemic circulation bear this marker. Antibodies to the CD4 antigen (e.g., OKT4) define the helper subgroup of human T cells (about 60–80% of the total T cells). These cells are not cytotoxic but rather aid in the regulation of B-cell responses and in cell-mediated reactions. They are the major regulatory cells in the immune system. These CD4+ cells respond to antigens complexed to MHCs of the class II type. The CD4+ subgroup of cells is particularly susceptible to the human immunodeficiency virus (HIV) of the acquired immunodeficiency syndrome (AIDS), with the percentage of this subset decreasing dramatically as this disease progresses. Further, these helper cells are necessary components of the autoimmune response seen in the experimental models of ocular inflammatory disease induced with retinal antigens (see discussion of autoimmunity later in this chapter). There is a subset of CD4+ cells that also bear IL-2 receptors (CD25) on their surface. In rodents, and possibly also in humans, some T-regulatory cells may bear the CD25 receptor (see below).

Antibodies to the CD8 antigen (i.e., OKT8) distinguish a population that includes cytotoxic T cells, making up about 20–30% of the total number of T cells. (In the older literature it was thought to harbor suppressor cells, but this is no longer thought to be the case). Antibodies directed against the CD8 antigen block class I histocompatibility-associated reactions.

Cytokines

Intercellular communication is in large part mediated by cytokines and chemokines (see below). Cytokines are produced by lymphocytes and macrophages, as well as by other cells. They are hormone-like proteins capable of amplifying an immune response as well as suppressing it. With the activation of a T lymphocyte, the production and release of various lymphokines will occur. One of the most important is IL-2, with a molecular weight of 15 000 Da in humans.

Table 1-2 Cytokines: An incomplete list

Type	Source	Target and Effect
Interferon-γ	T cells	Antiviral effects; promotes expression of MHC II Antigens on cell surfaces; increases MΦ tumor killing; inhibits some T-cell proliferation
Transforming growth factor-β	T cells, resident ocular cells	Suppresses generation of certain T cells; involved in ACAID and oral tolerance
Interleukin		
IL-1	Many nucleated cells, high levels in MΦ, keratinocyte, endothelial cells, some T and B cells	T- and B-cell proliferation; fibroblasts – proliferation, prostaglandin production; CNS – fever; bone and cartilage resorption; adhesion-molecule expression on endothelium
IL-2	Activated T cells	Activates T cells, B cells, MΦ, NK cells
IL-3	T cells	Affects hemopoietic lineage that is nonlymphoid eosinophil regulator; similar function to IL-5 GM-CSF
IL-4	T cells	Regulates many aspects of B-cell development, affects T cells, mast cells, and MΦ
IL-5	T cells, eosinophils	Affects hemopoietic lineage that is nonlymphoid, eosinophil regulator: similar function to IL-3 GM-CSF; induces B-cell differentiation into IgG- and IgM-secreting plasma cells
IL-6	MΦ T cells fibroblasts; endothelial cells, RPE	B cells – cofactor for Ig production; T cells – co-mitogen; proinflammatory in eye
IL-7	Stromal cells in bone marrow and thymus	Stimulates early B-cell progenitors; affects immature T cells
IL-8	NK cells, T cells	Chemoattractant of neutrophils, basophils, and some T cells; aids in neutrophils adhering to endothelium; induced by IL-1, TNF-α, and endotoxin
IL-9	T cells	Supports growth of helper T cells; may be enhancing factor for hematopoiesis in presence of other cytokines
IL-10	T cells, B cells, stimulated MΦ	Inhibits production of lymphokines by Th1 T cells
IL-11	Bone marrow stromal cells (fibroblasts)	Stimulates cells of myeloid, lymphoid, erythroid, and megakaryocytic lines; induces osteoclast formation; enhances erythrocytopoiesis, antigen-specific antibodies, acute-phase proteins, fever
IL-12	B cells, T cells	Induces IFN-γ synthesis: augments T-cell cytotoxic activity with IL-2; is chemotactic for NK cells and stimulates interaction with vascular endothelium; promotes lytic activity of NK cells; antitumor effects regulate proliferation of Th1 T cells but not Th2 or Th0
IL-13	T cells	Antiinflammatory activity as IL-4 and IL-10; down regulates IL-12 and IFN-α production and thus favors Th2 T-cell responses; inhibits proliferation of normal and leukemic human B-cell precursors; monocyte chemoattractant
IL-14	T cells	Induces B-cell proliferation, malignant B cells; inhibits immunoglobulin secretion
IL-15	Variety of cells	Stimulates proliferation of T cells; shares bioactivity of IL-2 and uses components of IL-2 receptor
IFN-α	Variety of cells	Antiviral
IFN-β	Variety of cells	Antiviral
IFN-γ	T and NK cells	Inflammation, activates MΦ
TGF-β	MΦ, lymphocytes	Depends on cell interaction
TNF-α	MΦ	Inflammation, tumor killing
TNF-β	T cells	Inflammation, tumor killing, enhanced phagocytosis

ACAID, anterior chamber-acquired immune deviation; CNS, central nervous system; GM-CSF, granulocyte macrophage colony-stimulating factor; IFN, interferon; MΦ, macrophage; NK, natural killer; RPE, retinal pigment epithelium; TFG, transforming growth factor; TNF, tumor necrosis factor.

The release of this lymphokine can stimulate lymphocyte growth and amplify or augment specific immune responses. Another lymphokine is IFN-γ, an important immunoregulator with the potent capacity to induce class II antigen expression on cells. TGF-β is a ubiquitous protein produced by many cells, including platelets and T cells; it appears to have the distinct ability to downregulate immune responses, and to play an important role in anterior chamber-acquired immune deviation (ACAID) and oral tolerance. The number of lymphokines that have been purified and for which effects have been described (see Table 1-2 for a partial list) continues to grow rapidly.

Table 1-3 Selected human leukocyte differentiation antigens (Incomplete list)

Cluster Designation	Main Cellular Distribution	Associated Functions
CD3	T cells, thymocytes	Signal transduction
CD4	Helper T cells	MHC class II coreceptor
CD8	Suppressor T cells, cytotoxic T cells	MHC class I receptor
CD11a	Leukocytes	LFA-1, adhesion molecule
CD11b	Granulocytes, MΦ	Mac-1 adhesion molecule
CD11c	Granulocytes, MΦ, T cells, B cells	α-Integrin, adhesion molecule
CD19	B cells	B-cell activation
CD20	B cells	B-cell activation
CD22	B cells	B-cell regulatory
CD25	T cells, B cells	α chain of IL-2 receptor (Tac) activation
CD28	T cells	Co-stimulatory T-cell marker
CD45	Leukocytes	Maturation
CD54	Endothelial, dendritic, and epithelial cells; activated T and B cells	ICAM-1, adhesion molecule; ligand of LFA-1 and Mac-1
CD56	NK cells	N-CAM, adhesion molecule
CD68	Macrophages	
CD69	NK cells, lymphocytes	Signal transmission receptor
CX3CR1	Monocytes	Chemoattractant
CXCR3	T cells	Cell maturation
CCR7	T cells	Migration to inflammation
CCR5	T cells	Chemokine receptor
CD8 – Co-receptor TRC during antigen stimulation with cytotoxic T-cells		

ICAM, intercellular adhesion molecule; IL, interleukin; LFA, lymphocyte function-associated molecule; MHC, major histocompatibility complex; N-CAM, neural cell adhesion molecule.

T-cell subsets

Helper T cells have been further subdivided, based on their functional characteristics, into several groups (**Fig. 1-2**). The first is the Th1 cell (**Fig. 1-3**). These cells show a cytokine profile of IFN-γ production. The cytokine profile of Th2 cells comprises IL-4, IL-5, IL-13 and perhaps TGF-β, and IL-10. In many animal models of human disease Th1 cells are associated with the initiation of disease, whereas Th2 cells are related to disease downregulation and allergy initiation, or are involved in parasitic diseases. But this story is still unclear. We know from experimental models of uveitis (see below), in which the autoaggressive cells that induce disease are the Th1 cells, that under certain conditions one can induce disease with Th2 cells (nature did not read the textbooks!). Indeed, yet another subset of cells that has been the center of great interest recently is that of the Th17 cell.[1] These cells produce proinflammatory cytokines including IL-17 (hence the name), IL-21 and 22. These cells develop in different environments depending on whether we look in the mouse or the human. In humans, IL-1, IL-6, and IL-23 appear to promote these cells. The cells play a role in host defense mechanisms against fungi and bacteria, and also in autoimmune disease. We have reported the presence of Th17 cells in the blood of sarcoidosis patients with uveitis.[2] Additionally, another human T-cell subset, NKT cells, also produce IL-17 and bear IL-23 receptors on their surface.[3]

One concept is that Th1 cells may initiate an immune response but the Th17 cells are involved in more chronic activity. Anti-IL-17 will almost certainly be an area of intense investigation in the coming years. An interesting question is whether Th1 cells and IL-17 are distinct cells, or are they rather a function of the immune environment, so that under certain circumstances they produce IL-17 and under others a Th1 repertoire? One still cannot answer that question in the human setting, but under experimental conditions it has been seen that Th17 cells may switch to a Th1 character, but that Th1 cells maintain that phenotype and do not change.[4] Also under experimental conditions in animals, when comparing these cells the nature of the intraocular inflammatory response was seen to be different. Th17 did not induce a

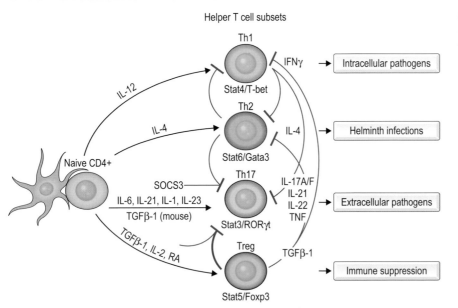

Helper T cell subsets

Figure 1-2. Helper T-cell subsets now recognized. (From: Zhi Chen, O'Shea JJ. Th17 cells: a new fate for differentiating helper T cells. Immunol Res 2008; 41: 87, with permission.)

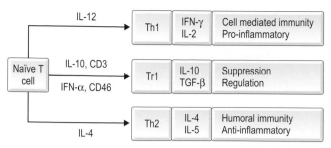

Figure 1-3. Development of three types of T cell participating in the immune response. Other T-cell types also exist, but are not shown. *(With kind permission from Springer Science & Business Media: From Th17 cells: a new fate for differentiating helper T cells. Zhi Chen – John J. O'Shea. Immunol Res (2008) 41:87–102.)*

Table 1-4 Cytokine repertoire of various CD4+ T cells

Cytokine	Tr1	Th0	Th1	Th2	Th17
IL-2	±	3+	3+	±	
IFN-γ	2+	2+	3+	±	
IL-4	–	2+	±	3+	
IL-5	2+	2+	±	3+	
IL-10	3+	1+	1+	2+	
TGF-β	3+	2+	2+	2+	
IL-17					3+
IL-22					2+

Based on findings in Roncarolo MG, Bacchetta R, Bordignon C, et al. Type 1 T regulatory cells. Immunol Rev 2001; 181: 68–71.

large lymphoid expansion and splenomegaly, as did Th1 cells; Th1 cells infiltrating the eye dissipate rapidly, whereas IL-17 cells remain; and markers on the surface of these infiltrating cells are different.[5]

IL-22 is part of the IL-17 group of cytokines produced during an inflammatory response.[6] Albeit made by lymphocytes, its receptors are present on epithelial cells. Thus it has been suggested that one of it major roles is to be the cross-talk lymphokine between resident tissue cells and infiltrating inflammatory cells, particularly T cells. This pro-inflammatory cytokine is found in the synovia of patients with rheumatoid arthritis and is upregulated in both Crohn's disease and ulcerative colitis.[7,8]

T-regulatory cells

It is clear that just as the immune system needs cells to initiate a response it needs cells to suppress or modify an immune response. One of the ways that need is met is with T-regulatory (Tr) cells.[9,10] It is hypothesized that these derive from a naive T cell under the influence of cytokines different from those of either Th1 or Th2 cells (see Fig. 1-3). T regs can be found in the thymus (u T regs) or in the peripheral circulation which can be induced (i T regs). Of interest is a report by Kemper and co-workers[11] of stimulating CD4+ cells with CD3 and CD46 (a complement regulator) and inducing Tr cells, that is, producing large amounts of IL-10, moderate amounts of TGF-β, and little IL-2. The literature is replete with information about different types of Tr cell and they have been reported in several organs, such as the gut, where peripheral immune tolerance needs to be induced.[12] Certain characteristics of many of these cells have been described (**Table 1-4**), and the underlying feature is their ability to produce IL-10 and TGF-β. They are capable of downregulating both CD4- and CD8-mediated inflammatory responses, requiring cell-to-cell contact. There are probably many types because nature usually provides redundancies. Of great interest are those that bear CD25 (the IL-2 receptor) on their cell surface. Much interest has centered on cells that have large numbers of these receptors on their surface ('bright cells'), with work suggesting that they are indeed 'negative regulatory' cells – that is, suppressor cells that can modify an immune response. Although the evidence is much clearer in mouse models, this area still is unfolding in human immunology, and it is not clear what the best markers for these cells are. Such an example is forkhead/winged helix transcription factor, or FoxP3,[13] thought to be a reliable marker in mice for the development and function of naturally occur-

ring T-regulatory cells, but its expression has been seen in T-effector cells (cells that induce inflammation) and so its value has been called into question, at least in humans.[14] When we evaluated the T cells of patients with ocular inflammatory disease, we found that the FoxP3 marker varied tremendously between patients and was not a very good indicator of poor T-regulatory function.[15]

An interesting observation is the increase in a subset of NK cells (so called CD56 'bright') after daclizumab therapy was noted; this subset makes large amounts of IL-10.[16] The implication of this increase in this cell population is that a regulatory cell is to be found there. The increase is seen when patients' disease is well controlled, and it has also been seen in multiple sclerosis patients receiving daclizumab therapy.

T-cell receptor

Much interest has centered on the T-cell receptor (TCR) (**Fig. 1-4**). T cells need to produce the TCR on their cell surface to recognize the MHC; this is part of the system that permits information transmitted to it by peptides presented on the APC. This complex interaction involves the MHC antigen on the APC surface, the peptide, either the CD4 or the CD8 antigen, and the TCR. The TCR is similar in structure to an immunoglobulin, having both an α and a β chain. The more distal ends of these chains are variable, and the hypervariable regions are termed V (variable) and J (joining) on the α chain and V, and D (diversity) regions on the β chain. Compared with the number of immunoglobulin genes, there are fewer V genes and more J genes in the TCR repertoire. It is logically assumed that the peptide, which has a special shape and therefore fits specifically in a lock-and-key fashion into the groove between the MHC and the TCR, would be the 'cement' of this union. In general that would be true, but 'superantigens,' which can bind to the sides of these molecules, can also bring them together and, under the right circumstances, initiate cellular responses. These superantigens are glycoproteins and can be bacterial products such as enterotoxins or viral products. It has been suggested that of all the possible combinations of gene arrangements that could possibly produce the variable region believed to cradle the peptide, certain genes within a family seem to be noted more frequently in autoimmune disease. One such group is the Vα family, with Vβ8.2 receiving much attention. A very small number of cells have a TCR made up not of α and β chains but rather γ and δ

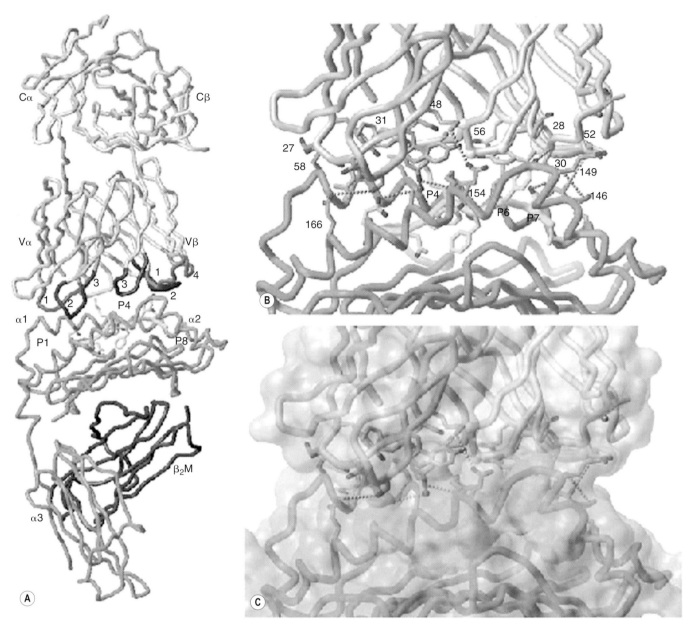

Figure 1-4. T-cell receptor in three dimensions to give an idea of the complexity of interaction. **A,** TCR is on top with various chains shown in different colors. Major histocompatibility antigen is below. **B,** Close-up of TCR MHC interphase. **C,** Molecular surfaces of interacting TCR, peptide, and MHC. *(From Garcia KC, Degano M, Pease LR, et al: Structural basis of plasticity in T cell receptor recognition of a self peptide-MHC antigen, Science 279:1166–1172 (20 Feb), 1998. Reprinted with permission from American Association for the Advancement of Science.)*

chains. These cells are usually CD4⁻ and CD8⁻, and their ability to interact with APCs is not great. They appear to be highly reactive to heat-shock proteins.

A state of suspended animation can be induced in T cells which is termed anergy. For T cells to be activated several signals need to be given: one through the TCR and the other through co-stimulatory receptors such as CD28; the third is the co-stimulant B7 linking to CD28 (which is on the T cell). If the TCR is activated but the co-stimulant is not, one sees a growth arrest in these cells: they simply stop functioning but do not die. A second way this can occur is when a weakly adherent peptide is linked to the TCR, even if co-stimulation occurs. It would seem to be a mechanism to prevent unwanted or nuisance immune responses. The full response takes place only if all the appropriate interactions have occurred.

Chemokines

This family of chemoattractant cytokines is characterized by its ability to induce directional migration of white blood cells. They will direct cell adhesion, homing, and angiogenesis. There are four major subfamilies of chemokines: CXC (nine of which are found on chromosome 4), CC (11 of which are found on chromosome 17), C (only one well-defined member, lymphotactin, on chromosome 11), and CX3C (fractalkine, on chromosome 16). The nomenclature is based on cysteine molecules. The CC chemokines have two adjacent cysteines at their amino terminus; the CXC chemokines have their N terminal cysteines separated by one amino acid; the C chemokines have only two cysteines, one at the terminal end and one downstream; the CX₃C chemokines have three amino acids between their two N terminal cysteines. Each chemokine family has special functions that affect different types of cell. An example of this fine specificity is seen within the CXC family. Those CXC chemokines with a Glu–Leu–Arg sequence near the end of the N terminus bind well to the CXCR2 on neutrophils. CXC chemokines not possessing that sequence are chemotactic for monocytes and lymphocytes. IL-8 can bind with either CXCR1 or CXCR2 (i.e., the chemokine receptors). Organisms have adapted to these chemokines as well. HIV gp120 will bind to CCR5 and CCR3, aiding its entry into the lymphocyte. This area is still evolving. Clearly, cell homing has importance in ocular inflammatory disease but probably in other conditions as well, such as diabetes and age-related macular degeneration, in which the immune components of the disease are just being explored but which may be important areas for therapeutic interventions.

Thymic expression and central immune tolerance

T-cell responses to an antigen are the basis of a large part of the ocular inflammatory process. For a T cell to 'recognize' an antigen it needs to bear on its surface a receptor that will combine with the antigen. The development of the T-cell receptor is a complex mechanism that involves the random recombination of at least three distinct gene segments that control the expression of the T-cell receptor. These T cells go through a selection process in the thymus. Immature cells from the bone marrow find their way into the thymus, rearranging their T-cell receptor components and at the same time expressing CD4 and CD8 co-receptor molecules. These cells move to a portion of the thymic cortex where they interact with stromal cells or dendritic cells bearing on their surface MHC molecules and self peptides. Thymocytes that fail to recognize the MHC complex are induced to die (apoptose). The T cells that have been selected will then migrate further into the thymus, coming into contact with dendritic cells expressing MHC molecules and self peptides. Here the cells that bind tightly to the MHC complex on dendritic cells are negatively selected and undergo programmed cell death (apoptosis). Only a very small fraction (3–5%) of the T-cell precursors that come into the thymus will emerge as mature T cells. The system is not perfect, and some autoresponsive cells escape the negative selection process, finding their way into the mature immune system. It is believed that they form the nidus of autoimmune responses. We can perhaps see evidence of this when we observe T-cell immune memory responses from normal individuals to the uveitogenic antigens from the back of the eye. The way the body deals with these cells falls under the rubric of peripheral tolerance. However, with regard to the thymus and how these observations affect the ocular immune response, we know that the thymus can often express organ-specific molecules such as insulin. Egwuagu and co-workers[17] have shown interesting findings in the thymus. It has been noted for some time that the susceptibility of some animal strains to uveitis after immunization with uveitogenic antigens depended on whether they expressed these antigens in the thymus. An example can be seen in **Figure 1-5**.

Four inbred strains of mice were evaluated for the expression in their thymus of two uveitogenic antigens (see below):

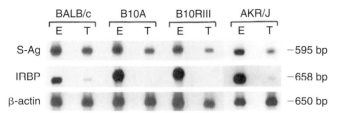

Figure 1-5. Transcription of S-antigen and IRBP genes (uveitogenic antigens) in eyes and thymuses of mouse strains. S-antigen and IRBP are abundant in the eyes of all animals and S-antigen is found in the thymuses of all four strains tested. However, IRBP was seen only in thymuses of two strains – BALBk and AKWJ – and not in those of B10.A or B10 RIII. The last two animals are susceptible to induction of uveitis with IRBP. *(From Egwuagu CE, Charukamnoetkanok P, Gery I: Thymic expression of autoantigens correlates with resistance to autoimmune disease, J Immunol 159:3109–3112, 1997.)* Copyright 1997, The American Association of Immunologists, Inc.)

interphotoreceptor retinoid-binding protein (IRBP) and S-antigen (arrestin). All four strains were resistant to the induction of uveitis when arrestin was used as the immunizing antigen, and all four expressed arrestin in their thymus. However, two of the four strains, B10.A and B10.RIII, were susceptible to uveitis induction when IRBP was used as the immunizing antigen. Of great interest was the fact that no IRBP mRNA could be detected using quantitative PCR assays in their thymus glands. These observations now include other rodents and primates.[18] In the Lewis rat, which is susceptible to both antigens, neither message is found in the thymus. For the rhesus monkey, which is susceptible to both S-antigen (S-Ag) and IRBP, no message is seen for IRBP and for S-Ag it is variable. These observations may provide an insight into the propensity for the disease in humans; thymuses removed from patients for various indications were investigated to see if these observations hold. Takase et al.[19] evaluated 18 human thymus samples taken from patients undergoing surgery for congenital heart disease. They found that there was indeed expression of the four antigens that can induce experimental uveitis (S-antigen, recoverin, RPE65 and interphotoreceptor retinoid-binding protein) in the thymi of the patients tested (none had uveitis). However, the expression of the various antigens was very variable, with some thymus samples showing strong expression whereas others did not. Many of the patients had peripheral T cells that responded to the S-antigen, but much less so to other antigens. The implication of these studies is that expression of these antigens in the thymus is very variable in humans, similar to what is seen in the differences between various rodent strains. Further, whereas the low expression and 'avidity' of the T cells to the antigen in the thymus may explain to some degree the finding of T cells in the blood that respond to the S-antigen, it clearly suggests that other mechanisms are also at work.

Recent work has identified the AIRE gene, the protein produced by which is expressed in a subset of medullary thymic epithelial cells. These cells are involved in the negative selection performed by thymic cells. AIRE appears to permit the expression of organ-specific autoantigens, thereby helping in the removal of autoaggressive cells. Loss of the AIRE gene leads to autoimmunity.[20] This is known to occur in humans and leads to autoimmune polyglandular syndrome (APS) type I, an autoimmune disease that is inherited in an autosomal recessive fashion. In addition to the adrenal insufficiency, mucocutaneous infections, and hypopara-thyoridism, these patients can manifest diabetes, Sjögren's syndrome, vitiligo, and uveitis.[21]

B cells

B cells make up the second broad arm of the lymphocyte immune response. Originating from the same pluripotential stem cell in the bone marrow as the T cell, the maturational process and role of the B cell are quite different. The term B cell originates from observations obtained from work with chickens, in which it was noted that antibody-producing cells would not develop if the bursa of Fabricius, a uniquely avian structure, was removed. The human equivalent appears to be the bone marrow. The B cell, under proper conditions, will develop into a plasma cell that is capable of secreting immunoglobulin. Therefore, its role is to function as the effector cell in humoral immunity. The unique characteristic of these cells is the presence of surface immunoglobulin on their cell membranes.

B-cells begin as a group of cells originating from stem cells designated as pro- or pre-B cells. The maturation process leading to a B cell is complex and not fully understood. What is clear is that various gene regions that control the B-cell's main product, immunoglobulins, are not physically next to each other. Through a process of translocation these genes align themselves next to each other, excising intervening genes. IL-7 is an important factor in the maturation process. B cells can be activated by their interaction with CD4+ T cells that express on their surface class II MHC antigens and CD40 ligand. B-cell activation will cause these cells to divide, usually in the context of T-cell interaction and cytokines elaborated by the T cell, including IL-4, IL-5, IL-6, IL-17 and IL-2.

Subgroups of B cells have been described. Naive, conventional (B2) B cells are found. Another type, memory B cells, live for long periods, are readily activated, and will produce immunoglobulin (Ig) isotypes other than IgM (see next section). These cells presumably play an important role in the anamnestic response of the organism. This is the very rapid antigen-specific immune response that occurs when the immune system encounters an antigen to which it has already been sensitized. Another subgroup consists of B1 (CD5+) lymphocytes, whose characteristics overlap with those of other B cells but which appear to be derived from a separate lineage and are very long-lived. These cells produce IL-10 and have been associated with autoantibody production. Chronic lymphocytic leukemias often derive from B1 cells.

B cells initially express surface IgM and IgD simultaneously, with differentiation occurring only after appropriate activation. Five major classes of immunoglobulin are identified on the basis of the structure of their heavy chains: α, γ, μ, δ, and ε, corresponding to IgA, IgG, IgM, IgD, and IgE (**Table 1-5**). The structure of the immunoglobulin demonstrates a symmetry, with two heavy and two light chains uniformly seen in all classes except IgM and IgA (**Fig. 1-6**). The production of immunoglobulin usually requires T-cell participation. Many 'relevant' antigens are T-cell dependent, meaning that the addition of antigen to a culture of pure B cells will not induce immunoglobulin production. However, polyclonal B-cell activators, such as lipopolysaccharide,

Table 1-5 Characteristics of human immunoglobulins

	IgG	IgA	IgM	IgE	IgD
Molecular weight (10^3)	150	150–300	900	190	180
Heavy chain	γ	α	μ	–	δ
Subclass	1,2,3,4	1,2	1,2	–	–
J chain	–	+	+	–	–
Crosses placenta	+	–	–	–	–
Serum half-life (days)	21	6	5	2	3
Complement activation	+	–	+	–	–
Serum concentration (mg/dL)	110	25	10	0.001	0.3
IN EYE					
Conjunctiva	Rich	Rich	Varies	Varies	Varies
Cornea	Moderate	Moderate	0	?	0
Aqueous	Low	Low	Low	?	0
Iris	Low	Low	Low	Varies	Varies
Choroid	Rich	Rich	Rich	Varies	Varies
Retina	Low	Low	Low	0	0
Vitreous	–	–	–	–	–

From Allansmith M. Unpublished data 1987. Used with permission.

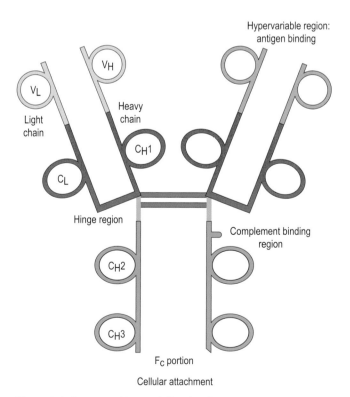

Figure 1-6. Structure of human IgG molecule.

pokeweed mitogen, dextran, and the Epstein–Barr virus (as well as other viruses), have the capacity to directly induce B-cell proliferation and immunoglobulin production. For a primary immune response B cells will produce IgM, which binds complement. With time – and if they encounter these antigens again – B cells will switch immunoglobulin production to IgG, usually during the primary response. This immunoglobulin class switching, which requires a gene rearrangement, is inherent in the B cell and is partly controlled by lymphokines. IL-4 has been associated with a switch to express IgG (in mouse IgG_1, in human IgG_4) and IgE, whereas IFN-γ controls a switch to IgG_{2a} and TGF-β to IgA.

Classes of Immunoglobulin

More IgA is made than any other immunoglobulin, much in the gut. IgG is the major circulating immunoglobulin class found in humans: it is synthesized at a very high rate and makes up about 75% of the total serum immunoglobulins. Plasma cells that produce IgG are found mainly in the spleen and the lymph nodes. Four subclasses of IgG have been identified in humans (G_1–G_4). G_1 and G_3 fix complement readily and can be transmitted to the fetus. The production of these subclasses is not random but reflects the antigen to which the antibody is being made. When doing tests in the serum or the chambers of the eye (aqueous or vitreous), we usually look at IgG production.

IgM is a pentamer made up of the typical antibody structure linked by disulfide bonds and J chains (**Fig. 1-7**). Only about one-fifteenth as much IgM as IgG is produced. Because of its size, it generally stays within the systemic circulation and, unlike IgG, will not cross the blood–brain barrier or the placenta. This antibody is expressed early on the surface of B cells. Therefore, initial antibody responses to exogenous pathogens, such as *Toxoplasma gondii*, are of this class. The observation of an IgM-specific antibody response helps to confirm a newly acquired infection. IgM has a complement-binding site and can mediate phagocytosis by fixing C3b, a component of the complement system.

One major role of both IgG and IgM is to interact with both effector cells and the complement system to limit the invasion of exogenous organisms. These immunoglobulins aid effector cells through opsonization, which occurs by the antibody coating an invading organism and assisting the phagocytic process. The Fc portion of the antibody molecule then can readily interact with effector cells, such as macrophages, thereby helping effectively resolve the infection. Persons with deficiencies in IgG and IgM are particularly prone to infection by pyogenic organisms such as *Streptococcus* and *Neisseria* species. In addition, both of these antibodies will activate the complement pathway, inducing cell lysis by that mechanism as well.

IgA is the major extravascular immunoglobulin, although it comprises only about 10–15% of the intravascular total. Two isotypes of IgA are noted: IgA_1 is more commonly seen intravascularly, whereas IgA_2 is somewhat more prevalent in the extravascular space. The IgA-secreting plasma cells are found in the subepithelial spaces of the gut, respiratory tract, tonsils, and salivary and lacrimal glands. IgA is an important component to the defense mechanism of the ocular surface, being found in a dimer linked by a J chain, a polypeptide needed for polymerization. In addition, a secretory component, a unique protein with parts of its molecule having no homology to other proteins, is needed for the IgA to appear in the gut and outside vessels. The secretory component is produced locally by epithelial cells that then form a complex with the IgA dimer/J chain (**Fig. 1-8**). This new complex is internalized by mucosal cells and then released on the apical surface of the cell through a proteolytic process. The amount of IgA within the eye is quite small. IgA can fix complement through the alternate pathway, and can serve as an opsonin for phagocytosis. IgA appears to exert its major role by preventing entry of pathogens into the internal environment of the organism by binding with the infectious agent. It may also impede the absorption of potential toxins and allergens into the body. Further, it can induce eosinophil degranulation.

IgE is slightly heavier than IgG because its heavy chain has an additional constant domain. Mast cells and basophils

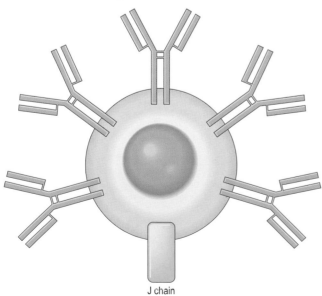

Figure 1-7. IgM pentamer with J chain.

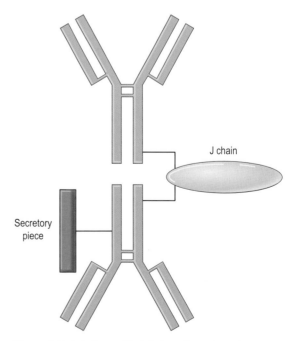

Figure 1-8. IgA dimer with J chain and secretory piece.

have Fc receptors for IgE, and IgE is thought to be one of the major mediators of the allergic or anaphylactoid reaction (see next section). It appears to be an important defense mechanism against parasites: one way IgE accomplishes this is to prime basophils and mast cells. Although its role in ocular surface disease has been well recognized, this has not been the case for intraocular inflammation.

IgD is found in minute quantities in the serum (0.5% of serum Ig). It is found simultaneously with IgM on B cells before specific stimulation. Little more is known about this antibody other than it is a major B-cell membrane receptor for antigen.

Antibodies directed toward specific antigens, particularly cell-surface antigens of the immune system, have provided the clinical and basic investigator with a powerful tool with which to identify various components of the immune system, as was described in the section on the T cell. The development of monoclonal antibodies using hybridoma technology has permitted the production of these immune probes in almost unlimited quantity. Immortalized myeloma cells can be fused with a B cell committed to the production of an antibody directed toward a relevant antigen. This is usually accomplished with the use of polyethylene glycol, which promotes cell membrane fusion. By careful screening, clones of these fused cells (i.e., hybrid cells or hybridomas) can be identified as producing the antibody needed. These can be isolated and grown, yielding essentially an unlimited source of the antibody derived from one clone of cells and directed against one specific determinant. Monoclonal antibodies have been raised against cell markers of virtually all cellular components of the immune system. Antibodies can now be 'humanized' so that only small parts of the variable end remains of mouse origin. The advantage to this is the reduced probability of an immune response to a foreign protein.

Other cells

Mast Cells

This large (15–20 μm) cell is intimately involved with type I hypersensitivity reactions (see next section). Its most characteristic feature is the presence of large granules in the cytoplasm. It is clear that there are subtypes of mast cells. In humans, mast cells are characterized by the presence or absence of the granule-associated protease chymase. It has been suggested that tryptase-positive, chymase-negative human mast cells are suggestive of mucosal mast cells found in the mouse. Mast cells contain a large number of biologically active agents, including histamine, serotonin, prostaglandins, leukotrienes, and chemotactic factors of anaphylaxis as well as cytokines and chemokines. Histamine is stored within the mast-cell granules. Once released into the environment, histamine can cause smooth muscle to contract and can increase small vessel permeability, giving the typical 'wheal and flare' response noted in skin tests. Serotonin, in humans, appears to have a major effect on vasoconstriction and blood pressure, whereas in rodents it may also affect vascular permeability. Prostaglandins, a family of lipids, are capable of stimulating a variety of biologic activities, including vasoconstriction and vasodilation. Leukotrienes are compounds produced de novo with antigen stimulation. Leukotriene B_4 is a potent chemotactic factor for both neutrophils and eosinophils, whereas leukotrienes C_4 and D_4, for example, enhance vascular permeability. At least two chemotactic factors of anaphylaxis attract eosinophils to a site of mast-cell degranulation, whereas other factors attract and immobilize neutrophils.

Mast-cell involvement in several external ocular conditions has been established. However, it is not yet clear what role this cell may play in intraocular inflammatory disorders. Mast cells are present in abundance in the choroid, and appear to be related to the susceptibility of at least one experimental model for uveitis (see discussion on autoimmunity). Human work supports the hypothesis that many cytokine-dependent processes are implicated in IgE-associated disorders. Many different cytokines and chemokines have been seen in mast cells. These include IL-4, IL-6, IL-8, tumor necrosis factor (TNF)-α, vascular endothelial growth factor (VEGF), and macrophage inflammatory protein (MIP)-1α.

All of these findings link the mast cell to a whole variety of immune processes. It can be speculated that when a mast cell degranulates in the choroid it also releases chemokines and lymphokines, which may be the initiating factor of what we describe as a T-cell-mediated disorder.

Eosinophils

These bilobed nucleated cells are about 10–15 μm in size and are thought to be terminally differentiated granulocytes. Their most morphologically unique characteristic is the approximately 200 granules that are highly acidophilic (taking up eosin in standard staining procedures) and which are found in the cytoplasm. They are almost entirely made up of major basic protein (molecular weight 9000 Da), but other toxic cationic granules include eosinophil-derived neurotoxia, eosinophil cationic protein, and eosinophil peroxidase. A minor percentage of these cells (5–25%) have IgG receptors, and about half may have complement receptors on their surface membranes, although it is not clear whether receptors for IgE are present. Eosinophils contain an abundant number of enzymes, which are quite similar in nature to those contained in neutrophils. Both cells contain a peroxidase and catalase, both of which can be antimicrobial, but eosinophils lack lysozymes and neutrophils lack the major basic protein. Eosinophils also contain several anti-inflammatory enzymes such as kininase, arylsulfatase, and histaminase. In addition, eosinophils produce growth factors such as IL-3 and IL-5, chemokines such as RANTES and MIP-1, cytokines such as TGF-α and TGF-β, VEGF, TNF-α, IL-1α, IL-6, and IL-8.

The eosinophil arises in the bone marrow from a myeloid progenitor, perhaps from a separate stem cell than neutrophils. The time spent in the systemic circulation is probably quite short, and the number seen on a routine blood smear is usually very low (1% or less of nucleated cells). These cells can be attracted to an area in the body by the release of mast-cell products and, once localized to an inflammatory site, are capable of performing several functions. The eosinophil may play an immunomodulatory role in the presence of mast-cell and basophil activation.

As mentioned, the cell contains the anti-inflammatory agents histaminase and arylsulfatase, capable of neutralizing the effect of histamine release and slow-reacting substance, both products of mast cells. Further, basophil function may be inhibited by prostaglandins E_1 and E_2, both produced by eosinophils. An additional immunomodulatory mechanism is the capacity of the eosinophil to ingest immunoreactive granules released by mast cells. An extremely important role played by these cells is in the response of the immune system to parasitic organisms. Eosinophils are seen in high numbers at the site of a parasitic infiltration and are known to bind tightly to the organism through receptors. Further, the release of the major basic protein granules or an eosinophil-produced peroxidase complexed with H_2O_2 and deposited on the parasite's surface membrane will lead to the death of the invading organism. Major basic protein may play a role in corneal ulceration in severe cases of allergy.

Neutrophils

Neutrophils are the most abundant type of white blood cell and it is clear that they play an important role in acute inflammation. They do not live as long as monocytes or lymphocytes, and are attracted to inflammatory sites by IL-8, interferon-γ, and C5a. One of their main functions is phagocytosis, in particular killing microbes using reactive oxygen species and hydrolytic enzymes. Whereas their role in innate immunity seemed clear, very provocative findings suggest a relationship with IL-17. IL-17 is made by not only by T cells and macrophages, but also by neutrophils. Further, IL-17 appears to mobilize lung neutrophils following a bacterial challenge.[22] This would therefore suggest that neutrophils are responding to immune responses from both the innate and the acquired side of the immune process.

Resident Ocular Cells

The interaction of the resident ocular cells with those of the immune system is a most provocative concept. It is clear that several cells of the eye, including RPE and Müller cells, either have functions similar to cells within the immune system or can be induced to bear markers that potentially permit them to participate in immune-mediated events. There are microglia in the retina that are of hematopoietic origin. One can speculate (but there is no in vivo proof) that the initial priming of the immune system may occur through this interchange, or that the continued recruitment of immune cells may be mediated through these mechanisms. The effects of immune cells and their products may also be important for certain ocular conditions, inasmuch as macrophages as well as T-cell products have a profound effect on fibrocyte growth and division, and the RPE and Müller cells may respond in like fashion. RPE, when activated, can act as efficient APCs. Numerous lymphokines are found in the eye, many of which are produced by ocular resident cells. As mentioned above, it is not clear whether there can be antigen presentation in the eye, but in experimental models these cells do modulate this process. We also know that resident ocular cells do modulate the ocular environment by eliciting molecules that alter the immune process (ACAID).

Complement system

The complement system is a cascade of soluble proteins that 'complement' the function of antibodies in the immune system. Each complement protein is a proteolytic enzyme that acts as a substrate for the enzymes that precede it in the cascade, and which then acts as a part of a proteolytic complex for the next protein in the cascade. The classic complement pathway begins when C1q, C1r, and C1s (parts of the first component of complement) interact with membrane-bound antigen–antibody complexes to form an enzyme that cleaves C4 into C4a and C4b. C4b binds to the cell membrane, followed by C2, which is then split by C1s to yield a complex called C4b,2a. This complex splits C3 into C3a and C3b, which then joins the complex to make C4b,2a,3b. This complex cleaves C5 into C5a and C5b. C5b then binds to the cell membrane, and C6, C7, and C8 bind to it. The resulting C5b,6,7,8 complex then leads to C9 polymerization into the membrane.

The alternate pathway of complement does not require antibody but can be activated directly by bacterial cell walls and is therefore a nonspecific defense mechanism. In this pathway a small amount of pre-existing C3b cleaves factor B into Ba and Bb. The bacterial cell wall or other membranes assist in this step. The resulting C3b,Bb complex then cleaves more C3, forming a C3b,Bb,3b complex which can then cleave C5, and the pathway proceeds as already described.

The result is the generation of chemotactic protein fragments (C5a), protein fragments that cause smooth muscle contraction (C3a and C5a), protein fragments that cause mast-cell degranulation (C5a), molecules that assist in neutrophil phagocytosis (C3b), and molecules that are capable of promoting cell lysis (C5b,6,7,8,9). The complement system is therefore involved in many of the effectors of the inflammatory response.

Complement has become an area of special focus because of its possible role in the pathogenesis of age-related macular degeneration (AMD). Complement factors have been found in the drusen of AMD eyes, suggesting that an immune response may have occurred after the activation of the complement cascade.[23] Several reports have appeared showing an association between a complement factor H variant and AMD.[24-26] These observations are most provocative and still need to be defined functionally. However, we have felt that it may be part of a larger series of mechanisms that collectively we have called the 'downregulatory immune environment' of the eye.[27] Indeed, this concept is now supported by the report that the CFH variant is associated with multifocal choroiditis, hence an alteration not unique to AMD.[28]

Cellular interactions: hypersensitivity reactions

Figure 1-9 is a simplified version of the myriad interactions that have been identified in the immune system's repertoire in the eye. Although many exceptions and alternative mechanisms (sometimes contradictory) have been proposed or partially demonstrated, certain useful basic concepts can be of help to the observer. The initiation of a response leading to immune memory requires antigen to be presented to T cells. Classically this is performed by dendritic cells (and perhaps macrophage cell lines) bearing the same class II (HLA-DR) antigens as the T cells. Other cells, however, may also be equally competent in performing this task. Potential candidates in the eye include the vascular endothelium, RPE, and Müller cells. Macrophages release factors such as IL-1 that are essential for the activation of the T cell. IL-1 also

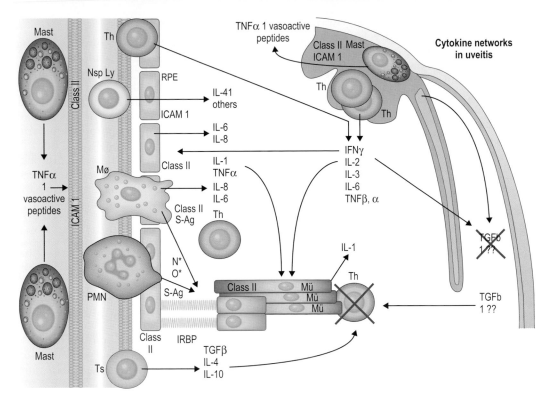

Figure 1-9. Schematic representation of (1) numerous interactions in the eye of cells of the immune system, and (2) cells resident in the eye. *(Courtesy Rachel Caspi, PhD.)*

may be necessary as a cell-membrane component for antigen presentation to occur.

The subsets of T cells, discussed earlier, cover a wide range of functions, from aiding B cells to produce antibody, to cell-mediated killing, to modulation of the immune response. A point worth bearing in mind is that T-cell recruitment is very much dependent on the release of factors (cytokines) that will help recruit and activate other initially uncommitted T cells. This seems to be a basic underlying mechanism for T-cell function.

Other cells also have a major impact on this T-cell–B-cell–macrophage axis. Mast-cell degranulation may assist the egress of immune cells into an organ, and the eosinophils, as well as neutrophils, will aid in killing and/or preparing pathogens for disposal by other parts of the immune system. T cells have a direct effect on mast-cell maturation in the bone marrow by the release of IL-3, whereas the T cell and other immune components have similar effects on other cells of the nonlymphoid series by the release of colony-stimulating factors.

Classic immune hypersensitivity reactions

Although it is not rare for any inflammatory response to involve several arms of the immune repertoire, it frequently appears that one arm of the system predominates. Inflammatory reactions were originally classified into four types or 'hypersensitivity reactions' by the British immunologists Philip Gell and Robin Coombs, with some recent additions.

Type I

This inflammatory reaction is mediated by antibodies, especially IgE. The binding of this antibody to mast cells or basophils results in the degranulation of these cells and the release of pharmacologically active products, as already mentioned. An ocular example of this reaction is hay fever. Typically a large amount of edema without structural damage is noted. The role for this immune mechanism in intraocular inflammatory disease is still unclear. It is not inconceivable that mast cells could play an ancillary role in some cases, but hard evidence is still lacking.

Type II

This type of reaction is mediated by cytotoxic antibodies and is thought to mediate hemolytic disorders, such as blood mismatch reactions and the scarring seen in ocular pemphigoid. It is clear that in ocular pemphigoid antibodies directed to the basement membrane of mucosal surfaces are present and may indeed be cytotoxic. One might consider the antibody effect of carcinoma or melanoma associated retinopathy to be a type II reaction. Intravitreal injections of human MAR IgG has been shown to alter retinal signaling.[29] Another ocular example may be the rare disorder acute anular outer retinopathy.[30] However, T cells can be noted to be infiltrating into the lesion in this disease. Some have suggested including in this category reactions termed antibody-dependent cell-mediated cytotoxicity, thereby making this category one that has a mixed mechanism.

Type III

This reaction is frequently referred to as an immune complex-mediated inflammatory response. The binding of antibody to an antigen – either fixed in tissue or free floating, that then deposits as a complex – can initiate the complement cascade, which in turn attracts cells capable of causing tissue damage. An example is the Arthus reaction, seen about 4 hours after the injection of antigen into the skin of a sensitized person or animal having substantial levels of circulating antibody directed to the antigen being injected locally. This hypersensitivity reaction had been suggested as being one of the major immune mechanisms leading to intraocular inflammatory disease, such as Behçet's disease. However, more recent evidence suggests that its role in the uveitic process is more limited. Phacoanaphylaxis is a disorder that appears to be immune complex driven, at least in part.

Type IV

This category of immune response is for those mediated solely by T cells. It is therefore termed a cell-mediated immune mechanism, rather than a humoral mechanism, as was the case for the other three types of hypersensitivity reactions. The positive skin test reaction noted 48 hours after a PPD test is placed in the skin is an example of a type IV hypersensitivity reaction. Granulomatous responses as seen in sarcoid are mediated by this mechanism, as well as sympathetic ophthalmia. In all of these cases the humoral arm of the immune system is thought not to play a significant role in the inflammatory reaction. To date, the evidence suggests that T-cell dysregulation or T cell-controlled inflammatory responses are an extremely important – perhaps even essential – mechanism for intraocular inflammatory disease.

Type V

This reaction has been added to the original four. In this reaction an antibody can act as a stimulant to a target cell or organ. An example is long-acting thyroid stimulator (LATS) antibody, a feature of Graves' disease. The LATS antibody is directed toward a portion of the TSH receptor in the thyroid and mimics the function of thyroid-stimulating hormone.

Concepts of disease pathogenesis

The potential mechanisms by which tissue damage is mediated by the immune system pose a question that has been hotly debated for some time. The debates are particularly vociferous because most arguments are difficult to support. However, recently these potential mechanisms have opened some of their secrets to observers, and the arguments of a previous generation are no longer acceptable. With our increased understanding of immune mechanisms comes the realization of the network's complexity: that the system has many alternative choices and that there is an extraordinary intertwining of events that appears to be necessary for the immune system to respond appropriately, as well as inappropriately. It still is conceptually valid to simplify these potential mechanisms, and in the following pages we attempt to do that – to provide the reader with concepts rather than numerous specific details. The understanding of these mechanisms is certainly an intellectually stimulating undertaking. However, it has a practical aspect as well. Therapeutic interventions will be increasingly specific, tailored to the problem at hand. Therefore, in the not-too-distant future, an understanding of the mechanisms of ocular inflammatory disease will be invaluable in choosing the appropriate therapy for the patient.

Immune characteristics of the eye

It seems reasonable to begin a section on immune mechanisms that may be responsible for intraocular inflammatory disease by reviewing the characteristics of the eye that might influence these responses. For years the eye was considered to be a 'privileged' immune site. The implication of this was that the immune system somehow ignored or was tolerant of the antigens in the eye. We think it appropriate to consider the eye as being indeed immune privileged, but in a different way than implied by the original notion. Although the characteristics to be reviewed are not always unique to the eye, the combination of all these factors does elevate this organ to a special relationship with the immune system.

Absence of lymphatic drainage

Like the brain, placenta, and testes, the eye has no direct lymphatic drainage, although in mice submandibular nodes do collect antigen from the eye.[31] The environment in which antigen presentation occurs plays an important role in the type of immune response the organism may mount. Experimentally, for example, antigen placed in an area with good lymphatic drainage will elicit an excellent immune response, with a measurable antibody response and cell-mediated immune response. However, the same antigen given intravenously may elicit a very different immune response, the ultimate response being immune tolerance (or anergy). Therefore this anatomic phenomenon may have a profound effect on the types of immune response elicited in the eye.

Intraocular microenvironment

It has been suggested that the eye has at least four ways to protect itself against unwanted or nuisance inflammatory processes. The first is having a barrier such as the blood–ocular barrier. The second is the presence of soluble or membrane-bound inhibitors that block the function of an organism. The third strategy is to kill an invading organism or cell that may be inducing an unwanted inflammation (by perhaps speeding up apoptosis or programmed cell death), and the fourth is to devise a method by which a state of tolerance is induced.[32] All of these barriers appear to exist in the eye.

Anterior Chamber-Associated Immune Deviation (ACAID)

This could be seen as an example of the fourth strategy mentioned above. The immune response elicited by antigen placement into the anterior chamber has interested immunologists for some time[33] and observations are constantly being added.[34] Allogeneic tissue implants (i.e., tissue from the same species but not an identical twin) in the anterior chamber were noted to survive longer than those placed in other orthotopic sites.[35] The placement of alloantigens into the anterior chamber of the eye has been noted to elicit a transient depression of cell-mediated immunity but an intact humoral response. This was initially called an F_1-lymphocyte-induced immune deviation.[36] A continued refinement and understanding of the phenomenon led to its being called ACAID.[37] The model has been further extended to include hapten-specific suppressor T-cell responses to syngeneic splenocytes that are coupled with azobenzenearsonate[38] (i.e., cell-bound antigens) and also has been obtained with soluble antigen alone,[39] such as histocompatibility and tumor antigens. In addition, the induction of ACAID can be enhanced by placing a cell line or tumor that is syngeneic to the MHC of the host,[40] and the capacity of the immune system to enhance or suppress tumor growth can be successfully manipulated by use of this phenomenon. Good antibody responses and cytotoxic T cells directed against the intraocularly placed tumor (or antigen) develop. However, although cells that mediate delayed hypersensitivity reactions do not form, antigen-specific suppressor cells do.

ACAID can be induced in primates,[41] rats, and mice.[39,42] An antigen-specific ACAID will develop with the injection of IRBP into the anterior chamber of rats or mice.[39,42] Of interest as well is the fact that the mice susceptible to IRBP-induced experimental autoimmune uveoretinitis (EAU) will not develop the disease if IRBP is injected into the eye before systemic immunization.[41]

Of prime import in ACAID is the presence of an intact ocular–splenic axis. The induction of suppressor T cells is enhanced when antigen processing bypasses the lymphatic drainage system normally present. There appears to be a unique processing of antigen in the dendritic cells of the eye. Cells then will carry the ACAID signal to the spleen for the activation of regulatory T cells. It has been reported that this signal in the blood was associated with F4/80+ macrophages, which populate the anterior uvea.[43] It appears that this signal is water soluble. Of interest is the fact that in vitro exposure of APCs to aqueous humor – or TGF-β – will confer ACAID-like properties on these cells.[44] Indeed, TGF-β appears to play one of the important roles in ACAID. Other investigators[45] have noted a soluble factor that could be transferred by serum alone. This apparent contradiction might reflect the different experimental methods that were used. It could, however, also reflect the fact that several mechanisms may exist for the induction of ACAID. Indeed, during the disruption of the normal mechanisms, as happens with the addition of INF-γ into the eye, prostaglandins may replace TGF-β as the mediator of suppression.[46] One might speculate on the following scenario: antigen enters into the anterior chamber and is taken up by APCs that live in the special environment of the eye. The APC brings the antigen to the spleen, secreting a chemokine (MIP-2) that will attract natural killer (NK) T cells. The NK T cells in turn will secrete IL-10 and TGF-β, both associated with a Th2 response. The T cells responding to this environment become regulatory cells that will suppress delayed hypersensitivity responses in the eye. In ACAID the afferent regulatory T cell is a CD4+ T cell, whereas the efferent regulator is a CD8+ T cell. The environment is such that lymphoid cells in the eye will not produce IL-12 or express CD40, important components of the immune response.[47] This is different from the tolerance that is induced when an antigen is given intravenously.[33]

The role of ACAID in clinical situations still needs to be evaluated; however, it is not difficult to speculate on its potential role in ocular tumors, as well as autoimmune and even infectious immune responses. This could be a mechanism by which nature attempts to limit unwanted inflammatory responses in the eye.[48]

Fas-Fas Ligand Interactions and Programmed Cell Death (Apoptosis)

Fas ligand (FasL) is a type II membrane protein that belongs to the TNF superfamily. It is found in the eye and can induce apoptotic cell death in cells that express Fas. Fas is part of the TNF receptor family and is found on lymphocytes. It is believed that apoptosis is one method of immune privilege in the eye. It should be added that others may not feel it is the only way that cell death can occur among invading auto-aggressive cells, but there is enough provocative evidence to suggest that it at least should be considered.[49] Organs that appear to be able to limit immune responses, such as the eye, testes, and brain, express FasL. Other organs, such as the liver and the intestine, express this antigen only during severe inflammatory processes. Gene therapy experiments performed on other organs where FasL is transferred can confer immune privilege. It is clear that the Fas-FasL works in concert with several factors. One cofactor appears to be TNF. Activated lymphocytes producing TNF will be more at risk to become apoptotic. Other mechanisms induce apoptosis through IL-2 activation of lymphocytes. These highly activated cells will ultimately die a programmed death. This raises the interesting question whether blockage of part of either the TNF system or the IL-2 circuitry, despite being beneficial on the one hand, could prevent apoptosis of these cells, thereby leaving them at a site of inflammation longer or circulating longer.

Resident Ocular Cells and Immune System

Although communication between resident organ cells and the immune system is not unique to the eye, the number of cells potentially capable of fulfilling this role in the eye is indeed remarkable. The list begins at the cornea with Langerhans' cells, and includes cells in the ciliary body that can express Ia antigens on their surfaces, the Müller cells, which are capable of profound effects on the immune response, and the RPE, with characteristics very similar to those of macrophages. Finally, the vascular endothelium of the eye, as in other organs, may be of great importance in regulating immune system activity.

Müller cells have been shown to have a profound affect on T cells.[50] Isolated pure cultures of rat Müller cells will downregulate the proliferative capabilities of S-Ag-specific T cells capable of inducing experimental uveitis. Cell-to-cell contact is needed to see this phenomenon. It is interesting to note that when Müller cells are killed with a specific poison, the disease induced by S-Ag immunization in rats appears to be worse than in rats with 'intact' retinal Müller cells in the retina.[51] Such experiments would suggest that Müller cells play a role similar to that of ACAID – that is, as part of the protective mechanisms that downregulate 'nuisance' inflammatory responses in the eye.

A very different story seems to emerge with both corneal endothelial cells and the RPE. Kawashima and Gregerson[52] reported that corneal endothelial cells block T-cell proliferation, but T-cell activation signals from an APC were not blocked. This inhibition was not neutralized by the addition of neutralizing antibodies to TGF-β$_1$ or TGF-β$_2$.

As mentioned, the RPE has many characteristics of macrophages. These cells have the capacity to migrate and engulf particles and have characteristics that strongly suggest a capacity to participate in the local immune response. The RPE has been shown to produce cytokines, the one of most note to date being perhaps IL-6,[53] a lymphokine capable of inducing intraocular inflammatory disease when injected into the eye. RPE cells, which express MHC class I antigens constitutively on their surface, can express class II antigens when activated[54] (see later discussion). Further, RPE cells in culture can act as APCs for S-Ag-specific T cells.[55] Here, then, it would appear that we have an example of an ocular resident cell capable of augmenting (or initiating?) an immune response in the eye, but there is no clinical proof to support this concept. However, we do have further experimental evidence that it could indeed happen. We have shown that the glucocorticoid-induced TNF-related receptor ligand (GITRL) is expressed constitutively at low levels on the RPE (and other ocular cells).[56] When GITRL expression is upregulated on RPE cells, the suppressive effects of the RPE on T-cell proliferation is abrogated and so is the production of TGF-β, an important contributor to the downregulatory environment. GITRL upregulation also induced proinflammatory cytokines in T cells.[57] Interestingly, GITR serves as a negative regulator for NK cell activation.[58] Indeed, one may argue that there are so many APCs, such as macrophages and dendritic cells, in the eye that it really does not seem reasonable to think that these ocular resident cells would initiate an immune response.

Cytokines and Chemokines and the Eye

A large number of cytokines, some produced locally by ocular resident cells and others by cells of the immune system, have been implicated in the ocular immune response. In addition to cytokines, numerous neuropeptides and other factors have been cited as being involved in the ocular immune response (see Fig. 1-9, which shows the complex nature of this response). As a result of numerous experiments, cytokines can be termed 'proinflammatory' or 'immunosuppressive' in the intraocular milieu (**Box 1-1**). Some cytokines have been noted to both stimulate and suppress the immune response, depending on the environment in which the cytokine is found. Instead of considering it contradictory, this phenomenon should be viewed as evidence of the complex immune response we are studying. IL-6 (produced locally), IL-2, and IFN-γ are perhaps the most important cytokines to be considered when an intraocular inflammatory response occurs. Foxman and co-workers[59] evaluated the simultaneous expression of several cytokines, chemokines, and chemokine receptors in the eye during an inflammatory episode. Of interest were the relatively high levels of chemokine activity in noninflamed eyes. For experimental autoimmune uveitis, IL-1α, IL-1β, IL-1 receptor antagonist, IL-6, and TNF-α were highly expressed (**Fig. 1-10**). Interferon-β is found in the serum of a large number of retinal vasculitis patients (including those with Behçet's disease).[60]

Box 1-1 Cytokines

PROINFLAMMATORY CYTOKINES

IL-1	TNF
IL-6	IL-2
IL-3	IL-8
IFN-γ	IL-4
IL-12	IL-17

ANTIINFLAMMATORY CYTOKINES

TGF-β	IL-4 (systemic)
IFN-γ	IL-10

The ocular downregulatory immune environment (DIE) appears to be rich in many factors, as already noted: in addition to TGF-β,[61,62] which has been localized to trabecular cells,[63] α-melanocyte-stimulating hormone,[64] calcitonin gene-related peptide,[65] and vasoactive intestinal peptide are found.[66] Other factors, such as hormones, may significantly affect the microenvironment. Sternberg and colleagues[67] have shown that rats not capable of mounting a major intrinsic cortisol response to trauma (or immunization with protein) are more prone to the development of autoimmune disorders. This observation is of further interest because the aqueous is deficient in cortisol-binding globulin; therefore this hormone could play a most important role in downregulating an immune response in the eye.[68]

Oral Tolerance

It seems reasonable to speak about an interesting approach to immunosuppression at this point because it is one that is dependent on the body's own immunosuppressive mechanisms. Oral tolerance has long been recognized as inducing systemic tolerance. It was first described in 1911 by Wells,[69] who prevented anaphylaxis in guinea pigs by feeding them egg protein. In 1946 Chase[70] showed that feeding the hapten dinitrofluorobenzene suppressed contact sensitivity. Information about positive mechanisms has been gained over the past few years.[71] Three possible immune mechanisms can be hypothesized: clonal deletion of autoaggressive cells, clonal anergy, and active suppression. Most information would suggest that active suppression is perhaps a predominant mechanism, but it is also clear that clonal anergy can be demonstrated under certain circumstances.[72,73] TGF-β appears to be the basic mediator of the active suppression seen after feeding. In studies using myelin basic protein, Miller and co-workers[74] showed that the epitopes of myelin basic protein triggering TGF-β after feeding were distinct from the encephalitogenic epitopes.

Oral tolerance has been shown to markedly alter the expression of S-Ag-induced EAU.[75] Feeding S-Ag to Lewis rats before immunization with this antigen suppressed the expression of EAU. Feeding of S-Ag even after immunization with S-Ag still was capable of suppressing EAU. Further, regulatory cells could be isolated from the spleen of fed animals. These are Th2 cells, cells that are capable of downregulating, as opposed to immune augmenting, Th1 cells. An intact spleen appears to be important in the development of this phenomenon.[76] It is of interest to note that nasal administration of retinal antigens can also suppress EAU.[77]

Because of these initial data and information being gathered from our collaborators working in the realm of other animal models and with patients having multiple sclerosis, we embarked on a pilot study in which we fed S-Ag to two patients with uveitis who were receiving immunosuppressive therapy for their disease. We hoped that we could induce immune tolerance and therefore stop or reduce their immunosuppressive therapy.[78] In one patient with pars planitis, oral prednisone was discontinued after the initiation of S-Ag feeding, and the therapeutic response was so dramatic that S-Ag feeding was stopped. This resulted in a recurrence of the disease. Restarting treatment with prednisone and then subsequent feeding of S-Ag resulted in a similar positive therapeutic response, and a double-masked study resulted from these initial findings (see Chapter 7). Feeding either

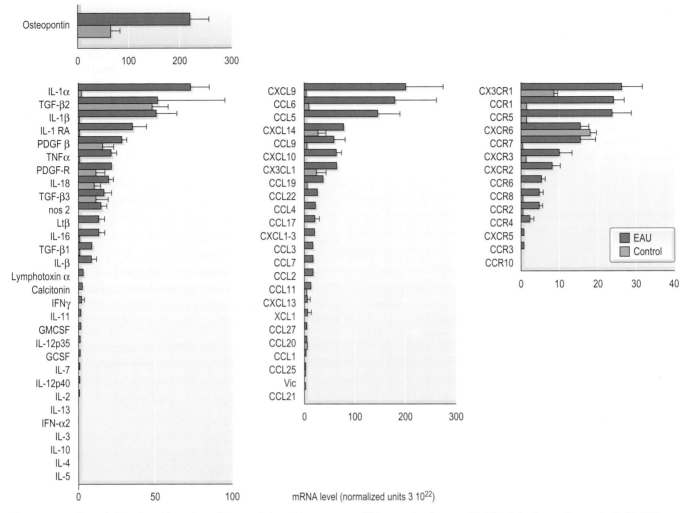

Figure 1-10. Upregulation of cytokines, chemokines, and chemokine receptor mRNA transcripts in eyes with EAU. Animals were immunized with IRBP to induce disease. *(From Foxman EF, Zhang M, Hurst SD, et al. Inflammatory mediators in uveitis: differential induction of cytokines and chemokines in Th1- versus Th2-mediated ocular inflammation. J Immunol 2002; 168: 2483–2492.* Copyright 2002, American Association of Immunologists.)

the antigen itself or an HLA-peptide that cross-reacts with S-Ag has shown promise.[79]

Choroidal circulation and anatomy

The choroid has a blood flow comparable only to that of the kidney. Therefore, systemic influences can be assumed to rapidly affect this portion of the eye. Indeed, the relatively large blood flow and its anatomy would act as a sort of trap for many bloodborne problems, most notably fungal disorders. Therefore most fungal lesions begin as a choroiditis.[80] The choroid has the capacity to function as a repository for immunoreactive cells, in the extreme taking on the anatomic structure of a lymph node (lymphoid hyperplasia). Therefore this organ can be the center for profound immune responses, as is the case in many disorders to be discussed. The high concentration of mast cells in the choroid may be one mechanism by which immunoreactive cells in the choroid could spread to other parts of the eye. The mast cell's release of immunoreactive factors could help T-cell egress and ingress from this compartment.

Retina

In addition to the uveitogenic antigens resident in its layers, the retina's being an 'extension of the brain' makes it particularly prone to certain neurotropic organisms. Examples include *T. gondii* and many viruses of the herpes family, which have a propensity for central nervous system tissue.

It is also important to remember that under normal circumstances the retinal vasculature has tight junctions, thus being impermeable to many molecules. Any perturbation, such as inflammation, that alters this permeability can result in a profound change in retinal functioning. Further, it is interesting to speculate that because the retina maintains a high degree of oxidative metabolism, the potential for the generation of oxygen radicals may lead to autotoxicity.

Immunogenetics

The capacity to respond to a specific immune stimulant is genetically determined. It has been noted that various mouse strains are variably susceptible to the same bacterial infection.[81] Another example of such a variable response is that seen against an allograft – that is, tissue taken from the same species but not from an identical twin or another animal of an inbred strain. The strength of the immune reaction against the allograft is in large part determined by antigens sitting on cell-surface membranes that are the products of genes classified as being in the MHC. The MHC region is termed the H-2 region in mice, and the histocompatibility lymphocyte antigen (HLA) region in humans. Immune response (IR) genes were discovered by Benacerraf and colleagues[82] in their experiments evaluating the immune response of guinea pigs to amino acid polymers. Breeding and cross-breeding led to the realization that a genetic region was responsible for this responsiveness or nonresponsiveness.[83] McDevitt and Chinitz[84] showed that antibody responses in mice to synthetic polypeptides were indeed linked to the MHC region. The observation that one region appeared to be responsible for both transplantation and general immune responses evoked enormous interest and led to the realization of the importance of this region. The HLA gene loci are found on chromosome 6 in humans. Three major classes of antigen are controlled by these genes.

Class I antigens

The class I antigens, which are proteins found on essentially all nucleated cells, are controlled by three loci in humans: A, B, and C. The class I molecule has a molecular weight of about 45 000 Da, is a glycoprotein, and is noncovalently linked to a β_2-microglobulin (**Fig. 1-11A and C**). The β_2-microglobulin molecule is not encoded within the MHC region but rather on chromosome 15, and is linked to the class I molecule at a later stage. A strong homology has been

shown between moieties of the class I molecule and immunoglobulins, suggesting similar early evolutionary paths. Class I molecules are quite heterogeneous, and several cell-surface membrane antigens controlled by each of the loci are defined. Complement-fixing cytotoxic antibodies can be raised against each variation, and these antigens are determined by serologic methods. The molecule will have an extracellular portion of the molecule, with the molecule extending through the membrane into the cytoplasm of the cell. Although the precise mechanisms are still unknown, it is known that the class I antigens participate in transplantation immunity by being the principal antigenic targets in allograft rejection. They also serve as recognition antigens for cytotoxic (CD8) T cells when they attack virally infected cells.

Class II and class III antigens

The class II antigens are produced by the HLA-D/DR locus.

There has been considerable debate as to whether the D/DR systems are the same. Some discrepancies in typing by means of the two methods have been noted in some non-white populations. Numerous alleles have been identified in the DR system. The test is performed on B cells by means of a complement-dependent microcytotoxicity assay and use of sera from multiparous women. The HLA-D/DR loci are

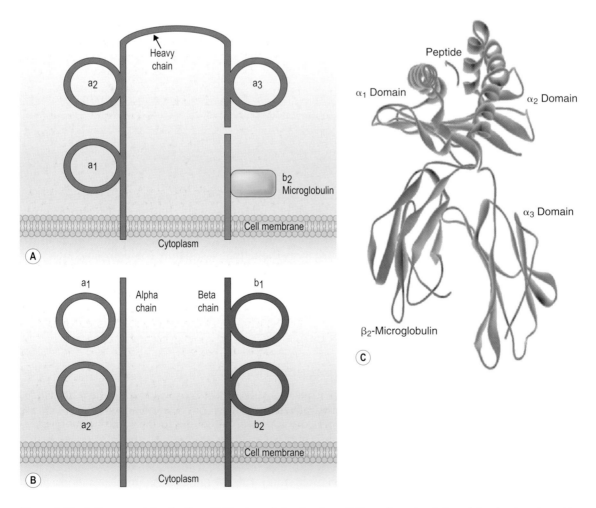

Figure 1-11. A, Structure of class I antigen. **B,** Structure of class II antigen. **C,** Three-dimensional view of class I antigen bound to peptide. *(From Lopez-Larrea C, Gonzalez S, Martinez-Borra J. The role of HLA-B27 polymorphism and molecular mimicry in spondyloarthropathy. Mol Med Today 1998; 4: 540–9.)*

thought to be the equivalent of the IR gene region already discussed. Further, the expression of cell-surface molecules these loci control has been given the generic term Ia antigens. The class II molecule is different from that of the class I. Here it is made up of an α chain with a molecular weight of 35 000 Da and a β chain of about 28 000 Da, which are noncovalently bound. No β_2-microglobulin is present (Fig. 1-11B).

The importance of the MHC gene products cannot be overstated, because large components of the immune response are histocompatibility restricted, meaning that immune cooperation will occur only if both components share identical D/DR antigens. B- and T-cell cooperation and T-cell cooperation with macrophages are such examples. This means that macrophages from one individual cannot present antigen to T cells from another unless they express the same class II antigens. In the case of the eye, the appearance of DR (or Ia) antigens on the cell surface of resident ocular cells (not usually thought of as part of the immune system) may indicate the potential for their role as accessory immune cells. Forrester and colleagues[85] found that the posterior uveal tract is richly populated with classic dendritic cells that constitutively express high levels of MHC II antigens. They further speculate about the important role in the interaction of resident ocular cells with the immune system, and by extension their initiation of autoimmune responses in the posterior pole.

Class III antigens produced within the MHC region are components of the complement cascade. Control of the levels of C1, C2, and C4 may also be encoded in this region.

Histocompatibility lymphocyte antigens

A logical adjunct to the recognition of the critical role the MHC region plays in the organism's immune response was the attempt to correlate certain disease processes with HLA antigens. There are several loci determining class I and II antigens (HLA A, B, C, DR, DQ, etc.). Each human has the capacity to express many different alleles. In the early days testing could not reveal that number in many persons, either because they had yet undetermined antigens or because they were homozygote for a specific allele. Associations have been made with certain diseases and HLA antigens. Brewerton and colleagues[86] were among the first to observe that an extremely high percentage of white patients with ankylosing spondylitis showed HLA-B27 positivity. The testing of other racial groups could not demonstrate as strong a correlation. Indeed, Khan and co-workers[87] demonstrated that HLA-B7 was associated with ankylosing spondylitis in African-Americans to a greater degree than was HLA-B27. One can infer from this and other studies that HLA associations may be different for various ethnic groups, and perhaps that different genes initiate responses that lead ultimately to a common pathway that we identify as disease. HLA allele distributions can vary dramatically from one ethnic group to another.[88] Therefore, identifying an HLA association in patients with a specific disease requires testing a large group of persons from the same gene pool who do not have the disease in question. This is done to determine the normal distribution of HLA antigens in that ethnic group. Only with this approach can it be determined whether a specific HLA antigen is more prevalent in a disease entity.

An example of such an HLA distribution can be seen from our studies dealing with birdshot retinochoroidopathy (**Table 1-6**) (see Chapter 25). One can see from Table 1-6 the distribution of alleles in both the white control and the white patient populations. Although not perhaps apparent initially, certain antigens may appear together more frequently than estimated by chance. This phenomenon is termed linkage disequilibrium. It indicates that certain HLA antigens appear consistently together more often than chance would allow. Such examples are HLA-A1, which is in known linkage disequilibrium with HLA-B8 and HLA-DR3; another would be HLA-A3 with HLA-B7 and HLA-DR2. In Table 1-6 it is HLA-A29 and HLA-B44. The percentage of patients bearing specific antigens can be seen, and the relative risk is calculated as follows:

$$\text{Relative risk} = \text{Antigen-positive patients} \times \text{Antigen-negative control subjects} / \text{Antigen-negative patients} \times \text{Antigen-positive control subjects}$$

The relative risk is an important indicator of the strength of the observation, because it indicates the increased risk for development of a given disease in persons having the antigen relative to those not carrying it. For birdshot retinochoroidopathy, it tells the observer that a white person who has the HLA-A29 antigen has an almost 50 times greater potential risk for developing this disease. Others have even calculated a higher relative risk for this disorder. Relative risks that are three to five times or less are usually of little practical help in determining risk. Some studies have used historic HLA data – that is, results obtained by others, perhaps at different institutions, possibly with different anti-HLA sera. It is clear that the use of such control subjects should be avoided if possible. Because of the great possible variation of HLA alleles in different groups, the use of control subjects of the same ethnic or racial group as that of patients in the disease group is essential.

Although mathematic programs exist to mix information gained from different ethnic or racial groups, the data obtained from these attempts are quite suspect. The basic rule poses real problems for those doing this type of research in countries with large numbers of citizens who are of mixed racial and ethnic parentage, such as Brazil, where great regional differences in HLA distribution are seen. Such problems also exist in India, where because of a strict caste system groups rarely intermarry, thereby creating a large number of 'mini-gene pools' in a society which, to an outsider, may appear homogeneous.

Ocular diseases have been evaluated extensively for their HLA associations (**Table 1-7**), some of which have large relative risks associated with them. The reader should always scrutinize the findings carefully, bearing in mind the aforementioned principles.

Why should there be an HLA association with certain diseases? The answer is that the reasons are unclear. The association may indeed reflect a specific immune response gene or one with which that gene is in linkage disequilibrium. Other concepts deal with HLA antigens and the exogenous environment. A provocative theory is one that was suggested by Botazzo and colleagues[89] some years ago. The reasoning behind this hypothesis is the requirement of class

Table 1-6 Distribution of HLA haplotypes in patients with birdshot retinochoroidopathy and in control subjects

HLA-A	Phenotype Frequency (%) Control Subjects (n = 418)	Patients (n = 20)	Exact p	Relative Risk HLA-A	HLA-A	Phenotype Frequency (%) Control Subjects (n = 418)	Patients (n = 20)	Exact p	Relative Risk HLA-A
1	24.4	20.0	0.7935	0.78	21	9.3	10.0	1.0000	1.08
2	52.6	35.0	0.1687	0.49	22	3.1	0.0	1.0000	0.00
3	27.3	15.0	0.3044	0.47	27	8.9	0.0	3.978	0.00
9	17.9	10.0	0.5493	0.51	35	19.4	15.0	0.7775	0.073
10	13.9	10.0	1.0000	0.69	37	2.4	0.0	1.0000	0.00
11	13.6	5.0	0.4955	0.33	38	7.4	5.0	1.0000	0.66
23	2.6	5.0	0.4335	1.95	39	4.3	5.0	0.5964	1.17
24	14.6	5.0	0.3337	0.31	40	12.0	10.0	1.0000	0.82
25	5.5	0.0	0.6147	0.00	42	0.5	0.0	1.0000	0.00
26	8.1	10.0	0.6751	1.26	44	25.4	45.0	0.6690	2.41
28	8.4	5.0	1.0000	0.58	45	1.9	5.0	0.3460	2.70
29	7.4	80.0	0.0000*	49.94	47	0.7	0.0	1.0000	0.00
30	5.5	0.0	0.6147	0.00	48	0.2	0.0	1.0000	0.00
31	4.3	0.0	1.0000	0.00	49	5.7	5.0	1.0000	0.86
32	9.3	10.0	1.0000	1.08	50	3.1	5.0	0.4855	1.64
33	1.4	0.0	1.0000	0.00	51	6.0	5.0	1.0000	0.83
36	0.2	0.0	1.0000	0.00	52	3.8	0.0	1.0000	0.00
HLA-B					53	3.4	0.0	1.0000	0.00
5	13.6	5.0	0.4955	0.33	54	1.0	0.0	1.0000	0.00
7	20.1	30.0	0.2676	1.70	55	0.7	0.0	1.0000	0.00
8	14.4	20.0	0.5133	1.49	**HLA-C1**				
12	27.5	50.0	0.0409†	2.64	1	8.4	5.0	1.0000	0.58
13	4.8	0.0	0.6147	0.00	2	9.1	10.0	0.7028	1.11
14	7.7	20.0	0.0719	3.02	3	25.4	10.0	0.1819	0.33
15	13.6	0.0	0.0911	0.00	4	20.6	15.0	0.7769	0.68
16	11.7	10.0	1.0000	0.84	5	5.7	10.0	0.3358	1.82
17	10.5	10.0	1.0000	0.94	6	5.5	5.0	1.0000	0.90
18	8.1	10.0	0.6751	1.26					

From Nussenblatt RB, Mittal KK, Ryan S, et al. Birdshot retinochoroidopathy – an association with HLA-A29 and immune responsiveness to retinal S-antigen. Am J Ophthalmol 1982; 94: 147–158. Used with permission.
*p < 0.0001.
†p < 0.05.

II antigens for antigen presentation and the initiation of the immune response. The inappropriate expression of class II coupled with other lapses of immune surveillance could lead to disease. A study that would support this notion was reported by Taurog and co-workers.[90] These authors produced rats transgenic for HLA-B27 and β_2-microglobulin, and found that the B27 transgene was expressed in a copy number-dependent fashion, and inflammatory disease depended on the expression of B27 above a critical threshold. The implication of essentially all theories is that

mechanisms to produce disease are multifactorial, and that exogenous and endogenous immune factors are needed. If not, disease expression would be far more common. A long series by Caspi and colleagues[91] of experiments in mice with experimentally induced uveitis supports this idea. From their observations, it is clear that the MHC plays a very important role in determining disease susceptibility. In mice certain permissive MHC types would include the $H-2^k$. However, the genetic background of the mice plays a very important role in determining the severity of the disease, so that a permissive MHC in a nonpermissive background will result in either very mild or no disease at all. Others have suggested that for some HLA antigens it is a question of molecular mimicry, with clones that escaped the negative and positive selection process in the thymus being activated by exogenous factors and ultimately attacking tissue when self peptide is presented in the context of HLA-B27 (**Fig. 1-12**). Molecular mimicry is an often used employed hypothesis in which

sequences from one antigen, whether from the host or from an invading organism, are very similar to sequences found in the proteins of the body. An immune response directed against the first antigen may thus be misdirected against the second. Therefore, an antigen derived from a pathogen may be similar to sequences of a structure in the eye, and the immune response initially directed against the pathogen will now be directed against the eye.

Single-nucleotide polymorphisms (SNPs)

An area that has received much attention is the genetic variations found normally in genes that mediate the immune response as opposed to those that control it. Any two random genomes are essentially identical: perhaps only 0.1% of the sequences will vary. Although this variance is due to several factors, the most common reason is SNPs, which are found throughout the genome, are stable, and are not considered mutations but rather normal (but relatively rare) variations from the norm. They are markers for different allelic forms of genes that can perform many different functions. For the purposes of this discusson, single-nucleotide changes can be found in genes whose products play an important role in the immune response, such as the cytokines. Indeed, one cytokine may have several SNP variations. Some SNPs do not appear to change the functioning of the protein at hand, but others appear to do so. An example would be an SNP in the promoter region of a cytokine that when stimulated produces either less or more of the given cytokine. One could imagine, then, that if population studies were performed as with HLA – that is, a disease group versus controls –SNPs might be identified more commonly in the disease

Table 1-7 Selected ocular diseases and their HLA associations

Disease	Antigen	Relative Risk
Acute anterior uveitis	HLA-B27 (W)	10
	HLA-B8 (AA)	5
Ankylosing spondylitis	HLA-B27 (W)	100
	HLA-B7 (AA)	
Complex-mediated disease	HLA-B51 (O) (?W)	4–6
Birdshot retinochoroidopathy	HLA-A29 (W)	49
Ocular pemphigoid	HLA-B12 (W)	3–4
Presumed ocular histoplasmosis	HLA-B7	(W)
Reiter's syndrome	HLA-B27 (W)	40
Rheumatoid arthritis	HLA-DR4 (W)	11
Sympathetic ophthalmia	HLA-A11 (M)	3.9
Vogt–Koyanagi–Harada disease	MT-3 (O)	74.5

AA, African-American; M, mixed ethnic study; O, Oriental; W, white.

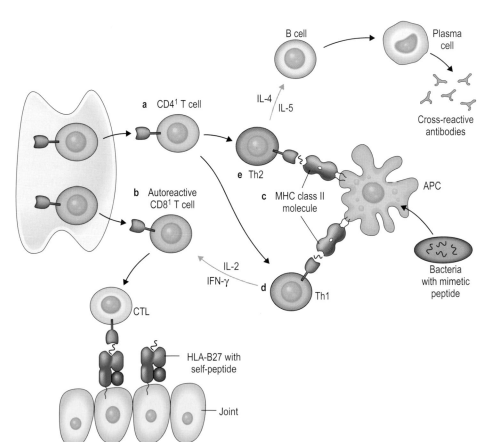

Figure 1-12. Molecular mimicry concept of autoimmunity as it may apply to HLA-B27. Clones of cells (a and b) escape positive and negative thymic selection described earlier in the chapter. They are capable of responding to autoantigens. These cells come into close contact with the antigen-processing cell (c), which has processed antigenic material from bacterium. Antigen mimics that of self-antigen. After antigenic information has been transferred, these cells are activated, becoming either Th1 or Th2 cells (e and d). They then elicit lymphokines, which produce a cell-mediated response against self-peptide linked to the HLA B27 or a B-cell/plasma-cell response, with antibodies also directed against the self-peptide. (*From Lopez-Larrea C, Gonzalez S, Martinez-Borra J, et al. The role of HLA-B27 polymorphism and molecular mimicry in spondyloarthropathy. Mol Med Today 1998; 540–9.*)

group and hence possibly associated with disease. This is indeed what has been done and is actively being done for many disorders, some of which are autoimmune and some neoplastic.[92] As mentioned above, variants of the CFH gene have been associated with age-related macular degeneration and multifocal choroiditis.

Epigenetics

The current understanding of epigenetics is 'the study of mechanisms that control somatically heritable gene expression status without changes in the underlying DNA sequence,[93] including DNA methylation/demethylation; histone modification (acetylation/deacetylation); chromatin modification; and control of transcription by noncoding RNAs (siRNA, miRNA). We are evaluating the involvement of DNA methylation in the immune system and the eye. DNA methylation has been shown to participate in the control of hematopoietic cell development. Comprehensive studies on DNA methylation in controlling cytokine expression in other immune cells, e.g., monocytes, NK cells and B cells, and genes with anti-inflammatory effect, e.g., IL-10 gene, are still lacking. This will be an area that will be very actively studied. It is hoped that such studies will help understand why a person with the same gene sequence has disease whereas another does not.

Immune complex-mediated disease

Type III hypersensitivity reactions were once thought to be the main mechanism of ocular inflammation. Immune complexes have a potentially important role in tissue destruction, but they may have an alternative role other than mediation of disease.

Immune complexes are formed by the association of an antibody with an autologous or exogenous antigen in the circulation, in the extravascular space, or on a cell surface. If the antibody molecule is of the IgM or IgG family, it has the capacity to bind to complement, thereby inducing tissue damage. The complexes often contain several immunoglobulin molecules and have a high molecular weight. One theory is that bivalent antigens are needed for the formation of immune complexes. Low levels of circulating immune complexes can be found in all normal persons. Immune complexes can function as an efficient way for the body to rid itself of unwanted tissue debris (or antigens), which is recognized more readily and removed more rapidly if bound to an antibody.

As mentioned, immune complexes can bind to tissue antigens, as in the kidney (an organ particularly prone to this type of immune-mediated damage), or to the vascular endothelium of many organs. With the fixing of complement, chemotactic factors could be released and neutrophils are attracted and activated. During this process they will release enzymes, which can degrade both proteins and collagen. This immune response will leave tissue damage, most frequently as areas of fibrinoid necrosis. In some models of immune complex-mediated disease of the lungs, TNF-α appears to be an important proinflammatory cytokine. This is mediated at least in part by the ability of TNF-α to upregulate the expression of adhesion molecules such as E-selectin and intercellular adhesion molecule (ICAM)-1. The addition of IL-4 or IL-10 not only affects the production of TNF-α but

also reduces nitric oxide production, protecting animals from immune complex-mediated lung injury.[94]

Several disorders have been hypothesized as being mediated by the type III hypersensitivity reaction. Serum sickness seen after the administration of a foreign protein is one of the classic examples. At least part of the pathologic process noted in patients with systemic lupus erythematosus kidney disease is thought to be mediated by this same mechanism, as is lens-induced endophthalmitis. Several infectious disorders are believed to have severe sequelae mediated by immune complexes as well. One such example is the severe renal disease seen after complexes form with soluble antigens of *Plasmodium falciparum*.

Gene expression profiling

Technology now permits the analysis of up- or downregulation in many genes at once. We were interested in characterizing gene expression in the monocytes from the blood of uveitis patients. Using a pathway specific cDNA microarray, we found that 67 inflammation- and autoimmune-associated gene products were differentially expressed in these cells. IL-22, IL-19, IL-20, IL-17 and IL-25 were highly expressed. We also found that there were four general patterns of gene expression, which were seen in related patients but did not necessarily correlate with clinical entities. Clearly multiple gene upregulation combinations can lead to the same clinical disease. This once again emphasizes how heterogeneous humans are.[95]

Tissue damage in the eye

The role of immune complex-mediated tissue damage in the eye still needs to be defined. Immune complexes can be demonstrated in the aqueous humor of patients with uveitis.[96,97] Circulating immune complexes have been reported in patients with Behçet's disease (see Chapter 26) and HLA-B27+ uveitis (see Chapter 19).[98,99] These and other findings have led some to speculate that immune complex-mediated tissue destruction could explain intraocular inflammatory disease, and that disease recurrence may be due to a repeated localization of immune complexes in the uveal tract.[100]

Experimentally one is able to induce inflammatory ocular disease by immune complex mediation. The placing of a foreign antigen (such as bovine serum albumin) into the eye, with a rechallenge some time later, will lead to an immune complex-mediated inflammatory response. Antigen–antibody complexes in the aqueous can be demonstrated only when the disease is active.[101] However, circulating immune complexes have not been shown to cause ocular inflammation.

Recent observations do not support the notion that immune complexes play a pivotal role in severe sight-threatening intermediate and posterior uveitis. In a review of iris specimens taken at the time of surgery from patients with uveitis, our laboratory noted no plasma cells nor evidence of immune complex-mediated disease (such as fibrinoid necrosis), but rather an influx of T cells.[102] Of particular note are the recent observations made concerning Behçet's disease, thought to be perhaps the most classic example of an immune complex-mediated uveitis. Anterior chamber paracentesis of well-established disease accompanied by hypopyon (see Chapter 26) reveals a large number of lymphocytes with a small number of neutrophils, the cell expected to predominate in an antigen–antibody reaction. A histologic review of a large number of globes from patients with complex-mediated disease failed to demonstrate evidence of immune complex-mediated disease. Of particular note was the pronounced perivasculitis and not fibrinoid changes of the retinal vasculature (DG Cogan, MD, personal communication, 1987). The deposition of complement and once again the lack of fibrinoid changes in the aphthous ulcers of these patients have led others also to conclude that other immune mechanisms were involved.[103] A final note is the observation by our group that circulating immune complexes either remained the same or increased in patients with immune complex-mediated disease whose condition was being therapeutically controlled with ciclosporin.[104]

The concept that the demonstration of immune complexes cannot be taken as prima facie evidence for an immune mechanism of destruction has begun to develop over the past few years. Kasp and colleagues[105] compared patients with retinal vasculitis who had circulating immune complexes and those who did not, and found that circulating immune complex formation seemed to protect against the more severe forms of retinal inflammatory disease. The possible explanation for this observation was that complexes seen in the group with the more favorable prognosis was made up of two antibodies, one harmful and the other produced by the body to neutralize the first. All assays for immune complexes rely on the detection of immunoglobulin aggregates.

It is important to remember that the hypervariable portion or idiotypic region of the immunoglobulin molecule – that part of the molecule directed against a specific antigen – can itself be an antigen for another immunoglobulin (the antiidiotypic antibody). This type of idiotypic–antiidiotypic complex has been recognized in several situations and may be a common immune mechanism. With the polyclonal response to a complex antigen, several idiotypic determinants may appear and be recognized as foreign, thereby initiating a response against these idiotypes. These antiidiotypes could also initiate an anti-antiidiotypic response, and so on. The importance of these observations is that this cascade can affect the immune response. de Kozak and Mirshahi[106] have shown that preimmunization with a monoclonal antibody directed against an epitope of the retinal S-Ag will protect animals from subsequent immunization with the retinal S-Ag. Another hypothesis is the induction of suppressor cells by antiidiotypic antibodies. This is the most probable explanation for a series of experiments by de Kozak and colleagues,[107] in which protection against EAU could be transferred with a lymph node preparation from antibody-immunized animals but not with the immunoglobulin fraction. Another possibility is the blocking effect of the second antibody, effectively removing the first antibody from circulation and preventing its intended effect on the immune response.

As mentioned above, an example of putative antibody mediated-ocular disease is cancer-related retinopathy. These patients produce antibodies that are believed to cross-react with their tumor and retinal elements, now thought to be the protein recoverin. The binding of the antibody to the retina will damage these elements and lead to poor vision.

T-cell responses and autoimmunity

On the basis of current concepts of autoimmunity and their apparent relevance to the eye, it seems appropriate to discuss T-cell mechanisms here as they appear to be inextricably intertwined. T-cell mechanisms are mediated not by the humoral route but rather through the direct contact of the T cell to the target cell or other immune cells, or through its release of lymphokines, thereby controlling the recruitment of other cells into the site of an immune response, these cells ultimately being the effector cells. In addition, T cells play a major suppressive role, both specific and nonspecific. Therefore dysregulation of this exquisite balance leading to autoimmunity would logically need to involve T cells.

Autoimmunity is an immune response directed against the host. This phenomenon is common and in the vast number of individuals does not lead to obvious disease. It is when these initial autoimmune mechanisms lead to tissue damage that we denote the outcome as autoimmune disease.[108] The mechanisms for autoimmune disease may vary considerably depending on the organ in question. Several mechanisms may lead ultimately to one final disease entity because of the relatively restricted way in which an organ is capable of responding to any immune response. Allison[109] and Weigle[110] both theorized that although sensitization may occur, the expression of disease would not be seen as long as the effector T cell is rendered 'tolerant' to the antigen in question. Such tolerance can occur if small amounts of the antigen are constantly circulating. This tolerant state is abrogated, however, if the effector T cell is now presented with a new moiety of the antigen, a situation which then leads to disease expression. Another hypothesis is that molecular mimicry is the initiating event (see earlier discussion of immunogenetics). The invading organism is quickly cleared, and the immune response is directed toward tissue components that are structurally similar. Another proposed mechanism is that nonspecific polyclonal activation of the immune system, either by virus or by immunostimulatory agents such as Gram-negative bacterial cell wall components, will overwhelm the normal regulatory mechanisms and permit 'forbidden clones' of cells to proliferate and cause tissue damage.

T-cell receptor and the expression of disease

As previously mentioned, much interest has centered on the antigen receptor expressed on the T-cell surface. The TCR has a complex structure, made up of several chains controlled by different genes. It has been suggested that a specific subfamily, the β chain of the TCR, is preferentially expressed on autoaggressive lymphocytes. In rats the Vβ8.2 subfamily epitope is expressed on a disproportionately large number of T cells capable of inducing EAU in naive animals.[111,112] Further work has refined this concept to a degree. It would appear that the Vβ8 family is expressed in these cells, but not necessarily exclusively. Egwuagu and co-workers[113] found that in rats the T cells invading the retina in S-Ag-induced EAU preferentially express Vβ8.2, but IRBP-immunized animals had in their retinas at an early stage of EAU T cells bearing both the Vβ8.2 and Vβ8.3 phenotypes. Further, in mice, Rao and colleagues[114] demonstrated a preferential usage of Vβ2, Vβ12, and Vβ15. These findings have both basic scientific and practical clinical implications. If it were true that one subfamily of Vβ8 was always expressed on T cells that are autoaggressive (i.e., induce autoimmune disease), then one could use this as a marker to identify such cells in the body, and, perhaps more importantly, these TCR peptide fragments could be used as a vaccinating agent to induce protection against all cells bearing this particular structure. Indeed, immunization (i.e., vaccination) with the Vβ8.2 fragments suppressed experimental autoimmune encephalomyelitis.[115] These results could not be reproduced in the experimental autoimmune uveitis model.[116] It is important to note that many questions still remain about the TCR-peptide–MHC complex. Structural biologic studies have not fully elucidated this relationship.[117] In one study,[118] in which the crystal structure of these relationships was evaluated, it was noted that the interface between the TCR and the peptide to which it is bound had minimal shape complementarity, and the β chain of the TCR, which is thought to determine the complementarity, had minimal interaction with the peptide. There was also a structural plasticity to the TCR once binding took place, suggesting a certain accommodation to different but similar proteins that it could or might bind with. In the evaluation of the crystal structure of an immunodominant sequence of myelin basic protein (which induces experimental allergic encephalomyelitis, a model of multiple sclerosis), the binding of the antigen in the TCR groove was found to be weak, and only a portion of the groove was occupied by the disease-inducing antigen.[119] Further studies indicated that 'cryptic' epitopes may be exposed under these circumstances, thereby explaining why these TCRs may escape selection in the thymus.

Ocular autoimmunity

The concept that the eye harbors autoimmune-inducing or uveitogenic materials has been suggested by many since the beginning of this century. It was the demonstration by Uhlenhuth[120] of autoantibody production to the lens that pioneered this whole area of investigation. Several investigators used homogenates from the eye which, when injected into an animal, appeared capable of inducing an intraocular inflammatory response. Particular tribute must be paid to Waldon Wacker and colleagues[121] working in Louisville, Kentucky, and to Jean-Pierre Faure and co-workers[122] working in Paris, France, for their zeal and scientific prowess in this area.

Uveitogenic antigens

The presence of uveitogenic antigens in the eye that are capable of inducing disease is an old concept, proposed as early as 1910 by Elschnig.[123] As we will see in some detail in the later section on autoimmunity, several antigens have been isolated that are capable of inducing ocular disease in rodents – in many respects similar to that seen in humans. This number of identifiable antigens capable of stimulating the immune system makes the eye unique, and suggests that the old concept of autoimmunity may be an important factor in ocular disease.

Retinal S-Antigen (Arrestin)

Wacker and colleagues reported the isolation, partial characterization, and immunologic properties of the retinal S-Ag

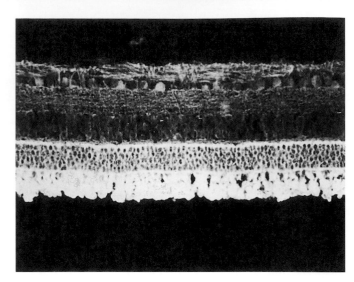

Figure 1-13. Distribution of retinal S-antigen in photoreceptor region. *(Courtesy of Waldon Wacker, PhD.)*

in 1977, with the French group soon after adding important new dimensions to this most important observation. The retinal S-Ag is one of the most potent of the uveitogenic antigens defined to date. This 48-kDa intracellular protein is localized to the photoreceptor region of the retina and the pineal gland in some species (**Fig. 1-13**). Preparations from various species demonstrate high levels of cross-reactivity, reflecting the fact that the molecule appears to be highly conserved through evolution. The S-Ag has a molecular weight of about 48 000 Da and contains a small amount of phospholipid. It is currently believed that S-Ag (or Arrestin)[124] has the ability to mediate rhodopsin-catalyzed adenosine triphosphate binding and to quench cyclic guanosine monophosphate phosphodiesterase (PDE) activation. It will bind to photoactivated phosphorylated rhodopsin, preventing the transducin-mediated activation of PDE.[125]

When injected in microgram quantities at a site far from the globe the S-Ag will cause an immune-mediated bilateral inflammatory response in the eye (EAU) (**Fig. 1-14**). The disease will begin as a retinitis in animals with angiotic retinae such as the monkey and the rat, with more choroidal involvement in animals with pauangiotic retinae such as the guinea pig (**Fig. 1-15**). Several S-Ag fragments have been shown to be pathogenic for Lewis rats.[126–129]

Interphotoreceptor Retinoid-Binding Protein

A second uveitogenic retinal antigen is IRBP. This 140-kDa molecule was identified, purified, and characterized by Wiggert and Chader,[130] and is believed to carry vitamin A derivatives between the photoreceptors and the RPE. It has four homologous domains.[131] Fox and colleagues[132] demonstrated that IRBP, purified to homogeneity, has potent uveitogenic properties, with disease induction occurring at dosages as low as 0.3 μg/rat. The course of the disease in the IRBP-induced EAU is shorter than that seen with S-Ag, and the meninges surrounding the pineal glands of animals immunized with IRBP showed inflammatory disease, whereas those receiving S-Ag did not. The disease induced in nonhuman primates with IRBP immunization shares similarities with that seen after S-Ag immunization, but has less vitreous inflammation and seems somewhat

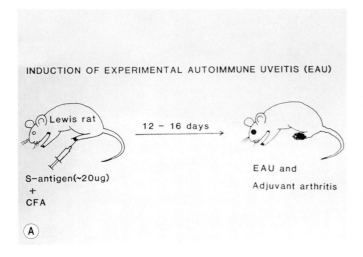

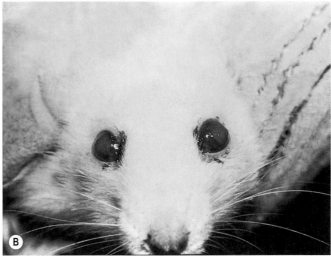

Figure 1-14. A, Active immunization scheme for induction of EAU. **B,** Appearance of rat immunized 2 weeks before with high dose of retinal S-antigen (arrestin). Bilateral panuveitis is clinically apparent.

more chronic[133] **(Fig. 1-16)**. Several IRBP fragments have been reported as being pathogenic for Lewis rats.[134–136] Recently Pennesi and colleagues[137] have created a transgenic mouse that has been humanized in terms of its HLA class II circuitry. This animal presented antigen using human HLA molecules and developed S-Ag-induced uveitis when it was resistant in the normal genotype.

Recoverin

Recoverin, a 23-kDa protein, is a calcium-binding protein that localizes to the retina and the pineal gland. This antigen has been shown to be the target of antibodies in the cancer-associated retinopathy syndrome.[138] Immunization of rats with as little as 10 μg of recoverin induced both uveitis and pinealitis.[139] The disease appears to be similar to that seen with S-Ag. EAU can be transferred to naive animals by lymph node cells from recoverin-immunized animals.

Bovine Melanin Protein

Bovine melanin protein is derived from choroid-containing remnants of adherent RPE. Broekhuyse and associates[140,141] reported that immunization was capable of inducing an autoimmune uveitis in rats. In the initial report, an anterior uveitis was the prominent aspect of the disease, with minimal choroidal involvement, and was therefore first called experimental autoimmune anterior uveitis. However, Chan and co-workers[142] showed choroidal disease to be a more constant finding. Broekhuyse and associates and Chan and co-workers have thus proposed the term experimental melanin protein-induced uveitis to describe this disorder.

Rhodopsin

High concentrations of rhodopsin will induce an S-Ag-like EAU.[143,144] A dose of 100–250 μg of the antigen is usually used, but this causes severe ocular disease and pinealitis, whereas lower doses give a concomitantly intermediate type of response. Opsin (rhodopsin's form in the light) seems to be less uveitogenic than rhodopsin.[145] Several fragments have been reported to be pathogenic in rat.[146]

Phosducin

Phosducin is a 33-kDa retinal protein that is thought to play a role in the phototransduction of rods.[147] It does not appear to be as potent as some of the other antigens mentioned: at a dose of 50 μg injected into a footpad, about 50% of the animals will develop disease. Patchy focal chorioretinal lesions with vitreitis and retinal vascular involvement have been reported.[148]

RPE 65

RPE 65 is a 61-kDa protein that is found specifically and abundantly in the RPE.[149] It is associated with the microsomal fraction of the RPE and appears to be highly conserved across vertebrates. It appears to play an important role in vitamin A metabolism. Mutations of RPE65 have been associated with Leber congenital amaurosis and retinitis pigmentosa.[150,151] It is interesting that immunization of rats with this antigen yielded a uveitis.[152] Although disease could be induced with the same dose of S-Ag (1 μg), the disease at higher doses was not as severe as that seen with S-Ag. Of interest was the fact that in this model a pinealitis was not seen, unlike that seen with S-Ag immunization. Strains of rat that usually are resistant to S-Ag-induced disease, such as the Brown Norway rat, did develop disease after immunization with RPE65.

Tyrosinase

Tyrosine proteins are found in melanocytes. It has been hypothesized for some time that melanocytic antigens were associated with the Vogt–Koyanagi–Harada syndrome (see Chapter 24). Two of these, tyrosinase-related proteins 1 (TRP1) and 2 (TRP2), have been isolated. TRP1 converts dihydroxyindole-2-carboxylic acid to Eu-melanin and TRP2 converts dopachrome to dihydoxyindol-2-carboxylic acid. Immunization with these antigens induced a severe anterior and posterior uveitis 12 days later,[153] and this continued for longer than a month, with in some animals a severe serous detachment and even lesions that appeared to resemble Dalen–Fuchs nodules. The lymphocytes of patients with Vogt–Koyanagi–Harada syndrome, when placed into culture with these antigens, will show strong immune memory.[154,155]

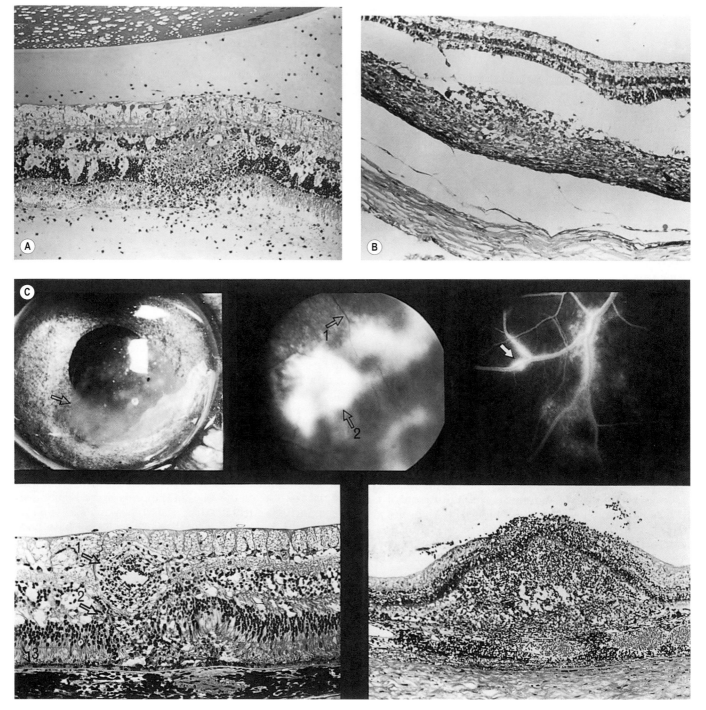

Figure 1-15. A, Retinitis seen in Lewis rat after immunization with retinal S-antigen. Inflammatory disease has destroyed normal retinal architecture. Severe anterior segment inflammatory response occurs when higher doses of antigen are used. **B,** S-antigen-induced inflammatory disease is more of a choroiditis when induced in pauangiotic animal, such as guinea pig. **C,** S-antigen-induced EAU in monkey. Note anterior chamber changes. Posterior retinal lesions, with fluorescein angiography showing periphlebitis. Histologic focal destruction of photoreceptor region, with perivasculitis. Lower right: Massive subretinal inflammatory response pushing retina upward. *(From Nussenblatt RB, Kuwabara T, de Monasterio RM. S-antigen uveitis in primates: a new model for human disease. Arch Ophthalmol 1981; 99: 1090–2.* Copyright 1981, American Medical Association.)

The S-Ag- and IRBP-induced models and the antigens themselves have been the ones best investigated to date.[156–158] The study of these immune-mediated models for human intraocular inflammatory disease has yielded information invaluable for our understanding of the human condition. Perhaps the most important observation was the dominant role of the T cell in this disorder. This was first reported when Salinas-Carmona and colleagues[159] noted that active immunization of nude rats (animals lacking an intact cell-mediated system) would not readily induce disease, whereas the heterozygote nude, having an intact T-cell circuitry, readily developed the disease. Further, transfer of splenic lymphocytes from S-Ag-immunized heterozygote animals to the nude rat (homozygote) did yield EAU.

However, if the T-cell fraction was removed from this cell transfer, the disease did not occur.

Further support for the mandatory role of the T cell was the development of uveitogenic T-cell lines from Lewis rats.[160,161] These IL-2 receptor + helper T cells will induce a disease that is identical histologically to that seen with active immunization.[162] The participation of other immune pathways in EAU has been examined. The transfer of hyperimmune serum containing anti-S-Ag antibodies to naive hosts will not induce disease. Immune complexes appear only in the reparative phase of the disease, suggesting that their appearance is one by which the immune system is down-regulating the response or clearing the debris left from the primary immune reaction.[163] The addition of cobra venom, a potent method by which the complement system will be depleted and therefore an excellent way to test the role of immune complexes in the mediation of disease, did not prevent the development of the posterior pole disease, but did dampen the anterior segment response.[164]

Mochizuki and co-workers[165] have noted that rat strain susceptibility to EAU induced with S-Ag was dramatically associated with the number of mast cells in the choroid, and de Kozak and colleagues[166] have shown that mast cells in the choroid degranulate just before the influx of T cells into the eye, thus suggesting that these cells 'open the door' into the eye for the T cells. This concept is especially provocative because Askenase and associates[167] have shown that mast-cell degranulation can be induced not only by IgE antibodies but also by T cells.

The changing patterns of cellular components and markers in the eye have given us a new understanding to this rapidly changing, finely orchestrated 'ballet.' Chan and colleagues[168] have shown that during the initial phase of S-Ag-induced EAU, helper T cells invade the eye, but later on it is the cytotoxic T subset that predominates (**Fig. 1-17**). This pattern has been seen in human disease as well. The widespread expression of class II antigens on several resident ocular cells is seen in EAU and in human uveitis, strengthening the observations seen in the animal model. It would also support the notion that these cells may be playing a role in the localized immune response (**Fig. 1-18**). The melanin

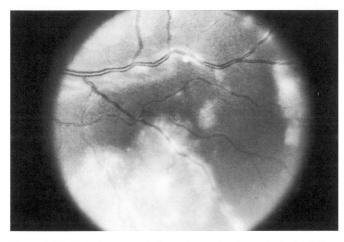

Figure 1-16. Posterior segment disease in monkey immunized with IRBP. Note deep retinal lesions and sheathing of retinal vessels.

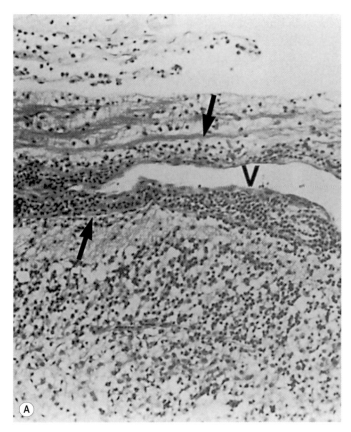

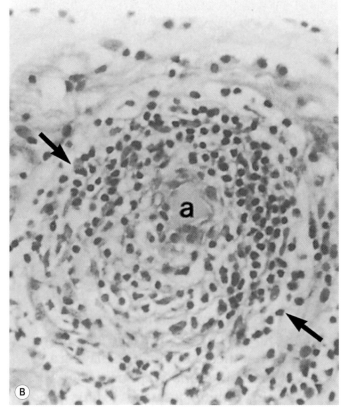

Figure 1-17. Photomicrographs of rat eye with EAU. **A,** Vessel (V) in cross-section demonstrating perivasculitis, with lymphocytes cuffing vessel along its route. **B,** Artery (a) with marked lymphocyte cuffing. *(Courtesy Chi Chan, MD.)*

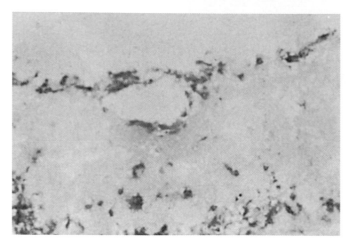

Figure 1-18. Immunohistochemical staining showing expression of Ia molecules on retinal endothelium of rat that has EAU.

protein-induced uveitis model has been noted to be characterized by a bilateral uveal infiltrate made up mostly of lymphocytes and monocytes, with most infiltrating T cells being CD4+. MHC class II antigens were expressed intraocularly. This model is suggestive of both the IRBP and the S-Ag models.[156–158]

Other Antigens

It is clear that other antigens can be the object of immune responses that result in an ocular inflammatory response. One other example is the anterior uveitis associated with myelin basic protein immunization. In addition to inducing changes in the central nervous system that is used as a model for multiple sclerosis, the anterior uveitis can be moderate and the immune response appears to target myelinated neurons in the iris. As with other models, CD4+ Th1 cells appear to mediate this disorder as well.[169–171]

Endotoxin and Other Bacterial Antigens

Another experimental model (but not autoimmune) is the injection into rats of the endotoxin lipopolysaccharide (LPS), a normal component of Gram-negative bacterial cell walls, at a site far from the globe. This will induce a relatively fleeting anterior segment inflammatory response characterized mostly by an infiltration of polymorphonuclear cells[172] and cytokine release.[173] This model has potential relevance because patients with ankylosing spondylitis[174] and uveitis[175] have been reported to have a higher incidence of *Klebsiella* organisms in their stool or infection with another Gram-negative bacterium during or shortly before the active portion of their disease than when their disease is quiet or compared with control subjects. Although these observations have not been universally corroborated, the findings do bring into question the potential role these Gram-negative organisms might play in immunomodulation. These antigens may activate complement without the participation of antibody. However, it is known that LPS can cause B-cell clonal expansion, bypassing the normal T-cell circuitry present to control such responses. The abundant B-cell response could cause large amounts of antibody formation and possibly immune complex formation, leading to an immune response. Either mechanism may be playing a role in the induction of anterior uveitis. One observation

was the demonstration of homology of six consecutive amino acids between HLA-B27 and *Klebsiella pneumoniae* nitrogenase residues, with autoantibodies against this residue being found in HLA-B27+ Reiter's syndrome and in patients with ankylosing spondylitis.[176]

Toll-like receptors, which are present on antigen-presenting cells, will bind to microbial products[177,178] and are considered critical for innate immunity activation. In other words, these microbial products are ligands to various toll-like receptors, activating the antigen-presenting cells to mature and perform efficiently, including the transfer of immune information to naive T cells. Fujimoto et al.[177,178] have shown that microbial products such as pertussis toxin are capable of enhancing or initiating pathogenic autoimmunity. This would suggest that infections, colds, etc, may play a sigfniciant role in initiating ocular immune responses.

Importance of Antigen Studies

This short synopsis concerning noninfectious ocular inflammatory animal models may convince the reader just how powerful a tool these models can be. The diseases induced have many features also seen in humans, allowing us to dissect the ocular immune response and drawing attention to the potential role of ocular resident cells in the immune response. Many of the clinical and pathologic alterations seen in the animal models are seen also in human disease. These models (particularly S-Ag and IRBP) have been excellent templates by which newer approaches to immunosuppression can be tested.[179–181]

Ciclosporin was first evaluated for ocular autoimmune disease with the use of the S-Ag-induced model of experimental uveitis. Experiments clearly demonstrated the efficacy of this agent in preventing the expression of disease in rats even if therapy was begun 1 week after immunization, at a time when immunocompetent cells capable of inducing disease are present.[182,183] Further, lymphocytes from the animals protected from EAU by ciclosporin therapy possessed immune memory for the antigen, giving positive in vitro proliferative responses to the S-Ag. Thus clonal deletion appears not to occur with ciclosporin therapy, but rather a shift in the immune kinetic occurs, so that the immune repertoire still functions but not in a synchronized manner. These initial observations led to the use of ciclosporin in human disease. Tacrolimus (FK506) has been evaluated in a similar fashion and found to be quite effective in preventing EAU, as was rapamycin, as well as the induction of tolerance with oral administration of the retinal S-Ag (see Chapter 7).

The continued evaluation of immunomodulation in EAU will lead to a variety of new therapeutic approaches because this model is increasingly used as a template to evaluate new therapies. Some of these strategies can be seen in **Figure 1-19**. Here the reader can see that numerous points of the immune system can be delineated and appropriate strategies employed. Microarray technology is being applied to these models to gain insight into gene activation in a way that could not be done before, that is, to observe hundreds and thousands of gene responses simultaneously (**Fig. 1-20**).

What is the potential role of the S-Ag or the other uveitogenic antigens found in the retina? This remains a matter of speculation. We have reported that patients with posterior and intermediate uveitis have exhibited in vitro cell-mediated proliferative responses to the S-Ag, not unlike those seen in the immunized animals.[184] It could be argued that these observations are epiphenomena and not relevant to the disease process. It is difficult to accept this hypothesis in view of the devastating disease induced by these antigens.

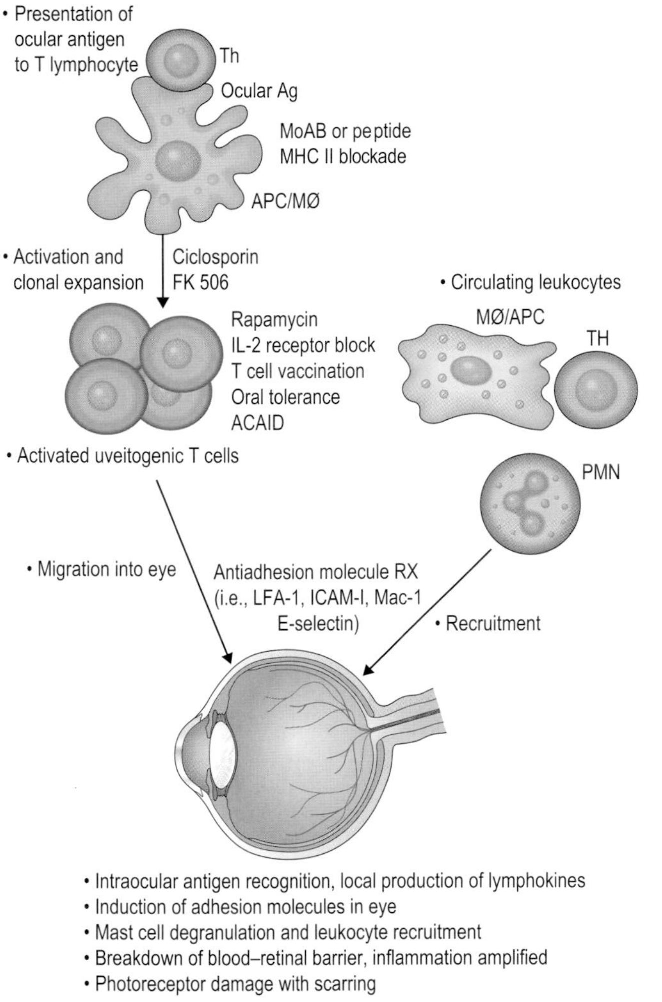

It is certainly possible that the initial event was not initiated by the S-Ag alone, but that the release of S-Ag followed an infectious process, whether viral or even toxoplasmic. It is also clear that the events leading to an 'autoimmune' uveitis are multifactorial.

Cell adhesion molecules and their role in lymphocyte homing and in disease

Cell-adhesion molecules (CAMs) are cell-surface glycoproteins important for the interaction of cells with other cells, and for the interaction of cells with the extracellular matrix. CAMs play an integral role in the development of the inflammatory response. These adhesion molecules are especially important for directing leukocytes to areas of inflammation. The upregulation of CAM expression on the vascular endothelium and surrounding area allows inflammatory cells to home to inflamed tissues.[185,186] CAMs are also involved in the interaction of lymphocytes and APCs, important for lymphocyte stimulation.

CAMs are divided into three structural groups: selectins, integrins, and the immunoglobulin gene superfamily. The selectins are a group of CAMs that appear to mediate the initial adhesion of inflammatory cells to the vascular endothelium, leading to a rolling of the cells along the vascular wall.[94] The integrins and members of the immunoglobulin supergene family then interact to form a more firm adherence between the leukocytes and the vascular endothelium, leading to transendothelial migration of the cells into the inflamed tissue.[187]

E-selectin, also known as endothelial leukocyte adhesion molecule-1 (ELAM-1, CD62E), mediates the attachment of polymorphonuclear leukocytes to endothelial cells in vitro and appears to be important in the recruitment of neutrophils in a local endotoxin response in the skin.[188] We investigated the expression of E-selectin in eyes with endotoxin-induced uveitis (EIU), a useful animal model for the study of acute ocular inflammation,[189] which is characterized by iris hyperemia, miosis, increased aqueous humor protein, and inflammatory cell infiltration into the anterior uvea and anterior chamber.[172,190–192] Inflammatory cells first enter the eye 6 hours after endotoxin injection, and the resultant uveitis peaks within 24 hours. EIU is thought to result from mediators released by activated cells, including macrophages, but the exact mechanism causing infiltration

Figure 1-19. Scheme showing induction of uveitis. Bullets (•) indicate what may be occurring based on evaluation of S-antigen uveitis model. *(Modified from Caspi RR, Nussenblatt RB. Natural and therapeutic control of ocular autoimmunity: rodent and man. In: Coutinho A, Kazatchkine MD, eds. Autoimmunity: physiology and disease. New York: Wiley-Liss, 1994.)*

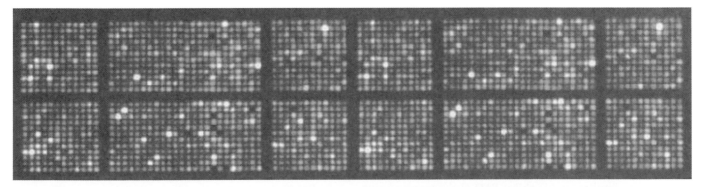

Figure 1-20. Microarray filter showing up- and downregulation of hundreds of genes evaluated at the same time. Dots on the filter have sequences of genes. By isolating RNA from cells and then using a reverse transcriptase, the complementary DNA can be obtained. The DNA can be placed on the complementary DNA structures on the microarray filter and thus genes that are active in a particular set of experiments can be identified. The technology can speed up information gathering enormously.

into the eye is not clearly defined. Recent data suggest that CAMs play an important role in the pathogenesis of this animal model of disease and that CAM expression is important for the recruitment of leukocytes into eyes with EIU.

ICAM-1 binds not only to Mac-1, but also to lymphocyte function-associated molecule-1 (LFA-1, CD11a/CD18), a second β_2-integrin expressed on all leukocytes predominantly involved in lymphocyte trafficking. A number of groups have studied how ICAM-1 and LFA-1 affect the development of EIU. In eyes with EIU in C3H/HeN mice, ICAM-1 is first expressed on the ciliary body epithelium 6 hours after endotoxin injection and, later, on the vascular endothelium of the ciliary body and iris and on the corneal endothelium.[193] Elner and colleagues[194] demonstrated the expression of ICAM-1 (CD54) on the corneal endothelium, and the expression of this cell adhesion molecule also appears to be important to the development of keratic precipitates. In experiments on Lewis rats we have seen that EIU can be prevented by treatment of animals with anti-ICAM-1 or anti-LFA-1 antibody at the time of endotoxin injection,[195] even when administered 6 hours after endotoxin injection when the eyes are already clinically inflamed. Rosenbaum and Boney[196] also showed that antibody to LFA-1 significantly reduced the cellular infiltrate associated with rabbit models of uveitis, but that vascular permeability was less affected. An ICAM neutralizing antibody can inhibit viral infection of the RPE by HTVL-1.[197]

The secretion of cytokines, particularly by infiltrating T lymphocytes, appears to regulate adhesion molecule expression. IFN-γ, IL-1, and TNF induce strong ICAM-1 expression at a transcriptional level, although the response to cytokines varies among cell types.[198–201] In vitro studies have shown that ICAM-1 expression on the cornea and RPE is upregulated by cytokines such as IL-1.[202,203] It is clear that one of the major effects of cytokines in the pathogenesis of EIU involves the upregulation of adhesion molecule expression.

CAMs have also been shown to play a critical role in the pathogenesis of EAU. We studied the expression of ICAM-1 and LFA-1 in B10.A mice with EAU.[204] ICAM-1 was first expressed on the vascular endothelium of the retina and ciliary body by 7 days after immunization, whereas infiltrating leukocytes expressing LFA-1 were not observed until 9 days after immunization, and clear histologic evidence of ocular inflammation did not occur until 11 days after immunization.

The effect of monoclonal antibodies against ICAM-1 and LFA-1 on the development of EAU has been examined. Ocular inflammation graded clinically at 14 and 21 days after immunization was significantly reduced in animals treated with anti-ICAM-1 ($p < 0.01$ at 14 and 21 days) or anti-LFA-1 antibody ($p < 0.01$ at 14 and 21 days). The inflammation graded histologically was also significantly reduced 21 days after immunization in animals treated with anti-ICAM-1 antibody ($p < 0.02$). Histologically graded inflammation was also reduced in animals treated with anti-LFA-1 antibody, but the difference did not reach statistical significance ($p < 0.10$). These data suggest that anti-adhesion molecule antibodies could inhibit EAU either by interfering with immunization and antigen sensitization or by blocking leukocyte homing and migration into the eye. These data indicate that antibodies against ICAM-1 and LFA-1 inhibit

EAU by interfering with both the induction and the effector phases of the disease. Adhesion molecules are also involved in the pathogenesis of lens-induced uveitis. Till and colleagues[205] showed that antibodies against adhesion molecules reduced ocular inflammation in lens-induced uveitis.

Recent studies in humans have also shown that cell-adhesion molecules are important in the development of ocular inflammation. We have shown that ICAM-1 is expressed in the retina and choroid of human eyes with posterior uveitis.[206] In addition, we demonstrated increased expression of ICAM-1 in corneas with allograft rejection.[207] Based on animal data, clinical trials are under way to examine the use of anti-adhesion molecule antibodies to treat inflammatory disease in humans. A recent phase I clinical trial in 18 patients who received cadaver donor renal allografts showed that immunosuppression with anti-ICAM-1 antibody resulted in significantly less rejection.[208] These data show not only that CAMs are involved in the pathogenesis of inflammation but also that drugs to block these adhesion molecules should provide effective therapy for inflammatory disease. In Chapter 7 we used Rapativa in the treament of patients with uveitis, with positive therapeutic effects.

Immune responses to invading viruses and parasites

The host's response to invading organisms is critical to its survival. Essentially all types of organism can invade the eye, and the response of the immune system will vary (**Table 1-8**).

Viral infections are of course of great concern to the ophthalmologist, particularly to those with a special interest in the anterior segment. However, the immune response to virus has taken on greater importance for those involved with intraocular inflammatory disease for both theoretic and practical reasons. Certain viruses have a particular propensity for retinal tissue, with herpes virus infections, particularly cytomegalovirus, being of ever-increasing concern.

The invasion of a virus into the organism leads to the mobilization of several aspects of the immune response. Antibody responses are abundant and may directly kill the virus. More frequently, however, cellular immune mechanisms appear to play a crucial role in eliminating the invader. T-cell responses against an invading virus have been well documented. The T-cell response is MHC restricted. The

Table 1-8 Immune mechanisms involved in infectious disease

Infectious Agent	Mode of Defense
Bacteria, virus	For neutralization, IgG with complement and neutrophils
Bacteria, virus	Gastrointestinal and respiratory infections: IgA, alternative complement pathway
Helminths	Intestinal IgE with mast cells
Pneumococci, encapsulated organisms	IgM, macrophages, and complement
Mycobacteria, virus	Cytotoxic T cells and perforin
Mycobacteria, virus, syphilis fungi	Macrophages and delayed-type hypersensitivity

T-cell is required to respond to a dual signal, that of the viral antigen and that of class I antigens sitting on a target cell membrane. NK cell activity is also seen to be directed against viral invasion. Found in the systemic circulation, these spontaneously cytotoxic cells are known also as large granular lymphocytes. NK cell activity is not MHC restricted, and virus-infected cells seem to be particularly vulnerable to this cell's attack, but the mechanism of recognition still remains unclear, though the cells are known to recognize certain viral antigens. These cells are thought to participate in antibody-dependent cell-mediated cytotoxicity, in which a specific antibody binds to the cell to enhance its destruction by cytotoxic cells. Macrophages also have important antiviral activity and will kill some engulfed virus particles. Others can be removed if macrophage activation is adequate.

The immune system is rapidly activated to efficiently handle a viral infection largely through the production of IFN. In response to a viral infection, both IFN-α and IFN-β are produced. The effect of IFN on a virally infected cell seems to be at least twofold: the production of a protein kinase, which inhibits viral protein synthesis, and the production of 2´,5´-adenylate synthetase, which inhibits viral RNA synthesis. In addition to this direct effect on the virus, the IFNs, because of their immunomodulatory properties,[209] profoundly affect the immune response as well. The appearance of class II MHC on cell-surface membranes could have an important effect on the rapidity of the immune response.

Because the immune response to the virus is largely cell mediated, any damage to this system could have grave consequences. This is the case with HIV infection, the virus that causes AIDS. This RNA virus, which has a marked propensity for Th cells, uses a reverse transcriptase to effectively incorporate its genetic library into that of the host cell. As the T cell becomes activated through antigen presentation by macrophages or other cells, the virus genome is also stimulated. The assembling and release of the HIV often lead to cell death. This virus then severely damages an important part of the immune system's mechanism for removing such infections. This has secondary repercussions in the body's attempt to clear other virus infections, such as cytomegalovirus.

Parasitic infections of the eye include many types of organism, from helminths to protozoa. The classically described response to parasitic infections is an eosinophilia. The release of the basic protein and other toxic products (see earlier discussion) from the eosinophil is thought to kill the organism. Certainly eosinophilia is characteristic of some forms of ocular parasitic infections, such as toxocariasis (see Chapter 16). However, for other infections, such as toxoplasmosis and onchocerciasis (see Chapters 14 and 17), this appears not to be the case. T cells seem to predominate in the eye in the more chronic forms of these diseases, and deficient T-cell functioning can lead to serious consequences. An example of this is the systemic and ocular toxoplasmic infection seen in patients with AIDS, in patients immunosuppressed because of neoplasms, or in those with iatrogenic suppression for graft survival.

Parasitic invaders have an additional capacity to evade immune surveillance. Immunosuppressive factors appear to be elaborated by the parasite, leading to a downgrading of macrophage and T-cell activity around it. Certain parasites cloak themselves in nonantigenic proteins, thereby avoiding immune attack. The cyst of *T. gondii* found in the eye is such an example, with the wall incorporating antigens from the host. Other parasites vary their antigenic appearance frequently to avoid the T-cell and macrophage-directed responses.

Suggested Readings

Gallin JI, Snyderman R, Fearon DT, et al, eds. Inflammation: basic principles and clinical correlates., Philadelphia: Lippincott Williams & Wilkins, 1999. (This edition is dedicated to Dr Ira Goldstein, a co-editor of a previous edition and one of my attendings in internal medicine many years ago: a very special person, a great loss to clinical immunology.)

Paul WE, ed. Fundamental immunology, 3rd edn. Philadelphia: Lippincott-Raven, 1999.

Paul WE, ed. Fundamental immunology, 6th edn. Philadelphia: Lippincott Williams & Wilkins, 2008.

References

1. Chen Z, O'Shea JJ. Th17 cells: a new fate for differentiating helper T cells. Immunol Res 2008; 41: 87–102.
2. Amadi-Obi A, Yu CR, Liu X, et al. TH17 cells contribute to uveitis and scleritis and are expanded by IL-2 and inhibited by IL-27/STAT1. Nature Med 2007; 13(6): 711–718.
3. Rachitskaya AV, Hansen AM, Horai R, et al. Cutting edge: NKT cells constitutively express IL-23 receptor and RORgammat and rapidly produce IL-17 upon receptor ligation in an IL-6-independent fashion. J Immunol 2008; 180(8): 5167–5171.
4. Shi G, Cox CA, Vistica BP, et al. Phenotype switching by inflammation-inducing polarized Th17 cells, but not by Th1 cells. J Immunol 2008; 181(10): 7205–7213.
5. Cox CA, Shi G, Yin H, et al. Both Th1 and Th17 are immunopathogenic but differ in other key biological activities. J Immunol 2008; 180(11): 7414–7422.
6. Ouyang W, Kolls JK, Zheng Y. The biological functions of T helper 17 cell effector cytokines in inflammation. Immunity 2008; 28(4): 454–467.
7. Andoh A, Zhang Z, Inatomi O, et al. Interleukin-22, a member of the IL-10 subfamily, induces inflammatory responses in colonic subepithelial myofibroblasts. Gastroenterology 2005; 129(3): 969–984.
8. Brand S, Beigel F, Olszak T, et al. IL-22 is increased in active Crohn's disease and promotes proinflammatory gene expression and intestinal epithelial cell migration. Am J Physiol Gastrointest Liver Physiol 2006; 290(4): G827–G838.
9. Piccirillo CA. Regulatory T cells in health and disease. Cytokine 2008; 43(3): 395–401.
10. Roncarolo MG, Bacchetta R, Bordignon C, et al. Type 1 T regulatory cells. Immunological Reviews 2001; 181: 68–71.
11. Kemper C, Chan AC, Green JM, et al. Activation of human CD4+ cells with CD3 and CD46 induces a T-regulatory cell 1 phenotype. Nature 2003; 421: 388–392.
12. Tsuji NM, Mizumachi K, Kurisaki J. Antigen-specific, CD4+CD25+ regulatory T cell clones induced in Peyer's patches. International Immunology 2003; 15: 525–534.

13. You, S, Alyanakian MA, Segovia B, et al. Immunoregulatory pathways controlling progression of autoimmunity in NOD mice. Ann N Y Acad Sci 2008; 1150: 300–310.

14. Roncarolo MG, Gregori S. Is FOXP3 a bona fide marker for human regulatory T cells? Eur J Immunol 2008; 38(4): 925–927.

15. Yeh S, Li Z, Forooghian F, et al. CD4+Foxp3+ T-regulatory cells in non-infectious uveitis. Arch Ophthalmol 2009 Apr; 127(4): 407–413.

16. Li Z, Lim WK, Mahesh SP, et al. Cutting edge: in vivo blockade of human IL-2 receptor induces expansion of CD56 (bright) regulatory NK cells in patients with active uveitis. J Immunol 2005; 174(9): 5187–5191.

17. Egwuagu CE, Charukamnoetkanok P, Gery I. Thymic expression of autoantigens correlates with resistance to autoimmune disease. J Immunol 1997; 159: 3109–3112.

18. Gery I, Egwuagu CE, Central tolerance mechanisms in control of susceptibility to autoimmune uveitic disease. Int Rev Immunol 2002; 21: 89–100.

19. Takase H, Yu CR, Mahdi RM, et al. Thymic expression of peripheral tissue antigens in humans: a remarkable variability among individuals. Int Immunol 2005; 17(8): 1131–1140.

20. Meloni A, Furcas M, Cetani F, et al. Autoantibodies against type I interferons as an additional diagnostic criterion for autoimmune polyendocrine syndrome type I. J Clin Endocrinol Metab 2008; 93(11): 4389–4397.

21. Devoss JJ, Shum AK, Johannes KP, et al. Effector mechanisms of the autoimmune syndrome in the murine model of autoimmune polyglandular syndrome type 1. J Immunol 2008; 181(6): 4072–4079.

22. Ferretti S, Bonneau O, Dubois GR, et al. IL-17, produced by lymphocytes and neutrophils, is necessary for lipopolysaccharide-induced airway neutrophilia: IL-15 as a possible trigger. J Immunol 2003; 170(4): 2106–2112.

23. Anderson DH, Mullins RF, Hageman GS, et al. A role for local inflammation in the formation of drusen in the aging eye. Am J Ophthalmol 2002; 134(3): 411–431.

24. Ng TK, Chen LJ, Liu DT, et al. Multiple gene polymorphisms in the complement factor H gene are associated with exudative age-related macular degeneration in Chinese. Invest Ophthalmol Vis Sci 2008; 49(8): 3312–3317.

25. Tuo J, Ning B, Bojanowski CM, et al. Synergic effect of polymorphisms in ERCC6 5′ flanking region and complement factor H on age-related macular degeneration predisposition. Proc Natl Acad Sci USA 2006; 103(24): 9256–9261.

26. Hageman GS, Anderson DH, Johnson LV, et al. A common haplotype in the complement regulatory gene factor H (HF1/CFH) predisposes individuals to age-related macular degeneration. Proc Natl Acad Sci USA 2005; 102(20): 7227–7232.

27. Nussenblatt RB, Ferris F, 3rd. Age-related macular degeneration and the immune response: implications for therapy. Am J Ophthalmol 2007; 144(4): 618–626.

28. Ferrara DC, Merriam JE, Freund KB, et al. Analysis of major alleles associated with age-related macular degeneration in patients with multifocal choroiditis: strong association with complement factor H. Arch Ophthalmol 2008; 126(11): 1562–1566.

29. Lei B, Bush RA, Milam AH, et al. Human melanoma-associated retinopathy (MAR) antibodies alter the retinal ON-response of the monkey ERG in vivo. Invest Ophthalmol Vis Sci 2000; 41(1): 262–266.

30. Tang J, Stevens RA, Okada AA, et al. Association of antiretinal antibodies in acute annular outer retinopathy. Arch Ophthalmol 2008; 126(1): 130–132.

31. Egan RM, Yorkey C, Black R, et al. Peptide-specific T cell clonal expansion in vivo following immunization in the eye, an immune privileged site. J Immunol 1996; 157: 2262–2271.

32. Ferguson TA, Green JM, Griffith TS. Cell death and immune privilege. Int Rev Immunol 2002; 21: 153–172.

33. Streilein-Stein J, Streilein JW. Anterior chamber associated immune deviation (ACAID): regulation, biological relevance, and implications for therapy. Int Rev Immunol 2002; 21: 123–152.

34. Stein-Streilein J. Immune regulation and the eye. Trends Immunol 2008; 29: 548–554.

35. Medawar P. Immunity to homologous grafted skin. III. The fate of skin homografts transplanted to brain, to subcutaneous tissue and to the anterior chamber of the eye. Br J Exp Pathol 1948; 29: 58–69.

36. Kaplan H, Streilein J. Immune response to immunization via the anterior chamber of the eye. I. F1-lymphocyte induced immune deviation. J Immunol 1977; 118: 809–814.

37. Streilein J, Neiderkom J. Induction of anterior chamber-associated immune deviation requires an intact, functional spleen. J Exp Med 1981; 153: 1058–1067.

38. Wetzig R, Foster C, Greene M. Ocular immune responses. I. Priming of A/J mice in the anterior chamber with azobenzenearsonate derivatized cells induces second-order-like suppressor T cells. J Immunol 1982; 128: 1753–1757.

39. Mizuno K, Clark A, Streilein J. Anterior chamber associate immunedeviation induced by soluble antigens. Invest Ophthalmol Vis Sci 1989; 30: 1112–1119.

40. Neiderkom J, Streilein J, Shadduck J. Deviant immune responses to allogeneic tumors injected intracamerally and subcutaneously in mice. Invest Ophthalmol Vis Sci 1981; 20: 355–363.

41. Eichhorn M, Horneber M, Streilein JW, et al. Anterior chamber associated immune deviation elicited via primate eyes. Invest Ophthalmol Vis Sci 1993; 342: 2926–2930.

42. Hara Y, Caspi R, Wiggert B, et al. Suppression of experimental autoimmune uveitis in mice by induction of anterior chamber associated immune deviation with interphotoreceptor retinoid binding protein. J Immunol 1992; 148: 1685–1692.

43. Wilbanks G, Streilein J. Studies on the induction of anterior chamber-associated immune deviation (ACAID). 1. Evidence that an antigen-specific, ACAID-inducing, cell-associated signal exists in the peripheral blood. J Immunol 1991; 146: 2610–2617.

44. Wilbanks G, Mammolenti M, Streilein J. Studies on the induction of anterior chamber-associated immune deviation (ACAID). III. Induction of ACAID depends upon intraocular transforming growth factor-beta. Eur J Immunol 1992; 22: 165–173.

45. Ferguson TA, Hayashi JD, Kaplan HJ. The immune response and the eye. III. Anterior chamber-associated immune deviation can be adoptively transferred by serum. J Immunol 1989; 143(3): 821–826.

46. Streilein J, Wilbanks G, Taylor A, et al. Eye-derived cytokines and the immunosuppressive intraocular microenvironment: a review. Curr Eye Res 1992; 11(suppl): 41–47.

47. Streilein JW, Masli S, Takeuchi M, Kezuka T. The eye's view of antigen presentation. Hum Immunol 2002; 63: 435–443.

48. Streilein J. Immune privilege as the result of local tissue barriers and immunosuppressive microenvironments. Curr Opin Immunol 1993; 5: 428–432.

49. Green DR, Ferguson TA. The role of FAS ligand in immune privilege. Nature Rev Mol Cell Biol 2001; 2: 917–924.

50. Caspi R, Roberge F, Nussenblatt R. Organ-resident, nonlymphoid cells suppress proliferation of autoimmune T-helper lymphocytes. Science 1987; 237: 1029–1032.

51. Chan C, Roberge F, Ni M, et al. Injury of Muller cells increases the incidence of experimental autoimmune uveoretinitis. Clin Immunol Immunopathol 1991; 59: 201–207.

52. Kawashima H, Gregerson D. Corneal endothelial cells block T cell

proliferation, but not T cell activation or responsiveness to exogenous IL-2. Curr Eye Res 1994; 13: 575–585.

53. Planck S, Dang T, Graves D, et al. Retinal pigment epithelial cells secrete interleukin-6 in response to interleukin-1. Invest Ophthalmol Vis Sci 1992; 33(1): 78–82.

54. Chan C, Detrick B, Nusenblatt R, et al. HLA-DR antigens on retinal pigment epithelial cells from patients with uveitis. Arch Ophthalmol 1986; 104: 725–729.

55. Percopo C, Hooks J, Shinohara T, et al. Cytokine-mediated activation of a neuronal retinal resident cell provokes antigen presentation. J Immunol 1990; 145: 4101–4107.

56. Kim BJ, Li Z, Fariss RN, et al. Constitutive and cytokine-induced GITR ligand expression on human retinal pigment epithelium and photoreceptors. Invest Ophthalmol Vis Sci 2004; 45(9): 3170–3176.

57. Mahesh SP, Li Z, Liu B, et al. Expression of GITR ligand abrogates immunosuppressive function of ocular tissue and differentially modulates inflammatory cytokines and chemokines. Eur J Immunol 2006; 36(8): 2128–2138.

58. Liu B, Li Z, Mahesh SP, et al. Glucocorticoid-induced tumor necrosis factor receptor negatively regulates activation of human primary natural killer (NK) cells by blocking proliferative signals and increasing NK cell apoptosis. J Biol Chem 2008; 283(13): 8202–8210.

59. Foxman EF, Zhang M, Hurst SD, et al. Inflammatory mediators in uveitis: differential induction of cytokines and chemokines in Th1- versus Th2- mediated ocular inflammation. J Immunol 2002; 168: 2483–2492.

60. Lee MT, Zhang M, Hurst SD, et al. Interferon-beta and adhesion molecules (E-selectin and s-intracellular adhesion molecule-1) are detected in sera from patients with retinal vasculitis and are induced in retinal vascular endothelial cells by Toll-like receptor 3 signalling. Clin Exp Immunol 2007; 147(1): 71–80.

61. Granstein R, Stszewski R, Knisely T, et al. Aqueous humor contains transforming growth factor-b and a small (<3500 daltons) inhibitor of thymocyte proliferation. J Immunol 1990; 144: 3021–3027.

62. Cousins S, Mccabe M, Danielpour D, et al. Identification of transforming growth factor beta as an immunosuppressive factor in aqueous humor. Invest Ophthalmol Vis Sci 1991; 32: 2201–2211.

63. Tripathi R, Li J, Borisuth N, et al. Trabecular cells of the eye express messenger RNA for transforming growth factor beta 1 and secrete this cytokine. Invest Ophthalmol Vis Sci 1993; 34: 2562–2569.

64. Taylor A, Streilein J, Cousins S. Identification of alpha-melanocyte stimulating hormone as a potential immunosuppressive factor in aqueous humor. Curr Eye Res 1992; 11: 1199–1206.

65. Wahlestedt C, Beding B, Ekman R, et al. Calcitonin gene-related peptide in the eye-release by sensory nerve stimulation and effects associated with neurogenic inflammation. Regulatory Peptides 1986; 16: 107–115.

66. Taylor A, Streilein J, Cousins S. Vasoactive intestinal peptide (VIP) contributes to the immunosuppressive activity of normal aqueous humor. J Immunol 1994; 153: 1080–1086.

67. Sternberg E, Hill J, Chrousos G, et al. Inflammatory mediator-induced hypothalamic–pituitary–adrenal axis activation is defective in streptococcal cell wall arthritis-susceptible Lewis rats. Proc Natl Acad Sci USA 1989; 153: 2374–2378.

68. Knisely TL, Hosoi J, Nazareno R, et al. The presence of biologically significant concentrations of glucocorticoids but little or no cortisol binding globulin within aqueous humor: relevance to immune privilege in the anterior chamber of the eye. Invest Ophthalmol Vis Sci 1994; 35: 3711–3723.

69. Wells H. Studies on the chemistry of anaphylaxis. III. Experiments with isolated proteins, especially those of hens' eggs. J Infect Dis 1911; 9: 147–151.

70. Chase M. Inhibition of experimental drug allergy by prior feeding of the sensitizing agent. Proc Soc Exp Biol Med 1946; 61: 257–259.

71. Weiner H, Friedman A, Miller A, et al. Oral tolerance: immunologic mechanisms and treatment of animal and human organ specific autoimmune diseases by oral administration of autoantigens. Ann Rev Immunol 1994; 12: 809–834.

72. Friedman A, Weiner H. Induction of anergy or active suppression following oral tolerance is determined by antigen dosage. Proc Natl Acad Sci USA 1994; 91: 6688–6692.

73. Gregerson D, Obritsch W, Donoso L. Oral tolerance in experimental autoimmune uveoretinitis. Distinct mechanisms of resistance are induced by low dose vs high dose feeding protocols. J Immunol 1993; 151: 5751–5761.

74. Miller A, Al-Sabbagh A, Santos L, et al. Epitopes of myelin basic protein that trigger TGF-beta release after oral tolerization are distinct from encephalitogenic epitopes and mediate epitope-driven bystander suppression. J Immunol 1993; 151: 7307–7315.

75. Nussenblatt R, Caspi R, Mahdi R, et al. Inhibition of S-antigen induced experimental autoimmune uveoretinitis by oral induction of tolerance with S-antigen. J Immunol 1990; 144: 1689–1695.

76. Suh E, Vistica B, Chan C, et al. Splenectomy abrogates the induction of oral tolerance in experimental autoimmune uveoretinitis. Curr Eye Res 1993; 12: 833–839.

77. Dick A, Cheng Y, Mckinnon A, et al. Nasal administration of retinal antigens suppresses the inflammatory response in experimental allergic uveoretinitis. A preliminary report of intranasal induction of tolerance with retinal antigens. Br J Ophthalmol 1993; 77: 171–175.

78. Nussenblatt R, De Smet M, Weiner H, et al. The treatment of the ocular complications of Behçet's disease with oral tolerization. In 6th International Conference on Behçet's disease. Amsterdam: Elsevier, 1993.

79. Thurau SR, Wildner G. Oral tolerance for treating uveitis – new hope for an old immunological mechanism. Prog Retinal Eye Res 2002; 21: 577–589.

80. Cogan D. Immunosuppression and eye disease. First Vail Lecture. Am J Ophthalmol 1977; 83: 777–788.

81. Shutze H, Gorer P, Finlayson M. The resistance of four mouse lines to bacterial infections. J Hyg 1936; 36: 37–49.

82. Benacerraf B, Green I, Paul W. The immune response of guinea pigs to hapten-poly-L-lysine conjugates as an example of the genetic control of the recognition of antigenicity. Cold Spring Harbor Symp Quant Biol 1967; 32: 569–575.

83. Bluestein HG, Green I, Benacerraf B. Specific immune response genes of the guinea pig. II. Relationship between the poly-L-lysine gene and the genes controlling immune responsiveness to copolymers of L-glutamic acid and L-tyrosine in random bred Hartley guinea pigs. J Exp Med 1971; 134: 471–481.

84. McDevitt H, Chinitz A. Genetic control of the antibody response: Relationship between immune response and histocompatibility (H-2) type. Science 1969; 163: 1207–1208.

85. Forrester J, Mcmenamin P, Holothouse I, et al. Localization and characterization of major histocompatibility complex class II-positive cells in the posterior segment of the eye: Implications for induction of autoimmune uveoretinitis. Invest Ophthalmol Vis Sci 1994; 35: 64–77.

86. Brewerton D, Hart, Nicholls FD, et al. Ankylosing spondylitis and HL-A27. Lancet 1973; i: 904.

87. Khan M, Kushner I, Braun WE. HLA-B7 and ankylosing spondylitis in American Blacks. N Engl J Med 1977; 297: 513.

88. Terasaki P. Histocompatibility testing 1980, in UCLA Tissue Typing Laboratory. Los Angeles: UCLA, 1980.

89. Bottazzo G, Pujol-Borrell R, Hanafusa T, et al. Role of aberrant HLA-DR expression and antigen presentation in induction of endocrine autoimmunity. Lancet 1983; ii: 1115–1119.

90. Taurog JD, Maika SD, Simmons WA, et al. Susceptibility to inflammatory disease in B27 transgenic rat lines correlates with the level of B27 expression. J Immunol 1993; 150: 4168–4178.

91. Caspi R, Grubbs B, Chan C, et al. Genetic control of susceptibility to experimental autoimmune uveoretinitis in the mouse model: Concomitant regulation by MHC and non-MHC genes. J Immunol 1992; 148: 2384–2389.

92. Shastry BS. SNP alleles in human disease and evolution. J Hum Genet 2002; 47: 561–566.

93. van der Maarel SM. Epigenetic mechanisms in health and disease. Ann Rheum Dis 2008 67(Suppl 3): 97–100.

94. Mulligan M, Varani J, Darne Ml, et al. Role of endothelial-leukocyte adhesion molecule 1 (ELAM-1) in neutrophil-mediated. J Clin Invest 1991; 88: 1396–1406.

95. Li Z, Liu B, Maminishkis A, et al. Gene expression profiling in autoimmune noninfectious uveitis disease. J Immunol 2008; 181(7): 5147–5157.

96. Derchnouchamps J, Vaerman J, Michiels J, et al. Immune complexes in the aqueous humor and serum. Am J Ophthalmol 1977; 84: 24–31.

97. Char D, Stein P, Masi R, et al. Immune complexes in uveitis. Am J Opthalmol 1979; 87: 678–681.

98. Lehner T, Almedida J, Levinsky R. Damaged membrane fragments and immune complexes in the blood of patients with Behçet's syndrome. Clin Exp Immunol 1978; 34: 206–212.

99. Vinje O, Miller P, Mellbye J. Immunological variables and acute phase reactants in patients with ankylosing spondylitis (Bechterew's syndrome) and their relatives. Clin Rheumatol 1984; 3: 501–513.

100. O'Connor G. Factors related to the initiation and recurrences of uveitis. XL Edward Jackson Memorial Lecture. Am J Ophthalmol 1983; 96: 577–599.

101. Howes EJ, Char D, Christenson M. Aqueous immune complexes in immunogenic uveitis. Invest Ophthalmol Vis Sci 1982; 23: 715–718.

102. Stevens GJ, Chan C, Wetzig R, et al. Iris lymphocytic infiltration in patients with clinically quiescent uveitis. Am J Ophthalmol 1987; 104: 508–515.

103. Poulter L, Lehner T, Duke O. Immunohistochemical investigations of recurrent oral ulcers and Behçet's disease. In: Lehner T, Barnes C, eds. Recent advances in Behçet's disease. London: Royal Society of Medicine Press, 1986; 123–128.

104. Nussenblatt R, Palestine A, Chan C, et al. Effectiveness of cyclosporine therapy for Behçet's disease. Arthritis Rheum 1985; 26: 671–679.

105. Kasp E, Graham E, Stanford M, et al. A point prevalence study of 150 patients with idiopathic retinal vasculitis: 2. Clinical relevance of antiretinal autoimmunity and circulating immune complexes. Br J Ophthalmol 1989; 73: 722–730.

106. de Kozak Y, Mirshahi M. Experimental autoimmune uveoretinitis: idiotypic regulation and disease suppression. Int Ophthalmol 1990; 14: 43–56.

107. de Kozak Y, Mirshahi M, Boucheix C, et al. Modulation of experimental autoimmune uveoretinitis by adoptive transfer of cells from rats immunized with anti-S antigen monoclonal antibody. Reg Immunol 1989; 2: 311–320.

108. Rose N, Bona C. Defining criteria for autoimmune diseases (Wetebsky's postulates revisited). Immunol Today 1993; 14: 426–430.

109. Allison A. Unresponsiveness to self antigens. Lancet 1971; ii: 1401–1403.

110. Weigle W. Recent observations and concepts in immunological unresponsiveness and autoimmunity. Clin Exp Immunol 1971; 9: 437–447.

111. Egwuagu C, Chow C, Beraud E, et al. T cell receptor beta-chain usage in experimental autoimmune uveoretinitis. J Autoimmunol 1991; 4: 315–324.

112. Gregerson D, Fling S, Merryman C, et al. Conserved T cell receptor V gene usage by uveitogenic T cells. Clin Immunol Immunopathol 1991; 58: 154–161.

113. Egwuagu C, Mahdi R, Nussenblatt R, et al. Evidence for selective accumulation of V beta 8+ T lymphocytes in experimental autoimmune uveoretinitis induced with two different retinal antigens. J Immunol 1993; 151: 1627–1636.

114. Rao N, Naida Y, Bell R, et al. Usage of T cell receptor beta-chain variable gene is highly restricted at the site of inflammation in murine autoimmune uveitis. J Immunol 1993; 150: 5716–5721.

115. Vandenbark A, Hashim G, Offner H. Immunization with a synthetic T-cell receptor V region peptide protects against experimental autoimmune encephalomyelitis. Nature 1989; 341: 541–544.

116. Kawano Y, Sasamoto Y, Kotake S, et al. Trials of vaccination against experimental autoimmune uveoretinitis with a T cell receptor peptide. Curr Eye Res 1991; 10: 789–795.

117. Bankovich AJ, Garcia KC. Not just any T cell receptor will do. Immunity 2003; 18: 7–11.

118. Garcia KC, Degano M, Pease LR, et al. Structural basis of plasticity in T cell receptor recognition of a self peptide-MHC antigen. Science 1998; 279: 1166–1172.

119. He XL, Radu C, Sidney J, et al. Structural snapshot of aberrant antigen presentation linked to autoimmunity: the immunodominant epitope of MBP complexed with I-A^u. Immunity 2002; 17: 83–94.

120. Uhlenhuth P. Zur Lehre von der Unterscheidung Verschiedener Eiweissarten mit Hilfe Spezifischer Sera. In: Festschrift zum 60 Geburtstag von Robert Koch. Jena: Fischer, 1903; 49–74.

121. Wacker W, Donoso L, Kalsow C. Experimental allergic uveitis. Isolation, characterization, and localization of a soluble uveitopathogenic antigen from bovine retina. J Immunol 1977; 119: 1949–1958.

122. Faure J. Autoimmunity and the retina. Curr Topics Eye Res 1980; 2: 215–302.

123. Elschnig A. Studien zur Sympathischen Ophthalmis. Die Antigen Wirkung des Augenpigmentes. Albrecht von Graefes Arch Ophthalmol 1910; 76: 509–546.

124. Pfister C, Dorey C, Vadot R, et al. Identite de la proteine dite '48k' qui interagit avec la rhodopsine illuminee dans les batonnets retiniens et de I' 'antigene S retinien' inducteur de l'uveo-retinite autoimmune experimentale. C R Acad Sci Paris 1984; 299: 261–265.

125. Pfister C, Chabre M, Plouet J, et al. Retinal S antigen identified as the 48k protein regulating light-dependent phosphodiesterase in rods. Science 1986; 228: 891–893.

126. Donoso L, Merryman C, Shinohara T, et al. S-antigen. Identification of the MAb A9-C6 monoclonal antibody binding site and the uveitopathogenic sites. Curr Eye Res 1986; 5: 995–1004.

127. de Smet M, Bitar G, Roberge F, et al. Human S-antigen: presence of multiple immunogenic and immunopathogenic sites in the Lewis rat. J Autoimmun 1993; 6: 587–599.

128. Gregerson D, Merryman C, Obritsch W, Donoso L. Identification of a potent new pathogenic site in human retinal S-antigen which induces experimental autoimmune uveoretinitis in LEW rats. Cell Immunol 1990; 128: 209–219.

129. Merryman C, Donoso L, Zhang X, et al. Characterization of a new, potent, immunopathogenic epitope in S-antigen that elicits T cells expressing V beta 8 and V alpha 2-like genes. J Immunol 1991; 146: 75–80.

130. Wiggert B, Chader GJ. Monkey interphotoreceptor retinoid-binding protein (IRBP): isolation, characterization, and synthesis. Prog Clin Biol Res 1985; 190: 89–110.

131. Borst D, Redmond T, Elser J, et al. Interphotoreceptor retinoid-binding, protein. Gene characterization, protein repeat structure, and its evolution. J Biol Chem 1989; 264: 1115–1123.

132. Fox G, Kuwabara T, Wiggert B, et al. Experimental autoimmune uveoretinitis (EAU) induced by retinal interphotoreceptor retinoid-binding protein (IRBP): Differences between

EAU induced by IRBP and by S-antigen. Clin Immunol Immunopathol 1987; 43: 256–264.

133. Hirose S, Kuwabara T, Nussenblatt R, et al. Uveitis induced in primates by interphotoreceptor retinoid-binding protein. Arch Ophthalmol 1986; 143: 79–83.

134. Donoso L, Merryman C, Sery T, et al. Human interstitial retinoid binding protein. A potent uveitopathogenic agent for the induction of experimental autoimmune uveitis. J Immunol 1989; 143: 79–83.

135. Kotake S, Redmond T, Wiggert B, et al. Unusual immunologic properties of the uveitogenic interphotoreceptor retinoid-binding protein-derived peptide R23. Invest Ophthalmol 1991; 146: 2995–3001.

136. Sanui H, Redmond T, Kotake S, et al. Identification of an immunodominant and highly immuopathogenic determinant in the retinal interphotoreceptor retinoid-binding protein (IRBP). J Exp Med 1989; 169: 1947–1960.

137. Pennesi G, Mattapallil MJ, Sun SH, et al. A humanized model of experimental autoimmune uveitis in HLA class II transgenic mice. J Clin Invest 2003; 111: 1171–1180.

138. Thirkill C, Tait R, Tyler N, et al. The cancer-associated retinopathy antigen is a recoverin-like protein. Invest Ophthalmol Vis Sci 1992; 33: 2768–2772.

139. Gery I, Chanaud NI, Anglade E. Recoverin is highly uveitogenic in Lewis rats. Invest Ophthalmol Vis Sci 1994; 35: 3342–3345.

140. Broekhuyse R, Kuhlmann E, Winkens H. Experimental autoimmune anterior uveitis (EAAU), a new form of experimental uveitis. I. Induction by a detergent-insoluble, intrinsic protein fraction of the retina pigment epithelium. Exp Eye Res 1991; 52: 465–474.

141. Broekhuyse R, Kuhlmann E, Winkens H. Experimental autoimmune anterior uveitis (EAAU). II. Dose-dependent induction and adoptive transfer using a melanin-bound antigen of the retinal pigment epithelium. Exp Eye Res 1992; 55: 401–411.

142. Chan C, Hikita N, Dastgheib K, et al. Experimental melanin-protein-induced uveitis in the Lewis rat. Immunopathologic processes. Ophthalmology 1994; 101: 1275–1280.

143. Schalken J, Winkens H, Van Vugt A, et al. Rhodopsin induced experimental autoimmune uveoretinitis in monkeys. Br J Ophthalmol 1989; 73: 68–172.

144. Schalken J, Winkens H, Van Vugt A, et al. Rhodopsin-induced experimental autoimmune uveoretinitis: dose-dependent clinicopathological features. Exp Eye Res 1988; 47: 35–145.

145. McMenamin P, Broekhuyse R, Forrester J. Ultrastructural pathology of experimental autoimmune uveitis: a review. Micron 1993; 24: 521–546.

146. Adamus D, Schmeid J, Hargrave P, et al. Induction of experimental autoimmune uveitis with rhodopsin synthetic peptides in Lewis rats. Curr Eye Res 1992; 11: 657–667.

147. Lee R, Fowler A, Mcginnis J, et al. Amino acid and cDNA sequence of bovine phosducin, a soluble phosphoprotein from photoreceptor cells. J Biol Chem 1990; 265: 15867–15873.

148. Dua H, Lee R, Lolley R, et al. Induction of experimental autoimmune uveitis by the retinal photoreceptor cell protein, phosducin. Curr Eye Res 1992; 11: 107–111.

149. Hamel CP, Tsilou E, Pfeffer BA, et al. Molecular cloning and expression of RPE65, a novel retinal pigment epithelium-specific microsomal protein that is post-transcriptionally regulated in vitro. J Biol Chem 1993; 268: 15751–15757.

150. Thompson DA, Gyurus P, Fleischer LL, et al. Genetics and phenotypes of RPE65 mutations in inherited retinal degeneration. Invest Ophthalmol Vis Sci 2000; 41: 4293–4299.

151. Morimura H, Fishman GA, Grover SA, et al. Mutations in the RPE65 gene in patients with autosomal recessive retinitis pigmentosa or Leber congenital amaurosis. Proc Natl Acad Sci USA 1998; 95: 3088–3093.

152. Ham DI, Gentleman S, Chan CC, et al. RPE65 is highly uveitogenic in rats. Invest Ophthalmol Vis Sci 2002; 43: 2258–2263.

153. Yamaki K, Kondo I, Nakmura H, et al. Ocular and extraocular inflammation induced by immunization of tyrosinase related protein 1 and 2 in Lewis rats. Exp Eye Res 2000; 71: 361–369.

154. Yamaki K, Gocho K, Hayakawa K, et al. Tyrosinase family proteins are antigens specific to Vogt–Koyanagi–Harada disease. J Immunol 2000; 165: 7323–7329.

155. Gocho K, Kondo I, Yamaki K. Identification of autoreactive T cells in Vogt–Koyanagi–Harada disease. Invest Ophthalmol Vis Sci 2001; 42: 2004–2009.

156. Caspi R. Experimental autoimmune uveoretinitis – rat and mouse. In: Cohen I, Miller A, eds. Autoimmune disease models: a guidebook. London: Academic Press, 1994; 57–81.

157. Caspi RR. Immune mechanisms in uveitis. Springer Semin Immunopathol 1999; 21: 113–124.

158. Caspi RR. Th1 and Th2 responses in pathogenesis and regulation of experimental autoimmune uveoretinitis. Int Rev Immunol 2002; 21: 197–208.

159. Salinas-Carmona M, Nussenblatt R, Gery I. Experimental autoimmune uveitis in the athymic nude rat. Eur J Immunol 1982; 25: 481–484.

160. Rozenszajn L, Muellenberg-Coulombre C, Gery I, et al. Induction of experimental autoimmune uveoretinitis (EAU) in rats by T cell lines. Immunology 1986; 57: 559–565.

161. Nussenblatt R, Palestine A, El-Saied M, et al. Long-term antigen specific and non-specific T-cell lines and clones in uveitis. Curr Eye Res 1984; 99–305.

162. Caspi R, Roberge F, Mcallister C, et al. T-cell lines mediating experimental autoimmune uveoretinitis (EAU) in the rat. J Immunol 1986; 136: 928–933.

163. Sakai J. Immune complexes in experimental autoimmune uveo-retinitis. Nippon Ganka Gakkai Zasshi 1982; 87: 1288–1299.

164. Marak GJ, Wacker W, Rao N, et al. Effects of complement depletion on experimental allergic uveitis. Ophthalmol Res 1979; 11: 97–107.

165. Mochizuki M, Kuwabara T, Chan C, et al. An association between susceptibility to experimental autoimmune uveitis and choroidal mast cell numbers. J Immunol 1984; 33: 1699–1701.

166. de Kozak Y, Sainte-Laudy J, Benveniste J, et al. Evidence for immediate hypersensitivity phenomena in experimental autoimmune uveoretinitis. Eur J Immunol 1981; 11: 612–617.

167. Askenase P, Rosenstein R, Ptak W. T-cells produce an antigen-binding factor with in vivo activity analogous to IgE antibody. J Exp Med 1983; 157: 862–873.

168. Chan C, Mochizuki M, Palestine A, et al. Kinetics of T-lymphocyte subsets in the eyes of Lewis rats with experimental autoimmune uveitis. Cell Immunol 1985; 96: 430–434.

169. Adamus G, Amundson D, Vainiene M, et al. Myelin basic protein specific T-helper cells induce experimental anterior uveitis. J Neurosci Res 1996; 44: 513–518.

170. Adamus G, Chan C. Experimental autoimmune uveitides: multiple antigens, diverse diseases. Int Rev Immunol 2002; 21: 209–229.

171. Jiang S, Arendt A, Hargrave PA, et al. Cryptic MCP epitope 1–20 is inducing autoimmune anterior uveitis without EAE in Lewis rats. Cell Immunol 2002; 217: 87–94.

172. Rosenbaum J, McDevitt HO, Guss RB, et al. Endotoxin-induced uveitis in rats as a model for human disease. Nature 1980; 286: 611–613.

173. De Vos A, Hoekzema R, Kijlstra A. Cytokines and uveitis, a review. Curr Eye Res 1992; 11: 581–597.

174. Ebringer A, Cowdell D, Cowling P. Sequential studies in ankylosing spondylitis. Ann Rheum Dis 1978; 37: 146–151.

175. Saari K. Acute anterior uveitis. In: Saari K, ed. Uveitis update. Amsterdam: Excerpta Medica, 1984; 79–90.

176. Schwimmbeck P, Yu D, Oldstone M. Autoantibodies to HLA B27 in the

sera of HLA B27 patients with ankylosing spondylitis and Reiter's syndrome. J Exp Med 1987; 166: 173–181.

177. Fujimoto C, Shi G, Gery I. Microbial products trigger autoimmune ocular inflammation. Ophthalmic Res 2008; 40(3–4): 193–199.

178. Fujimoto C, Shi G, Gery I, et al. Pertussis toxin is superior to TLR ligands in enhancing pathogenic autoimmunity, targeted at a neo-self antigen, by triggering robust expansion of Th1 cells and their cytokine production. J Immunol 2006; 177(10): 6896–6903.

179. Gery I, Mochizuki M, Nussenblatt R. Retinal specific antigens and immunopathogenic processes they provoke. In: Osborne N, Chader J, eds. Progress in retinal research. Oxford: Pergamon Press, 1986; 75–109.

180. Nussenblatt R. Proctor Lecture. Experimental autoimmune uveitis: Mechanisms of disease and clinical therapeutic indications. Invest Ophthalmol Vis Sci 1991; 32: 3131–3141.

181. Caspi R, Nussenblatt R. Natural and therapeutic control of ocular autoimmunity: rodent and man. In: Coutinho A, Kazatchkine M, eds. Autoimmunity: physiology and disease. New York: Wiley-Liss, 1994; 377–405.

182. Nussenblatt R, Rodrigues M, Wacker W, et al. Cyclosporin A. Inhibition of experimental autoimmune uveitis in Lewis rats. J Clin Invest 1981; 67: 1228–1231.

183. Nussenblatt R, Rodrigues M, Salinas-Carmona M, et al. Modulation of experimental autoimmune uveitis with cyclosporin A. Arch Ophthalmol 1982; 100: 1146–1149.

184. Nussenblatt R, Gery I, Ballintine E, et al. Cellular immune responsiveness of uveitis patients to retinal S-antigen. Am J Ophthalmol 1980; 89: 173–179.

185. Bevilacqua M, Stengelin S, Gimbrone M, et al. Endothelial leukocyte adhesion molecule-1: An inducible receptor for neutrophils related to complement regulatory proteins and lectins. Science 1989; 243: 1160–1164.

186. Luscinskas F, Brock A, Arnaout MJ. Endothelial-leukocyte adhesion molecule-1-dependent and leukocyte (CD11/CD18)-dependent mechanisms contribute to polymorphonuclear leukocyte adhesion to cytokine-activated human vascular endothelium. J Immunol 1989; 142: 2257–2263.

187. Springer T. Traffic signals for lymphocyte recirculation and leukocyte emigration: the multistep paradigm. Cell 1994; 76: 301–314.

188. Munro J, Pober J, Cotran R. Recruitment of neutrophils in the local endotoxin response: Association with de novo endothelial expression of endothelial leukocyte adhesion molecule-1. Lab Invest 1991; 64: 295–299.

189. Whitcup S, Wakefield D, Li Q, et al. Endothelial leukocyte adhesion molecule-1 in endotoxin-induced uveitis. Invest Ophthalmol Vis Sci 1992; 33: 2626–2630.

190. Ayo C. A toxic ocular action. New property of schwartzman toxins. J Immunol 1943; 46: 113–132.

191. Forrester J, Worgul B, Merriam GJ. Endotoxin-induced uveitis in the rat. Albrecht von Graefes Arch Klin Ophthalmol 1980; 213: 221–233.

192. Kogiso M, Tanouchi Y, Mimura Y, et al. Endotoxin-induced uveitis in mice. I. Induction of uveitis and role of T lymphocytes. Jpn J Ophthalmol 1992; 36: 281–290.

193. Whitcup S, Debarge L, Caspi R, et al. Monoclonal antibodies against ICAM-1 (CD54) and LFA-1 (CD11a/CD18) inhibit experimental autoimmune uveitis. Clin Immunol Immunopathol 1993; 67: 143–150.

194. Elner V, Elner S, Pavilack M, et al. Intercellular adhesion molecule-1 in human corneal endothelium: Modulation and function. Am J Pathol 1991; 138: 525–536.

195. Whitcup S, Hikita N, Shirao M, et al. Effect of monoclonal antibodies against ICAM-1 (CD54) an LFA-1 alpha (CD11a) in the prevention and treatment of endotoxin-induced uveitis (EIU). Invest Ophthalmol Vis Sci 1993; 34: 1143.

196. Rosenbaum J, Boney R. Efficacy of antibodies to adhesion molecules, CD11a or CD18, in rabbit models of uveitis. Curr Eye Res 1993; 12: 827–831.

197. Liu B, Li Z, Mahesh SP, et al. HTLV-1 infection of human retinal pigment epithelial cells and inhibition of viral infection by an antibody to ICAM-1. Invest Ophthalmol Vis Sci 2006; 47(4): 1510–1515.

198. Springer T. Adhesion receptors of the immune system. Nature 1990; 346: 425–434.

199. Springer T, Dustin M, Kishimoto T, Marlin S. The lymphocyte function-associated LFA-1, CD2, and LFA-3 molecules: cell adhesion receptors of the immune system. Ann Rev Immun 1987; 5: 223–252.

200. Dustin M, Springer T. Lymphocyte function-associated antigen-1 (LFA-1) interaction with intercellular adhesion molecule (ICAM-1) is one of at least three mechanisms for lymphocyte adhesion to cultured endothelial cells. J Cell Biol 1988; 107: 321–331.

201. Norris D. Cytokine modulation of adhesion molecules in the regulation of immunologic cytotoxicity of epidermal targets. J Invest Dermatol 1990; 95: 11S–120S.

202. Kaminska G, Niederkom J, McCulley J. Intercellular adhesion molecule-1 (ICAM-1) expression in normal and inflamed human cornea: induction by recombinant interferon gamma and interleukin-1. Ophthalmol Vis Sci 1991; 32(suppl): 677.

203. Liversidge J, Sewell H, Forrester J. Interactions between lymphocytes and cells of the blood–retina barrier: mechanisms of T lymphocyte adhesion to human retinal capillary endothelial cells and retinal pigment epithelial cells in vitro. Immunology 1990; 71: 390–396.

204. Whitcup S, Debarge L, Rosen H, et al. Monoclonal antibody against CD 11b/CD 18 inhibits endotoxin-induced uveitis. Invest Ophthalmol Vis Sci 1993; 34: 673–681.

205. Till G, Mulligan M, Lee S, et al. Adhesion molecules in experimental phacoanaphylactic endophthalmitis. Invest Ophthalmol Vis Sci 1992; 33(suppl): 795.

206. Whitcup S, Mulligan M, Lee S. Expression of cell adhesion molecules in posterior uveitis. Arch Ophthalmol 1992; 110: 662–666.

207. Whitcup S, Nussenblatt R, Price FJ, et al. Expression of cell adhesion molecules in corneal graft failure. Cornea 1993; 12: 475–480.

208. Haug C, Colvin RB, Delmonico FL, et al. A phase I trial of immunosuppression with anti-ICAM-1 (CD54) mAb in renal allograft recipients. Transplantation 1993; 55: 766–773.

209. Hooks J, Detrick B. Immunoregulatory functions of interferon. In: Torrence P, ed. Biological response modifiers. New York: Academic Press, 1985; 55–75.

Medical History in the Patient with Uveitis

Scott M. Whitcup

Key concepts

- A detailed medical history is the key to diagnosis in the majority of cases of uveitis.
- A uveitis medical history questionnaire provides a core of standardized information useful for diagnosis.
- Therapy should be targeted to not only address inflammation noted on examination, but also to treat symptoms that affect patient function or quality of life.
- Medical history is important in assessing response to therapy and side effects of medications.

The word 'diagnosis' comes from the Greek word meaning to distinguish and discern. Diagnosis encompasses both data collection and analysis of the compiled clinical information. The facts used in diagnosis come from a detailed medical history and a thorough physical examination. In the case of patients with uveitis, one must look beyond the eye for important diagnostic clues because the rheumatologic, infectious, and oncologic diseases that cause uveitis are often easier to diagnose after a careful medical history has been taken and a detailed physical examination has been performed. The ophthalmologist who does not examine the skin or joints of the patient with uveitis will miss the opportunity to correctly diagnose many cases. Observing the course of the disease as well as the response to therapy can also provide additional insights into identifying the correct causes of the disease.

A careful and detailed medical history is one of the keys to correct diagnosis in the patient with uveitis. It has been estimated that more than 90% of diagnoses can be made on the basis of the medical history alone. It is important not only to obtain a series of medical facts but also to form an impression about the overall course of the disease and its impact on the patient's quality of life. Are there defined disease episodes, or is the condition truly chronic? Is inflammation accompanied by pain and redness, or by floaters and visual loss? In chronic disease, the level of visual disability and discomfort that is tolerable for one patient is intolerable for another, and it is important to understand the patient's perspective before recommending therapy. In addition, some aspects of the disease can be modified by therapy but others cannot. By determining what is really bothering the patient, the physician can attempt to focus therapy on the most troublesome aspect of the disease. For example, some patients are troubled by mild conjunctival erythema and request treatment. Other patients do not like to use medications and tolerate mild redness. Importantly, the perception of visual loss differs greatly among patients. Even mild distortion in vision related to inflammation may interfere with the activities of some patients and warrant aggressive anti-inflammatory therapy. Only by fully understanding the patient and his/her relationship with the disease can the physician best counsel them and put the disorder into proper perspective.

Floaters and reduced vision are the two most common complaints of patients with inflammation of the vitreous, retina, and choroid. Most patients describe floaters as multiple small- or medium-sized spots that move as their eye moves. Other patients complain of blurred or reduced vision. In fact, when visual acuity is severely diminished, patients may be unable to visualize the floaters and may only complain of floaters as their vision starts to improve after therapy. A change in the pattern of floaters or visual impairment often signals a change in the underlying ocular disease, such as an increase in inflammation, the development of vitreous hemorrhage, or the condensation of the vitreous into a more organized opaque tissue. A careful history can also differentiate causes of brief visual impairment, such as vascular emboli, shifting subretinal fluid, or neurologic diseases such as migraine, from visual disability caused by ocular inflammatory disease.

A medical history should include a description of the patient, including age, gender, race, and occupation. The chief complaint should be succinctly stated, including the reason for the visit and the duration of the problem. The history of the present illness should then be documented, with the major symptoms in chronologic order and a definition of what makes those symptoms better or worse. A detailed past medical history, including family history, social history, and sexual history, is frequently omitted from the ophthalmic evaluation but is critical to the evaluation of the patient with uveitis. We find it extremely useful to have patients complete a uveitis medical history questionnaire before the examination; our questionnaire was developed in conjunction with Dr C. Steven Foster at the Massachusetts Eye and Ear Infirmary (see Appendix). The questionnaire is then reviewed with the patient during the medical history, when additional questions can be asked. The survey helps to guarantee that a core of medical information is gathered for all patients and that important medical questions are not neglected. However, the clinician should realize that completed questionnaires may contain errors. It is important to clarify patient responses and to ask verbally about important aspects of the history, even if the patient denied a symptom on the questionnaire. A study by Seltzer and McDermott[1] showed that 66% of patients who completed the same medical history questionnaire twice made at least one significant omission in their history.

Recently, electronic medical records (EMRs), also known as electronic health records (EHRs), have been incorporated into many clinical practices. The EMR can help address issues of missing records, missing critical information in the medical records, and poor legibility, and promote a more structured collection of data.[2] Some systems use speech recognition to assist in documenting the history. Finally, computerized algorithms may help clinicians improve both diagnosis and subsequent therapy. Unfortunately, despite the potential of EMRs, adoption rates have been slow.[3] Nevertheless, the use of this technology is increasing and should help both research and clinical care going forward.

Although uveitis rarely occurs within families, many forms of the disease, such as iritis associated with ankylosing spondylitis and birdshot retinochoroidopathy, have strong HLA associations that suggest an important inherited component. Thus it is important to recognize that autoimmune diseases may run in a family, and to document the occurrence of these diseases in other family members. Patients with uveitis may have relatives with diseases such as rheumatoid arthritis or systemic lupus erythematosus. Obtaining a social history is also important in the evaluation of the patient with uveitis. A patient's social situation can influence not only the type and severity of the diseases he/she acquires, but also the physician's ability to effectively treat the condition. Social problems can impede a patient's compliance with medical or surgical therapy. Furthermore, patients who are not able to take medication reliably or to comply with frequent laboratory monitoring of hematologic and renal status are not good candidates for immunosuppressive therapy that can impair the immune system.

References

1. Seltzer MH, McDermott JH. Inaccuracies in patient medical histories. Compr Ther 1999; 25: 258–264.
2. Bleeker SE, Derksen-Lubsen G, van Ginneken AM, et al. Structured data entry for narrative data in a broad specialty: patient history and physical examination in pediatrics. BMC Med Inform Decis Mak 2006; 6: 29.
3. Blumenthal D, Glaser JP. Information technology comes to medicine. N Engl J Med 2007; 356: 2527–2534.

APPENDIX

Sample Uveitis Questionnaire

FAMILY HISTORY

These questions refer to your parents, grandparents, children, grandchildren, brothers, sisters, aunts, and uncles.

Has anyone in your family had:

Cancer. . . . . Yes No
Diabetes . . . . Yes No
Allergies . . . . Yes No
Arthritis or rheumatism. . . . . Yes No
Syphilis. . . . . Yes No
Tuberculosis . . . . Yes No
Sickle cell disease or trait . . . . Yes No
Lyme disease. . . . . Yes No

Has anyone in your family had medical problems of the:

Eyes . . . . Yes No
Skin. . . . . Yes No
Kidneys . . . . Yes No
Lungs. . . . . Yes No
Stomach or bowel . . . . Yes No
Nervous system or brain . . . . Yes No

SOCIAL HISTORY

Age (years) _____
Current job _____
Have you lived outside of the US?. . . . . Yes No
If yes, where?
Have you ever owned a dog? . . . . Yes No
Have you ever owned a cat? . . . . Yes No
Have you ever eaten raw meat or
   uncooked sausage?. . . . . Yes No
Have you ever been exposed to sick animals?. . . . . Yes No
Do you drink untreated stream, well,
   or lake water?. . . . . Yes No
Do you smoke cigarettes? . . . . Yes No
How many alcoholic drinks do you have each day?
Have you ever used intravenous drugs?. . . . . Yes No
Have you ever taken birth control pills? . . . . Yes No
Have you ever had a bisexual or homosexual
   relationship?. . . . . Yes No

PERSONAL MEDICAL HISTORY

Are you allergic to any medications? . . . . Yes No
If yes, which medications?
Please list the medicines you are currently taking including nonprescription drugs such as aspirin, ibuprofen, antihistamines, etc.

_____
_____
_____
_____

MEDICAL HISTORY

Please list all eye operations you have had (including laser surgery) and the dates of the surgeries.

_____
_____
_____
_____

Please list all other operations you have had and the dates of the surgeries.

_____
_____
_____

Have you ever had any of the following illnesses?

Cancer. . . . . Yes No
Diabetes . . . . Yes No
Hepatitis. . . . . Yes No
High blood pressure . . . . Yes No

Have you ever had any of the following illnesses?

Anemia (low blood cell counts). . . . . Yes No
Pneumonia or pleurisy . . . . Yes No
Tuberculosis . . . . Yes No
Herpes (cold sores) . . . . Yes No
Chicken pox. . . . . Yes No
Shingles (zoster) . . . . Yes No
German measles (rubella). . . . . Yes No
Measles (rubeola) . . . . Yes No
Mumps . . . . Yes No
Chlamydia or trachoma . . . . Yes No
Syphilis. . . . . Yes No
Any other sexually transmitted disease . . . . Yes No
Leprosy . . . . Yes No
Leptospirosis. . . . . Yes No
Lyme disease. . . . . Yes No
Histoplasmosis. . . . . Yes No
Candidiasis or moniliasis . . . . Yes No
Coccidioidomycosis. . . . . Yes No
Sporotrichosis. . . . . Yes No
Cryptococcal infection. . . . . Yes No
Toxoplasmosis . . . . Yes No
Amoeba infection . . . . Yes No
Giardiasis . . . . Yes No
Toxocariasis . . . . Yes No
Cysticercosis . . . . Yes No
Trichinosis . . . . Yes No
Whipple's disease. . . . . Yes No
AIDS . . . . Yes No
Hay fever. . . . . Yes No
Allergies . . . . Yes No

Vasculitis. . . . . Yes No
Arthritis. . . . . Yes No
Rheumatoid arthritis . . . . Yes No
Lupus (systemic lupus erythematosus) . . . . Yes No
Scleroderma . . . . Yes No
Reiter's syndrome. . . . . Yes No
Colitis . . . . Yes No
Crohn's disease . . . . Yes No
Ulcerative colitis. . . . . Yes No
Behçet's disease . . . . Yes No
Sarcoidosis . . . . Yes No
Ankylosing spondylitis . . . . Yes No
Erythema nodosum . . . . Yes No
Temporal arteritis. . . . . Yes No
Multiple sclerosis . . . . Yes No
Serpiginous choroidopathy. . . . . Yes No
Fuchs' heterochromic iridocyclitis . . . . Yes No
Vogt–Koyanagi–Harada syndrome . . . . Yes No

General health

Chills. . . . . Yes No
Fevers (persistent or recurrent) . . . . Yes No
Night sweats. . . . . Yes No
Fatigue (tire easily) . . . . Yes No
Poor appetite . . . . Yes No
Unexplained weight loss. . . . . Yes No
Do you feel sick? . . . . Yes No

Neurologic

Frequent or severe headaches . . . . Yes No
Fainting. . . . . Yes No
Numbness or tingling in your body. . . . . Yes No
Paralysis or weakness in parts of your body . . . . . . Yes No
Seizures or convulsions. . . . . Yes No
Psychiatric conditions . . . . Yes No

Ears

Hard of hearing or deafness . . . . Yes No
Ringing or noises in your ears . . . . Yes No
Frequent or severe ear infections . . . . Yes No
Painful or swollen ear lobes . . . . Yes No

Nose and throat

Sores in your nose or mouth . . . . Yes No
Severe or recurrent nosebleeds . . . . Yes No
Frequent sneezing . . . . Yes No
Sinus trouble . . . . Yes No
Persistent hoarseness. . . . . Yes No
Tooth or gum infections . . . . Yes No

Skin

Rashes . . . . Yes No
Skin sores . . . . Yes No

Sunburn easily (photosensitivity) . . . . Yes No
White patches of skin or hair (vitiligo or
    poliosis) . . . . Yes No
Loss of hair. . . . . Yes No
Tick or severe insect bites . . . . Yes No
Painfully cold fingers. . . . . Yes No
Severe itching . . . . Yes No

Respiratory

Severe or frequent colds . . . . Yes No
Constant coughing. . . . . Yes No
Coughing up blood . . . . Yes No
Recent flu or viral infection . . . . Yes No
Wheezing or asthma attacks . . . . Yes No
Difficulty in breathing. . . . . Yes No

Cardiovascular

Chest pain . . . . Yes No
Shortness of breath . . . . Yes No
Swelling of your legs . . . . Yes No

Blood

Frequent or easy bruising . . . . Yes No
Frequent or easy bleeding. Yes No
Have you received blood transfusions? . . . . Yes No

Gastrointestinal

Trouble swallowing . . . . Yes No
Diarrhea . . . . Yes No
Bloody stools . . . . Yes No
Stomach ulcers. . . . . Yes No
Jaundice or yellow skin . . . . Yes No

Bones and joints

Stiff joints . . . . Yes No
Painful or swollen joints. . . . . Yes No
Stiff lower back . . . . Yes No
Back pain while sleeping or on
    awakening. . . . . Yes No
Muscle aches. . . . . Yes No

Genitourinary

Kidney problems . . . . Yes No
Bladder trouble . . . . Yes No
Blood in your urine. . . . . Yes No
Urinary discharge. . . . . Yes No
Genital sores or ulcers. . . . . Yes No
Prostatitis . . . . Yes No
Testicular pain . . . . Yes No
Are you pregnant? . . . . Yes No
Do you plan to become pregnant in the near
    future?. . . . . Yes No

Examination of the Patient with Uveitis

Scott M. Whitcup

Key concepts

- A thorough ophthalmic examination is critical for both diagnosis and assessing response to therapy.
- Use of standardized grading scales for assessing intraocular inflammation can improve patient management.
- Standard grading scales are available for anterior chamber cells and flare and vitreous cells and haze.
- A detailed examination of the peripheral retina can reveal pars plana exudates, signs of retinal vasculitis, Delen–Fuchs nodules, or other lesions suggesting active inflammation or infection.

The ocular examination of patients with uveitis is important not only to diagnose the disease correctly but also to determine the appropriate therapy. The examination will provide information that enables the examiner to generate a differential diagnosis and will allow the patient's subjective complaints to be placed into the framework of objective clinical findings. In addition, the baseline examination becomes an important yardstick against which treatment success or failure will be measured. Many inflammatory diseases are chronic and require potentially toxic therapy. Therefore, it is critical to accurately assess whether a patient is benefiting from treatment. This includes a thorough review of the patient's previous medical records and accurate assessment of the disease at each clinic visit. A complete review of the patient's medical records provides important information for planning new therapeutic approaches and guards against repeating therapies that were unsatisfactory in the past. Because a patient's medical record is valuable in assessing response to therapy, it is important to accurately record the presence or absence of important physical findings in a reproducible and standardized manner. Furthermore, because many of the ophthalmic findings in inflammatory disease, such as vitreous cells and haze, are evaluated only by subjective means, the examiner should strive to maintain internal consistency in grading the severity of the observations and to standardize these observations whenever possible. Importantly, standard grading scales should be used whenever possible. The use of standard scales provides consistency when different ophthalmologists are involved in the care of the patient over time. This also allows comparison of patients with those reported in the literature.

Visual acuity

Several factors can lead to reduced visual acuity in patients with uveitis or retinitis. A combination of corneal opacity, anterior chamber inflammation, cataract, and vitreous haze may exacerbate a disturbance in retinal function caused by retinal edema, necrosis, or scarring. In addition, optic nerve function may be compromised after inflammation or glaucoma. It is important for the clinician to determine the cause of diminished vision because the therapeutic approach will differ according to the cause. For example, it would be inappropriate to increase a patient's dose of prednisone to treat worsening vision that is due to a progressive posterior subcapsular cataract. Whatever type of visual acuity measurement is used, it must be performed under the same lighting conditions each time, otherwise the fluctuations induced by the testing environment will mask changes in vision caused by worsening disease or response to therapy. A best-corrected visual acuity measurement should be obtained either by refraction or at the very least with the use of a pinhole occluder. Near-vision measurement is also helpful because we have observed that an improvement in near vision can precede an improvement in distance vision by several weeks in patients with chronic macular edema.

The most common method to measure visual acuity is the Snellen eye chart. Like all eye charts, the Snellen chart tests a patient's ability to resolve high-contrast letters and is satisfactory if their vision is good. Unfortunately, the chart does not have enough sensitivity for patients with poor vision. There are no lines between 20/100 and 20/200 or between 20/200 and 20/400. In addition, there are too few letters on the lines above 20/100. Although an improvement in visual acuity from 20/200 to 20/125 may not be significant to the patient, the ability to measure this improvement is an important indicator that the current therapeutic approach is working. Because many patients with macular edema have a visual acuity of less than 20/80, initial improvement might be missed with use of a standard Snellen chart.

For these reasons, we have used the ETDRS chart initially developed for the evaluation of patients in the Early Treatment for Diabetic Retinopathy Study (ETDRS) (**Fig. 3-1**).[1] This chart has five letters per line starting with the 20/200 line, and every three lines represent a doubling of the visual angle. Therefore, improving from 20/40 to 20/20 represents the same level of improvement in visual function as 20/80 to 20/40. If patients cannot read the 20/200 line while sitting 4 m from the chart, they are moved to 1 m from the chart and the acuities are recorded as 5 over the appropriate

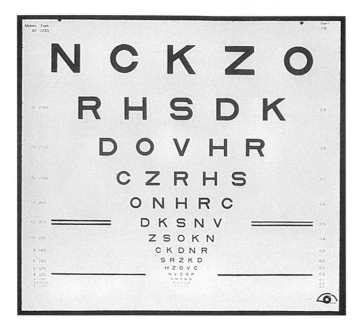

Figure 3-1. Visual acuity chart from Early Treatment of Diabetic Retinopathy Study (ETDRS). *(Courtesy Frederick Ferris, MD.)*

denominator, that is, 5/200. Because each line has five letters, the acuity can be expressed as the total number of letters read. The 1 and 4 m scales can be made continuous by adding 30 letters to the number read at 4 m. The scale of visual acuity is then linear and continuous from 5/200 (five letters) to 20/12.5 (95 letters).

A computerized method for testing visual acuity for clinical research has been developed as an alternative to the standard ETDRS testing protocol.[2] A multicenter study comparing this electronic visual acuity testing algorithm (E-ETDRS) was compared to the standard testing protocol and showed high test–retest reliability and good concordance with the standard ETDRS testing. This new method allows electronic capture of the data, eliminates computational errors, reduces testing time, and may help reduce technician bias.

External examination

As stated earlier, a detailed examination of the skin can provide useful diagnostic clues for the astute clinician. Not only should the skin of the lids be closely examined, but also the entire skin should be evaluated for presence of rashes, nodules, or vitiligo. We have diagnosed sarcoidosis on the basis of the presence of lid granulomas and of lesions on the extremities and chest, and we have diagnosed Kaposi's sarcoma based on characteristic vascular lesions on the upper eyelid. If any skin findings are noted, a consultation with a dermatologist and a skin biopsy should be considered.

Pupils and extraocular muscles

Evaluation of the pupils is frequently difficult in the patient with uveitis because of synechiae or chronic cycloplegic therapy. The inflamed pupil, even without synechiae, may not move well as a result of iris atrophy. When examination is possible, the status of the optic nerve can be assessed with the standard swinging flashlight test to detect an afferent pupillary defect.

Involvement of the extraocular muscles in intraocular inflammatory disease is unusual. Esotropia or exotropia resulting from long-standing visual loss may develop as a result of cataract, retinal, or optic nerve disease. The finding of a new vertical tropia or internuclear ophthalmoplegia should alert the physician to underlying diseases of the central nervous system that may be associated with causes of uveitis, such as multiple sclerosis, sarcoidosis, or non-Hodgkin's lymphoma.

Intraocular pressure measurement

Either elevated intraocular pressure or hypotony can occur as a result of intraocular inflammation. Goldmann applanation tonometry is usually sufficient to measure the intraocular pressure in patients with uveitis; however, fluorescein should not be instilled until the slit-lamp examination and ophthalmoscopy are completed, because fluorescein enters the eye and prevents an accurate assessment of the amount of flare in the anterior chamber. In addition, fluorescein may obscure the view of the posterior segment if the pupil is small, and may persist in the eye for more than 24 hours, especially in eyes with hypotonia and reduced aqueous flow. Therefore, applanation tonometry should either be performed under anesthetic without fluorescein, done with a pneumotonometer, or preferably, performed at the end of the examination.

Slit-lamp biomicroscopy

Conjunctiva

Conjunctival hyperemia is a common sign of acute anterior inflammation but is rare in chronic posterior segment disease. Usually conjunctival injection is uniform in the perilimbal region and represents ciliary body inflammation. The conjunctival injection of uveitis can be differentiated from conjunctivitis by the lack of involvement of the fornix and palpebral conjunctiva. Scleritis and episcleritis may occur in conjunction with some types of intraocular inflammation. Injected deep scleral vessels, a purple scleral hue, and severe pain distinguish true scleritis from more superficial inflammation. Scleritis associated with uveitis is often nodular and confined to a section of the globe, whereas ciliary body injection tends to involve the globe more diffusely. Some confusion may arise when a patient with intraocular inflammation develops an allergic reaction to topical medication. The eye becomes more painful and red during treatment, and this may be misinterpreted as worsening disease and failure of treatment. However, patients with a superimposed allergic reaction often develop itching, dermatitis, and significant conjunctival injection affecting the palpebral conjunctiva.

Cornea

Keratic Precipitates

Keratic precipitates (KPs) are the most commonly reported corneal finding in uveitis (**Fig. 3-2**). They are small

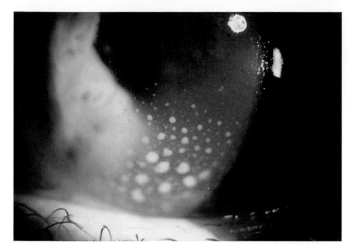

Figure 3-2. Granulomatous keratic precipitates present in patient with sarcoidosis.

aggregates of inflammatory cells that accumulate on the endothelial surface of the cornea. The presence of these deposits on the endothelium of the cornea can provide useful diagnostic information and indicates the current level of inflammatory activity. Also, in an eye without active anterior segment inflammation manifested by cells and flare, the presence of KPs tells the practitioner that the eye was previously inflamed.

KPs usually accumulate on the lower half of the cornea, often in a base-down triangle configuration; however, in some disorders, such as Fuchs' iridocyclitis, KPs may be present superiorly. The precipitates vary in size from flecks the size of cornea guttata to 1 mm in diameter. Because cornea guttata may be present in patients with uveitis, very fine small KPs can be distinguished by an inferior corneal location and slightly elongated shape. KPs can be easily seen with the slit lamp and direct or retroillumination. The small aggregates have been conventionally referred to as 'nongranulomatous,' whereas the larger, more greasy-appearing ones have been termed 'mutton-fat' or 'granulomatous.' These terms may be misleading because they imply a pathologic correlation that is rarely known. There is no objective way of defining granulomatous versus nongranulomatous KPs. The extreme instances are clear, but one may see both types coexisting in one patient at the same time, or see variations during the course of the disease or therapy. In general, the larger granulomatous aggregates are composed of macrophages and giant cells and occur in chronic inflammation, whereas the smaller nongranulomatous ones occur in acute inflammation and are more likely to be composed of neutrophils and lymphocytes. Nevertheless, there are a number of diseases typically associated with granulomatous KPs (see Box 4-3), and the presence of these precipitates can help in developing a differential diagnosis. In most inflammatory reactions, the neutrophil is the first cell present, and the transformed macrophages (epithelioid cells) and lymphocytes accumulate as the inflammation becomes more chronic. KPs therefore mimic the course of the inflammation in the tissue. For example, patients with documented pulmonary sarcoidosis may have acute anterior inflammatory episodes with small nongranulomatous KPs. If the inflammatory disease becomes chronic, the KP aggregates may become larger and more granulomatous. After the resolution of active inflammation, the KP aggregates may disappear completely or become smaller, translucent, or pigmented. KPs may also be washed away during intraocular surgery.

Other Corneal Findings

Other corneal findings can provide clues to the correct diagnosis. For example, corneal dendrites may be seen with uveitis as a result of herpes simplex virus infection. Interstitial keratitis may be associated with syphilis or Cogan's syndrome; the clinician should examine the cornea carefully because the presence of stromal ghost vessels extending more than several millimeters from the limbus may easily be overlooked. We have noted similar findings in the inferior cornea in patients with sarcoidosis. Finally, we have seen several patients with corneal grafts who were referred with conditions diagnosed as idiopathic uveitis. In a number of these the uveitis was actually caused by early allograft rejection.

Anterior chamber

The anterior chamber is easily examined with the slit lamp for signs of ocular inflammation. Because inflammatory cells do not arise in the aqueous, the presence of cells or increased protein (flare) in the anterior chamber is evidence of spillover from the inflamed iris or ciliary body. Not infrequently, a patient with recurrent iritis will come to the ophthalmologist complaining of pain, but because of a lack of cells or flare on examination will be told that there is no uveitis and that no therapy is needed. To the practitioner's dismay, the patient returns the next day with full-blown iritis. The explanation for this is that the inflammation begins in the iris and ciliary body, and only when sufficient inflammatory cells accumulate within these tissues do the cells begin to enter the aqueous and become visible to the clinician. Therefore, anterior chamber inflammation is a convenient but somewhat indirect measure of the inflammatory reaction in the iris and ciliary body.

Anterior chamber cells are primarily lymphocytes in most episodes of anterior uveitis, but a significant number of neutrophils may be present early in the course of disease. Anterior chamber cells are best seen by directing the slit-lamp beam obliquely across the eye and focusing posterior to the cornea. There is considerable variation among physicians on the grading of the number of cells. Because the cells represent an index of activity but not a direct measure of the active inflammation, we do not believe that the grading system must discriminate between small increments of disease. **Table 3-1** summarizes the system proposed by Hogan and colleagues,[3] the system proposed by Schlaegel that uses a wide beam with a narrow slit,[4] and our preferred system that uses a 1×1 mm slit beam. The smaller slit allows some resolution for more severe inflammation and less resolution at the milder end of the spectrum. We are most interested in quantifying anterior chamber cells during the early stages of acute inflammation when a change in cellularity may signal an early response to therapy, and when a lack of response might dictate a change in therapy. The problem with most classification systems is that it is impossible for clinicians to remember how many cells are associated with a trace grade of trace, occasional, or rare cells. Therefore we have modified our grading system: for grades of trace cells

Table 3-1 Grading of anterior chamber cells

Schlaegel*		Hogan†		Authors' Approach†		SUN Working Group	
Grade	Cells	Grade	Cells	Grade	Cells	Grade	Cells
–	–	0	0	0	0	0	<1
½+	Rare (normal)	Rare cells	1–2	–	–		
–	–	Occasional cell	3-7	–	–		
–	–	–	–	Trace‡	1–5	Trace	1–5
1+	Occasional cell	1+	7–10	1+‡	6–15	1+	6–15
1½+	2–7	1–2+	10–15	–	–		
2+	8–15	2+	15–20	2+	16–25	2+	16–25
2½+	16–30	–	–	–	–		
3+	Too many to count	3+	20–50	3+	26–50	3+	26–50
3½+	Too many to count	–	–	–	–		
4+	Most ever seen	4+	>50	4+	>50	4+	>50

Data from Schlaegel TF Jr. Essentials of uveitis. Boston: Little, Brown, 1967; 7; Hogan MJ, et al. Am J Ophthalmol 1959; 47: 155–70.
*Using a wide beam with a narrow slit.
†Using a 1 × 1 mm slit.
‡For grades of trace and 1+ the exact number of cells is recorded in parentheses, that is, 1+ (11).

(1–5) and 1+ cells (6–15 cells), I will put the exact number of cells counted in parentheses after the grade, for example 1+ (11) or trace (3). The grading scale we used was adopted at the First International Workshop discussing the standardization of uveitis nomenclature and published in 2005.[5] In many chronically inflamed eyes it may be impossible to eliminate every last cell, and these rare cells may not require treatment. Nevertheless, persistence of more than a rare cell may place the patient at increased risk for inflammatory complications and worsen the prognosis after cataract extraction.

It is also our experience that the size of the individual cells in the anterior chamber will decrease as the inflammation begins to resolve. This may occur before the number of cells actually decreases. A change from large activated lymphocytes to smaller cells may account for this clinical observation. It is important to differentiate inflammatory cells from other types of cell in the anterior chamber. Red blood cells, iris pigment cells, and malignant cells may be mistaken for inflammatory cells. The differentiation is especially difficult if a lymphoid malignancy is present: monoclonal antibody staining of cells obtained by paracentesis may be critical in identifying the type of cell.

Increased protein content in the anterior chamber is a manifestation of a breakdown of the blood–ocular barrier. When the slit beam is obliquely aimed across the anterior chamber, the ability to visualize the path of the beam is termed flare. There are approximately 7 g of protein/100 mL of blood, but only 11 mg of protein/100 mL of aqueous. A faint amount of flare is normal if a bright light is used. The amount of light scattering is proportional to the concentration of protein in a solution, and hence more flare indicates increased protein in the anterior chamber fluid. Flare can be clinically graded on a scale of 0–4+ using a grading scale published by Hogan and colleagues in 1959 (**Table 3-2**). This scale was adopted by the SUN Working Group with

Table 3-2 Grading of anterior chamber flare

Grade	Schlaegel[3]	Hogan et al.	SUN Working Group
0	Complete absence		None
½+	Faint (normal)	–	
1+	Very slight (normal)	Very slight	Faint
1½+	Mild	–	
2+	Mild to moderate	Moderate (iris and lens clear)	Moderate (iris and lens details clear)
3+	Moderate	Marked flare (iris and lens hazy)	Marked (iris and lens details hazy)
4+	Severe	Intense (fibrin, plastic aqueous)	Intense (fibrin or plastic aqueous)

Data from Schlaegel TF Jr. Essentials of uveitis. Boston: Little, Brown, 1967; 7; Hogan MJ, et al. Am J Ophthalmol 1959; 47: 155–70.

slight modification.[5] We have reserved the 4+ grade for leakage of protein so extensive that a fibrin clot is present. In addition to the subjective grading of flare, it is possible to more accurately measure the degree of light scattering and quantify the amount of protein. A technique described by Herman and colleagues[6] uses the principle that fluorescein in the anterior chamber will bind to albumin, and the amount of bound fluorescein will alter the polarization of fluorescein as measured by fluorophotometry. This method is able to quantify alterations in blood–ocular barrier leakage of albumin. A newer technique of objectively assessing aqueous flare measures the scattering of a laser beam projected across the anterior chamber. This laser flare meter is more fully described in Chapter 5.

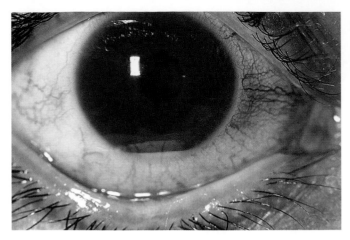

Figure 3-3. Hypopyon in patient with Behçet's disease.

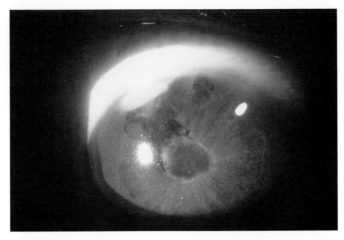

Figure 3-4. Posterior synechiae and closure of iridectomy.

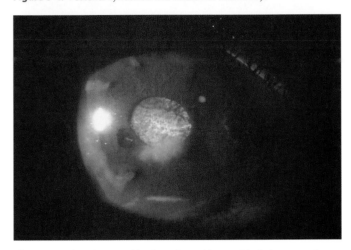

Figure 3-5. Anterior synechiae in patient with sarcoidosis demonstrating iris–cornea adhesions.

Some disagreement exists as to whether the presence of flare by itself, without cells or other signs of active inflammation, should be treated. In our opinion, without objective quantification of a change in the leakage across the blood–ocular barrier, chronic flare alone is not a sign of active inflammation. Damaged blood vessels may be leaky for a long time after the active inflammation has resolved. Continued treatment with drugs such as corticosteroids may do little to alter the repair of these vessels in the absence of active inflammation. There is no evidence that small amounts of increased protein in the anterior chamber are detrimental to the eye, and there appears to be no reason for continued therapy in this situation. Specifically, children with juvenile rheumatoid arthritis with flare but no cells should not be treated with topical corticosteroids. Therefore, flare should be considered a marker of inflammation but not necessarily a pathognomonic finding of active inflammation.

A hypopyon (**Fig. 3-3**) is a collection of leukocytes that settles in the lower angle of the anterior chamber. The cause of a hypopyon is unclear and is not related solely to the number of cells in the anterior chamber. It is also related to the presence of sufficient fibrin to cause the cells to clump and settle. Hypopyon is a dramatic but short-lived finding in ocular inflammation that has been associated with Behçet's disease, endophthalmitis, and rifabutin toxicity in patients with AIDS. A hypopyon may also occur sporadically in severe acute inflammation associated with many other types of uveitis.[7] Of course, a hypopyon frequently develops in patients with endophthalmitis, and infection should always be considered as a potential etiology. This is especially true in patients who have had recent intraocular surgery. However, a sterile hypopyon can also occur after intraocular surgery. Severe exacerbation of uveitis can occur after ocular surgery in patients with uveitis, especially if appropriate anti-inflammatory therapy is not given. Retained lens fragments can also precipitate severe intraocular inflammation and hypopyon.[8] A pseudohypopyon, composed of tumor cells or hemorrhagic debris, can occur in some of the masquerade syndromes (see Chapter 30) after vitreous hemorrhage. Finally, a hyphema can occur in eyes with uveitis, often due to neovascularization of the iris. Interestingly, a case of a pink hypopyon was noted in a patient with *Serratia marcescens* endophthalmitis.[9] Cytologic examination revealed no erythrocytes, and the pink color was due to the bacteria.

Iris

Inflammation is often accompanied by the release of mediators that promote fibrin deposition, clotting, and fibroblast proliferation, which are the probable causes of synechiae. Synechiae are adhesions between the iris and the lens capsule (posterior synechiae) (**Fig. 3-4**) or the iris and the cornea near the anterior chamber angle (peripheral anterior synechiae, PAS). The former are responsible for the development of pupillary block glaucoma, and the latter contribute to the development of obstruction of aqueous outflow. In general, the presence of synechiae indicates that the inflammation has been chronic or recurrent; however, these adhesions may occasionally develop within a few days in patients with severe inflammation. Although most peripheral anterior synechiae can be seen only by gonioscopy, some patients will develop more profound anterior adhesions (**Fig. 3-5**). Most posterior synechiae are located at the pupillary border, but patients with severe chronic inflammation can develop adhesions of the entire posterior iris surface to the anterior lens capsule. A fibrovascular membrane may develop in patients with long-standing and recurrent inflammation in whom the pupil size has been reduced to a few millimeters by posterior synechiae (**Fig. 3-6**). This membrane may be translucent and adherent to the surface of the lens and not apparent until cataract removal is attempted. The iris may

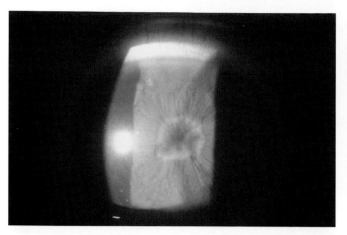

Figure 3-6. Posterior synechiae with fibrin membrane and totally occluded pupil.

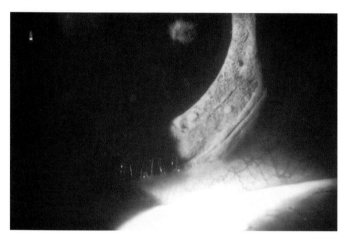

Figure 3-7. Busacca's nodules of iris in patient with Vogt–Koyanagi–Harada syndrome.

also become atrophic in certain uveitic conditions. For example, iris transillumination defects can be a clue to herpetic uveitis, especially when associated with corneal disease and persistent anterior uveitis.

Iris nodules are accumulations of inflammatory cells in the iris or on its surface. The Koeppe nodule develops on the pupillary border, whereas the Busacca's nodules occur on the iris surface (**Fig. 3-7**). Iris nodules tend to be found in diseases that have been termed granulomatous and are more specific for these conditions than are granulomatous KPs.

Anterior chamber angle

Because glaucoma is a frequent (and often the most severe) complication of uveitis, a thorough examination of the anterior chamber angle is indicated. The finding of neovascularization may indicate a need for panretinal photocoagulation. In addition, in patients with a uniocular uveitis examination of the angle may reveal an occult foreign body or ciliary body malignancy.

Lens

Many patients with uveitis develop cataracts because of underlying inflammation and the use of corticosteroids to treat the disease. Posterior subcapsular opacities are commonly seen early (**Fig. 3-8**), but the advanced cataract in

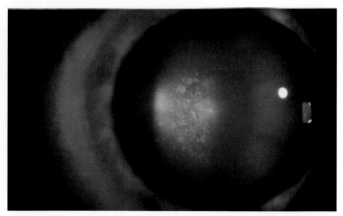

Figure 3-8. Posterior subcapsular cataract in patient with chronic recurrent anterior uveitis.

uveitis is frequently a complicated cataract with nuclear, cortical, and capsular opacities. It is important to determine how much of the diminished vision of a patient with uveitis is a result of a progressive cataract, because the therapy for cataract is surgical extraction and not increased immunosuppressive therapy. Cataract can also obscure the view of the vitreous, retina, and optic nerve, making the evaluation of patients with severe vision loss and dense cataracts difficult. In these patients, it is important to determine whether vision loss is due to the cataract, reversible ocular inflammatory disease, or an untreatable problem such as irreversible retinal or optic nerve atrophy. We have removed opaque cataracts in some patients in whom viewing the back of the eye was critical to determining whether systemic immunosuppressive therapy should be started. Electroretinography (ERG) can help determine whether the patient has residual visual function; however, dense cataract can also affect ERG recording. Evaluation of lens opacity and reduced vision is discussed in greater depth in Chapter 5 on diagnostic testing.

Vitreous

Inflammation in the vitreous, as in the anterior chamber, is characterized by increased cells and protein. The vitreous is rarely the source of the inflammatory cells, which instead arise from the choroid, retina, and ciliary body. However, in certain infections the focus of the inflammation may be in the vitreous. Both vitreous cells and haze are more difficult to quantify than aqueous cells and flare. The vitreous is larger, and cells or haze may be localized to only a part of the vitreous. Therefore, quantification may depend on how the eye was examined. For example, the anteroposterior location of small numbers of cells in a relatively clear vitreous can be determined with the use of the slit lamp, but in the severely inflamed eye the mid and posterior vitreous may be obscured by anterior vitreous cells and haze. Small pupil size, corneal opacity, and cataract will also make the grading process more difficult.

The grading of vitreous cells described by Kimura and colleagues[10] uses the Hruby lens to view the cells in retroillumination. The cells appear as black dots, and in some eyes it may be difficult to differentiate vitreal debris from active inflammatory cells. Debris is often pigmented and forms clumps that are larger than individual cells. We grade

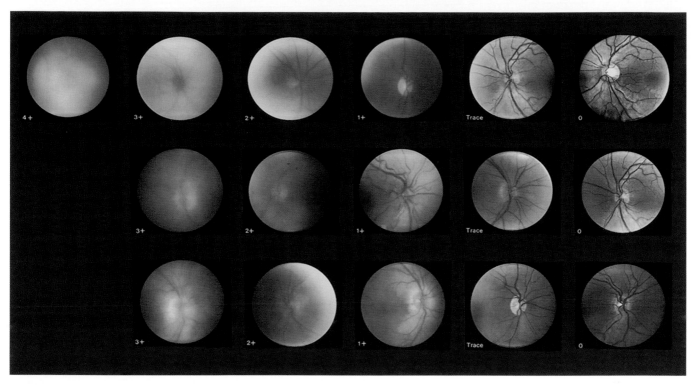

Figure 3-9. Grading of vitreous haze. *(From Nussenblatt RB, Palestine AG, Chan CC, et al. Standardization of vitreal inflammatory activity in intermediate and posterior uveitis. Ophthalmology 1985; 92: 467–71.)*

Table 3-3 Grading of vitreous cells with use of Hruby lens

Cells in Retroilluminated Field	Description	Grade
0–1	Clear	0+
2–20	Few opacities	Trace
21–50	Scattered opacities	1+
51–100	Moderate opacities	2+
101–250	Many opacities	3+
>251	Dense opacities	4+

overall vitreous cells and opacities in a manner similar to the scale devised by Kimura and colleagues (**Table 3-3**). We then note whether the major accumulation of cells is immediately behind the lens, in the anterior or posterior vitreous, or adjacent to a retinal lesion. Location of the cells is a function of both the ocular disease and its severity. The location of the cells is important in classifying the inflammation, but we have noted, for example, that patients with pars planitis, who usually have cells in the anterior vitreous, will develop many cells in the posterior vitreous if the inflammation is more severe. In many diseases, but especially in sarcoidosis and pars planitis, vitreous cells tend to aggregate into clumps called 'snowballs.' These snowballs settle in the inferior periphery near the retinal surface and are seen best with the indirect ophthalmoscope.

It is our strong opinion that vitreous haze is a better indicator of active inflammation than are vitreous cells, because it combines the optical effect of cellular infiltration and protein leakage. We have developed a grading scale based on the view of the optic disc and posterior retina with the use of the indirect ophthalmoscope and a 20 diopter lens

(**Fig. 3-9**).[11] It is important to mentally correct for lens opacities, anterior segment inflammation, and corneal disease; however, the use of the indirect ophthalmoscope prevents mild media opacities from interfering with the grading. The use of photographic standards makes this system more reproducible than other subjective grading systems. In practice it is useful to have the standard color photographs in the examining room. One can then examine the patient's eye and look at the grading chart to select the standard that best matches the degree of haze.

Vitreous strands, membranes, and areas of vitreoretinal traction are not uncommon in intermediate and posterior uveitis. They are best seen with the indirect ophthalmoscope, but may be studied in detail with a contact lens or a +90 diopter lens at the slit lamp. There is frequently a posterior vitreous detachment in patients with long-standing vitreous inflammation, as the fibrin in the vitreous contracts and pulls the posterior vitreous face forward. Recently, investigators have suggested that vitreous traction that causes an incomplete posterior vitreous detachment may be associated with the development of cystoid macular edema.[12]

Retina and choroid

Examination of the retina in inflammatory disease is best done with a combination of the indirect ophthalmoscope, the Hruby lens, the +90 diopter lens, and a mirrored contact lens. Because of coexisting vitreous inflammation, each of these has advantages and disadvantages. The indirect ophthalmoscope is ideal for defining the extent and height of retinal and choroidal lesions; it penetrates vitreous haze and other media opacities better than any other instrument. It is not good for defining the relative depth of a lesion within

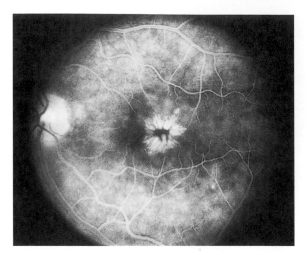

Figure 3-10. Fluorescein angiogram demonstrating cystoid macular edema caused by pars planitis.

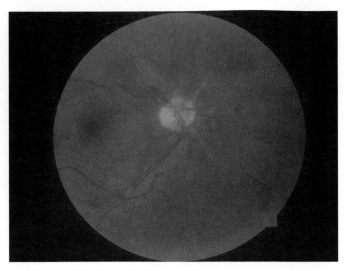

Figure 3-11. Retinal vascular sheathing in patient with idiopathic retinal vasculitis.

the retina or determining the presence of macular edema. The Hruby lens is somewhat better at penetrating haze than the +90 diopter or +78 diopter lenses, and is better for assessing macular edema. If the media is reasonably clear, the +90 diopter or +78 diopter lens, which provides an inverted view of the fundus, is ideal for viewing vascular abnormalities, intraretinal lesions, and vitreoretinal traction in the posterior retina. The midperiphery of the retina also can be seen with this lens, but the mirrored contact lens is more useful for the detailed examination of peripheral chorioretinal lesions.

Cystoid macular edema is a common retinal finding in patients with uveitis (**Fig. 3-10**). Although fluorescein angiography can more objectively document the presence of macular edema, clinical examination with the Hruby lens is easier, is cost-effective, and can be performed on each visit. In addition, examination with the Hruby lens allows the examiner to determine the extent of macular thickening associated with the edema. In the absence of vitreous haze, cystoid macular edema is easily seen. However, macular edema may be obscured by overlying vitreous haze and is best observed by viewing the macula with the light directed slightly to one side of the fovea. Cystoid macular edema may then be visualized by indirect illumination and will 'light up' in contrast to the surrounding retina. This technique also reduces light scattering from the vitreous. The surface of a cyst can sometimes be visualized as a subtle surface elevation, distinguishing it from a true macular hole. If the pupil is small, the viewing aperture will be reduced, and only a faint glimpse of the macular cysts will be seen by this method. Macular holes and lamellar holes as well as retinal pigment epithelial clumping are also commonly observed, and it is possible to see cloudy white areas of retinal edema without a classic cystoid pattern.

Retinal vascular alterations are also a common finding in patients with intermediate or posterior uveitis. Vascular sheathing of the arteries or veins, usually caused by infiltration of inflammatory cells around the vessels, is easily seen in the posterior pole (**Fig. 3-11**). Peripheral vascular sheathing is more subtle and may be missed if not specifically sought. Sheathing is often accompanied by vessel narrowing and sometimes by vascular obliteration. Peripheral vascular narrowing and obliteration are best evaluated with the

indirect ophthalmoscope, manifesting as an absence of small peripheral vessels. Acute vascular occlusion is accompanied by retinal edema, but old areas of vascular loss show only atrophic retina and retinal pigment epithelial stippling.

Retinal hemorrhages and cotton-wool spots frequently accompany retinal vasculitis, presumably related to the retinal ischemia produced by the inflammation. In addition, cellular retinal infiltrates can be observed in certain types of retinitis. These appear as white areas similar to cotton-wool spots but may be located deep within the retina compared to the superficial location of cotton-wool spots. In addition, active retinal infiltrates frequently have fuzzy edges, overlying vitreal cells, and surrounding retinal edema. Hard retinal exudates are relatively uncommon in inflammatory disease. It is possible that the retinal vessels do not leak large lipid-containing proteins from the plasma. When hard exudates are observed, they frequently occur between an area of retinal ischemia and an area of essentially normal retina. The presence of a subretinal neovascular membrane should be suspected if hard exudates, retinal edema, hemorrhage, or gray-white elevated lesions are seen.

Careful examination with the Hruby, +90 diopter, or contact lens is crucial in distinguishing a lesion that involves the neurosensory retina from lesions at the level of the retinal pigment epithelium or choroid. Examination of the edge of the lesion is often helpful in determining its depth and cause. At times it may still be difficult to know the location of an infiltrate without the aid of a fluorescein angiogram. Many lesions will have associated subretinal fluid or be covered by increased cellularity in the vitreous, and this should be documented. Exudative retinal detachments can be associated with a number of ocular inflammatory diseases, but are characteristic of specific conditions such as Vogt–Koyanagi–Harada syndrome (**Fig. 3-12**). The clinician, however, must carefully rule out a rhegmatogenous retinal detachment in these patients because treatment of a rhegmatogenous detachment will require surgical repair.

In addition to subretinal fluid, the subretinal space can be infiltrated with glial and retinal pigment epithelial cells that have proliferated as a consequence of the inflammation. These appear as plaques and bands of yellow-white tissue,

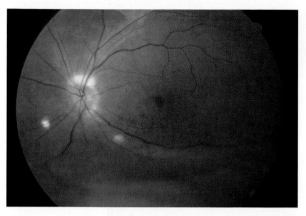

Figure 3-12. Exudative retinal detachment in a patient with Vogt–Koyanagi–Harada syndrome is seen inferior to the macula.

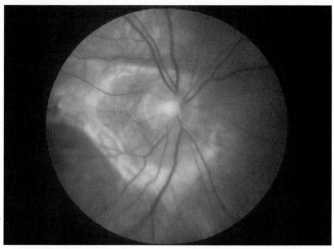

Figure 3-14. Large choroidal granuloma around optic disc in a patient with sarcoidosis.

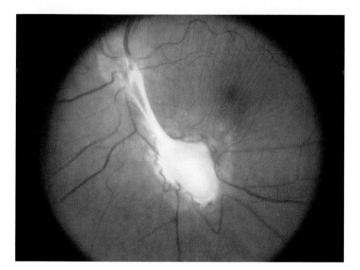

Figure 3-13. Dense fibrotic band extends from the optic disc to the inferior vascular arcade.

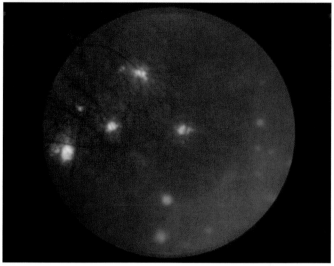

Figure 3-15. Dalen–Fuchs nodules are small, fairly discrete, yellow to white lesions that most commonly occur in the retinal periphery. The lesions are composed of collections of inflammatory cells between the retinal pigment epithelium and Bruch's membrane.

which for lack of a more specific term are often referred to as subretinal fibrosis. The inflammatory process stimulates the growth of fibroblasts and the metaplasia of the retinal pigment epithelium and possibly Müller cells. The bands of this tissue, combined with epiretinal and vitreoretinal bands, produce retinal traction and distortion (**Fig. 3-13**).

Choroidal lesions, with or without retinal involvement, are common in posterior inflammatory disease. When inflammatory lesions are deep and isolated to the choroid, they often appear as grayish-yellow elevated masses (**Fig. 3-14**). They are best seen with the indirect ophthalmoscope but may be missed because they can be subtle in both elevation and pigmentary change. One or more choroidal nodules may be present and can vary in size from 50 μm to 500 μm in diameter. Atrophic chorioretinal lesions with surrounding hyperpigmentation are a striking sign of inflammatory disease in the patient with uveitis. However, these lesions do not represent areas of active inflammation, and although they are the most prominent clinical feature of some diseases, they represent old inactive disease. Only active inflammation, not residual scarring, can be treated by drugs that modulate the immune response. Thus therapy is not indicated in patients with multiple chorioretinal scars without infiltrative lesions of the retina or choroid or active vitreitis. Although the appearance of inflammatory lesions of the

retina and choroid can vary greatly, some lesions have a characteristic presentation and can help in diagnosis. Dalen–Fuchs nodules tend to be small, discrete, deep, yellow-white chorioretinal lesions that may be associated with hyperpigmentation (**Fig. 3-15**). Dalen–Fuchs nodules are associated with sarcoidosis and sympathetic ophthalmia. The chorioretinal lesions associated with birdshot choroidopathy also have a characteristic appearance and distribution in the fundus, typically clustering nasal to the optic disc.

Examination of the retinal periphery and pars plana is an important part of the ocular examination of patients with uveitis. Pars plana snowbanking is the accumulation of a white fibroglial mass over the pars plana and adjacent retina (see Chapter 21). It is usually restricted to the inferior pars plana but may extend superiorly. Scleral depression is usually required to see the pars plana exudate, but in some patients the inflammatory mass may be large enough to be seen with the indirect ophthalmoscope without a lens (**Fig. 3-16**). Peripheral vitreous infiltrates lying on the retinal surface

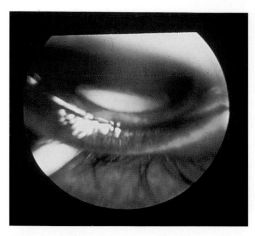

Figure 3-16. Exudate on pars plana (snowbank) in a patient with pars planitis. *(Courtesy Ronald Smith, MD.)*

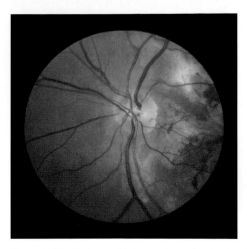

Figure 3-18. Optic neuritis in a patient with chorioretinitis.

Optic nerve

The optic nerve is a frequently overlooked cause of vision loss in patients with uveitis. Uveitis may affect the optic nerve in several ways. Disc hyperemia, papillitis, or papilledema may be seen in a number of uveitic conditions. Disc hyperemia may persist even in an eye with little clinically active inflammation elsewhere. Prominent disc hyperemia is frequently noted with Vogt–Koyanagi–Harada syndrome. Secondary glaucoma is one of the most common causes of irreversible vision loss in the uveitis patient. Neovascularization of the optic disc is a common finding in uveitis with retinal vasculitis, and can regress with anti-inflammatory therapy. Optic atrophy may develop in the presence of ocular inflammation or following diffuse loss of retinal tissue (**Fig. 3-17**). Granulomas may impinge on the optic nerve and optic disc in diseases such as sarcoidosis. Optic neuritis is observed in patients with uveitis (**Fig. 3-18**). Multiple sclerosis is associated with intermediate uveitis, and often manifests as optic neuritis. Examination of the optic disc with the Hruby lens or a +90 diopter lens, serial disc photographs, and electrophysiologic testing are often helpful in evaluating the patient with uveitis with visual loss.

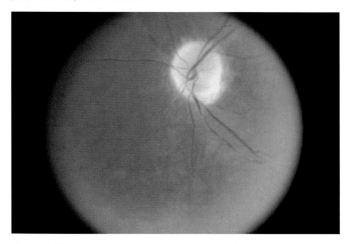

Figure 3-17. Optic atrophy in a patient with posterior uveitis. Thinning and occlusion of the retinal vessels can also be seen.

should not be interpreted as snowbanking. Peripheral neovascularization may be present within the snowbank, increasing the risk of vitreous hemorrhage. If the pars plana exudate is sparse and located only along the ora serrata, it may be difficult to identify unless immediate comparison is made with the ora serrata in other locations within the eye.

References

1. Ferris FL III, Kassoff A, Bresnick GH, et al. New visual acuity charts for clinical research. Am J Ophthalmol 1982; 94: 91–96.
2. Beck RW, Moke PS, Turpin AH, et al. A computerized method of visual acuity testing: adaptation of the early treatment of diabetic retinopathy study testing protocol. Am J Ophthalmol 2003; 135: 194–205.
3. Hogan MJ, Kimura SJ, Thygeson P. Signs and symptoms of uveitis. I. Anterior uveitis. Am J Ophthalmol 1959; 47: 155–170.
4. Schlaegel TF Jr. Essentials of uveitis. Boston: Little, Brown, 1967; 7.
5. Jabs DA, Nussenblatt RB, Rosenbaum JT. Standardization of uveitis nomenclature (SUN) Working Group. Standardization of uveitis

   nomenclature for reporting clinical data. Results of the First International Workshop. Am J Ophthalmol 2005; 140: 509–516.
6. Herman DC, McLaren JW, Brubaker RF. A method of determining concentration of albumin in the living eye. Invest Ophthalmol Vis Sci 1988; 29: 133–137.
7. Muccioli C, Belfort R Jr. Hypopyon in a patient with presumptive diffuse unilateral subacute neuroretinitis. Ocul Immunol Inflamm 2000; 8: 119–121.
8. Irvine WD, Flynn HW Jr, Murray TG, et al. Retained lens fragments after phacoemulsification manifesting as marked intraocular inflammation with hypopyon. Am J Ophthalmol 1992; 114: 610–614.

9. al Hazzaa SA, Tabbara KF, Gammon JA. Pink hypopyon: a sign of *Serratia marcescens* endophthalmitis. Br J Ophthalmol 1992; 76: 764–765.
10. Kimura SJ, Thygeson P, Hogan MJ. Signs and symptoms of uveitis. II. Classification of the posterior manifestations of uveitis. Am J Ophthalmol 1959; 47: 171–176.
11. Nussenblatt RB, Palestine AG, Chan CC, et al. Standardization of vitreal inflammatory activity in intermediate and posterior uveitis. Ophthalmology 1985; 92: 467–471.
12. Hikichi T, Trempe CL. Role of the vitreous in the prognosis of peripheral uveitis. Am J Ophthalmol 1993; 116: 401–405.

Development of a Differential Diagnosis

Scott M. Whitcup

Key concepts

- Diagnosis of uveitis is often challenging and developing an erudite differential diagnosis is a key to success.
- Classification of the uveitis is the first step and is guided by a serious of questions that can be answered from both the medical history and clinical examination.
- Classification of the uveitis and development of a list of potential diagnoses will help determine appropriate diagnostic testing, guide therapy, and help determine prognosis.
- Associated symptoms and signs are important sources of information and require a systemic review of symptoms and a detailed physical examination. Examination of the skin can be extremely rewarding in diagnosing uveitis. Referral to an internist, primary care physician, rheumatologist or other specialist is often required in the work-up of uveitis.

The correct diagnosis of uveitis is often challenging, not only for the general ophthalmologist but also for the uveitis specialist. Patients present with a plethora of ocular findings as well as associated systemic symptoms and signs. Ocular inflammation may be the initial presentation of an underlying systemic disease that, if undiagnosed and untreated, may lead to significant morbidity and even death. For example, we have seen a number of patients with intraocular lymphoma whose conditions were misdiagnosed and inappropriately treated as idiopathic uveitis. Even in patients with uveitis without an underlying systemic disease, misdiagnosis can lead to inappropriate therapy. A patient with fungal endophthalmitis who is thought to have sarcoidosis may be treated with corticosteroids, leading to an exacerbation of the infection, when appropriate antifungal therapy could be curative. In this chapter we review our diagnostic approach to patients with uveitis and present two cases to illustrate our approach.

Diagnosis is based largely on recognition of patterns that include findings from the medical history, clinical examination, and ordered tests, including laboratory tests and medical imaging. Medical experts are much better at recognizing the patterns consistent with medical diagnoses than are novices. Recent studies of memory suggest that this pattern recognition can be learned and takes practice. It should not be surprising, therefore, that doctors with many years of clinical practice are often better diagnosticians than less experienced care providers.

Much of what we know about memory and pattern recognition comes from the study of chess. In the 1960s De Groot[1,2] performed an intriguing study comparing the ability to recall chess patterns between players of varying abilities. A chessboard position, taken from a master game unknown to the subjects, was presented to participants for a short period varying from 2 to 15 seconds. Participants then had to reconstruct the board based on memory. The findings were dramatic. Grandmasters remembered board positions accurately, recalling an average of 93% of the pieces correctly after seeing the chess layout for only 2–5 seconds. The least experienced players only recalled about 50% of the pieces correctly. De Groot hypothesized that chess masters encode the positions of the pieces not as individuals but as groups. The data also suggest that the ability to recognize these patterns improves with experience, and can be learned with appropriate teaching and lots of practice.

The goal of this chapter is to provide the framework for clinicians to start collecting the information needed to form the disease patterns that help diagnose our patients. Knowing what questions to ask, what findings to look for, and what tests to order are all critical in seeing clear patterns from background noise. Every patient we see should help us fine tune our pattern recognition skills and allow us to better diagnose disease. First you need to collect the pieces of the puzzle that help us create the disease pattern. Second, you need to start putting the pieces together in ways that form several disease patterns. This is known as forming a differential diagnosis: identifying pieces of a puzzle that, when assembled, can form a handful of disease pictures. Finally, a specific diagnosis is made, often by ordering a key test that rules out all but one disease pattern. Recognizing potential disease patterns and forming a good differential diagnosis is the key to success.

Forming a differential diagnosis

The first step in developing a differential diagnosis for patients with inflammatory eye disease is to classify the uveitis in as detailed a fashion as possible. This can be achieved by systematically asking the eight questions listed in **Box 4-1**. You can then generate a list of possible diagnoses by combining the data obtained from the answers. Some of the information is obtained from the history, such as the age and demographics of the patient and associated systemic

Box 4-1 Classification of uveitis

1. Is the disease acute or chronic?
2. Is the inflammation granulomatous or nongranulomatous?
3. Is the disease unilateral or bilateral?
4. Where is the inflammation located in the eye?
5. What are the demographics of the patient?
6. What associated symptoms does the patient have?
7. What associated signs are present on physical examination?
8. What is the time course of the disease and response to previous therapy?

Box 4-2 Causes of acute and chronic uveitis

ACUTE UVEITIS

Most cases of anterior uveitis: idiopathic, ankylosing spondylitis, Reiter's syndrome, Fuchs' heterochromic iridocyclitis

Vogt–Koyanagi–Harada syndrome

Toxoplasmosis

White-dot syndromes: acute posterior multifocal placoid pigment epitheliopathy and multiple evanescent white-dot syndrome

Acute retinal necrosis

Postsurgical bacterial infection

Trauma

CHRONIC UVEITIS

Juvenile rheumatoid arthritis

Birdshot choroidopathy

Serpiginous choroidopathy

Tuberculous uveitis

Postoperative uveitis (*Propionibacterium acnes*, fungal)

Intraocular lymphoma

Sympathetic ophthalmia

Multifocal choroiditis

Sarcoidosis

Intermediate uveitis/pars planitis

symptoms. Other data, such as the type and anatomic location of the inflammation, are obtained from the ocular examination. Again, the need for information about systemic and neurologic signs necessitates a careful physical and neurologic examination of the patient by the ophthalmologist or by a consulting internist, internal medicine subspecialist, neurologist, or general medical practitioner.

Once the uveitis has been classified, a preliminary differential diagnosis should be generated. The answers to each of the questions in Box 4-1 will generate a list of possible diagnoses. The diagnoses that appear most frequently on these lists are then the most likely cause of the disorder. Ancillary examinations, including laboratory tests or specialized examinations such as radiography, electrophysiology, or a surgical procedure such as a diagnostic vitrectomy, can then be obtained to discern among the most likely diagnoses. In the next chapter on diagnostic testing, we show that the 'shotgun approach' of ordering every diagnostic test available will mislead the clinician into making the wrong diagnosis.

Classifying uveitis

1. Is the disease acute or chronic?

Acute occurrences of uveitis usually have a sudden onset and last up to 6 weeks. The most common causes are listed in **Box 4-2**. Most occurrences of anterior uveitis, such as HLA-B27-associated iritis and idiopathic anterior uveitis, fall into this category. Other diseases that typically cause acute uveitis include Vogt–Koyanagi–Harada syndrome, postoperative bacterial infection, toxoplasmosis, many of the 'white-dot syndromes,' such as acute posterior multifocal placoid pigment epitheliopathy (APMPPE) and multiple evanescent white-dot syndrome (MEWDS), and traumatic iritis. Although many diseases can cause acute uveitis, these are the conditions to consider first in the differential diagnosis. Chronic forms of uveitis have an insidious onset and typically last longer than 6 weeks. Other groups have defined a limited duration of uveitis as lasting 3 months or less, and persistent disease as lasting longer than 3 months.[3] Again, although many diseases can cause a uveitis that persists longer than 6 weeks, the uveitides that are characteristically chronic are listed in Box 4-2. Knowing whether the uveitis is acute or chronic is never sufficient to make a diagnosis, but it may aid in the diagnostic process.

2. Is the inflammation granulomatous or nongranulomatous?

The ocular examination offers a unique opportunity to determine the type of infiltrating inflammatory cells involved in the disease process without taking a biopsy sample for histologic analysis. In anterior uveitis, inflammatory cells attach to the corneal endothelium in conglomerates called keratic precipitates (KPs). The appearance of KPs has been used to classify the inflammatory process as granulomatous or nongranulomatous. The more common nongranulomatous type of KP is characterized by fine white collections of lymphocytes, plasma cells, and pigment. These precipitates can form in any disease and cause an anterior uveitis; the finding of nongranulomatous KPs does not help tremendously in the formulation of a differential diagnosis other than to alert the clinician that anterior inflammatory disease has occurred in the eye. Granulomatous KPs are large, greasy-appearing collections of lymphocytes, plasma cells, and giant cells (see Fig. 4-2). The finding of granulomatous KPs, also called 'mutton-fat' KPs, on slit-lamp examination can be a useful diagnostic clue. Patients with granulomatous KPs usually have a history of a chronic disease with an insidious onset, and frequently have posterior segment disease in addition to their anterior segment inflammation. Other ocular findings suggestive of granulomatous inflammation are iris nodules and choroidal granulomas. Importantly, the finding of granulomatous inflammation in the eye suggests a unique set of diagnostic possibilities that are listed in **Box 4-3**.

3. Is the disease unilateral or bilateral?

Although one eye may be affected first, uveitis resulting from most causes involves both eyes within the first several

Box 4-3 Causes of granulomatous inflammation in the eye

Sarcoidosis
Sympathetic ophthalmia
Uveitis associated with multiple sclerosis
Lens-induced uveitis
Intraocular foreign body
Vogt–Koyanagi–Harada syndrome
Syphilis
Tuberculosis
Other infectious agents

Box 4-4 Causes of unilateral uveitis

Sarcoidosis
Postsurgical uveitis
Intraocular foreign body
Parasitic disease
Acute retinal necrosis
Behçet's disease

Box 4-5 Causes of anterior uveitis

Idiopathic
Ankylosing spondylitis
Reiter's syndrome
Inflammatory bowel disease
Psoriatic arthritis
Behçet's disease
HLA-B27-associated disease
Juvenile rheumatoid arthritis
Fuchs' heterochromic iridocyclitis
Sarcoidosis
Syphilis
Glaucomatocyclitic crisis
Masquerade syndromes

months. Therefore, the history that the disease is both chronic and unilateral can help in diagnosing the condition. Diseases that frequently involve a single eye, even after months or years of the disorder, are listed in **Box 4-4**. Parasitic disease typically involves one eye, although some of the diseases, such as toxoplasmosis, occur bilaterally. Uveitis after ocular surgery or the presence of an intraocular foreign body is almost exclusively unilateral. The one disease that most ophthalmologists think of as a bilateral disease but which we see involving a single eye in a number of patients is sarcoidosis. Similarly, we have seen a number of patients with Behçet's disease that involved a single eye, especially those of Asian descent.

4. Where is the inflammation located in the eye?

It is important to determine the anatomic position of the inflammation within the eye. **Table 4-1** delineates three similar methods for the anatomic classification of intraocular inflammatory disease. We based our anatomic classification on the scheme proposed by the International Uveitis Study Group.[4] This was modified by the SUN Working Group by dividing the anatomic nomenclature into anterior, intermediate, posterior, and panuveitis and functions to both simplify and standardize the way the disease is described.[4] In addition to classifying uveitis as anterior, intermediate, or posterior uveitis or panuveitis, we note whether there is a predominant involvement of the cornea (keratouveitis), sclera (sclerouveitis), or retinal vasculature (retinal vasculitis) because these findings point to specific causes.

Anterior uveitis describes a disease limited predominantly to the anterior segment of the eye. Other terms used in the literature for anterior uveitis are iritis, iridocyclitis, and anterior cyclitis. The inflammation is characterized by conjunctival hyperemia, anterior chamber cell and flare, KPs, and

Table 4-1 Anatomic classification of uveitis

IUSG*	Tessler†	SUN Working Group[3]
–	Sclerouveitis	
–	Keratouveitis	
Anterior uveitis	Anterior uveitis	Anterior uveitis
Iritis	Iritis	Iritis
Anterior cyclitis	Iridocyclitis	Iridocyclitis
Iridocyclitis		Anterior cyclitis
Intermediate uveitis (formerly known as pars planitis)	Intermediate uveitis	Intermediate uveitis
Posterior cyclitis	Cyclitis	Pars planitis
Hyalitis	Vitritis	Posterior cyclitis
Basal retinochoroiditis	Pars planitis	Hyalitis
Posterior uveitis	Posterior uveitis	Posterior uveitis
Focal, multifocal, or diffuse choroiditis	Choroiditis	Focal, multifocal or diffuse choroiditis
Chorioretinitis or retinochoroiditis	Retinitis	Retinitis, chorioretinitis, or retinochoroiditis
Neuroretinitis	–	Neuroretinitis
Panuveitis	–	Panuveitis

*From Bloch-Michel E, Nussenblatt RB. International Uveitis Study Group recommendations for the evaluation of intraocular inflammatory disease. Am J Ophthalmol 1987; 103: 234–5.
†From Tessler HH. Classification and symptoms and signs of uveitis. In: Duane TD, Jaeger EA, eds. Clinical ophthalmology, vol 4. Philadelphia: JB Lippincott, 1987; 1–10.

iris abnormalities, including posterior synechiae and peripheral anterior synechiae. A mild cellular inflammatory response in the anterior vitreous is often seen. The common causes of anterior uveitis are listed in **Box 4-5**.

Intermediate uveitis is the anatomic diagnosis that causes the most confusion among ophthalmologists. However, the proper classification of a uveitis as intermediate is very important because an underlying cause for the disease can often be determined. Intermediate uveitis is characterized

Box 4-6 Causes of intermediate uveitis

Sarcoidosis
Inflammatory bowel disease
Multiple sclerosis
Lyme disease
Pars planitis*

*Not an etiologic diagnosis, but patients with intermediate uveitis of the par planitis subtype tend to have a worse prognosis.

Box 4-7 Causes of posterior uveitis

FOCAL RETINITIS
Toxoplasmosis
Onchocerciasis
Cysticercosis
Masquerade syndromes
MULTIFOCAL RETINITIS
Syphilis
Herpes simplex virus
Cytomegalovirus
Sarcoidosis
Masquerade syndromes
Candidiasis
Meningococcus
FOCAL CHOROIDITIS
Toxocariasis
Tuberculosis
Nocardiosis
Masquerade syndromes
MULTIFOCAL CHOROIDITIS
Histoplasmosis
Sympathetic ophthalmia
Vogt–Koyanagi–Harada syndrome
Sarcoidosis
Serpiginous choroidopathy
Birdshot choroidopathy
Masquerade syndromes (metastatic tumor)

Box 4-8 Causes of panuveitis

Syphilis
Sarcoidosis
Vogt–Koyanagi–Harada syndrome
Infectious endophthalmitis
Behçet's disease

by inflammation that primarily affects the vitreous and peripheral retina. Aggregates of inflammatory cells are frequently seen in the inferior vitreous and have been termed vitreous snowballs. Similarly, the accumulation of inflammatory cells and debris along the pars plana and ora serrata have been called snowbanks. A mild anterior uveitis often coexists, and cystoid macular edema is a frequent finding. The conditions associated with intermediate uveitis are listed in **Box 4-6**.

Disease limited to the posterior segment of the eye, particularly to the retina and choroid, is termed posterior uveitis. A large number of diseases cause posterior uveitis, so to further subdivide the disorders we classify posterior uveitis as predominantly a retinitis or choroiditis and as a focal or multifocal disease. The disorders that cause focal and multifocal retinitis and choroiditis are listed in **Box 4-7**. The term panuveitis is reserved for diseases that involve all segments of the eye, typically with a severe sight-reducing inflammatory response. The common causes of panuveitis are listed in **Box 4-8**.

Severe scleritis in association with uveitis is most frequently seen in patients with underlying connective tissue diseases such as rheumatoid arthritis and ankylosing spondylitis. Inflammatory bowel diseases, such as Crohn's disease and ulcerative colitis, also cause sclerouveitis. Finally, severe retinal vasculitis is associated with a subset of diseases that cause uveitis. Like scleritis, retinal vasculitis is often associated with underlying connective tissue disease. A full list of the disorders that cause retinal vasculitis can be found in Chapter 27.

5. What are the demographics of the patient?

Demographic information can lead the ophthalmologist to suspect certain types of uveitis, although there are always patients whose presentation varies from the usual age, gender, race, ethnic heritage, or social parameters characteristic of any particular disease. The age of the patient can be particularly useful in developing a differential diagnosis because certain causes of uveitis are more common among patients of specific age groups. A list of the diseases that occur more frequently in certain age groups is found in **Table 4-2**. One must be careful, however, not to rigidly apply these guidelines to patients. For example, although intraocular lymphoma is typically found in patients older than 65 years, we have seen patients with this disease in their 30s. Nevertheless, these guidelines are clearly useful, especially in diagnosing uveitis in children. Other demographic considerations in patients with uveitis are listed in **Table 4-3**.

6. What associated symptoms does the patient have?

As stated in Chapter 3, a thorough medical history is often the key to accurate diagnosis. Specific symptoms, both those relating to the eye and those suggesting systemic disease, should lead the clinician to suspect certain types of uveitis. We find that carefully defining a patient's symptoms is the most important step in determining the correct diagnosis. Many of the symptoms that suggest specific diagnoses are listed in **Table 4-4**. However, the enthusiasm to classify the patient within a diagnostic category may tempt the clinician to stretch the symptoms to fit a particular disease. For example, a patient who noted mild knee pain after playing basketball for the first time in 2 years should not be classified as having a chronic arthritis consistent with rheumatoid arthritis. Similarly, ringing in the ears after a 4-hour rock concert does not qualify as tinnitus suggestive of Vogt–Koyanagi–Harada syndrome. Importantly, the clinician must be careful not to suggest symptoms to the patient. Avoid asking questions such as 'You must have had some joint pain with this, haven't you?' Although it is important

Table 4-2 Age considerations in patients with uveitis*

Age (yr)	Diagnostic Considerations
<5	Juvenile rheumatoid arthritis Toxocariasis Postviral neuroretinitis (Retinoblastoma) (Juvenile xanthogranuloma) Leukemia
5–15	Juvenile rheumatoid arthritis Pars planitis Toxocariasis Postviral neuroretinitis Sarcoidosis Leukemia
16–25	Pars planitis Ankylosing spondylitis Idiopathic anterior uveitis Toxoplasmosis Sarcoidosis Acute retinal necrosis
25–45	Ankylosing spondylitis Idiopathic anterior uveitis Fuchs' heterochromic iridocyclitis Idiopathic intermediate uveitis Toxoplasmosis Behçet's disease Idiopathic retinal vasculitis Sarcoidosis White-dot syndromes Vogt–Koyanagi–Harada syndrome AIDS, syphilis Serpiginous choroidopathy
45–65	Birdshot retinochoroiditis Idiopathic anterior uveitis Idiopathic intermediate uveitis Idiopathic retinal vasculitis Behçet's disease Serpiginous choroidopathy Acute retinal necrosis
>65	Idiopathic anterior uveitis Idiopathic intermediate uveitis Idiopathic retinal vasculitis Serpiginous choroidopathy (Masquerade syndromes)

*Parentheses indicate noninflammatory diseases.

Table 4-3 Demographic considerations in uveitis

Factor	Disease Risks
Female	Pauciarticular juvenile rheumatoid arthritis, chronic anterior uveitis
Male	Ankylosing spondylitis, sympathetic ophthalmia
American black	Sarcoidosis
Native American	Vogt–Koyanagi–Harada syndrome
Midwestern American	Presumed ocular histoplasmosis
Japanese*	Vogt–Koyanagi–Harada syndrome Behçet's syndrome
Mediterranean ancestry	Behçet's syndrome
Central American	Cysticercosis, onchocerciasis
South American	Cysticercosis, toxoplasmosis
West African	Onchocerciasis
Intravenous drug user	Fungal endophthalmitis, AIDS
Promiscuous sexual activity	AIDS, syphilis
Frequent hiking in wooded areas	Lyme disease

*Not in Americans of Japanese extraction.

to interview patients about their medical history, the use of a standardized questionnaire helps ensure that symptoms are not missed or inappropriately suggested.

7. What associated signs are present on physical examination?

If it is rare to find ophthalmologists taking a detailed medical history in the office, it is almost unheard of for a detailed physical examination to be performed in the office. Unless you are prepared to do a thorough physical examination, it is probably more practical to refer patients to their primary care physician for this part of the evaluation. Nevertheless, it is fruitful for the ophthalmologist to examine a few things before making the referral. We have found that examination of the skin can be extremely rewarding in diagnosing uveitis. We have discovered sarcoid granulomas, rashes consistent with Lyme disease and syphilis, and Kaposi's sarcoma. A brief examination of the joints for signs of inflammation is also useful, and a screening neurologic examination is warranted, especially in patients who may have intraocular lymphoma, sarcoidosis, or Behçet's disease. Table 4-4 lists the systemic signs associated with specific uveitic conditions.

8. What is the time course of the disease and response to previous therapy?

The time course of the disease and the response to therapy can provide useful information in determining the cause. Is the disease responsive to antiinflammatory therapy? Does it require continued corticosteroid therapy? If so, how much corticosteroid is needed? Is the disease resistant to corticosteroid therapy? These questions can help the clinician determine the correct diagnosis. In general, infectious diseases may initially improve with antiinflammatory therapy but later worsen. Postoperative endophthalmitis caused by *Propionibacterium acnes* typically improves temporarily with topical or systemic corticosteroid therapy but then recurs. A temporary and partial response to therapy also suggests that the ocular inflammation may be associated with a chronic systemic disease such as sarcoidosis or a malignancy-like lymphoma. A long history of intermittent response to therapy tends to be more suggestive of a chronic noninfectious and nonmalignant disease, because both infection or malignancy often become evident after several years.

The old adage, 'When you hear hoofbeats, think of horses and not zebras,' also applies to the evaluation of the patient with uveitis. Common diseases are frequently the cause of uveitis even in cases that are difficult to diagnose. **Table 4-5** lists the most common causes of anterior and posterior uveitis from two published surveys of patients with uveitis.

Table 4-4 Systemic signs and symptoms in uveitis

Symptom or Sign	Possible Associated Conditions
Headaches	Sarcoidosis, Vogt–Koyanagi–Harada syndrome
Neurosensory deafness	Vogt–Koyanagi–Harada syndrome, sarcoidosis
Cerebrospinal fluid pleocytosis	Vogt–Koyanagi–Harada syndrome, sarcoidosis, acute posterior multifocal placoid pigment epitheliopathy, Behçet's syndrome
Paresthesia, weakness	Intermediate uveitis associated with multiple sclerosis, Behçet's syndrome, steroid myopathy
Psychosis	Vogt–Koyanagi–Harada syndrome, sarcoidosis, Behçet's disease, steroid psychosis, systemic lupus erythematosus
Vitiligo, poliosis	Vogt–Koyanagi–Harada syndrome
Erythema nodosum	Behçet's syndrome, sarcoidosis
Skin nodules	Sarcoidosis, onchocerciasis
Alopecia	Vogt–Koyanagi–Harada syndrome
Skin rash	Behçet's syndrome, sarcoidosis, viral exanthem, syphilis, herpes zoster, psoriatic arthritis, Lyme disease
Oral ulcers	Behçet's syndrome, inflammatory bowel disease
Genital ulcers	Behçet's syndrome, Reiter's syndrome, sexually transmitted diseases
Salivary or lacrimal gland swelling	Sarcoidosis, lymphoma
Lymphoid organ enlargement	Sarcoidosis, AIDS
Diarrhea	Whipple's disease, inflammatory bowel disease
Cough, shortness of breath	Sarcoidosis, tuberculosis, malignancy
Sinusitis	Wegener's granulomatosis
Systemic vasculitis	Behçet's syndrome, sarcoidosis, relapsing polychondritis
Arthritis	Behçet's syndrome, Reiter's syndrome, sarcoidosis, juvenile rheumatoid arthritis, rheumatoid arthritis, Lyme disease, inflammatory bowel disease, Wegener's granulomatosus, systemic lupus erythematosus, other connective tissue diseases
Sacroiliitis	Ankylosing spondylitis, Reiter's syndrome, inflammatory bowel disease
Chemotherapy or other immunosuppression	Cytomegalovirus retinitis, *Candida* retinitis, other opportunistic organisms

Table 4-5 Common causes of anterior and posterior uveitis

Diagnosis	Perkins et al. (%)*	Henderly et al. (%)†
ANTERIOR UVEITIS		
Idiopathic anterior uveitis	32.7	12.1
HLA-B27-associated anterior uveitis	–	3.0
Juvenile rheumatoid arthritis	5.1	2.8
Fuchs' heterochromic iridocyclitis	6.3	1.8
Ankylosing spondylitis	5.7	1.5
Reiter's syndrome	5.2	1.0
Inflammatory bowel disease	2.9	0.3
Syphilis	1.2	0.8
Intraocular lens-related anterior uveitis	–	1.0
POSTERIOR UVEITIS		
Toxoplasmic retinochoroiditis	9.2	7.0
Idiopathic retinal vasculitis	4.6	6.8
Idiopathic posterior uveitis	6.9	3.7
Ocular histoplasmosis	–	3.5
Toxocariasis	2.9	2.6
Serpiginous choroidopathy	–	2.0
Acute posterior multifocal placoid pigment epitheliopathy	–	1.8
Acute retinal necrosis	–	1.3
Birdshot choroidopathy	–	1.2
Intraocular lymphoma	1.1	1.2

*Data from Perkins ES, Folk J. Uveitis in London and Iowa. Ophthalmologica 1984; 36: 189.
†Data from Henderly DE, Genstler AJ, Smith RE, et al. Changing patterns of uveitis. Am J Ophthalmol 1987; 103: 131–6.

Case 4-1

A 42-year-old white woman presented with a 10-year history of bilateral uveitis treated intermittently with topical and systemic corticosteroids and a chief complaint of blurred vision that was worse in the left eye. A detailed medical history was significant for sinusitis and depression. On examination, her visual acuity was 20/50 in the right eye and 20/100 in the left. Slit-lamp biomicroscopy showed mutton-fat KPs in the left eye. There were trace vitreous cells and haze in the right eye and 2+ vitreous cells and haze in the left eye. There were peripheral retinal vasculitis and cystoid macular edema in both eyes (**Fig. 4-1**). Physical examination revealed no rash, joint findings, or other abnormalities. Neurologic examination was normal.

Most clinicians will find it difficult to derive an erudite differential diagnosis from simply reading this case history, but by classifying the uveitis with the eight questions previously outlined, lists of possible diagnoses can be generated. By comparing these lists, the most likely diagnoses can then be identified. Question 1 asks whether the disease is acute or

Once the above questions are answered, lists of possible diagnoses are generated. By determining the diagnoses that appear most frequently, a final list of the most likely conditions responsible for the patient's uveitis is generated. The clinician can then order diagnostic studies to discern among them. The following cases will help to illustrate the process of developing a differential diagnosis in the patient with uveitis.

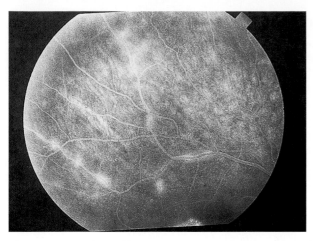

Figure 4-1. Late phase of fluorescein angiogram showing staining of blood vessel walls and leakage of dye from peripheral retinal vasculature.

chronic. Because the patient has a 10-year history of disease, the uveitis is clearly chronic and this is associated with the diseases listed in Box 4-2. The patient has mutton-fat KPs, suggesting that the uveitis is granulomatous, and this suggests the list of diagnoses shown in Box 4-3. The disease is bilateral, which does not point to a specific set of diseases; however, with prominent vitritis and peripheral retinal vasculitis, the anatomic classification of an intermediate uveitis does suggest a specific set of possible diseases to the clinician (Box 4-6). The patient is white and in the 24–45-year age range, suggesting the diagnoses shown in Table 4-2. As seen in Table 4-4, a complaint of sinusitis suggests a possible diagnosis of Wegener's granulomatosis, but the patient had no specific findings on physical examination.

In summary, the uveitis can be classified as a chronic, granulomatous, bilateral, intermediate uveitis in a middle-aged white woman with intermittent response to topical and systemic corticosteroids. The lists containing possible diagnoses for this patient are shown in **Box 4-9**. If you compare these lists, the most frequently mentioned disorders include sarcoidosis, other causes of intermediate uveitis such as multiple sclerosis and inflammatory bowel disease, and other chronic disorders such as Behçet's disease and Wegener's granulomatosis. Diagnostic tests were then ordered to discern between the most likely disorders. Results of a diagnostic evaluation for sarcoidosis and Wegener's granulomatosis, including a chest X-ray, serum angiotensin-converting enzyme level, antineutrophil cytoplasmic antibody test, and CT scan of the sinuses, were normal. However, an MRI scan of the brain revealed lesions consistent with a diagnosis of multiple sclerosis. The patient later developed an episode of lower extremity weakness followed by a second episode of paresthesia that extended to the level of the umbilicus that was diagnostic of this disease.

Case 4-2

A 73-year-old white woman presented with blurred vision in both eyes that had been present during the previous year. The patient first noted floaters in the left eye 1 year ago, but did not see an ophthalmologist until 3 months earlier, when she was

---

Box 4-9 Lists of diagnoses generated for Case 4-1

Chronic, granulomatous, bilateral, intermediate uveitis in a middle-aged white woman with intermittent response to topical and systemic corticosteroids

CHRONIC UVEITIS
Juvenile rheumatoid arthritis
Birdshot choroidopathy
Serpiginous choroidopathy
Tuberculous uveitis
Postsurgical uveitis (*Propionibacterium acnes*, fungal)
Intraocular lymphoma
Sympathetic ophthalmia
Multifocal choroiditis
Sarcoidosis
Intermediate uveitis/pars planitis
INTERMEDIATE UVEITIS
Sarcoidosis
Inflammatory bowel disease
Multiple sclerosis
Lyme disease
Pars planitis
GRANULOMATOUS INFLAMMATION IN EYE
Sarcoidosis
Sympathetic ophthalmia
Uveitis associated with multiple sclerosis
Lens-induced uveitis
Intraocular foreign body
Vogt–Koyanagi–Harada syndrome
Syphilis
Tuberculosis
Other infectious agents
AGE 25–45 YR
Ankylosing spondylitis
Idiopathic anterior uveitis
Fuchs' heterochromic iridocyclitis
Intermediate uveitis
Toxoplasmosis
Behçet's disease
Idiopathic retinal vasculitis
Sarcoidosis
White-dot syndromes
Vogt–Koyanagi–Harada syndrome
AIDS
Syphilis
Serpiginous choroidopathy
ASSOCIATED SYMPTOMS AND SIGNS
Sinusitis – Wegener's disease

---

found to have a slight decrease in visual acuity in the left eye and bilateral mild vitritis. Over the next 3 months her vision decreased in both eyes, and she was referred to the National Eye Institute. She had a history of type II diabetes mellitus controlled with oral hypoglycemic agents, and of rheumatic fever as a child. She also complained of weight loss and unsteady gait. She lived in a wooded area in Glen Falls, New York.

On examination, visual acuity was 20/50 in the right eye and 20/125 in the left. Anterior segment examination was normal, but there were 2+ vitreous cells and 1+ vitreous haze in both

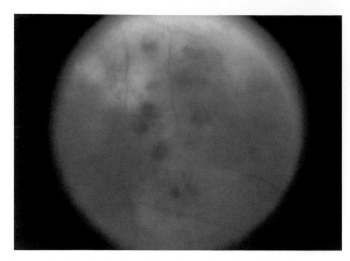

Figure 4-2. Fundus photograph showing yellow subretinal infiltrates, retinal hemorrhage, and retinal edema in eye with 20/125 visual acuity and moderate vitritis.

eyes. Funduscopic examination revealed punctate yellow subretinal infiltrates in both eyes and retinal hemorrhage and edema in the left eye (**Fig. 4-2**). Physical examination revealed ataxia.

Again, this patient's condition presents difficulty in diagnosis, but with the approach detailed in Case 4-1 a differential diagnosis can be readily developed. The disease is chronic and the inflammation nongranulomatous. It is a bilateral disease and is classified as a multifocal retinitis. Therefore the patient is classified as having a chronic, nongranulomatous, bilateral, multifocal retinitis. She is an elderly white woman, and the history of living in a wooded area suggests a demographic susceptibility to Lyme disease. Her symptom of weight loss suggests the possibility of an underlying malignancy, malnutrition, or possible gastrointestinal disease, and the unsteady gait alerts the clinician to the possibility of neurologic disease. The diagnoses generated by this classification are shown in **Box 4-10**. As you can see, the most frequently listed diagnoses include sarcoidosis, infectious diseases, and the masquerade syndromes, most notably intraocular lymphoma.

Our first concern was that the patient had an underlying malignancy. Systemic evaluation was unrewarding, and a vitrectomy showed no malignant cells. However, two measurements of serum angiotensin-converting enzyme levels were elevated at 81 U/L and 101 U/L (normal range 8–52 U/L), and a bronchoscopy confirmed the diagnosis of sarcoidosis.

We hope that this chapter will provide the clinician with a pragmatic approach to generating a differential diagnosis. This will then permit the ophthalmologist to order the appropriate tests to discern among the most likely possibilities. As you will see in Chapter 5, the alternative shotgun approach of indiscriminately ordering every diagnostic test in the book may be both expensive and misleading.

Box 4-10 Lists of diagnoses generated for Case 4-2

Chronic, nongranulomatous, bilateral, multifocal retinitis in an elderly white woman
CHRONIC UVEITIS
Juvenile rheumatoid arthritis
Birdshot choroidopathy
Serpiginous choroidopathy
Tuberculous uveitis
Postsurgical uveitis (*Propionibacterium acnes*, fungal)
Intraocular lymphoma
Sympathetic ophthalmia
Multifocal choroiditis
Sarcoidosis
Intermediate uveitis/pars planitis
GRANULOMATOUS INFLAMMATION IN THE EYE
Sarcoidosis
Sympathetic ophthalmia
Uveitis associated with multiple sclerosis
Lens-induced uveitis
Intraocular foreign body
Vogt–Koyanagi–Harada syndrome
Syphilis
Tuberculosis
Other infectious agents
MULTIFOCAL RETINITIS
Syphilis
Herpes simplex virus
Cytomegalovirus
Sarcoidosis
Masquerade syndromes
Candida
Meningococcus
AGE >65 YR
Idiopathic anterior uveitis
Idiopathic intermediate uveitis
Idiopathic retinal vasculitis
Serpiginous choroidopathy
Masquerade syndromes
Sarcoidosis
DEMOGRAPHIC CONSIDERATIONS
Patient lives in an area endemic for Lyme disease

References

1. de Groot AD. Thought and choice in chess. The Hague: Mouton Publishers 1965.
2. de Groot AD, Gobet F. Perception and memory in chess. Studies in the heuristics of the professional eye. Assen: Van Gorcum, 1966.
3. Jabs DA, Nussenblatt RB, Rosenbaum JT. Standardization of Uveitis Nomenclature (SUN) Working Group. Standardization of uveitis nomenclature for reporting clinical data. Results of the First International Workshop. Am J Ophthlamol 2005; 140: 509–516.
4. Bloch-Michel E, Nussenblatt RB. International Uveitis Study Group recommendations for the evaluation of intraocular inflammatory disease. Am J Ophthalmol 1987; 103: 234–235.

Diagnostic Testing

Scott M. Whitcup

Key concepts

- Mistakes in ordering and interpreting diagnostic tests can lead to misdiagnosis and inappropriate therapy.
- Diagnostic tests should be ordered to narrow down the differential diagnosis.
- Clinicians must know the sensitivity and specificity of the diagnostic test to avoid misinterpretation of the results.
- A few diagnostic tests are both highly sensitive and highly specific and may therefore be useful as a screening test for patients with many forms of uveitis. The FTA-ABS test for syphilis is an example of a diagnostic test often used as a general screening for patients with uveitis.
- Assessing the likelihood of disease before the diagnostic test is crucial in determining the likelihood of disease after either a positive or a negative diagnostic test.
- Tests including fluorescein angiography and ocular coherence tomography are helpful in assessing response to therapy.
- Some diagnostic tests, such as bone mineral density studies, help to limit side effects of therapy and are now part of the standard care of patients on systemic antiinflammatory therapy.

What diagnostic tests should you order in the evaluation of the patient with uveitis? This is one of the most difficult questions we are asked. It is clear, however, that a nonselective approach to testing is costly and inefficient and provides information that is often irrelevant or, worse yet, that may lead to an incorrect diagnosis and inappropriate therapy. It is important to understand how to interpret diagnostic data because this information will help the clinician to order the appropriate tests.

Why does the clinician order diagnostic tests? Usually diagnostic tests are ordered to aid in making the correct diagnosis. Unfortunately, many clinicians are overly influenced when positive or negative results for a diagnostic test come back from the laboratory. A clinical example will serve to illustrate this point. A 34-year-old African-American woman from Texas presents with an intermediate uveitis in both eyes that has been present for the past 7 months. There is no history of rash, arthritis, or fever, but the patient does complain of wheezing and shortness of breath on exertion.

The ophthalmologist orders a battery of diagnostic tests, including a serologic test for Lyme disease that has a positive result. Of course, the ophthalmologist is ecstatic in diagnosing the patient's condition and treats her with a 2-week course of ceftriaxone. There are only three problems with this scenario: the patient probably does not have Lyme disease, did not need the expensive 2-week course of intravenous antibiotics, and more likely has sarcoidosis that is not being treated!

Before one can appropriately interpret the results of a diagnostic test, three pieces of information are needed. First, one needs to know the sensitivity of the diagnostic test (**Fig. 5-1**). This is calculated by dividing the number of patients who actually have the disease and who on testing have a positive result, by the total number of patients with the disease who are tested. Another name given to patients with a disease who have a positive test result is true positives: they have a positive test result and actually have the disease. Patients who have the disease but who have a negative test result are called false negatives. Many of the commonly used serologic tests for Lyme disease have a sensitivity of 90%. What does that mean? It means that if 100 patients with Lyme disease were tested, 90 would have a positive result (true positives), but 10 would have a negative result (false negatives). Furthermore, many diagnostic tests have varying sensitivities based on the stage of the disease. For example, Lyme serologies are less sensitive during the acute stage of the disease.

The second piece of information you need to have to interpret a diagnostic test result is the specificity (Fig. 5-1). The specificity of a diagnostic test is calculated by dividing the number of patients who do not have the disease in question and who have had an appropriately negative test result, by the total number of people without the disease who are tested. People who do not have the disease and who have a negative test result are called true negatives. Similarly, people who do not have the disease but who have a positive test result anyway are called false positives. In the case of the serologic test for Lyme disease, the specificity is also 90%. This means that if 100 patients without Lyme disease take this test, 90 will have an appropriately negative result, but 10 will have a misleading positive result!

Pretest likelihood of disease

The third and critical piece of information needed for test interpretation is often ignored by many doctors. This piece of information is called the pretest likelihood of the disease

	Disease present	Disease absent
Test positive	True positives (a)	False positives (b)
Test negative	False negatives (c)	True negatives (d)

Figure 5-1. Sensitivity and specificity of diagnostic tests. Sensitivity = a/a + c. Specificity = d/b + d.

and is defined as the chance that the patient has a particular disease before the diagnostic test is ordered. The pretest likelihood can be based on a number of factors, such as the patient's history and physical examination and the incidence of a particular disease in that area. This is the figure that most depends on the clinician's prowess and ability: the more accurate the physician's calculation of the pretest likelihood of disease, the more accurate the subsequent interpretation of the test result will be.

What is the pretest likelihood of Lyme disease in the case of the 34-year-old woman from San Antonio with intermediate uveitis who has no other symptoms and signs of Lyme disease and who does not live in an area endemic for the disease? The prevalence of Lyme disease in San Antonio, Texas, is probably less than 1 in 1000, and with no other evidence of the disease the pretest likelihood of the disease would probably be less than this. But let us be generous and say that the pretest likelihood of this patient having Lyme disease is 1 in 1000 or 0.1%. How do we interpret her positive test result for Lyme disease?

The likelihood that the diagnosis of Lyme disease is correct in this patient can be calculated because we now have the sensitivity of the test (90%), the specificity of the test (90%), and the pretest likelihood of the disease (0.1%). This calculation of what is called the post-test likelihood of disease is carried out with the use of a formula derived by the mathematician Bayes and is called Bayes' theorem. The standard form of Bayes' theorem states the following:

$$\text{Post-test probability} = \frac{\text{Pretest probability} \times \text{sensitivity}}{\begin{array}{l}(\text{Pretest probability} \times \text{sensitivity})\\ + (1 - \text{pretest probability})(1 - \text{specificity})\end{array}}$$

Bayes' theorem has been understood for two centuries but has only been applied to clinical reasoning over the past 30 years.[1–5] Although formulas may appear daunting to some clinicians, computer programs and nomograms have been developed to help the clinician interpret the data.[6,7] So what is the likelihood that our patient has Lyme disease, given her positive laboratory test result? With Bayes' theorem the chance that she has Lyme disease is still only 0.9%, or a chance of 9 out of 1000! Although this represents an almost 10-fold increase in likelihood compared with the pretest likelihood, because there was a very small chance that she had Lyme disease before the test, she still probably does not have the disease. Knowing that the post-test likelihood of the patient having Lyme disease is less than 1%, the clinician probably would not opt to treat her with antibiotics.

Diagnostic tests are also not as useful if there is a very strong likelihood that a patient has the disease before the test is ordered. If this same patient came from Lyme, Connecticut, had a history of a tick bite followed by an erythematous, round rash, and now presented with an

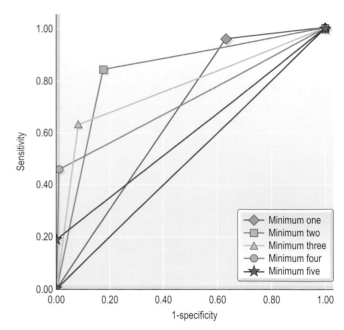

Figure 5-2. Receiver operating characteristic (ROC) curve for the requirement for each additional number of ocular features required to make a diagnosis of ocular sarcoidosis. The area under the ROC curve is greatest (0.84) for requiring a minimum of two ocular features to make the diagnosis, with a sensitivity of 84.0% and a specificity of 83.0%. *(From Asukata Y, Ishihara M, Hasumi Y, et al. Guidelines for the diagnosis of ocular sarcoidosis. Ocul Immunol Inflamm 2008; 16: 77–81, with permission.)*

intermediate uveitis and arthritis, even without testing she would probably have a greater than 99% chance of having the disease. Even if the result of her serologic test for Lyme disease was negative, after applying Bayes' theorem the patient would still have about a 99% chance of having the disease!

Diagnostic tests are most helpful when the pretest likelihood of the disease is about 50%. For our patient with intermediate uveitis, if after our initial assessment we thought that her chance of having Lyme disease was 50%, a positive serologic test result would increase the post-test likelihood of the disease to 90%. So in this case, we start with a 50 : 50 chance of Lyme disease but end up with Lyme disease being by far the most likely diagnosis.

Receiver operating characteristic (ROC) curve

Many diagnostic tests involve establishing a numerical cut-off, above which a patient is felt to have a 'positive' test and hence is more likely to have the disease. Where you set that cut-off affects the sensitivity and specificity of the test and determines the number of false positive and false negative test results. Unless a test is 100% sensitive and 100% specific, the more sensitive it is the more likely you are to get false positives. The sensitivity of a test can be graphed against 1-specificity of the test to obtain what is called the receiver operating characteristic (ROC) curve (**Fig. 5-2**). The performance of a diagnostic test can be quantified by calculating the area under the ROC curve. Importantly, the ability of two continous variables to diagnose a disease can be distinguished by comparing the two ROC curves and the area under these curves, and determining whether this difference is statistically significant.[8,9] If so, the test with the greater area under the ROC curve may be more discriminating.

It is also important to critically assess the quality of the data underlying the sensitivity and specificity numbers you use.[10] Data usually come from a number of clinical trials that use the given test. A meta-analysis of these studies can be used to assess diagnostic test accuracy by graphing the results on the ROC curve.

So now that you have the knowledge to analyze data, it should be easy to interpret your patients' test data, right? Unfortunately, it is not that easy. It is difficult to obtain the sensitivities and specificities for many of the common diagnostic tests we order. Many laboratories are considering providing a nomogram listing the post-test likelihood of the disease for differing pretest likelihoods because they already know the current sensitivity and specificity for that test. But how do we know the sensitivity or specificity of a chest X-ray for the diagnosis of sarcoidosis, or of a diagnostic vitrectomy for intraocular lymphoma? These figures are difficult to obtain and may vary tremendously from institution to institution. More and more, however, articles are being published on the sensitivity and specificity of diagnostic procedures and tests. In addition, the clinician can do the calculations on the basis of hypothetical numbers. For example, one might ask this question: given a 95% sensitivity and a 95% specificity for a test in a patient who I think has a 10% chance of having the disease, what is the post-test likelihood of the disease? It is surprising how much such calculations can help you to decide on a diagnostic or therapeutic approach to patients with complicated conditions. Rosenbaum and Wernick[3] have written a review on how to apply Bayes' theorem to the evaluation of patients with uveitis, and this should be useful to many clinicians.

Diagnostic tests for uveitis

After your initial differential diagnosis is generated, diagnostic tests should be ordered to help discern among the most likely disorders. Remember that diagnostic tests will have the most utility in confirming or rejecting diagnoses that start with about a 50% chance of being correct. **Table 5-1** and **Box 5-1** list the common diagnostic tests useful for the evaluation of patients with uveitis. In addition to helping the clinician make the correct diagnosis, diagnostic tests are ordered in two other clinical settings. The first of these involves ordering tests to help the practitioner exclude the diagnosis of tumor and infection, because these disorders require specific therapy and would be exacerbated by antiinflammatory treatment. The second is to determine why a patient's vision has decreased and whether this change is reversible. In eyes with complicated uveitis, the reasons for poor vision may be multifactorial, and the clinician needs as much information as possible.

The number of diagnostic tests available to the ophthalmologist has increased tremendously over the last decade. Many tests are expensive yet yield little useful information; others are critical for the appropriate management of patients. These tests can be arbitrarily grouped into laboratory tests, imaging techniques, skin testing, surgical specimens, and ancillary ophthalmic tests. Many of the tests listed in Table 5-1 and Box 5-1 are more thoroughly discussed in later chapters on specific diseases; however, several points for each group of diagnostic tests deserve comment here.

Table 5-1 Laboratory tests in uveitis

Tests	Conditions/Comments
Angiotensin-converting enzyme	Sarcoidosis; may be elevated in children without sarcoidosis
Antiphospholipid Ab (lupus anticoagulant and anticardiolipin Ab)	Thrombosis, CNS disease, and spontaneous abortions in patients with systemic lupus erythematosus
ANA	Systemic lupus erythematosus and other rheumatic diseases
Antifungal Ab	Fungal disease
ANCA	Wegener's granulomatosis (cANCA)
Polyarteritis nodosa (pANCA)	
Antitoxoplasma Ab	Toxoplasmosis
Antiviral Ab	Viral infection
Calcium	Sarcoidosis
Chlamydia complement-fixation test	Chlamydia
C-reactive protein	Underlying inflammatory disease (i.e., rheumatic disease)
Cultures	Bacterial, fungal, mycobacterial, and viral diseases
Erythrocyte sedimentation rate	Underlying systemic diseases (i.e, rheumatic disease, malignancy)
Complete blood cell count	Underlying systemic disease
HIV ELISA	HIV
HTLV-1	HTLV-1 infection
HLA typing	(Specific HLA types associated with specific diseases)
Immune complexes	Rarely useful
Liver function tests	Sarcoidosis, hepatitis
Lumbar function for cell count	APMPPE, VKH, Infection, Malignancy
Lumbar puncture for CSF VDRL	Syphilis
Lumbar puncture for culture and Gram stain	Infection
Lumbar puncture for cytology	CNS lymphoma
Lyme serology	Lyme disease (be aware of false-positive results)
Rheumatoid factor (RF)	Rheumatoid arthritis; girls with JRA and uveitis often RF negative but ANA positive
Stool for ova and parasites	Parasitic disease
T-cell subsets	(Low CD4+ count predisposes patient for opportunistic infections)
Thyroid function tests	Increased incidence of thyroid disease in patients with uveitis
Urinalysis	(Blood suggests rheumatic disease)
VDRL/FTA-ABS	Syphilis

Ab, Antibody; ANA, antinuclear antibody; APMPPE, acute posterior multifocal placoid pigment epitheliopathy; CNS, central nervous system; CSF, cerebrospinal fluid; ELISA, enzyme-linked immunosorbent assay; HIV, human immunodeficiency virus; HTLV, human T-cell leukemia/lymphoma virus; JRA, juvenile rheumatoid arthritis; VKH, Vogt–Koyanagi–Harada syndrome.

Box 5-1 Other diagnostic tests in uveitis

IMAGING TESTS

CT scan of head
CT scan of sinuses
Gallium scan
Hand X-ray
MRI of head
Sacroiliac X-ray
SKIN TESTING
Allergy testing
Anergy testing
Behçetin
Histoplasmin
Pathergy
PPD

ANCILLARY OPHTHALMIC TESTING

Color vision testing
Contrast sensitivity
Electroretinogram
Electrooculogram
Fluorescein angiography
Indocyanine green angiography
Laser interferometry
Laser flare photometry
Manifest refraction
Optical coherence tomography
Ultrasound of orbit
Ultrasound of retina
Visual evoked potentials
Visual field testing

BIOPSY SPECIMENS

Conjunctiva
Lacrimal gland
Aqueous humor
Vitreous
Choroid and retina
Skin

Laboratory tests

Laboratory tests usually are the first diagnostic tests that most physicians order. Although we have emphasized that laboratory tests should not be routinely used to screen patients with uveitis for disease, and that tests should be ordered only to discern among likely diagnoses, there is one exception: practically all patients with uveitis should be tested for syphilis. There are a number of factors that support the use of laboratory tests to screen for syphilis in most patients with uveitis. Syphilis remains a common cause of uveitis and is easily treatable. Patients with untreated ocular syphilis often have devastating visual outcomes. Importantly, the fluorescent treponemal antibody absorption (FTA-ABS) test for syphilis is both extremely sensitive and specific. For patients with late syphilis – the stage of disease – associated with uveitis, the sensitivity and specificity of the FTA-ABS test are both 99%. With this combination of a treatable, common disease; poor outcome in untreated patients; and a highly sensitive and specific diagnostic test with little

risk and moderate cost, screening becomes useful. It is important to note, however, that other laboratory tests for syphilis are not as good for screening for late syphilis (see Chapter 10). The Venereal Disease Research Laboratory (VDRL) test, for example, has a sensitivity of only 70% for late syphilis. Therefore the clinician should insist on an FTA-ABS test in evaluation of the patient with uveitis. Also, the incidence of syphilis in patients with AIDS is increasing.[11,12] As a result, all patients with syphilis who have uveitis should also be tested for human immunodeficiency virus (HIV) infection, and vice versa.

A number of tests are used for research purposes but are commercially available. Many practitioners order these tests but do not know what to do with the results when they come back. Standardization of many of these tests is subpar, and many of these tests are better left unordered. One example is testing for circulating immune complexes. Circulating immune complexes were first thought to be the mechanism underlying the destruction of the eye in various forms of uveitis. Tests for circulating immune complexes were ordered, and if present they were assumed to be the cause of the disease. However, it is no longer clear that immune complexes are the cause of many occurrences of uveitis. Circulating immune complexes are found in many persons, and the evidence to date suggests that their presence in ocular inflammatory disease may be protective rather than destructive (see Chapter 1).

A number of laboratory tests are used in the evaluation of patients with possible rheumatic diseases.[13] Acute-phase reactants include a number of proteins produced by the liver in reponse to stress, and signal underlying inflammation. The most commonly used tests for acute-phase reactants are the erythrocyte sedimentation rate (ESR) and C-reactive protein (CRP). Rheumatoid factor (RF) is an autoantibody against the Fc portion of human IgG. The test is relatively sensitive for rheumatoid arthritis, and may also be positive in patients with other rheumatic diseases, including Sjögren's syndrome and systemic lupus erythematosis (SLE). However, RF may also be positive in patients with chronic inflammatory diseases or malignancy and is also seen in normal subjects. Antinuclear antibodies are another test indicative of underlying connective tissue diseases. They are extremely senstive for SLE, and depending on the immunofluorescence pattern of the test, can indicate specific disorders such as polymyositis, dermatomyositic, or CREST (calcinosis, Raynaud's phenomenon, esophogeal dysmotility, sclerodactyly, and telangiectasis).

The antineutrophil cytoplasmic antibody (ANCA) test has been very helpful in the diagnosis of Wegener's granulomatosis, a systemic vasculitis characterized by a necrotizing granulomatous vasculitis of the upper and lower respiratory tracts, a focal necrotizing glomerulonephritis, and systemic small vessel vasculitis involving a number of organ systems, and in follow-up of patients with this disease. Ocular involvement including uveitis, scleritis, and retinal vasculitis occurs in about 16% of patients.[14–16] Young[17] described 98 patients with uveitis tested for the presence of ANCAs by an indirect immunofluorescence method and found a positive ANCA test result in patients with chronic uveitis from various causes. A cytoplasmic pattern of staining (cANCA) is felt to be more specific for Wegener's granulomatosis than a peripheral pattern (pANCA). Soukasian and colleagues[18] reported that ANCA test results were positive in seven patients with scleritis caused by Wegener's granulomatosis but negative in 54 patients with other ocular inflammatory diseases; this suggests that the test is both sensitive and specific. High specificity of the cANCA test for Wegener's granulomatosis in patients with ocular inflammatory disease has been reported by other investigators as well.[19] The ANCA test may also be useful in guiding immunosuppressive therapy. Failure of ANCA titers to revert to normal levels may be associated with an increased risk of relapse.[20] These patients may benefit from more aggressive immunosuppressive therapy.

Image analysis

Although newer techniques provide the practitioner with high-resolution images, simple radiographic techniques, such as skull X-rays to evaluate patients with suspected congenital toxoplasmosis for calcifications, should not be overlooked. Chest X-rays should be obtained in patients suspected of having sarcoidosis or tuberculosis. A computed tomography (CT) or magnetic resonance imaging (MRI) scan of the brain is indicated for patients with possible intraocular lymphoma (see Chapter 30). In contrast, sinus radiographs are frequently ordered as part of the evaluation of patients with uveitis; however, it is not clear that this test is helpful on a routine basis. Patients with a history of sinus disease and uveitis may have an underlying systemic vasculitis such as Wegener's granulomatosis, but in these patients an ANCA test, consultation with an otolaryngologist, and possibly a CT scan of the sinuses may be more appropriate and useful than sinus radiographs.

Skin testing

Skin testing is often neglected by the practitioner, but these simple tests can give the observer a large amount of information. The purified protein derivative (PPD) and histoplasmin skin tests are easily performed and give important clinical data. The PPD test is important in the evaluation of the patient with uveitis with a history suggesting tuberculosis. In addition, patients should have a PPD test before they are given immunosuppressive therapy, because if the PPD test result is positive these patients will require antituberculous therapy before immunosuppressive therapy is begun. Patients with a history of possible tuberculosis or a positive reaction to a tuberculosis skin test should be tested with a lower-strength PPD, such as a 1 test unit dose, instead of the usual 5 test unit dose. If these test results are negative, then the higher test dose can be given. The histoplasmin skin test is useful in evaluating patients with presumed ocular histoplasmosis syndrome; however, the test may activate an old, inactive histoplasmosis lesion and should be avoided in patients with macular lesions.

Skin testing can also be used to document anergy. Patients with sarcoidosis are typically anergic and should have depressed responses to skin testing with control antigens such as tetanus. Systemic corticosteroid administration sometimes reverses anergy in these patients, whereas ciclosporin may prevent type IV hypersensitivity reactions in the skin and yield a negative result to the skin test. In the past, the Kveim test was commonly performed for sarcoidosis, but the result was very dependent on the batch of Kveim antigen that was used. Currently, Kveim antigen cannot be obtained, and the test is no longer used. The Behçetin skin test is also infrequently performed. In this test, patients with suspected Behçet's disease are stuck with a sterile needle, and the skin is observed or samples are biopsied for evidence of a type IV reaction. The hypothesis is that patients with Behçet's disease will display a positive delayed hypersensitivity response to the needlestick (pathergy). Although the test is rarely performed, a history of skin reactions to phlebotomy draws or after intravenous line placements may suggest pathergy and the diagnosis of Behçet's disease.

Allergy testing was at one time a very important component in the evaluation of the patient with uveitis. The relevance of atopy or a specific allergy to uveitis is not clear. Hard evidence showing that type I hypersensitivity reactions are a major, underlying force in intraocular inflammatory disease is lacking: only anecdotal information suggests perhaps a secondary role.[21] As a result, we only occasionally order allergy testing for our patients.

Tissue samples

The diagnosis of many forms of uveitis is based on the history and the typical appearance of the ocular disease. Nevertheless, the definitive diagnosis of many occurrences of uveitis requires histologic confirmation. No oncologist or radiation therapist would agree to treat a patient with presumed intraocular lymphoma without a tissue diagnosis. Similarly, the definitive diagnosis of sarcoidosis also requires histologic confirmation. In many other instances, analysis of ocular fluid or tissue can provide a wealth of information to the clinician. The information is, however, only as good as the evaluation of the specimen. It is imperative that the tissue is processed expeditiously by a person experienced in a variety of histologic and immunologic techniques, including immunohistochemical staining.

The evaluation of intraocular fluid is of great potential value. A condition for which the analysis of intraocular fluids has aided the clinician in diagnosis is toxoplasmosis. Problems arise when atypical lesions are noted in a patient with low levels of circulating antitoxoplasma antibody. Desmonts[22] proposed that local (that is, intraocular) production of specific antitoxoplasmosis antibody strongly suggests an active ocular lesion as a result of toxoplasmosis. To demonstrate local production of antibody, the specific antibody in the eye is measured relative to the total amount of globulin in the eye. This led Desmonts to calculate the antibody coefficient (C). The formula for determining this value is:

$$C = \text{Antibody titer} \frac{\text{Aqueous humor}}{\text{Serum}} \times \text{Immunoglobulin} \frac{\text{Serum}}{\text{Aqueous humor}}$$

Ideally, the antibody coefficient should be 1.0. A coefficient from 2 to 7 is compatible with local production of specific antibody, but a coefficient greater than 8 is considered highly suggestive of local production. An example of the use of this formula is presented in **Box 5-2**.

Similar evaluations have been performed to look for local antibody production to virus. Timsit and colleagues[23] detected herpes simplex virus (HSV) antibodies in the

---

Box 5-2 Analysis of aqueous humor for antibody

A = Inverse titer of specific IgG in aqueous

B = Total IgG in aqueous

X = Inverse titer of specific IgG in serum

Y = Total IgG in serum

If (A/B)/(X/Y) > 1, then there is local antibody production within the eye, suggesting intraocular infection

EXAMPLE:

Aqueous titer to toxoplasmosis = 1:200; aqueous IgG = 0.1 g/dL

Serum titer to toxoplasmosis = 1:400; serum IgG = 3 g/dL

Therefore: A/B = 60, suggesting that uveitis is due to toxoplasmosis

---

aqueous of half of patients with clinically confirmed herpes keratouveitis. Kaplan and colleagues[24] found antibodies against either HSV or vesicular stomatitis virus in the aqueous of four of 20 patients with idiopathic uveitis. Samples may, however, become contaminated with peripheral serum. Further, local production of specific antibody may be related to a polyclonal B-cell activation totally unrelated to the virus in question. Clearly, these methods require further refinement, and only with continued attempts at such refinement can this technique help in the diagnosis of intraocular inflammatory disease. Although this approach is not generally used in the United States, it is commonly used by many specialists in Europe.[25]

Diagnostic vitrectomy is mostly used to evaluate the possibility of either infection or malignancy. Intraocular inflammation as a result of autoimmune disease may look similar to the inflammation after infection. In patients with a history of postsurgical uveitis, a diagnostic vitrectomy and anterior chamber tap are often warranted. Recently, a number of slow-growing bacteria have been identified as causes of chronic insidious postsurgical uveitis. One of these organisms, *Propionibacterium acnes*, is described in detail in the chapter on postsurgical uveitis (see Chapter 18) and the chapter on masquerade syndromes (see Chapter 30). Davis and colleagues[26] reported on 84 eyes in 78 patients who underwent pars plana vitrectomy for diagnostic purposes. The preoperative diagnosis was either infection or malignancy. Vitreous testing led to a diagnosis in 48 of 78 patients. When the preoperative indication was compared with the final clinical diagnosis, the efficiency of the diagnostic procedure of cytologic evaluation, flow cytometry, and bacterial or fungal culture was 67%, 79%, and 96%, respectively. Margolis and colleagues[27] reviewed 45 eyes of 44 consecutive patients with posterior segment inflammation who underwent pars plana vitrectomy for diagnostic purposes. The vitreous analysis, which included culture, cytologic analysis, and flow cytometry, identified a specific cause in nine (20%) of the 45 eyes. In addition, visual acuity improved in 60%.

Many clinicians routinely obtain samples for biopsy from the conjunctiva and lacrimal gland in the search for histologic evidence of sarcoidosis. Most studies, however, report disappointing results with random 'blind biopsies'.[28] We suggest obtaining a biopsy sample from the conjunctiva only if a specific lesion is noted, and of the lacrimal glands only if they are clinically enlarged or show increased uptake on a gallium scan. We have, however, found that biopsy of skin lesions can be extremely helpful to the clinician. We have made the diagnosis of sarcoidosis in numerous patients on the basis of a noncaseating granuloma found on skin biopsy.

Finally, we have performed chorioretinal biopsy in patients with severe posterior uveitis that caused severe visual loss in one eye and threatened the other eye despite therapy. This technique is more fully described in the chapter on the role of surgery in the diagnosis and treatment of uveitis (see Chapter 8).

Ancillary ophthalmic tests

Electrophysiology

Electrophysiologic testing can help to determine the cause of visual loss in some patients with uveitis, but in general rarely leads to a specific diagnosis. Both the electroretinogram (ERG) and the electrooculogram (EOG) can be altered in many of the inflammatory disorders of the retina and choroid. Experiments in the 1960s showed that the ERG was altered in animals with experimental uveitis.[29] Clinical studies also showed altered ERGs in patients with uveitis.[30] Because of the general lack of specificity, the electroretinogram will only tell the observer if significant widespread damage has occurred, and to date we are not aware of changes noted on the electroretinogram or on the electrooculogram that are specific for entities within the broad category of posterior uveitis. Feurst and colleagues[31] reported that the electroretinograms of patients with birdshot retinochoroidopathy show a loss of blue cone responses in the dark-adapted state (see Chapter 25). We have noted a loss of blue cone responses not only in birdshot retinochoroidopathy,[32] but also in other posterior uveitis entities. This may reflect a general effect of the immune response on the retina's electrophysiologic responsiveness. Because it is difficult to assess the clinical response to therapy in some patients with birdshot retinochoroidopathy, a number of uveitis specialists use ERG monitoring to assess the progression of disease and response to therapy.[33-35]

One problem with the use of electrophysiology in assessing some forms of uveitis is that the pathology is limited to the macula. As a result, the ERG may be relatively normal. The use of multifocal ERG allows the assessment of function in the central retina.[36,37] The multifocal ERG may also be used to assess changes with therapy.[38]

Laser interferometry

Early in our therapeutic studies we wanted to know whether we could predict which patients with uveitis might improve with immunosuppressive therapy. We had noted that there was a discrepancy between the visual acuity obtained with the standard Snellen and later the Early Treatment Diabetic Retinopathy Study (ETDRS) eye charts and the laser interferometer. The visual acuity obtained with the laser interferometer is often better than that measured with eye charts. We hypothesized that these differences might be caused by potentially reversible macular changes as a result of the ongoing inflammatory disease. In a prospective study of 26 patients treated with ciclosporin for endogenous intermediate and posterior uveitis, we noted an improvement in 86% of patients in whom the laser interferometer predicted a

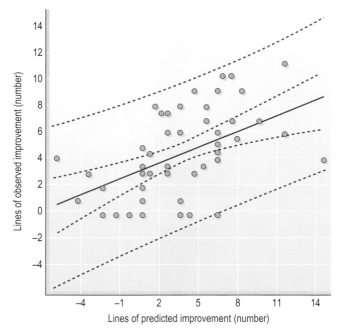

Figure 5-3. Linear regression plot of number of lines of predicted improvement using laser interferometer (slope = 0.40, intercept = 2.96) and observed improvement after ciclosporin therapy (R = 0.53). Outer dotted lines represent 95% confidence limits. *(From Palestine AG, Alter GJ, Chan CC, et al. Laser interferometry and visual prognosis in uveitis. Ophthalmology 1985; 92: 1567–9.)*

three-line or better improvement in vision compared with the standard measurement of visual acuity (**Fig. 5-3**). In contrast, only 52% of the patients in whom laser interferometry showed less than a three-line improvement later showed improvement with ciclosporin therapy. There was a moderate correlation between the predicted number of lines of improvement with the laser interferometer and the number of lines actually improved with therapy (R = 0.59, $p < 0.001$). We therefore perform a laser interferometry visual acuity determination on all patients with uveitis having poor vision. If the laser interferometry acuity is better than the visual acuity measured on an ETDRS chart, we expect to see an improvement in visual acuity with therapy even in patients with cystoid macular edema.

Fluorescein angiography

Fluorescein angiography is an invaluable aid in evaluating the numerous changes in uveitic eyes. The alterations seen are variable and frequently require the observer to evaluate the angiogram for some time before a satisfactory interpretation is made. Some of the more frequently noted ocular changes that are highlighted with fluorescein angiography are listed in **Box 5-3**. Corresponding stereo photographs may be helpful in establishing the level at which the pathologic condition in the eye is occurring.

Macular edema is one of the major causes of reduced vision in many types of intraocular inflammatory disease. The cause of this is not absolutely known. We assume, logically, that it is due to a swelling of the retinal layers, which disrupts the intimate association of the retinal elements that results in crisp vision or distorts the alignment of the photoreceptors. However, we know that patients with angiographic evidence of mild or moderate macular edema can have good visual acuity. Further, we have been most struck

Box 5-3 Major fluorescein angiographic findings in uveitis
Cystoid macular edema
Subretinal neovascular membranes
Disc leakage
Late staining of retinal vessels
Neovascularization of retinal vessels
Retinal vascular capillary dropout and reorganization
Retinal pigment epithelium perturbations

that patients can have an improvement of vision after therapeutic intervention, yet the fluorescein angiogram shows no change in the leakage of fluorescein. Because late leakage seen on angiography is not strongly correlated with a drop in vision, we explored other possible alterations that might be evaluated with fluorescein angiography. We hypothesized that retinal thickening and not the leakage of fluorescein into the retina was one of the major causes of the decrease in vision. We measured the amount of retinal thickening with the use of standard angiographic photos taken early in the angiogram (**Fig. 5-4**).[39] We noted a strong correlation between retinal thickening and the visual acuity of these eyes (**Figs 5-5 and 5-6**). The amount of dye leakage in the late phase of the angiogram did not, however, correlate well with visual acuity. More recently, the OCT has been used to assess macular edema in patients with uveitis. Nevertheless, useful information about the vascular morphology and the presence of vasculitis can best be assessed by fluorescein angiography.

In reading the angiogram, it is important to look at the early frames to best visualize the microvasculature surrounding the fovea. To best enhance the stereo effect, we have found it useful to use a 'map reader'. If one wishes to compare sequential fluorescein angiograms, the photos must be taken with the Allan separator always set at the same value. Differences in the separator settings can induce an artificial increase or decrease in the height of lesions noted when the photos are viewed with the stereo viewer.

Many inflammatory eye diseases are thought to be associated with abnormalities in choroidal blood flow. Unfortunately, the excitation and fluorescence of fluorescein dye are absorbed and scattered by the retinal pigment. In addition, fluorescein dye rapidly leaks from the fenestrated vessels of the choriocapillaris, leading to a diffuse background choroidal fluorescence. Both of these factors combine to obscure a detailed analysis of the choroidal blood flow with fluorescein angiography.

Indocyanine green

Indocyanine green (ICG) is a water-soluble tricarbocyanine dye that was first used to measure cardiac output.[40] Unlike fluorescein, ICG is almost completely bound to plasma proteins and does not leak from normal retinal or choroidal vessels. Importantly, the pigment of the retinal pigment epithelium and neurosensory retina does not significantly block the choroidal fluorescence when ICG dye is illuminated with infrared light. ICG fluorescence is also more easily detected through hemorrhage. As a result, ICG angiography, which is recorded on either infrared photography or video angiography, is a useful tool for demonstrating abnormalities of

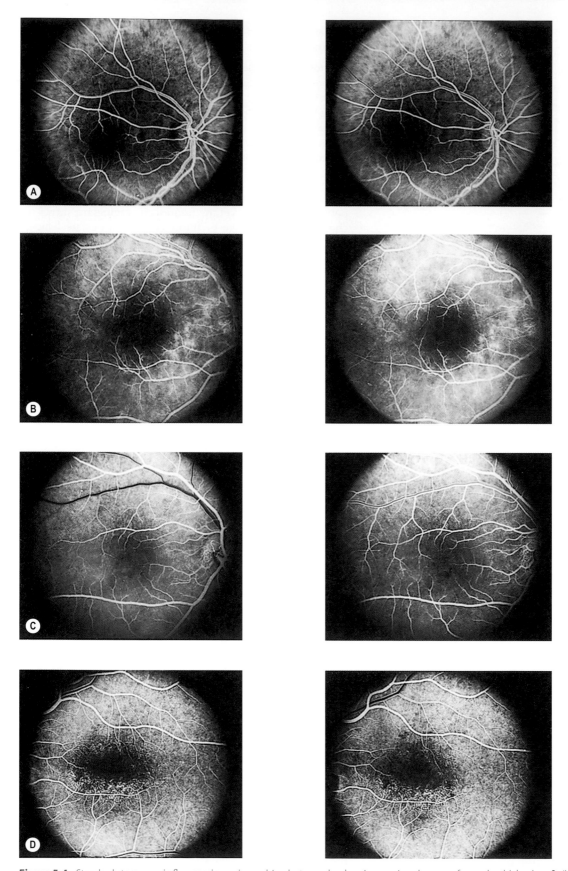

Figure 5-4. Standard stereoscopic fluorescein angiographic photographs showing varying degrees of macular thickening. **A,** 'Normal'. **B–D,** In order of increasing macular thickening. A strong light source should be placed under photographs, and macular thickening can be best evaluated using 'map reader' (Air Photo Supply, model PS-2 stereo viewer), which will yield maximum stereopsis. *(From Nussenblatt RB, Kaufman SC, Palestine AG, et al. Macular thickening and visual acuity. Ophthalmology 1987; 94: 1134–9.)*

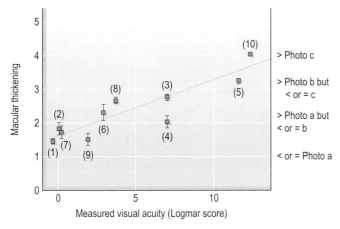

Figure 5-5. Mean (±1 standard error) of 13 gradings of macular thickening for eyes with cystoid macular edema (11 because of uveitis, two because of diabetes). Simple linear regression showed significant relationship between mean thickening and actual visual acuity. *(From Nussenblatt RB, Kaufman SC, Palestine AG, et al. Macular thickening and visual acuity. Ophthalmology 1987; 94: 1134–9.)*

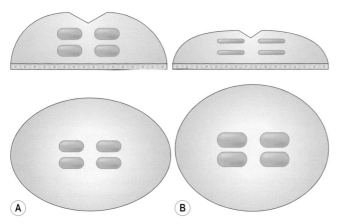

Figure 5-6. Proposed scheme as to why fluorescein leakage may appear to be same but macular thickening may have decreased, resulting in improvement in visual acuity. **A,** During an acute episode of uveitis, cystic spaces are filled with fluid and the macula is thickened. **B,** With therapy there is a reduction in macular thickening but the amount of leakage will appear to be the same if the angiogram is reviewed in standard fashion. *(From Nussenblatt RB, Kaufman SC, Palestine AG, et al. Macular thickening and visual acuity. Ophthalmology 1987; 94: 1134–9.)*

choroidal blood flow, including choroidal neovascular membranes.[41–44]

ICG angiography has now been used to study patients with a number of uveitic conditions. In patients with serpiginous choroiditis, ICG angiography has demonstrated blockage of choroidal fluorescence in active areas of lesions with return of the normal choroidal fluorescence as the inflammation subsided.[45] In addition, the chorioretinal lesions associated with birdshot choroiditis are often difficult to observe clinically or to document with fluorescein angiography. However, Krupsky and colleagues[46] showed that ICG angiography was superior to fluorescein angiography in demonstrating these lesions that appeared as hypofluorescent areas, suggesting loss of the choriocapillaris. Herbort and colleagues[47,48] have used ICG angiography to assess disease activity in several forms of uveitis, including VKH and Behçet's disease. Researchers are also using ICG angiography to compare active and quiescent chorioretinal lesions in patients with uveitis, and it is hoped that this technique

will provide new insight into the pathophysiology of a number of uveitic disorders.

Laser flare photometry

Although standardized schemes for assessing anterior chamber cells and flare have been described in the literature, grading differs tremendously between clinicians and even for the same grader over time. A laser device has been developed to assess flare in the anterior chamber of the eye and should standardize the grading of anterior chamber inflammation; objective grading of flare is extremely useful in determining response to therapy.[49,50] Furthermore, it is difficult to detect the induced flare caused by small amounts of protein in the aqueous humor resulting from early breakdown of the blood–aqueous barrier. After cataract surgery, for example, it would be nice to predict which eyes were at risk of developing uveitis and cystoid macular edema. The laser flare photometer is more sensitive than the eye in detecting flare and may be useful in predicting which eyes are at risk for developing worsening inflammatory disease, and possibly identifying eyes that require more aggressive antiinflammatory therapy. In one study of 30 uveitis patients, outflow facility was significantly reduced in patients with elevated flare photometry results.[51] An association between laser flare photometry values and complications of uveitis has also been reported.[52] However, randomized clinical trials have not demonstrated that increasing therapy to decrease laser flare photometry values improves clinical outcomes compared to basing therapy on clinical assessment.[53]

Optical coherence tomography

Optical coherence tomography (OCT) allows the noninvasive assessment of retinal thickness. This technique may be useful in assessing retinal edema in patients with uveitis and response to therapy. In a recent study, Antcliff and associates[54] compared OCT and fluorescein angiography in 58 patients with uveitis and suspected cystoid macular edema (CME). One hundred and eight eyes had similar results by both OCT and fluorescein angiography; 67 eyes had CME and 41 eyes had no CME. In 10 eyes subretinal fluid was detected by OCT but not by fluorescein angiography. Five of these eyes had CME detected by fluorescein angiography but not by OCT. Three other eyes had CME detected by fluorescein angiography but not by OCT. The authors concluded that OCT is as effective as fluorescein angiography for detecting CME but is superior for demonstrating axial distribution of fluid. Similar to fluorescein angiography, the accuracy of the measurements is affected by small pupil size and media opacity.

Since the last edition of this book there have been improvements in OCT technology and a number of new studies assessing the use in uveitis. OCT is useful for detecting macular edema and assessing response to therapy.[55] Reductions in macular thickness in patients with uveitic CME can be detected on OCT within a week of corticosteroid therapy **(Fig. 5-7)**. OCT may be useful in detecting retinal pathology in other forms of posterior uveitis.[56] Finally, spectral-domain OCT may provide additional information and be useful in assessing uveitic eyes, especially when hazy media obscures clinical examination.[57]

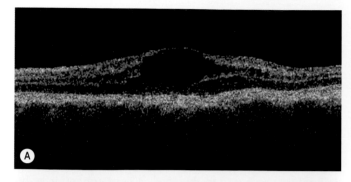
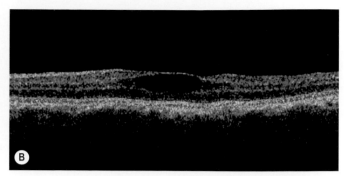
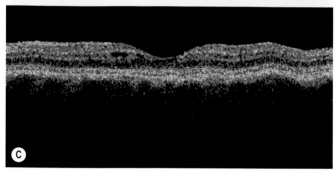

Figure 5-7. Ocular coherence tomography (OCT) of the retina from a patient with intermediate uveitis and recurrent cystoid macular edema. **A,** A thickened macular with a large cystoid space. **B,** Two months after a subtenon injection of triamcinolone, there is improvement; however, the OCT shows residual retinal thickening with cystic changes. **C,** With continued therapy the OCT shows further improvement in retinal thickening associated with an improvement in visual acuity. *(Courtesy of Ralph Levinson, MD.)*

High-frequency ultrasound biomicroscopy and multifrequency ultrasound

High-frequency ultrasound biomicroscopy (UBM) allows detailed imaging of the anterior segment of the eye, ciliary body, pars plana, and peripheral vitreous. Because many patients with uveitis have severe media opacity that impairs the clinician's ability to examine these structures clinically, UBM can allow assessment of inflammatory lesions not otherwise visible. In our experience, UBM is useful in selected patients with uveitis. UBM also can help in assessing inflammation in patients with severe media opacity, in assessing the placement of an intraocular lens to see whether it may be contributing to inflammation, and in evaluating causes of hypotony because it can provide detailed information on the anatomy of the ciliary body. Recently, Tran and colleagues[58] retrospectively reviewed UBM findings from 111 eyes in 77 patients with uveitis. They noted that UBM findings contributed to the diagnosis or had an impact on treatment in 43% of patients. In a study of seven eyes in five patients with intermediate uveitis, ultrasound examination with both 50- and 20-MHz frequency probes were able to detect snowbanks and may be useful in eyes with small pupils or dense vitritis to assess disease activity.[59]

Fundus autofluorescence

Liebman and Leigh described autofluorescence of visual receptors in an aritcle in Nature in 1969.[60] More recently, autofluorescence has been used to assess pathologic changes to the retinal pigment epithelium that are thought to be associated with clinically relevant changes in function. Autofluorescence may be useful in assessing changes to the RPE that may be missed with other imaging modalities. The technique has been used to assess patients with a number of retinal conditions, including age-related macular degeneration and uveitis. For example, focal accumulation of autofluorescent material was shown at the level of the RPE in patients with central serous chorioretinopathy.[61] Autofluorescence was also used to show more widespread involvement of the RPE than previously documented in patients with multifocal choroiditis and panuveitis.[62]

Other diagnostic tests

Polymerase chain reaction (PCR)

Since its initial description by Saiki and colleagues,[63] the polymerase chain reaction (PCR) has become one of the most commonly used techniques in biomedical research. It provides a simple way to amplify a specific fragment of DNA, and this technique has proved useful for the study of genetic diseases and the detection of infectious agents. Pertinent to the field of uveitis, PCR has also been used to detect viruses, bacteria, and parasites in the eye.[64]

To start the PCR four components are combined: (1) target DNA, (2) primers (short strands of DNA that tag the section of target DNA to be copied, (3) polymerase (the enzyme that catalyzes gene replication), and (4) nucleotides. The PCR is based on the consecutive repetition of three reactions. First, the target DNA is denatured by heating the test tube to 95°C. Second, primers are annealed to a targeted strip of DNA as the temperature of the test tube is reduced. Finally, in the third step of the PCR polymerase triggers the synthesis of a new DNA molecule between the primers. These three steps of the reaction are then repeated

Box 5-4 FDA-Approved PCR tests for infectious agents associated with uveitis

HIV-1
Hepatitis C virus
Mycobacterium tuberculosis
Neiserria gonorrhea
Chlamydia trachomatis
Aspergillus galactomannan

consecutively during 30–40 cycles and controlled by the raising and lowering of the temperature of the test tube.

At the end of the PCR, the amount of target DNA is increased by 1 million- to 1 billion times. However, the extreme sensitivity of the technique requires very strict laboratory procedures to prevent carryover of positive substrate between samples that could lead to false-positive results. The PCR can be used to detect DNA fragments in many types of specimens including cells, body fluids, and paraffin-embedded sections. The PCR is currently being used to identify the DNA of infectious agents in the eye, because, as we have seen, the interpretation of serologic tests is often misleading. Before PCR can be carried out, the sequence of the target DNA (specific for the organisms in question) must be available, and the appropriate primers must then be synthesized. Viral DNA has been identified by PCR in eyes with a number of disorders including acute retinal necrosis.[65] We currently use the PCR in our laboratory to diagnose ocular toxoplasmosis.[66,67]

The US Food and Drug Administration has approved nucleic acid amplification tests for the detection of a number of infectious agents that can also cause uveitis (**Box 5-4**). PCR tests are now commercialy available for *Mycobacterium tuberculosis*.[68] Initially, these tests were only indicated for use in patients with respiratory specimens that produced negative results on acid-fast bacilli smears. These tests are now thought to be a reasonable adjunctive test in all patients with presumed tuberculosis. Of course, these tests should not replace the standard acid-fast bacilli smear or mycobacterial cultures, and should only be interpreted in the context of other clinical information. Unfortunately, these commercial tests have not been well studied for the diagnosis of tuberculosis from ocular specimens, although there are studies showing that PCR can detect *Mycobacterium tuberculosis* from the vitreous in some patients.[69,70] There are now commercially available PCR tests for other infectious agents that can cause uveitis. FDA-approved tests to detect *Niesseria gonorrheae*, *Chlamydia trachomatis*, HIV, hepatitis C virus, and *Aspergillus* can now be ordered. Importantly, noncommercial PCR testing can be useful in elucidating infectious causes of uveitis. *Tropheryma whipplei* was identified by PCR from the vitreous of a patient with uveitis associated with Whipple's disease.[71] To date, PCR is still predominantly a research tool. Because of its exquisite sensitivity, the chances of false-positive results are significant. In addition, a small piece of DNA found in the eye of a patient may represent a remnant from an infection that occurred long ago and may be totally unrelated to the patient's current illness. Nevertheless, the use of PCR will continue to proliferate in ophthalmic research, and it will probably be available clinically in the near future to detect infectious agents in ocular specimens.

Rapid tests for herpes simplex and herpes zoster

Currently, biopsy specimens, including cells obtained from anterior chamber taps, are tested for herpesvirus with the use of a direct fluorescent antibody test after 48 hours and 5 days of growth. Enzyme-linked immunosorbent assays, which give almost immediate diagnostic information, are available. However, problems with sensitivity and specificity arise and need to be thoroughly investigated before these tests can be used routinely in clinical practice.

Bone mineral density studies

Historically, clinical tests including laboratories tests and imaging studies were performed to make a diagnosis or to assess the efficacy of therapy. Diagnostic tests are now used to monitor treatment toxicity. As we have stated, corticosteroids remain the mainstay of therapy for uveitis. Unfortunately, researchers have shown that corticosteroids can promote osteoporosis. One study showed that patients receiving prednisone at a dose greater than 7.5 mg/day lost 10–15% of trabecular bone in the lumbar spine within 1 year.[72] At prednisone doses greater than 30 mg/day bone loss increased to 30–50%. In one study of corticosteroid-induced osteoporosis in patients with uveitis, seven symptomatic fractures occurred in 129 patients during treatment.[73] Bone mineral density studies can accurately assess bone loss in patients treated with corticosteroids. If there is a reasonable chance for chronic steroid use, bone mineral density studies should be performed within 3 months of the start of systemic corticosteroid therapy and annually thereafter. If these studies show osteoporosis, patients may benefit from antiresorptive agents such as calcitonin, alendronate, etidronate, or risedronate.

Genetic testing for steroid-induced glaucoma

Glaucoma is a major cause of visual loss in patients with uveitis. Glaucoma occurs in many patients with uveitis in the presence of active inflammation. In addition, glaucoma can occur as a side effect of corticosteroid use. To date, it has not been possible to predict which patients with uveitis are at greatest risk for glaucoma. Stone and coworkers[74] analyzed sequence-tagged site content and haplotype sharing between families affected with chromosome 1q-linked open-angle glaucoma to prioritize candidate genes for mutation screening. These researchers identified a gene encoding a trabecular meshwork protein (TIGR) associated with glaucoma. Polansky and associates[75] showed that glucocorticoids and oxidative stress stimuli induced TIGR in cultures of human trabecular meshwork cells, suggesting a mechanism of action for both corticosteroid-induced glaucoma and uveitic glaucoma. Clinical testing for genes associated with glaucoma, such as TIGR, may help clinicians predict which patients are at greatest risk for developing glaucoma, but to date is not routinely used in clinical practice.

Neurologic tests

The eye is a part of the brain, and many forms of uveitis have associated central nervous system involvement. Because the eye can be a window to the brain and provide insight into neurologic disease, evaluation of the brain and cerebrospinal fluid can give important clues to the underlying cause of ocular inflammatory disease. For example, lumbar puncture is useful in evaluating patients with possible Vogt–Koyanagi–Harada syndrome or intraocular lymphoma.

References

1. Griner PF, Mayewski RJ, Mushlin AL, et al. Selection and interpretation of diagnostic tests and procedures: principles and applications, Ann Intern Med 1981; 94: 553–600.

2. Rembold CM, Watson D. Posttest probability calculation by weights: a simple form of Bayes' theorem, Ann Intern Med 1988; 108: 115–120.

3. Rosenbaum JT, Wernick R. The utility of routine screening of patients with uveitis for systemic lupus erythematosus or tuberculosis, Arch Ophthalmol 1990; 108: 1291–1293.

4. Warner HR, Toronto AF, Veasey LG, et al. A mathematical approach to medical diagnosis: application to congenital heart disease. JAMA 1961; 177: 177–183.

5. Warner HR, Toronto AF, Veasy LG. Experience with Bayes' theorem for computer diagnosis of congenital heart disease. Ann NY Acad Sci 1964; 115: 558–567.

6. Fagan TJ. Nomogram for Bayes' theorem. N Engl J Med 1975; 293: 257.

7. Gorry GA, Barnett GO. Sequential diagnosis by computer. JAMA 1968; 205: 849–854.

8. Cassoux N, Giron A, Bodaghi B, et al. IL-10 measurement in aqueous humor for screening patients with suspicion of primary intraocular lymphoma. Invest Ophthalmol Vis Sci 2007; 48: 3253–3259.

9. Asukata Y, Ishihara M, Hasumi Y, et al. Guidelines for the diagnosis of ocular sarcoidosis. Ocul Immunol Inflamm 2008; 16: 77–81.

10. Leeflang MMG, Deeks JJ, Gatsonis C, et al, on behalf of the Cochrane Diagnostic Test Accuracy Working Group. Systematic reviews of diagnostic test accuracy. Ann Intern Med 2008; 149: 889–897.

11. Passo MS, Rosenbaum JT. Ocular syphilis in patients with human immunodeficiency virus infection. Am J Ophthalmol 1988; 106: 1–6.

12. Tramont EC. Syphilis in the AIDS era. N Engl J Med 1987; 316: 1600–1601.

13. Quan T, Kan I, Craft JE. Diagnostic tests in rheumatic diseases. In: Goldman L, Ausiello D, eds. Cecil Textbook of Medicine. Philadelphia: WB Saunders, 2004;1627–1630.

14. Fauci AS, Haynes BF, Katz P, et al. Wegener's granulomatosis: prospective clinical and therapeutic experience with 85 patients for 21 years. Ann Intern Med 1983; 98: 76–85.

15. Nolle B, Specks U, Ludemann J, et al. Anticytoplasmic autoantibodies: their immunodiagnostic value in Wegener's granulomatosis. Ann Intern Med 1989; 111: 28–40.

16. Cohen-Tervaert MD, van der Woude FJ, Fauci AS, et al. Association between active Wegener's granulomatosis and anticytoplasmic antibodies. Arch Intern Med 1989; 149: 2461–2465.

17. Young DW. The antineutrophil antibody in uveitis. Br J Ophthalmol 1991; 75: 208–211.

18. Soukasian SH, Foster CS, Niles JL, et al. Diagnostic value of anti-neutrophil cytoplasmic antibodies in scleritis associated with Wegener's granulomatosis. Ophthalmology 1992; 99: 125–132.

19. Nolle B, Coners H, Guncker G. ANCA in ocular inflammatory disorders. Adv Exp Med Biol 1993; 336: 305–307.

20. Power WJ, Rodriguez A, Neves RA, et al. Disease relapse in patients with ocular manifestations of Wegener granulomatosis. Ophthalmology 1995; 102: 154–160.

21. Bloch-Michel E, Timsit JC. Uveitis with allergy to candidin. Ophthalmologica 1985; 191: 102–106.

22. Desmonts G. Definitive serological diagnosis to ocular toxoplasmosis. Arch Ophthalmol 1966; 76: 839–853.

23. Timsit JC, Fortier B, Pontet F, et al. Value of the immunoenzyme method (ELISA) in determining serum and aqueous humor antiherpes immunoglobulin levels (apropos of 155 cases). J Fr Ophtalmol 1982; 5: 669–674.

24. Kaplan HJ, Lee FK, Waldrep JC, et al. Viral antibodies in the aqueous humor in idiopathic uveitis. In: Saari KM, ed. Uveitis update. Amsterdam: Excerpta Medica 1984; 437–442.

25. Kijlstra A, Breebaart AC, Baarsma GS, et al. Aqueous chamber taps in toxoplasmic chorioretinitis. Doc Ophthalmol 1986; 64: 53–58.

26. Davis JL, Miller DM, Ruiz P. Diagnostic testing of vitrectomy specimens. Am J Ophthalmol 2005; 140: 822–829.

27. Margolis R, Brasil OF, Lowder CY, et al. Vitrectomy for the diagnosis and management of uveitis of unknown cause. Ophthalmology 2007; 114: 1893–1897.

28. Weinreb RN, Tessler H. Laboratory diagnosis of ophthalmic sarcoidosis. Surv Ophthalmol 1984; 28: 653–664.

29. Takata H. Electroretinographic studies of experimental uveitis. (III). Characteristics of B- and C-potential of 'inflammation type ERG'. Nippon Ganka Kiyo 1963; 14: 409–415.

30. Ourgaud AG, Haudiquet G, Tassy AF. Clinical study and ERG (oscillatory potential) in Vogt–Koyanagi–Harada syndrome. Bull Soc Ophthalmol Fr 1966; 66: 470–475.

31. Feurst DJ, Tessler HH, Fishman GA, et al. Birdshot retinochoroidopathy. Arch Ophthalmol 1984; 102: 214–219.

32. Gasch AT, Smith JA, Whitcup SM. Birdshot retinochoroidopathy. Br J Ophthalmol 1999; 83: 241–249.

33. Zacks DN, Samson CM, Lowenstein J, et al. Electroretinograms as an indicator of disease activity in birdshot retinochoroidopathy. Graefes Arch Clin Exp Ophthalmol 2002; 240: 601–607.

34. Holder GE, Robson AG, Pavesio C, et al. Electrophysiological characterisation and monitoring in the management of birdshot chorioretinopathy. Br J Ophthalmol 2005; 89: 709–718.

35. Sobrin L, Lam BL, Liu M, et al. Electroretinographic monitoring in birdshot chorioretinopathy. Am J Ophthalmol 2005; 140: 52–64.

36. Kretschmann U, Schlote T, Stubiger N, et al. Multifocal electroretinography in acquired macular dysfunction. Klin Monatsbl Augenheilkd 1998; 212: 93–100.

37. Kretschmann U, Bock M, Gockeln R, et al. Clinical applications of multifocal electroretinography. Doc Ophthalmol 2000; 100: 99–113.

38. Stubiger N, Besch D, Deuter CM, et al. Multifocal ERG changes in patients with ocular Behçet's disease during therapy with interferon alpha 2a. Adv Exp Med Biol 2003; 528: 529–532.

39. Nussenblatt RB, Kaufman SC, Palestine AG, et al. Macular thickening and visual acuity. Ophthalmology 1987; 94: 1134–1139.

40. Fox IJ, Wood EH. Indocyanine green: physical and physiologic properties. Proc Mayo Clin 1960; 35: 732–744.

41. Kogure K, David NJ, Yamanouchi U, et al. Infrared absorption angiography of the fundus circulation. Arch Ophthalmol 1970; 83: 209–214.

42. Flower RW, Hocheimer BF. A clinical technique and apparatus for simultaneous angiography of the separate retinal and choroidal circulations. Invest Ophthalmol 1973; 12: 248–261.

43. Flower RW, Hochheimer BF Indocyanine green dye fluorescence and infrared absorption choroidal angiography performed simultaneously with fluorescein angiography. Johns Hopkins Med J 1976; 138: 33–42.

44. Destro M, Puliafito CA. Indocyanine green videoangiography of choroidal neovascularizations. Ophthalmology 1989; 96: 846–853.

45. Bischoff P. Bedeutung der infrarotangiographie fur die differentialdiagnostik der aderhauttumoren. Klin Mbl Augenheilkd 1985; 186: 187–193.

46. Krupsky S, Friedman E, Foster CS, et al. Indocyanine green angiography in choroidal diseases. Invest Ophthalmol Vis Sci 1992; 33(suppl): 723.

47. Herbort CP, Mantovani A, Bouchenaki N. Indocyanine green angiography in Vogt–Koyanagi–Harada disease: angiographic signs and utility in patient follow-up. Int Ophthalmol 2007; 27: 173–182.

48. Klaeger AJ, Tran VT, Hiroz CA, et al. Use of ultrasound biomicroscopy, indocyanine green angiography and HLA-B51 testing as adjunct methods in the appraisal of Behçet's uveitis. Int Ophthamol 2004; 25: 57–63.

49. Shah SM, Spalton DJ, Taylor JC. Correlations between laser flare measurements and anterior chamber protein concentrations. Invest Ophthalmol Vis Sci 1992; 33: 2878–2884.

50. Guex-Crosier Y, Pittet N, Herbort CP. Evaluation of laser flare-cell photometry in the appraisal and management of intraocular inflammation in uveitis. Ophthalmology 1994; 101: 728–735.

51. Ladas JG, Yu F, Loo R, et al. Relationship between aqueous humor protein level and outflow facility in patients with uveitis. Invest Ophthalmol Vis Sci 2001; 42: 2584–2588.

52. Gonzales CA, Ladas JG, Davis JL, et al. Relationships between laser flare photometry values and complications of uveitis. Arch Ophthalmol 2001; 119: 1763–1769.

53. Davis JL, Dacanay LM, Holland GN, et al. Laser flare photometry and complications of chronic uveitis in children. Am J Ophthalmol 2003; 135: 763–771.

54. Antcliff RJ, Stanford MR, Chauhan DS, et al. Comparison between optical coherence tomography and fundus fluorescein angiography for the detection of cystoid macular edema in patients with uveitis. Ophthalmology 2000; 107: 593–597.

55. Sivaprasad S, Ikeji F, Xing W, et al. Tomographic assessment of therapeutic response to uveitis macular oedema. Clin Exp Ophthalmol 2007; 35: 719–723.

56. Gallagher MJ, Yilmaz T, Cervantes-Castaneda RA, et al. The characteristic features of optical coherence tomography in posterior uveitis. Br J Ophthalmol 2007; 91: 1680–1685.

57. Gupta V, Gupta P, Singh R, et al. Spectral-domain cirrus high-definition optical coherence tomography is better than time-domain stratus optical coherency tomography for evaluation of macular pathologic features in uveitis. Am J Ophthalmol 2008; (in press)

58. Tran VT, LeHoang P, Herbort CP. Value of high-frequency ultrasound biomicroscopy in uveitis. Eye 2001; 15: 23–30.

59. Doro D, Manfre A, Deligianni V, et al. Combined 50- and 20-MHz frequency ultrasound imaging in intermediate uveitis. Am J Ophthalmol 2006; 141: 953–955.

60. Liebman PA, Leigh RA. Autofluorescence of visual receptors. Nature 1969; 221: 1249–1251.

61. von Ruckmann A, Schmidt KG, Fitzke FW, et al. Serous central chorioretinopathy. Acute autofluorescence of the pigment epithelium of the eye. Ophthalmologe 1999; 96: 6–10.

62. Haen SP, Spaide RF. Fundus autofluorescence in multifocal choroiditis and panuveitis. Am J Ophthalmol 2008; 145: 847–853.

63. Saiki RK, Gelfand DH, Stoffel S, et al. Primer-directed enzymatic amplification of DNA with a thermostable DNA polymerase. Science 1988; 239: 487–491.

64. Van Gelder RN. Applications of polymerase chain reaction to diagnosis of ophthalmic disease. Surv Ophthalmol 2001; 46: 248–258.

65. Forster DJ, Dugel PU, Frangieh GT, et al. Rapidly progressive outer retinal necrosis in the acquired immunodeficiency syndrome. Am J Ophthalmol 1990; 110: 341–348.

66. Chan CC, Palestine AG, Li Q, et al. Diagnosis of ocular toxoplasmosis by the use of immunocytology and the polymerase chain reaction. Am J Ophthalmol 1994; 117: 803–805.

67. Brezin AP, Egwuagu CE, Burnier M Jr, et al. Identification of *Toxoplasma gondii* in paraffin-embedded sections by the polymerase chain reaction. Am J Ophthalmol 1990; 110: 599–604.

68. Update: nucleic acid amplification tests for tuberculosis, MMWR Morbid Mortal Wkly Rep 2000; 49: 593–594.

69. Therese KL, Jayanthi U, Madhavan HN. Application of nested polymerase chain reaction (nPCR) using MPB 64 gene primers to detect *Mycobacterium tuberculosis* DNA in clinical specimens from extrapulmonary tuberculosis patients. Indian J Med Res 2005; 122: 165–170.

70. Matos K, Muccioli C, Belfort R Jr, et al. Correlation between clinical diagnosis and PCR analysis of serum, aqueous, and aqueous and vitreous samples in patients with inflammatory eye disease. Arq Bras Oftalmol 2007; 70: 109–114.

71. Rickman LS, Freeman WR, Green WR. Brief report: uveitis caused by *Tropheryma whippelii* (Whipple's bacillus), N Engl J Med 1995; 332: 363–366.

72. Lukert BP, Raisz LG. Glucocorticoid-induced osteoporosis. Rheum Dis Clin North Am 1994; 20: 629–650.

73. Jones NP, Anderton LC, Cheong FM, et al. Corticosteroid-induced osteoporosis in patients with uveitis. Eye 2002; 16: 587–593.

74. Stone EM, Fingert JH, Alward WL, et al. Identification of a gene that causes primary open angle glaucoma. Science 1997; 275: 668–670.

75. Polansky JR, Fauss DJ, Chen P, et al. Cellular pharmacology and molecular biology of the trabecular mesh-work inducible glucocorticoid response gene product. Ophthalmologica 1997; 211: 126–139.

Evidence-Based Medicine in Uveitis

Scott M. Whitcup

Key concepts

- All published literature does not have equal import.
- All medical literature, including this book, must be read critically.
- Whenever possible, treatment decisions should be based on evidence-based medicine. Evidence-based medicine is defined as the conscientious, explicit and judicious use of current best evidence in making decisions about the care of individual patients.
- The best evidence usually comes from well-conducted, randomized clinical trials; however, there are relatively few randomized clinical trials in uveitis, although the number is increasing.
- It is important to understand the strength or level of evidence supporting treatment decisions.

The practice of medicine is based on applying what we have learned from our medical training in addition to the knowledge gained by reading books and articles and attending scientific conferences. It is our hope, for example, that the book you are reading will assist you in the care of patients with uveitis. However, all medical literature, including our book, must be read critically. Much of the information that appears to be irrefutable scientific dogma is actually based on inconclusive data derived from a handful of patients. Because the recommendations are in print and stated by seemingly reputable authorities, they are often followed blindly. It is frequently useful to thoroughly review the original references on which various therapeutic approaches are based; what you find may surprise you.

There is a growing movement to basing treatment decisions on evidence-based medicine. Evidence-based medicine is defined as the conscientious, explicit and judicious use of current best evidence in making decisions about the care of individual patients.[1] Evidence-based medicine has been divided into two types: evidence-based guidelines and evidence-based individual decision making. In each case, the goal is to base therapy on the best evidence available. A number of classifications for the quality of evidence have been proposed. One commonly used stratification was developed by the US Preventative Services Task Force and is detailed in **Table 6-1**). An assessment of the quality of the information in the literature is critical in determining the best treatment for our patients.

When treatment recommendations are made in published guidelines or in the literature, they can also be categorized by the level of evidence on which the information is based. The US Preventative Services Task Force uses the categories listed in **Table 6-2**.

When you read the medical literature, it is important to determine the experimental methods used in the various studies. Sometimes this information can be discerned from the title of the paper; at other times the Methods section must be read. Occasionally the study method is not stated in the paper: if this is the case, the article is probably not worth reading. Many of the clinical studies in the literature are retrospective, meaning that the data were collected from previous patient visits. Retrospective studies can provide valuable information but are usually limited by the quality and thoroughness of the patient records. A patient's symptoms and clinical findings, although present, are often not recorded. For example, if there is no comment in a patient's record about vitreous haze, does this mean that vitreous haze was absent or that it was present but not recorded in the note? Fortunately, most ophthalmic notes contain a core of data including visual acuity, intraocular pressure, and results of anterior segment and retinal examination. Nevertheless, prospective studies, when specific data are collected during patient visits on specifically designed case report forms, are less prone to errors.

Study design

There are four basic clinical studies: case series, case–control studies, cohort studies, and randomized clinical trials.[2] The case report or case series is probably the weakest method of deriving clinical data. Case series are usually retrospective reviews that list the clinical findings of patients with a specific disease. Case series can illustrate the variety of clinical manifestations of diseases and provide information about diagnosis, management, and prognosis. However, in addition to the problem of data missing from patient records, the reader should be aware of other pitfalls that may jeopardize the value of the report. First, the disease or condition may not be adequately defined. If patients with sympathetic ophthalmia are inadvertently included in a series of patients with Vogt–Koyanagi–Harada syndrome, the findings and conclusions may be altered. Second, the patient population reported may be dissimilar from that in the clinician's practice. Frequently uveitis specialists see patients with more severe diseases because these are the ones referred to their practice. Therefore, a uveitis specialist may report that the

Table 6-1 US Preventative Services Task Force classification for the quality of scientific information in the literature

Level I	Evidence obtained from at least one properly designed randomized controlled trial
Level II-1	Evidence obtained from well-designed controlled trials without randomization
Level II-2	Evidence obtained from well-designed cohort or case-control analytic studies, preferably from more than one center or research group
Level II-3	Evidence obtained from multiple time series with or without the intervention. Dramatic results in uncontrolled trials might also be regarded as this type of evidence
Level III	Opinions of respected authorities, based on clinical experience, descriptive studies, or reports of expert committees

Table 6-2 US Preventative Services Task Force classification for treatment recommendations

Level A	Good scientific evidence suggests that the benefits of the clinical service substantially outweighs the potential risks. Clinicians should discuss the service with eligible patients
Level B	At least fair scientific evidence suggests that the benefits of the clinical service outweighs the potential risks. Clinicians should discuss the service with eligible patients
Level C	At least fair scientific evidence suggests that there are benefits provided by the clinical service, but the balance between benefits and risks are too close for making general recommendations. Clinicians need not offer it unless there are individual considerations
Level D	At least fair scientific evidence suggests that the risks of the clinical service outweigh potential benefits. Clinicians should not routinely offer the service to asymptomatic patients
Level I	Scientific evidence is lacking, of poor quality, or conflicting, such that the risk versus benefit balance cannot be assessed. Clinicians should help patients understand the uncertainty surrounding the clinical service

visual prognosis for a given disease, such as sarcoidosis, is poor. If this report is based on a series of patients composed of referred patients with end-stage disease, it may be biased. Be especially wary of retrospective reviews that make global dogmatic statements on the basis of a few patients. Finally, case series have no control group for comparison. If a report states that depression was found in 35% of patients with uveitis, it is not clear that this represents a causal relationship. Visual loss and not uveitis may be the cause of depression. It would be important to know how many patients with other ocular diseases that cause visual loss (a control group) have depression. For example, the same percentage of patients with visual loss from retinal degenerations may also be depressed.

The case–control study is a second type of clinical study in which the investigator compares a group of patients with a given condition to a control group without the condition. The records of both groups are then compared to see whether certain factors were more likely to occur in one group than in the other. The classic example of a case–control study would be to examine patients with lung cancer and a group without the disease and determine their smoking history. It is then possible to compute an odds ratio that determines the relative risk for a given condition such as lung cancer, given a specific factor such as smoking. Case–control studies, albeit more powerful than case series, are prone to bias, many relying on a retrospective review of patients' records to determine the differences in a number of clinical parameters between cases and controls. Additional bias arises from the method of choosing the case and control subjects. Despite the potential bias, case–control studies are becoming more common in the literature because they are easy to carry out, especially with the computerization of clinical records. In addition, they are often the only feasible method available to study rare disorders.

A cohort study identifies two groups or 'cohorts' of patients, for example one cohort that receives a certain treatment and one cohort that does not. The groups are then followed prospectively for the development of a specific outcome. However, because the treatments are not assigned randomly, it is possible that the two groups differ in important parameters. For example, if you followed two groups of patients with glaucoma, one treated with medications and one treated surgically, you may falsely conclude that surgical therapy is inferior for treating glaucoma because these patients had a worse visual outcome. However, it may be that the patients treated medically had milder disease and better initial visual acuity than patients who received surgical therapy.

Pharmaceutical drug development includes a number of clinical studies, but the final determination of safety and efficacy is based predominantly on pivotal randomized, controlled clinical trials. Clinical studies during the development of a new medication are divided into four phases. Phase I clinical trials are the initial safety trials of a new medicine and are usually conducted in normal volunteers. The trials can be open label, for which patients and investigators are unmasked to the treatment allocation. Multiple doses may be tested in a phase I trial, often starting with the lowest dosage and escalating to higher dosages if tolerated. Phase II trials are designed to study the safety and efficacy of a new medication. These trials are often double-masked, in which neither patients nor investigators know what treatment is being administered. Classically these are called double-blind studies; however, in ophthalmology we prefer the term double-masked, because it is difficult to get a patient with an eye disease to enroll in a study with double-blind in the title. Phase II trials typically have more patients than phase I trials and are conducted in patients with the disease, but still may examine several dosages or treatment regimens. The phase III clinical trial is the pivotal clinical trial for the approval of the medication. These are almost always larger randomized clinical trials comparing the new medication to the standard treatment or to placebo. The US Food and Drug Administration (FDA) almost always requires two phase III trials with corroborative findings before approving a new drug. Studies conducted after a medicine is approved and marketed are called phase IV trials. These are conducted in patient populations for which the medicine is intended, and may compare the medicine to currently available therapies.

The randomized clinical trial provides the most powerful evidence about the value of a new therapy or diagnostic approach.[3] Because patients enrolled into the study are randomly assigned into a specific group, if there are sufficient numbers of patients the groups are usually equivalent

Box 6-1 Components of a randomized clinical trial

- Study approved by Institutional Review Board (IRB) and appropriate informed consent obtained from patients
- Disease well defined with specific diagnostic criteria
- Patient population well defined with specific inclusion and exclusion criteria
- Patients randomly assigned to new treatment and control treatment according to standardized and documented procedures
- Patients and investigators appropriately masked from treatment assignment
- Sample size accurately determined to control for type I and type II errors
- Outcome measures specified, and minimum differences to be considered as clinically important, detailed
- Procedures for the conduct of the trial well detailed
- Timing of study visits and collection of data strictly specified and monitored
- Statistical analysis plan specified before locking of the database and unmasking of treatment assignments. Results of an intent to treat analysis, in which all randomly assigned patients are included in the analysis provided, even if additional analyses performed

clinically. From an ethical standpoint, randomized clinical trials should compare treatments when the investigator is unsure which therapy is better. The situation where both treatment approaches have equivalent merits is termed clinical equipoise.[4,5]

Even randomized controlled trials need to be designed appropriately and well conducted to ensure meaningful results. Key issues in the design and conduct of randomized clinical trials are listed in Box 6-1. The investigators should have performed previous studies in the area and include people with appropriate training in the conduct and analysis of the study. The primary outcome of the study should be clearly stated, even if multiple outcomes are examined. The procedure for enrolling patients should be clearly delineated and state the inclusion and exclusion criteria. In addition, the therapy should be clearly stated, and the control group should be clinically appropriate. For example, if one were designing a trial to study the benefits of phacoemulsification as a technique for cataract surgery, it would be clinically inappropriate to compare this technique to intracapsular cataract extraction because extracapsular cataract surgery is the more frequently performed procedure.

It is extremely important that the paper include a discussion of sample size calculation. Sample size is based not only on the event rate expected in the two groups but also on the level of protection against type I and type II errors. A type I error occurs when the study falsely concludes that the therapies tested are different when in fact they are the same. A type II error occurs when the study falsely concludes that there is no difference between the therapies when in fact a difference exists. Many randomized clinical trials in the literature are underpowered. This means that the potential for a type II error is high: sometimes 30% or higher. In these studies a conclusion that there was no statistically significant difference between the two groups is meaningless: there could in fact be a big difference between the two groups, but not enough patients were tested to show that difference.

Here is an example of an underpowered study. If we wanted to test the hypothesis that the two sides of a quarter are different, we could flip the coin a number of times and record the results. If you flipped the coin three times (similar to enrolling three patients) and got heads each time, you might falsely conclude that the two sides were the same: both sides had a head on. The chance that you would reach this wrong conclusion would, however, diminish as you increased the number of times you flipped the coin! You would then have more power to show a difference between the two sides of the coin and thus have more protection against a type II error. Remember that studies can never definitively prove that two treatments are the same. No matter how many times you flip a coin and only see heads, there is still some chance that there was a tail on the other side that did not come up. Nevertheless, if you flip the coin enough times or enroll enough patients in a trial, the chance of this type II error becomes increasingly unlikely.

The data in randomized trials should be appropriately collected, and patients should have a reasonably high level of adherence to protocol procedures with few missed data or loss to follow-up. Observers should be masked to the treatments that patients receive. Statistical methods should be appropriate for the data and the tables and figures easily read. Finally, it is important that the authors' conclusions are supported by the data and do not exceed the evidence. There are many examples in the literature where results in a narrowly defined patient population are inappropriately generalized to broader patient groups.

Clinical trials in uveitis

Unfortunately, most of the uveitis literature is composed of case series and case reports. As stated above, these studies can provide useful information but are highly prone to bias and lack a control population for comparison of the findings. Despite their superior strength as a clinical design, few case–control studies or cohort studies of patients with uveitis have been conducted. Even rarer are randomized controlled clinical trials of therapies for patients with uveitis.[6] Most of the published randomized clinical trials in uveitis focus on postoperative inflammation. Comparatively few randomized trials have studied therapies for other forms of uveitis. Part of the explanation for this stems from difficulties that arise when patients with this disorder are studied. Many forms of uveitis are rare; therefore, it is difficult to recruit enough patients to fulfill the sample size requirements. It is important that the observers are masked to the therapy, which may be difficult if surgical treatment is compared with medications. Patients with uveitis often have underlying systemic diseases that make it difficult for them to follow a predetermined therapeutic protocol because their other diseases often require systemic therapy.

Nevertheless, randomized clinical trials can be conducted in patients with uveitis. In these trials it is important to collect data in a standardized fashion. We record visual acuity according to a standard protocol with the use of ETDRS charts.[7] Inflammatory activity is similarly recorded with standardized methods, such as grading scales for vitreous haze or laser interferometry for anterior chamber haze.[8] Well-conducted randomized clinical trials are not only important in illustrating the safety and efficacy of new treatments, but also in better defining the natural history of the disease. We will undoubtedly learn more about the underlying natural history of inflammatory eye disease through the analysis of data from randomized studies.

Many large randomized clinical trials are conducted as part of the drug approval process. Unfortunately, few medications have been developed specifically for the treatment of uveitis. As a result, most of the therapies administered in clinical practice are used off label. More recently, there has been an interest in obtaining regulatory approval of medications for nonsurgical and noninfectious uveitis, and this has led to larger, randomized clinical trials. Sustained-release fluocinolone acetonide implants were shown to significantly reduce uveitis recurrences in patients with noninfectious posterior uveitis.[9] Additional randomized clinical trials assessing several new therapies for intermediate and posterior uveitis are currently in progress, and publications of these studies should follow and add to our understanding of the disease.

The National Eye Institute has conducted several small randomized clinical trials in patients with uveitis. In one study, ciclosporin was compared with prednisolone for the treatment of endogenous uveitis.[10] In this trial, 28 patients were randomly assigned to treatment with ciclosporin and 28 were randomly assigned to treatment with prednisolone. Although no statistically significant difference was found between the primary outcomes of visual acuity or vitreous haze of patients in the two groups, because of the small numbers it would be wrong to conclude that the two therapies were the same. The authors were careful not to state that the study proved that the two therapies were equivalent, and instead suggested that because similar outcomes were achieved, ciclosporin could be considered as an alternative to corticosteroid therapy. Because the randomized clinical trial is often the best source of useful clinical information, some of the randomized clinical trials on uveitis or other inflammatory eye diseases sponsored by the National Institutes of Health are listed in **Box 6-2**. Many important randomized clinical trials have also been conducted on the ocular complications of AIDS, and these trials are described in Chapter 11.

Box 6-2 Examples of National Institutes of Health – funded randomized clinical trials in inflammatory eye diseases

1. Argon laser photocoagulation for ocular histoplasmosis. Results of a randomized clinical trial. Arch Ophthalmol 1983; 101: 1347–57.
2. Endophthalmitis Vitrectomy Study Group. Results of the Endophthalmitis Vitrectomy Study. A randomized trial of immediate vitrectomy and of intravenous antibiotics for the treatment of postoperative bacterial endophthalmitis. Arch Ophthalmol 1995; 113: 1479–96.
3. Wilhelmus KR, Gee L, Jauck WW, et al. for the Herpetic Eye Disease Study Group. Herpetic Eye Disease Study (HEDS). A controlled trial of topical corticosteroids for herpes simplex stromal keratitis. Ophthalmology 1994; 101: 1883–96.
4. Herpetic Eye Disease Study Group. A controlled trial of oral acyclovir for iridocyclitis caused by herpes simplex virus. Arch Ophthalmol 1996; 114: 1065–72.
5. Nussenblatt RB, Gery I, Weiner HL, et al. Treatment of uveitis by oral administration of retinal antigens. Results of phase I/II randomized masked trial. Am J Ophthalmol 1997; 123: 583–92.
6. Nussenblatt RB, Palestine AG, Chan CC, et al. Randomized, double-masked study of ciclosporin compared to prednisolone in the treatment of endogenous uveitis. Am J Ophthalmol 1991; 112: 138–46.
7. Whitcup SM, Csaky KG, Podgor MJ, et al. A randomized, masked, cross-over trial of acetazolamide for cystoid macular edema in patients with uveitis. Ophthalmology 1996; 103: 1054–63.
8. Beck RW, Cleary PA, Anderson MM Jr, et al. for the Optic Neuritis Study Group. A randomized, controlled trial of corticosteroids in the treatment of acute optic neuritis. N Engl J Med 1992; 326: 581–8.
9. Buggage RR, Levy-Clarke G, Sen HN, et al. A double-masked, randomized study to investigate the safety and efficacy of daclizumab to treat the ocular complications related to Behçet's disease. Ocul Immunol Inflamm 2007; 15: 63–70.
10. Smith JA, Thompson DJ, Whitcup SM, et al. A randomized, placebo-controlled, double-masked clinical trial of etanercept for the treatment of uveitis associated with juvenile idiopathic arthritis. Arthritis Rheum 2005; 53: 18–23.

References

1. Sackett DL, Rosenberg WM, Gray JA, et al. Evidence based medicine: what it is and what it isn't. Br Med J 1996; 312: 71–72.
2. Sackett DL, Haynes RB, Tugwell P. Clinical epidemiology: a basic science for clinical medicine. Boston: Little, Brown, 1985; 224–229.
3. Meinert CL, Tonascia S. Clinical trials design, conduct, and analysis. New York: Oxford University Press, 1986; 274–275.
4. Freedman B. Equipoise and the ethics of clinical research. N Engl J Med 1987; 317: 141–145.
5. Johnson N, Lilford RJ, Brazier W. At what level of collective equipoise does a clinical trial become ethical? J Med Ethics 1991; 17: 30–34.
6. Okada AA. Noninfectious uveitis: a scarcity of randomized clinical trials. Arch Ophthalmol 2005; 123: 682–683.
7. Ferris FL III, Kassoff A, Bresnick GH, et al. New visual acuity charts for clinical research. Am J Ophthalmol 1982; 94: 91–96.
8. Nussenblatt RB, Palestine AG, Chan CC, et al. Standardization of vitreal inflammatory activity in intermediate and posterior uveitis. Ophthalmology 1985; 92: 467–471.
9. Jaffe GJ, Martin D, Callanan D, et al. Fluocinolone Acetonide Uveitis Study Group. Fluocinolone acetonide implant (Retisert) for noninfectious posterior uveitis: thirty-four-week results of a multicenter randomized clinical study. Ophthalmology 2006; 113: 1020–1027.
10. Nussenblatt RB, Palestine AG, Chan CC, et al. Randomized, double-masked study of cyclosporine compared to prednisolone in the treatment of endogenous uveitis. Am J Ophthalmol 1991; 112: 138–146.

Philosophy, Goals, and Approaches to Medical Therapy

Robert B. Nussenblatt

Key concepts

- Therapy must be geared to the anatomic position of the inflammatory process; topical medication will not treat posterior pole disease.
- Corticosteroid therapy can be used in acute situations, but steroid-sparing therapies must be added by 3 months if it is clear that continued therapy is needed.
- Establish goals that should be met with therapy. If not met, consider altering therapy.
- Patients needing immunosuppressive therapy need to be advised as to possible problems related to the therapy and expectations, and need to be carefully monitored for adverse affects.

This chapter represents in some ways the very heart of the treating physician's role. How do you choose the best therapeutic agent for your patient? This decision is often tension provoking because patients requiring the types of therapy under discussion usually have bilateral sight-threatening disease, are afraid, and are depending on the physician to choose a therapeutic intervention that will quickly restore their vision. Often the task is fraught with difficulties, which must be explained to the patient. It is truly a partnership. The more the patient knows about the physician's goals and concerns, the more the patient can help. It is fair to say that in recent years enormous advances have occurred in our understanding of how to use many of the drugs under discussion. There has been a recent shift in interest to the use of intraocular therapy and also to more specific therapies, such as the use of monoclonal antibodies that target specific parts of the immune cascade. Animal models have helped us better understand underlying mechanisms, which has led to a more rational decision-making process.[1] Further, pharmacology is a burgeoning area with real hope for the future; indeed, other, yet untapped, sources may also provide new immunosuppressive drugs to the growing armamentarium.[2] At present there may not be any one ideal drug, but treating physicians have some latitude in their choices. However, each of the agents discussed in this chapter is a powerful medication that must be evaluated with care and respect.

Goals and philosophy

In the treatment of uveitis the decision to intervene with any therapeutic agent should be based on both a thorough clinical evaluation and philosophic guidelines. In general, the approach to therapy should take into account at least the following considerations.

Pain, photophobia, and discomfort

Symptom relief is an important goal for several reasons. The first and foremost is, of course, the ethical imperative of the physician. However, practical considerations should not be overlooked. Pain relief helps in the establishment of a good patient–physician relationship, which is of primary importance in what is frequently a long therapeutic course with ups and downs. A second practical reason is that once pain relief is obtained the patient is able to cooperate more readily. The ability to examine the patient's ocular condition in greater detail and to obtain more reliable test results, particularly visual acuity, is of immeasurable help to the physician.

Degree and location of inflammatory disease

The type and frequency of administration of any therapeutic choice depend on the physician's evaluation of how 'serious' the inflammatory disease is and what ocular structures are being affected. For instance, if the sequela of an intraocular inflammation is limited to posterior synechiae, then the use of topical mydriatics and corticosteroids may be a reasonable approach to therapy. However, disease that is more posteriorly located would need to be approached by means of quite different strategies. If alternative therapies are available, the physician needs to decide which one to start initially. In addition, if vital structures, such as the macula, are involved, more aggressive immunosuppressive therapy may need to be used, even though the potential for side effects may be greater.

Evaluation of visual acuity and prospect of reversibility

In most cases of inflammatory disease involving the intermediate and posterior portions of the globe an alteration in the patient's visual acuity is the reason for therapeutic intervention. It is also the major reason that the patient consults the physician – in the hope that therapy will positively affect the condition. It is therefore imperative that the physician attempts to define as clearly as possible why the vision has decreased. On this decision will hinge the therapeutic approach. Has the vision decreased because of recently developed macular edema, or because the patient's cataract progressed as a result of recurrent bouts of anterior uveitis?

Or have both occurred? Does the patient need a cataract extraction only? Is this surgery needed to better follow the effects of long-term immunosuppressive therapy? The physician must constantly question his or her decisions, seeking to confirm the original hypothesis, because these patients frequently have multifactorial reasons for vision changes. The use of various tests in the clinic can help in this evaluation, but the ultimate decision still lies with the treating physician.

Before embarking on any therapy that has a significant risk for the patient, the physician must weigh this inherent risk against any benefits. It is therefore necessary to decide whether any or all of the visual alteration is due to irreversible changes. Is there a macular hole so that the vision may never be better than 20/200, or should surgery be considered? Have subretinal neovascularization and the resultant scarring left little hope for good vision despite a possible surgical procedure? It is wrong to begin therapy if no reasonable hope for visual improvement exists. In addition, when does one commence therapy? Although the answer is highly variable, it is always based on the physician's belief that the side effects of the therapeutic intervention are outweighed by the potential good. It is the physician's duty to desist from inappropriate therapy as much as it is to institute beneficial treatment. There are generally pressures on the physician for action that make him or her more readily accepting of therapeutic intervention. Why not try? Often this is acceptable, but patients need to know if they are facing unfavorable odds, which makes their input in deciding if treatment should be given even more important.

Follow-up procedures and standardization of observations

It is imperative that a reasonable time be allotted to evaluate whether a specific therapy is effective. We have found that up to 3 months is a reasonable period in which to evaluate whether an acute problem will improve. One should remember that ocular changes due to uveitis may resolve slowly, and the observer must use changes – sometimes subtle – in the ocular examination to determine whether to continue therapy. The patient should adhere to a regular follow-up schedule and should know whom to contact if an emergency arises. At the start of systemic immunosuppressive therapy patients should be examined at least weekly. These initial weekly examinations can later be replaced by visits every 2 weeks, with the patient eventually returning monthly for the initial half year. The physician needs to preset the definition of a therapeutic 'success' and adhere to these criteria. Just as it is unwise to stop or alter therapy too soon, it is not reasonable to continue therapy if the minimal criteria for success are not met. Such criteria may include an increase of vision, a decrease in the amount of vitreous haze, a decrease in the number of cells in the anterior chamber, or a decrease in the photophobia the patient is having.

With the criteria that determine successful treatment there is a presupposition that tests are performed in a standard manner and that test results reflect a change in the ocular status rather than the fact that a different person performed the test. Standardization of observations is critical to the successful evaluation of these patients' condition. We have taken great pains to standardize our visual acuity assessment and the evaluation of ocular inflammation.

One eye or two

We generally avoid the use of systemic drugs in patients who have unilateral chronic uveitis and no underlying systemic disease. In our experience it is rare that unilateral disease justifies long-term therapy, but it certainly happens. In the patient with sight remaining in only one eye, a value judgment needs to be made concerning whether local therapy should be used before systemic therapy is employed.

General health and age of patient

The very basic considerations of patient health and age must play a role in deciding what sort of therapy to use. We thoroughly evaluate all patients and examine therapeutic alternatives before starting systemic therapy, especially in children. The secondary effects of systemic immunosuppressive agents, such as steroids, can have a major and lifelong impact on a growing child. A diagnosis of diabetes may be a relative contraindication for systemic corticosteroid therapy, whereas uncontrolled hypertension or renal disease may make ciclosporin a poor therapeutic choice. The physician must be always aware that most of these therapies have significant systemic and local effects.

Patient reliability, preferences, and understanding

The patient has come for expert advice concerning what frequently is a sight-threatening disorder that is often irreversible. Time should be spent with the patient, who deserves an explanation of ocular (and systemic) findings, the seriousness of these findings, the type of therapy warranted, and the possible positive and adverse effects. We have found that the fully informed patient provides invaluable aid to the treating physician. Obtaining informed written consent may be a requirement under certain circumstances, such as with experimental therapies. Patients with uveitis usually require long-term care, and the more the patient understands medical concerns, uncertainties, and possible therapeutic alternatives early on, the easier is the treating physician's task.

Nonsurgical therapeutic options

Corticosteroids

The corticosteroid family of medications has been the mainstay of therapy for ocular inflammatory disease since its introduction by Gordon in the early 1950s.[3] Its use in ophthalmology began soon after its introduction into the medical armamentarium.[4] The synthetic compounds usually used by the physician are variations of the compounds normally found in the body, and they profoundly affect many aspects of the organism's physiology. The synthetic preparations available to the physician were developed because of their particularly effective mediation of one aspect of these hormones' effects: immunosuppression. The treating physician should be totally at ease with the various therapeutic strategies available.

Mode of Action

In humans, corticosteroids are not considered to be cytotoxic agents. Human immune cells are not susceptible to lysis by corticosteroid administration, even at the higher dosages usually employed, unlike some of the agents to be covered in this chapter. Mice, rats, and rabbits are considered to be corticosteroid-sensitive animals, with their lymphocytes showing a marked tendency toward lysis after the administration of corticosteroids. Therefore, extrapolation from animal experiments must take place only after careful evaluation.

The mechanism of entry into the cell by steroids has been evaluated by means of several systems. The underlying point for the action of all the steroid hormones is the need for cellular receptors. The steroid is met at the cell surface by the appropriate receptor and then complexes with it in the cytoplasm of the cell. This complex then migrates to the nucleus, where it exerts its effect on DNA transcription, leading to changes in RNA production. These RNA alterations result in changes in protein production and cell function. In steroid-sensitive animals, such as the rat, cells with steroid receptors will be lysed. However, in humans this is not the case, and in vivo and in vitro testing is therefore needed to fully evaluate the effect of the hormone on the system in question.

The effects of steroids on the immune system are both local and systemic. Essentially all cellular components are affected. On the systemic level, a profound change is seen particularly with neutrophils and lymphocytes (**Fig. 7-1**). For lymphocytes, Clamen[5] and Fauci[6] showed that a large number of the lymphocytes in the intravascular space continuously recirculate with the extravascular lymphocyte pool in organs such as the bone marrow, spleen, and lymph nodes. The addition of steroids induces a change in the recirculation pattern, with a large number of T cells, particularly the helper T subset, sequestered out of the intravascular circulation. This phenomenon results in a break in the recruitment of immunoreactive cells to the site of the inflammatory reaction. The effect on neutrophils appears to be quite striking as well. Steroid therapy induces a larger number of neutrophils to be produced by the bone marrow. In addition to this increased production, the circulating half-life of these cells on reaching the intravascular space is prolonged. Concomitant with these effects is an impeding of neutrophil migration from this space to the site of inflam-

mation. Decreases in the number of circulating monocytes, eosinophils, and basophils have also been observed.

Although the changes in the immune system are profound, it is important to remember that they are temporary. Fauci[7] demonstrated that T-cell subsets return to essentially the presteroid ingestion state after about 24 hours. This observation is most important in developing a strategy for the treatment of an acutely active inflammatory condition, whether in the eye or elsewhere.

Profound effects on cell function have been noted with the addition of a steroid. The effects on the various immune cell populations include a decrease in bactericidal activity, a decrease in delayed hypersensitivity reactions, a decrease in lymphokine production, and changes in immediate hypersensitivity reactions. In addition, steroid administration has a profound effect on local resident cells in an organ, particularly the vascular endothelium. A reduction in the leakage of fluid during an inflammatory episode from the capillary endothelium results from steroid administration, thereby reducing tissue swelling. Further, during an inflammatory response there is a decrease in the amount of intracellular fluid taken in by cells, thereby reducing cell swelling and avoiding the resultant decrease in function and ultimate lysis. The effect of steroids on lysosome membranes, thought at one time to be an important stabilizing factor, now remains unclear.

Other effects of steroids are beginning to become clear. Among the many factors involved in uveitis are the matrix metalloproteinases (MMPs). MMPs are a class of proteolytic enzymes that influence tissue architecture. Their products have been implicated in a wide range of physiologic and pathologic processes and diseases. MMPs have been described in the pathogenesis of blood–retinal barrier breakdown and increased vascular permeability. Furthermore, MMPs also have been shown to play a role in the breakdown of the blood–brain barrier and increased vascular leakage in experimental animal encephalomyelitis. Inflammatory cells themselves may also modulate the production of some MMPs, with some cytokines stimulating and others inhibiting their production. Some steroids, such as anecortave acetate, an angiostatic steroid which is presently under evaluation, inhibit the expression of some MMPs involved in angiogenesis.

Preparations, Dosage Schedules, and Complications

Many steroid preparations are now available. It should be remembered that they have varying potencies, and therefore sometimes quite different concentrations of each drug need to be used (**Table 7-1 and Fig. 7-2**).

Topical application of corticosteroids is an excellent way to treat certain uveitides. Our own preference has been the use of prednisolone formulations for severe intraocular inflammatory disease. The basis for this choice is not scientific but rather the result of usage and convenience, and hence knowing what to expect with this formulation. Although studies do show differences in corneal penetration between phosphate and acetate preparations of steroids, we have not noted a major difference in efficacy between the two preparations for treating active inflammation. When the diagnosis is made, it is imperative that initial treatment of the uveitis be aggressive. We frequently ask the patient to administer his or her drops every hour while awake. One

Glucocorticoids	
Antiinflammatory effects	
Neutrophils	Inhibit neutrophil migration ↓ Neutrophil adherence to vascular endothelium ↓ Bactericidal activity of neutrophils
Immunosuppressive effects	
Mononuclear phagocytes	↓ Chemotaxis ↓ Clearance of antibody coated particles ↓ Production of Il-1 and TNFα
Lymphocytes	Redistribution of T lymphocytes (CD4.CD8) Inhibit T lymphocyte activation → ↓ proliferation and lymphokine production Inhibit Ig production by B cells (high dose)

Figure 7-1. Antiinflammatory effects of corticosteroids.

Table 7-1 Relative potencies of corticosteroids

Preparation	Systemic Equivalent (mg)	Antiinflammatory Potency
Hydrocortisone	20	1.0
Cortisone	25	0.8
Prednisolone	5	4.0
Prednisone	5	4.0
Dexamethasone	0.75	26
Methylprednisolone	4	5
Triamcinolone	4	5
Betamethasone	0.6	33

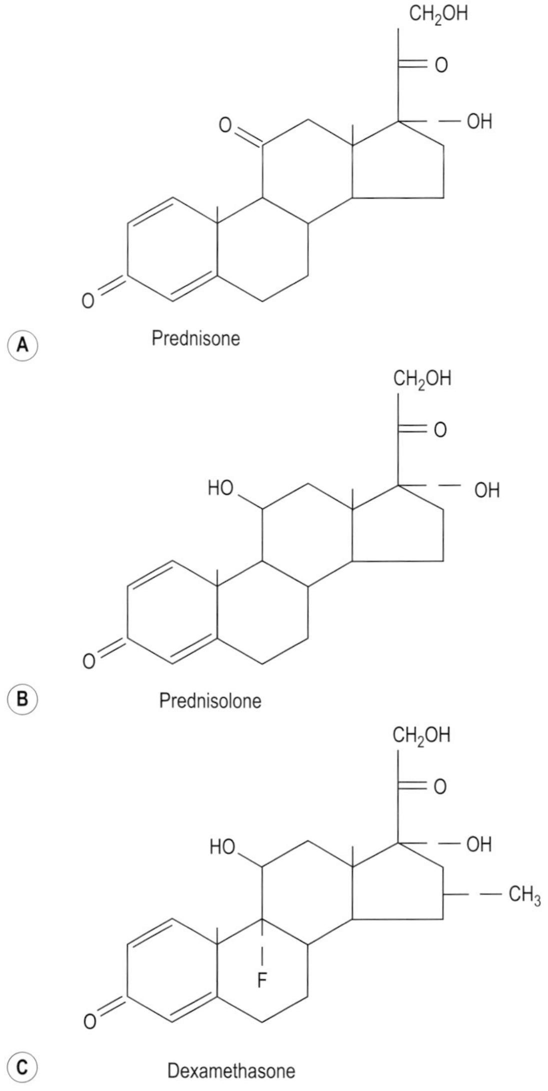

A   Prednisone

B   Prednisolone

C   Dexamethasone

Figure 7-2. Structures of more commonly used corticosteroids.

can even consider asking patients to begin their topical therapy by taking a drop every 15 minutes for the first hour, as a sort of loading dose. Our opinion is that 'failures' of this therapy are often due to infrequent dosing schedules. Further, the longer the duration and the more chronic the disease, the more difficult it often is to bring under control. Once a dosing schedule has been found to be effective, as

evidenced by a reduction in the flare and cells in the eye, we then see the patient often (every 2–3 days to once a week) and begin a very slow tapering of the drops. The schedule for tapering is unique to each patient, but persons who have had numerous attacks may need to receive one or two drops a day for weeks or even months.

A second option is to inject the corticosteroid periocularly. This method, which permits a relatively high concentration of material to be given rapidly, is an effective way to treat particularly severe inflammatory conditions. There is the general choice between long-acting preparations (in a depot vehicle) and shorter-acting soluble preparations. These injections can be given every 1–2 weeks for short periods. In addition to treatment of severe anterior segment disease in general, this is a useful approach for unilateral disease, at the time of surgery on an uveitic eye, and for patients in whom the systemic effects of steroids should be avoided. We have found this to be an effective way to treat cystoid macular edema, even in children, although the procedure may require that young children receive general anesthesia. In one study[8] 25 of 28 eyes given a sub-Tenon's injection of 40 mg triamcinolone had improved vision at 6 weeks post injection. In another study by Bui Quoc and colleagues,[9] 61 patients with uveitis were given one or more periocular injections of triamcinolone. Intraocular pressure elevation was seen in 21% of patients and 52% of patients were thought to have effective therapy based on angiographic changes and an improvement in visual acuity.

Several approaches to periocular injections have been suggested, and it probably is best to use the approach with which one feels the most comfortable. The approach from the superotemporal aspect of the globe, as described by Schlaegel,[10] is thought to reduce the possibility of penetration of the globe and to place the medication under Tenon's capsule and in the region of the macula. Freeman and coworkers[11] demonstrated that the temporal approach is efficient for placing the injected steroid close to the macula. Using any of these approaches, we rarely need to systemically premedicate an adult. Topical anesthetics are liberally used, and the area in which the injection is to be given (such as the superotemporal aspect of the globe) is further anesthetized with a cotton swab soaked in topical anesthetic (either 4% lidocaine or cocaine). If there are no contraindications, we generally inject triamcinolone (Kenalog) 40 mg in 1 mL because this preparation appears to cause less fibrosis. Some practitioners have suggested mixing the steroid preparation with a local anesthetic. We generally do not do this because the increased volume needed increases the pain of the procedure. An alternate approach that has become popular is to inject the steroid preparation directly through the lower lid or the inferior fornix (using a 25-gauge needle) while the patient looks upward. After the injection, for the patient's comfort, we put a patch on the eye and give a mild analgesic. We have rarely found the need to inject the steroid anteriorly over the pars plana/peripheral retina, a technique that is thought to increase the chance of steroid-induced ocular hypertension. If the procedure is performed on an outpatient basis, the person will be observed for some time (30–90 minutes) to be sure there are no untoward problems. We will use periocular injections over a 4–12-week interval, giving a series of two to four injections before declaring this method ineffective (**Fig. 7-3**). Finally, anecortave acetate, a corticosteroid that has been modified so that its corticosteroid activity has been eliminated, is also injected periocularly. The interest in this molecule is related to its retardation of blood vessel growth through inhibition of endothelial cell migration.[12]

An additional local approach that has attracted great attention is the intraocular administration of corticosteroids.

To date this route of administration has been achieved using three approaches. The first is the direct injection, usually of triamcinolone (2–4 mg), into the vitreous; the second is the use of a soluble pledget placed into the anterior or posterior chamber; and the third is placement of a slow-release fluocinolone acetonide-containing implant into the eye.

Intravitreal steroid injections have been reported to be effective for many intraocular problems, including choroidal neovascularization, CME secondary to uveitis, diabetes, central vein occlusion, and pseudophakia.[13-15] In one study[15] in which 2 mg of triamcinolone were injected into uveitic eyes with cystoid macular edema, five of six eyes showed a reduction in macular thickening in 1 week based on optical coherence tomographic measurements. Two of the five eyes could be maintained afterward with periocular injections. However, only a moderate improvement in visual acuity was seen despite the return of the macula to its anatomically normal configuration. In one 40-patient randomized study[16] comparing orbital floor injection of steroid versus intravitreal injections for CME, foveal thickness increased with orbital floor injections but decreased with intravitreal injections, with CME improving in that group in 50% of patients. However, at 6 months there was no difference in the best

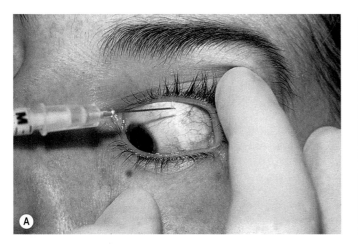

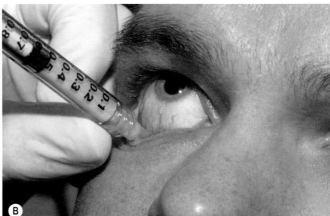

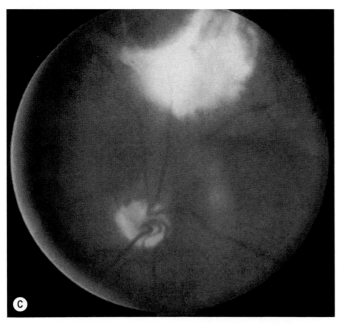

Figure 7-3. A, Temporal approach to giving periocular injection. **B,** Inferior fornix approach. *(Courtesy Dr Roxana Ursea.)* **C,** Although the possibility is markedly reduced if precautions are taken, perforation of the globe can occur, as seen here.

corrected vision between the two groups. This perhaps underlines the issue that repeat injections are necessary for a sustained release, an approach that is being used less and less. The positives and negatives of this approach continue to be discussed, particularly with the significant increase in intraocular pressure and cataract formation.[17] Regression of iris neovascularization has been reported using this approach as well.[18] In one study of 113 patients treated with intravitreal triamcinolone for subretinal neovascularization, 30% developed an increase in intraocular pressure >5 mmHg within the first 3 months.[19] In addition to an increase in pressure, a clinical picture resembling an endophthalmitis was reported, with the normal concern as to whether it was sterile or infectious. Further, the triamcinolone preparations currently being used contain alcohol, which has an unknown effect on the retina. An intraocular preparation free of such components is now available.

Fluocinolone acetonide (FA) intravitreous implants have been evaluated in several studies, and the results of a 3-year clinical trial have recently been published.[20] In this study 110 patients received a 0.59 mg FA implant and 168 received a 2.1 mg FA implant, all placed intravitreously. Uveitis recurrence was reduced to 4%, 10%, and 20% during the 1, 2, and 3 year periods for the 0.59 mg implant. More implanted eyes had an improvement in vision than did nonimplanted eyes. However, glaucoma surgery was required in 40% of the implanted eyes, compared to 2% of the nonimplanted eyes. Additionally, 93% of the phakic eyes that were implanted needed cataract surgery, whereas only 20% of the nonimplanted eyes needed this surgery. The Retisert implant is FDA approved for use in uveitis. However, questions remain as to the overall use of this approach in uveitis patients.[21] Because of equipoise in the community as a whole, the Multicenter Uveitis Steroid Treatment (MUST) trial was initiated. This is a phase IV randomized controlled clinical trial comparing two treatments, the FA implant versus standard therapy, for patients with vision-threatening noninfectious intermediate uveitis, posterior uveitis, or panuveitis. It is projected that the study will be complete in late 2011.

Ozurdex. Ozurdex is a sustained-release biodegradable intravitreal implant containing dexamethasone. The implant is placed in the vitreous using a 22-gauge applicator and the biodegradable polymers break down into H_2O and CO_2 as dexamethasone is released. A clinical study comparing applicator and surgical placement of Ozurdex found that patients receiving applicator placement had a similar efficacy but a slightly lower rate of certain adverse effects than did those receiving surgical placement.[22]

Ozurdex is currently FDA approved for macular edema associated with retinal vein occlusion and is also being developed for both diabetic macular edema and uveitis. A recent study demonstrated that Ozurdex was well tolerated and produced improvements in visual acuity, macular thickness, and fluorescein leakage in patients with persistent macular edema despite laser treatment or medical therapy. Eligible causes of macular edema in this study were diabetic retinopathy, retinal vein occlusion, uveitis, and Irvine-Gass syndrome.[23] In a subgroup analysis of patients in this study who had macular edema due to either Uveitis or Irvine-Gass syndrome,[24] those receiving the 700 mg Ozurdex implant had significantly greater improvement in visual acuity than

did controls up to 6 month following a single application. Ozurdex was well tolerated, with no cases of endophthalmitis. The number of patients with an increase in intraocular pressure (IOP) ≥10 mmHg at any visit during the 6-month trial was 12% in the 350 µg Ozurdex group, 17% in the 700 µg Ozurdex group, and 3% in the control group. No patients required surgical treatment for glaucoma.[23]

Secondary Effects

The topical application of steroid induces an increase in IOP in a significant number of persons. This should be monitored closely. It has been our experience that some patients with uveitis are extremely sensitive to steroid therapy, with dramatic increases in IOP noted even when topical steroids are administered on a very modest schedule. The reactivation of corneal herpes simplex infection can occur with topical steroid therapy. This is of even greater import in those patients undergoing corneal grafting, as a large proportion of these persons are undergoing this procedure because of corneal herpes.

The periocular injection of steroid has secondary effects unique to the procedure as well. (1) Although periocular steroid injections are an effective therapy for childhood uveitis, they may require general anesthesia, with the potential inherent side effects. (2) Possible penetration of the globe with the needle should be a constant concern to the ophthalmologist.[25] (3) Continued periocular injections can induce orbital problems, such as proptosis of the globe and fibrosis of the extraocular muscles. (4) Retinal and choroidal occlusions after a posterior sub-Tenon's injection given to treat cystoid macular edema have been reported.[26] (5) Severe or intractable glaucoma can occur after periocular injections. This can become particularly problematic when a depot injection has been used. In such cases the depot may need to be removed surgically, which is sometimes a major undertaking. In a retrospective review of 64 patients, Levin and colleagues[27] found that in nonglaucomatous eyes a history of a steroid-induced increase in intraocular pressure is a relative contraindication to injection. In another study of 53 patients who had a total of 162 posterior sub-Tenon's steroid injections, an increase in IOP was seen in 36%.[28] (6) Reactions to the vehicle in which the steroid injection has been placed can also occur (**Fig. 7-4**). (7) In patients with scleritis and ocular toxoplasmosis, periocular injections can be problematic. In the former the injections could potentially inhibit new collagen growth to a point where perforation of the globe may occur. This theory is being questioned by some. With toxoplasmosis, the acutely high intraocular steroid dose may effectively prevent the body's normal antitoxoplasma mechanisms, thereby causing an exacerbation of the ocular disease. Intraocular steroid injections or implants may also result in elevations of IOP in a large proportion of patients. The complications of intraocular steroid placement are just beginning to be reported. As mentioned earlier, they include increased IOP, endophthalmitis, and much rarer but always potential problems after any penetrating injury to the globe (i.e., vitreous hemorrhage and retinal detachment).

Systemic corticosteroids remain the initial drug of choice for most patients with severe bilateral endogenous sight-threatening uveitis. The striking exception to this rule is patients with Behçet's disease (see Chapter 26). When initi-

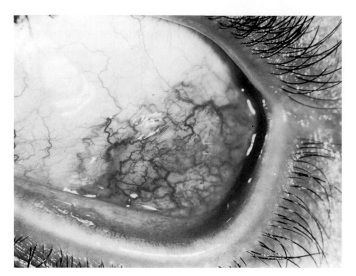

Figure 7-4. Allergic response in conjunctiva after periocular injection of steroid. The patient underwent skin testing and was found to have a profound allergic response to the vehicle.

Table 7-2 Common immunosuppressive agents used systemically to control intraocular inflammatory disease

Agent	Usual Dosage*
Prednisone	Oral: 1–2 mg/kg/day
Methylprednisolone	IV pulse: 1 g over 1–2 h
Intraocular triamcinolone	Intravitreal: 2–4 mg
Antimetabolites	
Methotrexate	Oral: 7.5–15 mg weekly; can be given intramuscularly
Azathioprine weight/day	Oral: 50–150 mg daily, 1–1.5 mg/kg, but up to 2.5 mg/kg body
Mycophenolate mofetil	Oral: 1 g twice per day
Alkylating agents	
Cyclophosphamide	Oral: 50–100 mg daily, up to 2.5 mg/kg body weight/day
	IV pulse: 750 mg/m² (adjusted to kidney function and white blood cell count)
Chlorambucil	Oral: 0.1–0.2 mg/kg/day
Ciclosporin	Oral: up to 5 mg/kg/day, usually given with prednisone, 10–20 mg/day
FK506	Oral: 0.10–0.15 mg/kg body weight/day
Daclizumab	IV or SC: 1–2 mg/kg
Etanercept	SC: 25 mg twice weekly; children 0.4 mg/kg twice weekly
Infliximab	SC: 3–10 mg/kg
Interferon-α	SC: 3–6 × 10⁶ IU qd × 1 mo, then qod; 3 × 10⁶ IU three times per week

*It is important to note that the dosages should ultimately be determined by a treating physician with experience using these medications on the basis of the medical state of the patient in question. Further, not all of these medications (or the route of therapy indicated) have been approved by various governmental agencies (i.e., U.S. Food and Drug Administration) for use in patients with uveitis. Therefore the physician needs to inquire about their specific use.

ating systemic steroid therapy, one should keep in mind several considerations. It is imperative that the treating physician (to the best of his or her ability) rule out the possibility of infection or malignant disease as a cause for the intraocular inflammation. Uppermost is the clinical impression, based on the ocular examination, that there is an inflammatory response that requires systemic therapy. It is also important for the practitioner to set standards by which to decide whether the therapy is successful or not. A detailed explanation should be given to the patient before starting therapy. The subject matter should include duration of therapy, goals, and side effects.

We generally find it advisable to begin therapy with prednisone 1–1.5 mg/kg/day (**Table 7-2**). The relatively high dose and daily therapy appear to increase the efficacy of this approach, which takes into account the known effects of corticosteroids in humans, already described. The high doses of corticosteroids should be maintained until one sees a clinical effect, but it is clear that the treating physician must set a reasonable time limit to decide whether this form of therapy is truly worthwhile. If it is determined that the corticosteroids are having a beneficial effect, then a slow reduction of the therapeutic dose needs to be established. A too-rapid reduction can lead to recurrence. The slow-tapering plan permits the treating physician to see if the reduction will cause a reactivation, which frequently manifests as a mild ocular inflammation and perhaps a minimal decrease in visual acuity. Some patients may need only a periodic short course of systemic steroids, whereas others require long-term maintenance therapy. Antacids or other antiulcer medications and calcium supplements can be given to patients, particularly those receiving long-term therapy. We routinely give ranitidine, 150 mg once or twice a day, to all our patients receiving oral prednisone for any length of time.

Alternate-day therapy is certainly a logical goal to aim for because side effects of such administration are much less than those with daily dosing. Fauci[7] has suggested that one way to attain this is to double the daily maintenance dosage and then slowly reduce the alternate-day dosage by 5 mg until zero is reached. In our experience those patients with severe inflammatory disease or persistent macular edema often do not do well with alternate-day therapy, but it still remains a logical goal. It is important to stress the method outlined by Fauci, because it has been our experience in ophthalmology that the plan is rarely followed. If a patient is taking prednisone 20 mg/day and the decision has been made to attempt an alternate-day approach, then the treating physician needs to double the daily amount of prednisone from 20 to 40 mg/day and then begin a slow taper every other day.

How long does one treat? What is a reasonable long-term dosage? These are not easy questions to answer. Each patient's requirements, capacities, and willingness for treatment are very different. Obviously the best dosage of steroid is none at all. However, being realistic, we believe that a reasonable daily adult maintenance dose is from 10 to 20 mg of prednisone, or as low a dose as is possible. This of course varies from patient to patient. For many patients with severe inflammatory disease we commonly see undertreatment, with therapy lasting only for 3–4 weeks followed by a rapid taper. Unfortunately, this therapeutic approach is wishful thinking and will not work in many patients. We will not consider lowering the steroid dosage below 10–20 mg unless the ocular disease appears quiescent for an extended period, usually about 3 months. In some diseases, such as sympathetic ophthalmia (see Chapter 23), we have elected to treat with maintenance dosages for at least a year, fearing a recurrence if therapy were stopped earlier. As a general tapering schedule, if the dose of prednisone is >40 mg/day, then one can reduce by 10 mg/day every 1–2 weeks; if the dose is between 20 and 40 mg/day, one can reduce by 5 mg/day every 1–2 weeks; if the dose is between 10 and 20 mg/day, one can reduce by 2.5 mg/day every 1–2 weeks; and if the dose is <10 mg, one can reduce by 1–2.5 mg/day every 1–4 weeks.[29] As soon as it is clear that long-term (i.e., >3 months) therapy will be needed, we begin to think about adding a second agent (see below).

Intravenously administered 'pulse' corticosteroid therapy can also be employed. We have used this approach in patients who have a severe bilateral process that needs to be treated as rapidly as possible, administering 1 g of methyl-prednisolone intravenously and repeating daily for 3 days. Patients are hospitalized and examined by an internist before the administration of this therapy. It is not yet clear whether this method indeed renders better results than does giving a high dose of oral prednisone, such as 80 mg/day, but in our experience it certainly reverses an acute process very rapidly. This approach has been used to treat the Vogt–Koyanagi–Harada syndrome as well as the ocular manifestations of Behçet's disease.[30]

The potential side effects of corticosteroids should be familiar to those giving the medication. Some of the more common secondary problems are seen in **Box 7-1**. Other adverse reactions have included nonketotic hyperosmolar coma in young nondiabetic patients receiving systemic corticosteroids for a short time,[31] and central serous retinopathy.[32]

The effects of long-term corticosteroid administration are a constant concern. Polito and coworkers[33] studied the growth of 10 boys with glomerulonephritis who received prednisone (1.2 mg/kg) every other day for at least 2 consecutive years. They found that in six patients the peak growth velocity was delayed after age 15. However, after 16 years of age the growth velocity was significantly higher than expected and permitted these patients to reach their genetic height potential. We have also gained a heightened sensitivity to the development of osteoporosis with corticosteroid therapy. Corticosteroids affect many aspects of bone health, including calcium homeostasis, and sex hormones, which are inhibitors of bone formation, enhancing osteoclast-mediated bone resorption and reducing osteoblast-mediated bone formation.[34] The effects of steroids can be seen within the first 6 months of therapy. The prevalence of vertebral fractures in patients with asthma treated with corticosteroids for at least 1 year is 11%.[34] Most experts will recommend 800 IU of vitamin D daily as well as 1500 mg of calcium. Exercise is important, and hormone replacement therapy can be considered in menopausal women. Finally, antiresorptive agents such as alendronate, etidronate, and risedronate should be considered, particularly if bone density studies demonstrate osteoporosis or if patients are receiving long-term steroid therapy.

Box 7-1 Secondary effects of corticosteroid therapy

FLUIDS, ELECTROLYTES
Sodium retention, potassium loss
Fluid retention
Hypokalemic alkalosis
Hyperosmolar coma

MUSCULOSKELETAL
Muscle weakness
Steroid myopathy
Osteoporosis
Aseptic necrosis of femoral and humeral heads
Tendon rupture

GASTROINTESTINAL
Nausea
Increased appetite
Peptic ulcer
Perforation of small and large bowel
Pancreatitis

DERMATOLOGIC
Poor wound healing
Easy bruisability
Increased sweating

NEUROLOGIC
Convulsions
Headaches
Hyperexcitability
Moodiness
Psychosis

ENDOCRINE
Menstrual irregularities
Cushingoid state
Suppression of growth in children
Hirsutism
Suppression of adrenocortical pituitary axis
Diabetes

OPHTHALMIC
Cataracts
Glaucoma
Central serous retinopathy
Activation of herpes (topical)

OTHER
Weight gain
Thromboembolism

A question that must be constantly asked is whether the desired effect warrants the potential or real side effects. There is no easy answer, and a dialogue between the patient and the physician is the only way this question can be addressed. Although corticosteroids remain the mainstay of therapy for uveitis, the condition in some patients is resistant to steroids. For those receiving long-term steroid therapy the risk of developing unacceptable side effects at the dosages that need to be given to control the disease are real. In those patients other immunomodulatory agents are added as steroid-sparing agents so that lower steroid doses (or none at all) can be used.

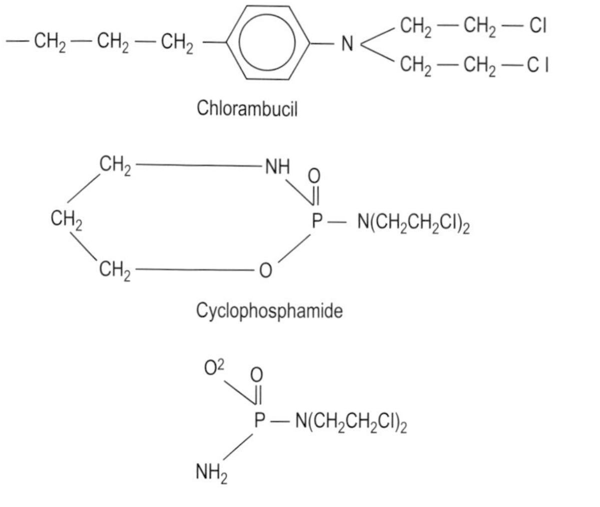

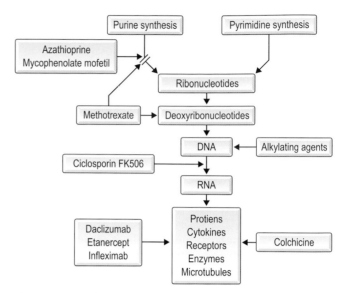

Figure 7-5. Structure and active moiety of the two most-used alkylating agents.

Figure 7-6. Site of action of several agents used to treat ocular inflammatory disease.

The combination of steroids with these agents provides reasonable and effective regimens for some patients and is discussed next. Although we may often begin therapy with corticosteroids, we will add a steroid-sparing agent if more than 3–4 months of significant amounts of steroids (15–20 mg) are needed to control the ocular inflammation. This philosophic shift to multiple agents sooner rather than later represents an important change in our therapeutic strategy.

Cytotoxic agents

It is curious to note that cytotoxic agents have their roots in instruments of destruction, namely chemical warfare. Although mustard gas was synthesized earlier, its use during World War I, with the resultant lymphopenia and lymphoid aplasia, led to the evaluation of this family of agents for therapeutic purposes. On a practical basis, two major categories of cytotoxic agent are used today in the treatment of ocular inflammatory disease: alkylating agents, such as chlorambucil and cyclophosphamide (**Fig. 7-5**), and antimetabolites, such as azathioprine and methotrexate (see Fig. 7-8). They have been used by physicians for several decades, but their true efficacy in many ocular disorders remains unclear; however, more information has recently been gained in their use for other putative autoimmune diseases. The physician treating severe sight-threatening disease should be aware of these agents and how they may fit into the general scheme of nonsurgical therapy for uveitis. Although, when viewed as a group, they are associated with serious side effects, the role they play as steroid-sparing or -replacing agents cannot be denied.[35,36]

Alkylating agents

Mode of Action

The alkylating agents have the ability to undergo reactions that result in the formation of covalent links (alkylation) of neutrophilic substances. In interacting with DNA strands alkylating agents are thought to interact with the 7-nitrogen guanine (**Fig. 7-6**).[37] This cross-linking of DNA would result in the inability of the cell's DNA to properly separate during division, ultimately leading to the death of the cell.

Nitrogen mustards are unstable compounds, and alterations in their structures were invariably tried to increase stability. An aromatic modification of mustard gas is chlorambucil (see Fig. 7-5), a compound stable enough to be given by mouth. Cyclophosphamide is yet another modification, with a cyclic phosphamide group added. For cyclophosphamide to become an active agent it must be metabolized in the liver's microsomal system. It is theorized that phosphoramide mustard (see Fig. 7-5) is the most active of the metabolites.

The effect of alkylating agents on the immune system is rather profound. Higher doses are thought to more acutely affect B-cell function than T-cell function, but long-term lower dosages may have an equal or even greater effect on T-cell function. Paradoxically, administration of alkylating agents to animals can result in the loss of suppressor cells, something that is certainly not advisable for patients with a poorly controlled immunoregulatory system. The alkylating agents are thought to be more potent in inducing a response than are the antimetabolites. However, with greater efficacy comes more potential for adverse secondary effects. These agents are thought to mediate ocular inflammatory disease through the killing of clones of cells that are causing damage in the eye. This may be occurring at some central location (e.g., lymph node or bone marrow) or at the end organ itself. The response is not specific and will theoretically affect any actively dividing cell.

Indications and Dosages

Buckley and Gills[38] reported the efficacy of cyclophosphamide therapy in the treatment of intermediate uveitis. In addition, alkylating agents have been frequently used in the treatment of Behçet's disease.[39] The recommendations of the International Uveitis Study Group for the use of cytotoxic agents were decided upon in the early 1980s. Although somewhat dated, their basic concepts still seem to hold true. Treatment of Behçet's disease was one absolute recommendation, because corticosteroid therapy was not thought to adequately control the retinal/retinal vascular disease frequently observed in these patients. In general, alkylating agents are indicated for severe bilateral sight-threatening endogenous uveitis. Again, it cannot be overly stressed that the treating physician must be confident that the disease being treated does not have an infectious component. Further, the physician should consider therapy only if there is vision to save. It should not be considered in end-stage disease just to be sure that 'everything was tried.' The potential side effects of these agents necessitate a good reason for their administration. The patient must be well informed of the physician's intentions and expectations, as well as of any possible side effects. It is probably reasonable to ask the patient to sign a consent form. In addition, an internist should examine the patient to be sure that there is no systemic contraindication for therapy, and to help in the dosing and follow-up. Although this therapeutic approach is used in generalized life-threatening autoimmune diseases in children, we have not used it in pregnant women or children with uveitis because of the concern of the potential long-term side effects of these drugs. If these drugs are used in younger persons, the physician should discuss the side effects in depth. One important consideration is the possibility that the medication may induce azoospermia, and banking of sperm before the initiation of therapy might be considered. Harvesting of ova, although performed less frequently, might also be considered.

For cyclophosphamide, adult patients can start at about 2 mg/kg/day by mouth, with the usual starting dose for a rapid effect being between 150 and 200 mg/day (see Table 7-2). The drug should be taken on an empty stomach because it can be activated in the gastrointestinal tract if taken with food. The white blood cell count with differential must be monitored constantly, beginning with a baseline value. One may begin to see a drop in the white blood cell count within a few days to a week. Once this occurs, the dosage may be reduced by 25–50 mg, the object being a white blood cell count that stabilizes at no lower than 3000/mm^3. The total neutrophil count should not fall to less than 1500–2000/mm^3. Nevertheless, the dosage used should be based predominantly on the therapeutic effect of the drug on ocular inflammation.

Pulse cyclophosphamide (see Table 7-2) has been widely used in the treatment of systemic collagen vascular disease, such as the renal disease associated with systemic lupus erythematosus. This approach to therapy is thought to carry fewer risks than everyday oral therapy. Hoffman and associates[40] found that intermittent cyclophosphamide therapy combined with steroid therapy yielded a long-term failure rate of 79% in patients with Wegener's granulomatosis. We also have not found this approach to be particularly effective, as breakthroughs of disease activity tend to occur between therapeutic courses. Rosenbaum[41] reported that in 11 patients with uveitis treated with pulse cyclophosphamide, five benefited but only two had a sustained improvement without the use of additional immunosuppressive therapy. Rosenbaum concluded that most patients with uveitis do not experience a prolonged benefit from this therapeutic approach. Systemic steroids can be administered along with the alkylating agent. This permits one to use lower dosages of both and thus avoid some of the side effects of both.

Godfrey and colleagues[42] have used chlorambucil to treat several disorders, including Behçet's disease and sympathetic ophthalmia. This medication can be administered on an outpatient basis. The total dose is usually between 6 and 12 mg/day. We generally give a lower initial dose (2 mg) to be sure that there are no idiosyncratic responses and then increase the dose. As with cyclophosphamide, the white blood cell count and differential must be constantly monitored.

A somewhat different approach was discussed by Tessler and Jennings,[43] who reported the use of high-dose short-term chlorambucil in the treatment of Behçet's disease and sympathetic ophthalmia. These authors believed that they induced remission in all patients, using an average total dose of 2.2 g over 23 weeks for the patients with Behçet's disease and a total of 0.9 g over 11 weeks for the patients with sympathetic ophthalmia.

Secondary Effects

A wide range of side effects has been reported with alkylating agents.[44] For these particular agents, leukopenia is a major effect, yielding immunosuppression. Thrombocytopenia and anemia also occur. An increased incidence of infection, particularly viral, is another great concern. Interstitial fibrosis of the lungs, testicular atrophy, and hemorrhagic cystitis are associated with cyclophosphamide therapy, the latter being a relative indication for discontinuation of the drug. Renal toxicity has been attributed to the metabolites of alkylating agents,[45] and visual disturbances have been reported with high doses of cyclophosphamide.[46] Teratogenicity is a major concern, and cyclophosphamide is excreted in breast milk.

Because sterility is a real concern for those receiving alkylating agents, semen can be banked and oocytes cryopreserved. Recently, a gonadotropin-releasing hormone (GnRH) agonist has been used to preserve ovarian function in patients receiving cyclophosphamide (Cytoxan)[47] and treatment for lymphoma.[48] This treatment induces a menopause-like state, in essence returning the ovaries to a prepubertal state; prepubertal ovaries are thought to be more resistant to the gonadotoxic effects of alkylating agents. Although this treatment is effective, there is a potential loss of bone density because of a relative estrogen deficiency. For those under 16 years of age the use of a GnRH agonistic analog is not recommended because of its unknown effect on bone development.

Perhaps the most disquieting adverse effects seen with these agents are those that may occur after long-term therapy. The first is the potential for secondary malignancy.[44] Secondary urinary bladder cancer seems to occur in patients who have hemorrhagic cystitis. Of course the underlying disorder being treated may also predispose some patients to the development of these disorders, particularly myeloproliferative and lymphoproliferative neoplasms. A second troublesome observation is the finding of chromosomal damage with extended cyclophosphamide therapy.[49] In the review of Hoffman and colleagues'[50] 158 patients with Wegener's granulomatosis, a series of disturbing complications ascribed to cyclophosphamide therapy were reported: 73 patients had 140 serious infections that required hospitalization and intravenous antibiotic therapy; 43% had cystitis, 2.8% had bladder cancer, and 2% had myelodysplasia. Of the women treated, 57% ceased menstruating for 1 year, with test results supporting the diagnosis of ovarian failure. There was a calculated 24-fold increase in malignant conditions and a calculated 33-fold increase in bladder cancer, occurring 7 months to 10 years after the medication was stopped. In a longitudinal cohort study in patients with rheumatoid arthritis with a 20-year follow-up, 119 patients treated with cyclophosphamide between 1968 and 1973 were compared with 119 patients who did not receive cyclophosphamide. An increased risk of malignancy was seen in the cyclophosphamide group (relative risk 1.5%).[51] Of interest were the nine bladder malignancies seen in the cyclophosphamide group versus none for those not receiving cyclophosphamide. Three of those malignancies occurred 14, 16, and 17 years after cyclophosphamide was stopped. Lane and colleagues[52] reviewed 543 charts of patients with uveitis and compared those receiving corticosteroids with those receiving immunosuppression. No difference was noted.

It should be added that during the past few years, because of the aforementioned complications, alkylating agent therapy has been used less and less by internists for the treatment of putative autoimmune diseases. However, the anecdotal evidence certainly suggests a positive therapeutic effect in curtailing severe intraocular inflammatory disease. For life-threatening systemic vasculitis or in some patients with sight-threatening retinal vasculitis cyclophosphamide may be a most effective medication. Also, in the Third World this sort of therapy is readily available and relatively cheap, two very important considerations. As with many other problems in medicine, this class of drugs presents a dual-edged sword, and their use should be considered only after long reflection.

Many recommendations for cytotoxic agent therapy that the reader will find in the literature were written before the use of ciclosporin, tacrolimus (FK506), or monoclonal antibody therapy entered into clinical practice, as well as before the use of low-dose methotrexate or azathioprine. In our approach, cytotoxic agents are often used last – after corticosteroids, ciclosporin, and monoclonal antibody therapy – for sight-threatening intraocular inflammatory disease. We would use cytotoxic agents if the side effects of steroid or ciclosporin were simply intolerable, but the patient clearly was having an excellent therapeutic response to immunosuppressive therapy. We would make every effort to avoid using alkylating agents in children, as the long-term effects of these agents sometimes make the risk difficult to justify ethically. It should be stressed that until recently no comparative clinical trials have been attempted to evaluate the true efficacy of these agents in the treatment of uveitis, nor are most of these agents listed in the *Physicians' Desk Reference* as indicated for the therapy of uveitis. There is, however, no reason to doubt that in some conditions these agents may be effective: for example, they have an apparent profound positive effect on the ocular manifestations of Behçet's disease[39]; Tabbara,[53] however, has questioned that assessment.

In our experience, mostly with the alkylating agents, cytotoxic drugs have not been as effective in controlling severe inflammatory conditions such as Behçet's disease as had been previously suggested. We have had patients with Behçet's disease discontinue ciclosporin therapy because of toxicity and then have a very poor therapeutic result with an alkylating agent, necessitating a third therapeutic approach. However, others seem to have done well. Although alkylat-

ing agents are tolerated reasonably well, the side effects, such as leukopenia, may last for some time even after discontinuance of the medication. We therefore advise caution when clinicians use these agents. The ophthalmologist should have someone well versed in this therapeutic approach actively involved in the care of the patient, should set strict goals in terms of the therapeutic effect that must be reached, and should avoid using these agents in children unless forced to do so, and then only with the in-depth understanding and permission of both the parents and the child. Locally administered methotrexate (or other agents) may prove to be a useful therapeutic approach to neoplastic disease with only a local reactivation in the eye.

Antimetabolites

In this category of medications, azathioprine and mycophenolate mofetil, which alter purine metabolism, and methotrexate, a folate analog, are the three most widely used (**Fig. 7-7**).

Azathioprine

Mode of Action

Azathioprine (Imuran) is thought to be a prodrug. Upon metabolism it is converted into the active agent 6-mercaptopurine. Azathioprine is better absorbed, causes less gastrointestinal disturbance, and is less likely to be inactivated by liver enzymes than is 6-mercaptopurine. Once converted to its active form, it is thought to affect DNA and RNA metabolism by being converted to 6-thioinosine-5-phosphate (T-IMP) by the enzyme hypoxanthine guanine phosphoribosyltransferase. T-IMP is probably incorporated into nucleic acids, thus leading to false codes being generated. It appears that azathioprine has a greater effect on the afferent arm of the immune response when it is given before the antigenic challenge.

Indications and Dosages

For putative autoimmune diseases such as rheumatoid arthritis, the suggested dosage of azathioprine is about 1–2.5 mg/kg/day,[54,55] the average dose being 50–100 mg daily, given as one dose or in divided doses[56] (see Table 7-2).

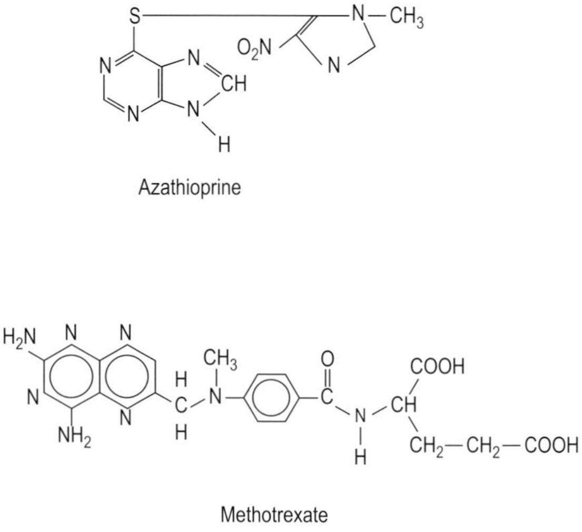

Figure 7-7. Structures of two antimetabolites.

The combination of azathioprine with low-dose steroid has been used in the treatment of uveitis by Andrasch and colleagues,[57] with about half of their 22 patients showing a positive therapeutic effect and the others having either no response or severe adverse effects. Other authors have used the drug for the treatment of sympathetic ophthalmia, the Vogt–Koyanagi–Harada syndrome, and pars planitis.[58] More than half of the patients with Behçet's disease whom Aoki and Sugiura[59] treated with azathioprine appeared to have an improvement of their ocular disease. Yazici and coworkers[60] showed in a double-masked study that azathioprine (2.5 mg/kg/day) was superior to placebo in the prevention of new eye disease associated with Behçet's disease. Hooper and Kaplan[61] used an initial dosage of azathioprine of 1.5 mg/kg/day combined with steroid and ciclosporin for sight-threatening serpiginous choroidopathy (see Chapter 28). Certain drugs, such as allopurinol, can interfere with the metabolism of 6-mercaptopurine, and the dosage of the agent must be reduced accordingly.

In a recent subgroup analysis of the SITE study (see the last paragraph of this chapter) 145 patients were who were treated with azathioprine as a sole immunosuppressive agent were evaluated.[62] It was noted to be moderately effective as a single steroid-sparing agent for control of disease and its steroid-sparing value. It required months to achieve a treatment goal and was tolerated by most patients. It appeared useful for patients with intermediate uveitis.

Secondary Effects

Antimetabolites can have serious side effects,[44] but in the past few years the use of lower doses has prevented these from occurring or has made them more tolerable. For azathioprine, perhaps the most problematic acute adverse effects are leukopenia, thrombocytopenia, and gastrointestinal disturbances. Of great long-term concern is that chronic immunosuppression increases the risk of neoplasia. Connell and colleagues[63] studied the risk of neoplasia in 755 patients with inflammatory bowel disease who were treated with azathioprine. These patients received a dose of 2 mg/kg/day for a median of 12.5 months, and no cases of non-Hodgkin's lymphoma were reported. There appeared to be no difference in cancer frequency among 86 patients with chronic ulcerative colitis who received azathioprine and 180 matched patients who did not. It appears that the risk of neoplasia is lower in those patients treated for autoimmune disorders, such as rheumatoid arthritis, than in those receiving therapy for the prevention of transplantation rejection.

Mycophenolate mofetil

Mycophenolate mofetil (CellCept) is an agent becoming more and more frequently used.[64] It has a molecular weight of 433.5 Da and metabolizes to mycophenolic acid, which reversibly inhibits inosine monophosphate dehydrogenase, inhibiting a pathway of guanosine nucleotide synthesis without incorporation into DNA. It affects both T and B cells and interferes with cellular adhesion to vascular endothelium. In animal models mycophenolate mofetil has prolonged the survival of allogeneic transplants. This agent has been used in preventing the expression of experimental autoimmune uveitis (EAU) (30 mg/kg/day) even after immunization, but at higher doses (60 mg/kg/day).[65] It was first used in humans in combination with corticosteroids and ciclosporin for the prevention of organ rejection after allogeneic renal transplants. Mycophenolate mofetil is taken on an empty stomach and has high oral bioavailability. It may be considered a reasonable alternative to either azathioprine or methotrexate therapy. Several small studies have reported good results with mycophenolate mofetil.[66,67] Kilmartin and colleagues[66] treated nine patients with uveitis with mycophenolate mofetil and saw an improvement in eight of them, with a follow-up of 10–36 weeks. These patients suffered from ciclosporin toxicity. In a study evaluating the National Eye Institute experience, 60 patients were treated with mycophenolate mofetil and it was found to be moderately effective.[68] In Baltatzis and colleagues'[69] report of 54 patients it was an effective steroid-sparing agent in 54% of cases and was used also as a monotherapy. In their report, Larkin and Lightman[67] also treated some patients with scleritis and reported success. Additionally the National Eye Institute's experience with this drug in scleritis has been reported.[70] In this small study, mycophenolate mofetil was found to be a useful steroid-sparing agent in patients with controlled scleritis but not as an effective adjunctive agent for patients with active scleritis. Others have found it also to be a very useful steroid-sparing agent with a manageable side-effects profile.[71] In a recent retropective report it appeared to reduce ocular inflammation more rapidly than did methotrexate.[72]

The dose of mycophenolate mofetil is usually 1 g orally twice daily. Some patients have received up to 3 g/day (1.5 g twice daily), but there does not seem to be an increased therapeutic effect although toxicity may increase. The most common adverse event appears to be gastrointestinal effects, with as many as 31% of patients reporting this problem. In two smaller reports of patients with uveitis, in addition to nausea, patients complained of myalgia, fatigue, and headache. In patients receiving transplants other problems have been noted, such as leukopenia, nonmelanoma skin cancers, and opportunistic infections, but these patients are usually heavily immunosuppressed.[66,67,73–75]

Methotrexate

Mode of Action

Methotrexate is a folate analog, differing from folic acid only in that a hydrogen atom and hydroxyl group have been replaced by a methyl and amino group. Folate analogs are known to have profound effects on cellular metabolism by inhibiting dihydrofolate reductase activity. This enzyme is imperative for the production of tetrahydrofolate, an important coenzyme in cell metabolism. Tetrahydrofolate is needed for the production of thymidylate, an essential component of DNA, and mediates the production of purine nucleotides, also needed for RNA metabolism. Methotrexate demonstrates time-specific characteristics in that, under certain experimental conditions, an augmented immune response may be noted if the drug is given before antigenic challenge. Several effects on the immune system have been enumerated. Methotrexate has been shown to have an antiproliferative effect on endothelial cells,[76] can reduce the synthesis of leukotriene B4 in neutrophils,[77] has been shown to reduce the concentration of interleukin-1β in synovial fluid,[78] and can suppress cell-mediated immunity.[79] An added action of methotrexate is its inhibition of histamine release.

Indications and Dosages

Several dosage schedules have been suggested, with a weekly oral or intramuscular dose of 7.5–25 mg given until a therapeutic response is noted (see Table 7-2). Patients need to be told to abstain from all alcohol consumption. Cyclitis and sympathetic ophthalmia have been reported to improve with the administration of this agent, but Behçet's disease and iridocyclitis have not.[80] Holz and colleagues[81] reported the use of low-dose methotrexate in the treatment of 14 patients with uveitis. Using a regimen of either 40 mg given intravenously once weekly followed by 15 mg/wk given orally, or 15 mg of oral methotrexate only, they found an improvement of visual acuity in 11 of the patients and an improvement in inflammatory disease in all. However, using the low dose of 12.5 mg/week of methotrexate, Shah and colleagues[82] found that 16 patients with assorted ocular inflammatory conditions (including intermediate uveitis (nine patients) and retinal vasculitis (three patients)) had a reduction in inflammatory activity and most of those could taper or discontinue their steroid therapy. However, when one looks at the success rate for those patients with chronic uveitis, only five of the nine showed a response, and improvement in visual acuity was not used as the criterion for success. Of the three patients with retinal vasculitis, an improvement from moderate to mild disease was seen in two, and the other one had no improvement. Most practitioners will usually not treat acute uveitis in adults with methotrexate alone. Usually it is used as a steroid- or ciclosporin-sparing agent as reported by Dev and coworkers[83] in treating sarcoid uveitis. Pascalis and associates[84] used all three – corticosteroids, ciclosporin, and methotrexate – with good results in patients with uveitis. Methotrexate is well tolerated in children and is used extensively. Even in a disorder such as rheumatoid arthritis for which methotrexate monotherapy has been shown to be effective, the addition of ciclosporin has been shown to produce significant clinical improvement in some patients.[85] One combination to be particularly careful of is methotrexate and leflunomide. Weinblatt and colleagues[86] reported serious liver disease in a patient receiving this combination. In a subgroup analysis of the SITE study (see the final conclusions of this chapter below), methotrexate was evaluated in 534 patients with uveitis. Adding methotrexate to an anti-inflammatory regimen was often effective in the management of anterior uveitis, sometimes effective for scleritis, but less often effective for intermediate, posterior or panuveitis.[87]

Methotrexate has been used periocularly for the treatment of malignant conditions. Rootman and Gudauskas[88] used subconjunctival injections of methotrexate, cytarabine, and corticosteroids to successfully treat a leukemic infiltrate into the eye. Methotrexate has been used intravitreally to treat intraocular B-cell lymphoma.[89] Good responses have been seen using 400 μg/0.1 mL. These injections can be repeated, but care must be taken because reflux at the side of the intravitreal injection can damage limbal stem cells.

Secondary Effects

The secondary effects of methotrexate are legion,[29,44] but more recent use of lower doses has given this agent a new therapeutic life. Severe toxic reactions have been reported with this medication, although usually at higher doses. Marked depression of the white blood cell count and thrombocytopenia can occur. Hepatotoxicity (liver atrophy, cirrhosis, and even necrosis) is one of the most worrisome side effects.[90] Up to one-third of those receiving long-term weekly doses of methotrexate will have elevated serum aminotransferase levels.[91] Liver enzyme levels twice normal warrant withholding or stopping the medication; the levels usually return to normal rapidly. Zachariae and coworkers[92] have reported that cirrhosis developed in 25% of patients with psoriasis who received long-term low-dose methotrexate therapy. The age of the patient and the duration of therapy are both independent predictors of possible toxicity. When to perform a liver biopsy still remains a controversial question. It has been suggested that a liver biopsy should be considered in patients before methotrexate therapy is begun if there is a history of excessive alcohol consumption, abnormal results of liver function tests, or chronic hepatitis. Liver biopsy should also be considered during therapy if elevated liver function test results persist or a decrease in the serum albumin concentration is seen.[36]

Another concern is an acute pneumonitis that can be accompanied by fever, progressive shortness of breath, and cough in 1–5% of patients treated with methotrexate.[93–95] This appears to be due to a drug hypersensitivity reaction, and it can occur early or late in the course of therapy. Because an X-ray film may reveal interstitial and alveolar infiltration, sometimes bronchoalveolar lavage is needed to rule out an infectious process such as *Pneumocystis carinii* pneumonia. In most patients the reaction disappears with discontinuation of therapy.

Methotrexate may also impair renal function. The agent has been noted in the tears of patients receiving high-dose therapy.[96] Methotrexate can have a high rate of toxicity, but this appears to be partly dose related. In the low-dose study of Holz and colleagues,[81] slight elevations of transaminase levels were noted in four of 13 patients, partial alopecia in two, and nausea in three. A disturbing report from Zimmer-Galler and Lie[97] described a patient with rheumatoid arthritis treated with low-dose methotrexate for 16 months who developed blurred vision. This was noted to be due to choroidal nodules, which ultimately were shown to be a large B-cell non-Hodgkin's lymphoma. It is always difficult to distinguish the underlying propensity of patients with autoimmune disease for developing neoplasms from a real risk from the therapy.

Methotrexate is teratogenic and may foster malformations in children whose fathers are receiving the medication. Therefore it should not be used during pregnancy, and birth control should be used for some time after the medication is stopped.

Ciclosporin

Mode of Action

Ciclosporin is a natural product of several fungi. It was first investigated because of its potential antibiotic qualities, and is indeed antibacterial but with a most limited spectrum. It was the unique immunomodulatory properties first observed by Jean Borel at Sandoz Ltd, Basel, Switzerland, that altered immunotherapy principles and therapeutics in a profound way. Ciclosporin A, now termed ciclosporin (Sandimmune), is a neutral lipophilic cyclic endecapeptide with an unique

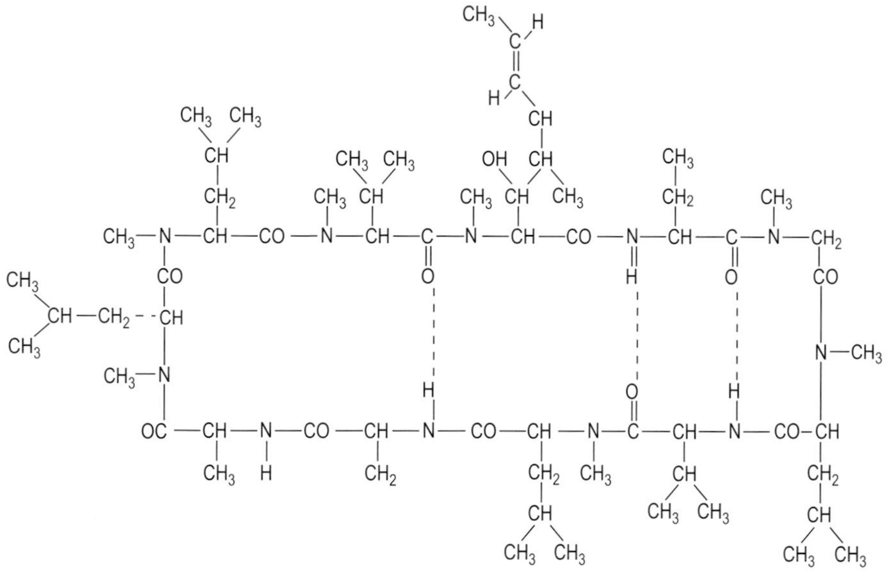

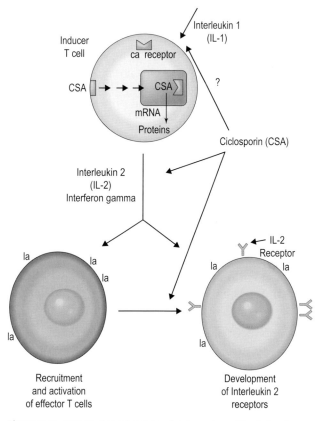

Figure 7-8. Structure of ciclosporin (Sandimmune).

amino acid side chain at the C1 position (**Fig. 7-8**). It is one of a large family of ciclosporins, some naturally occurring and some synthetically produced. This uncharged molecule, with a molecular weight of 1202 Da, is insoluble in water. The original preparation for human use was an olive oil solution with 12.5% ethanol, which was taken by mouth with either milk or juice. The absorption of this oral preparation was variable, ranging from 4% to 60%, with probably about one-third of the agent usually absorbed.[98,99] The agent is concentrated in lipid-containing tissues such as breast, pancreas, liver, lymphoid tissue, and kidney. We found about 40% of the plasma concentration in the aqueous of patients with quiescent uveitis under therapy with ciclosporin and undergoing cataract surgery.[100] Ciclosporin tablets are now available.

The agent is metabolized in the liver by the cytochrome P450 microsomal enzyme system. The ring structure is maintained throughout the metabolic process, with only 0.1% of the drug not undergoing metabolic changes. At least 15 metabolic products of ciclosporin are known. The parent structure appears to be the most active form. Drugs that interfere with cytochrome P450 activity will slow ciclosporin metabolism and will affect ciclosporin levels. Ketoconazole is one such agent, permitting a reduction by up to 90% of the oral dose of ciclosporin.[101] Other medications that inhibit ciclosporin metabolism include oral contraceptives, androgens, and erythromycin.

Ciclosporin has been demonstrated to have a far more restricted effect on the immune system than any other immunosuppressive agent or other monoclonal antibodies. Although theoretically ciclosporin would affect any cell with its binding protein, its major clinical effect is actively directed against the factors that promote T-cell activation and recruitment. The exact point at which ciclosporin intervenes in this scheme is debated (**Fig. 7-9**). It appears that ciclosporin enters the cell and is bound to an immunophilin (cyclophilin) meeting it at the cell membrane, similar to the action seen with corticosteroids. It then is escorted into the nucleus, where it affects messenger ribonucleic acid (mRNA) production and ultimately protein synthesis. Although the mechanism still remains to be definitely

Figure 7-9. Proposed mechanisms of ciclosporin on T-cell circuitry.

shown, much has been elucidated.[102] Ciclosporin blocks the activation of genes in T cells.[103] One intriguing notion is that ciclosporin binds to proteins binding to the interleukin (IL)-2 (IL-2) enhancer (such as NF-AT and octamer-associated protein), which helps in the activation of the transcription of the IL-2 gene. These sites have been shown to be sensitive to ciclosporin.[104]

On the basis of several in vitro systems, different observations have been made concerning the mode of action of ciclosporin. Larsson[105] reported that ciclosporin blocked the acquisition of IL-2 receptors and thereby prevented resting

89

cells from becoming activated and responding to IL-2. This theme has been less emphasized in the more recent literature. Others, such as Bunjes and coworkers,[106] have suggested that ciclosporin affects the release of IL-2 but that the acquisition of these receptors was not inhibited by ciclosporin. The blockage of ciclosporin production was noted by Kaufman and colleagues[107] in a T-cell hybridoma that produces IL-2 but does not bear IL-2 receptors. It may be that ciclosporin's mode of action depends on the state of T-cell activation and the type of stimulus for T-cell activation.[108] It is clear, however, that ciclosporin was unique in mediating its action through the T-cell circuitry.

The T cell most affected seems to be the inducer T-cell subset. We have noted that recruitment of inducer T cells into the draining lymph node of a site of S-antigen immunization is markedly diminished with ciclosporin administration. Shifts in the kinetic T- and B-cell response are also noted when animals are given ciclosporin.

Dosages and Indications

The dosage schedule for ciclosporin administration has undergone much change.[109] In our early studies[110] on the use of ciclosporin in ocular inflammatory disease patients were given an initial dose of 10 mg/kg/day, which at the time was thought to be rather modest inasmuch as often two to two and a half times this dose was being given to treat recipients of whole organ transplants. However, it became clear that dose-induced renal alterations made this starting dose no longer acceptable (see later discussion of toxicity). Studies have suggested that a lower initiating dose of ciclosporin may not induce any or at least considerably lessen the possibility of renal toxicity[111] (to be discussed). It is usually suggested that ciclosporin be given at a starting dose of 5 mg/kg/day (**Fig. 7-10**; see also Table 7-2), either as a single dose or as a twice-daily regimen. The twice-daily regimen is more commonly employed to avoid large spikes in serum ciclosporin levels, which may predispose the patient to renal toxicity. A recommended maximum dose of 7 mg/kg/day can be considered in special cases, such as children or patients with documented low ciclosporin serum levels. Ciclosporin is often used in combination with prednisone,

usually at 10–20 mg/day, but for short periods at even higher levels.

A relative contraindication for the initiation of therapy is poorly controlled hypertension or a history of renal disease accompanied by reduced creatinine clearance or both. In addition, older patients (over 55 years of age) must be evaluated particularly closely because they lack an adequate renal reserve. If the patient is currently being treated with cytotoxic agents, we would discontinue the medication for at least 1 month before ciclosporin is given. Those taking steroids orally continue to do so, with a slow taper to the 10–20 mg/day range. The ocular response to ciclosporin may be relatively slow (weeks to months), but preset goals should be established and should be met by about 3 months of therapy. The serum creatinine level should not be permitted to rise to 30% over baseline. Optimal decreases in ciclosporin dosages are usually between 50 and 100 mg/day at a time. Stopping the medication abruptly is ill advised because a rebound of the ocular disease may ensue.

The question of how long one needs to treat patients with ciclosporin is somewhat open-ended. It appears that an immunologically tolerant state is not induced with this medication, and therefore an extended therapeutic course is indicated in most patients. We have stopped the medication in some patients with no recurrence of their disease, which may be explained by the fact that the disease has run its course.

On the basis of our early observations,[110,112,113] ciclosporin was used in patients with active bilateral sight-threatening noninfectious uveitis who were unable to tolerate systemic corticosteroid therapy at a moderate dose (>25 mg of prednisone) necessary for the treatment of their intraocular inflammatory disease.[114] Of special interest was the particularly positive clinical effect seen in patients with Behçet's disease who were treated with this medication.[115] This has been supported by a randomized, masked study in Japan[116] and in a study carried out by Diaz-Llopis and colleagues,[117] who found that with a dose of 5 mg/kg/day and a maintenance dose of 2 mg/kg/day, a good response was seen in 86% of patients, with a disappearance of attacks in 43%. This appears to be the one disease in which ciclosporin might be considered as an initial therapeutic agent combined with a moderate amount of prednisone, but only if specific criteria are met (see Chapter 26).

Several reports support the use of ciclosporin in various types of intraocular inflammatory disease. Ciclosporin is now usually used in conjunction with another immunosuppressive agent, probably most frequently with corticosteroids. Towler and coworkers[118] treated 13 patients with chronic intraocular inflammation with a mean ciclosporin dosage of 4.1 mg/kg/day, combined when needed with 15 mg or less of prednisone per day. They found that 10 patients had improved visual acuity, and in the other three acuity remained stable. One patient needed to return to an alternative form of immunosuppression. Secchi and colleagues,[119] in an open, noncontrolled, multicenter long-term study of the use of ciclosporin, found it useful in the treatment of patients with posterior and intermediate uveitis, reducing the number and severity of attacks while improving visual acuity and reducing inflammation. Leznoff and coworkers[120] reported a therapeutically positive response with ciclosporin in patients with sympathetic ophthalmia, as well as in a patient with a corneal transplant, but a

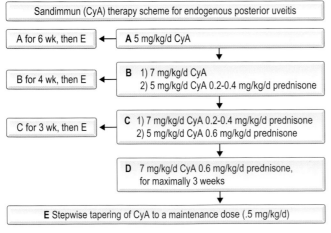

Figure 7-10. Therapeutic scheme for treatment of sight-threatening bilateral endogenous uveitis with ciclosporin. *(Reproduced with permission from Ben Ezra D, Nussenblatt RB, Timonen P: Optimal use of Sandimmune in endogenous uveitis. With kind permission of Springer Science & Business Media.)*

questionable response in patients with intermediate uveitis and serpiginous choroiditis. Pascalis and colleagues[84] reported the use of ciclosporin (initial dose of 5 mg/kg/day) combined with fluocortolone and low-dose methotrexate in treating 32 patients with difficult-to-control noninfectious uveitis. They noted that 20 patients had a return to normal visual acuity, and all had a disappearance of ocular inflammatory activity. The follow-up period was from 6 to 18 months, during which they noted no signs of hepatic or renal toxicity. Ciclosporin is well tolerated by children,[121] with Walton and coworkers reporting improvement in 64% or stabilization in 75% of eyes treated in children and adolescents with uveitis. Hesselink et al.[122] felt that the smaller dose used now reduced the efficacy of ciclosporin. This may be true, but the medication remains a very useful addition to the armamentarium. A recent subgroup analysis of the SITE study (see last paragraph of this chapter) evaluated 373 patients starting ciclosporin montherapy.[123] As was noted in our randomized study, about half gained sustained complete control of their inflammation by 1 year. The authors felt that, along with corticosteroid therapy, ciclosporin was modestly effective for controlling ocular inflammation. Adult dosing, based on the results of this study, ranged from 150 to 250 mg/day. Other agents were probably preferable for patients over the age of 55.

Like corticosteroids, ciclosporin has been placed into slow-release implants. Gilger and coworkers[124] reported that ciclosporin implants decreased the severity of experimental uveitis in horses. A pilot study at the National Eye Institute was initiated to evaluate the safety of such a device and to elicit observations to determine its effectiveness. The implants were tolerated in the small number of patients treated, but a marked therapeutic effect was not seen.[125] Most patients continued to have cystoid macular edema and required systemic immunosuppressive therapy. Slow-release ciclosporin implants will probably be continued to be investigated, but at present they appear to be directed towards treating ocular surface disease.

A topical preparation of ciclosporin is now commercially available and has been shown to be effective in treating moderate to severe dry eye.[126] Although perhaps important for treatment of immune diseases involving the ocular surface, this method of application does not result in significant amounts of drug entering the eye because of the physical properties of the medication. Therefore, topical application does not appear to a useful therapeutic approach for severe intermediate and posterior uveitis in the formulations currently available.

Secondary Effects

Table 7-3 lists the secondary effects we have noted with ciclosporin. However, these were observed when ciclosporin was administered as the sole immunosuppressive agent at 10 mg/kg/day, which we no longer do. At lower doses of ciclosporin the secondary effects noted by our patients have diminished considerably. When these side effects do occur, they are usually well tolerated by this group of highly motivated patients. However, the two secondary problems that cause the most concern for the treating physician are hypertension and renal toxicity. Depending on one's definition of renal toxicity, it develops in as many as 75–100% of patients treated with ciclosporin.[100,127] It is not clear what the inci-

Table 7-3 Secondary effects associated with administration of ciclosporin (10 mg/kg/day) in patients with uveitis

Effects	Incidence (%)
Symptoms	
Paresthesia/hyperesthesia	40
Epigastric burning	20
Fatigue	24
Hypertrichorism	20
Gingivitis	20
Reduced appetite	5
Breast tenderness/fibroadenoma	8
Hidradenitis	4
Signs	
Hypertension	24
Mild anemia	24
Hyperuricemia	20
Increased sedimentation rate	75
Abnormal liver function tests	6
Renal toxicity	?
No opportunistic infections or lymphoma	

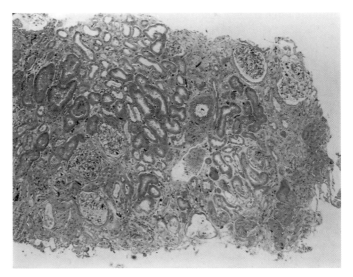

Figure 7-11. Renal biopsy from patient receiving ciclosporin for uveitis. Interstitial fibrosis and marked patchy loss of renal tubules suggest toxicity due to this agent. Serum creatinine level was within normal limits at the time of biopsy.

dence of irreversible renal toxicity will be with the lower dosage of ciclosporin now recommended. At a higher dosage the alterations we noted on renal biopsy, after an average of 2 years of therapy, were renal tubular atrophy and interstitial fibrosis, with the glomeruli remaining mainly intact. Renal vascular alterations can also appear[127] (**Fig. 7-11**). These alterations were noted histologically when the mean serum creatinine level of the patients undergoing biopsy was 1.5 mg/dL, within the upper limits of normal. It would appear that there is a reversible and irreversible component to the renal toxicity induced by ciclosporin. It may be that the starting dose of 10 mg/kg/day sets into motion the mechanisms leading ultimately to the changes noted histologically. Some have found that changes in renal function can develop even at lower starting doses of ciclosporin.[128] However, most recent reports from investigators treating autoimmune conditions (other than uveitis) with lower starting and maintenance doses of ciclosporin have been heartening because little or no alteration in renal function associated with this agent has been noted.[111] Feutren and Mihatsch[129] reviewed 192 renal biopsy specimens from patients treated with ciclosporin for a variety of conditions, including diabetes mellitus, Sjögren's syndrome, and uveitis. It was found that three independent variables distinguished the 41 patients with ciclosporin-induced nephropathy from those free of nephropathy: a higher initial dose of ciclosporin, a larger maximal increase in the serum creatinine concentration above baseline, and age. Therefore it has been suggested that to reduce the risk of nephropathy a dose of 5 mg/kg/day should be used, and serum creatinine levels should not rise more than 30% over the patient's baseline level. Also, a retrospective analysis of 1663 patients who had undergone renal transplantation and were receiving long-term ciclosporin therapy demonstrated that progressive toxic nephropathy did not occur.[130] The addition of bromocriptine[131] to the regimen permits the use of a lower dose of ciclosporin, with the hope that a similar therapeutic result with less toxicity would be achieved. However, this approach is not being used. Ciclosporin interacts with many agents, and one must be very cognisant of this. The concomitant use of NSAIDS with ciclosporin will almost ensure decreased renal function. Other medications that can interact with ciclosporin can be seen in **Box 7-2**.

We and others[132,133] have reported that ciclosporin can be found in the anterior chamber of patients receiving systemic medication, and in the CSF as well. A recent report by Mora et al.[130] suggested that tear-fluid levels of ciclosporin correlated with systemic levels of the medication.

Opportunistic infections have not been a major problem in patients with uveitis treated with ciclosporin. Certainly,

Box 7-2 Some medications that may interact pharmokinetically with ciclosporin

Amiodarone
Carbamazepine
Clarithromycin
Corticosteroid
Diltiazem
Doxycyclin
Erythromycin
Fluconazole
Itraconazole
Ketoconazole
Nicardipine
Nifedipine
Phenytoin
Protease inhibitors
Rifampin
Verapamil
Theophylline

some risk is present if patients receive other immunosuppressive agents combined with ciclosporin. A trend was observed toward less renal toxicity in patients who received combined ciclosporin/steroid therapy rather than ciclosporin alone.[134] We have noted that patients with uveitis treated with ciclosporin demonstrate appropriate immune responses both to new antigens and to old ones requiring a 'recall' response.[135] Therefore, vaccination can apparently be performed on patients treated with this medication, but pre- and post-immunization titers should be checked. Further, to date, no lymphomas or other ciclosporin-related neoplasms have been seen in our patients. The incidence of lymphoma observed in graft recipients treated with ciclosporin was 0.3%.[100] Most disease develops in the first few months and has mainly been associated with multiple-drug regimens. Ciclosporin may cause CNS changes: the most common we have seen are tremors (at higher dosages). It has been suggested that Behçet's patients receiving ciclosporin may develop CNS problems, but that was not seen in the original randomized study in Japan. However, it has been reported to cause headache, mood alterations, and rarely leukoencephalopathy, seizures, visual disurbances, psychiatric problems, and motor and speech disturbances.[136]

Tacrolimus

Mode of Action

Tacrolimus (FK506), an immunosuppressive agent with a molecular weight of 822 Da, was isolated from the broth of *Streptomyces tsukubaensis*[137,138] (**Fig. 7-12**) and is believed to have essentially the same mechanism of action as ciclosporin.[102] One difference is that the immunophilin that binds with tacrolimus is FK506-binding protein (FKBP) instead of cyclophilin. It suppresses the formation of mRNA for IL-2, as does ciclosporin, but at an effective in vitro therapeutic concentration about 100 times less than that of ciclosporin.[138] Using a dose 10–30 times smaller than that of ciclosporin, tacrolimus was found to be effective in preventing the development of experimental autoimmune uveitis in rats[139] as well as in monkeys.[140] However, the toxic effects (see later discussion) are seen at therapeutic doses, so that the decreased therapeutic dosage appears to have little benefit. It is metabolized by the cytochrome P450 system.

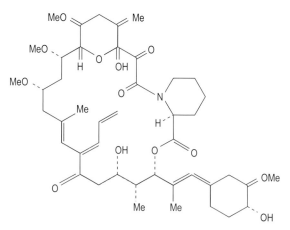

Figure 7-12. Structure of tacrolimus (FK506). *(From Schreiber SL, Crabtree GR. The mechanism of action of ciclosporin A and FK506. Immunol Today 1992; 13: 136.)*

Indications and Dosages

An open-label clinical trial to evaluate the use of tacrolimus was performed in Japan; 53 patients (most with Behçet's disease) were treated at varying doses, and about three-quarters were thought to have benefited.[141] A review of patients with Behçet's disease alone[142] confirmed these initial observations. A daily dose of 0.10–0.15 mg/kg body weight/day has been suggested to be appropriate. Sloper and co-workers[143] reported their experience with tacrolimus, treating six patients with uveitis refractory to ciclosporin. Five of the six patients had a two-line or more improvement. Kilmartin and colleagues[144] reported on seven patients with uveitis treated with tacrolimus, with two being withdrawn from therapy and the other five continuing. An initial dose of 0.05 mg/kg/day has generally been used in the treatment of uveitis, whereas for use in transplant recipients doses of 0.10–0.15 mg/kg/day have been used. Concentrations in the blood need to be monitored.

Secondary Effects

With essentially the same mechanism of action as ciclosporin, one might assume similar secondary effects for tacrolimus. Adverse affects include renal impairment, noted in 28% of patients reported by Mochizuki and colleagues.[141] Neurologic symptoms, including tremors, headache, ophthalmoplegia, and meningitis-like symptoms, have been noted. Gastrointestinal symptoms, usually manifested as nausea, loss of appetite, and abdominal pain, can occur. Hyperglycemia was reported by Mochizuki and colleagues[141] in 13% of patients. In a report comparing the nephrotoxic effects of tacrolimus and ciclosporin in liver transplant recipients,[145] the early development of severe nephrotoxicity was noted only in some patients receiving tacrolimus.

Lx 211 (Voclosporin)

With ciclosporin being the first, efforts have begun to evaluate the next generation of calcineurin inhibitors for uveitis and other ophthalmic indications.[146] This molecule has a modification of the functional group on the amino acid residue at position 1 of the parent molecule (**Fig. 7-13**). This was designed to affect the metabolism of the new molecule. It is felt that this change gives the molecule a more predict-able pharmacokinetic profile, greater biologic activity and less toxicity.[146] Voclosporin's therapeutic effectiveness has been tested in the EAU model and was found to effectively suppress the expression of EAU; it also inhibited lymphocyte proliferation from these animals.[147] At present Lx211 is being evaluated in three phase III trials, with over 500 patients enrolled worldwide. The results should be made known sometime in 2009.

Rapamycin

Mode of Action

Rapamycin (Rapamune, Sirolimus) is a macrolide immunosuppressant purified from isolates of *Streptomyces hygroscopicus* collected on Rapa Nui (Easter Island).[148] It blocks the proliferative signals of transduction in T cells[149,150] (**Fig. 7-14**). This blockage has been shown to prevent the expression of IL-2, IL-4, and IL-6. Of great interest and potential therapeutic importance is the fact that rapamycin's effect occurs much later in the cell cycle (G_1 to S-phase transition) than that of either ciclosporin or tacrolimus. Rapamycin appears not to inhibit the expression of IL-2 receptors and IL-2 production, but may interfere with the cell's ability to respond to interleukins, such as IL-2 and IL-4.[149,151] Rapamycin is bound in the cytoplasm to the same immunophilin as tacrolimus (FKBP), and therefore these two agents will competitively inhibit each other if placed in the same environment.

Indications and Dosages

Rapamycin has been used in a small number of patients with uveitis, as well those undergoing renal transplantation[152,153] at a dose of 2 mg/day. Because it is bound by the same cytoplasmic receptor as tacrolimus, the two agents should not be given together. Rapamycin has been shown to be very effective in inhibiting the induction of EAU in Lewis rats[154] and in completely inhibiting transfer of EAU[155] at a dose of 0.1 mg/kg/day given as a continuous intravenous infusion. Studies have shown that ciclosporin and rapamycin may have a synergistic effect in vitro on T lymphocytes.[156] The combination of ciclosporin 2 mg/kg/day (one-fifth the normal dose) plus intravenously administered rapamycin 0.01 mg/kg/day (one-tenth the normal therapeutic dose) will act synergistically to prevent the expression of EAU.[157]

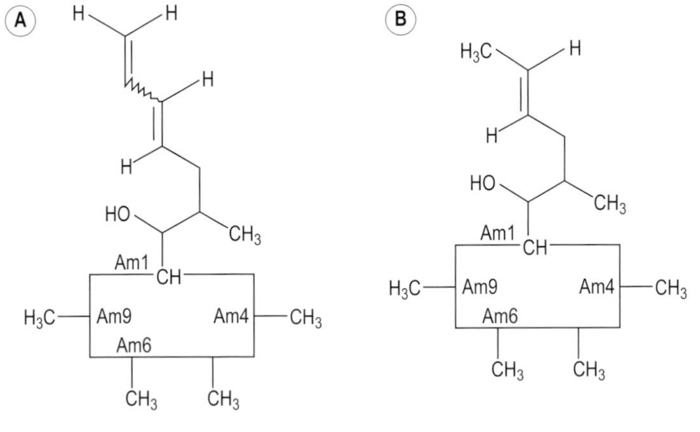

Figure 7-13. **A,** Structure of Lx 211, compared with **B** ciclosporin. *(From Anglade E, et al. Next-generation calcineurin inhibitors for ophthalmic indications. Exp Opin Invest Drugs 2007; 16: 1525–40.)*

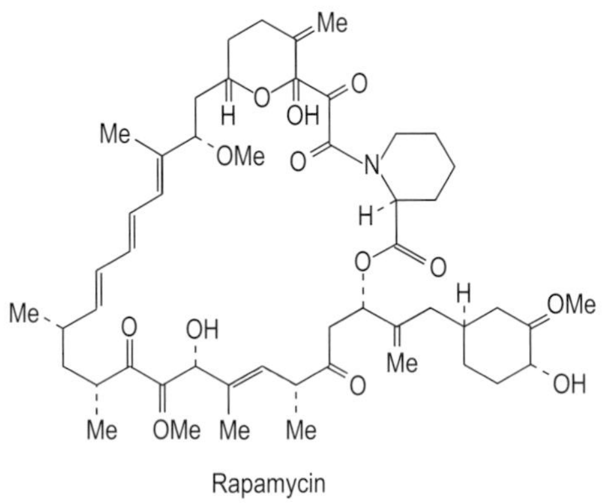

Rapamycin

Figure 7-14. Structure of rapamycin. *(From Schreiber SL, Crabtree GR. The mechanism of action of ciclosporin A and FK506. Immunol Today 1992; 13: 136.)*

There is great interest in the possible role of rapamycin in inducing peripheral immune tolerance.

Toxicity

At a therapeutic dosage of 0.1 mg/kg/day animals have been reported to lose weight.[150] Of concern have been reports of myocardial toxicity in rats.[158] However, these have occurred at relatively high doses of the drug. Gastrointestinal vasculitis has been noted in dogs.[159] In some patients diarrhea and a pneumonitis have been associated with the administration of the drug. It is hoped that with combined rapamycin and ciclosporin therapy the markedly lowered doses may provide adequate immunosuppression with minimal or no risk of toxicity. Even better, it is theoretically possible that rapamycin combined with a monoclonal antibody such as daclizumab (see below) may induce peripheral tolerance.

Antibodies and monoclonal antibodies

Antibodies and monoclonal antibodies directed against various parts of the immune cascade have been used more and more extensively in the treatment of uveitis in humans.[160,161] (**Table 7-4**). These antibodies have been used for some time in other areas of medicine. Anti-T-cell monoclonal antibodies, such as OKT3, have been recognized as effective immunosuppressive agents,[162] and their use to prevent renal graft rejection has become well established.[163] Many regimens for the prevention of graft rejection call for OKT3 monoclonal antibody therapy, followed by other immunosuppressive therapy. It was reported that two patients who underwent renal transplantation suffered marked visual loss after OKT3 therapy.[164] In the one patient tested the results of the electroretinogram were flat.

More and more antibodies directed against specific receptors to lymphokines on T cells and other players in the immune system have been developed and evaluated. Other biologic agents, alemtuzumab and anakinra, have been used

in limited case reports for ocular inflammatory diseases, although others have been used more extensively. One of the prime targets for such therapy has been the IL-2/IL-2 receptor complex. The 55-kDa Tac subunit is expressed on T and B cells after lymphokine or antigen activation. Monoclonal antibodies directed against the 55-kDa Tac subunit have been developed. These anti-Tac antibodies have been reported to be effective in prolonging allograft survival in monkeys and humans[165,166] and in reducing the incidence of graft-versus-host disease in humans.[167] Initial problems dealt with immune reactions against a foreign protein (i.e., mouse-produced antibody), but technology now has permitted these antibodies to be 'humanized' (**Fig. 7-15**) so that essentially they are not recognized as 'foreign.'[168] Another area of prime interest is the TNF/TNF receptor complex.

Adhesion molecules (see Chapter 1) are an area of great interest both for the basic researcher and those interested in interventional studies. Injections of anti-Mac-1 antibodies have been shown to inhibit endotoxin-induced uveitis.[169] Using several models of ocular inflammation, Rosenbaum and Boney[170] demonstrated that the time of administration was important. Whitcup and coworkers[171] have shown that monoclonal antibodies directed against intercellular adhesion molecule-1 (ICAM-1) and lymphocyte function-associated molecule-1 inhibited EAU. Antibodies against ICAM-1 are being used to prevent allograft rejection and to treat rheumatoid arthritis in humans.

Daclizumab

The IL-2 receptor (IL-2R) system is a well-characterized lymphokine receptor system that plays a central role in the induction of immune responses. High-affinity IL-2R complexes are expressed on activated lymphoid cells. They consist of three subunits (α, β, and γ), each capable of binding IL-2. The 70-kDa IL-2R and 64-kDa IL-2R subunits are normally expressed on most resting T, B, natural killer

Table 7-4 Examples of biologic products*

Agent	Proprietary	Target	Mode	Application
Infliximab	Remicade	TNF-α	Chimeric	RA, Crohn's, uveitis
Daclizumab	Zenapax	CD25/IL-2	Humanized	Transplantation, uveitis
Basiliximab		CD25/IL-2	Chimeric	Transplantation
Etanercept	Enbrel	TNF-α	Fusion protein	RA, JIA
Efalizumab	Raptiva	CD11a	Humanized	Psoriasis, uveitis
Adalimumab	Humira	TNF-α	Humanized	RA, Crohn's, uveitis
Muromonab-CD3	OKT3	CD3	Murine	Organ transplant rejection
Alemtuzumab	Campath-1H	CD52	Humanized	Leukemia/lymphoma
Ibritumomab	Zevulin	CD20	Murine + chelator + radioactive subs.	Lymphoma
Rituximab	Rituxin	CD20	Chimeric	Lymphoma, RA
Omalizumab	Xolair	IgE-Fc Binding Domain	Humanized	Mostly Asthma
Tocilizumab	Actemra	IL-6R	Humanized	Under review – RA
Nimotuzumab	BIOMAb EGFR	EGFR inhibitor	Humanized	Glioma (India)
Abatacept	Orencia	CTLA-4	Fusion Protein	Rheumatoid Arthritis

*The reader needs to be aware of the most recent rules and regulations concerning these medications. The information here is merely meant to give examples and is by no means complete or suggestive of therapeutic approaches.

Monoclonal Antibodies

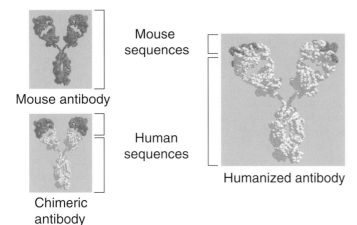

Mouse antibody

Mouse sequences

Chimeric antibody

Human sequences

Humanized antibody

Figure 7-15. Monoclonal antibodies are usually derived in mice. Giving such an antibody to humans induces an immune response against it because it is seen as foreign. Some antibodies are chimeras, which reduces the foreign antigen load to some degree. Most antibodies now are 'humanized' with very few of the original amino acids left, which permits the necessary conformational integrity of the antibody. *(Courtesy Protein Design Laboratories.)*

(NK) and lymphokine-activated killer cells, which mediate signaling and receptor internalization. The 55-kDa IL-2 (p55, Tac, or CD25) subunit, on the other hand, is expressed by most T, B, and NK cells only after they have been activated by interaction with an antigen or with IL-2. The Tac subunit associated with the IL-2R β-γ subunits forms the high-affinity IL-2R complex. Thus expression of the Tac subunit marks a critical step in the activation of all T cells that are major contributors to both allograft destruction and autoimmune disorders. Caspi and associates[169] demonstrated the presence of high-affinity IL-2 receptors in animal models of uveitis (see Chapter 1). Additionally, IL-2 receptors can be demonstrated on the surface of human cells in patients with uveitis. The humanized anti-Tac monoclonal antibody (daclizumab, Zenapax) is a recombinant monoclonal immunoglobulin of the human immunoglobulin (Ig) G_1 isotype. The recombinant genes encoding daclizumab are a composite of human (90%) and murine (10%) antibody sequences. Therefore, the antibody is 'humanized' by combining the complementarity-determining regions and other selected residues of the murine anti-Tac antibody with the framework and constant regions of the human IgG_1 antibody. It is hoped that daclizumab can suppress the autoreactive T cells, which play a critical role in the development of intraocular inflammation in patients with uveitis. There are no known toxicities specific to daclizumab, although administration of such a foreign protein could cause an allergic or anaphylactic reaction. Some of the reactions that may have been associated with daclizumab in a small number of patients were shortness of breath and low blood pressure.

A trial of daclizumab at the National Eye Institute, which has been going on for several years,[172,173] suggests that there is a benefit from daclizumab therapy for the treatment of noninfectious uveitis. This observation is based on outcomes from a small group of patients. In the original study, nine of 10 participants with uveitis treated with daclizumab infu-

sions every 4 weeks were successfully tapered off their standard immunosuppressive regimens and subsequently continued to receive daclizumab, with maintenance or improvement of their visual acuity. After 4 years seven of these 10 patients continued to receive the drug. Patients initially received infusions and currently receive a subcutaneous preparation of the medication once a month. Adverse effects possibly but not clearly related to daclizumab recorded in this study included cutaneous lesions, edema, upper extremity neuralgia, upper respiratory tract infections such as colds and bronchitis, and herpes zoster. One patient in this study, after 4 years of monthly daclizumab therapy, was found to have a small, low-grade renal cell carcinoma that was surgically removed. This patient was initially withdrawn from further daclizumab treatments, but subsequently the treatment was restarted. Further studies have included a small multicenter study examining the possibility of treatment with subcutaneously administered daclizumab without an infusion as induction therapy. Preliminary data suggest that de novo subcutaneous daclizumab therapy yields very good serum levels for an extended period, permitting a taper of other immunosuppressive agents. It would appear that this approach is useful in treating disease that is controlled: that is, daclizumab is given when patient's disease is controlled with 'standard' immunosuppression, which then can be tapered, leaving daclizumab as the only agent. Papaliodis and colleagues[174] have reported that daclizumab was an effective therapeutic agent for some of their patients. We noted that patients with active intraocular inflammatory disease did not respond as well as those with quiet disease who then were switched to daclizumab therapy. We performed a small study treating patients with active intermediate and posterior uveitis who initially received 8 mg/kg of daclizumab followed 2 weeks later by 4 mg/kg, after which a standard dose of daclizumab was administered monthly. By 4 weeks, four of the five patients showed a two-step decrease in vitreous haze, with the fifth patient meeting that step at week 20. Vision at enrollment was 69.2 ETDRS letters, and following treatment was 78.2 letters (p < 0.12).[175]

Etanercept

Etanercept (Enbrel) is engineered to contain two identical soluble tumor necrosis factor (TNF) receptors that have been fused with the Fc domain of human IgG_1. This molecule binds to and inactivates TNF. In support of the use of this medication in the treatment of human disease is the finding that TNF-α is found during the acute phase of experimental autoimmune uveoretinitis.[176] Additionally, TNF-α levels are higher in both the aqueous and the serum of patients with uveitis compared with those of control subjects.[177] Interestingly, the serum levels were significantly higher than the aqueous levels and correlated with recurrent uveitis. In the clinical realm etanercept has been used extensively in the treatment of patients with rheumatologic disorders. In one randomized study, patients with persistently active rheumatoid arthritis despite methotrexate therapy did significantly better when etanercept was added to their regimen (25 mg subcutaneously twice weekly).[178] In a study treating children with polyarticular juvenile rheumatoid arthritis, patients' joints responded statistically far better to etanercept (0.4 mg/kg subcutaneously twice weekly) than to placebo.[179] No differences in adverse effects were noted. The effect of this medication and the next (infliximab) seems not to be as clear. Smith and colleagues[180] evaluated 16 patients, 14 receiving etanercept and two receiving infliximab for either eye inflammation or joint disease. Eight patients had rheumatoid arthritis, three had juvenile rheumatoid arthritis, and three had uveitis without joint disease. All of the 12 with articular disease saw benefits with either medication; however, only six of 16 (38%) of those with uveitis had any benefit. It was the conclusion of the authors that other TNF inhibitors, particularly Remicade, may be better at controlling associated inflammatory arthritis than uveitis.

The major concern associated with this agent is infection. Patients who have received etanercept have developed serious infections, including sepsis, and several have died from their infections within 2–16 weeks of initiation of therapy. Etanercept should not be used in patients with active infections, whether chronic or acute or localized or generalized, and it should be discontinued if a patient develops a serious infection. Live vaccines should not be given. The most frequent adverse events reported in clinical trials were injection site reactions (37%), infections (35%), and headaches (17%). Malignancies were rare;[181] autoantibody development has been reported, although clinical symptoms of a lupus-like syndrome are rare. As with infliximab, there is concern regarding the possible reactivation of tuberculosis. Fonollosa et al.[182] reported that a tuberculous uveitis appeared in a patient receiving etanercept for rheumatoid arthritis.

Infliximab (Remicade)

Infliximab is a mouse-derived chimeric monoclonal antibody directed against TNF-α. It interferes with the binding of TNF to the two known receptors – TNFr1, which binds to soluble TNF, and TNFr2, which binds membrane-bound TNF. One group of authors[183] reported giving five patients with Behçet's disease one infliximab infusion, with a marked resolution of disease within 24 hours and 'complete' suppression by 7 days (see also the review by Sfikakis[184]). It is difficult to assess the value of this treatment because the authors reported that ocular inflammatory disease went into remission after 7 days, which is what could occur during the natural course of Behçet's disease. Here only a comparison of the number of attacks could really help to assess the value of this approach (see Chapter 26). However, more reports have appeared strongly suggesting that these initial observations may be valid. Indeed, criteria for the use of infliximab in Behçet's disease have been published, suggesting its use if first-line agents are not effective.[185] Pipitone et al.[186] reported the usefulness of this agent in treating neuro-Behçet's. Seven patients with HLA-B27-associated anterior uveitis were treated with infliximab (10 mg/kg);[187] six of the seven responded, but relapses were seen in four after a median of 5–6.4 months. It has been used for active scleritis with good results.[188] There have numerous reports using this medication in childhood uveitis and other types of intermediate and posterior uveitis as well as retinal vasculitis. As with all studies authors claim success (we do that too!). It is clear from the number of articles that there should be a real therapeutic effect. However, the caveat is always that without a controlled trial we just cannot measure its real effect, in either the short or the long term.

As with etanercept, the major concern with infliximab is an increased risk of infection, in particular tuberculosis[189] (including its unmasking), with one calculation being a risk of 70 in 147 000 cases. Ten instances of life-threatening *Histoplasmosis capsulatum* infection have also been reported, nine in patients receiving infliximab and one in a patient receiving etanercept.[190] It has been suggested that signaling through the TNF2 receptor may be crucial in host defenses against intracellular pathogens such as tuberculosis. In addition, the use of infliximab may enhance brain lesions associated with multiple sclerosis. These changes were noted on magnetic resonance images.[191] However, in one patient with neurosarcoidosis, infliximab therapy was thought to be beneficial.[192] An aseptic meningitis and lupus-like syndromes have been reported, as has been a retrobulbar optic neuritis.[193] Although methotrexate-associated pneumonitis is seen in 1% of patients, Kramer and associates[194] reported pulmonary toxicity in three of 50 patients (6%) receiving a stable dose of methotrexate and infliximab. Malignancies are rare.[181]

Adalimumab (Humira)

Adilimumab is a fully human anti-TNF-α monoclonal antibody (IgG$_1$) that blocks the interaction of TNF-α with p75 and p55 cell surface receptors. It has been evaluated in a several trials in rheumatoid arthritis, including studies combining it with methotrexate. It has been licensed for use in rheumatoid arthritis and psoriatic arthritis, and has been reported to be useful in the treatment of Behçet's disease,[195,196] VKH (one case),[197] and childhood uveitis.[198,199] Humanized monoclonal antibodies are theoretically superior to those that are chimeric. However, whether this agent will show equal therapeutic effectiveness to infliximab still remains to be seen. To date no cases of tuberculosis have been reported with this agent, but its use should be avoided in patients with multiple sclerosis.[161]

Efalizumab (Raptiva)

We and others have seen that adhesion molecules play an important role in the ocular immune response. CD11a and CD 18 are subunits of LFA-1, a T-cell surface molecule important in T-cell activation, T-cell migration into sites of inflammation, and cytotoxic T-cell function. LFA-1 interacts with ICAM-1 on the vascular endothelial cells at targeted sites to regulate cell trafficking and migration. Binding to CD11a on lymphocytes blocks the interaction between LFA-1 and ICAM-1, thereby interrupting lymphocyte migration and inflammation. The blockage is reversible and does not deplete T cells. We have shown that interference with adhesion molecule function, including CD11a, positively altered the course of disease in animals with experimentally induced uveitis.[171] Efalizumab is a humanized immunoglobulin (Ig) G$_1$ version of the murine efalizumab monoclonal antibody MHM24, which recognizes human and chimpanzee CD11a. Efalizumab blocks T cell-dependent functions mediated by LFA1, including inhibition of the mixed lymphocyte response to heterologous lymphocytes and adhesion of human T cells to keratinocytes. Efalizumab has been approved by the FDA for the treatment of adults with moderate to severe chronic plague psoriasis,[200] which is believed to be a T cell-mediated disease. It is a subcutaneous injection that is given weekly, the usual dose being 0.7 mg/kg initially and then 1 mg/kg. We evaluated the safety and possible effectiveness of efalizumab in treating uveitic macular edema. Six patients received weekly subcutaneous injections for an extended period, during which no serious side effects were noted. Best visual acuity improved by over six letters in the worst eye, together with reductions in macular thickness.[201] Recently two cases of progressive multifocal leukoencephalopathy (PML) have been reported in older patients with plaque psoriasis who received efalizumab for many years. Although other medications have been associated with this complication, it is not yet clear how this will affect the further use of this medication for uveitis. One possible approach taken for other medications is to reserve this for short-term use in order to effect a quick therapeutic response. However, as of this writing, sales of Raptiva in the United States have been suspended.

Rituximab (Rituxan)

Rituximab is a genetically engineered chimeric murine/human monoclonal IgG$_1$ κ antibody directed against the CD20 antigen. . The Fab domain of rituximab binds to the CD20 antigen on B lymphocytes, and the Fc domain recruits immune effector functions to mediate B-cell lysis in vitro, leading to B-cell depletion. Rituximab has an approximate molecular weight of 145 kDa. It has been used to treat a number of hematologic processes, including B-cell lymphoma and primary central nervous system lymphoma.[202,203] It will certainly be used for the treatment of primary intraocular lymphoma as there are preliminary reports suggesting usefulness. There are also studies reporting its use in ocular adnexal lymphomas.[204,205] It has been reported to have a positive therapeutic effect in rheumatoid arthritis and other autoimmune diseases.[206] The recommended dose is 375 mg/m^2 as an intravenous infusion, weekly for four to eight doses for non-Hodgkin's lymphoma and two-1000 mg intravenous infusions separated by 2 weeks for rheumatoid arthritis (for rheumatoid arthritis it was given intravenously at days 0 and 15 and was combined with methotrexate 10–25 mg/week). Glucocorticoids, administered as methylprednisolone 100 mg intravenously or its equivalent 30 minutes prior to each infusion, are recommended to reduce the incidence and severity of infusion reactions. In rheumatoid arthritis, treatment with rituximab induced depletion of peripheral B lymphocytes, with all patients demonstrating near complete depletion within 2 weeks after receiving the first dose of Rituxan. The majority of patients showed peripheral B-cell depletion for at least 6 months, followed by subsequent gradual recovery after that time. A small proportion of patients (4%) had prolonged peripheral B-cell depletion lasting more than 3 years after a single course of treatment. In RA studies, total serum immunoglobulin levels, IgM, IgG, and IgA were reduced at 6 months, with the greatest change observed in IgM. However, mean immunoglobulin levels remained within normal levels over the 24-week period. Small numbers of patients experienced reductions in IgM (7%), IgG (2%), and IgA (1%) levels below the lower limit of normal. The clinical consequences of a reduction in immunoglobulin levels in RA patients treated with rituximab are unclear.

This raises a very interesting question as to mechanism, as anti-T-cell therapy has been the dominant approach in the past. B cells may be acting at multiple sites in the autoimmune/inflammatory process, including through the production of rheumatoid factor (RF) and other autoantibodies, antigen presentation, T-cell activation, and/or proinflammatory cytokine production; alternatively, it may be inducing peripheral immune tolerance. It has been used in the treatment of anterior uveitis, Behçet's disease and Wegener's granulomatosis.[207–209]

Anakinra (Kineret)

Anakinra is a recombinant human interleukin-1 receptor antagonist (IL-1RA) that binds to interleukin-1 type 1 receptors. In doing so it downregulates the proinflammatory effects of IL-1. It has been shown to effectively treat the clinical expression of experimentally induced uveitis in mice.[210] Reports of its use in patients with ocular inflammation have appeared. This includes pediatric uveitis patients with CINCA syndrome (chronic infantile neurologic, cutaneous, and articular [211] and the Blau's syndrome, a pediatric granulomatous arthritis associated with the NOD2 gene).[212]

Alemtuzumab (Campath-1H)

This is an anti-CD52 monoclonal antibody that targets T and B lymphocytes. It has been used to treat a variety of hematologic disorders, including myelodysplastic syndrome, aplastic anemia, chronic lymphocytic leukemia, and T-cell leukemias/lymphomas.[213–215] Dick et al.[216] reported its use for severe ocular inflammation in 10 patients with a variety of ophthalmic inflammatory diagnoses, including Wegener's granulomatosis, retinal vasculitis, sympathetic ophthalmia and Behçet's disease. All patients showed an initial improvement, and remission was seen in eight. No serious adverse events were noted during a short follow-up period.[216]

Abatacept (Orencia)

This medication is a fusion protein that consists of the extracellular domain of the human cytotoxic T-lymphocyte-associated antigen 4 (CTLA-4) and a modified Fc portion of an immunoglobulin G$_1$ molecule. It binds to the ligand of CTLA-4 and is used in the treatment of rheumatoid arthritis and juvenile idiopathic arthritis. Its use to date in the treatment of uveitis is very limited, with one paper published so far.[217] It can be used alone or in conjunction with disease-modifying antirheumatic drugs (DMARDs) such as methotrexate, but not with a TNF-α inhibitor. Studies showed that patients receiving abatacept and Remicade had considerably higher rates of infection compared to controls. It is also not recommended in patients with chronic obstructive pulmonary disease, again because of the risk of infection. It may increase the risk of lymphoma and possibly lung carcinoma. Just how useful this medication may be in the treatment of uveitis remains to be seen.

Intravenous immunoglobulin therapy

Intravenous immunoglobulin (IVIg) therapy has been used in the treatment of a few patients with ocular inflammatory disease, including ocular cicatrical permphigoid, VKH, and birdshot retinopathy,[218–220] and in patients with cancer-associated retinopathy.[221] IVIg was initially intended for the treatment of patients with immunodeficiencies. It is a preparation that is almost completely intact IgG, including all IgG subclasses as seen in normal human plasma. It is a pooled

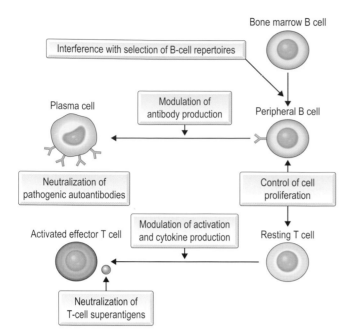

Figure 7-16. Effects of IVIg on the immune system. *(Reproduced with permission from Immunomodulation of Autoimmune and Inflammatory Diseases with Intravenous Immune Globulin Michel D. Kazatchkine, M.D., and Srini V. Kaveri, D.V.M., Ph.D, New England Medical Journal Vol. 345, No. 10 September 6, 2001. Copyright 2001 Massachusetts Medical Society. All rights reserved.)*

material made up from 7–10 000 donors[218] and has slowly found a place in the treatment of putative immune-mediated disorders such as Guillain–Barré syndrome, Kawasaki disease, and juvenile dermatomyositis. The mechanism of its action is speculative (**Fig. 7-16**)[222] and several have been suggested, such as a blockage of B-cell responses, inhibition of phagocytosis, and alteration of cytokine production.[223] Recently it has been suggested that immunoglobulins may neutralize C3a and C5a of the complement cascade, also known as anaphylotoxins.[224] It has been reported to prevent the expression of experimental autoimmune uveitis.[225] Rosenbaum and colleagues[220] treated 10 patients with IVIg, five of whom appeared to have a clear clinical benefit. Patients received 0.5 g/kg body weight/day (infused over 4 hours) for 3 consecutive days on a monthly basis, ultimately changing to an every-3-month schedule. Guy and Aptsiauri[221] reported using IVIg in three patients with carcinoma-associated retinopathy. One patient had increased visual acuity within 24 hours of the first dose, one had an improvement in visual fields but no increase in vision, and one had no improvement. Some concerns that have been raised include the problem of infection despite surveillance. Hepatitis C infection was ascribed to this form of therapy, and we still are concerned about disorders caused by prions. Uveitis has been described in patients after IVIg infusions for immune-mediated (nonocular disorders),[226] and there is a risk of thrombosis, including retinal vein thrombosis. Finally, IVIg should not be given to patients with an isolated IgA deficiency because they develop allergic responses to preparations that contain IgA.

Oral tolerance

Oral tolerance is an approach that has received much clinical interest. A discussion of some of the basic mechanisms leading to the clinical application mentioned here can be found in Chapter 1. Feeding of antigens has been reported to be effective in the treatment of multiple sclerosis and rheumatoid arthritis.[227,228] In a pilot study this approach was applied to two patients with uveitis, one with pars planitis and one with the ocular complications of Behçet's disease.[229] The patients who entered into this study had lymphocytes demonstrating in vitro proliferative responses to the retinal S-antigen. The patient with pars planitis had been treated with prednisone and was able to stop his medication completely once he began the feeding with 30 mg of S-antigen three times a week. Of interest is the fact that because of the maintenance of good visual acuity with the feeding, continued oral dosing of the retinal S-antigen was stopped, in the hope that long-standing tolerance had been achieved. However, the patient had a reactivation of his disease. He was treated with systemic steroids and S-antigen feedings were begun again; he ultimately needed no further medication because his disease abated, and he was left with a visual acuity of 20/20 and 20/25 in each eye. After these observations, a randomized phase I/II masked trial to evaluate the effect and safety of the oral administration of retinal antigens was undertaken.[230] Patients with uveitis were randomly assigned to receive either bovine retinal S-antigen alone, a mixture of soluble retinal antigens alone, retinal S-antigen and retinal soluble antigens, or placebo. Although the time to the primary endpoint (time to ocular inflammatory disease) was not statistically significant for any of the groups, the group that received the purified S-antigen alone appeared to be able to be tapered off their immunosuppressive medication more successfully compared with either the placebo group ($p = 0.08$) or either group receiving multiple soluble antigens. No toxic effects attributable to any treatment were observed (**Fig. 7-17**).

This approach is beginning to attract attention once again.[231] Thurau and Wildner[232] used as antigen for uveitis a 14 amino acid sequence of HLA-B antigens that was seen to mimic retinal S-antigen. The underlying logic for this choice is different from using the retinal S-antigen found in the eye. Here it is hypothesized that because of low avidity, T cells that can bind to this antigen sequence escape the normal clearing mechanisms in the thymus and enter into the systemic circulation. Under certain circumstances these cells can enter the eye and are then activated by antigens in the eye that mimic the original antigen, in the eye perhaps S-antigen, thereby producing a auveitis (**Fig. 7-18**.) Thurau and Wildner would suggest that this could explain the association between HLA class I antigens and uveitis. This approach has been used in a limited number of patients,[233] and a larger proof of concept study is planned.

Interferon-α

Interferon-α is used for its antitumor and antiviral actions, but the exact mechanism for either is not known other than it inhibits tumor growth and viral replication. One report has suggested that IFN-α may inhibit inflammatory processes by enhancing IL-10 production, an event that may be negative in a patient with AIDS but very beneficial in one with an excessive sterile inflammatory response.[234] It has been used in the treatment of the ocular complications of Behçet's disease and multiple sclerosis.[235] Several reports suggest that treatment with IFN-α will diminish or com-

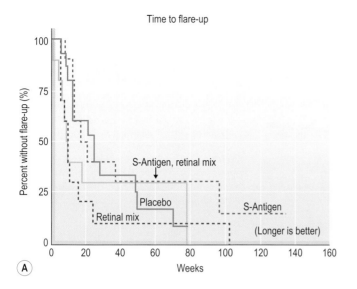

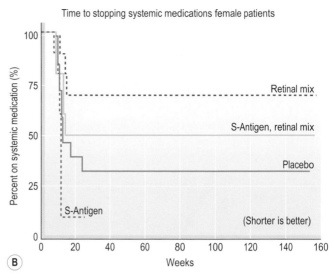

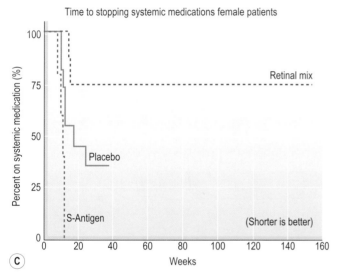

Figure 7-17. Results of the oral administration of bovine S-antigen to patients with uveitis tapering off their immunosuppressive agents. The power of this phase I/II study could definitively demonstrate efficacy. Results are shown as Kaplan–Meier curves. **A,** The time to flare up (i.e., longer is better) was longer in the patients receiving pure S-antigen, whereas those receiving multiple antigens (the retinal mix) did the worst, even when compared with placebo. **B,** Time to stopping medications. Here shorter is better, and the reverse of **A** is seen. Those patients receiving the purified S-antigen alone appeared to be tapered off their immunosuppressive medication more successfully than those given placebo ($p = 0.08$); the retinal mix group did the worst. **C,** Tapering of medications for the female patients. All of these patients receiving S-antigen were tapered off their standard medication. It is unclear why patients receiving multiple antigens should do so much worse, but other studies have now shown this phenomenon. No toxic effects were attributable to the medication. (*Modified from Nussenblatt RB, et al. Treatment of uveitis by oral administration of retinal antigens: results of a phase I/II randomized masked trial. Am J Ophthalmol 1997; 123: 684–7.*)

pletely stop all attacks (see Chapter 26). Kötter and colleagues[236] used an initial dose of 6 × 106 IU subcutaneously daily and then 3 × 106 IU every day for 1 month, followed by 3 × 106 IU subcutaneously every other day. This group saw an improvement in all seven patients treated. Pivetti-Pezzi and coworkers[237] and Wechsler and associates[238] used a dose of 3 × 106 IU three times a week. Pivetti-Pezzi and coworkers[237] saw a 50% reduction of ocular relapses. There have been numerous reports suggesting the usefulness of this approach, from treating nerve-head neovascularization[239] in Behçet's disease to performing intraocular surgery under IFN-α therapy.[240] All patients had a flu-like illness during therapy, and a Behçet's disease-like retinopathy has been associated with IFN-α. It is interesting that the use of IFN for Behçet's disease is far more common in Europe than in North America. The FDA further warns that the α interferons cause or aggravate fatal or life-threatening neuropsychiatric, autoimmune, ischemic, and infectious disorders. Controlled trials will be needed to resolve this difference and see whether the potential advantages outweigh the potential risks.

In summary, the general approach to the use of immunosuppressive agents is to choose the smallest amount histori-cally considered effective for the anatomic area affected (**Fig. 7-19**). However, it is important to establish control of the disease early with sufficient medication and to taper the medication after the inflammation resolves. Topical steroids for anterior segment disease can be most effective if given frequently. Periocular administration of steroids is often overlooked, but it is effective for the patient with unilateral disease or cystoid macular edema, and for the child in whom one wishes to avoid the secondary effects of systemic corticosteroid administration. The use of intraocular steroid (injection or device) may change our therapeutic paradigm significantly. Systemic corticosteroid administration is still the mainstay of therapy in sight-threatening bilateral intermediate and posterior endogenous uveitis, but a second (and sometimes third) agent needs to be started once it is clear that immunosuppressive therapy needs to be continued for an extended period. Both azathioprine (Imuran) and methotrexate, which are being used more frequently in both children and adults, are reasonable steroid- or ciclosporin-sparing agents. The role of monoclonal antibody therapy remains to be seen, and just where intraocular steroid or immunosuppressive therapy will fit also needs evaluation. We generally reserve cytotoxic agents for therapeutic failures

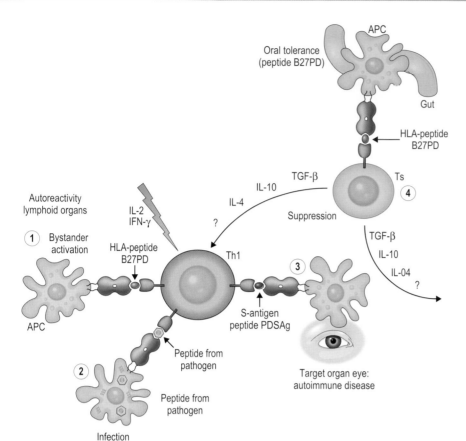

Figure 7-18. Hypothesis explaining role of B27PD: how it may induce uveitis through molecular mimicry. T cells that have a low affinity for MHC will escape to the peripheral circulation. They can be activated when they meet either the original antigen or one that mimics it. In this case if would be the retinal S-antigen in the eye or an antigen from an organism that is invading. These activated T cells will then attack the retina. Feeding B27PD antigen is hypothesized to induce antigen-specific downregulatory cells which will suppress the effector cells. *(From Thurau SR, Wildner G. An HLA-peptide mimics organ-specific antigen in autoimmune uveitis: its role in pathogenesis and therapeutic induction of oral tolerance. Autoimmun Rev 2003; 2: 171–6.)*

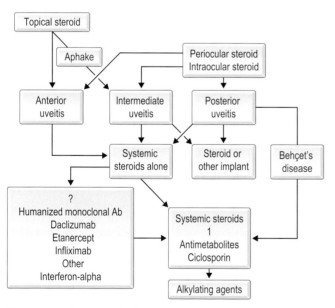

Figure 7-19. Primary medical therapies for endogenous uveitis.

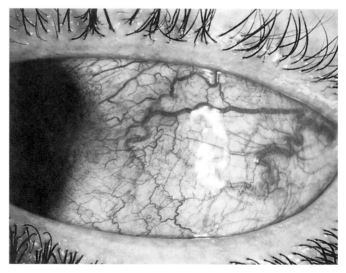

Figure 7-20. Practitioners must always reevaluate their therapeutic approach if no response or a worsening of the condition is seen. This patient was treated with high doses of immunosuppressive agents for scleritis. Therapy worsened the condition. The patient had a large ringlike toxoplasmosis lesion in the retinal periphery, which was severe enough to cause secondary scleritis. Appropriate therapy led to disappearance of the lesion.

with the aforementioned agents. We would not use alkylating agents in children except under the most exceptional of circumstances. It is imperative that the therapeutic approach be reevaluated if the patient's clinical course worsens (**Fig. 7-20**). What is clear is that we now have many more options to offer our patients needing immunosuppressive therapy, and I am sure that these will increase dramatically in the next few years.

Antiviral therapy

It seems appropriate to mention the more frequently used agents for severe intraocular inflammatory disease due to virus. Perhaps in part pushed by the AIDS epidemic, the development of new antiviral agents, particularly against the herpes family of viruses, has been most impressive, and many agents have been introduced in the recent past.[241] This development underlines the increasing importance of better diagnostic testing to rapidly identify the invading virus, which is still sometimes difficult to do and often based on clinical impressions. The importance of rapid, precise diagnosis will take on an even greater importance as the armamentarium against these organisms continues to increase and become more specific.

Aciclovir

The development of aciclovir as an effective antiviral agent stems from the increased understanding of how the herpes family of viruses enters a cell and usurps the cell's control over itself. Nucleosides are needed for the building of new DNA. Nucleosides and aciclovir (**Fig. 7-21**) must be triphosphorylated to be incorporated into a DNA chain. These reactions are mediated by kinases. The diphosphate and triphosphate forms of the nucleoside and aciclovir are mediated through cellular kinases, but the initial phosphorylation of aciclovir is mediated through a kinase (thymidine kinase) specified by the herpesvirus gene. This enzyme is found only in infected cells. The human cellular kinase phosphorylates aciclovir to a very minimal degree, and therefore the drug is most active in those cells that are infected. Aciclovir will take its place in the growing DNA chain, but unlike the nucleoside it lacks a sugar of its own and therefore the DNA chain is terminated at this point. In addition, the DNA polymerase is bound at this point and unable to be used elsewhere. Although aciclovir is highly

effective against herpes simplex virus, it is known that herpesviruses can develop drug resistance through mutational changes in the viral DNA polymerase, making aciclovir triphosphate a poorer substrate. Further, some viruses may mutate and develop a different type of thymidine kinase. In a similar fashion, aciclovir is a very poor substrate for the kinase elaborated by cytomegalovirus. Ganciclovir, dihydroxypropoxymethylguanine (**Fig. 7-22**), a molecule that closely resembles aciclovir is, however, very effective against this member of the herpes family (see later discussion).

For documented herpes simplex or zoster infections, the drug that is currently recommended for immunocompetent patients is aciclovir or its derivatives. The drug can initially be given intravenously to obtain high tissue levels. The initial dose is 5 mg/kg every 8 hours for a patient with a normal serum creatinine level. Renal function should be followed up, and the dose should be adjusted accordingly. Aciclovir can be given orally as well, but its oral absorption is not especially good. For herpes simplex infections, the recommended dose by mouth is 200 mg five times a day. For herpes zoster, higher concentrations are needed and four tablets (800 mg) taken five times a day is recommended. Intravenous aciclovir can suppress renal function, and hydration should be well maintained. Oral aciclovir is usually well tolerated with few significant side effects.

Ganciclovir

Ganciclovir is similar to aciclovir but is a much more effective substrate for cytomegalovirus (CMV). It has been shown to be effective in the treatment of CMV retinitis.[242] Generally, for the induction phase of therapy an initial intravenous dose of 5 mg/kg every 12 hours is given for 14 or 21 days. In the past patients were wedded to this therapy once it had begun, and an indwelling catheter (i.e., Hickman catheter) was placed to facilitate administration. The administration time has an impact on the patient's quality of life. Ganciclovir is not frequently nephrotoxic, but like aciclovir is excreted by the kidneys, and the dose should be adjusted for renal function. Bone marrow depression is problematic if patients are taking antiretroviral agents, such as azidothymidine (AZT), with similar toxicity. Ganciclovir causes significant granulocytopenia, and the dose must be reduced or the drug stopped to keep the absolute granulocyte count at >500–1000/mm³, or granulocyte-stimulating factors can be given. Ganciclovir may have significant testicular toxicity. After the

Acyclovir

Ganciclovir

Figure 7-21. Structures of aciclovir and ganciclovir. Minimal change in the structure of ganciclovir permits it to be considerably more effective against cytomegalovirus infections.

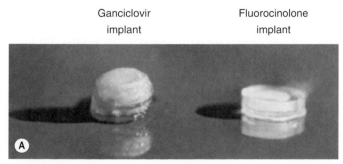

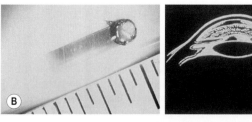

Ganciclovir implant

Fluorocinolone implant

Figure 7-22. A, Comparison of ganciclovir and steroid intraocular devices. *(From Jaffe GJ, et al. Fluocinolone acetonide sustained drug delivery device to treat severe uveitis. Ophthalmology 2000; 107: 2024–33.)* The steroid device is thinner. **B,** Position in vitreous after suturing into sclera at pars plana. *(Courtesy Chiron Corp.)*

induction period, a maintenance dose is given, usually 10 mg/kg/day, adjusted to any renal pathologic condition.

Intravitreal injections of ganciclovir are effective in delaying the progression of CMV retinitis.[243] The injections are initially given twice a week and then weekly. There is an associated risk of endophthalmitis, retinal detachment, and vitreous hemorrhage.[244] An intraocular slow-release device for ganciclovir has been developed[245] (Fig. 7-19). Two rates of release were developed, a 2 µg/h device (with an approximate life span of 4 months) and a 1 µg/h device (with an approximate life span of 8 months). The 2 µg/h device was evaluated in a consecutive case series and was shown to halt CMV progression in 27 patients – or 90% of the 30 eyes into which it was implanted.[246] A randomized controlled trial evaluating the 1 µg/h device showed efficacy in 26 patients (30 eyes).[247]

In that study the median time to progression of CMV retinitis in eyes with the device was 226 days; 12 implants were exchanged for new devices. A final visual acuity of 20/25 or better was obtained in 34 of 39 eyes. The estimated risk of development of CMV in the contralateral eye was 50% over the course of the study, and systemic CMV was documented in 31% of these patients who were not receiving systemic antiviral therapy. Of note was the fact that in the patient group studied, seven late retinal detachments and one retinal tear without detachment occurred. Future studies will certainly deal with the retinal detachment risk and the use of the device in conjunction with oral systemic medications for the prophylactic treatment of patients with CMV infection, either viscerally or in the contralateral eye. The use of local therapy clearly benefits the patient's quality of life, because the hours of intravenous infusion previously needed are avoided. However, the lack of systemic coverage and HAART therapy have to be considered in the treatment strategy.[248]

An oral form of ganciclovir has been developed[249] and has been shown to impede the development of CMV retinitis. Valganciclovir is a monovalyl ester prodrug that is rapidly hydrolyzed to the active form – ganciclovir. Several studies have looked at various combination of the oral formulation compared with the intravenous preparation in the treatment of CMV retinitis. Earlier work looked at the use of an oral formulation combined with a ganciclovir implant.[250] Martin and coworkers,[251] in a randomized controlled trial, compared 160 patients with AIDS and CMV retinitis receiving either valganciclovir or intravenous ganciclovir as induction therapy. Patients were either induced with standard intravenous ganciclovir doses or received valganciclovir 900 mg twice daily orally for 3 weeks as an induction therapy, and then 900 mg daily for maintenance. Orally administered valganciclovir appeared to be as effective as intravenous ganciclovir for induction treatment, and was a convenient and effective maintenance regimen as well.

Valaciclovir

Valciclovir hydrochloride is the hydrochloride salt of the L-valyl ester of the antiviral drug aciclovir. It is given orally and is almost completely converted to aciclovir and L-valine in the intestine and the liver. It has antiviral activity against herpes simplex virus types I and II and herpes zoster, as does aciclovir. After ingestion, about one half of valaciclovir becomes available as aciclovir. The recommended dose of valaciclovir for the treatment of herpes zoster is 1 g orally three times per day. Therapy should be initiated as soon as symptoms and signs appear. For initial episodes of genital herpes the dose recommended is 1 g twice per day for 10 days, and for recurrent disease 500 mg twice per day for 3 days. Overdosing of the drug can lead to acute renal failure.

Famciclovir

Famciclovir is the prodrug of penciclovir. It is an orally administered drug and essentially all is converted to the active antiviral compound, penciclovir. Penciclovir has strong inhibitory effects against herpes simplex virus types 1 and 2, as well as varicella zoster. Tyring and coworkers[252] carried out a study of 454 patients with ophthalmic zoster of the trigeminal nerve. In this study patient were randomized to either oral famciclovir 500 mg three times daily or oral aciclovir 800 mg five times a day for 7 days. The two drugs appeared to demonstrate similar efficacy and famciclovir was well tolerated. Because the drug is cleared in the kidney, dosage must be appropriately reduced for patients with reduced renal function. There are no well-controlled studies in pregnant women. Although testicular toxicity was noted in rodents, studies in normal males did not show a change in sperm count or motility. Urticaria, hallucinations, and confusion have been reported by patients taking the drug.

Foscarnet

Foscarnet (trisodium phosphonoformate) is a pyrophosphate analog that has been shown to be effective in the initial treatment of CMV infection as well as for infections caused by other herpes family viruses in patients undergoing renal and bone marrow transplantation.[253] Although foscarnet is effective, herpes simplex viruses resistant to it already have been reported.[254] Foscarnet is also effective against HIV when it is added to infected cultures.[255] Initially, a continuous intravenous infusion was used in treating CMV infections,[242,256] but now therapy starts with induction doses that are given twice daily, and then a maintenance dose is given once a day (see Table 7-2).[257] In a randomized comparative trial, retinitis progressed after 13 weeks with immediate foscarnet therapy versus 3.2 weeks in those receiving no treatment.[258] As with ganciclovir, the drug is generally administered through an indwelling central line. In a study comparing the efficacy of ganciclovir versus foscarnet, the two drugs appeared to be equivalent in controlling CMV retinitis and maintaining visual acuity.[259] However, this study found that there was a longer survival among the patients receiving foscarnet than in those receiving ganciclovir (12.6 months versus 8.5 months).[260] Foscarnet has been shown to be a useful salvage therapy in patients with CMV retinitis who are intolerant of or whose disease is resistant to ganciclovir.[258,261] Foscarnet has an associated nephrotoxicity, as well as metabolite alterations, that requires constant surveillance with eventual dosage reduction. Foscarnet has been licensed by the Food and Drug Administration (FDA) for the treatment of CMV retinitis.

Alternate means of administering foscarnet have been reported. Gumbel and coworkers[262] have reported the use of liposome-encapsulated foscarnet, and Sarraf and colleagues[263] have used transscleral iontophoresis to deliver foscarnet into the rabbit eye. The evaluation of intravitreal injections of foscarnet into rabbit eyes showed that intermittent injections appeared not to induce retinopathy.[264,265] Diaz-Llopis and colleagues[266] injected foscarnet (in a dose of 2400 µg) into the vitreous of 11 patients (15 eyes). Eight eyes had active CMV retinitis, the rest being in a quiescent stage of disease. These eyes received biweekly injections over a 3-week induction period, which was followed by weekly injections, as did the eyes that were in a quiescent stage. A total of 304 injections were given with a mean follow-up period of 16 weeks, and all eyes appeared to respond therapeutically over the period of the study.

Combined ganciclovir and foscarnet

This approach to therapy was increasingly used, particularly as patient survival lengthened and the possibility of viral resistance increased. Jacobson and coworkers[267] evaluated this approach in 29 patients with AIDS and found that combination therapy appeared to provide better in vivo antiviral activity in suppressing CMV replication than did monotherapy. Weinberg and colleagues[268] treated seven patients (nine eyes) with combination therapy. All of these patients had had progression of their retinitis with a monotherapy regimen, and many were intolerant of the induction doses usually given. The authors found that combination therapy was fairly well tolerated and prolonged the interval to progression. A Studies of Ocular Complications of AIDS (SOCA) randomized study[269] found that the time to progression in the group receiving combination therapy was statistically significantly longer than the time to progression seen in patients receiving either foscarnet or ganciclovir.

Cidofovir

Cidovofir (Vistide), 1-(S)-[3-hydroxy-2-(phosphonylmethoxy)propyl] cytosine dihydrate, is a nucleotide analog that has a broad spectrum of action against herpesviruses. The intracellular metabolite of cidofovir inhibits DNA polymerases from herpesviruses at a 50-fold lower concentration than that needed to inhibit human α-DNA polymerase. The metabolite has a very long half-life of 30 hours.[270,271] Cidofovir has been shown to have good anti-CMV activity, with a median infective dose (ID_{50}) for murine CMV of 0.02 µg/mL compared to 0.3 µg/mL for ganciclovir. This anti-CMV medication should be given only intravenously. It suppresses CMV replication by inhibiting viral DNA synthesis. Cidofovir must be administered with probenecid. There have been clinical trials to show the effectiveness of cidofovir in the treatment of CMV retinitis.[272] The recommended induction dose for patients with a serum creatinine level <1.5 mg/dL, a calculated creatinine clearance level >55 mL/min, and a urine protein level of <100 mg/dL (<2+ proteinuria) is 5 mg/kg body weight given intravenously over 1 hour. It is given once a week for 2 consecutive weeks. A maintenance dose for patients with the renal status mentioned above is 5 mg/kg given every 2 weeks. Renal impairment is the major concern. Acute renal failure may occur even after a few infusions. Cidofovir is contraindicated for treatment of patients receiving other nephrotoxic medications. Intraocular instillation of cidofovir may lead to severe hypotony.

Uveitis after cidofovir administration has been well established.[273]

Fomivirsen

Fomivirsen (Vitravene) is a 21-base phosphorothioate oligodeoxynucleotide which is complementary to mRNA of the major immediate early region proteins of human cytomegalovirus. When placed into the eye, it is slowly cleared with a half-life of about 55 hours in humans.[274] It is not detected in the systemic circulation after intravitreal placement. A series of studies using this drug (which is only available for intravitreal administration) has been reported.[275–277] In one randomized controlled study that used a 165 µg intravitreal fomivirsen dose given weekly three times followed by every other week therapy the time to progression of peripheral retinal lesions of CMV infection was shown to be significantly greater than with deferred therapy. The time to progression was similar to that reported with systemically administered anti-CMV therapy. Two other clinical trials using a 330 µg dose also showed positive results. The evaluation of these studies was complicated by the use of highly active antiretroviral therapy (HAART) and oral ganciclovir.[276] A report evaluating the safety profile of the medication[277] showed that ocular complications were not trivial, with rates calculated from 4.06 to 8.35 events per person-year, depending on the dose used. Ocular inflammation was the most commonly seen event (0.87 event/person-year for the FDA-approved dosing schedule), followed by a pigment retinopathy (0.21 event/person-year), and a transient elevation of intraocular pressure was noted. A good review of these studies puts them into perspective.[278] The fomivirsen dosing schedule is better than that for intraocular injections of either ganciclovir or foscarnet, both of which need to be given as multiple injections per week initially followed by weekly injections. Fomivirsen requires a weekly loading schedule followed by every other week therapy. Probably it should be used in conjunction with systemic anti-CMV medication to prevent disease in the other eye.

In summary, in immunocompetent persons aciclovir remains a reasonable choice for infections caused by the herpesvirus family. There are several other choices, but cost may be a concern. However, aciclovir is, at best, weakly effective against CMV infections, including retinitis. This concern was much greater before the HAART era. It is clear that the number of patients with AIDS in the United States presenting with CMV retinitis has dramatically decreased, but it still occurs. Most patients with CMV retinitis (in whom HAART has usually failed but who are immunosuppressed iatrogenically) begin therapy with systemic ganciclovir rather than foscarnet, despite a randomized study to show that survival is longer with the latter. The reasons for this are complex, but they include the facts that increased intravenous hydration is needed to prevent foscarnet-induced renal toxicity; that most physicians still have more experience with ganciclovir; that foscarnet requires more monitoring; and that patient complaints are more frequent with foscarnet, a problem that may reflect the treating physician's lack of experience with the drug. Patients respond differently to these medications, and some trial and error is unavoidable. The use of colony-stimulating factor to boost granulocyte production and generally overcome bone marrow toxicity helps in administration of ganciclovir at adequate dosages while antiretroviral therapy is continued. Long-term therapy, once available only through a central line placed to continue intravenous therapy, now includes a ganciclovir implant and oral anti-CMV medication. The introduction of sustained-release devices that deliver ganciclovir at a rate that provides therapeutic doses to the eye for up to 8 months has, in our experience, had a profoundly positive effect on the lifestyle of patients. Avoiding the need for daily infusions of drug has been important for these patients. There was of course a tradeoff: these patients were not being treated for the prevention of CMV infection elsewhere, such as in the contralateral eye. The use of oral ganciclovir (and other oral anti-CMV agents that may be developed) may be one alternative therapy that could be coupled with the local device.

Colchicine

Mode of Action

Colchicine, or acetyltrimethylcolchicinic acid, has poorly understood antiinflammatory characteristics. Colchicine suppresses lactic acid production in leukocytes and reduces phagocytosis. In addition, it also reduces polymorphonuclear cell migration.

Indications and Dosages

Heightened polymorphonuclear cell migration is a characteristic of patients with Behçet's disease (see Chapter 26) and may be a cause of the repeated ocular attacks seen in that disorder. Colchicine has been used in the treatment of Behçet's disease. It should be stressed that this agent is not employed to treat the active inflammatory condition but rather is used prophylactically in the person with multiple ocular attacks to reduce the frequency of these attacks, which can lead to blindness. This approach has not met with universal approval, being more popular in Japan than in other countries with a high incidence of this disease, such as Turkey. Many believe that this agent is not effective in treating white patients. Its use might be considered in those fairly rare patients with Behçet's disease who have unilateral involvement and in whom one may not feel fully justified in using more powerful immunosuppressive agents. The average dose of oral colchicine is 0.6 mg twice daily. Some clinicians have suggested that higher dosages may be helpful, but this is based on anecdotal information. Its effect on Behçet's disease has been at best marginal in our experience.

Secondary Effects

Gastrointestinal reactions such as abdominal pain, diarrhea, nausea, and vomiting are quite common. Prolonged administration may cause bone marrow depression, with thrombocytopenia and aplastic anemia. Colchicine is contraindicated in pregnant women because it can harm the fetus.

Mydriatic and cycloplegic agents

The use of mydriatic and cycloplegic agents is an important adjunct to antiinflammatory or immunosuppressive therapy. The major indication for the use of dilating agents is the presence of a 'significant' anterior chamber inflammatory response. In those patients the addition of mydriatics helps

prevent the development of posterior synechiae and, in the extreme, iris bombe. Further, cycloplegia will make the patient more comfortable and helps ensure that the treating physician has an unhindered view of the media and fundus. We generally do not use long-term dilating agents, such as atropine, except postoperatively. Use of the shorter-acting agents, such as tropicamide (Mydriacyl), helps to keep the iris moving and hence reduces the possibility of posterior synechiae. One medication possibly to be avoided in patients with uveitis is cyclopentolate (Cyclogyl), as this has been shown to be an effective chemoattractant for leukocytes.[279] Therefore, the addition of this medication to the therapeutic regimen may prove problematic.

Antitoxoplasmosis therapy

The therapeutic approach to treating ocular toxoplasmosis ideally consists of a combination of medications. Sulfadiazine (or trisulfapyrimidines, a mixture of sulfadiazine, sulfamerazine, and sulfamethazine) prevents the conversion of para-aminobenzoic acid to folic acid, which is needed for the carbon metabolism of the *Toxoplasma* organism, and in humans it is particularly needed for erythropoiesis (**Fig. 7-23**). Pyrimethamine (Daraprim) blocks the conversion of folic acid to folinic acid. A combination of these agents has been found to be synergistic in the killing of *Toxoplasma*. Sulfadiazine can be given as a 1–2 g loading dose, followed by 0.5–1 g orally four times daily. This is given in conjunction with a loading dose of 50–75 mg of pyrimethamine, followed by 25 mg twice daily. The therapy should be given for 3–4 weeks. Folic acid-containing vitamins should be stopped during this treatment period. Because of the potentially serious depression of erythropoiesis that can be a consequence of pyrimethamine therapy, leucovorin, 3–5 mg, is given orally or intramuscularly two or three times a week. We obtain a baseline white blood cell count with differential and a platelet count, and weekly thereafter. We give the leucovorin for 1 week after stopping the pyrimethamine. If there is a decrease in the platelet count (<100 000/mm³) or the appearance of hypersegmented polymorphonuclear lymphocytes, we discontinue the pyrimethamine. Pyrimethamine crosses the blood–brain barrier and is also used in the treatment of congenital toxoplasmosis. Sulfadiazine availability had been very limited in the United States, with clinicians needing to contact the Centers for Disease Control and Prevention in Atlanta, Georgia, for access. This situation has now been remedied, and the drug is now readily available.

Clindamycin has been shown to be effective in killing the *Toxoplasma* organism[280] and has the added advantage of

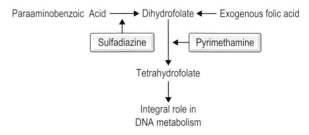

Figure 7-23. Effects of sulfadiazine and pyrimethamine on carbon metabolism in *Toxoplasma* and in humans.

being readily absorbed into ocular tissues. It can be used as a therapeutic substitute for pyrimethamine. Evidence suggests that a synergistic effect may be seen when clindamycin is combined with sulfadiazine.[281] We have used clindamycin 150–300 mg four times daily orally or subconjunctivally combined with the aforementioned sulfadiazine regimen. We treat for 3–4 weeks. We have noted that a large number of patients have suffered enough gastrointestinal distress as a result of this medication to warrant a reduction in the dosage or discontinuation of treatment. A pseudomembranous colitis is a serious side effect of this medication. Clindamycin does not cross the blood–brain barrier and is not effective for the treatment of congenital toxoplasmosis or encephalitis due to *Toxoplasma*. However, it has recently been used intravitreally to treat active toxoplasmosis in a pregnant woman.[282] It should be remembered that this agent has not received FDA approval for this specific indication.

Another medication that has received much attention is atovaquone (Mepron). This hydroxynaphthoquinone has potent antiprotozoal activity. It appears to uncouple mitochondrial electron transport and in doing so inhibits pyrimidine and nucleic acid synthesis in the cell. In one animal study,[283] atovaquone (50 mg/kg/day) given for 15 days significantly extended the lifespan of mice inoculated intraperitoneally with *Toxoplasma gondii* from 9 days to 26 days. Of great interest is the report of studies suggesting that the drug might have activity against *Toxoplasma* cysts.[284] This finding has a significant theoretic value because recurrences are thought to be due to the breaking down of cysts, but recurrences after therapy have been seen and therefore, albeit unproven, it is highly unlikely that cysts are being killed in patients' eyes. Patients with AIDS who have toxoplasmic encephalitis have been treated with atovaquone.[285] The oral dose of atovaquone to date has been 750 mg four times daily. The medication seems to have been well tolerated, even when given concomitantly with AZT or didanosine. Most patients showed stabilization or improvement of their disease for at least some period. We had the opportunity to report the improvement of toxoplasmic retinitis in a patient with AIDS (before the HAART era) after the initiation of atovaquone 750 mg four times daily.[286] Other patients with ocular toxoplasmosis (those with AIDS and immunocompetent patients) have now been treated in the United States as well as in France and Brazil. Patients appear to tolerate the medication well, and observations indicate a therapeutic effect.

Other medications that have been used in the treatment of toxoplasmosis include minocycline, spiramycin, and sulfasoxazole. Minocycline positively alters the clinical course of toxoplasmosis in animals.[287] Spiramycin has been used with some success to treat ocular toxoplasmosis in humans.[288] However, recurrences are very common. It is used in Latin America as a prophylactic agent because it is tolerated reasonably well; its prophylactic efficacy is yet to be evaluated, if indeed it is useful in such a role. Trimethoprim-sulfamethoxazole is perhaps less effective against *Toxoplasma* than either sulfadiazine or trisulfapyrimidine, but nonetheless has been used in the treatment of ocular toxoplasmosis.[289] Tetracycline can be considered for patients in whom the more standard therapies cannot be used. Spiramycin, clarithromycin, and azithromycin have also been used to treat toxoplasmosis, but the numbers of patients reported on to date are not large enough to measure their effectiveness.[290,291]

The use of corticosteroids as the sole therapeutic agent for toxoplasmosis is never indicated. However, there is a role for their judicious use in some patients in combination with antitoxoplasmosis therapy (see Chapter 14).

Other therapeutic approaches

Immunostimulators

This therapeutic approach was quite popular several years ago for the treatment of endogenous uveitis. Levamisole was thought to boost immune responses and might therefore be useful in the treatment of uveitis. Others suggested the use of transfer factor, a leukocyte dialysate that was capable of transferring antigen-specific (such as purified protein derivative) type IV hypersensitivity responses from a sensitized organism to a nonsensitized one. Transfer factor had been used to treat patients with cutaneous candidiasis. In uveitis the suggestion is that an exogenous factor to which the patient is unable to mount an immune response is causing the disease. All information to date suggests that patients with endogenous uveitis are fully immunocompetent, but rather there is a perturbation of their immunoregulatory system. One could frankly argue that the addition of an immunostimulatory agent may exacerbate the problem.

Plasmapheresis

The removal from the bloodstream of toxic products is a concept that originated in the work performed by Abel and coworkers in 1914.[292] The first therapeutic success using plasmapheresis was for macroglobulinemia.[293] The rationale for this approach is that soluble products in the blood could be readily removed, and so it was tried in diseases such as systemic lupus erythematosus, in which immune complexes were thought to play an important role in pathogenesis. The exact mechanism of action of plasmapheresis remains speculative. It is possible that even if humoral mechanisms are less important in intraocular inflammatory disease, this approach could remove cytokines important for the propagation or perpetuation of disease. Its role in uveitis still is not clear. It has been reported as being effective in treating the acute attacks of Behçet's disease,[294] but its continued use is unwieldy, and although initial success may be seen, a rebound of the disease may occur with time. Therefore, to maintain a more prolonged clinical effect, most studies have resorted to adding corticosteroids or cytotoxic agents.[293]

Nonsteroidal antiinflammatory agents

Prostaglandin inhibitors are well known to the ophthalmic community. They have been suggested to be therapeutically helpful for various ocular conditions, including aphakic macular edema.[295] Some reports suggested that indomethacin reduces the severity and recurrences of anterior uveitis when used in conjunction with corticosteroids. Although isolated reports discussed the use of these agents in the treatment of uveitis,[296] they have not been demonstrated to be effective as sole agents in the treatment of endogenous intraocular inflammatory disease. Herbort,[297] however, has looked extensively at the use of diclofenac in the treatment of capsulotomy inflammatory responses after Nd:YAG laser treatment. He reported that an effective therapeutic end-point could be achieved with a combination of dexamethasone acetate 0.1% (Maxidex drops), diclofenac drops 0.1% (Voltaren-Ophtha), and systemic diclofenac (Voltaren). Diclofenac may be useful as a sole agent in treating post-operative cataract inflammation.

It is gratifying to be able to finish this chapter with epidemiologic data concerning the use of immunosuppressive agents over a long period of time. The Systemic Immunosuppressive Therapy for Eye Diseases study (SITE) was able to evaluate the use of immunosuppressive agents in uveitis by collecting data from several centers with long-term experience in the use of these agents in the treatment of these patients.[298] This retrospective cohort study wished to evaluate the risk overall and cancer mortality in uveitis patients treated with immunosuppressive agents: it included 7957 patients, 2340 of whom had received immunosuppressive therapy during the follow-up period, which entailed over 66 000 person-years. The results suggested that the use of azathioprine, methotrexate, mycophenolate mofetil, ciclosporin, dapsone, and systemic corticosteroids did not increase the overall incidence of cancer nor cancer mortality. Cyclophosphamide was not seen to increase overall mortality but did tend to increase overall cancer mortality, although its use can be justified short term in difficult-to-treat sight-threatening conditions.[299] Although the numbers were too small for a more definitive finding, TNF inhibitors may increase overall and cancer mortality. This important study is the first step in obtaining long-term data about the use of these medications.

Caution: The drugs discussed in this chapter may have an important role in the treatment of various types of intraocular inflammatory disease. The reader should be reminded that not all of the drugs described here have been approved by the FDA for use in the treatment of uveitis. Others may be available under study protocols. It is the practitioner's duty to inquire as to the status of any medication and how the drug can be used within an accepted framework. It is also important to remember that some agents have been reported to induce uveitis (**Box 7-3**).

Box 7-3 Medications possibly causing uveitis (according to Micromedex)

Brimonidine
Cidofovir
Demecarium
Deserpidine
Diethylcarbamazine
Echothiophate
Formivirsen
Ganciclovir
Gentian violet
Immunoglobulin
Indinavir
Influenza vaccine
Isoflurophate
Latanoprost
Metipranolol
Pamidronate
Pyrethrum extract/piperonyl butoxide
Rescinnamine
Rifabutin
Ritonavir
Streptokinase
Terbinafine
Trimethoprim
Varicella vaccine

It is important to remember that many of the agents listed have a single or very few case reports associated with the event(s). Others seem more commonly associated with uveitis.

References

1. Nussenblatt RB. Bench to bedside: new approaches to the immunotherapy of uveitic disease. Int Rev Immunol 2002; 21(2–3): 273–289.
2. Wen S, Gao R, Hu Z. Comparison of Chinese traditional therapy combined with Western medicine and Western medicine alone in the treatment of uveitis. Yen Ko Hsueh Pao 1991; 7: 205–208.
3. Gordon D. Prednisone and prednisolone in ocular disease. Am J Ophthalmol 1956; 41: 593–600.
4. Hench P, Kendall E, Slocumb C. The effect of a hormone of the adrenal cortex (17-hydroxy-11-dehyrocorticosterone: compound E) and of pituitary adrenocorticotropic hormone on rheumatoid arthritis. Proc Staff Meet Mayo Clin 1949; 24: 181–197.
5. Clamen H. Anti-inflammatory effects of corticosteroids. Clin Immunol Allergy 1984; 4: 317–329.
6. Fauci AS, Dale DC, Balow JE. Glucocorticosteroid therapy: mechanisms of action and clinical considerations. Ann Intern Med 1976; 84(3): 304–315.
7. Fauci A. Alternate-day corticosteroid therapy. Am J Med 1978; 64: 729–731.
8. Tanner V, Kanski JJ, Frith PA. Posterior sub-Tenon's triamcinolone injections in the treatment of uveitis. Eye 1998; 12: 679–685.
9. Bui Quoc E, Bodaghi B, Adam R, et al. Hypertonie cortisonique apres injection sous-tenonienne de triamcinolone acetonide au cours de l'uveite. J Fr Ophtalmol 2002; 25: 1048–1056.
10. Schlaegel TJ. Essentials of Uveitis. 1969, Boston: Little, Brown and Company. pp 41–42.
11. Freeman W, Green R, Smith R. Echographic localization of corticosteroids after periocular injection. Am J Ophthalmol 1987; 103: 281–288.
12. Penn JS, Rajaratnam VS, Collier RJ, et al. The effect of an angiostatic steroid on neovascularization in a rat model of retinopathy of prematurity. Invest Ophthalmol Vis Sci 2001; 42: 283–290.
13. Cunningham MA, Edelman JL, Kaushal S. Intravitreal steroids for macular edema: the past, the present, and the future. Surv Ophthalmol 2008; 53(2): 139–149.
14. Martidis A, Duker JS, Puliafito CA. Intravitreal triamcinolone for refractory cystoid macular edema secondary to birdshot retinochoroidapthy. Arch Ophthalmol 2001; 119: 1380–1383.
15. Antcliff RJ, Spalton DJ, Stanford MR, et al. Intravitreal triamcinolone for uveitic cystoid macular edema: an optical coherence tomography study. Ophthalmology 2001; 108: 765–772.

16. Roesel M, Tappeiner C, Heinz C, et al. comparison between intravitreal and orbital floor triamcinolone acetonide after phacoemulsification in patients with endogenous uveitis. Am J Ophthalmol 2008; 147: 406–412.

17. van Kooij B, Rothova A, de Vries P. The pros and cons of intravitreal triamcinolone injections for uveitis and inflammatory cystoid macular edema. Ocul Immunol Inflamm 2006; 14(2): 73–85.

18. Jonas JB, Hayler JK, Sofker A, et al. Regression of neovascular iris vessels by intravitreal injection of crystalline cortisone. J Glaucoma 2001; 10: 284–287.

19. Wingate RJB, Beaumont PE. Intravitreal triamcinolone and elevated intraocular pressure. Aust NZ J Ophthalmol 1999; 27: 431–432.

20. Callanan DG, Jaffe GJ, Martin DF, et al. Treatment of posterior uveitis with a fluocinolone acetonide implant: three-year clinical trial results. Arch Ophthalmol 2008; 126(9): 1191–1201.

21. Yeh S, Nussenblatt RB. Fluocinolone acetonide for the treatment of uveitis: weighing the balance between local and systemic immunosuppression. Arch Ophthalmol 2008; 126(9): 1287–1289.

22. Haller JA, Dugel P, Weinberg DV, et al. Evaluation of the safety and performance of an applicator for a novel intravitreal dexamethasone drug delivery system for the treatment of macular edema. Retina 2009; 29(1): 46–51.

23. Kuppermann BD, Blumenkranz MS, Haller JA, et al. Randomized controlled study of an intravitreous dexamethasone drug delivery system in patients with persistent macular edema. Arch Ophthalmol 2007; 125(3): 309–317.

24. Williams GA, Haller JA, Kuppermann BD, et al. Treatment of uveitic macular edema with a dexamethasone posterior-segment drug delivery system. Am J Ophthalmol 2009; 147(6): 1048–1054, 54 e1–e2.

25. Piccolino FC, Pandolfo A, Polizzi A, et al. Retinal toxicity from accidental intraocular injection of depo-medrol. Retina 2001; 22: 117–119.

26. Moshfeghi DM, Lowder CY, Roth DB, et al. Retinal and choroidal vascular occlusion after posterior sub-tenon triamcinolone injection. Am J Ophthalmol 2002; 134: 132–134.

27. Levin DS, Han DP, Dev S, et al. Subtenon's depot corticosteroid injections in patients with a history of corticosteroid-induced intraocular pressure elevation. Am J Ophthalmol 2002; 133: 196–202.

28. Lafranco Dafflon M, Tran VT, Guex-Crosier Y, et al. Posterior sub-tenon's steroid injections for the treatment of posterior ocular inflammation: indications, efficacy and side effects. Graefe's Arch Clin Exp Ophthalmol 1999; 237: 289–295.

29. Jabs DA, Rosenbaum JT, Foster CS, et al. Perspective. Guidelines for the use of immunosuppressive drugs in patients with ocular inflammatory disorders: recommendations of an expert panel. Am J Ophthalmol 2000; 130: 492–513.

30. Reed JB, Morse LS, Schwab IR. High-dose intravenous pulse methylprednisolone hemisuccinate in acute Behcet retinitis. Am J Ophthalmol 1998; 125: 410–411.

31. Fujikawa L, Meisler D, Nozik R. Hyperosmolar hyperglycemic nonketotic coma. A complication of short-term systemic corticosteroids. Ophthalmology 1983; 90: 1239–1242.

32. Wakakura M, Ishikawa S. Central serous chorioretinopathy complicating systemic corticosteroid treatment. Br J Ophthalmol 1984; 68: 329–331.

33. Polito C, La Manna A, Papale MR, et al. Delayed pubertal growth spurt and normal adult height attainment in boys receiving long-term alternate-day prednisone therapy. Clin Pediatr 1999; 38: 279–285.

34. American College of Rheumatology Task Force on Osteoporosis Guidelines, Recommendations for the prevention and treatment of glucocorticoid-induced osteoporosis. Arthritis Rheum 1996; 39: 1791–1801.

35. Hemady R, Tauber J, Foster C. Immunosuppressive drugs in immune and inflammatory ocular disease. Surv Ophthalmol 1991; 35: 369–385.

36. Cash J, Klippel J. Second-line drug therapy for rheumatoid arthritis. N Engl J Med 1994; 330: 1368–1375.

37. Dorr R, Fritz W. Cancer Chemotherapy Handbook. 1980, New York: Elsevier.

38. Buckley CI, Gills JJ. Cyclophosphamide therapy of peripheral uveitis. Arch Intern Med 1969; 124: 29–35.

39. Mamo J, Azzam S. Treatment of Behcet's disease with chlorambucil. Arch Ophthalmol 1970; 84: 446–450.

40. Hoffman G, Kerr G, Leavitt R, et al. Treatment of Wegener's granulomatosis with intermittent high-dose intravenous cyclophosphamide. Am J Med 1990; 89: 403–410.

41. Rosenbaum J. Treatment of severe refractory uveitis with intravenous cyclophosphamide. J Rheumatol 1994; 21: 12–125.

42. Godfrey W, Epstein W, O'Connor GR, et al. The use of chlorambucil in intractable idiopathic uveitis. Am J Ophthalmol 1974; 78: 415–428.

43. Tessler H, Jennings T. High-dose short-term chlorambucil for intractable sympathetic ophthalmia and Behcet's disease. Br J Ophthalmol 1990; 74: 353–357.

44. Nashel D. Mechanisms of action and clinical applications of cytotoxic drugs in rheumatic disorders. Med Clin North Am 1985; 69: 817–840.

45. DeFronzo R, Braine H, Colvin OM, et al. Water intoxication in man after cyclophosphamide therapy. Ann Intern Med 1973; 78: 861–869.

46. Kende G, Sirkin S, Thomas PR, et al. Blurring of vision, a previously indescribed complication of cyclophosphamide therapy. Cancer 1979; 44: 69–71.

47. Slater, CA, Liang MH, McCune JW, et al. Preserving ovarian function in patients receiving cyclophosphamide. Lupus 1999; 8: 3–10.

48. Blumenfeld Z, Avivi I. Trying to preserve ovarian function in the face of chemotherapy. Fertil Steril 1999; 71: 773–774.

49. Reeves B, Casey G, Harris H, et al. Long-term cytogenetic follow-up study of patients with uveitis treated with chlorambucil. Carcinogenesis 1985; 6(11): 1615–1619.

50. Hoffman G, Kerr G, Leavitt R, et al. Wegener's granulomatosis: an analysis of 158 patients. Ann Intern Med 1992; 116: 488–498.

51. Radis CD, Kahl LE, Baker GL, et al. Effects of cyclosphosphamide on the development of malignancy and on long-term survival of patients with rheumatoid arthritis. A 20-year followup study. Arthritis Rheum 1995; 38: 1120–1127.

52. Lane L, Tamesis R, Rodriguez A, et al. Systemic immunosuppressive therapy and the occurrence of malignancy in patients with ocular inflammatory disease. Ophthalmology 1995; 102: 1530–1535.

53. Tabbara K. Chlorambucil in Behcet's disease, a reappraisal. Ophthalmology 1983; 90: 906–908.

54. Urowitz M, Hunter T, Bookman M, et al. Azathioprine in rheumatoid arthritis: A double-blind study comparing full dose to half dose. J Rheumatol 1974; 1: 274–281.

55. Woodland J, Chaput-de-Saintonge D, Evans SJ, et al. Azathioprine in rheumatoid arthritis: Double-blind study of full versus half doses versus placebo. Ann Rheum Dis 1981; 40: 355–359.

56. O'reilly T. Azathioprine in the treatment of refractory rheumatoid arthritis. J Ir Med Assoc 1977; 70: 344–346.

57. Andrasch R, Pirofsky B, Burns R. Immunosuppressive therapy for severe chronic uveitis. Arch Ophthalmol 1978; 96: 247–251.

58. Newell F, Krill A, Thomson A. The treatment of uveitis with 6-mercaptopurine. Am J Ophthalmol 1966; 61: 1250–1255.

59. Aoki K, Sugiura S. Immunosuppressive treatment of Behcet's disease. Mod Probl Ophthalmol 1976; 16: 309–313.

60. Yazici H, Pazarli H, Barnes CG, et al. A controlled trial of azathioprine in Behcet's syndrome. N Engl J Med 1990; 322: 281–285.

61. Hooper PL, Kaplan HJ. Triple agent immunosuppression in serpiginous

choroiditis. Ophthalmology 1991; 98: 944–950.

62. Pasadhika S, Gerald AF, Rando A, et al. Azathioprine for ocular inflammatory diseases. Am J Ophthalmol 2009. In Press.

63. Connell W, Kamm M, Dickson M, et al. Long-term neoplasia risk after azathioprine treatment in inflammatory bowel disease. Lancet 1994; 343: 1249–1252.

64. Zierhut M, Stubiger N, Siepmann K, et al. MMF and eye disease. Lupus 2005; 14(Suppl 1): s50–s54.

65. Chanaud NPI, Vistica BP, Eugui E, et al. Inhibition of experimental autoimmune uveoretinitis by mycophenolate mofetil, an inhibitor of purine metabolism. Exp Eye Res 1995; 35: 429–434.

66. Kilmartin DJ, Forrester JV, Dick AD. Rescue therapy with mycophenolate mofetil in refractory uveitis. Lancet 1998; 352: 35–36.

67. Larkin G, Lightman S. Mycophenolate mofetil. A useful immunosuppressive in inflammatory eye disease. Ophthalmology 1999; 106: 370–374.

68. Sen HN, Suhler EB, Al-Khatib SQ, et al. Mycophenolate mofetil for the treatment of scleritis. Ophthalmology 2003; 110: 1750–1755.

69. Baltatzis S, Tufail F, Vredeveld BA, \et al. Mycophenolate mofetil as an immunomodulatory agent in the treatment of chronic ocular inflammatory disorders. Ophthalmology 2003; 110(5): 1061–1065.

70. Sen HN, Suhler EB, Al-Khatib SQ, et al. Mycophenolate mofetil for the treatment of scleritis. Ophthalmology 2003; 110: 1750–1755.

71. Thorne JE, Jabs DA, Qazi FA, et al. Mycophenolate mofetil therapy for inflammatory eye disease. Ophthalmology 2005; 112(8): 1472–1477.

72. Galor A, Jabs DA, Leder H, et al. Comparison of antimetabolite drugs as corticosteroid-sparing therapy for noninfectious ocular inflammation. Ophthalmology 2008; 115(10): 1826–1832.

73. Sollinger HW. US renal transplant mycophenolate mofetil study group. Mycophenolate mofetil for the prevention of acute rejection in primary cadaveric renal allograft recipients. Transplantation 1995; 60: 225–232.

74. European mycophenolate mofetil cooperative study group. Placebo controlled study of mycophenolate mofetil combined with cyclosporin and corticosteroids for prevention of acute rejection. Lancet 1995; 345: 1321–1325.

75. The tricontinental mycophenolate mofetil renal transplantation study group. A blinded, randomized clinical trial of mycophenolate mofetil for the prevention of acute rejection in cadaveric renal allograft recipients.

Transplantation 1996; 61: 1029–1037.

76. Cronstein B. Molecular mechanism of methotrexate action in inflammation. Inflammation 1992; 16: 411–423.

77. Sperling R, Benincaso A, Anderson RJ, et al. Acute and chronic suppression of leukotriene B4 synthesis ex vivo in neutrophils from patients with rheumatoid arthritis beginning treatment with methotrexate. Arthritis Rheum 1992; 35: 376–384.

78. Thomas R, Carroll G. Reduction of leukocyte and interleukin-1 beta concentrations in the synovial fluid of rheumatoid arthritis patients treated with methotrexate. Arthritis Rheum 1993; 36: 1244–1254.

79. Olsen N, Murray L. Antiproliferative effects of methotrexate on peripheral blood mononuclear cells. Arthritis Rheum 1989; 32: 378–385.

80. Wong V. Immunosuppressive therapy of ocular inflammatory diseases. Arch Ophthalmol 1969; 81: 628–637.

81. Holz F, Krastel H, Breitbart A, et al. Low-dose methotrexate treatment in noninfectious uveitis resistant to corticosteroids. Ger J Ophthalmol 1992; 1: 142–144.

82. Shah S, Lowder CY, Schmitt MA, et al. Low-dose methotrexate therapy for ocular inflammatory disease. Ophthalmology 1992; 99: 1419–1423.

83. Dev S, McCallum RM, Jaffe GJ. Methotrexate treatment for sarcoid-associated panuveitis. Ophthalmology 1999; 106: 111–118.

84. Pascalis L, Pia G, Aresu G, et al. Combined cyclosporin A-steroid-MTX treatment in endogenous non-infectious uveitis. J Autoimmun 1993; 6: 467–480.

85. Tugwell P, Pincus T, Yocum D, et al. Combination therapy with cyclosporine and methotrexate in severe rheumatoid arthritis. N Engl J Med 1995; 333: 137–141.

86. Weinblatt ME, Dixon JA, Falchuk KR. Serious liver disease in a patient receiving methotrexate and leflunomide. Arthritis Rheum 2001; 43: 2609–2611.

87. Gangaputra S, Newcomb CW, Liesegang TL, et al. Methotrexate for ocular inflammatory disease. Ophthalmology 2009; In Press.

88. Rootman J, Gudauskas G. Treatment of ocular leukemia with local chemotherapy. Cancer Treat Rep 1985; 69: 119–122.

89. Smith JR, Rosenbaum JT, Wilson DJ, et al. Role of Intravitreal methotrexate in the management of primary central nervous system lymphoma with ocular involvement. Ophthalmology 2002; 109: 1709–1716.

90. Rothenberg S, Iqbal M, da Costa M. Effect of folate compounds on the accumulation of methotrexate and the activity of dihydrofolate reductase in liver, kidney, and small intestine of the mouse. J Pharmacol Exp Ther 1982; 223: 631–634.

91. Furst D, Erikson N, Clute L, et al. Adverse experience with methotrexate during 176 weeks of a longterm prospective trial in patients with rheumatoid arthritis. J Rheumatol 1990; 17: 1628–1635.

92. Zachariae H, Kragballe K, Sogaard H. Methotrexate induced liver cirrhosis: studies including serial liver biopsies during continued treatment. Br J Dermatol 1980; 102: 407–412.

93. Hargreaves M, Mowat A, Benson M. Acute pneumonitis associated with low dose methotrexate treatment for rheumatoid arthritis: report of five cases and review of published reports. Thorax 1992; 47: 628–633.

94. Carroll G, Thomas R, Phatouros CC, et al. Incidence, prevalence and possible risk factors for pneumonitis in patients with rheumatoid arthritis receiving methotrexate. J Rheumatol 1994; 21: 51–54.

95. Cannon GW, Finck BK, Simpson KM, et al. Methotrexate induced pulmonary disease during treatment of rheumatoid arthritis in large clinical trials (abstract). Arthritis Rheum 2000; 43(suppl 9): 341.

96. Doroshow J, Locker GY, Gaasterland DE, et al. Ocular irritation from high-dose methotrexate therapy: Pharmacokinetics of drug in the tear film. Cancer 1981; 48: 2158–2162.

97. Zimmer-Galler I, Lie J. Choroidal infiltrates as the initial manifestations of lymphoma in rheumatoid arthritis with low-dose methotrexate. Mayo Clin Proc 1994; 69: 258–261.

98. Beveridge T, Gratwohl A, Michot F, et al. Cyclosporin A: Pharmacokinetics after a single dose in man and serum levels after multiple dosing in recipients of allogeneic bone-marrow grafts. Curr Ther Res 1981; 30: 5–18.

99. Beveridge T, Pharmacokinetics and metabolism of cyclsporin A. In: Cyclosporin A, White D, eds. 1982, Elsevier Biomedical Press: New York. p. 35–44.

100. Nussenblatt R, Palestine A. Cyclosporine: immunology, pharmacology, and therapeutic uses. Surv Ophthalmol 1986; 31: 159–169.

101. de Smet M, Rubin BI, Whitcup SM, et al. Combined use of cyclosporine and ketoconazole in the treatment of endogenous uveitis. Am J Ophthalmol 1992; 113: 687–690.

102. Schreiber S, Crabtree G. The mechanism of action of cyclosporin A and FK506. Immunol Today 1992; 13: 136–142.

103. Cross S, Halden NF, Lenardo MJ, et al. Functionally distinct NF-kappa B binding sites in the immunoglobulin kappa and IL-2 receptor alpha chain genes. Science 1989; 244: 466–469.

104. Granelli-Piperno A, Nolan P, Inaba K, et al. The effect of immunosuppressive agents on the induction of nuclear factors that bind to sites on the interleukin 2 promoter. J Exp Med 1990; 172: 1869–1872.

105. Larsson E. Cyclosporin A and dexamethasone suppress T-cell responses by selectively acting at distinct sites of the triggering process. J Immunol 1980; 124: 2828–2833.

106. Bunjes D, Hardt C, Röllinghoff M, et al. Cyclosporin A mediates immunosuppression of primary cytotoxic T cell responses by impairing the release of interleukin 1 and interleukin 2. Eur J Immunol 1981; 11: 657–661.

107. Kaufman Y, Chang AE, Robb RJ, et al. Mechanism of action of cyclosporin A: Inhibition of lymphokine secretion studied with antigen-stimulated T-cell hybridomas. J Immunol 1984; 133: 3107–3111.

108. DosReis G, Shevach E. Effect of cyclosporin on T-cell function in vitro: The mechanism of suppression of T cell proliferation depends on the nature of the T cell stimulus as well as the differentiation state of the responding T cell. J Immunol 1982; 129: 2360–2367.

109. Nussenblatt R. The expanding use of immunosuppression in the treatment of non-infectious ocular disease. J Autoimmun 1992; 5(suppl A): 247–257.

110. Nussenblatt R, Palestine A, Chan C. Cyclosporin A therapy in the treatment of intraocular inflammatory disease resistant to systemic corticosteroids and cytotoxic agents. Am J Ophthalmol 1983; 96: 275–282.

111. Miescher P, Favre H, Chatelanat F, et al. Combined steroid-cyclosporin treatment of chronic auto-immune diseases. Clinical results and assessment of nephrotoxicity by renal biopsy. Klin Wochenschr 1987.

112. Nussenblatt R, Palestine AG, Rook AH, et al. Treatment of intraocular inflammatory disease with Cyclosporin A. Lancet 1983; ii: 235–238.

113. Nussenblatt R, Palestine A, Chan C. Cyclosporine therapy for uveitis: long term followup. J Ocul Pharmacol 1985; 1: 369–381.

114. de Smet M, Nussenblatt R. Clinical use of cyclosporine in ocular disease. Int Ophthalmol Clin 1993; 33: 32–45.

115. Nussenblatt R, Palestine A, Chan C, et al. Effectiveness of cyclosporin therapy for Behçet's disease. Arthitis Rheum 1985; 28: 671–679.

116. Masuda K, Nakajima A, Urayama A, et al. Double-masked trial of cyclosporin versus colchicine and long-term open study of cyclosporin in Behçet's disease. Lancet 1989; 1(8647): 1093–1096.

117. Diaz-Llopis M, Cervera M, Menezo J. Cyclosporin A treatment of Behçet's disease: a long-term study. Curr Eye Res 1990; 9(suppl): 17–23.

118. Towler H, Whiting P, Forrester J. Combination low dose cyclosporin A and steroid therapy in chronic intraocular inflammation. Eye 1990; 4(pt3): 514–520.

119. Secchi A, De Rosa C, Pivetti-Pezzi P, et al. Open noncontrolled multicenter long-term trial with cyclosporin in endogenous non-infectious uveitis. Ophthalmologica 1991; 202: 217–224.

120. Leznoff A, Shea M, Binkley KE, et al. Cyclosporine in the treatment of nonmicrobial inflammatory ophthalmic disease. Can J Ophthalmol 1992; 27: 302–306.

121. Walton RC, Nussenblatt RB, Whitcup SM. Cyclosporine therapy for severe sight-threatening uveitis in children and adolescents. Ophthalmology 1998; 105: 2028–2034.

122. Hesselink DA, Baarsma GS, Kuijpers RW, et al. Experience with cyclosporine in endogenous uveitis posterior. Transplant Proc 2004; 36(2 Suppl): 372S–377S.

123. Kacmaz R, Austin H, Balow J, et al. Cyclosporine for ocular inflammation. N Engl J Med 1986; 314: 1293–1298.

124. Gilger BC, Malok E, Stewart T, et al. Effect of an intravitreal cyclosporine implant on experimental uveitis in horses. Vet Immunol Immunopathol 2000; 76: 239–255.

125. Feutren G, Mihatsch M. Risk factors for cyclosporine-induced nephropathy in patients with autoimmune diseases. International Kidney Biopsy Registry of Cyclosporine in Autoimmune Diseases. N Engl J Med 1992; 326: 1654–1660.

126. Sall K, Stevenson OD, Mundorf TK, et al. Two multicenter, randomized studies of the efficacy and safety of cyclosporine ophthalmic emulsion in moderate to severe dry eye disease. CsA Phase 3 Study Group. Ophthalmology 2000; 107(4): 631–639.

127. Palestine A, Austin HA 3rd, Balow JE, et al. Renal histopathologic alterations in patients treated with cyclosporine for uveitis. N Engl J Med 1986; 314: 1293–1298.

128. Deray G, Benhmida M, Le Hoang P, et al. Renal function and blood pressure in patients receiving long-term, low-dose cyclosporine therapy for idiopathic autoimmune uveitis. Ann Intern Med 1992; 117: 578–583.

129. Feutren G, Mihatsch M. Risk factors for cyclosporine-induced nephropathy in patients with autoimmune diseases. International Kidney Biopsy Registry of Cyclosporine in Autoimmune Diseases. N Engl J Med 1992; 326: 1654–1660.

130. Burke JJ, Pirsch JD, Ramos EL, et al. Long-term efficacy and safety of cyclosporine in renal-transplant recipients. N Engl J Med 1994; 331: 358–363.

131. Palestine A, Nussenblatt R, Gelato M. Therapy for Human Autoimmune Uveitis with low-dose Cyclosporine plus Bromocriptine. Transplant Proc 1988; (suppl 4 June): 131–135.

132. Tabbara KF, Gee SS, Alvarez H. Ocular bioavailability of cyclosporine after oral administration. Transplant Proc 1988; 20(2 Suppl 2): 656–659.

133. Palestine AG, Nussenblatt RB, Chan CC. Cyclosporine penetration into the anterior chamber and cerebrospinal fluid. Am J Ophthalmol 1985; 99(2): 210–211.

134. Whitcup SM, Salvo ECJ, Nussenblatt RB. Combined cyclosporine and corticosteroid therapy for sight-threatening uveitis in Behçet's disease. Am J Ophthalmol 1994; 118: 39–45.

135. Palestine A, Roberge F, Charous BL, et al. The effect of cyclosporine on immunization with tetanus and keyhole limpet hemocyanin (KLH) in humans. J Clin Immunol 1985; 5: 115–121.

136. Chang SH, Lim CS, Low TS, et al. Cyclosporine-associated encephalopathy: a case report and literature review. Transplant Proc 2001; 33(7–8): 3700–3701.

137. Mochizuki M, Masuda K, Sakane T, et al. A clnical trial of FK506 in refractory uveitis. Am J Ophthalmol 1993; 115: 763–769.

138. Tocci M, Matkovich DA, Collier KA, et al. The immunosuppressant FK506 selectively inhibits expression of early T cell activation genes. J Immunol 1989; 143: 718–726.

139. Kawashima H., Fujino Y, Mochizuki M. Effects of a new immunosuppressive agent, FK506, on experimental autoimmune uveoretinitis in rats. Invest Ophthalmol Vis Sci 1988; 29: 1265–1271.

140. Fujino Y, Mochizuki M, Chan CC, et al. FK506 treatment of S-antigen induced uveitis in primates. Curr Eye Res 1991; 10: 679–690.

141. Mochizuki M, Masuda K, Sakane T, et al. A clnical trial of FK506 in refractory uveitis. Am J Ophthalmol 1993; 115: 763–769.

142. Mochizuki M. Japanese-FK506-Study-Group. Refractory Uveitis in Behçet's Disease. Proceedings of the 6th International Conference on Behçet's Disease. In: Wechsler B, Godeau P, eds. 1993, Excerpta Medica: Amsterdam. p. 655–660.

143. Sloper CML, Powell RJ, Dua HS. Tacrolimus (F506) in the treatment of posterior uveitis refractory to cyclosporine. Ophthalmology 1999; 106: 723–728.

144. Kilmartin DJ, Forrester JV, Dick AD. Tacrolimus (FK506) in failed cyclosporin A therapy in endogenous posterior uveitis. Ocul Immunol Inflamm 1998; 6: 101–109.

145. Porayko M, Textor SC, Krom RA, et al. Nephrotoxic effects of primary immunosuppression with fk506 and cyclosporine regimens after liver transplantation. Mayo Clin Proc 1994; 69: 105–111.

146. Anglade E, Yatscoff R, Foster R, et al. Next-generation calcineurin inhibitors for ophthalmic indications. Exp Opin Invest Drugs 2007; 16(10): 1525–1540.

147. Cunningham MA, Austin BA, Li Z, et al. LX211 (voclosporin) suppresses experimental uveitis and inhibits human T cells. Invest Ophthalmol Vis Sci 2009; 50(1): 249–255.

148. Sehgal S, Baker H, Vezina C. Rapamycin (AY-22,989), a new antifungal antibiotic. II. Fermentation, isolation, and characterization. J Antibiotics 1975; 28: 727–732.

149. Dumont F, Staruch MJ, Koprak SL, et al. Distinct mechanisms of suppression of murine T cell activation by the related macrolides FK-506 and Rapamycin. J Immunol 1990; 144: 251–258.

150. Bierer E, Mattila PS, Standaert RF, et al. Two distinct signal transmission pathways in T lymphocytes are inhibited by complexes formed between immunophilin and either FK506 or rapamycin. Proc Natl Acad Sci USA 1990; 87: 9231–9235.

151. Henderson, D, Naya I, Bundick RV, et al. Comparison of the effects of FK-506, cyclosporin A and rapamycin on IL-2 production. Immunology 1991; 73: 316–321.

152. Gonwa TA, Hricik DE, Brinker K, et al. Improved renal function in sirolimus-treated renal transplant patients after early cyclosporine elimination. Transplantation 2002; 74: 1560–1567.

153. Nussenblatt RB, Coleman H, Jirawuthiworavong G, et al. The treatment of multifocal choroiditis associated choroidal neovascularization with sirolimus (rapamycin). Acta Ophthalmol Scand 2007; 85(2): 230–231.

154. Roberge F, Xu D, Chan CC, et al. Treatment of autoimmune uveoretinitis in the rat with rapamycin, an inhibitor of lymphocyte growth factor signal transduction. Curr Eye Res 1993; 12: 197–203.

155. Roberge F, Kozhich Alexander, Chan Chi-Chao, et al. Inhibition of cellular transfer of experimental autoimmune uveoretinitis by Rapamycin. Ocul Immunol Inflamm 1993; 1: 269–273.

156. Kahan B, Gibbons S, Tejpal N, et al. Synergistic interactions of cyclosporine and rapamycin to inhibit immune performances of normal human peripheral blood lymphocytes in vitro. Transplantation 1991; 51: 232–239.

157. Martin D, DeBarge LR, Nussenblatt RB, et al. synergistic effect of rapamycin and cyclosporin a in the treatment of experimental autoimmune uveoretinitis. J Immunol 1995; 154: 922–927.

158. Whiting P, Woo J, Adam BJ, et al. Toxicity of rapamycin – a comparative and combination study with cyclosporine at immunotherapeutic dosage in the rat. Transplantation 1991; 52: 203–208.

159. Calne R, Collier DS, Lim S, et al. Rapamycin for immunosuppression in organ allografting. Lancet 1989; 2: 227–232.

160. Jap A, Chee SP. Immunosuppressive therapy for ocular diseases. Curr Opin Ophthalmol 2008; 19(6): 535–540.

161. Yeh S, Nussenblatt RB. Biologic therapies for retinal disease: infliximab, adalimumab, etanercept, daclizumab, and others. In: Nguyen QD, Mieler WF, eds. Retinal Pharmacotherapy: Elsevier, in press.

162. Chatenoud L, Bach J-F. Anti-T-cell Monoclonal Antibodies as Immunosuppressive Agents., in Immunopharmacology in Autoimmune Diseases and Transplantation. In: Rugstad H, Endresen L, Forre O, eds. 1992, Plenum Press: New York. p. 189–203.

163. O'Connell P, Corpier C, Steele A, et al. Monoclonal Antibody Therapy. In: Thomson A, ed. Immunology in Renal Transplantation. London: Edward Arnold, 1993.

164. Dukar O, Barr C. Visual loss complicating OKT3 monoclonal antibody therapy. Am J Ophthalmol 1993; 115: 781–785.

165. Brown P, Parenteau GL, Dirbas FM, et al. Anti-Tac-H, a humanized antibody to the interleukin 2 receptor, prolongs primate cardiac allograft survival. Proc Natl Acad Sci USA 1991; 88(7): 2663–2667.

166. Soulillou JP, Cantarovich D, Le Mauff B, et al. Randomized controlled trial of a monoclonal antibody against the interleukin-2 receptor (33B3.1) as compared with rabbit antithymocyte globulin for prophylaxis against rejection of renal allografts. N Engl J Med 1987; 322: 1175–1182.

167. Blaise D, Olive D, Hirn M, et al. Prevention of acute GVHD by in vivo use of anti-interleukin-2 receptor monoclonal antibody (33B3.1): a feasibility trial in 15 patients. Bone Marrow Transplant 1991; 8: 105–111.

168. Queen C, Schneider WP, Selick HE, et al. A humanized antibody that binds to the interleukin 2 receptor. Proc Natl Acad Sci USA 1989; 86: 10029–10033.

169. Whitcup S., DeBarge LR, Rosen H, et al. Monoclonal antibody against CD11b/CD18 inhibits endotoxin-induced uveitis. Invest Ophthalmol Vis Sci 1993; 34: 673–681.

170. Rosenbaum JT, Boney RS. Efficacy of antibodies to adhesions molecules, CD11a or CD18, in rabbit models of uveitis. Curr Eye Res 1993; 12: 827–831.

171. Whitcup SM, DeBarge LR, Caspi RR, et al. Monoclonal antibodies against ICAM-1 (CD54) and LFA-1 (CD11a/CD18) inhibit experimental autoimmune uveitis. Clin Immunol Immunopathol 1993; 67: 143–150.

172. Nussenblatt RB, Fortin E, Schiffman R, et al. Treatment of noninfectious intermediate and posterior uveitis with the humanized anti-Tac mAb: a phase I/II clinical trial. Proc Natl Acad Sci USA 1999; 96: 7462–7466.

173. Nussenblatt RB, Thompson DJ, Li Z, et al. Humanized anti-interleukin-2 (IL-2) receptor alpha therapy: long term results in uveitis patients and preliminary safety and activity data for establishing parameters for subcutaneous administration. 2003; 21(3): 283–293.

174. Papaliodis GN, Chu D, Foster CS. Treatment of ocular inflammatory disorders with daclizumab. Ophthalmology 2003; 110(4): 786–789.

175. Yeh S, Wroblewski K, Buggage R, et al. High-dose humanized anti-IL-2 receptor alpha antibody (daclizumab) for the treatment of active, non-infectious uveitis. J Autoimmun 2008; 31(2): 91–97.

176. Kim HS, Yoon SK, Joo C. The expression of multiple cytokines and inducible nitric oxide synthase in experimental melanin-protein-induced uveitis. Ophthalmic Res 2001; 33: 329–335.

177. Santos Lacomba M, Marcos Martín C, Gallardo Galera JM, et al. Aqueous humor and serum tumor necrosis factor-alpha in clinical uveitis. Ophthalmic Res 2001; 33: 251–255.

178. Weinblatt M, Kremer JM, Bankhurst AD, et al. A trial of etanercept, a recombinant tumor necrosis factor receptor:Fc fusion protein, in patients with rheumatoid arthritis receiving methotrexate. N Engl J Med 1999; 340: 253–259.

179. Lovell DJ, Criannini EH, Reiff A, et al. Etanercept in children with polyarticular juvenile rheumatoid arthritis. Pediatric Rheumatology Collaborative Study Group. New England Journal of Medicine 2000; 342: 763–769.

180. Smith JR, Levinson RD, Holland GN, et al. Differential efficacy of TNF inhibition in the management of uveitis and associated rheumatic disease. Arthritis Rheum 2001; 45: 252–257.

181. Brown SL, Greene MH, Gershon SK, et al. Tumor necrosis factor antagonist therapy and lymphoma development. Arthritis Rheum 2002; 46: 3151–3158.

182. Fonollosa A, Segura A, Giralt J, et al. Tuberculous uveitis after treatment with etanercept. Graefes Arch Clin Exp Ophthalmol 2007; 245(9): 1397–1399.

183. Sfikakis PP, Theodossiadis PG, Katsiari CG, et al. Effect of infliximab on sight-threatening panuveitis in Behcet's disease. Lancet 2001; 358: 295–296.

184. Sfikakis PP. Behcet's disease: a new target for anti-tumour necrosis factor treatment. Ann Rheum Dis 2002; 61(Suppl 2): ii51–ii53.

185. Sfikakis PP, Markomichelakis N, Alpsoy E, et al. Anti-TNF therapy in the management of Behcet's disease – review and basis for

recommendations. Rheumatology (Oxford) 2007; 46(5): 736–741.

186. Pipitone N, Olivieri I, Padula A, et al. Infliximab for the treatment of Neuro-Behcet's disease: a case series and review of the literature. Arthritis Rheum 2008; 59(2): 285–290.

187. El-Shabrawi Y, Hermann J. Anti-tumor necrosis factor-alpha therapy with infliximab as an alternative to corticosteroids in the treatment of human leukocyte antigen B27-associated acute anterior uveitis. Ophthalmology 2002; 109: 2342–2346.

188. Sen HN, Sangave A, Hammel K, et al. Infliximab for the treatment of active scleritis. Can J Ophthalmol 2009; 44: e9–e12.

189. Liberopoulos EN, Drosos AA, Elisaf MS. Exacerbation of tuberculous enteritis after treatment with infliximab. Am J Med 2002; 113: 615.

190. Lee J-H, Slifman NR, Gershon SK, et al. Life-threatening histoplasmosis complicating immunotherapy with tumor necrosis factor alpha antagonists infliximab and etanercept. Arthritis Rheum 2002; 46: 2565–2570.

191. van Oosten BW, Barkhof F, Truyen L, et al. Increased MRI activity and immune activation in two multiple sclerosis patients treated with the monoclonal anti-tumor necrosis factor antibody cA2. Neurology 1996; 47: 1531–1534.

192. Pettersen JA, Zochodne DW, Bell RB, et al. Refractory neurosarcoidosis responding to infliximab. Neurology 2002; 59: 1660–1661.

193. Foroozan R, Buono LM Sergott RC, et al. Retrobulbar optic neuritis associated with infliximab. Arch Ophthalmol 2002; 120: 985–987.

194. Kramer N, Chuzhin Y, Kaufman LD, et al. Methotrexate pneumonitis after initiation of infliximab therapy for rheumatoid arthritis. Arthritis Rheum 2002; 47: 670–671.

195. Mushtaq B, Saeed T, Situnayake RD, et al. Adalimumab for sight-threatening uveitis in Behcet's disease. Eye 2007; 21(6): 824–825.

196. van Laar JA, Missotten T, van Daele PL, et al. Adalimumab: a new modality for Behcet's disease? Ann Rheum Dis 2007; 66(4): 565–566.

197. Diaz-Llopis M, García-Delpech S, Salom D, et al. Adalimumab therapy for refractory uveitis: a pilot study. J Ocul Pharmacol Ther 2008; 24(3): 351–361.

198. Tynjala P, Kotaniemi K, Lindahl P, et al. Adalimumab in juvenile idiopathic arthritis-associated chronic anterior uveitis. Rheumatology (Oxford) 2008; 47(3): 339–344.

199. Vazquez-Cobian LB, Flynn T, Lehman TJ. Adalimumab therapy for childhood uveitis. J Pediatr 2006; 149(4): 572–575.

200. Gordon KB, Papp KA, Hamilton TK, et al. Efalizumab for patients with moderate to severe plaque psoriasis: a randomized controlled trial. JAMA 2003; 290(23): 3073–3080.

201. Faia LJ, Yeh S, Nussenblatt B, et al. Efalizumab (Raptiva) for the treatment of macular edema associated with intermediate or posterior uveitis in 08-PP-30018478-AAO. 2008: Am Acad Ophthalmol Abstract Book.

202. Hoang-Xuan K, Camilleri-Broet S, Soussain C. Recent advances in primary CNS lymphoma. Curr Opin Oncol 2004; 16(6): 601–606.

203. Bosly A, Keating MJ, Stasi R, et al. Rituximab in B-cell disorders other than non-Hodgkin's lymphoma. Anticancer Drugs 2002; 13(Suppl 2): S25–S33.

204. Rigacci L, Nassi L, Puccioni M, et al. Rituximab and chlorambucil as first-line treatment for low-grade ocular adnexal lymphomas. Ann Hematol 2007; 86(8): 565–568.

205. Ferreri AJ, Ponzoni M, Martinelli G, et al. Rituximab in patients with mucosal-associated lymphoid tissue-type lymphoma of the ocular adnexa. Haematologica 2005; 90(11): 1578–1579.

206. Gurcan HM, Keskin DB, Stern JN, et al. A review of the current use of rituximab in autoimmune diseases. Int Immunopharmacol 2009; 9(1): 10–25.

207. Tappeiner C, Heinz C, Specker C, et al. Rituximab as a treatment option for refractory endogenous anterior uveitis. Ophthalmic Res 2007; 39(3): 184–186.

208. Onal S, Kazokoglu H, Koc A, et al. Rituximab for remission induction in a patient with relapsing necrotizing scleritis associated with limited Wegener's granulomatosis. Ocul Immunol Inflamm 2008; 16(5): 230–232.

209. Sadreddini S, Noshad H, Molaeefard M, et al. Treatment of retinal vasculitis in Behcet's disease with rituximab. Mod Rheumatol 2008; 18(3): 306–308.

210. Lim WK, Fujimoto C, Ursea R, et al. Suppression of immune-mediated ocular inflammation in mice by interleukin 1 receptor antagonist administration. Arch Ophthalmol 2005; 123(7): 957–963.

211. Teoh SC, Sharma S, Hogan A, et al. Tailoring biological treatment: anakinra treatment of posterior uveitis associated with the CINCA syndrome. Br J Ophthalmol 2007; 91(2): 263–264.

212. Arostegui JI, Arnal C, Merino R, et al. NOD2 gene-associated pediatric granulomatous arthritis: clinical diversity, novel and recurrent mutations, and evidence of clinical improvement with interleukin-1 blockade in a Spanish cohort. Arthritis Rheum 2007; 56(11): 3805–3813.

213. Nabhan C. The emerging role of alemtuzumab in chronic lymphocytic leukemia. Clin Lymphoma Myeloma 2005; 6(2): 115–121.

214. Osterborg A, Mellstedt H, Keating M. Clinical effects of alemtuzumab (Campath-1H) in B-cell chronic lymphocytic leukemia. Med Oncol 2002; 19(Suppl): S21–S26.

215. Dearden C. The role of alemtuzumab in the management of T-cell malignancies. Semin Oncol 2006; 33(2 Suppl 5): S44–S52.

216. Dick AD, Meyer P, James T, et al. Campath-1H therapy in refractory ocular inflammatory disease. Br J Ophthalmol 2000; 84(1): 107–109.

217. Angeles-Han S, Flynn T, Lehman T. Abatacept for refractory juvenile idiopathic arthritis-associated uveitis- a case report. J Rheumatol 2008; 35(9): 1897–1898.

218. Tellier Z. Human immunoglobulins in intraocular inflammation. Ann NY Acad Sci 2007; 1110: 337–347.

219. Cassoux N, Haroun O, George F, et al. Effect of intravenous immunoglobulin (IVIg) in the treatment of birdshot retinochoroidopathy (Abstract). Invest Ophthalmol Vis Sci 1996; 37: S369.

220. Rosenbaum JT, George RK, Gordon C. The treatment of refractory uveitis with intravenous immunoglobulin. Am J Ophthalmol 1999; 127: 545–549.

221. Guy J, Aptsiauri N. Treatment of paraneoplastic visual loss with intravenous immunoglobuli: report of 3 cases. Arch Ophthalmol 1999; 117: 471–477.

222. Kazatchkine MD, Kaveri SV. Immunomodulation of autoimmune and inflammatory diseases with intravenous immune globulin. N Engl J Med 2001; 345(10): 747–755.

223. Dalakas MC. Intravenous immune globulin therapy for neurologic diseases. Ann Intern Med 1997; 126: 721–730.

224. Basta M, Van Goor F, Luccioli S, et al. F(ab)'2-mediated neutralization of C3a and C5a anaphylatoxins: a novel effector function of immunoglobulins. Nat Med 2003; 9(4): 431–438.

225. Saoudi A, Hurez V, de Kozak Y, et al. Human immunoglobulin preparations for intravenous use prevent experimental autoimmune uveoretinitis. Int Ophthalmol 1993; 5: 1559–1567.

226. Ayliffe W, Haeney M, Roberts SC, et al. Uveitis after antineutrophil cytoplasmic antibody contamination of immunoglobulin replacement therapy. Lancet 1992; 339: 558–559.

227. Weiner H, Mackin GA, Matsui M, et al. Double-blind pilot trial of oral tolerization with myelin antigens in multiple sclerosis. Science 1993; 259(5099): 1321–1324.

228. Trentham D, Dynesius-Trentham RA, Orav EJ, et al. Effects of oral administration of type II collagen on rheumatoid arthritis. Science 1993; 261(5129): 1727–1730.

229. Nussenblatt R, de Smet M, Weiner HL, et al. The treatment of the ocular complications of Behcet's disease with oral tolerization., in Behcet's Disease.

Proceedings of the 6th International Conference on Behcet's Disease. Wechsler B, Godeau P, eds. 1993, Excerpta Medica: Amsterdam. p. 641–646.

230. Nussenblatt RB, Gery I, Weiner HL, et al. Treatment of uveitis by oral administration of retinal antigens: results of a phase I/II randomized masked trial. Am J Ophthalmol 1997; 123: 684–687.

231. Faria AM, Weiner HL. Oral tolerance: therapeutic implications for autoimmune diseases. Clin Dev Immunol 2006; 13(2–4): 143–157.

232. Thurau SR Wildner G. An HLA-peptide mimics organ-specific antigen in autoimmune uveitis: its role in pathogenesis and therapeutic induction of oral tolerance. Autoimmun Rev 2003; 2(4): 171–176.

233. Thurau SR, Fricke H, Burchardi C, et al. Long-term follow-up of oral tolerance induction with HLA-peptide B27PD in patients with uveitis. Ann NY Acad Sci 2004; 1029: 408–412.

234. Curreli S, Romerio F, Secchiero P, et al. IFN-alpha2b increases interleukin 10 expression in primary activated human CD8(+) T cells. J Interferon Cytokine Res 2002; 22: 1167–1173.

235. Mackensen F, Max R, Becker MD. Interferon therapy for ocular disease. Curr Opin Ophthalmol 2006; 17(6): 567–573.

236. Kotter I, Eckstein AK, Stübiger N, et al. Treatment of ocular symptoms of Behcet's disease with interferon alfa 2a: a pilot study. Br J Ophthalmol 1998; 82: 488–494.

237. Pivetti-Pezzi P, Accorinti M, Pirraglia MP, et al. Interferon alpha for ocular Behcet's disease. Acta Ophthalmol Scand 1997; 75: 720–722.

238. Wechsler B, Bodaghi B, Huong DL, et al. Efficacy of interferon alfa-2a in severe and refractory uveitis associated with Behcet's disease. Ocul Immunol Inflamm 2000; 4: 293–301.

239. Tugal-Tutkun I, Onal S, Altan-Yaycioglu R, et al. Neovascularization of the optic disc in Behcet's disease. Jpn J Ophthalmol 2006; 50(3): 256–265.

240. Krause L, Altenburg A, Bechrakis NE, et al. Intraocular surgery under systemic interferon-alpha therapy in ocular Adamantiades-Behcet's disease. Graefes Arch Clin Exp Ophthalmol 2007; 245(11): 1617–1621.

241. Naesens L, De Clerq E. Recent developments in herpesvirus therapy. Herpes 2001; 8: 12–16.

242. Palestine A, Stevens G Jr, Lane HC, et al. Treatment of cytomegalovirus retinitis with dihydroxy propoxymethyl guanine. Am J Ophthalmol 1986; 101: 95–101.

243. Cantrill H, Henry K, Melroe NH, et al. Treatment of cytomegalovirus retinitis with intravitreal ganciclovir: long term results. Ophthalmology 1989; 96: 367–374.

244. Cochereau-Massin I, Lehoang P, Lautier-Frau M, et al. Efficacy and tolerance of intravitreal ganciclovir in cytomegalovirus retinitis in acquired immune deficiency syndrome. Ophthalmology 1991; 98: 1348–1353.

245. Smith T, Pearson PA, Blandford DL, et al. Intravitreal sustained-release ganciclovir. Arch Ophthalmol 1992; 110: 255–258.

246. Anand R, Nightingale SD, Fish RH, et al. Control of cytomegalovirus retinitis using sustained release of intraocular ganciclovir. Arch Ophthalmol 1993; 111: 223–227.

247. Martin D, Parks DJ, Mellow SD, et al. Treatment of cytomegalovirus retinitis with an intraocular sustained-release ganciclovir implant: A randomized controlled clinical trial. N Engl J Med 1994.

248. Martin DF, Parks DJ, Mellow SD, et al. Use of the ganciclovir implant for the treatment of cytomegalovirus retinitis in the era of potent antiretroviral therapy: recommendations of the International AIDS Society-USA panel. Am J Ophthalmol 1999; 127(3): 329–339.

249. Spector S, Busch DF, Follansbee S, et al. Pharmacokinetic, safety, and antiviral profiles of oral ganciclovir in persons infected with human immunodeficiency virus: a phase I/II study. AIDS Clinical Trials Group, and Cytomegalovirus Cooperative Study Group. J Infect Dis 1995; 171: 1431–1437.

250. Martin DF, Kuppermann BD, Wolitz RA, et al. Oral ganciclovir for patients with cytomegalovirus retinitis treated with a ganciclovir implant. N Engl J Med 1999; 340: 1063–1070.

251. Martin DF, Sierra-Madero J, Walmsley S, et al. A controlled trial of valganciclovir as induction therapy for cytomegalovirus retinitis. N Engl J Med 2002; 346(15): 1119–1126.

252. Tyring S, Engst R, Corriveau C, et al. Famciclovir for ophthalmic zoster: a randomised aciclovir controlled study. Br J Ophthalmol 2001; 85(5): 576–581.

253. Ringden O, Wilczek H, Lönnqvist B, et al. Foscarnet for cytomegalovirus infections. Lancet 1985; i: 1503.

254. Safrin S, Kemmerly S, Plotkin B, et al. Foscarnet-resistant herpes simplex virus infection in patiens with AIDS. J Infect Dis 1994; 169: 193–196.

255. Sandstrom E, Kaplan JC, Byington RE, et al. Inhibition of human T-cell lymphotropic virus type III in vitro by phosphonoformate. Lancet 1985; i: 1480.

256. Le Hoang P, Girard B, Robinet M, et al. Comparative study of foscarnet and DHPG in the treatment of CMV retinitis in AIDS. Invest Ophthalmol Vis Sci 1988; 29 (suppl 3) (in press).

257. Le Hoang P, Girard B, Robinet M, et al. Foscarnet in the treatment of cytomegalovirus retinitis in acquired immune deficiency syndrome. Ophthalmology 1989; 6: 865–873.

258. Palestine AG, Polis MA, De Smet MD, et al. A randomized controlled trial of foscarnet in the treatment of cytomegalovirus retinitis in patients with the acquired immunodeficiency syndrome. Ann Intern Med 1991; 115: 665–673.

259. AIDS-research-group. and AIDS-clinical-trials-group. Foscarnet-Ganciclovir cytomegalovirus retinitis trial. 4. Visual outcomes. Studies of ocular complications of AIDS research group in collaboration with the AIDS clinical trials group. Ophthalmology 1994; 101: 1250–1261.

260. AIDS-research-group. and AIDS-clinical-trials-group. Mortality in patients with the acquired immunodeficiency syndrome treated with either foscarnet or ganciclovir for cytomegalovirus retinitis. N Engl J Med 1992; 326: 213–220.

261. Jacobson M, Wulfsohn M, Feinberg JE, et al. Phase II dose-ranging trail of foscarnet salvage therapy for cytomegalovirus retinitis in AIDS patients intolerant of or resistant to gancilovir (ACTG protocol 093). AIDS clinical trials group of the National Institute of Allergy and Infectious Diseases. AIDS 1994; 8: 451–459.

262. Gumbel H, Rückert DG, Cinatl J, et al. In vitro anti-human cytomegalovirus activity of liposome-encapsulated foscarnet. Ger J Ophthalmol 1994; 3: 5–8.

263. Sarraf D, Equi RA, Holland GN, et al. Transscleral iontophoresis of foscarnet. Am J Ophthalmol 1993; 115: 748–754.

264. Turrini B, Tognon MS, De Caro G, et al. Intraviteal use of foscarnet: retinopathy of repeated injections in the rabbit eye. Ophthalmic Res 1994; 26: 110–115.

265. Berthe P, Baudouin C, Garraffo R, et al. Toxicologic and pharmacokinetic analysis of intravitreal injections of foscarnet, either alone or in combination with ganciclovir. Invest Ophthalmol Vis Sci 1994; 35: 1038–1045.

266. Diaz-Llopis M, España E, Muñoz G, et al. High dose intravitreal foscarnet in the treatment of cytomegalovirus retinitis in AIDS. Br J Ophthalmol 1994; 78: 120–124.

267. Jacobson M, Kramer F, Bassiakos Y, et al. Randomized phase I trial of two different combination foscarnet and ganciclovir chronic maintenance therapy regimens for AIDS patients with cytomegalovirus retinitis. AIDS clinical trials group protocol 151. J Infect Dis 1994; 170: 189–193.

268. Weinberg D, Murphy R, Naughton K. Combined daily therapy with intravenous ganciclovir and foscarnet for patients with recurrent cytomegalovirus retinitis. Am J Ophthalmol 1994; 177: 776–782.

269. SOCA Research Group in collaboration with AIDS Clinical trial

group. Combination foscarnet and gancyclovir therapy vs monotherapy for the treatment of relapsed cytomegalovirus retinitis in patients with AIDS: the cytomegalovirus retinitis retreatment trial. Arch Ophthalmol 1996; 114: 23–33.

270. Bronson J, Ghazzouli I, Hitchcock MJ, et al. Synthesis and antiviral activity of the nucleotide analogue(S)-1-[3-hydroxy-2-(phosphonylmethoxy)propyl]cytosine. J Med Chem 1989; 32: 1457–1463.

271. Hitchcock M, Woods K, Bronson J, et al. Intracellular metabolism of the anti-herpes agent, (S)-1-[3-hydroxy-2-(phosphonylmethoxy)propl]cytosine (HPMPC). Mol Pharm 1992; 41: 197–202.

272. The Studies of Ocular Complications of AIDS Research Group in Collaboration with the AIDS Clinical Trials Group. Cidofovir (HPMPC) for the treatment of cytomegalovirus retinitis in patients with AIDS: the HPMPC Peripheral Cytomegalovirus Retinitis Trial. Ann Intern Med 1997; 126: 264–274.

273. Cochereau I, Doan S, Diraison MC, et al. Uveitis in patients treated with intravenous cidofovir. Ocul Immunol Inflamm 1999; 7: 223–229.

274. Geary RS, Henry SP, Grillone LR. Fomivirsen. Clinical pharmacology and potential drug interactions. Clin Pharmacokinet 2002; 41: 255–260.

275. The Vitravene Study Group. A randomized controlled clinical trial of intravitreous fomivirsen for treatment of newly diagnosed peripheral cytomegalovirus retinitis in patients with AIDS. Am J Ophthalmol 2002; 133: 467–474.

276. The Vitravene Study Group. Randomized dose-comparison studies of intravitreous fomivirsen for treatment of cytomegalovirus retinitis that has reactivated or is persistently active despite other therapies in patients with AIDS. Am J Ophthalmol 2002; 133: 475–483.

277. The Vitravene Study Group. Safety of intravenous fomivirsen for treatment of cytomegalovirus retinitis in patients with AIDS. Am J Ophthalmol 2002; 133: 484–498.

278. Jabs DA, Griffiths PD. Editorial. Fomivirsen for the treatment of cytomegalovirus retinitis. Am J Ophthalmol 2002; 133: 552–556.

279. Tsai E, Till G, Marak GJ. Effects of mydriatic agents on neutrophil migration. Ophthalmic Res 1988; 20: 14–19.

280. Tate G, Martin R. Clindamycin in the treatment of ocular toxoplasmosis. Can J Ophthalmol 1977; 12: 188–195.

281. Tabbara K, O'Connor G. Treatment of ocular toxoplasmosis with clindamycin and sulfadiazine. Ophthalmology 1980; 87: 129–134.

282. Martinez CE, Zhang D, Conway MD, et al. Successful management of ocular toxoplasmosis during pregnancy using combined intraocular clindamycin and dexamethasone with systemic sulfadiazine. Int Ophthalmol 1999; 22: 85–88.

283. Hudson A, Randall AW, Fry M, et al. Novel anti-malarial hydroxynaphthoquinones with potent broad spectrum anti-protozoal activity. Parasitology 1985; 90: 45–55.

284. Araujo F, Huskins J, Remington J. Remarkable in vitro and vivo activities of 566C80 against tachyzoites and tissue cysts of Toxoplasma gondii. Antimicrob Agents Chemother 1991; 35: 293–299.

285. Kovacs J, O'Neil D, Feuerstein I, et al. Efficacy of 566C80 in the treatment of toxoplasmosis in patients with AIDS. Lancet 1992; 340: 637–638.

286. Lopez J, de Smet MD, Masur H, et al. Orally administered 566C80 for treatment of ocular toxoplasmosis in a patient with the acquired immunodeficiency syndrome. Am J Ophthalmol 1992; 113: 331–333.

287. Rollins D, Tabbara KF, Ghosheh R, et al. Minocycline in experimental ocular toxoplasmosis in the rabbit. Am J Ophthalmol 1982; 93: 361–365.

288. McCabe R, Remington J. Toxoplasmosis., Tropical and Geographical Medicine. In: Warren K, Mahoud A, eds. 1994, McGraw-Hill: New York. p. 281.

289. Opremcak EM, Scales DK, Sharpe MR. Trimethoprim-sulafmethoxazole therapy for ocular toxoplasmosis. Ophthalmology 1992; 99: 920–925.

290. Brun-Pascaud M, Rajagopalan-Levasseur P, Chau F, et al. Drug evaluation of concurrent Pneumocystis carinii, Toxoplasma gondii, and Mycobacterium avium complex infections in a rat model. Antimicrob Agents Chemother 1998; 42: 1068–1072.

291. Siegfried Gagne S. Toxoplasmosis. Prim Care Update Ob/Gyn 2001; 8: 122–126.

292. Abell JJ, Rowntree LG, Turner BB. Plasma removal with return of corpuscles. J Pharm Exp Ther 1914; 5: 920–925.

293. Skoog W, Adams W, Plasmapheresis in a case of Waldenström's macroglobulinemia. Clin Res 1959; 7: 96.

294. Saraux H, Hoang Le, Audebert A-A, et al. Interet de la plasmapherese dans le traitement du syndrome de Behcet. Bull Soc Ophthalmol Fr 1982; 41–44.

295. Yanuzzi L. A perspective on treatment of aphaki cystoid macular edema. Surv Ophthalmol 1984; 28 (suppl): 540–553.

296. Monthey K. Nonsteroid anti-inflammatory drugs in the treatment of intermediate uveitis. Dev Ophthalmol 1992; 23: 158–162.

297. Herbort C. Uveoscleritis after excessive neodymium:YAG laser posterior capsulotomy. J Cataract Refract Surg 1994; 20(1): 80–81.

298. Kempen J, Daniel E, Dunn JP, et al. Risk of overall and cancer mortality among patients with ocular inflammation treated with immunosuppressive therapy: retrospective cohort study. Br Med J 2009; In Press.

299. Kempen JH, Gangaputra S, Daniel E, et al. Long-term risk of malignancy among patients treated with immunosuppressive agents for ocular inflammation: a critical assessment of the evidence. Am J Ophthalmol 2008; 146(6): 802–812 e1.

Role of Surgery in the Patient with Uveitis

Robert B. Nussenblatt

Key concepts

- Inflammatory disease needs to be clinically quiescent for at least 3 months before elective surgery is considered.
- Adequate immunosuppressive therapy perioperatively is very important.
- Surgery needs to be considered when there is something to save, not when the disease is end-stage.

Despite even optimal medical therapy, structural damage will develop in many eyes with chronic inflammation, which can be repaired only by surgical intervention. In the past, surgery was often attempted hesitantly because of a high incidence of complications, including uncontrolled inflammation, hypotony, and phthisis. Two advances have contributed to safer surgical intervention in these eyes. The first is improved control of inflammation with steroids or other drugs, and the second is the rapid advancement in microsurgical techniques that has improved our ability to operate on the anterior segment, vitreous, and retina.[1] In this chapter principles of ophthalmic surgery as they apply to the inflamed eye, both for therapy and for diagnosis, are discussed. However, the anatomic alterations in eyes with severe uveitis are unique, and the approach to each eye often must be determined individually.

Considerations

In general, the indications for proceeding with surgery need to be more carefully considered in eyes with uveitis. Because of the possible increased risks, surgery is frequently not justified for eyes with slightly reduced – but functional – vision which are not in danger of visual loss from a surgically repairable problem. On the other hand, we have observed many eyes in which surgery was delayed for so long that potentially treatable problems became hidden behind cataract or vitreous haze. Vision was then permanently lost because of the attempt to use surgery conservatively; vision might have been saved if the inflammatory disease and its complications could have been directly viewed and treated. There is a tendency to not operate on an eye with dense opacities and light perception vision while unseen and untreated inflammation causes further permanent damage to the retina. In the end the eye does go blind, but there was

a point in the course of the disease at which the potential benefits of surgical intervention, even if low, outweighed the resultant risk of nonintervention. In addition to visual rehabilitation, surgical procedures in eyes with uveitis are performed as part of a diagnostic evaluation. The relative risks versus the potential benefits are considered here.

Except for the few situations in which it is necessary to operate on an acutely inflamed eye, surgery should be performed when the inflammation is quiescent. However, in some patients it is impossible to clear every cell from the anterior chamber or vitreous. Furthermore, in patients with dense cataracts and primarily vitreoretinal inflammation it is impossible accurately to assess the activity of the disease behind the opacity. Therefore, an attempt should be made to reduce the inflammation as much as possible but not to delay surgery while the patient endures a long-term visual handicap because the inflammation never becomes completely quiescent. If the inflammatory activity cannot be assessed, the eye may be treated prophylactically for a few days as though active inflammation were present.

In our opinion, corticosteroids are still the best drugs for the control of inflammation in the perioperative period. In a small study of 20 patients randomly selected to receive prednisone or ciclosporin before cataract surgery, we found that three of 10 patients treated with ciclosporin – but none of the steroid-treated patients – had severe postoperative inflammation that necessitated a change in medication to the other drug. Corticosteroids work at multiple points in the inflammatory process, as described in Chapter 7, and are able to affect inflammation mediated by neutrophils and macrophages as well as that by lymphocytes. Therefore, they may prevent nonspecific postoperative inflammation that may occur in a previously inflamed eye as well as inhibit the more specific pathways of inflammation. We prefer to begin steroid therapy on the day before or the day of surgery if the patient is not already receiving the drug, and if there is no evidence of active inflammatory disease. Some practitioners prefer to start steroid therapy several days before the scheduled surgical intervention. If there is no strong contraindication this may not be unreasonable in some patients, although it should be remembered that the effects of the daily steroid are gone 24 hours later. Usually a dose of 1 mg/kg/day of steroid is adequate. In addition, we give a subconjunctival corticosteroid injection at the time of surgery. If the patient has a history of severe intraocular inflammation, we also give an intravenous dose of corticosteroids, such as 50–100 mg of methylprednisolone, at the time of surgery. The goal is clearly to prevent severe postoperative inflammation.

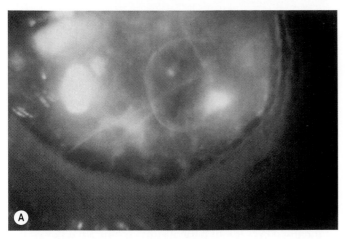
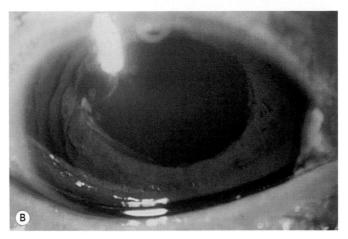

Figure 8-1. A, Uveitic eye after extracapsular cataract extraction (phacoemulsification) and intraocular lens placement. The postoperative inflammatory response was severe, with the development of fibrin in the anterior chamber. **B,** Clinical improvement occurred 24 hours after injection with tissue plasminogen activator. *(Courtesy Rubens Belfort Jr, MD, Sao Paulo, Brazil.)*

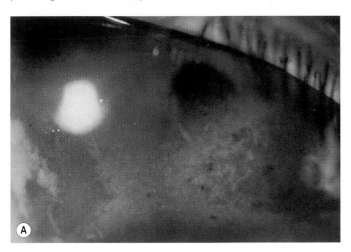
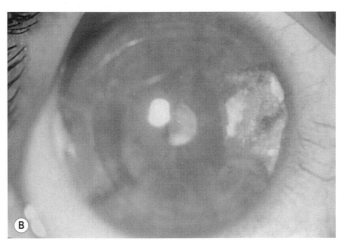

Figure 8-2. A, Band keratopathy in 6-year-old boy with bilateral uveitis. **B,** Same eye 2 days after excimer laser surgery performed under topical anesthesia. *(Courtesy Rubens Belfort Jr, MD, Sao Paulo, Brazil.)*

The surgeon should be aware that with the aforementioned perioperative therapy the eye may appear relatively quiet for the first few days after surgery, but the inflammation may increase a few days later. It is therefore critical to examine patients with uveitis daily during the first 5–7 days after surgery. In young patients and those with sarcoidosis we have specifically noted marked postoperative flares of inflammation accompanied by significant fibrin and protein within the eye. At times the fibrin is so dense that it mimics vitreous bands, and the retina cannot be viewed. Tissue plasminogen activator can be used to clear severe fibrin accumulation in the anterior chamber (**Fig. 8-1**). After surgery these eyes frequently have hypotony, and although they appear to be in imminent danger of phthisis, continued treatment with steroids combined with patience usually results in marked clearing within 3–5 days without apparent additional ocular damage.

Removal of band keratopathy

Calcium hydroxyapatite accumulates in Bowman's membrane of the cornea in some patients with sarcoidosis or juvenile rheumatoid arthritis and occasionally in younger patients with a chronic uveitis such as pars planitis. Its location may be related to the local pH of the interpalpebral cornea. It can be removed by chelation if it is located centrally and interferes with vision because of opacity or glare, or if it is the cause of recurrent corneal erosions. Although chelation with 1–2% ethylenediaminetetraacetic acid (EDTA) can be performed under local anesthesia, the age of most patients with this condition makes general anesthesia necessary. Our procedure is to use a sterile 1.7% solution of EDTA in water or saline applied to the cornea with cotton or a cellulose applicator. Gentle pressure and movement of the applicator result in removal of the corneal epithelium and gradual solubilization of the calcium deposits. This procedure can take up to 30 minutes and often must be performed before intraocular surgery. Occasionally, resistant deposits must be gently removed with a spatula or Tooke knife, but this may cause scarring of Bowman's membrane and should be avoided in the visual axis. The eye is then patched until the epithelial defect heals. Band keratopathy has also been removed with the excimer laser (**Fig. 8-2**). It should remembered that eyes with uveitis may have recurrences of the band even years after the removal of the calcium.[2] Further, the procedure may very rarely induce a severe inflammatory response, as was reported in one patient.[3]

Corneal transplantation

Although keratitic precipitates involve the corneal endothelial surface, endothelial decompensation is rare in our experience in patients with chronic uveitis. Thus corneal transplantation is rarely performed in this group because of corneal edema, but it may be necessary in patients with corneoscleral melting in association with systemic inflammatory disease and intraocular inflammation, or in patients with herpetic keratouveitis. If the intraocular inflammation has been severe, there may be coexistent glaucoma or cataract. The primary goal before corneal transplantation in these patients is to control the immune process, or the newly grafted tissue will melt as well. The ongoing inflammatory response suggests that the risk for rejection of a cornea transplant in any patient with active uveitis is high because there are already large numbers of cells in the eye that could present corneal antigens to the immune system and participate in the rejection event. Certain severe manifestations of immune-mediated ocular surface disease, such as vernal keratoconjunctivitis, can lead to limbal stem cell deficiency, and before a penetrating keratoplasty is considered the ocular surface environment needs to be addressed. The treating physician should be aware of drugs being given for other indications that may induce a uveitis and risk graft survival. Richards and co-workers[4] described such a case of a patient receiving alendronate sodium for osteoporosis. The uveitis resolved after cessation of the drug.

Cataract surgery

Much information has been acquired during recent years concerning cataract extraction in uveitic eyes.[5] Although there is not yet an absolute consensus on the most ideal method of cataract removal, we are moving closer to that goal and some basic tenets are being established. Individual patients and various disorders often require different approaches. Summaries of procedures performed 20–30 years ago suggested that the outcome of cataract surgery in eyes with uveitis was poor, and that phthisis occurred frequently. This is clearly no longer the case in our experience, nor in that of other investigators, thanks largely to new technologies and approaches. Today, intracapsular cataract extraction is rarely if ever performed. The theoretic advantage of not leaving residual lens material in the eye seems to be outweighed by the larger incision and higher incidence of retinal detachment and cystoid macular edema. We reserve intracapsular extraction for mature lenses in eyes with phacoantigenic uveitis or phacogenic glaucoma, or in eyes with lenses that are dislocated or mobile because of loosened ciliary processes.

Extracapsular extraction, either via irrigation/aspiration or – now almost always – with phacoemulsification, is now the centerpoint of the discussion. These approaches have the advantages of smaller incisions and less manipulation of the iris. Reports support the use of phacoemulsification over an expression/irrigation system. Several studies[6–8] have shown less postoperative inflammation in eyes undergoing phacoemulsification. Chee and colleagues[9] looked at this question in uveitic eyes prospectively, comparing the two methods, and found that the eyes with phacoemulsification invariably had less inflammation. We expect to see good results for all patients with uveitis upon whom we operate. However, we do see complications. Postoperative hyphema is not uncommon in inflamed eyes. Postoperatively one might see the formation of posterior synechiae to the capsule, pupillary block glaucoma, the inability to remove vitreous debris, haze and vitreoretinal traction, and possible opacification of the posterior capsule. We have also observed patients in whom a neodynium:yttrium–aluminum–garnet (Nd:YAG) laser capsulotomy leads to an exacerbation of inflammation. Herbort[10] reported the case of a patient in whom a severe and recurrent scleritis and uveitis developed after an Nd:YAG capsulotomy was performed 18 months after cataract extraction. Also, laser-induced iris punctures often close off readily in inflamed eyes. In all patients undergoing surgery we wish to see the ocular inflammatory process well controlled for at least 3 months (and preferably 6).

The surgeon may encounter challenging technical problems. If the pupil is less than 2–3 mm the surgeon is likely to encounter a dense fibrin membrane across it. To widen the pupillary aperture we often use disposable iris retractors in the four quadrants. In rare eyes the pupil will not dilate until this membrane is cut with a Van Ness scissors after sodium hyaluronate (Healon) has been administered. Posterior synechiae not only may be present at the pupillary border but also may extend over the entire surface of the lens. These extensive adhesions cannot be easily broken with an iris spatula, but with the aid of a sector iridectomy and pupillary membrane sectioning an adequate anterior capsulotomy can be performed. In addition, an anterior surgical approach should be avoided if there are peripheral anterior synechiae extending onto clear cornea, because the surgical incision may not enter the anterior chamber but instead go through the iris into the posterior chamber. With the use of iris retractors we have been able to perform phacoemulsification on many uveitic eyes requiring surgery. Many of these patients are young, and phacoemulsification time is quite low. Most of the nucleus can be removed by aspiration.

The surgeon should expect uveitic eyes to bleed from the conjunctiva, Tenon's capsule, the corneoscleral wound, and the iris. Even eyes that have been quiet for several months appear to have an increased tendency to bleed during or after surgery. Bleeding can be controlled by careful cautery, by tamponade with the irrigating solution, and by patience. Entering into the anterior chamber through a scleral tunnel or clear cornea still is discussed. The clear cornea approach has a certain advantage if glaucoma surgery is contemplated.

It is imperative to restate that one needs to use any means necessary to bring the eye's inflammatory disease under strict control. Some would mandate even the absence of every cell, which for us is sometimes most difficult to obtain, but the message is one we fully support. The disease must be controlled, and it must be controlled for an extended period – usually 3–6 months – before we would consider surgical intervention. The patient should be informed about the possible need for continued and even more aggressive immunosuppressive therapy to control the disease postoperatively. An extracapsular cataract extraction (phacoemulsification) and placement of the intraocular lens (IOL) in the bag would be our preferred approach. We would prefer to make

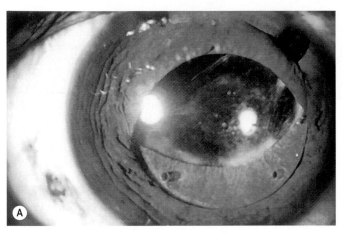
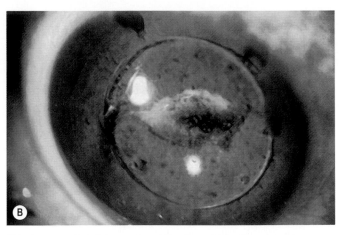

Figure 8-3. Uveitic eye that underwent cataract surgery and posterior chamber IOL placement. **A,** Inferior portion of lens has migrated anterior to lens plane. **B,** The whole lens is now forward. This 'iris capture' occurred without marked inflammatory disease. *(Courtesy Rubens Belfort Jr, MD, Sao Paulo, Brazil.)*

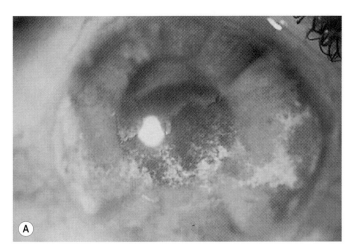
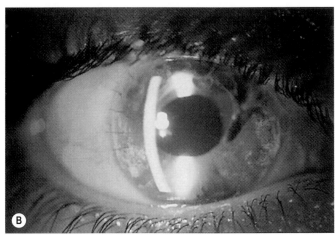

Figure 8-4. When his disease was quiescent, an 11-year-old boy with anterior uveitis underwent cataract extraction and IOL placement. **A,** After multiple YAG capsulotomies and EDTA treatments, a persistent anterior chamber reaction required topical steroid therapy. **B,** After IOL removal and normalization of intraocular pressure, inflammation was absent, steroid therapy had been discontinued, and visual acuity was 20/100. *(Courtesy Rubens Belfort Jr, MD, Sao Paulo, Brazil.)*

a small as an incision as possible, and various techniques are reported in the literature.[11] This is often followed by a curtailed anterior vitrectomy. This sort of approach is outlined by Walker and colleagues.[12] The decision as to whether to place an IOL continues to be debated, and although there are no strict rules (how can there be in medicine?), certain guidelines have evolved. Patients with chronically active granulomatous disease seem to cause us the most concern. Iris capture (**Fig. 8-3**)[13] is also a real concern (but we see this less and less), and patients with posterior synechiae have a greater risk for occurrence of this problem as well as the capsule contraction syndrome postoperatively.[14]

Much interest has been shown in surface-modified lenses and the possibility of their reducing the postoperative inflammatory response. Percival and Pai[15] placed a heparin surface-modified one-piece lens into the posterior chamber of 36 patients with cataracts associated with previous or chronic recurrent uveitis. They found that recurrent inflammatory disease was present, including an acute postoperative fibrin reaction, but the heparin coating appeared to provide a cell-free IOL surface in most eyes (**Figs 8-4 and 8-5**). Reports suggest that heparin modification does not provide a signifi-

cant benefit.[16] Alio and colleagues,[17] in a prospective study of cataract surgery in uveitic eyes, compared four different types of IOL. Using hydrophobic acrylic, silicone, polymethylmethacrylate (PMMA), and heparin surface-modified PMMA lenses, they concluded that the acrylic IOLs had a better visual outcome and lower complication rate, whereas both acrylic and heparin surface-modified PMMA lenses had the lowest relapse rates. Elgohary et al.[18] found that YAG capsulotomies were more common in older patients, but there were generally fewer problems in patients receiving prophylactic systemic steroid with either plate-haptic silicone lenses or three-piece silicone lenses than with PMMA. Others have suggested the use of acrylic lenses.[19] Angle-supported lenses have been associated with anterior and intermediate uveitedes.[20]

The eyes of patients with juvenile idiopathic arthritis (JIA) deserve separate comment.[21] These eyes have not been considered good candidates for IOLs. The reason for this is the potential of the lens to act as a scaffold for the development of membranes in eyes with low-grade chronic disease that is often difficult to control. We have generally not placed an IOL in children with uveitis. Lundvall and Zetterstrom[22] reported their experience with 10 eyes in seven children. With a follow-up of 1–5 years, they reported that most eyes had visual acuities between 20/20 and 20/50. Glaucoma developed in three eyes. In a 5-year follow-up of 17 children (20 eyes) with chronic uveitis undergoing cataract extraction,[23] an almost equal number of patients with JRA and without underwent IOL placement or pars plana removal of the lens. Of interest in this study reported by BenEzra and Cohen[23] was the finding that 5 years after surgery, only two of nine eyes in the JRA group retained a visual acuity of 6/9 or better. Most of the other eyes had a visual acuity of 6/240. However, in the group without JRA, 11 eyes (54.5%) retained a visual acuity of 6/12 or better. A child's inflammatory response can be exuberant, causing serious difficulties postoperatively. However, recent studies suggest that this approach is being questioned. Kotaniemi et al.[24] reported that 64% of 36 JIA eyes receiving an implant had visual acuities of 20/40 or better. A list of recent results reported where intraocular lenses are placed is seen in **Table 8-1**. Woreta et al.[25] reported on the risk factors for ocular complications in 75 JIA patients undergoing surgery, and found that 67%

had ocular complications. Eyes with more than 1+ flare, a history of previous intraocular surgery, and posterior synechiae all had a higher risk of poorer vision postoperatively. It would seem that the degree of activity, control of disease and secondary anatomic alterations due to the uveitis may be important considerations.

Results from the literature support the notion that IOL placement in uveitic eyes can result in a positive outcome.[8,26] Pleyer and colleagues[27] reported in a 5-year series that 71% of 28 eyes receiving an IOL had a postoperative visual acuity of 0.5 or better, compared to 54% of the 24 eyes that were aphakic. Because this was not a randomized study it is difficult to compare the relative 'success' rates. Foster and colleagues[28] reported that in 20 uveitic eyes extracapsular cataract extraction with posterior chamber IOL and pars plana vitrectomy, if needed, produced 20/100 or better visual acuity in 60% of the eyes operated on. Tessler and Farber,[29] comparing IOL placement with no IOL placement in uveitic eyes, believed that IOLs appeared to be relatively safe in patients with what was described as chronic iridocyclitis. However, a comment[30] and our interpretation of the paper would indeed suggest that the data would argue for the reverse – that is, eyes with IOLs had a poorer postoperative result. As Tessler and Farber stated, only a larger study could definitively settle this question. In a study of 89 patients (106 eyes) Hazari and colleagues[31] reported that eyes receiving an IOL had a better visual outcome than those not receiving an IOL. It should be noted that eyes that did not have an improvement in visual acuity had persistent uveitis, a problem that the practitioner must be continuously aware of. Kim and colleagues[32] reported a recurrence of Behçet's disease in a patient that necessitated IOL exchange and vitrectomy, with a resultant poor visual outcome. It appears that eyes with Fuchs' heterochromic iridocyclitis do well after cataract surgery and IOL placement.[33]

Akova and Foster,[34] in a retrospective analysis of their patients with sarcoidosis, found that of 102 patients, 14 (21 eyes) had surgery because of visual acuity of 20/100 or less. In stressing the need for absolute control of the intraocular inflammatory disease, they found that 19 of the 21 patients

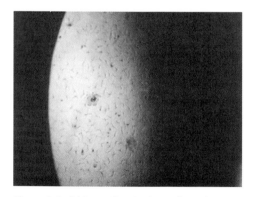

Figure 8-5. With retroillumination, cells can be seen to accumulate on the anterior surface of IOLs in uveitic eyes. Elongated cell bodies of smaller cells suggest macrophages. Larger cells with more substantial cytoplasm also appear.

Table 8-1 Studies of primary lens implantation in pediatric uveitic cataracts. (From: Zaborowski AG, Quinn AG, Dick AD, et al. Cataract surgery in pediatric uveitis. J Pediatr Strabismus 2008; 45(5): 270–8; with permission)

Author	No. of Patients	No. of Study Eyes	Uveitic Diagnosis	Age at Surgery (yrs)	Follow-up (yrs)	Summary of BCVA at Latest Follow-up
BenEzra & Cohen (2000)[33]	10	10	5 JIA, 5 non-JIA	4 to 17	5	JIA: <20/200 in 4 of 5; Non-JIA: <20/200 2 of 5, >20/30 in 2 of 5
Lundvall & Zetterström (2000)[50]	7	10	All 'typical of JIA'	3.5 to 10 (mean = 6.5)	1 to 5.2 (mean = 2.3)	20/50 to 20/20 in 8 of 10 eyes
Lam et al. (2003)[20]	5	6	All JIA	7 to 12 (median = 8.5)	1.4 to 5.8 (median = 3.6)	≥20/40 in all
Petric et al. (2005)[49]	6	7	All JIA	5 to 14 (median = 8)	2.2 to 5 (mean = 4)	≥20/40 in all
Kotaniemi & Penttila (2006)[48]	25	36	All JIA	Mean 4.5	0.1 to 11 (mean = 3.3)	≥20/40 in 64% 20/40 to 20/60 in 11%, <20/60 in 25%
Namet et al. (2007)[18]	18	19	10 JIA, 9 non-JIA	4 to 24 (mean = 14.3)	0.3 to 14 (mean = 3.9)	≥20/40 in 13, <20/40 in 6

BCVA = best-corrected visual acuity; JIA = juvenile idiopathic arthritis.

received IOLs, and that 61% of the eyes had a stable visual acuity of 20/40 or better. In eyes that did not have a dramatic improvement in visual acuity, retinal pathologic conditions such as cystoid edema and epiretinal membranes, as well as glaucomatous optic nerve disease, were found.

As mentioned above, JRA is a disorder in which IOL placement has not been recommended. In a review of 16 eyes in 10 patients with JRA, Fox and colleagues[35] found that after pars plana lensectomy and vitrectomy the short-term visual acuity was 20/70 or better in 13 eyes (81%), but a longer follow-up showed that the final visual acuity was 20/70 or better in nine of them (56%). This drop was attributed to glaucoma and retinal disease such as cystoid edema.

There are other challenges that the uveitic eye can present to the surgeon. One is operating on an eye with long-standing exudative detachments. Secchi[36] reported good results in these eyes with total lens removal combined with anterior vitrectomy and placement of a scleral fixation lens.

Complications from the cataract surgery or sequelae from the ongoing inflammation must be expected, particularly when an IOL has been placed.[37,38] Posterior capsule opacification is seen frequently. When Dana and colleagues[39] compared rates of posterior capsule opacification between 78 patients with uveitis and 106 patients without uveitis undergoing cataract surgery, the rates were comparable when an adjustment was made for the younger age of the patients with uveitis. In a report by Estafanous and colleagues[7] of 39 uveitic eyes needing surgery, posterior capsular opacification was seen in 24 eyes (62%), with 12 of these (31%) needing Nd:YAG capsulotomy. Of these patients 41% had a recurrence of their disease. If cystoid macular edema was present before surgery, it will most probably be there after the surgery and will need to be addressed. Epiretinal membrane formations can be seen. Lenses do need to be explanted, even after the best preoperative consideration by the surgeon. In a report by Foster and colleagues[40] of 19 patients whose lenses were explanted, a perilental membrane was the reason in eight, low-grade inflammation in eight, a cyclitic membrane leading to hypotony in one, retinal detachment in one, and vitreous hemorrhage in one.

Pars plana lensectomy, usually combined with vitrectomy, has been used by several authors to remove a cataract, reshape the pupil, and remove vitreous opacities and vitreoretinal traction in one operation.[41–45] The operation can be performed using the standard technique: three 1-mm incisions 3 or 3.5 mm posterior to the limbus. Trauma to the trabecular meshwork is avoided. Usually the use of disposable iris retractors will provide the surgeon with an adequate view initially, until the lens has been removed. However, if this is not the case, the pupillary aperture can be enlarged with the vitrectomy instrument to be round and large enough to examine the retina after surgery. However, this technique can provoke bleeding from the edge of the iris. In addition, more conjunctiva can be left undisturbed for use in a future filtering operation. The main disadvantage is the removal of the posterior capsular barrier. Some surgeons have advocated keeping the anterior capsule intact to use as a possible support if a secondary implant is considered. We have had no experience with this approach. The possibility of retinal detachment shortly after surgery is less than 1% in our experience. This operation is difficult to perform in patients over 50 years of age because,

in our experience, the lens nucleus becomes rather hard, making it more difficult to remove. It has been suggested by several authors that pars plana vitrectomy reduces or eliminates recurrences of inflammation because it removes an antigen load from the vitreous. This has not been our experience. However, removal of the vitreous can reduce the accumulation of cells and haze during an episode of inflammation, but the vision will still be affected by a new inflammatory episode. We therefore prefer to perform this operation in patients younger than 50 who have had vitreitis as part of their ocular inflammation, especially if the vitreous and retina cannot be visualized preoperatively because the pupil is small or there are other structural alterations in the anterior chamber.

Our technique for pars plana lensectomy/vitrectomy is to make three radial conjunctival incisions. These are cleaned down to bare sclera, and scleral incisions are made 3 mm posterior to the limbus. An infusing cannula is inserted in one incision but is not turned on. An ultrasonic fragmenting instrument and an irrigating needle are introduced into the lens, and the lens material is removed within the capsular bag, using both the fragmenting instrument and the vitrectomy instrument. An alternative is to place the light pipe under the lens to help visualization. Entry into the eye must be parallel to the iris or the posterior capsule will be broken prematurely. After the lens material is removed, the vitreous cutter is used to remove the lens capsule and anterior vitreous and to reshape the pupil. A vitrectomy is then performed to remove opacities and any tractional abnormalities.

Results for cataract surgery have been reported to be favorable with both an anterior chamber approach and entry through the pars plana. Results depend more on previous damage from the inflammation than from surgical complications. Praeger and colleagues[46] reported excellent improvement after extracapsular surgery in patients with JRA. Mackensen and Loeffler[47] reported that in 86 patients with chronic iridocyclitis who underwent extracapsular surgery, inflammation was reduced by 70% and recurrences by 94%. Vision improved in most patients. In a study by Smith and colleagues[41] 12 patients with chronic uveitis who underwent pars plana lensectomy/vitrectomy had improved vision, but cystoid macular edema impaired the acuity in most of them. Girard and colleagues[42] reported that 5-year remissions of uveitis occurred in all of their 23 patients, and 21 had improved vision after pars plana surgery. In the 39 patients Petrilli and coworkers[43] studied after pars plana surgery, 23% had vision better than 20/40, and 56% had vision worse than 20/100; 18% had cystoid macular edema. Other authors have had similar experiences.[44,45] In our experience the average vision after surgery in patients with long-standing chronic inflammation was 20/100 (**Fig. 8-6**). Phthisis occurred in approximately 2% of the eyes, and 90% of the patients had improved vision.

Hypotony is often mentioned as a contraindication for cataract removal in these patients. However, if the cataract is dense and vision limited to hand movements or worse, surgery by the pars plana route can be considered in eyes with intraocular pressures <3 mmHg. It can be useful in treating cases of hypotony where bands are creating traction on the ciliary body and resulting in reduced aqueous production. We have seen that removal of these tractional forces will cause an increase in intraocular pressure – not

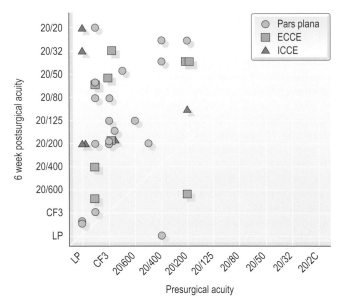

Figure 8-6. Change in visual acuity after cataract removal in patients with uveitis.

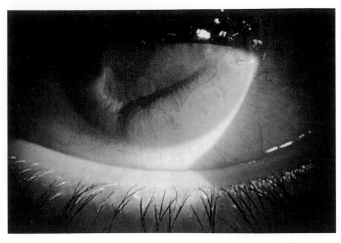

Figure 8-7. Slit-lamp photograph of patient with uveitis and pupillary block glaucoma. Iris bombé, due to broad iris–lens synechiae, localized from the 3- to the 6-o'clock position.

enormous, but enough to achieve a more reassuring pressure. Yu et al.[48] reported similar results in patients with JIA.

Although phthisis may result, we have observed five eyes with preoperative hypotony in which there was an increase in intraocular pressure of several mmHg after pars plana lensectomy/vitrectomy. In many eyes with posterior inflammation there is a dense anterior hyaloid that may be associated with ciliary body traction. Removal of this traction may result in improved ciliary body function.

Glaucoma surgery

Secondary glaucoma that cannot be controlled by medical therapy is sometimes a consequence of severe anterior segment inflammation. It is important to differentiate between pupillary block glaucoma and secondary angle closure by peripheral anterior synechiae. The two processes may coexist in the eye with uveitis. Active inflammation may suppress ciliary body function and also reduce trabecular filtration. Thus intraocular pressure in the actively inflamed eye may be higher or lower than in the uninflamed eye. Although patients with long-standing chronic inflammation have poor outflow, increased inflammation will lead to reduced aqueous production and a pressure decrease. If treatment with corticosteroids is accompanied by an increase in pressure, it does not necessarily mean that the patient is a 'steroid responder.'

It may be difficult to distinguish pupillary block glaucoma in a patient with chronic inflammation and posterior synechiae that involve the entire lens surface. These patients do not show a classic iris bombé pattern but may have a subtle shallowing of the anterior chamber with a low, peripheral iris bombé. The iris elevation may be localized only to areas where the iris and the lens are not adherent (**Fig. 8-7**). If the diagnosis is suspected but unclear, a laser iridectomy will confirm it and also be therapeutic. If the laser iridectomy fails to lower the intraocular pressure, pupillary block can be ruled out as a mechanism.

Filtering surgery such as a trabeculectomy is less successful in patients with ongoing uveitis because of the younger age of such patients, and because the inflammatory mediators promote fibrous tissue growth and closure of the filtering bleb. An alternative surgical approach, that of deep sclerectomy using various implants, has been reported be useful in treating uveitic glaucoma.[49] A normal response on the part of the treating physician is frequently to practice restraint because of the problems inherent in operating on uveitis patients. An insidious loss of visual function due to the glaucoma can ensue even with excellent control of the uveitis. The operation should be performed when the eye is quiet at a site where surgery has not previously been performed. Because these eyes frequently need repeated surgical procedures, combining a filtering operation (often with mitomycin C) with cataract removal, if appropriate, seems justified to reduce the number of possible interventions.[50]

Drugs such as 5-fluorouracil (5-FU) and mitomycin C are used to improve the success of filtering surgery by slowing the growth of fibrous tissue. Patitsas and colleagues[51] used 5-FU combined with filtering surgery to treat patients with both uveitis and glaucoma. They found that intraocular pressure was controlled in 71% of 21 eyes over a median of 35 months. Control was better achieved in phakic eyes (90%) than in aphakic or pseudophakic (55%) eyes. Complications that have been associated with 5-FU use occurred. Towler and coworkers[52] reported their experience with 50 uveitic glaucomatous eyes in 43 consecutive patients. They observed an 82% success rate at 1 and 2 years and a 67% success rate at 5 years by applying 5-FU (25 mg/mL) for 5 minutes to the area of the bleb. In another report by Ceballos et al.[53] 44 eyes in 44 patients were treated with local application of either mitomycin C or 5-FU. A complete success was defined as an intraocular pressure of 21 mmHg or less in a patient taking no other antiglaucoma medication. In this study, the success rates at 2 years were 39% in males and 71% in females, and 74% in whites but only 55% in blacks. Over half of the patients developed cataracts or saw their cataracts progress, and 25% needed repeat surgery. Although 5-FU therapy may keep the bleb open during the initial few weeks, months, or years after surgery, recurrent inflammation could still threaten to destroy a functional filtering bleb. Indeed,

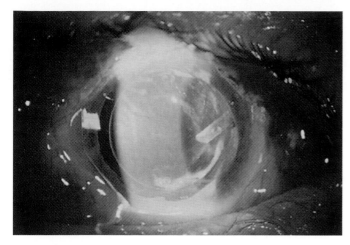

Figure 8-8. Uveitic eye with secondary glaucoma that could not be controlled with maximum medication or trabeculectomy surgery. The tube from a single-plate Molteno implant can be seen in the anterior chamber at the 2-o'clock position.

there has been one report of an idiosyncratic anterior granulomatous uveitis in a patient who received one injection of subconjunctival 5-FU.[54]

Alternative approaches in children include a modified goniotomy or trabeculodialysis. Kanski and McAllister[55] reported on 23 such operations and found a 60% success rate in patients with JRA. However, in only five patients could control be achieved without additional antiglaucoma medication. Williams and colleagues[56] reported a success rate in 56% of 25 uveitic eyes undergoing trabeculodialysis, with aphakic eyes doing no worse than those that were phakic. Ultrasonic filtering surgery has not yet been used in enough patients with uveitis to determine whether this approach may be helpful.

The approach that has gained the most use in uveitis patients is an aqueous draining device. In the past we used the Molteno implant (**Fig. 8-8**). Although in our experience patients can demonstrate an intraocular inflammatory response combined with hypotony during the first days after surgery, on a long-term basis there appears to be good control of the intraocular pressure. Hill and coworkers[57] reviewed the cases of 45 patients with both uveitis and glaucoma and found that an aqueous drainage device was more likely to control the intraocular pressure in those who had significant, immediate, or chronic postoperative inflammation. However, they also believed that trabeculectomy produced surprisingly good results as well. Freedman and Rubin[58] have also reported good results with a single-plate Molteno implant. More recently we have used the Baerveldt implant,[59] and recently there have been several reports using using the Ahmed valve.[60,61] Long-term results with the Ahmed valve in uveitis patients have been reported.[62] At 4 years, 74% of patients needed glaucoma medication and the complication rate was 12%/person-year. The visual acuity loss was 4%/person-year. The results suggested it to be safe and moderately effective.

Another alternative is the Schocket implant. Although results with this procedure were reported to compare favorably with those from use of the Molteno implant,[63,64] it has not been used in the uveitic eyes with glaucoma we have dealt with at the National Eye Institute.

If the aforementioned surgical approaches fail, one can try to reduce aqueous formation. Cyclocryotherapy and laser destruction are both possible methods of achieving this. Cryotherapy is now very rarely (if ever) used. Cyclocryotherapy is performed in sequential treatments 4–8 weeks apart. One begins by treating from the 6- to the 8-o'clock positions with 1-minute freezes. If this fails to lower the pressure after several weeks, six more clock-hour positions are treated, with three of the clock hours overlapping the first treatment. Further treatments may be required, but these need to be approached cautiously. The operation is accompanied by significant postoperative pain and does not work immediately. Preoperative anterior chamber paracentesis has been suggested to prevent an immediate cryotherapy-induced rise in intraocular pressure. Laser destruction of the ciliary processes allows more careful titration of the destructive process but requires a widely dilated pupil so that the ciliary body can be visualized and directly treated. Such dilation is difficult to achieve in patients with chronic uveitis, and this approach may carry a risk of sympathetic ophthalmia.

It has been estimated that about 18% of uveitic eyes or almost 20% of patients with uveitis will develop secondary glaucoma.[65] A smaller percentage will ultimately need surgery. Providing this care is surely a challenge. One should consider glaucoma surgery while there is vision to save and not wait until it is an end-stage procedure. Usually the choice is between trabeculectomy with a locally applied antimetabolite and a drainage instrument such as a Molteno, Ahmed, or Baerveldt device. Much will depend on whether surgery was performed previously, the state of the conjunctiva, and the preference of the glaucoma specialist. Generally we would use a drainage device, the Baerveldt first. A valved device would be considered if there was a history of hypotony or evidence of poor aqueous production and almost complete angle closure by peripheral anterior synechiae. If a trabeculectomy is contemplated, then mitomycin C would be used.

Treatment of vitreoretinal disease

Significant vitreous opacities, areas of vitreoretinal traction, or epiretinal membranes sometimes develop in patients who have severe posterior inflammation, and newer techniques have permitted these problems to be approached with a reasonable hope of success.[66] Lens fragments after cataract surgery can be a source of ongoing inflammation and should be promptly removed.[67] If the opacities and membranes appear to be the major source of a decrease in vision, or if there is a significant tractional retinal detachment, then vitrectomy without lensectomy is indicated. In general, the surgical management of these eyes does not differ from that of eyes with vitreous opacities or traction from other causes. Vitrectomy is now often combined with phacoemulsification, and in addition there has been recent interest in using 25-gauge vitrectomy units, with many reporting good results.[68,69]

The value of vitrectomy alone as a therapeutic tool for intraocular inflammatory disease remains problematic.[70] Bacskulin and Eckardt[71] found in 13 children with uveitis who underwent vitrectomy, either alone or combined with lensectomy, that their disease was easier to treat, and in some there was resolution of macular edema. We have found that vitrectomy is useful in helping to observe the posterior pole and thus follow the course of disease, and the procedure appears to make it easier for steroid to penetrate intraocularly. However, we have not found it to be an effective therapy when used alone, as had been suggested by Kaplan[72] and Stavrou et al.[73] who found that in 44% of 43 eyes there was an improvement in the course of intermediate uveitis. Bovey and colleagues[74] performed vitrectomy or cataract extraction or both in 30 eyes and found an improvement in visual acuity but no decrease in the inflammatory process, nor did Nolle[75] and Eckardt in nine patients with multifocal chorioretinitis who underwent vitrectomy. Guttfleisch et al.[76] performed pars plana vitrectomy coupled with intravitreal injections of triamcinolone to treat cystoid macular edema. CME improved in 58% of patients in the first 6 weeks, but the effect was transient, with 85% of patients additionally showing cataract progression, and increases in intraocular pressure seen in over one-quarter of 19 patients treated. Indeed, a small randomized comparing vitrectomy (n = 12) to medical therapy (n = 11) for CME showed that in the vitrectomized group CME improved in four patients, remained unchanged in seven, and worsened in one.[77] In a very good review of 44 interventional case series involving 1575 patients, Becker and Davis[78] found that in 39 articles the visual acuity of vitrectomized uveitic eyes improved in 68% of cases, was unchanged in 20%, and was worse in 12%. The findings of CME in patients halved. The devil is in the details. When evaluating these findings so many factors complicate the interpretation that is most difficult to arrive at a reasonable clinical conclusion. One possible exception to this is reported salutary effect of vitrectomy on juvenile uveitis.

The prognosis for visual improvement after removal of the epiretinal membrane is worse in eyes with uveitis than in eyes with idiopathic membranes.[79] Retinal detachment is surprisingly not that uncommon in these patients. In one review of 1387 patients,[80] 43 (46 eyes) had a retinal detachment (3.1% of the total). It was most frequently associated with panuveitis and eyes with infectious disease. The uveitis was active in almost one half of the patients studied. In addition, after repair of a rhegmatogenous retinal detachment by standard scleral buckling procedures there is probably a higher risk of proliferative vitreoretinopathy (PVR) in eyes with ongoing chronic inflammation, because the inflammatory mediators stimulate fibrous tissue proliferation. It was seen in 30% of the patients reported by Kerkhoff and associates.[80] The development of PVR usually necessitates additional surgery with membrane stripping and gas–fluid exchange. After this procedure, control of the inflammation is critical or the membranes may reform. Re-attachment occurs in a small minority of patients after one operation, whereas anatomic reattachment occurs in close to 90% of patients, and the final vision is poor (20/200 or worse in close to three-quarters of patients).[80]

Serous detachment is a commonly faced problem in uveitis and is almost always treated medically. However, there are stubborn cases that may simply not respond to therapy, either for physical reasons such as traction or for reasons that are unclear. Surgical drainage can be contemplated, often with reattachment succeeding.[81] Another type of drainage reported in the literature is puncture of cystoid macular edema lesions. This may flatten the cyst but will not result in an improvement of vision.[82]

The repair of giant retinal tears that may complicate viral retinitis, such as acute retinal necrosis or cytomegalovirus retinitis, is not always best managed by scleral buckling. The retina in these diseases has become necrotic and areas may be ischemic. The use of a high buckle might increase this ischemia, leading to retinal neovascularization. An alternative solution has been to perform a pars plana vitrectomy and to reattach the retina with gas or silicone oil tamponade and laser photocoagulation.[83]

Laser treatment

Lasers can be used to perform peripheral iridectomies and posterior capsulotomies, to cut pupillary membranes, to clear deposits off the anterior surface of an IOL, and to treat retinal or subretinal neovascularization. The use of the laser, however, does not eliminate the possibility of inducing inflammation.

In the anterior segment either the YAG or the argon laser can be used to perform an iridotomy. Although the procedure is probably technically easier with the YAG laser, there is the theoretic possibility that the incidence of hyphema from the vascular, inflamed iris may be greater after YAG than after argon laser treatment because the YAG laser does not coagulate tissue. This comparison has not been studied in patients with uveitis. Posterior capsulotomy is easily performed with the YAG laser unless there has been a significant fibrous reaction or calcification as a result of the inflammation. Pupillary membranes can occasionally be so dense that the laser procedure becomes very long, necessitates the use of high energies, or cannot be successfully performed at all (**Fig. 8-9**). In addition, although an uncomplicated capsulotomy can be performed with only a few bursts of laser energy – and at the time of the procedure it appears that little has been disrupted within the eye – the energy delivered by the YAG laser does alter the blood–aqueous barrier.[84] We have observed several patients with chronic uveitis who have had severe flares of inflammation associated with a marked temporary decrease in acuity 1 day after YAG laser capsulotomy.

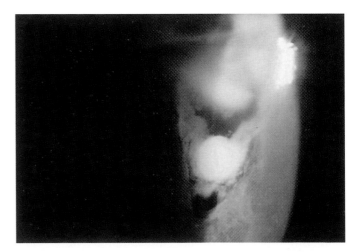

Figure 8-9. YAG laser membrane disruption in a patient with dense pupillary membrane after cataract surgery.

In rabbits, the application of the YAG laser to the iris induced intraocular production of interleukin (IL)-6, IL-8, and tumor necrosis factor-α as well as nitric oxide.[85] Timolol appeared to reduce the production of all these mediators of inflammation except for nitric oxide. Therefore, use of the YAG laser in patients with severe inflammatory disease should be treated with the same concern as an invasive surgical procedure, and the patient should be pretreated with corticosteroids to prevent recurrence of the inflammation.

Photocoagulation of the retina for surface or subretinal neovascularization may also be accompanied by bouts of inflammation. Panretinal or sector argon photocoagulation for surface neovascularization is indicated if the new vessels have not regressed with antiinflammatory therapy. Patients with sarcoidosis and neovascularization of the optic disc often show regression of the vessels with steroid therapy. In contrast, patients with retinal neovascularization due to Behçet's disease rarely show resolution because the retinal ischemia remains even when the eye is quiet. These eyes usually respond to panretinal photocoagulation. Retinal laser therapy may lead to increased intraocular inflammation, not only because of the alterations in the blood–retinal barrier related to the laser energy but also because there may be significant amounts of retinal antigens released during the destruction of the retina. We have seen one patient who had previous ocular procedures in the right eye but developed sympathetic ophthalmia in both eyes shortly after a retinal hole in the left eye was treated with laser. The Dalen–Fuchs nodules began around the site of laser therapy and expanded to involve the rest of that eye. This implies that the release of antigen in an already primed patient triggered an autoimmune response.

Subretinal neovascular membranes are seen in uveitis, as in the presumed ocular histoplasmosis syndrome, multifocal choroiditis, and serpiginous choroidopathy. Because alterations in Bruch's membrane are widespread in some types of uveitis, these membranes can occur in a variety of locations. If the neovascular membrane is at the posterior pole, argon laser has been used, but its use is decreasing. Photodynamic therapy (PDT) has been reported to have been used in several uveitis studies. Reports describing the use of PDT in mutifocal choroiditis suggest that some patients may benefit from this approach,[86,87] whereas in Vogt–Kanagi–Harada syndrome (VKH) the development of subretinal fibrosis is a concerning factor.[88] Others did not report it useful in a very small number of younger patients with uveitis.[89] Others have combined PDT with immunosuppressive therapy, either intravitreal or systemic steroid, with an improvement in vision of 13 letters for 15 months. These are very small studies, but I would consider adequate immunosuppressive therapy in these patients although overwhelming data are lacking. However, Tatar et al.[90] found that specimens of age-related macular degeneration membranes taken from eyes receiving PDT demonstrated an infiltrate of leukocytes and macrophages and enhanced proliferative activity. They recommended antiinflammatory therapy as an adjunct. For these reasons we would consider anti-VEGF (vascular endothelial growth factor) therapy first. Bevacizumab therapy can have a significant effect on the membrane, but we would try immunosuppressive therapy first or together with the anti-VEGF therapy. In one report Tran et al.[91] found that leakage stopped in three eyes but reduced in seven, so we still need to improve our approach to this sequela of uveitis.

In extramacular lesions the physician must balance the potential visual loss from the membrane with the potential increase in inflammation that could result from the therapy. If treated, the response to therapy would not be expected to differ from the response in other, more common causes of the subretinal membranes. Another concern is the effect of repetitive PDT on the already damaged retinal pigment epithelium (RPE) of an uveitic eye. Data on feeder vessel therapy is still lacking.

Photodynamic therapy

PDT has entered into standard ophthalmic practice for the treatment of age-related macular degeneration.[92,93] In the 2-year follow-up of a randomized study, 53% (213 patients) of the 407 patients receiving Visudyne lost fewer than 15 letters than did 38% (78 patients) of 207 receiving placebo. It appears that those patients with a classic choroidal neovascular lesion (i.e., the neovascular lesion makes up more than 50% of the lesion) appeared to fare the best. We are seeing more and more reports of PDT being applied to lesions associated with inflammatory conditions, such as VKH[94] and multifocal choroiditis.[95] Initial reports are reasonably favorable, but the long-term effectiveness of this therapy is being questioned, as the histopathology of PDT eyes does not show permanent closure of subretinal vessels.[96] In addition there is the concern of the long-term affects of PDT on the RPE. The most frequently reported side effects (in some 10–20% of patients) associated with PDT therapy have been headaches, reactions at the site of the injection, and visual disturbances. Patients have complained of blurred and reduced vision as well as visual field defects. Within 7 days of therapy a severe drop in vision (i.e., four lines or more) has been reported in a smaller number of patients (1–4%), with a partial recovery occurring in many. Photosensitivity reactions can occur if patients are exposed to significant sunlight.

Diagnostic surgery

Surgical procedures frequently are the only method of distinguishing a disease of presumed autoimmune etiology from an infectious or malignant ocular process. The clinical appearance of many ocular infections and some malignant conditions is not always diagnostic. For example, a patient with cytomegalovirus retinitis may have lesions that are consistent with those of Behçet's disease during a certain period in the disease course. The overall courses of the two diseases are different, but at the time the physician examines the patient the two may appear similar. In this example, a careful history would probably suggest that, if the patient were immunosuppressed, a viral retinitis was more likely than an autoimmune disease. Infection with *Propionibacterium acnes* (see Chapter 9) and large cell lymphoma of the vitreous (see Chapter 30) are other examples of diseases that are not autoimmune but whose effects may appear similar. In addition, if an infectious or malignant process is suspected, the appropriate therapy usually cannot begin until the diagnosis is confirmed by histologic or microbiologic examination.

The indication for any intraocular diagnostic procedure in an inflamed eye is that, in the physician's experience, the course of the uveitis or its appearance is not typical for the suspected autoimmune disease and that an infectious or malignant process is suspected. It is unusual for such a suspicion to be strong at the time of the first examination. However, as the patient's disease fails to respond to therapy in an expected manner, the physician begins to suspect that the original diagnosis may be incorrect and other diagnoses need to be considered. Once these alternate diagnoses are proposed, the appropriate diagnostic surgical procedure may be the only way to reliably exclude these possibilities.

Anterior chamber paracentesis

Anterior chamber paracentesis is an easily performed technique that yields a small amount of fluid for analysis. The procedure can be performed under local anesthesia. The eye can be fixed by a forceps firmly holding the limbus and is then entered with a 30-gauge needle on a tuberculin syringe; at least 200–250 μL of fluid can usually be obtained. A small hyphema may occur if the eye is actively inflamed, but this will resolve as the anterior chamber rapidly reforms. This small amount of fluid must be handled carefully using a plan established for handling the specimen before the procedure is begun. In general, we spin the fluid, separate the cells, and prepare slides for immunohistologic examination. The supernatant can then be analyzed for antibodies and cytokines, and PCR is now commonly performed. Serum should be obtained for comparison on the same day if antibodies are to be compared. However, if an infectious organism is suspected the unspun fluid must be cultured. Because of the small amount of fluid, only one or two types of culture can be set up, and the clinician must select the tests that will be most helpful. If too many tests are attempted, the amount of fluid may produce negative results because of inadequate sample size.

We will generally use aqueous for PCR and cytokine studies. We will use it less commonly for antibody measurement. IL-10:IL-6 ratios have proved to be useful screening tests when primary intraocular lymphoma is suspected.[97] PCR has become very widely used, particularly for DNA viruses and other infectious organisms, and we are beginning to use it with a better understanding of its strengths and weaknesses. In one report evaluating PCR performed on both aqueous and vitreous for a possible infectious process, the predictive value of a positive test was 98.7% and that of a negative test was 67.9%.[98]

If an infection is suspected, the vitreous provides more material for culture. In addition, even in postoperative endophthalmitis, the vitreous has a higher yield of positive culture results and more types of cultures can be set up with the material. However, if you need to use an aqueous specimen, it should be cultured in its entirety if an infectious organism is suspected and there is no other sample. Otherwise, it should be centrifuged at approximately 1000 rpm and the supernatant carefully removed. The cells that remain can be resuspended in 50–100 μL of buffered saline, and samples of 10–15 μL can be placed on gelatinized glass slides. This provides a sufficient number of slides for monoclonal antibody studies or other special stains. In pseudophakia or aphakia and after a vitrectomy, a communication between the vitreous cavity and the anterior chamber exists and the aqueous specimen may show positive results for lymphomatous cells.

Vitreous specimens may be obtained either by vitrectomy or by direct vitreous aspiration. Vitreous aspiration has been reported by others to be adequate for diagnostic purposes in the majority of patients considered, except for a few in whom other tests needed to be performed.[99] We try to avoid diagnostic difficulties, even for a few patients, and therefore prefer to perform a vitrectomy because more material can be obtained, and the posterior ocular structures can be better visualized after the surgery. In addition, this procedure provides more control over the amount of vitreous traction produced during surgery. In some situations it is useful to obtain an undiluted vitreous sample. This can be accomplished by aspirating the vitreous directly with a syringe and needle, or by using the vitrectomy instrument on low suction without turning on the infusion until 0.5–1 mL of fluid is obtained. This latter method prevents pulling on the vitreous base and prevents prolonged hypotony in the eye. The sample can be aspirated directly into a syringe. If a lymphoma is suspected we put a small amount of culture fluid (such as RPMI medium 1640) into the vitrectomy cassette. This is immediately sent to the laboratory before the surgical procedure has been completed. When one uses the vitreous fluid that is diluted with irrigating solution, it is sometimes useful to pass a portion through a Millipore filter. The Millipore filter can be cut up to culture for fungus or can be studied by the cytologist. Direct application onto gelatinized slides is also useful for cytologic study and monoclonal antibody staining. If the cells are trapped in cut pieces of dense vitreous, a portion of the sample can be incubated with hyaluronidase to digest the vitreous and free the cells. The cells can be also cultured or typed by immunohistologic or cell-sorting techniques. The fluid can be analyzed for antibodies or cytokines,[100] and as mentioned above PCR can be performed. These findings can be a valuable diagnostic tool in adjusting therapy.[98,101]

Chorioretinal biopsy

Occasionally neither aqueous nor vitreous specimens will provide a useful answer. Certain pathogens may not 'spill over' into the vitreous if the disease involves the retina or choroid only. For example, cytomegalovirus, which is difficult to culture from the vitreous, can be cultured from or seen on electron microscopic examination of the retina. In diseases in which vision is threatened and where the physician seems sure that continuation of the present therapy will not be effective, it may be reasonable to consider a chorioretinal biopsy.[102,103] This procedure provides a small piece of tissue which, if handled carefully, can provide a diagnosis. This procedure is probably useful only when the diagnostic possibilities include diseases for which there is a specific therapy. In general, it has been performed in patients with progressive chorioretinal lesions of unknown cause.[104] The indications for the biopsy include macula-threatening lesions unresponsive to therapy, or suspicion of either a malignant process or an infection. In the eyes on which we have performed chorioretinal biopsy, the preoperative visual acuity was 20/200 or worse.

Our procedure for chorioretinal biopsy is similar to that described by Peyman and colleagues,[105] except that we have not used an external support ring and we perform the vitrectomy before the biopsy incision. If the vitrectomy is completed first, the localization of an area of active disease to be biopsied is more accurate. A biopsy specimen of normal retina or retina in which the disease is quiescent will rarely provide diagnostic information. A flap-door approach rather than a full-thickness eye wall resection is used. A scleral flap (6 6 mm) is made, beginning 4 mm from the limbus and hinged posteriorly (**Fig. 8-10**). As thick a flap as possible is made. The inner bed is surrounded by diathermy. An inner rectangle of remaining sclera, choroid, and retina (4×2–3 mm) is removed with a microblade and sharp Van Ness scissors. The blade must be inserted fully to sever the retina cleanly. The specimen should be gripped in only one corner with fine-toothed forceps so the tissue is not damaged.

It is important to attempt to keep the specimen together so that the correct anatomic relationships are preserved. After the specimen is removed, any vitreous around the wound is removed. The scleral flap is then sutured over the bed with nylon suture, and the eye reinflated with either air or balanced salt solution. This procedure is used to obtain a biopsy specimen from a process involving the peripheral retina near the ora serrata. The incision may be moved somewhat posteriorly to obtain tissue anterior to the equator. It is not suitable for lesions found in the posterior pole.

An alternate method of biopsy is endoretinal biopsy. This has been used by Freeman and colleagues[83] to obtain a specimen from the edge of detached retina during retinal re-attachment procedures. If the retina is detached with a large tear, an intraocular scissors can be used to obtain a sample of the tissue. If the retina is not detached, a piece could conceivably be removed from the eye after photocoagulation without disturbing the choroid.

Cole et al.[106] described a technique using intense endodiode laser therapy around the 2×2 mm area that is cut out with a 20 gauge vertical cutting intraocular scissors (**Fig. 8-11**). The advantage of this approach is that biopsies could be performed more posteriorly than with the ab externo approach mentioned above. The retinal or chorioretinal biopsy specimen should be divided as shown in **Figure 8-12**. This permits culture, histologic examination, and monoclonal antibody studies, and maximizes the chance of gleaning useful information. There is sufficient specimen for only limited numbers of cultures, and therefore the piece should be sent for either viral or fungal culturing. Because most fungal pathogens that involve the choroid and retina can be cultured from the vitreous – but in viral retinitis viral cultures of the vitreous may indicate negative results because of neutralizing antibodies or low viral shedding – we prefer to send most specimens for viral studies if an infectious cause is suspected. The PCR can be used for retinal tissue as well. Additional studies using monoclonal antibodies can aid in identifying the type of fungus or virus that is present, and

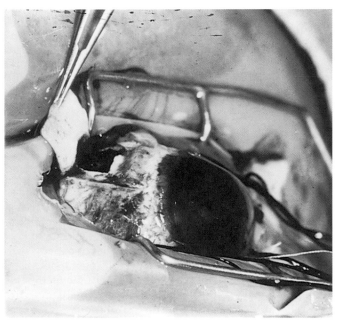

Figure 8-10. Scleral flap incision during chorioretinal biopsy procedure of lesion near ora serrata.

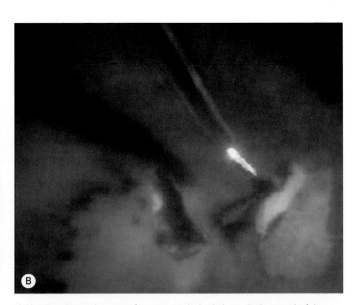

Figure 8-11. An ab interno approach to perform a combined retinal and choroidal biopsy. **A,** Application of intense endodiode laser. **B,** Removal of the biopsy site. *(From Cole CJ, Kwan AS, Laidlaw DAH, Aylward GW. A new technique of combined retinal and choroidal biopsy. Br J Ophthalmol 2008; 92: 1357–1360; with permission from BMJ Publishing Group Ltd)*

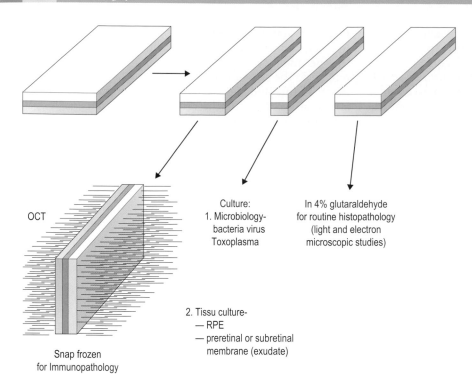

Figure 8-12. Schematic drawing of approach to subdivide and analyze chorioretinal biopsy specimen.

OCT

Culture:
1. Microbiology-
   bacteria virus
   Toxoplasma

In 4% glutaraldehyde
for routine histopathology
(light and electron
microscopic studies)

2. Tissu culture-
   — RPE
   — preretinal or subretinal
     membrane (exudate)

Snap frozen
for Immunopathology

the results may be available much sooner than the time needed to culture the organism.

Careful handling of ocular specimens obtained for diagnostic purposes is essential if they are to be of use. Advance planning and notification of the laboratories that will be involved in processing the specimen are useful in ensuring that the specimen is expected and will be processed correctly.

Subretinal surgery

Interest has centered on the development of new surgical and diagnostic techniques for subretinal (submacular) surgery (**Fig. 8-13**). The implications of these techniques would seem to go beyond the surgery itself and will also influence future work in RPE transplantation. The removal of subfoveal neovascular membranes[107] in the eyes of patients with the presumed ocular histoplasmosis syndrome paved the way for an exciting new area of therapy (**Fig. 8-14**). This is in contrast to patients with age-related maculopathy, who have not consistently had such an improvement in vision. Thomas and colleagues[108] found that after subretinal surgery in eyes with the ocular histoplasmosis syndrome, visual acuity was stabilized or improved in 56 eyes (83%), whereas 20/40 or greater was achieved in 21 eyes (31%) (mean follow-up 10.5 months). The results are quite different in eyes with age-related maculopathy, in which visual acuity was improved in five of the eyes operated on (12%) and 20/40 or better visual acuity occurred in two (5%), with a mean follow-up of 15 months. Of interest is Gass's hypothesis[109] that the membranes removed from patients with histoplasmosis grew in the subsensory retinal space and not under the RPE as did those from patients with age-related maculopathy. In addition, the membranes from patients with histoplasmosis are covered with a redundant layer of RPE, and therefore removal may aid in the normal apposition of the retinal elements. The question remains as to how widely applicable subretinal surgery will be for patients with uveitis in general. Recurrence rates of membranes still need to be determined. However, removal of the membrane alone may not be sufficient to restore vision, as defective RPE cells, as well as damaged or lost photoreceptors, may be the major problem. This may then represent just the first step of a whole series of rehabilitation measures that will be needed.

Case 8-1

A middle-aged African-American man with a history of glaucoma and cataract surgery in his right eye had reduced vision in that eye and, subsequently, in the left eye. Ocular examination showed peripheral choroidal detachments, as well as multiple subretinal yellow-white lesions strewn throughout the fundus. HLA typing showed HLA-A29 positivity. An extensive workup failed to help in making a diagnosis, except that the patient showed purified protein derivative positivity and a monoclonal band in the urine. The differential diagnosis included miliary tuberculosis, lymphoma, other systemic neoplastic metastases, an undetected infectious process, and birdshot retinochoroidopathy. After extensive discussion, it was believed that a chorioretinal biopsy was indicated. The results of the biopsy showed the ocular condition to be reactive lymphoid hyperplasia, which resolved with oral prednisone therapy. (For a more detailed description of this case, see Cheung MK, Martin DF, Chan CC, et al. Diagnosis of reactive lymphoid hyperplasia by chorioretinal biopsy. Am J Ophthalmol 1994; 118: 457–62.)

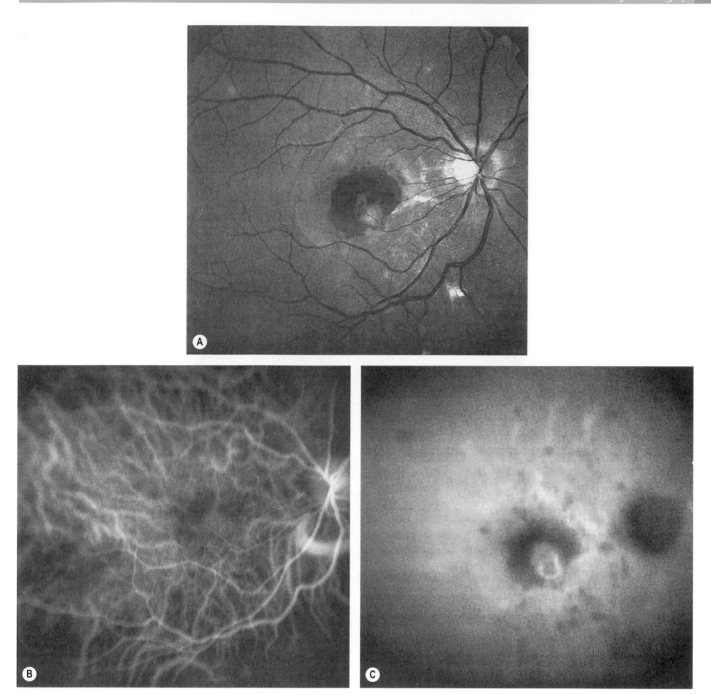

Figure 8-13. Indocyanine green (ICG) angiogram showing position of submacular neovascular net. **A,** Fundus photograph showing submacular hemorrhage with marked reduction in visual acuity. Because of the presence of blood, the fluorescein angiogram was difficult to interpret. **B,** ICG early photograph shows feeder vessel to net. **C,** Later photograph outlines the extent of the net, which was successfully treated with laser photocoagulation and not removed by surgery.

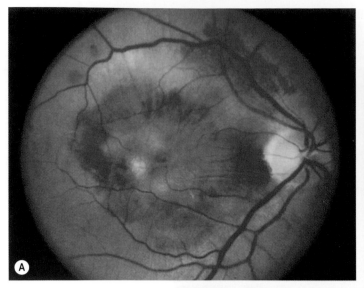
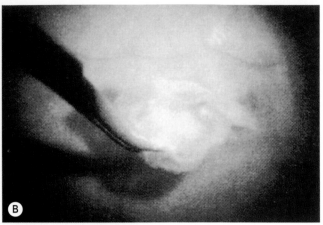
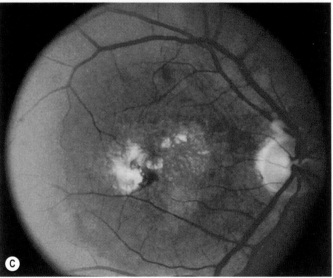

Figure 8-14. A, Subretinal neovascular lesion in the macular region. **B,** Removal of lesion with special subretinal forceps. **C,** Fundus as it appears after surgery. *(Courtesy Antonio Capone Jr, MD and Daniel Martin, MD, Emory University, Atlanta, GA.)*

References

1. Arevalo JF, Garcia-Amaris RA. The role of vitreo-retinal surgery in children with uveitis. Int Ophthalmol Clin 2008; 48: 153–172.

2. Najjar DM, Cohen EJ, Rapuano CJ, et al. EDTA chelation for calcific band keratopathy: results and long-term follow-up. Am J Ophthalmol 2004; 137(6): 1056–1064.

3. Babu K, Murthy KR. Hypopyon uveitis following band keratopathy removal in ankylosing spondylitis – a case report. Ocul Immunol Inflamm 2006; 14: 57–58.

4. Richards JC, Wiffen SJ. Corneal graft rejection precipitated by uveitis secondary to alendronate sodium therapy. Cornea 2006; 25: 1100–1101.

5. Foster C, Rashid S. Management of coincident cataract and uveitis. Curr Opin Ophthalmol 2003; 14: 1–6.

6. Ram J, Kaushik S, Brar GS, et al. Phacoemulsification in patients with Fuchs' heterochromic uveitis. J Cataract Refract Surg 2002; 28: 1372–1378.

7. Estafanous MF, Lowder CY, Meisler DM, et al. Phacoemulsification cataract extraction and posterior chamber lens implantation in patients with uveitis. Am J Ophthalmol 2001; 131: 620–625.

8. Meier FM, Tuft SJ, Pavesio CE. Cataract surgery in uveitis. Ophthalmol Clin North Am 2002; 15: 365–373.

9. Chee SP, Ti SE, Sivakumar M, et al. Postoperative inflammation: extracapsular cataract extraction versus phacoemulsification. J Cataract Refract Surg 1999; 25: 1280–1285.

10. Herbort CP. Uveoscleritis after excessive neodynium YAG laser posterior capsulotomy. J Cataract Refract Surg 1994; 20: 80–81.

11. Kamoi K, Mochizuki M. Phaco dislocation technique in young patients with uveitis. J Cataract Refract Surg 2008; 34: 1239–1241.

12. Walker J, Rao NA, Ober RR, et al. A combined anterior and posterior approach to cataract surgery in patients with chronic uveitis. Int Ophthalmol 1993; 17: 63–69.

13. Belfort R, Nussenblatt RB. Surgical approaches to uveitis. Int Ophthalmol Clin 1990; 30: 314–317.

14. Davison JA. Capsule contraction syndrome. J Cataract Refract Surg 1993; 19: 582–589.

15. Percival SP, Pai V. Heparin-modified lenses for eyes at risk for breakdown of the blood–aqueous barrier during cataract surgery. J Cataract Refract Surg 1993; 19: 760–765.

16. Tabbara KF, Al-Kaff AS, Al-Rajhi AA, et al. Heparin surface-modified intraocular lenses in patients with inactive uveitis or diabetes. Ophthalmology 1998; 105: 843–845.

17. Alio JL, Chipont E, BenEzra D, et al. Comparative performance of intraocular lenses in eyes with cataract and uveitis. J Cataract Refract Surg 2002; 28: 2096–2108.

18. Elgohary MA, McCluskey PJ, Towler HM, et al. Outcome of phacoemulsification in patients with uveitis. Br J Ophthalmol 2007.

19. Van Gelder RN, Leveque TK. Cataract surgery in the setting of uveitis. Curr Opin Ophthalmol 2009; 20: 42–45.

20. Leccisotti A. Iridocyclitis associated with angle-supported phakic intraocular lenses. J Cataract Refract Surg 2006; 32: 1007–1010.

21. Zaborowski AG, Quinn AG, Dick AD. Cataract surgery in pediatric uveitis. J Pediatr Ophthalmol Strabismus 2008; 45: 270–278.

22. Lundvall A, Zetterstrom C. Cataract extraction and intraocular lens implantation in children with uveitis. Br J Ophthalmol 2000; 84: 791–793.

23. BenEzra D, Cohen E. Cataract surgery in children with chronic uveitis. Ophthalmology 2000; 107: 1255–1260.

24. Kotaniemi K, Penttila H. Intraocular lens implantation in patients with juvenile idiopathic arthritis-associated uveitis. Ophthalmic Res 2006; 38: 318–323.

25. Woreta F, Thorne JE, Jabs DA, et al. Risk factors for ocular complications and poor visual acuity at presentation among patients with uveitis associated with juvenile idiopathic arthritis. Am J Ophthalmol 2007; 143(4): 647–655.

26. Foster CS, Fong LP, Singh G. Cataract surgery and intraocular lens implantation in patients with uveitis. Ophthalmology 1989; 96: 281–288.

27. Pleyer U, Pawlikowska J, Zierhut M, et al. Clinical aspects, follow-up and results of cataract extraction in uveitis. Ophtalmologie 1992; 89: 295–300.

28. Foster RE, Lowder CY, Meisler DM, et al. Combined extracapsular cataract extraction, posterior chamber intraocular lens implantation, and pars plana vitrectomy. Ophthalmic Surg 1993; 24: 446–452.

29. Tessler HH, Farber MD. Intraocular lens implantation versus no intraocular lens implantation in patients with chronic iridocyclitis and pars planitis. Ophthalmology 1993; 100: 1206–1209.

30. Anderson T. IOLs in uveitis patients. [Letter to the editor.] Ophthalmology 1994; 101: 625–626.

31. Hazari A, Sangwan VS. Cataract surgery in uveitis. Indian J Ophthalmol 2002; 50: 103–107.

32. Kim CY, Kang SJ, Lee SJ, et al. Opacification of a hydrophilic acrylic intraocular lens with exacerbation of Behcet's uveitis. J Cataract Refract Surg 2002; 28: 1276–1278.

33. Daus W, Schmidbauer J, Buschendorff P, et al. Results of extracapsular cataract extraction with intraocular lens implantation in eyes with uveitis and Fuchs' heterochromic iridocyclitis. Ger J Ophthalmol 1992; 1: 399–402.

34. Akova YA, Foster RE. Cataract surgery in patients with sarcoidosis associated uveitis. Ophthalmology 1994; 101: 473–479.

35. Fox GM, Flynn Jr HW, Davis JL, et al. Causes of reduced visual acuity on long-term follow-up after cataract extraction in patients with uveitis and juvenile rheumatoid arthritis. Am J Ophthalmol 1993; 114: 708–714.

36. Secchi AG. Cataract surgery in exudative uveitis: effectiveness of total lens removal, anterior vitrectomy, and scleral fixation of PC IOLs. Eur J Ophthalmol 2008; 18: 220–225.

37. Carlson AN, Stewart WC, Tso PC. Intraocular lens complications requiring removal or exchange. Surv Ophthalmol 1998; 42: 417–440.

38. Harper SL, Foster CS. Intraocular lens explantation in uveitis. Int Ophthalmol Clin 2000; 40: 107–116.

39. Dana MR, Chatzistefanou K, Schaumberg DA, et al. Posterior capsule opacification after cataract surgery in patients with uveitis. Ophthalmology 1997; 104: 1387–1393.

40. Foster C, Stavrou P, Zafirakis P, et al. Intraocular lens removal from patients with uveitis. Am J Ophthalmol 1999; 128: 31–37.

41. Smith RE, Kokoris N, Nobe JR, et al. Lensectomy-vitrectomy in chronic uveitis. Trans Am Ophthalmol Soc 1983; 81: 261–275.

42. Girard LJ, Rodriguez J, Mailman ML, et al. Cataract and uveitis management by pars plana lensectomy and vitrectomy by ultrasonic fragmentation. Retina 1985; 5: 107–114.

43. Petrelli AM, Belfort Jr R, Abreu MT, et al. Ultrasonic fragmentation of cataract in uveitis. Retina 1986; 6: 61–65.

44. Diamond JG, Kaplan HJ. Uveitis: effect of vitrectomy combined with lensectomy. Ophthalmology 1979; 86: 1320–1328.

45. Dangel ME, Stark WJ, Michels RG. Surgical management of cataract associated with chronic uveitis. Ophthalmic Surg 1983; 14: 145–152.

46. Praeger DL, Schneider HA, Sakowski Jr AD, et al. Kelman procedure in the treatment of complicated cataract of the uveitis of Still's disease. Trans Am Ophthalmol Soc UK 1976; 96: 168–172.

47. Mackensen G, Loeffler K. Cataract extraction in chronic iridocyclitis: long term followups. Klin Monatsbl Augenheilkd 1983; 183: 7–9.

48. Yu EN, Paredes I, Foster CS. Surgery for hypotony in patients with juvenile idiopathic arthritis-associated uveitis. Ocul Immunol Inflamm 2007; 15: 11–17.

49. Al Obeidan SA, Osman EA, Al-Muammar AM, et al. Efficacy and safety of deep sclerectomy in uveitic glaucoma. Int Ophthalmol 2009: Oct; 29(5): 367–372. Epub 2008.

50. Park UC, Ahn JK, Park KH, et al. Phacotrabeculectomy with mitomycin C in patients with uveitis. Am J Ophthalmol 2006; 142(6): 1005–1012.

51. Patitsas CJ, Rockwood EJ, Meisler DM, et al. Glaucoma filtering surgery with postoperative 5-fluorouracil in patients with intraocular inflammatory disease. Ophthalmology 1992; 99: 594–599.

52. Towler HMA, McCluskey P, Shaer B, et al. Long-term followup of trabeculectomy with intraoperative 5-fluorouracil for uveitis related glaucoma. Ophthalmology 2000; 107: 1822–1828.

53. Ceballos EM, Beck AD, Lynn MJ. Trabeculectomy with antiproliferative agents in uveitis glaucoma. J Glaucoma 2002; 11: 189–196.

54. Mohan M, Kumar H, Rana S. Acute granulomatous iritis following 5-fluorouracil therapy for failed trabeculectomy. Indian J Ophthalmol 1991; 39: 125–126.

55. Kanski JJ, McAllister JA. Trabeculodialysis for inflammatory glaucoma in children and young adults. Ophthalmology 1985; 92: 927–930.

56. Williams RD, Hoskins HD, Shaffer RN. Trabeculodialysis for inflammatory glaucoma: a review of 25 cases. Ophthalmic Surg 1992; 23: 36–37.

57. Hill RA, Nguyen QH, Baerveldt G, et al. Trabeculectomy and Molteno implantation for glaucomas associated with uveitis. Ophthalmology 1993; 100: 903–908.

58. Freedman J, Rubin B. Molteno implants as a treatment for refractory glaucoma in black patients. Arch Ophthalmol 1992; 109: 1417–1420.

59. Ceballos EM, Parrish RKI, Schiffman JC. Outcome of Baerveldt glaucoma implants for the treatment of glaucoma. Ophthalmology 2002; 109: 2256–2260.

60. Da Mata A, Burk SE, Netland PA, et al. Management of uveitic glaucoma with Ahmed glaucoma valve implantation. Ophthalmology 1999; 106: 2168–2172.

61. Rachmiel R, Trope GE, Buys YM, et al. Ahmed glaucoma valve implantation in uveitic glaucoma versus open-angle glaucoma patients. Can J Ophthalmol 2008; 43(4): 462–467.

62. Papadaki TG, Zacharopoulos IP, Pasquale LR, et al. Long-term results of Ahmed glaucoma valve implantation for uveitic glaucoma. Am J Ophthalmol 2007; 144(1): 62–69.

63. Smith MF, Sherwood MB, McGorray SP. Comparison of the double-plate Molteno drainage implant with the Schocket procedure. Arch Ophthalmol 1992; 110: 1246–1250.

64. Omi CA, De Almeida GV, Cohen R, et al. Modified Schocket implant for refractory glaucoma: experience of 55 cases. Ophthalmology 1991; 98: 211–214.

65. Takahashi T, Ohtani S, Miyata K, et al. A clinical evaluation of uveitis-associated secondary glaucoma. Japanese Journal of Ophthalmology 2002; 46: 556–562.

66. Freeman WR. Application of vitreoretinal surgery to inflammatory and infectious disease of the posterior segment. Int Ophthalmol Clin 1992; 32: 15–33.

67. Chen CL, Wang TY, Cheng JH, et al. Immediate pars plana vitrectomy improves outcome in retained intravitreal lens fragments after phacoemulsification. Ophthalmologica 2008; 222(4): 277–283.

68. Soheilian M, Mirdehghan SA, Peyman GA. Sutureless combined 25-gauge vitrectomy, phacoemulsification, and posterior chamber intraocular lens implantation for management of uveitic cataract associated with posterior segment disease. Retina 2008; 28: 941–946.

69. Androudi S, Ahmed M, Fiore T, et al. Combined pars plana vitrectomy and phacoemulsification to restore visual acuity in patients with chronic uveitis. J Cataract Refract Surg 2005; 31(3): 472–478.

70. Rothova A. Inflammatory cystoid macular edema. Curr Opin Ophthalmol 2007; 18: 487–492.

71. Bacskulin A, Eckardt C. Results of pars plana vitrectomy in chronic uveitis in childhood. Ophthalmologie 1993; 90: 434–439.

72. Kaplan HJ. Surgical treatment of intermediate uveitis. In: Boke WRF, Manthey KF, Nussenblatt RB, eds. Intermediate uveitis. Basel: Karger, 1992; 185–189.

73. Stavrou P, Baltatzis S, Letko E, et al. Pars plana vitrectomy in patients with intermediate uveitis. Ocul Immunol Inflamm 2001; 9: 141–151.

74. Bovey EH, Gonvers M, Herbort CP. Pars plana vitrectomy in uveitis. Klin Monatsbl Augenheilkd 1992; 200: 464–467.

75. Nolle B, Eckardt C. Vitrectomy in multifocal chorioretinitis. Ger J Ophthalmol 1993; 2: 14–19.

76. Gutfleisch M, Spital G, Mingels A, et al. Pars plana vitrectomy with intravitreal triamcinolone: effect on uveitic cystoid macular oedema and treatment limitations. Br J Ophthalmol 2007; 91(3): 345–348.

77. Tranos P, Scott R, Zambarakji H, et al. The effect of pars plana vitrectomy on cystoid macular oedema associated with chronic uveitis: a randomised, controlled pilot study. Br J Ophthalmol 2006; 90(9): 1107–1110.

78. Trittibach P, Koerner F, Sarra GM, et al. Vitrectomy for juvenile uveitis: prognostic factors for the long-term functional outcome. Eye 2006; 20(2): 184–190.

79. Michels RG. Vitrectomy for macular pucker. Ophthalmology 1984; 91: 1384–1388.

80. Kerkhoff FT, Lamberts QJ, van den Biesen PR, et al. Rhegmatogenous retinal detachment and uveitis. Ophthalmology 2003; 110: 427–431.

81. Galor A, Lowder CY, Kaiser PK, et al. Surgical drainage of chronic serous retinal detachment associated with uveitis. Retina 2008; 28(2): 282–288.

82. Singh RP, Margolis R, Kaiser PK. Cystoid puncture for chronic cystoid macular oedema. Br J Ophthalmol 2007; 91: 1062–1064.

83. Freeman WR, Henderly DE, Wan WL, et al. Prevalence, pathophysiology, and treatment of rhegmatogenous retinal detachment in treated cytomegalovirus retinitis. Am J Ophthalmol 1987; 103: 527–536.

84. Forster RK, Zachary IG, Cottingham Jr AJ, et al. Further observations on the diagnosis, cause and treatment of endophthalmitis. Am J Ophthalmol 1976; 81: 52–56.

85. Er H, Doganay S, Evereklioglu C, et al. Effects of L-NAME and timolol on aqueous IL-1beta, IL-6, IL-8, TNF-alpha, and NO levels after Nd:YAG laser iridotomy in rabbits. Eur J Ophthalmol 2002; 12: 281–286.

86. Parodi MB, et al. Photodynamic therapy for juxtafoveal choroidal neovascularization associated with multifocal choroiditis. Am J Ophthalmol 2006; 141: 123–128.

87. Gerth C, Spital G, Lommatzsch A, et al. Photodynamic therapy for choroidal neovascularization in patients with multifocal choroiditis and panuveitis. Eur J Ophthalmol 2006; 16(1): 111–118.

88. Nowilaty SR, Bouhaimed M. Photodynamic therapy for subfoveal choroidal neovascularisation in Vogt–Koyanagi–Harada disease. Br J Ophthalmol 2006; 90: 982–986.

89. Lipski A, Bornfeld N, Jurklies B. Photodynamic therapy with verteporfin in paediatric and young adult patients: long-term treatment results of choroidal neovascularisations. Br J Ophthalmol 2008; 92: 655–660.

90. Tatar O, Adam A, Shinoda K, et al. Influence of verteporfin photodynamic therapy on inflammation in human choroidal neovascular membranes secondary to age-related macular degeneration. Retina 2007; 27(6): 713–723.

91. Tran TH, Fardeau C, Terrada C, et al. Intravitreal bevacizumab for refractory choroidal neovascularization (CNV) secondary to uveitis. Graefes Arch Clin Exp Ophthalmol 2008; 246(12): 1685–1692.

92. Bressler NM. Photodynamic therapy of subfoveal choroidal neovascularization in age-related macular degeneration with verteporfin: two-year results of 2 randomized clinical trials – Tap report 2. Arch Ophthalmol 2001; 119: 198–207.

93. Anon. Guidelines for using verteporfin (visudyne) in photodynamic therapy to treat choroidal neovascularization due to age-related macular degeneration and other causes. Retina 2002; 22: 6–18.

94. Farah ME, Costa RA, Muccioli C, et al. Photodynamic therapy with verteporfin for subfoveal choroidal neovascularization in Vogt-Koyanagi-Harada syndrome. Am J Ophthalmol 2002; 134: 137–139.

95. Spaide RF, Freund KB, Slakter J, et al. Treatment of subfoveal choroidal neovascularization associated with multifocal choroiditis and panuveitis with photodynamic therapy. Retina 2002; 22: 545–549.

96. Moshfeghi DM, Kaiser PK, Grossniklaus HE, et al. Clinicopathologic study after submacular removal of choroidal neovascular membranes treated with verteporfin ocular photodynamic therapy. Am J Ophthalmol 2003; 135: 343–350.

97. Cassoux N, Giron A, Bodaghi B, et al. IL-10 measurement in aqueous humor for screening patients with suspicion of primary intraocular lymphoma. Invest Ophthalmol Vis Sci 2007; 48(7): 3253–3259.

98. Harper TW, Miller D, Schiffman JC, et al. Polymerase chain reaction analysis of aqueous and vitreous specimens in the diagnosis of posterior segment infectious uveitis. Am J Ophthalmol 2009; 147(1): 140–147 e2.

99. Lobo A, Lightman S. Vitreous aspiration needle tap in the diagnosis of intraocular inflammation. Ophthalmology 2003; 110: 595–599.

100. Davis JL, Solomon D, Nussenblatt RB, et al. Immunocytochemical staining of vitreous cells: indications, techniques, and results. Ophthalmology 1992; 99: 250–256.

101. Baarsma GS, Luyendijk L, Kijlstra A, et al. Analysis of local antibody production in the vitreous humor of patients with severe uveitis. Am J Ophthalmol 1991; 112: 147–150.

102. Martin DF, Chan CC, de Smet MD, et al. The role of chorioretinal biopsy in the management of posterior uveitis. Ophthalmology 1993; 100: 705–714.

103. Lim LL, Suhler EB, Rosenbaum JT, et al. The role of choroidal and retinal biopsies in the diagnosis and management of atypical presentations of uveitis. Trans Am Ophthalmol Soc 2005; 103: 84–91; discussion 91–92.

104. Lafaut BA, Hanssens M, Verbraeken H, et al. Chorioretinal biopsy in the diagnosis of intraocular lymphoma: a

case report. Bull Soc Belge Ophtalmol 1994; 252: 67–73.

105. Peyman GA, Juarez CP, Raichand M. Full-thickness eye-wall biopsy: long term results in 9 patients. Br J Ophthalmol 1981; 65: 723–726.

106. Cole CJ, Kwan AS, Laidlaw DA, et al. A new technique of combined retinal and choroidal biopsy. Br J Ophthalmol 2008; 92(10): 1357–1360.

107. Thomas MA, Kaplan HJ. Surgical removal of subfoveal neovascularization in the presumed ocular histoplasmosis syndrome. Am J Ophthalmol 1991; 111: 1–7.

108. Thomas MA, Dickinson JD, Melberg NS, et al. Visual results after surgical removal of subfoveal choroidal neovascular membranes. Ophthalmology 1994; 101: 1384–1396.

109. Gass JDM. Biomicroscopic and histopathologic considerations regarding the feasibility of surgical excision of subfoveal neovascular membranes. Am J Ophthalmol 1994; 118: 285–298.

Bacterial and Fungal Diseases

Scott M. Whitcup

Key concepts

- Infection remains a common cause of uveitis. Better diagnostic tests are helping to identify specific microbial agents as the cause of a number of uveitic conditions such as Whipple's disease.
- Prompt diagnosis is critical so that appropriate antiinfective therapy can be started.
- Many diagnostic tests for infectious causes of uveitis mislead the clinician and lead to inappropriate therapy.
- Clinicians should know the sensitivity and specificity of the diagnostic tests ordered for infectious causes of uveitis. Clinicians must also know the pretest likelihood of disease to adequately interpret results (see Chapter 5).
- Ocular involvement from tuberculosis occurs in about 1–2% of patients but remains difficult to diagnose. Active tuberculosis can occur as a complication of immunusuppressive therapy with anti-cytokine therapy.
- Histoplasmosis is the fungal disease most commonly associated with uveitis.
- Risk factors for fungal infections of the eye include ocular surgery, immunosuppression, systemic mycotic infections, intravenous drug use, and ocular trauma.

Introduction

The next two chapters will focus on uveitis caused by ocular infection due to bacteria or fungus. Although a number of infectious agents can invade the eye and lead to ocular inflammation, we will concentrate on the most common bacterial and fungal causes of uveitis, including leprosy, tuberculosis, syphilis, and other related spirochetal diseases, Lyme disease, relapsing fever, leptospirosis, brucellosis, candidal infections, and aspergillosis. The spirochetal diseases, as a group, are discussed in detail in Chapter 10. Postsurgical bacterial and fungal endophthalmitis are also discussed in Chapter 18.

Half a century ago, bacterial diseases such as tuberculosis and syphilis were thought to cause the majority of cases of uveitis. Even today, a number of infectious diseases remain important causes of uveitis. Because specific antimicrobial therapy can be curative and prevent long-term visual sequelae, early diagnosis of infectious causes of uveitis should be a priority for all practitioners. Further, as immunosuppressive therapy can exacerbate an underlying infection, leading to blindness and rarely even death, diagnosing and treating an infectious cause of uveitis can be both sight saving and life saving.

Infections may elicit a uveitis by a number of pathogenic mechanisms. Direct infection of ocular tissues usually leads to an inflammatory response manifested by signs and symptoms of uveitis. Injection of bacterial endotoxins at sites far from the eye will also elicit intraocular inflammation in the absence of ocular infection. Endotoxins generate a number of harmful biologic effects, including fever, hypotension, disseminated coagulation, and shock. In the same year that Murray Shear elucidated the basic structure of endotoxin, Ayo[1] demonstrated that a single intravenous injection of endotoxin could induce ocular inflammation, and this inflammatory response was ascribed to 'Schwartzman toxins.' Although this endotoxin-induced uveitis (EIU) was easily elicited in dogs, cats, and rabbits, smaller laboratory animals were resistant to development of the disease. In 1980, Rosenbaum and colleagues[2] demonstrated EIU in Lewis rats after intravenous, intraperitoneal, or intrafootpad injection of lipopolysaccharide (LPS), and Forrester and colleagues[3] showed EIU after intraocular LPS injection in Columbia–Sherman rats. More recently, EIU has also been described in C3H/HeN mice.[4] EIU is now a useful animal model for the study of acute ocular inflammation and is characterized by iris hyperemia, miosis, increased aqueous humor protein concentration, and inflammatory cell infiltration into the anterior uvea and anterior chamber (**Fig. 9-1**). Inflammatory cell infiltration into the vitreous in the area of the optic nerve head also occurs. As you will see in the chapter on anterior uveitis (Chapter 19), uveitis can follow bacterial infections such as bacterial dysentery, and the mechanism of some of these occurrences may be the result of an immunologic response to endotoxin.

Leprosy

Leprosy was the first documented bacterial infection in humans. The etiologic agent of leprosy, *Mycobacterium leprae*, is a Gram-positive intracellular bacillus that was first identified by Hansen in 1874;[5] however, the disease has been a scourge to society for thousands of years. It is found predominantly in the developing world, but it is estimated that from 10 to 15 million people have leprosy[6] and that from 500 000 to 700 000 persons have been blinded by this condition.[7] The organisms have a tropism for parts of the body

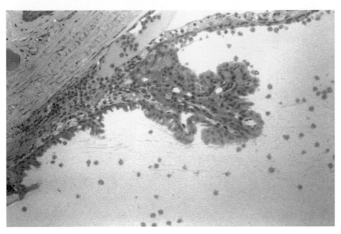

Figure 9-1. Histologic section of anterior chamber of mouse with endotoxin-induced uveitis shows infiltration with neutrophils, macrophages, and occasional lymphocytes. (Hematoxylin and eosin, ×200.)

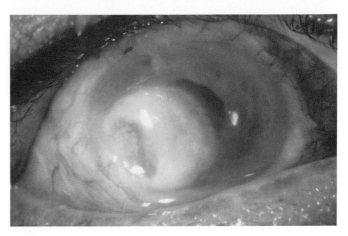

Figure 9-2. Severe bacterial corneal ulcer in patient with leprosy. (*Courtesy R. Christopher Walton, MD.*)

with low temperatures, particularly organs of ectodermal origin such as skin, peripheral nerves, nasal mucosa, and the eye. The mode of transmission of leprosy remains unclear. Although most of the population is exposed to the bacillus in endemic areas, more than 90% are immune to the disease and do not develop symptoms. Leprosy is often divided into two major subtypes: tuberculoid and lepromatous. In patients with tuberculoid leprosy, the organism induces a strong cell-mediated immune response, and few organisms are found invading organ tissues. Little immunity follows the infection in patients with lepromatous leprosy, and a plethora of organisms are found throughout the body. Borderline forms of the disease also exist in some classification systems.[8]

Clinical findings

From 50% to 70% of patients with leprosy have the tuberculoid form, which tends to be localized to the skin and nerves.[9] The disease in these patients is characterized by granuloma formation and the absence of a large number of bacilli because of their active cell-mediated immune response. The skin test with lepromin is highly positive (Mitsuda reaction). The lepromatous form of the disease is characterized by a severe generalized condition with massive bacterial infection. In contrast to patients with tuberculoid leprosy, these patients have a poor cellular immune response, and macrophages are predominantly found on histologic examination. Intraocular inflammatory disease occurs more commonly in this form of leprosy. In addition, the severe disfiguring changes of the limbs and face are associated with lepromatous leprosy. In patients with borderline groupings of leprosy, a sudden shift to the lepromatous state can occur.

A list of the ocular complications of leprosy is given in **Box 9-1**. In one study, over half of patients with multibacillary leprosy had ocular involvement.[10] Structural damage to the eyelids, poor lid closure as a result of facial nerve involvement, and impaired corneal sensation often lead to exposure of the cornea. Loss of the temporal portion of the eyebrows (madarosis) is a typical finding and a stigma to those affected. It is important to remember, however, that trachoma can exist in the same population with leprosy and can compound the external disease in these patients.[11] The keratitis

Box 9-1 Ocular manifestations of leprosy

Prominent corneal nerves
Decreased corneal sensitivity
Madarosis
Ectropion
Entropion
Episcleritis/scleritis
Trichiasis
Glaucoma
Cataract
Blocked nasolacrimal ducts
Pterygium
Conjunctivitis
Granulomatous anterior uveitis
Iris pearls
Iris atrophy
Facial nerve palsy (tuberculoid leprosy)
Ptosis
Exposure keratitis
Orbicularis oculi weakness
Lagophthalmos
Trigeminal nerve involvement
Corneal anesthesia
Lid lesions and deformities (lepromatous leprosy)
Choroidal lesions

associated with leprosy starts superiorly and first appears as subepithelial chalky infiltrates surrounded by gray stromal opacifications.[12] Corneal exposure predisposes patients to development of corneal ulcers (**Fig. 9-2**) that are often difficult to manage.

Intraocular inflammatory disease is a known complication of leprosy. In a retrospective study of 531 leprosy patients, 4% had iritis.[13] The organisms can directly invade the iris and ciliary body, and chronic anterior uveitis is commonly seen in these patients. If the uveitis is not aggressively treated, cataract and hypotony frequently result. Less frequently, patients present with an acute anterior uveitis. In a study of 100 patients with leprosy in Brazil, 72 had ocular complications.[14] Seventeen had a chronic anterior uveitis, whereas only two had an acute anterior uveitis. In a study

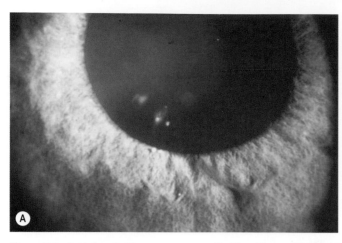
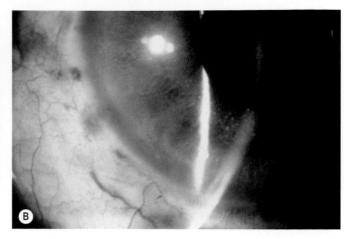

Figure 9-3. A, Iris 'pearl' of leprosy seen as small white object on iris edge. In **B,** many of these can be seen just right of the slit beam. *(Courtesy Khalid Tabbara, MD.)*

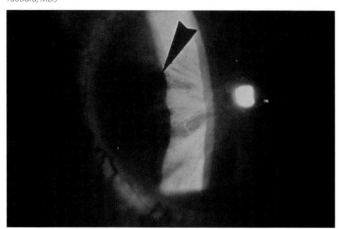

Figure 9-4. Multiple areas of iris atrophy (arrowhead) in patient with iritis caused by leprosy. *(Courtesy Fernando Orefice, MD.)*

in Nepal, 8% of patients with tuberculoid leprosy had uveitis, whereas 16% of patients with lepromatous leprosy had anterior chamber inflammatory disease.[15] Spaide and colleagues[16] found that uveitis was uncommon in leprosy patients in the United States, which possibly reflects the results of more aggressive treatment with antilepromatous and antiinflammatory agents. Granulomas form in the iris and appear as iris 'pearls' on the anterior surface (**Fig. 9-3**). Iris atrophy also occurs in many patients (**Fig. 9-4**).

Although less common, changes to the retina have been described in patients with leprosy. Patients with long-standing lepromatous leprosy can have large numbers of organisms that invade not only the anterior segment but also the adjoining peripheral pars plana and retina. Pars planitis has been reported in patients with leprosy.[17] Chovet and colleagues[18] demonstrated segmental vasculitis in the posterior pole on fluorescein angiography in patients with lepromatous disease. Blindness can occur from a number of the ocular complications of leprosy.

Immunology and pathology

Humans are the only natural host for *M. leprae*. After entering the host, the organism reproduces in mononuclear cells, particularly skin histiocytes. The doubling time for the organisms is extraordinarily long – about 20 days – and

attempts to culture the organism in a cell-free environment have not been successful. Some work has centered on the use of the nine-banded armadillo as an experimental model.[19] This animal has a low basal temperature that seems to permit large numbers of *M. leprae* to propagate.

The immune characteristics of patients with this disorder have been extensively studied. Imbalances in T cells,[20] antigen-specific suppressor T cells,[21] and defective production of monocyte-activating cytokines have all been described.[22] CD4+ T cells predominate in tuberculoid lesions, but CD8+ T cells are almost exclusively found in lepromatous lesions.[23] Family studies with HLA typing have suggested that there is an HLA-linked recessive gene that may predispose patients to the tuberculoid form of the disease.[24]

The reactional states of leprosy have been divided into two categories: type I and type II. The type I reaction is also known as the reversal reaction and is a delayed hypersensitivity response directed against bacillary antigens. The type II reaction is also known as erythema nodosum leprosum and is an immune-complex reaction. Patients with the reversal reaction (type I) may be more likely to present with orbicularis oculi weakness and lagophthalmos.[25]

Therapy

Dapsone, rifampin, and clofazimine are the principal antileprosy agents used. The World Health Organization recommends multidrug treatment regimens because of the existence of dapsone-resistant strains of *M. leprae*.[26] More aggressive therapy may be warranted in patients with multibacillary disease. The use of thalidomide has been useful in patients with recurring and persistant erythema nodosum leprosum.[27] Attempts to develop a vaccine are currently under way. Ocular care of patients with leprosy requires careful management of the external disease, including surgical management of eyelid deformities and judicial use of ocular lubrication. If intraocular surgery is planned, great care must be taken to be sure that the eye has no active inflammation.

Tuberculosis

Guyton and Woods identified tuberculosis (TB) as the most common underlying disease in the vast majority of patients with granulomatous uveitis seen by them in the 1940s.[27a] It is now clear that many of these patients actually had other conditions, such as ocular histoplasmosis, that caused the uveitis. Although the rates of incidence, mortality, and morbidity from TB have declined since the 1940s, 25 000–30 000 new cases are still reported annually in the United States.[28] For a time, reported cases of TB rose predominantly because of infection of patients with AIDS and immigration from endemic countries.[29] However, 25 313 cases of TB (9.8 cases per 100 000 population) were reported to the Centers for Disease Control and Prevention in 1993, a 5.1% decrease from 1992.[30] Since then, the number of cases has continued to decline. In 2007, 13 293 cases of TB were reported in the United States.[31] More recently, activated tuberculosis has been associated with the use of anti-cytokine therapy, including anti-TNF treatments.[32] As patients with uveitis with associated autoimmune disease are more commonly treated with anti-TNF drugs, tuberculosis may again return as a more common cause of uveitis, even in the developing world.

Systemic disease

Infection in the United States is transmitted predominantly in aerosolized droplets. Most patients develop an asymptomatic, self-limited pneumonia that usually heals with granuloma formation. Sensitization develops 2–10 weeks after infection and is manifested by a positive skin test to an extract of the tuberculous bacillus (purified protein derivative, PPD). The granulomas usually calcify and remain inactive. However, onset of symptoms can occur after a breakdown of the patient's immune system associated with age, disease, or the use of immunosuppressive therapy for other conditions.

Ocular disease

Ocular involvement occurs in about 1–2% of patients with TB.[33] The ocular manifestations of TB are listed in **Box 9-2**. TB can involve both the anterior and posterior segments of the eye as well as the ocular adnexa and orbit. In miliary TB tubercles can be seen in the choroid, giving the impression of a unifocal or multifocal choroiditis (**Fig. 9-5**). There has been debate about whether at least some cases of serpiginous choroiditis may be caused by tuberculosis.[34,35] Choroidal tubercles have also been associated with the development of subretinal neovascularization.[36] More rarely, tubercles occur in the anterior chamber and may elicit a severe inflammatory response (**Fig. 9-6**). In addition, tubercle formation of the lids conjunctiva, cornea, and sclera have been reported.[37] Granulomatous iritis is the inflammatory condition most often associated with TB.[38] Coles[39] wrote that TB should be suspected not only in cases of granulomatous uveitis but also in cases of intense nongranulomatous anterior uveitis of short duration, mild relapsing uveitis, or chronic smoldering inflammatory disease.

Interstitial keratitis and phlyctenular keratoconjunctivitis are common findings in patients with ocular TB; however, they are not thought to result from direct invasion of organisms but instead to represent an immunologic response to the mycobacteria. Eales' disease, a disorder characterized by retinal vasculitis and vitreous hemorrhage, is also associated with TB (see Fig. 27-2, A and B). Finally, optic nerve involvement and cataracts have also been reported in patients with

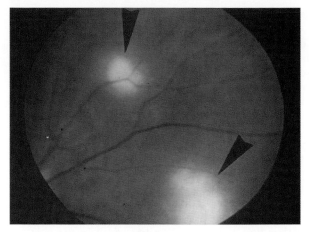

Figure 9-5. Two large choroidal lesions (arrowheads) caused by miliary tuberculosis. *(Courtesy Fernando Orefice, MD.)*

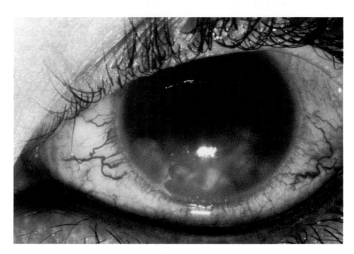

Figure 9-6. Patient with systemic tuberculosis who presented with a large floccular mass in anterior chamber. *(Courtesy Roberto Neufeld, MD.)*

Box 9-2 Ocular manifestations of tuberculosis

Tubercle formation of eyelids
Conjunctivitis
Interstitial keratitis
Anterior uveitis
Scleritis
Choroidal granulomas
Posterior uveitis
Retinal vasculitis

ocular TB.[33,37] A number of infectious and noninfectious disorders may cause ocular disease similar to TB. For example, the retinal periphlebitis that results from TB can mimic the ocular disease associated with sarcoidosis and syphilis. Finally, an underlying immunosuppressive state, such as AIDS, should always be considered in patients with ocular TB.

Diagnosis

The diagnosis of ocular TB is usually difficult to make. We have spent countless hours debating the diagnostic approach to patients with possible TB-associated uveitis. Definitive diagnosis requires the identification of *Mycobacterium tuberculosis* organisms in ocular tissues or fluids, but samples are often difficult to obtain, and biopsy may be hard to justify in a patient who has only a small chance of having the disease. Patients with suspected ocular TB should have a systemic evaluation for evidence of the disease. A chest X-ray should be obtained and tuberculin skin tests performed. If the clinical findings support a diagnosis of TB, a complete course of antituberculosis therapy should be considered. In a study in Japanese patients with intraocular inflammation, 26 of 126 had a positive tuberculin skin test result.[40] Ten of these 26 patients had clinical findings consistent with TB and had a favorable response to antituberculosis therapy.

An intermediate-strength tuberculin skin test should be used for most patients. However, if a patient has a history of TB or has had a positive PPD test result in the past, an intermediate-strength PPD may cause a severe dermatologic response and a lower-strength one should be used. The PPD test is not 100% sensitive or specific for the disease. One patient with numerous tubercle bacilli in the eye was reported to have a negative PPD test result and no systemic manifestations of disease.[41] Importantly, a positive PPD test result in a patient with uveitis does not mean that the uveitis is caused by TB, because TB is a very rare cause of inflammatory eye disease. In fact, without other signs of TB, a positive PPD test result in a patient with uveitis is probably more misleading than helpful. Interferon-γ-release assays are new alternatives to the tuberculin skin test. These new assays, especially QuantiFERON-TB Gold, have excellent specificity and are unaffected by BCG vaccination.[42]

Although many patients with ocular TB will have evidence of systemic disease, TB infection limited to specific organs, including the eye, may occur. Microscopic examination of ocular tissues or fluids may show bacilli; however, culture is more sensitive. The polymerase chain reaction (PCR) has also been used to diagnose TB infection,[43] but in most laboratories this is currently only experimental.

Therapy

Because of the development of treatment-resistant TB, recommended treatment regimens have become more aggressive. Previously the recommended treatment was regimens of isoniazid and ethambutol for 1.5 to 2 years. Since the late 1960s, however, a number of studies have demonstrated that short-course treatment regimens can be effective. Most regimens contain isoniazid and rifampin for 9 months. A third drug – ethambutol, streptomycin, or pyrazinamide – was usually added for the first 3 months to prevent resistance. Most regimens now include at least a 2-month course of four drugs, including isoniazid, rifampin, pyrazinamide, and ethambutol, followed by an additional 4 months of isoniazid and rifampin. Clearly, therapy should be administered by a practitioner well versed in the current treatment recommendations.[44,45]

The difficult decision is whether antituberculous therapy is warranted for the patient with uveitis compatible with TB, no evidence of systemic disease, and a positive PPD test result. Schlaegel and Weber[46] have recommended an isoniazid therapeutic test for these patients. This involves giving isoniazid at 300 mg/day and examining the patient every week. If ocular inflammation improves after 1–2 weeks of therapy, the patient is considered to have a positive test response. Schlaegel and Weber suggested that these patients should then receive a full course of therapy. There are several problems with this test, however. From a practical point of view, many patients with presumed tuberculous uveitis are concomitantly treated with corticosteroids, which makes it difficult to determine whether the antituberculous or the antiinflammatory therapy had the principal effect. The disease course may wax and wane; therefore, improvement may be due to the natural course of the disorder and be unrelated to antituberculous drugs. Importantly, a randomized double-masked study of isoniazid in the treatment of uveitis showed no significant difference between the treated and placebo groups.[47] Our current recommendation is to treat patients with uveitis and a positive PPD test result only if there are other findings to support the diagnosis of TB. The addition of antitubercular therapy to corticosteroids in uveitis patients with underlying latent or manifest TB appears to reduce the recurrences of uveitis.[48] Although hematogenous seeding of organisms from the lung is the most common mode of ocular infection, results on the chest X-ray may be normal, and disease is occasionally limited to a specific organ. A history of exposure to TB, a history of inadequately treated TB, a positive PPD test result with a large area of induration, or positive culture results all greatly increase the likelihood of disease. Once a decision to treat is made, the patient should receive at least two drugs for at least 3–6 months before a decision about efficacy is made.

Other bacterial infections

Brucellosis

Brucellosis is a bacterium that infects the genitourinary tract of cattle (*Brucella abortus*) and pigs (*Brucella suis*). Humans become infected after exposure to infected animals or contaminated meat or dairy products. The disease in humans is characterized by fever, chills, headache, arthralgias, lymphadenopathy, and splenomegaly. Diagnosis can be difficult but is based on positive blood cultures or cultures of usually sterile fluids. Serologic tests are available for brucellosis and assist with the diagnosis.

In one case series, ocular manifestations associated with brucellosis were reported in 26% of the patients.[49] In another study of 1551 patients with brucellosis, 52 (3.4%) had ocular involvement.[50] The organism has been reported to affect all the ocular structures, but optic nerve involvement appears to be the most serious ocular manifestation.[51] **Box 9-3** lists the ocular manifestations of the disease. Uveitis has been described in patients with brucellosis. Recurrent iritis, localized thickening of the iris, and multiple irregular choroidal exudates associated with little inflammation and retinal detachment have all been ascribed to brucellosis.[52,53] Walker and colleagues[54] published the case of a patient with brucellosis who had well-circumscribed lesions in the periphery of the choroid (**Fig. 9-7**). *Brucella* organisms have never been cultured from the eye in uveitis[53] although a high *Brucella* agglutination titer was noted in the vitreous specimen of a patient with ocular brucellosis.[55] With current health measures, including pasteurization, the incidence of this disease has declined dramatically.

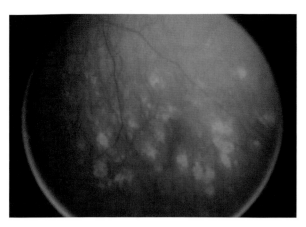

Figure 9-7. Well-circumscribed lesions in periphery of choroid in patient with brucellosis. *(Courtesy Narsing A. Rao, MD.)*

Box 9-3 Ocular manifestations of brucellosis

Disc edema
Optic neuritis
Keratitis
Corneal ulcers
Conjunctivitis
Chronic anterior uveitis
Multifocal choroiditis
Eyelid edema
Dacryoadenitis
Episcleritis
Posterior uveitis
Cranial nerve palsies
Endophthalmitis
Retinal detachment

Antimicrobial therapy for brucellosis is aimed and eradicating active infection, treating symptoms, and preventing recurrence. The standard treatment involves streptomycin and doxycycline. It is not clear whether antibiotic therapy is helpful for uveitis associated with brucellosis. Nevertheless, therapy with combinations of tetracyclines, cephalosporins, and other antibiotics appears effective for systemic disease and is indicated for patients with possible brucellosis-associated uveitis.

Whipple's disease

Whipple's disease is a chronic infectious disease caused by *Tropheryma whipplei*. The disorder is characterized by malabsorption that causes chronic diarrhea. Anterior uveitis and vitritis have been rarely reported in patients with Whipple's disease.[56] However, because antibiotic therapy can effectively treat this disease, it is important to diagnose Whipple's disease in patients with uveitis who have gastrointestinal symptoms. *Tropheryma whipplei* DNA has been found in the stool and saliva of patients with the disease using PCR, and may be of value in analyzing other specimens, including aqueous humor.[57,58]

Treatment and prognosis

Before treatment with antibiotics was possible, Whipple's disease was a fatal disorder. Antibiotics that cross the

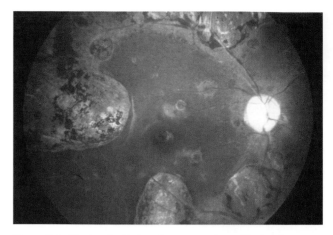

Figure 9-8. Chorioretinal lesions in young patient with chronic granulomatous disease. Macular involvement resulted in decreased visual acuity.

blood–brain barrier are felt to have lower recurrence rates, and many recomment oral administration of tremethoprim-sulfamethaxazole twice a day for 1–2 years.[59] This therapy is often preceded by parenteral administration of streptomycin together with penicillin G or with ceftriaxone. The prognosis is usually good, if the disease is diagnosed promptly and treated appropriately. Patients with a neurologic recurrence, however, have a poor prognosis and may require additional antibiotic and immunotherapy such as interferon-γ.[60]

Chronic granulomatous disease

Chronic granulomatous disease (CGD) is an inherited disorder that predisposes affected children to pyogenic infections. Currently, an X-linked recessive and an autosomal recessive form of the disease have been identified. A number of ocular findings are associated with this disease, including blepharokeratoconjunctivitis with pannus formation and inflammatory chorioretinal lesions that lead to extensive scarring (**Fig. 9-8**).[61] We recently found chorioretinal lesions in seven of 19 patients (37%) with X-linked CGD but in none of six patients with autosomal recessive disease. Three of the patients with chorioretinal lesions had visual acuity <20/400 and abnormal electrooculograms. Usually by the time these lesions are discovered in young children, who rarely complain of problems with their vision, there is no active inflammatory disease. It is unclear whether treatment with corticosteroids or antibiotics alters the course of the lesions; however, therapy is probably indicated if acute inflammatory disease is noted. In any event, sight-threatening disease is a frequent complication of CGD and appears to be associated with the X-linked form of the disease; periodic eye examinations are warranted in these patients.[62,63]

Fungal disease

The most common fungal disease associated with uveitis is histoplasmosis. Ocular histoplasmosis and presumed ocular histoplasmosis syndrome are described in Chapter 15 on ocular histoplasmosis. In general, fungal infection of the choroid, retina, and vitreous occurs in several types of

14. Shields JA, Waring GO III, Monte LG. Ocular findings in leprosy. Am J Ophthalmol 1974; 77: 880–890.

15. Brandt F, Malla OK. Ocular findings in leprous patients: a report of a survey in Malunga/Nepal. Albrecht von Graefes Arch Klin Exp Ophthalmol 1981; 217: 27–34.

16. Spaide R, Nattis R, Lipka A, et al. Ocular findings in leprosy in the United States. Am J Ophthalmol 1985; 100: 411–416.

17. Vedy J, Graveline J. Précis d'ophtalmologie tropicale, Marseille, 1979, Diffusion Generale de Librairie, p 125.

18. Chovet M, Metge P, Fauxpoint B, et al. Uvéite posté lépreuse. Bull Soc Ophtalmol Fr 1976; 12: 1215–1217.

19. Kircheimer WF, Storrs EE. Attempts to establish the armadillo (Drasypus novemcentus Linn.) as a model for study of leprosy. Int J Lepr 1971; 39: 693–702.

20. Wallach D, Cottenot F, Bach M-A. Imbalances in T-cell subpopulations in lepromatous leprosy. Int J Leprosy 1982; 50: 282–290.

21. Stoner GL, Atlaw T, Touw J, et al. Antigen-specific suppressor cells in subclinical leprosy infection. Lancet 1981; 2: 1372–1377.

22. Horwitz MA, Levis WR, Cohn ZA. Defective production of monocyte-activating cytokines in lepromatous leprosy. J Exp Med 1984; 159: 666–678.

23. Van Voorhis WC, Kaplan G, Nunes Sarno E, et al. The cutaneous infiltrates of leprosy: cellular characteristics and the predominant T-cell phenotypes, N Engl J Med 1982; 307: 1593–1597.

24. De Vries RRP, van Eden W, van Rood JJ. HLA-linked control of the course of M. leprae infection. Leprosy Rev 1981; 52(suppl): 109–119.

25. Daniel E, Koshy S, Rao GS, et al. Ocular complications in newly diagnosed borderline lepromatous and lepromatous leprosy patients: baseline profile of the Indian cohort. Br J Ophthalmol 2002; 86: 1336–1340.

26. WHO Study Group. Chemotherapy of leprosy for control programmes. WHO Tech Rep Ser 1982; 675.

27. Walker SL, Waters MF, Lockwood DN. The role of thalidomide in the management of erythem nodosum leprosum. Lepr Rev 2007; 78: 197–215.

27a. Guyton JS, Woods AC. Etiology of uveitis: a clinical study of 562 cases. Arch Ophthalmol 1941; 26: 986–1018.

28. Glassroth J, Robins AG, Snider DE. Tuberculosis in the 1980s. N Engl J Med 1980; 302: 1441–1450.

29. Barnes PF, Bloch AB, Davidson PT, et al. Tuberculosis in patients with human immunodeficiency virus infection. N Engl J Med 1991; 324: 1644–1650.

30. Centers for Disease Control and Prevention. Expanded tuberculosis surveillance and tuberculosis

morbidity, United States 1993, MMWR Morbid Mortal Wkly Rep 1994; 43: 361–366.

31. Trends in tuberculosis – United States, 2007. MMWR Morb Mortal Wkly Rep 2008; 21: 281–285.

32. Giles JT, Bathon JM. Serious infections associated with anticytokine therapies in the rheumatic diseases. J Intens Care Med 2004; 19: 320–334.

33. Donahue HC. Ophthalmologic experience in a tuberculosis sanatorium. Am J Ophthalmol 1967; 64: 742–748.

34. Ustinova EI, Zhuravleva LV, Bataev VM, Khokkanen VM, Zavarzin Lul. Experience in the differential diagnosis of peripapillary 'geographic' choroid disease and tuberculous chorioretinitis. Vestn Oftalmol 1990; 106: 43–46.

35. Mackensen F, Backer MD, Wiehler U, et al. QuantiFERON TB-Gold – A new test strengthening long-suspected tuberculous involvement in serpiginous-like choroiditis. Am J Ophthlamol 2008; (in press).

36. Massaro D, Katz S, Sachs M. Choroidal tubercles: a clue to hematogenous tuberculosis. Ann Intern Med 1964; 60: 231–241.

37. Helm CJ, Holland GN. Ocular tuberculosis. Surv Ophthalmol 1993; 38: 229–256.

38. Darrell RW. Acute tuberculous panophthalmitis. Arch Ophthalmol 1967; 78: 51–54.

39. Coles RS. Uveitis associated with systemic disease. Surv Ophthalmol 1963; 8: 377–392.

40. Morimura Y, Okada AA, Kawahara S, et al. Tuberculin skin testing in uveitis patients and treatment of presumed intracoular tuberculosis in Japan. Ophthalmology 2002; 109: 851–857.

41. Smith RE. Tuberculoma of the choroid, discussion. Ophthalmology 1980; 87: 257–258.

42. Pai M, Zwerling A, Menzies D. Systemic Review: T-cell-based assays for the diagnosis of latent tuberculosis infection: an update. Ann Intern Med 2008; 149: 177–184.

43. Musial CE, Tice LS, Stockman L, et al. Identification of mycobacteria from culture by using the Gen-Probe Rapid Diagnostic System for Mycobacterium avium complex and Mycobacterium tuberculosis complex, J Clin Microbiol 1988; 26: 2120–2123.

44. Schlaegel TF Jr, O'Connor GR. Tuberculosis and syphilis. Arch Ophthalmol 1981; 99: 2206–2207.

45. Blumberg HM, Burman WJ, Chaisson RE, et al. American Thoracic Society/ Centers for Disease Control and Prevention/Infectious Diseases Society of America: Treatment of tuberculosis. Am J Respir Crit Care Med 2003; 167: 603–662.

46. Schlaegel TF Jr, Weber JC. Double-blind therapeutic trial of isoniazid in 344 patients with uveitis. Br J Ophthalmol 1969; 53: 425–427.

47. Oksala A, Salminen A. Leptospiral uveitis. Acta Ophthalmol 1956; 34: 185–194.

48. Bansal R, Gupta A, Gupta V, et al. Role of anti-tubercular therapy in uveitis with latent/manifest tuberculosis. Am J Ophthalmol 2008; (in press).

49. Gungur K, Bekir NA, Namiduru M. Ocular complications associated with brucellosis in an endemic area. Eur J Ophthalmol 2002; 12: 232–237.

50. Rolando I, Olarte L, Vilchez, et al. Ocular manifestations associated with brucellosis: a 26-year experience in Peru. Clin Infect Dis 2008; 1: 1338–1345.

51. Puig-Solanes M, Heatley J, Arenas F, et al. Ocular complications in brucellosis. Am J Ophthalmol 1953; 36: 675.

52. Tabbara KF, al Kassimi H. Ocular brucellosis. Br J Ophthalmol 1990; 74: 249.

53. Rolando I, Carbone A, Haro D, et al. Retinal detachment in chronic brucellosis. Am J Ophthalmol 1985; 99: 733.

54. Walker J, Sharma OP, Rao NA. Brucellosis and uveitis. Am J Ophthalmol 1992; 114: 374–375.

55. Akduman L, Or M, Hasanreisoglu B, et al. A case of ocular brucellosis: importance of vitreous specimen. Acta Ophthalmol (Copenhagen) 1993; 71: 130–132.

56. Selsky EJ, Knox DL, Maumanee AE, et al. Ocular involvement in Whipple's disease. Retina 1984; 4: 103–106.

57. Fenollar F, Laouira S, Lepidi H, et al. Value of Tropheryma whipplei quantitative polymerase chain reaction assay for the diagnosis of Whipple disease: usefulness of saliva and stool specimens for first-line screening. Clin Infect Dis 2008; 47: 659–667.

58. Nubourgh I, Vandergheynst F, Lefebvre P, et al. An atypical case of Whipple's disease: case report and review of the literature. Acta Clin Belg 2008; 63: 107–111.

59. Fenollar F, Puechal X, Raoult D. Whipple's disease. N Engl J Med 2007; 356: 55–66.

60. Schneider T, Stallmach A, von Herbay A, et al. Treatment of refractory Whipple disease with interferon-γ. Ann Intern Med 1998; 129: 857–877.

61. Palestine AG, Meyers SM, Fauci AS, et al. Ocular findings in patients with neutrophil dysfunction. Am J Ophthalmol 1983; 95: 598–604.

62. Parks DJ, Walton RC, Cheung MK, et al. Sight-threatening complications of chronic granulomatous disease. Ophthalmology 1994; 101(suppl): 132.

63. Goldblatt D, Butcher J, Thrasher AJ, et al. Chorioretinal lesions in patients and carriers of chronic granulomatous disease. J Pediatr 1999; 134: 780–783.

64. Narndran N, Balasubramaniam B, Johnson E, et al. Five-year retrospective review of guideline-based management of fungal endopthalmitis. Acta Ophthalmol 2008; 86: 525–532.

65. Abe F, Tateyama M, Shibuya H, et al. Disseminated fungal infection. Acta Pathol Jpn 1984; 34: 1201–1208.

66. Edwards JE, Foos RY, Montgomerie JZ, et al. Ocular manifestations of candida septicemia: review of seventy-six cases of hematogenous candida endophthalmitis. Medicine (Baltimore) 1974; 53: 47–75.

67. Gallo J, Playfair J, Gregory-Roberts J, et al. Fungal endophthalmitis in narcotic abusers. Med J Aust 1985; 142: 386–388.

68. Cohen M, Edwards JE Jr, Hensley TJ, et al. Experimental hematogenous *Candida albicans* endophthalmitis: electron microscopy. Invest Ophthalmol Vis Sci 1977; 16: 498–511.

69. Blumenkranz MS, Stevens DA. Therapy of endogenous fungal endophthalmitis. Arch Ophthalmol 1980; 98: 1216–1220.

70. Goodman DF, Stern WH. Oral ketoconazole and intraocular amphotericin B for treatment of postoperative *Candida parapsilosis* endophthalmitis. Arch Ophthalmol 1987; 105: 172–173.

71. Naidoff MA, Green WR. Endogenous Aspergillus endophthalmitis occurring after kidney transplant. Am J Ophthalmol 1975; 79: 502–509.

72. Roney P, Barr CC, Chun CH, et al. Endogenous *Aspergillus* endophthalmitis, Rev Infect Dis 1986; 8: 955–958.

73. Young RC, Bennett JE, Vogel CL, et al. Aspergillosis: the spectrum of the disease in 98 patients. Medicine (Baltimore) 1970; 49: 147–173.

74. Sihota R, Agarwal HC, Grover AK, et al. Aspergillus endophthalmitis. J Ophthalmol 1987; 71: 611–613.

75. Glasgow BJ, Brown HH, Foos RY. Miliary retinitis in coccidioidomycosis. Am J Ophthalmol 1987; 104: 24–27.

76. Hiles DA, Font RL. Unilateral intraocular cryptococcosis with unilateral spontaneous regression. Am J Ophthalmol 1968; 65: 98–108.

77. Goldstein BG, Buellner H. Histoplasmic endophthalmitis: a clinicopathologic correlation. Arch Ophthalmol 1983; 101: 774–777.

78. Font RL, Jakobiec FA. Granulomatous necrotizing retinochoroiditis caused by *Sporotrichum schenkii*. Arch Ophthalmol 1976; 94: 1513–1519.

79. Font RL, Spaulding AG, Green WR. Endogenous mycotic panophthalmitis caused by *Blastomyces dermatitidis*. Arch Ophthalmol 1967; 77: 217–222.

80. Shah KB, Wu TG, Wilhelmus KR, et al. Activity of voriconazole against corneal isolates of *Scedosporium apiospermum*. Cornea 2003; 22: 33–36.

81. Harnard P, Hamard H, Nghou S. Leber's idiopathic stellate neuroretinitis: Apropos of 9 cases. J Fr Ophthahlmol 1994; 116–123.

82. Shoari M, Katz B. Recurrent neuroretinitis in an adolescent with ulcerative colitis. J Neuro-ophthalmol 2005; 25: 286–288.

Spirochetal Diseases

Scott M. Whitcup

Key concepts

- Spirochetal disease includes a historical and clinical gamut of infections causing uveitis, including syphilis, endemic syphilis, Lyme disease, relapsing fever, and leptospirosis.
- Ocular findings can occur in primary, secondary, latent, and tertiary syphilis.
- The VDRL test can be falsely negative, especially in later stages of the disease, and a more sensitive and specific test such as the FTA-ABS test should be considered when evaluating patients with possible syphilitic uveitis.
- Lyme serology should be ordered in patients with a history or findings consistent with the disease. False positive results are common when the test is ordered in patients with an extremely low likelihood of Lyme disease.
- Antibiotic regimens for spirochetal disease change frequently. Consulting a physician well versed in treating these diseases is important to ensure the appropriate drug, dose, route, and length of treatment.

Spirochetal infections and the eye

This chapter focuses on uveitis caused by spirochetes. This comprises a variety of infectious diseases with ocular manifestations, including syphilis, bejel, pinta, yaws, Lyme disease, relapsing fever, and leptospirosis. The ocular manifestations of syphilis have been known for well over a century, whereas Lyme disease was first described in the 1970s. The first section of this chapter is devoted to treponemal infections, of which syphilis is by far the most common and important to the practicing ophthalmologist. Syphilis remains an important cause of eye disease and blindness in the United States, and is diagnosed with increasing frequency in patients with acquired immunodeficiency syndrome (AIDS). Sections on endemic syphilis (bejel) and nonvenereal treponemal infections (yaws and pinta) are also included.

The second part of the chapter contains sections on two infections caused by spirochetes of the genus *Borrelia* and a section on leptospirosis. Although the cause of syphilis was identified at the beginning of the 20th century, the causative agent for Lyme disease was not discovered until 1982.

Interestingly, Lyme disease and syphilis share many clinical features and should be considered together in the differential diagnosis of infectious diseases with ophthalmic involvement. The chapter also reviews relapsing fever, an additional infection caused by *Borrelia* that is often misdiagnosed. Leptospirosis is discussed at the end of the chapter and may be an important cause of uveitis of unknown etiology.

Spirochetes

Definition

Spirochetes are a phylum of bacteria characterized by long, helically coiled cells. These bacteria have lengthwise flagella called axial filaments that allow the spirochetes to move. There are three groups of spirochetes implicated in human disease: *Treponema*, which cause syphilis and the nonvenereal treponematoses; *Borrelia*, which cause relapsing fever and Lyme disease; and *Leptospira*, which cause leptospirosis.

Venereal treponemal diseases

Syphilis

Etiology and Epidemiology

Syphilis was originally called the *great pox*, but it acquired its current name from the title character of a poem written in 1530 by the Veronese physician and poet Girolamo Fracastoro. Syphilis has also been called the *great imitator*, because of the myriad symptoms and signs in its repertoire and its ability to mimic numerous other illnesses. Although clinical descriptions of syphilis date back at least half a millennium, it was not until 1905 that Schaudin and Hoffman[1] isolated the spirochete *Treponema pallidum* from skin lesions of patients with syphilis.

After initial infection there is both a humoral and a cellular immune response. In 1910, Wasserman introduced a complement fixation test to detect nonspecific antibodies that react against cardiolipins, and these antibodies are commonly found in patients with syphilis. The next milestone in the history of syphilis was the use of arsenic derivatives to treat the disease. The *coup de grâce* in the war against syphilis came in 1943 with the discovery of penicillin, which is still the mainstay of therapy today.[2] In the late 1980s there was a substantial increase in primary and secondary syphilis and an increased incidence of congenital syphilis, especially in the inner cities.[3] In 1986, only 57 cases of congenital syphilis were reported in New York City, but in 1989 more than 1000 cases were documented.[4] With focused efforts to reduce syphilis in the United States, in 2000 the rate of primary and secondary syphilis was 2.1 cases per 100 000 population, the lowest since reporting began in 1941.[5] From 2001 to 2004, rates increased to 2.7 cases per 100 000 population. Approximately 84% of cases occurred in men. Primary and secondary syphilis incidence also varied by race/ethnicity. The incidence of primary and secondary syphilis in 2004 was 9.0 per 100 000 population among blacks, 1.6 among whites, 3.2 among Hispanics, 1.2 among Asian/Pacific Islanders, and 3.2 among American Indian/Alaska Natives. Syphilis is also a problem in patients co-infected with human immunodeficiency virus (HIV). These patients may not mount a serologic response to the treponemal infection and thus elude diagnosis. In addition, standard therapy may be insufficient to eradicate the infection in these immunocompromised patients.[6,7]

T. pallidum is a spirochete that is approximately 0.01–0.02 μm wide and 5–20 μm long. Although it cannot survive long out of the body, it can be cultured and remains viable for several days. Syphilis is transmitted almost exclusively by sexual contact, including sexual intercourse, orogenital and anorectal contact, and occasionally kissing. The disease is most infectious in patients with untreated primary syphilis or secondary syphilis with skin lesions. Disease can also be transmitted by patients with early latent syphilis, especially if they have mucocutaneous involvement; however, disease in patients with late latent syphilis and tertiary syphilis is not infectious. Congenital syphilis occurs with transplacental spread of the spirochete. Interestingly, infection with syphilis does not confer lasting immunity, especially if treatment is received early in the course of the disease.

T. pallidum can penetrate intact mucous membranes or abraded skin. The period of incubation varies from 10 to 90 days, but averages 3 weeks.[8] Before primary skin lesions appear, the spirochete spreads via the lymphatics to the bloodstream, from which it then disseminates.

As with many of the spirochetal diseases, the clinical course of syphilis is divided into stages: primary, secondary, and tertiary syphilis (**Box 10-1**).

Clinical Manifestations

Primary syphilis. The chancre is the predominant lesion of primary syphilis. It appears about 4 weeks after infection and heals in about 1–2 months in untreated individuals. The lesion begins as an erythematous papule at the inoculation site and later erodes to form a painless ulcer. Multiple chancres can occur, especially in patients coinfected with HIV.[9] Serous fluid from these lesions is teeming with spirochetes.

Box 10-1 Syphilis – key features

- Caused by the spirochete *Treponema pallidum*
- Transmitted almost exclusively by sexual contact
- Congenital syphilis occurs with transplacental spread of the spirochete
- Disease is divided into stages: primary, secondary, latent, and tertiary
- Tertiary syphilis is subdivided into three subgroups: benign tertiary syphilis, cardiovascular syphilis, and neurosyphilis
- If untreated, syphilis will disseminate

Lesions occur on the penis, anus, and rectum in men and on the cervix, vulva, and perineum in women. Small lesions may also occur on the lips, tongue, buccal mucosa, and skin, and chancres of the eyelids and conjunctiva have also been described.[10]

Secondary syphilis. If untreated, disease in patients with primary syphilis will progress to secondary syphilis 4–10 weeks after the initial manifestations of the disease. One of the unique characteristics of syphilis is that it always disseminates.[11] The skin is involved in about 90% of patients with secondary syphilis. A generalized rash is characteristic of secondary syphilis and may be maculopapular or pustular. The rash commonly occurs on the flexor and volar surfaces of the body, typically the palms and the soles. The rash usually resolves without scarring, but some patients are left with areas of hyper- or hypopigmentation. Mucous membranes become eroded, forming erythematous patches. Condylomata lata is another characteristic dermatologic manifestation of secondary syphilis. The papules develop at the mucocutaneous junctions and in moist areas of the skin, and appear as dull pink or gray hypertrophic lesions. Systemic symptoms of secondary syphilis include fever, malaise, headache, nausea, anorexia, and joint pain.[12] A generalized lymphadenopathy is found in both primary and secondary syphilis. Syphilitic infiltration of the kidneys, liver, and gastrointestinal tract also occurs in secondary syphilis, and about 10% of patients have ocular involvement. Anterior uveitis is the predominant eye finding in early secondary syphilis and may be the most common ocular lesion in syphilis.[13] Some patients may demonstrate a cerebrospinal fluid (CSF) pleocytosis, and a few of these patients experience acute syphilitic meningitis with headache, neck stiffness, cranial nerve palsies, and disc edema.

Latent syphilis. In the first year after initial infection, patients may have recurrences of infectious mucocutaneous lesions. This period of the disease is called *early latent syphilis*. The late latent phase of syphilis occurs after 1 year of infection, and during this stage of the disease infectious relapses are rare. Most patients who have not been treated remain in this late latent phase of the disease; however, about 30% go on to experience tertiary syphilis.

Tertiary syphilis. Tertiary syphilis is also called *late syphilis* and is often subdivided into three groups: benign tertiary syphilis, cardiovascular syphilis, and neurosyphilis.

Benign tertiary syphilis. The gumma is the typical lesion of benign tertiary syphilis and is a chronic granulomatous lesion that heals with scarring and fibrosis. It is a rare finding in the penicillin era and responds rapidly to treatment. Gummas tend to develop in the skin and mucous membranes, but can occur in almost any tissue and have even been found in the choroid of the eye.[14]

Cardiovascular syphilis. The lesions of cardiovascular syphilis include aortitis and aortic aneurysms, aortic valvular insufficiency, and narrowing of the coronary ostia. Disease starts about 5–10 years after infection, but symptoms of cardiovascular syphilis may not be clinically evident for more than 20 years.

Neurosyphilis. This condition is said to occur in 5–10% of untreated patients with syphilis. Asymptomatic neurosyphilis is found in some patients who have a positive CSF Venereal Disease Research Laboratory (VDRL) test result but no symptoms of central nervous system (CNS) disease. In addition, invasion of the CNS by *T. pallidum* may be more common in early syphilis than once thought. Lukehart and colleagues[15] isolated *T. pallidum* from the CSF in 12 of 40 (30%) patients with untreated primary and secondary syphilis, and an additional four patients, in whom no *T. pallidum* was isolated, had reactive CSF on the VDRL test. Neurosyphilis can occur at any time in the course of the disease. Uveitis and hearing loss are more common in the earlier stages.[15a]

One type of neurosyphilis, meningovascular syphilis, presents as an aseptic meningitis that can occur at any time after primary syphilis. Unilateral or bilateral cranial nerve palsies are common, and headache, neck stiffness, dizziness, lassitude, and blurred vision occur. The classic neuro-ophthalmic finding of neurosyphilis is the Argyll Robertson pupil.[16] This is a small, irregular pupil that is unreactive to light but normally reactive to accommodation; it is commonly seen in cases of meningovascular syphilis in which the base of the brain is involved. If the spinal cord is involved patients may experience bulbar symptoms, muscle weakness and wasting, and slowly progressive spastic paraplegia with bladder incontinence.

T. pallidum may also invade the substance of the brain. Parenchymatous neurosyphilis is a meningoencephalitis with progressive loss of cortical function. Patients can experience altered mental status and even syphilitic psychosis, with irritability, reduced memory, poor judgment, confusion, and delusions. Seizures may occur. On neurologic examination patients demonstrate tremors of the mouth and tongue, hyperreflexia, and in some cases extensor plantar responses. Pathologically, the brain parenchyma is infiltrated with spirochetes, and the meninges are inflamed and thickened. The CSF is hypercellular and has a positive VDRL test result. Cranial nerve palsies, however, are uncommon, and optic atrophy is rare. Although pupillary abnormalities may be seen, a complete Argyll Robertson pupil is not characteristic. Neurosyphilis should still be considered in the differential diagnosis of advanced neurologic disease with generalized paresis, although this finding is rare in the United States.

Tabes dorsalis is a form of neurosyphilis with involvement of the posterior columns and the posterior roots of the spinal cord, resulting in pain, ataxia, sensory changes, reduced tendon reflexes, and ocular findings. Severe stabbing pain in the lower extremities heralds this form of neurosyphilis. Unsteadiness and a wide-based gait develop later, followed by hyperesthesia and paresthesia. Incontinence and impotence are other common sequelae. Charcot's arthropathy occurs in large joints devoid of sensation that are prone to destructive changes. Argyll Robertson pupils are frequent in this form of neurosyphilis, and optic atrophy is commonly found.

Congenital syphilis. Congenital syphilis results from the transplacental transmission of *T. pallidum* from the mother to the fetus. Untreated primary or secondary syphilis is almost invariably transmitted to the fetus, whereas transmission in later stages of the disease occurs less frequently.

Congenital syphilis is preventable with proper treatment of the mother; therefore, all expectant mothers should have a VDRL test at the beginning and near the end of pregnancy. In fact, screening at the time of delivery is now mandatory in the State of New York.[5]

Signs and symptoms of early congenital syphilis may not appear until several days after birth, and Dorfman and Glaser[17] stated that the diagnosis of congenital syphilis may be missed if serologic tests are not performed for both the mother and her infant at the time of delivery. A generalized rash develops and resembles the rash of secondary syphilis, except that in the infant the rash may be vesicular or bullous. Rhinitis (also called the snuffles), jaundice, hepatosplenomegaly, anorexia, and pseudoparalysis may also be found. Osteochondritis and pathologic fractures are common, and radiographic changes on bone films are present in more than 90% of patients. Chorioretinitis is often evident in the first few months of life.

Congenital syphilis may mimic other congenital infections, such as rubella, cytomegalovirus infection, and toxoplasmosis. A positive serologic test result for syphilis may be caused by passive transfer of antibody from the mother; therefore, diagnosis of congenital syphilis is based on a positive fluorescent treponemal antibody absorption (FTA-ABS) test and a rising VDRL titer. Results of serologic tests performed in infants and their mothers may be negative at the time of delivery if syphilis is acquired toward the end of the pregnancy.

After 2 years the child is described as having late congenital syphilis. Like syphilis in adults, late congenital syphilis may remain latent with few sequelae, although cardiovascular involvement does occur, and meningovascular syphilis with neurologic manifestations, including eighth cranial nerve deafness, is common. Acute syphilitic meningitis, generalized paresis, and tabes dorsalis are less common. Interstitial keratitis is the classic ophthalmic sign of congenital syphilis, occurring in 10% of patients.

Deformities of the permanent teeth occur after early syphilitic infection. The characteristic Hutchinson teeth are notched, thin, upper incisors with abnormal spacing. Hutchinson's triad is the occurrence of Hutchinson's teeth, interstitial keratitis, and deafness, but the occurrence of all three in the same patient is unusual. The bone lesions of early congenital syphilis tend to progress in late congenital syphilis, with the development of syphilitic arthritis. Finally, gummas may develop in the subcutaneous tissue and produce ulcerative skin lesions.

Ocular Manifestations

Table 10-1 lists some of the more common eye manifestations of the different stages of syphilis. Ophthalmic manifestations of primary syphilis are limited to chancres of the eyelid and the conjunctiva. A primary syphilitic lesion in the lacrimal gland is extremely rare but has been reported.[18]

The eyelids are commonly involved in the rash of secondary syphilis, and blepharitis and loss of lashes and eyebrows are common. Conjunctivitis mimicking trachoma has also been seen in secondary syphilis, but dacryocystitis and dacryoadenitis are rare. Keratitis, iris nodules (**Fig. 10-1**), iridocyclitis, episcleritis, and scleritis have all been reported in secondary syphilis. Late in the secondary stage, chorioretinitis and vitritis may develop (**Fig. 10-2A**). A diffuse

Table 10-1 Ocular manifestations of syphilis

PRIMARY SYPHILIS
Chancres of the eyelid and conjunctiva

SECONDARY SYPHILIS
Blepharitis
Madarosis
Conjunctivitis
Dacryocystitis
Dacryoadenitis
Keratitis
Iris nodules
Iridocyclitis
Episcleritis
Scleritis
Chorioretinitis
Vitritis
Neuroretinitis
Disc edema
Exudative retinal detachment
Perivasculitis

TERTIARY SYPHILIS
Gummas of the eyelids
Unilateral interstitial keratitis
Punctate stromal keratitis
Bilateral periostitis of the orbital bone
Episcleritis
Scleritis
Anterior and posterior uveitis
Chorioretinitis
Vasculitis
Venous and arterial occlusive disease
Exudative retinal detachment
Macular edema
Neuroretinitis
Vitritis
Pseudoretinitis pigmentosa
Chorioretinal neovascular membrane
Lens dislocation
Argyll Robertson pupil
Oculomotor palsies

CONGENITAL SYPHILIS
Bilateral interstitial keratitis
Pigmentary retinitis
Glaucoma
Keratouveitis

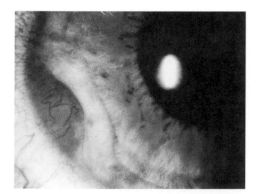

Figure 10-1. Iris nodule caused by syphilis. *(From Case records of the Massachusetts General Hospital. Weekly clinicopathological exercises. N Engl J Med 1984; 310: 972–81.)*

neuroretinitis may occur and is often localized to the peripapillary area.[19] This is followed by a pigmentary retinopathy similar in appearance to retinitis pigmentosa. Disc edema (**Fig. 10-3**), exudative retinal detachment, and perivasculitis are less common findings.[20–22]

The gummas of tertiary syphilis can involve the eyelids, and if extensive can cause destructive ulceration, but gummatous dacryoadenitis and infiltration of the lacrimal sac have only rarely been reported. Conjunctival vascular changes occur, but gummas of the conjunctiva almost never occur. As seen in secondary syphilis, syphilitic blepharitis with madarosis is common. A diffuse bilateral periostitis is the most common orbital finding of tertiary syphilis. Uniocular interstitial keratitis is the most common corneal finding in tertiary syphilis, but punctate stromal keratitis can occur with iritis. Episcleritis and scleritis occur, but discrete gummas of the sclera are rare. Uveitis is a common finding in late tertiary syphilis. Halperin and colleagues[23] stated that the main posterior segment complications of acquired syphilis include chorioretinitis, vasculitis, venous and arterial occlusive disease, retinal detachment with choroidal effusion, macular edema, neuroretinitis, optic neuritis, vitritis (Fig. 10-2A), and pseudoretinitis pigmentosa (Fig. 10-2B). Choroidal neovascular membranes and subretinal fibrosis (**Fig. 10-4**) can also occur. A posterior placoid chorioretinitis has been described in late latent syphilis.[23a] Vitreous opacities are common, and lens dislocation has been reported in many patients.

The most typical manifestation of congenital syphilis is bilateral interstitial keratitis, which appears later in life. A pigmentary retinitis and glaucoma can also occur as a result of congenital syphilitic keratouveitis.

The Argyll Robertson pupil and disc edema are most commonly seen in meningovascular syphilis, along with oculomotor palsies and other pupillary abnormalities. Later in the course of meningovascular syphilis, optic atrophy occurs. A complete Argyll Robertson pupil is rare in cases of general paresis, but, as with optic atrophy, is more common in cases of tabes dorsalis.

Diagnosis

The diagnosis of syphilis is based on the clinical history, physical examination, and laboratory tests. Although darkfield examination or immunofluorescent staining of mucocutaneous lesions can lead to the prompt diagnosis of primary, secondary, and early congenital syphilis, most physicians order serologic tests to make or confirm a diagnosis. There are both nontreponemal and treponemal tests. Confusion often arises in determining whether a VDRL test should be ordered rather than an FTA-ABS test, and in the interpretation of the results. In this section the various diagnostic tests for syphilis are explained, and a strategy for ordering tests is outlined (**Box 10-2**).

Darkfield microscopy can be used to identify spirochetes present in tissue fluids. *T. pallidum* is difficult to distinguish from other spirochetes, and so darkfield examination requires expertise. In clinical practice, greater reliance is placed on the serologic test for syphilis.

The two most commonly used screening tests for syphilis are the VDRL test and the rapid plasma reagin (RPR) test. Both of these are nontreponemal reaginic tests. Infection with *T. pallidum* stimulates nonspecific antibodies against

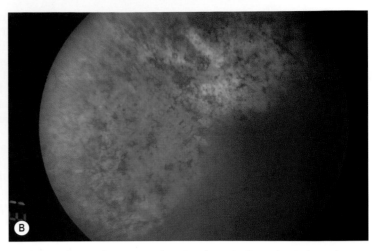

Figure 10-2. Fundus photograph of a patient with uveitis associated with syphilis. **A** shows a dense vitritis obscuring the optic disc and retinal vasculature. **B** shows the same patient following treatment with intravenous penicillin. The vitritis and retinal infiltrates have resolved, revealing the pigmentary retinopathy characteristic of ocular syphilis.

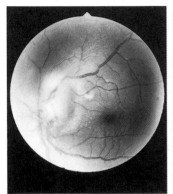 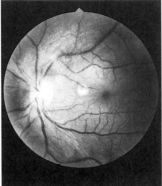

Figure 10-3. A, Patient with acquired syphilis who presented with papillitis and retinitis. **B,** The findings resolved following treatment with intravenous antibiotics. *(Courtesy Phuc Le Hoang, MD.)*

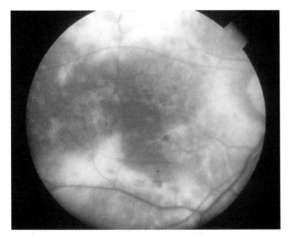

Figure 10-4. Extensive subretinal fibrosis caused by ocular syphilis. *(Courtesy Rubens Belfort Jr, MD.)*

cardiolipin. The VDRL test quantitates these antibodies by use of slide flocculation. The VDRL test is well standardized, and the result is reported as reactive, weakly reactive, borderline, or nonreactive. The rapid plasma reagin test is a similar assay for detecting anticardiolipin antibody.

Box 10-2 Diagnosis of syphilis – key points

- Diagnosis is based on clinical history, physical examination, and laboratory tests
- There are both nontreponemal and treponemal tests for syphilis
- Nontreponemal tests are often used to screen for syphilis. The two most common screening tests are the Venereal Disease Research Laboratory (VDRL) test and the rapid plasma reagin (RPR) test
- Treponemal tests are more sensitive in diagnosing patients with latent or late syphilis and more specific than the VDRL. The most commonly used treponemal test is the fluorescent treponemal antibody absorption (FTA-ABS) test

---

The sensitivity and the specificity of the VDRL test vary, depending on the stage of disease (**Table 10-2**). The VDRL test starts to become positive about 1–2 weeks after the appearance of the primary chancre and is positive in 99% of patients with secondary syphilis.[24] In later stages of the disease, however, the VDRL test reactivity decreases, and only about 70% of patients with cardiovascular syphilis or neurosyphilis have a positive VDRL test result. In addition, the VDRL test often becomes nonreactive after treatment for syphilis.

The serologic tests for syphilis are not 100% specific, and false-positive results can occur, especially in patients with other spirochetal diseases and connective tissue diseases (**Table 10-3**). Any weakly reactive or reactive VDRL test needs to be confirmed with a more specific test. The tests used for this purpose are the treponemal tests for syphilis, such as the *T. pallidum* agglutination tests (TPHA and MHA-TP) or the more commonly used FTA-ABS test. The *T. pallidum* immobilization test is almost completely specific for syphilis, but is expensive and difficult to perform and therefore rarely used. The microhemagglutination–*T. pallidum* (MHA-TP) assay for antibodies to *T. pallidum* is another specific test for syphilis but is also used less frequently than the FTA-ABS test. In the FTA-ABS test, the patient's serum is absorbed with extracts of nonpathogenic treponemes to remove possible

Table 10-2 Patients with positive results to VDRL and FTA-ABS tests

Percentage of patients with positive results				
Late or latent syphilis				
Test				
	Primary syphilis	*Secondary syphilis*	*Treated disease*	*Untreated disease*
VDRL	70	99	1	70
FTA-ABS	85	100	98	98

VDRL, Venereal Disease Research Laboratory; FTA-ABS, fluorescent treponemal antibody absorption.

Table 10-3 Causes of false-positive serologic test results for syphilis

SPIROCHETAL INFECTIONS
Endemic syphilis (bejel)
Yaws and pinta
Leptospirosis
Lyme disease
Relapsing fever

OTHER INFECTIONS
Chancroid
Chickenpox
Hepatitis
HIV infection
Infectious mononucleosis
Leprosy
Lymphogranuloma venereum
Malaria
Measles
Mycoplasma pneumonia
Pneumococcal pneumonia
Rickettsial disease
Scarlet fever
Subacute bacterial endocarditis
Tuberculosis
Trypanosomiasis

NONINFECTIOUS CAUSES
Blood transfusions
Chronic liver disease
Connective tissue disease
Narcotic addiction
Pregnancy
Vaccination

cross-reacting antitreponemal antibody that is not specific for *T. pallidum*. The absorbed serum is then made to react against *T. pallidum*, and specific antibodies are detected by the addition of fluorescein-labeled antihuman γ-globulin. Results are reported as nonreactive or as 1+ to 4+ positive, based on the intensity of the fluorescence.

A weakly reactive FTA-ABS test may not be reproducible. The FTA-ABS test is more sensitive than the VDRL test at all stages of syphilis, but it is more expensive and difficult to perform. The FTA-ABS test is also not entirely specific for syphilis, because false-positive results are seen in patients with systemic lupus erythematosus, biliary cirrhosis, and some connective tissue diseases, such as rheumatoid arthritis (see Table 10-3).

Because serologic tests for syphilis may take several weeks to become reactive, immediate diagnosis requires demonstration of treponemes in tissue fluid by darkfield microscopy. The VDRL test is an excellent screening test for patients with later primary syphilis and secondary syphilis. The sensitivity of the VDRL test is 99% for patients with secondary syphilis; however, all positive results should be confirmed with an FTA-ABS test.

Because the sensitivity of the VDRL test may be only 70% in patients with latent or late syphilis, both VDRL and FTA-ABS tests should be ordered if a later stage of disease is suspected. From the ophthalmic standpoint, many patients with uveitis or disc edema are suspected of having late syphilis, and many uveitis specialists and neuro-ophthalmologists routinely order both VDRL and FTA-ABS tests in the evaluation of these patients. As stated above, in the United States, testing for syphilis has consisted of initial screening with an inexpensive nontreponemal test, with subsequent testing of reactive specimens with a treponemal test. Some clinical laboratories have started using automated treponemal tests and then retest reactive results with a nontreponemal test.[24a] It is not clear what the recommendations are for patients who test positive with the treponemal test and then negative for the nontreponemal test. If not previously treated, these patients should probably be treated for late latent syphilis.

In addition, all patients who may have had syphilis for more than a year should have a lumbar puncture for CSF examination. A cell count, differential count, protein determination, and VDRL test should be performed on the CSF to look for evidence of neurosyphilis. As stated previously, CNS invasion by *T. pallidum* may be common in early syphilis.[15] The finding of CNS involvement is important because the recommended therapy is different from that for patients without CNS involvement. Serologic tests for neurosyphilis can also be confusing. The CSF-VDRL is insensitive but highly specific. A CSF serologic diagnosis is usually based on production of local antitreponemal antibodies, and an intrathecal *T. pallidum* antibody index can be calculated.

Infants born with congenital syphilis have positive VDRL and FTA-ABS test results from the passive transfer of immunoglobulin (Ig) G antibodies across the placenta; therefore, an IgM FTA-ABS test is used to diagnose congenital syphilis because IgM antibodies do not cross the placenta, and a positive test result would indicate actual infection in the infant.[25]

Patients with undiagnosed interstitial keratitis should be suspected of having late congenital syphilis. A thorough history of previous therapy should be elicited, and patients should then undergo VDRL and FTA-ABS tests and a CSF examination. If the CSF VDRL test result is positive, some experts recommend that the patient be treated as for latent syphilis (**Table 10-4**). Patients with a positive serum VDRL or FTA-ABS result but negative CSF findings are treated as for primary or secondary syphilis.

Finally, newer diagnostic techniques may be helpful in diagnosing syphilis in patients with ocular manifestations of syphilis. The polymerase chain reaction (PCR) may be used to detect *T. pallidum* in ocular specimens such as aqueous humor.

Prognosis

Most patients recover without long-term sequelae if syphilis is recognized and treated early. If untreated, about 25% of

Table 10-4 Treatment of syphilis

PRIMARY AND SECONDARY SYPHILIS

Procaine penicillin, 2.4 million units IM daily, and probenecid, 1 g PO qd × 14 days or benzathine penicillin G, 2.4 million units IM in a single dose (although treatment failures have been reported)

If penicillin allergies exist, treat with doxycycline, 100 mg PO bid × 15 days or tetracycline 500 mg PO qid for 15 days. (Ceftrizone and azithromycin have also been used)

LATENT AND TERTIARY SYPHILIS, INCLUDING NEUROSYPHILIS

Aqueous crystalline penicillin G, 3–4 million units IV q 4 h × 10–14 days or benzathine penicillin G, 2.4 million units IM given weekly × 3. (Ceftriaxone and amoxicillin also have been used)

CONGENITAL SYPHILIS IN THE INFANT

Procaine penicillin, 50 000 units/kg/day IM × 10 days, or aqueous crystalline penicillin G, 50 000 units/kg/day IV in two divided doses × 10 days.

these patients have one or more relapses with mucocutaneous lesions. Eventually, most untreated patients remain in a latent stage of the disease; however, about one-third go on to experience tertiary syphilis. Benign tertiary syphilis occurs in about 15% of untreated patients. Cardiovascular syphilis occurs in 10% of these, and CNS involvement is seen in about 8% of untreated patients.

Treatment

General recommendations. Although guidelines for the treatment of syphilis exist, controversy persists. Before treating a patient with syphilis one should refer to the most current recommendations for therapy, and consultation with an infectious disease specialist may be helpful. Coinfection with HIV should be ruled out because standard therapy may be insufficient to eradicate disease in these patients. Recommendations for therapy are based on the stage of disease and are presented in Table 10-4.[24] Riedner and colleagues evaluated the efficacy of treating primary or latent syphilis with a single oral dose of 2 g azithromycin or a single intramuscular dose of 2.4 million units of penicillin G benzathine.[26] Cure rates were 97.7% for patients in the azithromycin group and 95.0% in the penicillin G benzathine group, achieving the prescribed criteria for equivalence.

Unfortunately, the ideal therapy for patients with uveitic syphilis has not been determined. Virulent *T. pallidum* infection has been reported to persist in the eye despite treatment with penicillin; therefore, many experts suggest that patients with any ocular inflammation secondary to syphilis be treated as for neurosyphilis, even if the CSF findings are normal.

In addition to treating the patient, the physician has a responsibility to report the disease to the local health department to ensure that all sexual contacts over at least the past 3 months are contacted, examined, and treated as necessary.

Patients with syphilis should have the VDRL test repeated at 3, 6, and 12 months after treatment because titers should become nonreactive within a year after successful therapy. In addition, patients with CSF involvement should have repeated CSF examinations at 6-month intervals for at least 3 years. Patients should be re-treated if clinical evidence of

syphilis occurs, if a previously nonreactive VDRL test again becomes reactive, or if an initially high-titer VDRL test does not decrease fourfold within a year.

Finally, patients receiving therapy for syphilis, especially intravenous therapy, should be monitored for a Jarisch–Herxheimer reaction. This is a hypersensitivity response to treponemal antigens. The reaction may exacerbate pre-existing ocular inflammation, such as uveitis and interstitial keratitis; prophylaxis with corticosteroids may help in some cases.

Approach to Syphilis in Patients with AIDS

Recognition of concurrent infection with HIV in patients with syphilis is important to the clinician because the diagnostic and therapeutic approach to syphilis may differ in these patients. Numerous reports suggest that uncharacteristic clinical manifestations of syphilis may occur in patients with concomitant HIV infection.[27,28] Unusual cases of ocular syphilis in HIV-infected patients with findings of panuveitis and retinal detachment have been reported, and some authors have stated that the incidence of ocular complications of syphilis may be increased in HIV-infected patients.[29–31] In addition, acute retinal necrosis and acute retinitis have been associated with syphilis in patients coinfected with HIV.[21,29] Despite some unique symptoms and signs, these patients usually also experience the characteristic clinical manifestations of syphilis. Patients with both HIV infection and syphilis may have an accelerated course with a greater likelihood of uveitis and progression to neurosyphilis.[27,30,32] In the study by Berry and colleagues[6] there was no difference in the detection of *T. pallidum* in the CSF in patients with or without concurrent HIV infection; nevertheless, it appears that treatment failures are more common in HIV-infected patients.[6,33,34] In addition, serologic evidence of syphilis may be delayed. Hicks and colleagues[35] reported on a patient with AIDS and skin manifestations consistent with secondary syphilis in whom the VDRL and FTA-ABS results were negative on two separate occasions. A skin biopsy demonstrated spirochetes with Warthin–Starry staining of the tissue, and the patient's VDRL and FTA-ABS test results later became positive, suggesting a delayed immunologic response.

Although patients with HIV infection and syphilis have more symptoms of CNS involvement, such as acute syphilitic meningitis and hearing loss, many of them do not have positive CSF VDRL test results and may manifest only CSF leukocytosis or elevated CSF protein concentration, findings that are seen in HIV patients without syphilis.[36] These findings have prompted some clinicians to treat all patients with concurrent HIV infection and syphilis with high-dose antibiotic therapy to cover the possibility of CNS involvement. The Centers for Disease Control and Prevention in Atlanta is currently studying the question of appropriate antibiotic therapy for patients with syphilis and concurrent HIV infection. For now, recommendations include the careful evaluation of all patients with syphilis for underlying HIV infection. Patients with AIDS should also be monitored for clinical signs of syphilis, and the diagnosis should be pursued despite negative serologic results early in the course of the disease.

Patients with syphilis and HIV infection should have a lumbar puncture to look for evidence of neurosyphilis.

Because treatment failures are common, some infectious disease consultants suggest that all patients be treated with a regimen adequate for neurosyphilis. After treatment, a VDRL test is suggested every month for at least 3 months, with close observation for evidence of recurrence.[37]

Nonvenereal treponematoses

Endemic syphilis

Etiology and Epidemiology

Endemic syphilis, yaws, and pinta are three nonvenereal treponemal infections that are spread by body contact and are endemic in certain geographic areas. Endemic syphilis, also known as *bejel*, is caused by *T. pallidum* II, a spirochete that is morphologically and serologically indistinguishable from the *T. pallidum* that causes syphilis. Bejel is endemic in many arid countries, mostly in the Middle East and Africa.[38]

Clinical Manifestations

The onset of bejel usually occurs in childhood and typically presents with a mucous patch on the buccal mucosa. Mucosal lesions are followed by papulosquamous and erosive papular lesions of the trunk and extremities. Latency can occur if the early stages of the disease are not treated. Periostitis of the bones of the legs and gummatous lesions of the nose and soft palate are seen in later stages. Neurologic and cardiovascular involvement and congenital transmission of endemic syphilis are uncharacteristic. Similarly, chancres, which are typical of primary syphilis, are not found as early signs of endemic syphilis.

Ocular Manifestations

Although neurologic involvement is uncharacteristic of endemic syphilis, ocular manifestations have been reported. Tabbara and colleagues[39] studied 17 patients with clinical and serologic findings that were consistent with endemic syphilis who also had ocular complaints. Ocular findings included uveitis in nine patients, optic atrophy in six, and chorioretinal scars in six. Additional findings are presented in **Table 10-5**.

Diagnosis

Serologic tests do not distinguish endemic syphilis from venereal syphilis. Both the VDRL and FTA-ABS results are typically positive in endemic syphilis, and spirochetes can be isolated from skin lesions. Differentiation of venereal and nonvenereal syphilis is therefore made on clinical grounds.

Table 10-5 Ocular manifestations of endemic syphilis

Anterior uveitis
Iris atrophy
Cataract
Vitreous opacity
Optic atrophy
Choroiditis
Chorioretinitis
Attenuated retinal arterioles
Patchy choroidal atrophy

Prognosis

Most patients with bejel respond well to antibiotic therapy. The prognosis of untreated bejel is unknown. Patients can experience neurologic or cardiovascular sequelae late in the course of their disease; however, symptoms are usually mild in comparison with those of tertiary syphilis.

Treatment

Patients with early lesions are treated with one dose of penicillin G benzathine, 1.2 million units, given intramuscularly. Treatment of all household members and other close personal contacts is recommended. Patients with late manifestations of endemic syphilis are treated with two doses of penicillin separated by 7 days. After treatment most patients become seronegative, and they should be monitored for this development.

Yaws and pinta

Yaws, also called *frambesia*, is a nonvenereal treponematosis that is endemic in humid countries near the equator.[40] After an incubation period of 3–4 weeks, the first manifestation of the disease is a skin papule, often on the lower extremities. The lesion enlarges, ulcerates, and becomes crusted, often with regional lymphadenitis. A secondary, generalized rash occurs as the initial lesion heals. Soft granulomas then erupt on the face, legs, and buttocks, often at mucocutaneous junctions. Hyperkeratotic lesions also develop and may occur on the soles of the feet. Later in the course of the disease, periostitis, exostoses of the maxillary bone, juxta-articular nodules, and gummatous skin lesions may appear.

Pinta is the third nonvenereal treponematosis and is endemic among the Native Americans of Mexico, Central America, and South America. Similar to yaws, pinta begins as a small papule at the inoculation site, with regional lymphadenitis followed by a generalized maculopapular eruption. One to several years after healing of the initial skin lesion, large blue or brown macules are found over the extremities, face, and neck. They later become depigmented and may be misdiagnosed as vitiligo. Again, as in yaws, hyperkeratotic lesions are found on the soles of the feet.

Ocular Manifestations

Smith and coworkers[41] headed a cooperative study to determine whether neuro-ophthalmic involvement occurs in late yaws or pinta. A group of 71 patients with late yaws, 11 with late pinta, and 41 matched, positive, and negative control subjects were examined. Ocular and neurologic abnormalities were not found in patients with late pinta, although one had a bilateral interstitial keratitis. Nevertheless, several patients with late yaws had neuro-ophthalmic abnormalities, including light-near dissociation of the pupillary response, perivascular pigmentation, sheathing of the retinal vessels, and moderate optic atrophy. Central nervous system involvement in yaws is also supported by the isolation of treponemes from aqueous humor as well as CSF abnormalities in 24.9% of 902 patients.[42]

Diagnosis

As in endemic syphilis, spirochetes may be isolated from skin lesions at the site of inoculation. Two weeks after inoculation, both the VDRL and FTA-ABS test results are positive, and the diagnosis of yaws and pinta is based on clinical findings in the setting of positive syphilis serologic findings.

Prognosis

Yaws may undergo spontaneous clinical and serologic resolution at any stage of the disease without therapy; however, antibiotic treatment improves the cure rate. Untreated patients may experience periarticular ulcers causing crippling contractures and osteomyelitis. Patients with untreated pinta experience depigmented patches of the skin, which may lead to social ostracization, the major consequence of pinta.

Treatment

Penicillin is the preferred drug to treat yaws and pinta. The treatment recommendations are outlined in the section on endemic syphilis.

Borrelia infection

Lyme disease

Etiology and Epidemiology

In the spring and summer of 1975, a group of children living in Lyme, Connecticut, presented with an inflammatory arthropathy similar to that in juvenile rheumatoid arthritis.[43] A characteristic rash was associated with the illness, as were neurologic and cardiac abnormalities. In 1977 Steere and others[43] labeled this illness Lyme disease. Epidemiologic studies implicated ticks as the vector for the disease, but the etiologic agent remained elusive.

Similar rashes called erythema migrans or erythema chronicum migrans had been associated with tick bites and systemic disease in Europe, and spirochete-like structures had been found in skin specimens from several patients.[44] In the United States, evidence was accumulating that patients with Lyme disease who were treated with penicillin fared better than untreated patients. A tick-borne organism was suspected as the causative agent, and in 1982, Burgdorfer and coworkers[45] found spirochetes in *Ixodes dammini* ticks while looking for the cause of Rocky Mountain Spotted Fever in their Montana laboratory. Spirochetes were later isolated from patients with Lyme disease in the United States, as well as from patients in Europe with erythema migrans and Bannwarth's syndrome (a chronic lymphocytic meningitis associated with erythema chronicum migrans).[46] The previously unrecognized spirochete was isolated by Burgdorfer and Barbour[47] and was named *Borrelia burgdorferi*.

Along with *Leptospira* and *Treponema*, *Borrelia* belongs to the eubacterial phylum of spirochetes.[48] These organisms are usually more loosely coiled than other spirochetes, but if coiled, they have a corkscrew appearance and look exactly like *T. pallidum*. *Borrelia* species are easy to isolate from infected ticks but difficult to isolate from infected patients. *B. burgdorferi* is transmitted by certain *Ixodes* ticks. In the United States, the preferred host for the larval and nymphal forms of the tick is the white-footed mouse,[49] whereas the preferred host for the adult form of the tick is the white-tailed deer.[50] The ticks have now been found on at least 30 species of animal and 49 species of bird.[51] Lyme disease also occurs in domestic animals, including cats, dogs, and horses. *Ixodes* ticks are 'multitalented' and transmit babesiosis and tularemia in addition to Lyme disease.

From 1980 to 1988, 13 795 cases of Lyme disease were reported in the United States.[52] During 1992–2006 a total of 248 074 cases of Lyme disease were reported in the 50 states, the District of Columbia, and US territories.[53] The annual count increased 101% from 9908 cases in 1992 to 19 931 cases in 2006. Most of the cases were reported from 10 states (Connecticut, Delaware, Massachusetts, Maryland, Minnesota, New Jersey, New York, Pennsylvania, Rhode Island, and Wisconsin).[53] Lyme disease is thought to be the most common vector-borne infection in the US, and it has been reported throughout the world, especially North America, Europe, and Asia. The rapid spread of the disease has been attributed to an increase in forested areas that house the tick-infested deer and to the migration of susceptible residents into these areas. For example, during a 7-year period 35% of 190 residents living adjacent to a nature preserve in Ipswich, Massachusetts, acquired Lyme disease.[54] The number of cases continues to grow as awareness of the disease by both physicians and patients increases.

Clinical Manifestations

Lyme disease is usually described as occurring in stages (**Box 10-3**). Early infection is divided into stage 1 (local) and stage 2 (disseminated). Late infection is categorized as stage 3 (persistent). After infection, the spirochete spreads locally in the skin in 60–80% of patients and causes the characteristic rash, erythema migrans,[51,55] which is an oval or anular erythematous lesion with expanding borders that usually fades within 3–4 weeks in untreated patients but may recur later in the disease (**Fig. 10-5**). Patients recall being bitten by a tick about half of the time. Specific antibody to *B. burgdorferi* is often lacking at this stage of the disease, during which patients may have minor flu-like constitutional symptoms and regional lymphadenopathy. The most common ocular finding in early Lyme disease is conjunctivitis.[55]

Stage 2 disease occurs within days to weeks after infection, during which time the spirochete can spread to many organs via the blood, causing a multitude of signs and symptoms. These systemic manifestations are mainly characterized by cardiac and neurologic involvement, although patients may experience secondary anular skin lesions. Neurologically, patients have severe headache and mild stiffness of the neck. The CSF is normal early on in the disease but later reveals a lymphocytic pleocytosis with a cell count in the range of $100/mm^3$, elevated protein concentration, and normal glucose concentration.[56] Peripheral neuropathies, intermittent arthralgia, and musculoskeletal pain are common, and unilateral and bilateral Bell's palsy is the most common cranial neuropathy.[57]

Box 10-3 Lyme disease – key features

- Caused by the spirochete *Borrelia burgdorferi*
- Transmitted in the *Ixodes dammini* tick
- Disease is divided into stages. Early infection is divided into stage 1 (local) and stage 2 (disseminated). Late infection is categorized as stage 3 (persistent)
- After infection the spirochete spreads locally in the skin in 60–80% of patients, causing the characteristic erythema migrans rash
- Conjunctivitis is the most common ocular finding in early Lyme disease

---

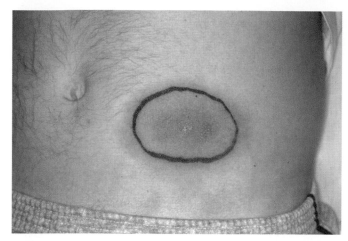

Figure 10-5. Characteristic lesions of erythema migrans associated with Lyme disease.

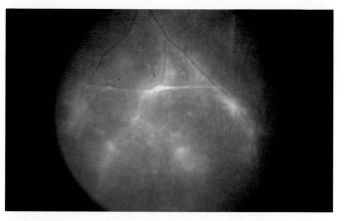

Figure 10-6. Retinal vasculitis in a patient with ocular Lyme disease. Sheathing of peripheral retinal vessels and mild vitritis are seen in this patient on this fluorescein angiogram. The patient also had a scleritis. The ocular findings resolved after treatment with intravenous ceftriaxone.

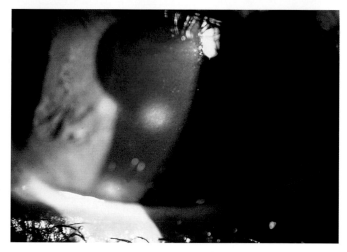

Figure 10-7. Multiple intrastromal lesions of Lyme keratitis. (*Courtesy of Ernest Kornmehl, M.D., From Albert & Jacobiec, Principles and Practices of Opthalmology, Copyright Elsevier.*)

From 4% to 8% of patients have cardiac involvement with fluctuating atrioventricular block.[58] Fewer patients have been reported with acute myopericarditis. About 6 months after infection patients can acquire oligoarticular arthritis with a white blood cell count in joint fluid of 500–110 000/mm³. Other manifestations of stage 2 Lyme disease include hepatitis, nonproductive cough, microscopic hematuria or proteinuria, and orchitis.[51] The ocular findings most commonly reported in stage 2 disease are conjunctivitis and uveitis.

Stage 3 infection is characterized by prolonged episodes of arthritis. Chronic neurologic manifestations include ataxia, chronic encephalomyelitis, spastic paraparesis, and dementia. Patients often have chronic fatigue, and erythema migrans can occur late in the disease. Bilateral keratitis is described as a characteristic finding in late infection.[57-61]

Transplacental transmission of *B. burgdorferi* has been reported in two infants whose mothers had Lyme disease in the first trimester of pregnancy,[62-64] although a study of 463 infants from endemic or nonendemic areas showed no association between congenital malformations and the presence of detectable antibody to *B. burgdorferi* in cord blood.[65]

Ocular Manifestations

In initial reports, the only consistently reported ocular finding in Lyme disease was transient conjunctivitis, occurring in 11% of persons with stage 1 disease.[55] Other ocular findings reported in the early stages of disease include episcleritis, iridocyclitis with posterior synechiae, and retinal vasculitis (**Fig. 10-6**).[66,67] Steere and associates[68] reported on a case of a 45-year-old woman who, 4 weeks after the onset of erythema migrans, experienced unilateral iritis followed by panophthalmitis; spirochetes were found in specimens of vitreous debris obtained at surgery.

In March 1987, Bertuch and associates[59] reported on three patients with ocular findings of Lyme disease. The first patient presented with bilateral Bell's palsy and late-occurring optic neuritis. The other two patients experienced patchy intrastromal infiltrates of the cornea from Bowman's layer to Descemet's membrane. These corneal infiltrates caused reduced vision but no pain, and occurred late in the course of disease. Dramatic resolution of the keratitis occurred after treatment with topical corticosteroids, suggesting an immune mechanism rather than a direct infection

with the spirochete. Baum and associates[60] reported three patients who acquired bilateral keratitis long after Lyme disease was diagnosed and treated, and also noted the effectiveness of topical corticosteroid therapy. Since then, several other papers have documented keratitis late in the course of Lyme disease (**Fig. 10-7**).[61,66,67,69-72]

Less common ocular findings associated with Lyme disease have also been reported in single case reports. Bialasiewicz and associates[73] described a patient with meningeal symptoms and diffuse choroiditis, cystoid macular edema, and exudative retinal detachments initially misdiagnosed as Vogt–Koyanagi–Harada disease. Immunofluorescence results for Lyme disease were positive, and the patient improved markedly after treatment with doxycycline. Koch and associates[74] reported retinal pigment epithelial detachments in a man with neuroborreliosis. Scholes and Teske[75] tested 19 patients with intermediate uveitis for Lyme disease, and seven of 19 patients had positive antibody titers, suggesting a possible association between Lyme disease and pars planitis. Copeland and associates[76] reported on two patients with intermediate uveitis that was only partially responsive to steroids who were later diagnosed with Lyme disease after positive Lyme titers were obtained. The uveitis

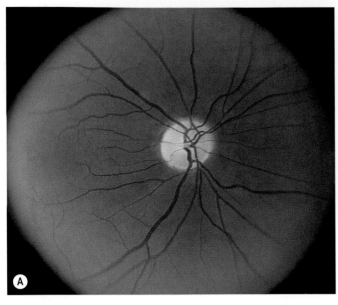 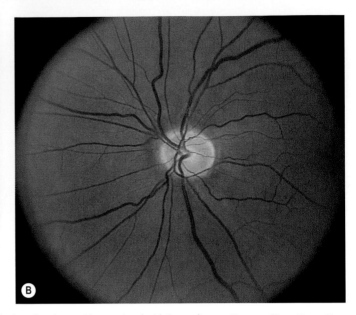

Figure 10-8. A, Right and **B,** left optic nerve demonstrating pallor after resolution of optic neuritis associated with Lyme disease. *(Courtesy of Ernest Kornmehl, M.D., From Albert & Jacobiec, Principles and Practices of Opthalmology, Copyright Elsevier.)*

in both patients cleared rapidly with systemic antibiotic treatment. In a report by Winward and colleagues,[77] patients with intermediate uveitis associated with Lyme disease demonstrated more significant anterior segment inflammation. Subsequent studies confirmed the presence of significant posterior segment inflammation, especially vitritis and retinal vasculitis, in some cases of Lyme disease.[71,72,78,79]

Neuro-ophthalmic findings in Lyme disease are common.[44,80] Involvement of the CNS by Lyme disease causes cranial nerve palsies. Unilateral and bilateral Bell's palsies are the most common cranial nerve palsies and often result in exposure keratitis. Diplopia due to sixth, fourth, and third cranial nerve palsies can occur. Wu and associates[81] described a 7-year-old child who had bilateral disc edema in association with Lyme disease. A similar patient was described by Jacobson and Frens[82] and was diagnosed with a pseudotumor cerebri syndrome associated with Lyme disease. Optic disc edema may be the sole presenting sign of Lyme disease.[83] Other reported neuro-ophthalmic manifestations of Lyme disease include optic neuritis (**Fig. 10-8**), cortical blindness, and orbital myositis.[84,85–87] The association of some of these ocular findings with Lyme disease stems from one or two case reports in which the diagnosis of Lyme disease was based predominantly on positive serologic findings. Because serologic results for Lyme disease may be falsely positive, some of the cases may have been wrongly diagnosed.[88] A list of the ophthalmic manifestations associated with Lyme disease is presented in **Table 10-6**.

Diagnosis

Techniques for the diagnosis of Lyme disease are not ideal. A patient with a history of a tick bite who later experiences erythema migrans most surely has Lyme disease; however, a tick bite is recalled in only about 50% of cases, and a pathognomonic rash may be overlooked or may not occur in a significant number of patients. Erythema migrans is the only clinical sign of clear diagnostic value; however, earlobe lymphocytoma, meningoradiculoneuritis (Garin–Bujadoux–Bannwarth syndrome), and acrodermatitis chronica atrophi-

Table 10-6 Ocular manifestations of lyme disease

EARLY INFECTION
Conjunctivitis
Episcleritis
Posterior scleritis
Iridocyclitis
Retinal vasculitis
Optic disc edema
Panophthalmitis
Choroiditis
Pars planitis
Exudative retinal detachment
Retinal pigment epithelial detachment
Exposure keratitis
Diplopia
Cortical blindness
Orbital myositis

LATE INFECTION
Keratitis
Episcleritis

cans may be of some diagnostic value.[89] Because of the difficulty of culturing *B. burgdorferi* from patients, laboratory diagnosis is made by serologic findings. Most patients have elevated antibody titers to *B. burgdorferi* several weeks after infection. Both immunofluorescent assays and enzyme-linked immunosorbent assays (ELISAs) are used in the diagnosis of Lyme disease, although the ELISA is more sensitive in all stages of the disease. Unfortunately, serologic testing has not been standardized, and interlaboratory variability is significant, although improving.[90–92] The sensitivity of the ELISA for Lyme disease in several laboratories approaches 90% after the first few weeks of infection. Many laboratories confirm positive ELISA results with Western blot assays. Nevertheless, the clinician must be aware of false-negative and false-positive results. False-negative results occur during the first few weeks of infection, when antibody titers may be low and may be missed by serologic tests of lower sensitivities. Early antibiotic therapy may also cause false-negative test results, and cases of seronegative Lyme disease have been reported.[93]

False-positive results may also occur as a result of cross-reaction between *B. burgdorferi* and other spirochetes, such as *T. pallidum*. Cross-reactivity between a Lyme immunofluorescence assay test and an FTA-ABS test is reported in 11–54% of patients.[94-96] In a study by Hunter and coworkers,[97] 22% of patients with Lyme disease had a reactive FTA-ABS test at a dilution of 1 : 5, but all of these samples were negative at a dilution of 1 : 10. Nevertheless, the rapid plasma reagin test and the microhemagglutination–*T. pallidum* test are usually negative in patients with Lyme disease.[94] False-positive results have also been reported in many autoimmune disorders, Rocky Mountain Spotted Fever, infectious mononucleosis, and neurologic disorders.[96,98-100] Importantly, in most areas of the United States the prevalence of Lyme disease is low. Even with a sensitivity and a specificity of 90%, the predictive value of a positive ELISA for Lyme disease is probably less than 20% in patients with a clinical picture atypical for the disease.

A fourfold increase in serial anti-*B. burgdorferi* IgM antibody levels in patients with a clinical history compatible with Lyme disease remains the most specific laboratory indicator, but this increase is not often documented by serial tests. Western blot analysis and PCR[101,102] are increasingly used for the diagnosis.

Recommendations for laboratory screening for Lyme disease include obtaining an ELISA using both an IgM-specific and IgG-specific antiimmunoglobulin or a polyvalent antiimmunoglobulin.[98] Persistence of the specific IgM response throughout infection is an unusual feature of the antibody response seen in some patients with Lyme disease, and may be secondary to an impairment in the helper T-cell function needed to switch from IgM to IgG production.[103] All positive or equivocal results by ELISA should be confirmed by Western blotting.[104,105] Because the clinical appearances of Lyme disease and syphilis are similar, a rapid plasma reagin test and an FTA-ABS test should be performed on all patients tested for Lyme disease, and infectious mononucleosis should also be considered as a possible cause of false-positive results. Finally, the importance of pursuing a history of tick bites, residence in or travel to areas with endemic Lyme disease, rash, chronic joint complaints, or facial nerve palsy cannot be overemphasized.

The literature is now replete with articles stressing the overdiagnosis of Lyme disease.[104-106] In cases of ocular inflammation without a clinical history of tick bite, characteristic rash, arthritis, or neurologic complaints, the likelihood is extremely low that Lyme disease is the cause of the inflammation. In such cases, serologic testing is probably not indicated.[107,108] Cases of uveitis in endemic areas with suspicious nonocular symptoms should be evaluated with ELISA. As mentioned earlier, positive ELISA results should be confirmed with Western blotting, and in certain cases ocular samples may be obtained for PCR, cytologic study, or culture.[109,110] More recently, PCR has been used to help diagnose ocular Lyme disease.[110a]

Prognosis

From 10% to 40% of patients with untreated erythema chronicum migrans progress to stage 2 Lyme disease; 3–10%

Table 10-7 Treatment of lyme disease

EARLY INFECTION

Adults

Doxycycline 100 mg PO bid × 14–21 days *OR*
Amoxicillin 500 mg PO tid × 14–21 days
If penicillin allergic use cefuroxime axetil 500 mg PO bid

Children

Amoxicillin 50 mg/kg/day divided into three doses (maximum 500 mg/dose)

SEVERE UVEITIS OR NEUROLOGIC ABNORMALITIES OR ARTHRITIS

Ceftriaxone 2 g/day IV × 14–21 days

of patients experience chronic arthritis, acrodermatitis chronica atrophicans, or neurologic disease. Once it occurs, arthritis does not always respond to antibiotic therapy. Similarly, it is not known whether neurologic involvement is prevented by oral antibiotic therapy for early Lyme disease.

Treatment

Recommendations for the treatment of Lyme disease were reviewed by the Infectious Diseases Society of America[104] and can be found in **Table 10-7**. Patients with mild ocular disease may respond well to oral antibiotics, but in cases of more severe ocular manifestations, such as posterior uveitis, intravenous antibiotic therapy with ceftriaxone is probably the treatment of choice, if prolonged treatment is required. Some data suggest that prior treatment with corticosteroids may predispose the patient to antibiotic failure; therefore, the use of topical corticosteroids should be limited to patients with anterior segment inflammation who are also being treated with antibiotics.[77,111] Topical corticosteroids are also used to treat Lyme keratitis.[60] If the suspicion for Lyme disease is high a therapeutic trial of antibiotics seems warranted, even in seronegative patients. Finally, chemoprophylaxis and vaccine development continue to be pursued despite early disappointments.[89]

Relapsing fever

Etiology and Epidemiology

Relapsing fever is an acute infectious disease caused by spirochetes of the genus *Borrelia* and characterized by recurrent bouts of fever separated by relatively asymptomatic periods.[112,113] Relapsing fever is divided into two epidemiologic types: epidemic, or louse-borne, and endemic, or tick-borne (**Box 10-4**). Epidemic relapsing fever is transmitted from person to person by the human body louse *Pediculus humanus*, which has previously ingested blood infected with *Borrelia recurrentis*.[114] Infection occurs when the hemolymph from infected body lice contaminates abraded or even normal skin, usually from scratching, when lice are crushed and come into contact with previously excoriated bites. The epidemic form of relapsing fever is found in parts of Africa, South America, and China where crowding, poor sanitation, and famine foster louse infestation.[112]

Endemic relapsing fever was first documented in the United States in 1915 after five persons contracted the disease in Bear Creek Canyon, Colorado.[115] This form of the disease is caused by at least 15 species of *Borrelia*, and the tick vectors have now been identified as several species of the genus *Ornithodorus* with a rodent reservoir.[112,116]

Box 10-4 Relapsing fever – key features

- Caused by spirochetes of the genus *Borrelia*
- Two epidemiologic types: epidemic (louse-borne) and endemic (tick-borne)
- Characterized by recurrent bouts of fever separated by relatively asymptomatic periods
- Eye pain, blurred vision, and photophobia are often seen with disease onset
- Diagnosis is usually based on finding *Borrelia* on thick smear of blood during a febrile episode
- Mortality reported in 2–5% of treated patients and up to 40% of untreated patients

Table 10-8 Ocular manifestations of relapsing fever

Conjunctivitis
Subconjunctival and retinal hemorrhages
Iridocyclitis (usually after several relapses of the disease)
Vitritis
Ptosis (secondary to facial nerve paralysis)
Mydriasis
Optic neuritis
Retinal venous occlusion

Transmission to humans occurs when infected saliva from the tick contaminates the site of the bite. In the United States, tick-borne relapsing fever occurs mostly in western states, usually between May and September.[117]

Clinical Manifestations

After inoculation, the spirochetes multiply in the blood and invade most tissues of the body. Onset of the disease occurs 3–12 days after infection and is marked by fever (temperature up to 39–40°C), chills, severe headache,[113] and commonly eye pain, blurred vision, and photophobia. Other symptoms include myalgias and joint pain, meningismus, anorexia, abdominal pain, nonproductive cough, and neurologic symptoms, including facial paralysis and altered mental status. Hepatosplenomegaly, jaundice, myocarditis, and heart failure sometimes occur late in the disease. The course of louse-borne relapsing fever tends to be more severe than that of tick-borne relapsing fever. Bleeding is common in both forms of the disease and often manifests as purpura, petechiae, or epistaxis.[118] Subconjunctival and retinal hemorrhages have been described. In more severe cases of relapsing fever, gastrointestinal or cerebral hemorrhage and disseminated intravascular coagulation may result in death.

The initial attack of relapsing fever lasts 3–6 days and is followed by an afebrile period of 6–9 days. Defervescence may be accompanied by hypotension. Relapses tend to become shorter and less severe as the disease progresses. Mortality in relapsing fever ranges between 2 and 5% in treated cases and as high as 40% in untreated cases.[113]

Eye pain and photophobia are common, and conjunctivitis and iridocyclitis have both been reported in approximately 15% of cases of relapsing fever, usually after several relapses.[119] Cases of more severe uveitis with vitritis have been reported, but they apparently respond well to therapy.[120] Neuro-ophthalmic manifestations of relapsing fever are mostly limited to ptosis caused by paralysis of the facial nerve, but pupillary dilatation and optic neuritis have also been documented. Retinal venous occlusion with retinal hemorrhage and exudate has been documented in one case.[112]

Ocular Manifestations

The ocular manifestations of relapsing fever are listed in **Table 10-8**.

Diagnosis

Definitive diagnosis of relapsing fever is based on the presence of *Borrelia* on a thick smear of peripheral blood obtained during a febrile episode. *Borrelia* species are best seen with Giemsa's or Wright's stain.[113] Repeated smears or use of an acridine orange fluorescent stain increases the sensitivity of the smears.[113,121] If direct methods of diagnosis fail, blood from the patient may be injected into mice or rats, and the blood from these animals may then be examined for spirochetes.

Immunofluorescence assays and ELISAs are being developed, but serologic findings are not yet useful in diagnosing relapsing fever.[115] The description of a specific antigen may facilitate the serologic detection of *Borrelia* responsible for relapsing fever, in contrast to the *B. burgdorferi* of Lyme disease.[122] Nonspecific laboratory abnormalities include anemia, elevated erythrocyte sedimentation rate, platelet count <150 000/mm³, and prolonged bleeding time. Serologic results for syphilis may be positive in as many as 10% of patients tested. In patients with CNS involvement, analysis of the CSF usually reveals a pleocytosis with an elevated protein concentration but a normal glucose level.[113]

Prognosis

Ninety-five percent of patients with relapsing fever recover with therapy, but if untreated, louse-borne relapsing fever is often fatal. Rare complications include respiratory disease, nephritis, endocarditis, neurologic disease, and bleeding diatheses. Uveitis may lead to permanent visual disability.

Treatment

The treatment of choice for tick-borne relapsing fever in adults is tetracycline, 500 mg orally, every 6 hours for 7–10 days. Penicillin, erythromycin, and chloramphenicol are also effective. In louse-borne relapsing fever the treatment of choice in adults is one 500 mg dose of erythromycin, given orally or intravenously. Ceftriaxone is effective against *Borrelia* species and may be used intravenously to treat relapsing fever. Vancomycin may or may not be of value because of the possible persistence of organisms in the CNS.[123] Therapy should be given during the early part of a febrile episode to diminish the possibility of a Jarisch–Herxheimer reaction,[124] which is caused by the release of a nonendotoxin pyrogen as *Borrelia* species are killed, and is characterized by rigors, fever, and elevated blood pressure, followed by hypotension and possible shock.

Leptospirosis

Etiology and Epidemiology

Leptospirosis is a zoonosis caused by spirochetes of the genus *Leptospira* whose natural reservoir is wild animals, mostly rodents. Weil[125] first recognized a severe form of leptospirosis as a distinct clinical entity in 1886, and the spirochetal cause of Weil's disease was discovered by Inada and coworkers in 1915.[126] Leptospirosis can affect domestic animals, including livestock and dogs. Humans are an accidental host, acquiring the disease through contact with infected urine, tissues, or water. The spirochetes invade humans through abraded skin, mucous membranes, or the conjunctiva, although penetration through intact skin occasionally occurs. The disease is often occupational, occurring in farmers, veterinarians, and abattoir workers.[127,128] Most cases of leptospirosis in the United States are acquired during water sports and occur predominantly in young adult men in the late summer and early fall.[126,128] Although the exact incidence remains unknown, since 1970 physicians have reported 40–120 cases annually to the Centers for Disease Control and Prevention.[129] However, these figures are probably an underestimate: active surveillance programs report a fivefold increase in the incidence of leptospirosis.[130]

Two hundred and seven different leptospiral serovars have been identified, with pathologic leptospires belonging to the species *Leptospira interrogans*.[127] Only 40–120 cases of leptospirosis are reported annually, but because the signs and symptoms of the disease are not distinct, many cases go undiagnosed. Once inside the host, leptospires enter the bloodstream, can penetrate tissues, and are found in almost all organs within 24 hours. The mechanism by which leptospires cause tissue damage is not entirely clear; however, serovar-specific lipopolysaccharide has been identified in the aqueous humor of patients with leptospiral uveitis, suggesting a causative role for endotoxin in this disease.[130a]

Clinical Manifestations

The incubation period for leptospirosis ranges from 2 to 26 days, with the usual period extending from 7 to 13 days. The disease is often biphasic; the first or leptospiremic phase is abrupt in onset and characterized by severe frontal, bitemporal, or retro-orbital headaches; fever and chills; and severe muscle aches (**Box 10-5**). Conjunctival suffusion is a characteristic finding that usually appears on the third or fourth day of the disease, but is frequently overlooked.[131,132] Hepatosplenomegaly and jaundice are uncommon in the first stage, but occur later in the course of more severe forms of the disease. The leptospiremic phase lasts from 4 to 9 days, with recurrent fever spikes exceeding a temperature of 39°C.

For 8–10 days after infection leptospires can be isolated from blood and CSF, but disappear as defervescence takes place and the patient enters the second or immune phase of the disease. The immune phase of leptospirosis begins on the 6th to the 12th day of the illness and corresponds to the time when antibodies appear in the serum. The clinical course of the immune phase is variable, and some patients experience few symptoms. However, high fever and meningismus may occur in half of patients, and examination of CSF after the 7th day after infection reveals pleocytosis in 50%, often with a mildly elevated protein level. Other manifestations of the disease include encephalitis; optic neuritis; cranial nerve paresis involving the sixth, seventh, and eighth cranial nerves; and peripheral neuropathies. Spontaneous abortion may result from leptospirosis acquired during pregnancy.

Ocular Manifestations

The ocular manifestations of leptospirosis are listed in **Table 10-9**. Ocular findings have been reported in 3–92% of patients,[133] bulbar and palpebral conjunctival hyperemia with engorged conjunctival and episcleral vessels being the most common and characteristic. This hyperemia usually occurs without discomfort, lacrimation, or discharge; however, if ocular discharge is present, it can harbor leptospires and can be a source of further infection.[134] In an outbreak of leptospirosis among 74 athletes participating in triathlons, 43% reported eye pain, and 26% had red eyes.[135] Uveitis is a common finding in leptospirosis. In a series of 73 patients with uveitis associated with leptospirosis, panuveitis was seen in 106 eyes (95.5%), retinal periphlebitis in 57 (51.4%), and hypopyon in 14 (12.6%).[136]

Interestingly, leptospirosis may be an important cause of recurrent uveitis in horses and is a leading cause of blindness in these animals. During a 7-year period, horses seropositive for leptospirosis were 13.2 times more likely to have uveitis than were seronegative animals.[137] A study from India reported leptospiral antibodies in 15 of 15 patients with acute panuveitis and retinal vasculitis during a post-monsoon period.[138] Panuveitis with papillitis has been reported in a case of leptospirosis.[139]

Weil's disease

A severe form of leptospirosis, Weil's disease, occurs with jaundice, azotemia, hemorrhages, anemia, persistent fever, and altered mental status. Renal and hepatocellular dysfunction usually occurs on the 3rd to 6th day after infection. Mortality from leptospirosis occurs only in patients with jaundice and approaches 15% in younger patients and 30% in patients over 60 years of age.

In Weil's disease with hepatic involvement scleral icterus is present, and in patients with severe disease subconjunctival and retinal hemorrhages may occur. Less commonly, during the immune phase of the disease with CNS involvement, patients may acquire palpebral herpes, optic neuritis,

---

Box 10-5 Leptospirosis – key features

- Caused by spirochetes of the genus Leptospira
- Natural reservoir is wild animals, mostly rodents
- Humans acquire disease through contact with infected urine, tissues, or water
- Disease is divided into two phases: leptospiremic and immune
- Ocular findings occur in 3–92% of patients. Conjunctival suffusion is the characteristic finding in the leptospiremic phase. Retinal findings are common in the immune phase

---

Table 10-9 Ocular manifestations of leptospirosis

LEPTOSPIREMIC PHASE
Conjunctival suffusion

IMMUNE PHASE
Iridocyclitis
Optic neuritis
Facial nerve palsy
Palpebral herpes
Posterior uveitis (with retinal exudates)
Scleral icterus
Subconjunctival hemorrhages
Retinal hemorrhages

and facial nerve paresis. Between 10% and 44% of patients with leptospirosis experience uveitis,[140] which is typically an acute, often bilateral, iridocyclitis with fine keratic precipitates, posterior synechiae, occasional vitreous opacities, and rarely retinal exudates. Patients often have blurred vision and mild ocular irritation, but respond well to treatment with mydriatics and topical steroids. More severe cases of uveitis have been reported and may occur long after the disease has appeared to subside. Barkay and Garzozi[132] reported on 16 patients with predominantly anterior uveitis secondary to leptospirosis with positive serologic results. Leptospirosis should be considered as a possible cause of uveitis of unknown cause, especially in patients with occupational or recreational risk factors for the disease.

Diagnosis

The white blood cell count is normal to slightly elevated in most cases of leptospirosis; values >15 000 cells/mm³ suggest the presence of hepatic disease. Differential counts usually reveal >70% neutrophils, a finding that may differentiate leptospirosis from viral infection. In patients with liver involvement, intravascular hemolysis may cause anemia and elevated serum bilirubin levels.

A definitive diagnosis of leptospirosis requires isolation of the spirochete from a clinical specimen, usually blood or CSF, or seroconversion (a fourfold or greater rise in antibody titer) in the presence of clinical illness. The organism is present in blood and CSF for only 8–10 days after infection, and the spirochete quickly disappears as antibodies appear in the serum. The leptospires can be identified by darkfield examination, but this technique requires expertise. Leptospiruria occurs during the immune phase, although leptospires are easily confused with cellular debris in urine sediment. Tissue samples may also be examined, but tissue analysis for leptospires is predominantly limited to postmortem examination. Detection of leptospira DNA by PCR in the aqueous humor of a patient with uveitis has been reported.[141]

In practice, laboratory diagnosis of leptospirosis is usually made serologically. The macroscopic slide agglutination test uses a boiled suspension of leptospires and is used mostly as a screening test. The microscopic agglutination test uses live or formalin-treated antigens, is more specific, and can be used to determine both antibody titer and serotype. Sensitive and specific complement fixation tests and ELISAs for the detection of IgM antibody against leptospiral antigens have been developed. They are both inexpensive and easy to use and are playing an increasing role in the diagnosis of leptospirosis. Agglutinins appear on the 6th to 12th day of illness, and the maximum titer is reached during the 3rd and 4th weeks. Early treatment with antibiotics may delay or suppress development of the antibody response, but if initial serologic test results are negative the tests should be repeated 2 weeks later.

Prognosis

Patients with anicteric leptospirosis usually recover uneventfully within 2–6 weeks, although convalescence may extend up to 1 month. Death occurs in 5–30% of untreated patients and is usually attributable to acute renal failure. Uveitis occurs in 10% of patients from 2 weeks to 1 year after initial infection, but the prognosis for these patients is generally good.

Table 10-10 Treatment of leptospirosis

MILD INFECTION
Doxycycline 100 mg PO bid × 7 days *OR*
Amoxicillin 500 mg PO q6h × 7 days *OR*
Ampicillin 500–750 mg PO q6h × 7 days

MODERATE TO SEVERE INFECTION
Penicillin G 1.5 million units IV q6h × 10 days *OR*
Ampicillin 0.5–1g IV q6h × 10 days *OR*
Ceftriaxone 1g IV qd × 10 days

SEVERE UVEITIS OR NEUROLOGIC ABNORMALITIES OR ARTHRITIS
Ceftriaxone 2 g/day IV × 14–21 days

Treatment

Recommendations for the treatment of leptospirosis can be found in **Table 10-10**. Chemotherapeutic trials were conducted during outbreaks of leptospirosis in military personnel training in Panama. Doxycycline, 200 mg orally once a week and at the end of training, prevented infection.[142] Antibiotics have been shown to reduce disease complications if they are given by the fourth day of infection; however, administration is still recommended for severe infections, even if diagnosis is made after 4 days after infection.

In severe cases of leptospirosis, recommended therapy is penicillin G, 1.5 million units, or ampicillin, 500–1000 mg, administered intravenously every 6 hours for 10 days. Intravenous ceftriaxone has also been used to treat severe leptospirosis. Less severe cases may be treated with a 7-day course of doxycycline, 100 mg orally twice a day; ampicillin, 500–750 mg orally every 6 hours; or amoxicillin, 500 mg orally every 6 hours.[143,144] Supportive therapy is given for renal failure, hypotension, and hemorrhage.

Prevention of leptospirosis centers on the elimination of large animal reservoirs of disease, including livestock and pets. In fact, cattle-associated leptospirosis is a problem in the British Isles, and at least 4% of all British dairy farmers are at risk for infection.[128]

The ophthalmologist must be diligent in pursuing the clinical history for evidence of previous or persistent low-grade infection that is suggestive of leptospirosis when evaluating patients with a uveitis of unknown cause, especially in dairy farmers. Because many cases are unrecognized, it is not possible to state definitively how many cases of uveitis are secondary to leptospirosis; however, one report indicated that only 17% of 483 proven cases of leptospirosis were initially diagnosed correctly.[145] In an editorial, Watt[146] suggested that a history of water or animal contact in a patient with severe myalgias and conjunctival suffusion suggests the presence of leptospirosis, particularly in someone returning from travel in Asia or Latin America. The ophthalmologist can confirm the diagnosis by sending a serum sample to a reference laboratory for the microscopic agglutination test or for an ELISA for leptospirosis.

Case 10-1

A 59-year-old HIV-positive white man developed a sudden decrease in vision in both eyes. Visual acuity was 20/400 OU. Examination revealed bilateral hypopyons (see **Fig. 10-9**), dense

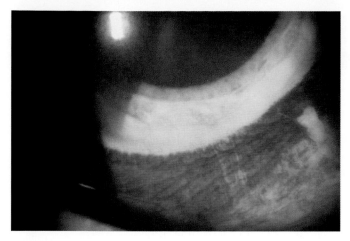

vitritis, and patchy areas of retinal infiltrates in both eyes (see Fig. 10-2A). The patient was referred to the National Institutes of Health with a presumed diagnosis of cytomegalovirus retinitis. Laboratory evaluation at the National Institutes of Health revealed positive VDRL and FTA-ABS test results. A diagnosis of syphilis was made, and the patient was treated with intravenous penicillin G. Within 2 weeks visual acuity improved to 20/40 OU. The retinal infiltrates also resolved, and the patient was left with a pigmentary retinopathy characteristic of resolved syphilitic retinitis (see Fig. 10-2B).

Figure 10-9. Hypopyon uveitis in a patient with syphilis (see Case 10-1).

References

1. Schaudin FR, Hoffman E. Vorlüfger Berichtüber das Vorkommen von Spirochaeten in syphilitschen Krankheitsproducten und bei Papillomen. Arb Gesundheitsamte 1905; 22: 527.
2. Mahoney JF, Arnold RC, Harris A. Penicillin treatment of syphilis: A preliminary report. J Vener Dis Inform 1943; 24: 355–357.
3. Continuing increase in infectious syphilis – United States. MMWR Morb Mortal Wkly Rep 1988; 37: 35–38.
4. Congenital syphilis – New York City, 1986–1988. MMWR Morb Mortal Wkly Rep 1989; 38: 825–829.
5. Primary and secondary syphilis – United States, 2003–2004. MMWR Morb Mortal Wkly Rep 2005; 55: 269–273.
6. Berry CD, Hooton TM, Collier AC, et al. Neurologic relapse after benzathine penicillin therapy for secondary syphilis in a patient with HIV infection. N Engl J Med 1987; 316: 1587–1589.
7. Johns DR, Tierney M, Felsenstein D. Alteration in the natural history of neurosyphilis by concurrent infection with the human immunodeficiency virus. N Engl J Med 1987; 316: 1569–1572.
8. Sparling PF. Natural history of syphilis. In: Holmes KK, Per-Anders M, Sparling PF, Wiesner PJ, eds. Sexually transmitted diseases. New York: McGraw-Hill, 1990, p 214.
9. Chapel TA. The variability of syphilitic chancres. Sex Transm Dis 1978; 5: 68–70.
10. Pulido JS, Corbett JJ, McLeish WM. Syphilis. In: Gold DH, Weingeist TA, eds. The Eye and Systemic Disease. Philadelphia, JB Lippincott, 1990, p 234.
11. Tramont EC. Syphilis in adults: From Christopher Columbus to Sir Alexander Fleming to AIDS. Clin Infect Dis 1995; 21: 1361–1371.
12. Chapel TA. The signs and symptoms of secondary syphilis. Sex Transm Dis 1980; 7: 161–164.
13. Woods AC. Syphilis of the eye. Am J Syph Gonorrhea Vener Dis 1943; 27: 133–186.
14. Wilhelmus KR. Syphilis. In: Insler MS, ed. AIDS and Other Sexually Transmitted Diseases and the Eye. Orlando, FL, Grune & Stratton, 1987, pp 73–104.
15. Lukehart SA, Hook EW, Baker-Zander SA, et al. Invasion of the central nervous system by *Treponema pallidum*: Implications for diagnosis and treatment. Ann Intern Med 1988; 109: 855–862.
15a. Marra CM. Update on neurosyphilis. Curr Infect Dis Rep 2009; 11: 127–134.
16. Lowenfeld IE. The Argyll Robertson pupil, 1869–1969: A critical survey of the literature. Surv Ophthalmol 1969; 14: 199–299.
17. Dorfman DH, Glaser JH. Congenital syphilis presenting in infants after the newborn period. N Engl J Med 1990; 323: 1299–1302.
18. Duke-Elder S. System of Ophthalmology, vol XIII, The Ocular Adnexa, Part II, Lacrimal, Orbital, and Paraorbital Diseases. St. Louis, CV Mosby, 1974, p 615.
19. Arruga J, Valentines J, Mauri F, et al. Neuroretinitis in acquired syphilis. Ophthalmology 1985; 92: 262–270.
20. Morgan CM, Webb RM, O'Connor GR. Atypical syphilitic chorioretinitis and vasculitis. Retina 1984; 4: 225–231.
21. Mendelsohn AD, Jampol LM. Syphilitic retinitis. A cause of necrotizing retinitis. Retina 1985; 4: 221–234.
22. Jumper JM, Machemer R, Gallemore RP, et al. Exudative retinal detachment and retinitis associated with acquired syphilitic uveitis. Retina 2000; 20: 190–194.
23. Halperin LS, Lewis H, Blumenkranz MS, et al. Choroidal neovascular membrane and other chorioretinal complications of acquired syphilis. Am J Ophthalmol 1989; 108: 554–562.
23a. Tsimpida M, Low LC, Posner E, et al. Acute syphilitic posterior placoid chorioretinitis in late latent syphilis. Int J STD AIDS 2009; 20: 207–208.
24. Tramont EC. *Treponema pallidum* (syphilis). In: Mandell GL, Bennett JE, Dolin R, eds. Mandell, Douglas and Bennett's Principles and Practice of Infectious Diseases, 6th ed. New York, Churchill Livingstone, 2005, pp 2768–2785.
24a. Syphilis testing algorithms using treponemal tests for initial screening – Four laboratories, New York City, 2005–2006. MMWR Morb Mortal Wkly Rep 2008; 57: 872–875.
25. Guidelines for the prevention and control of congenital syphilis. MMWR Morb Mortal Wkly Rep 1988; 37(Suppl 1): 1–13.
26. Riedner G, Rusizoka M, Todd J, et al. Single-dose azithromycin versus penicillin G benzathine for the treatment of early syphilis. N Engl J Med 2005; 353: 1236–1244.
27. Johns DR, Tierney M, Felsenstein D. Alterations in the natural history of neurosyphilis by concurrent infection with the human immunodeficiency virus. N Engl J Med 1987; 316: 1569–1572.
28. Tramont EC. Syphilis in the AIDS era. N Engl J Med 1987; 316: 1600–1601.
29. Stoumbos VD, Klein ML. Syphilitic retinitis in a patient with acquired immunodeficiency syndrome-related complex. Am J Ophthalmol 1987; 103: 103–104.
30. Passo MS, Rosenbaum JT. Ocular syphilis in patients with human immunodeficiency virus infection. Am J Ophthalmol 1988; 106: 1–6.

31. Levy JH, Liss RA, Maguire AM. Neurosyphilis and ocular syphilis in patients with concurrent human immunodeficiency virus infection. Retina 1989; 9: 175–180.

32. Zaidman GW. Neurosyphilis and retrobulbar neuritis in a patient with AIDS. Ann Ophthalmol 1986; 18: 260–261.

33. Markowitz DM, Beutner KR, Maggio RP, et al. Failure of recommended treatment for secondary syphilis. JAMA 1986; 255: 1767–1768.

34. Richards BW, Hessburg TJ, Nussbaum JN. Recurrent syphilitic uveitis. [Letter] N Engl J Med 1989; 320: 62.

35. Hicks CB, Benson PM, Lupton GP, et al. Seronegative secondary syphilis in a patient infected with the human immunodeficiency virus (HIV) with Kaposi sarcoma. Ann Intern Med 1987; 107: 492–495.

36. Hollander H. Cerebrospinal fluid normalities and abnormalities in individuals infected with human immunodeficiency virus. J Infect Dis 1988; 158: 855–858.

37. Recommendations for diagnosing and treating syphilis in HIV-infected patients. MMWR Morb Mortal Wkly Rep 1988; 37: 600–608.

38. Pace JL, Csonka GW. Endemic non-venereal syphilis (bejel) in Saudi Arabia. Br J Vener Dis 1984; 60: 293–297.

39. Tabbara KF, Al Kaff AS, Fadel T. Ocular manifestations of endemic syphilis (bejel). Ophthalmology 1989; 96: 1087–1091.

40. Smith JL. Neuro-ophthalmological study of late yaws: I. An introduction to yaws. Br J Vener Dis 1971; 47: 223–225.

41. Smith JL, David NJ, Indgin S, et al. Neuro-ophthalmological study of late yaws and pinta: II. The Caracas project. Br J Vener Dis 1971; 47: 226–251.

42. Roman GC, Roman LN. Occurrence of congenital, cardiovascular, visceral, neurologic, and neuro-ophthalmologic complications in late yaws: a theme for future research. Rev Infect Dis 1986; 8: 760–770.

43. Steere AC, Malawista SE, Snydman DR, et al. Lyme arthritis: An epidemic of oligoarticular arthritis in children and adults in three Connecticut communities. Arthritis Rheum 1977; 20: 7–17.

44. MacDonald AB. Lyme disease: A neuro-ophthalmologic view. J Clin Neuroophthalmol 1987; 7: 185–190.

45. Burgdorfer W, Barbour AG, Hayes SF, et al. Lyme disease: A tick-borne spirochetosis? Science 1982; 216: 1317–1319.

46. Berger BW, Kaplan MH, Rothenberg IR, et al. Isolation and characterization of the Lyme disease spirochete from the skin of patients with erythema chronicum migrans. J Am Acad Dermatol 1985; 13: 444–449.

47. Barbour AG. Isolation and cultivation of Lyme disease spirochetes. Yale J Biol Med 1984; 57: 521–525.

48. Barbour AG, Hayes SF. Biology of *Borrelia* species. Microbiol Rev 1986; 50: 381–400.

49. Levine JF, Wilson ML, Spielman A. Mice as reservoirs of the Lyme disease spirochete. Am J Trop Med Hyg 1985; 34: 355–360.

50. Wilson ML, Adler GH, Spielman A. Correlation between abundance of deer and that of the deer tick, *Ixodes dammini* (Acari: Ixodidae). Ann Entomol Soc Am 1986; 23: 172–176.

51. Steere AC. Lyme disease. N Engl J Med 1989; 321: 586–596.

52. Tsai TS, Bailey RE, Moore PS. National surveillance of Lyme disease 1987–1988. Conn Med 1986; 53: 324–326.

53. Surveillance for Lyme Disease – Unites States, 1992–2006. MMWR Morb Mortal Wkly Rep 2008; 57(SS10): 1–9.

54. Lastavica CC, Wilson ML, Berardi VP, et al. Rapid emergence of a focal epidemic of Lyme disease in coastal Massachusetts. N Engl J Med 1989; 320: 133–137.

55. Steere AC, Bartenhagen NH, Craft JE, et al. The early clinical manifestations of Lyme disease. Ann Intern Med 1983; 99: 76–82.

56. Pachner AR, Steere AC. The triad of neurologic manifestations of Lyme disease: Meningitis, cranial neuritis, and radiculoneuritis. Neurology 1985; 35: 47–53.

57. Clark JR, Carlson RD, Sasaki CT, et al. Facial paralysis in Lyme disease. Laryngoscope 1985; 95: 1341–1345.

58. Steere AC, Batsford WP, Weinberg M, et al. Lyme carditis: Cardiac abnormalities of Lyme disease. Ann Intern Med 1980; 93: 8–16.

59. Bertuch AW, Rocco E, Schwartz EG. Eye findings in Lyme disease. Conn Med 1987; 51: 151–152.

60. Baum J, Barza M, Weinstein P, et al. Bilateral keratitis as a manifestation of Lyme disease. Am J Ophthalmol 1988; 105: 75–77.

61. Orlin SE, Lauffer JL. Lyme disease keratitis. Am J Ophthalmol 1989; 107: 678–680.

62. Schlesinger PA, Duray PH, Burke BA, et al. Maternal–fetal transmission of the Lyme disease spirochete, *Borrelia burgdorferi*. Ann Intern Med 1985; 103: 67–69.

63. Weber K, Bratzke HJ, Neubert U, et al. *Borrelia burgdorferi* in a newborn despite oral penicillin for Lyme borreliosis during pregnancy. Pediatr Infect Dis J 1988; 7: 286–289.

64. Markowitz LE, Steere AC, Benach JL, et al. Lyme disease during pregnancy. JAMA 1986; 255: 3394–3396.

65. Williams CL, Benach JL, Curran AS, et al. Lyme disease during pregnancy: A cord blood serosurvey. Ann NY Acad Sci 1988; 539: 504–506.

66. Aaberg TM. The expanding ophthalmologic spectrum of Lyme disease. Am J Ophthalmol 1989; 107: 77–80.

67. Flack AJ, Lavoie PE. Episcleritis, conjunctivitis, and keratitis as other manifestations of Lyme disease. Ophthalmology 1990; 97: 973–975.

68. Steere AC, Duray PH, Kauffmann DJ, et al. Unilateral blindness caused by infection with the Lyme disease spirochete, *Borrelia burgdorferi*. Ann Intern Med 1985; 103: 382–384.

69. Kornmehl EW, Lesser RL, Jaros P, et al. Bilateral keratitis in Lyme disease. Ophthalmology 1989; 96: 1194–1197.

70. deLuise VP, O'Leary MJ. Peripheral ulcerative keratitis related to Lyme disease. [Letter] Am J Ophthalmol 1991; 111: 244–245.

71. Suttorp-Schulten MSA, Kuiper H, Kijlstra A, et al. Long-term effects of ceftriaxone treatment on intraocular Lyme borreliosis. Am J Ophthalmol 1993; 116: 571–575.

72. Karma A, Seppala I, Mikkila H, et al. Diagnosis and clinical characteristics of ocular Lyme borreliosis. Am J Ophthalmol 1995; 119: 127–135.

73. Bialasiewicz AA, Ruprecht KW, Naumann GOH, et al. Bilateral diffuse choroiditis and exudative retinal detachments with evidence of Lyme disease. Am J Ophthalmol 1988; 105: 419–420.

74. Koch F, Augustin AJ, Boker T. Neuroborreliosis with retinal pigment epithelium detachments. Ger J Ophthalmol 1996; 5: 12–15.

75. Scholes GN, Teske M. Lyme disease and pars planitis. Ophthalmology 1989; 107(Suppl): 126.

76. Copeland RA Jr, Nozik RA, Shimokaji G. Uveitis in Lyme disease. Ophthalmology 1989; 107(Suppl): 127.

77. Winward KE, Smith JL, Culbertson WW, et al. Ocular Lyme borreliosis. Am J Ophthalmol 1989; 108: 651–657.

78. Leys AM, Schonherr U, Lang GE, et al. Retinal vasculitis in Lyme borreliosis. Bull Soc Belge Ophthalmol 1995; 259: 205–214.

79. Vine AK. Retinal vasculitis. Semin Neurol 1994; 14: 354–360.

80. Logigian EL, Kaplan RF, Steere AC. Chronic neurologic manifestations of Lyme disease. N Engl J Med 1990; 323: 1438–1444.

81. Wu G, Lincoff H, Ellsworth RM, et al. Optic disc edema and Lyme disease. Ann Ophthalmol 1986; 18: 252–255.

82. Jacobson DM, Frens DB. Pseudotumor cerebri syndrome associated with Lyme disease. Am J Ophthalmol 1989; 107: 81–82.

83. Federowski JJ, Hyman C. Optic disk edema as the presenting sign of Lyme disease. Clin Infect Dis 1996; 23: 639–640.

84. Scott IU, Silva-Lepe A, Siatkowski RM. Chiasmal optic neuritis in Lyme disease. Am J Ophthalmol 1997; 123: 136–138.

85. Schecter SL. Lyme disease associated with optic neuropathy. Am J Med 1986; 81: 143–145.

86. Reik L Jr, Burgdorfer W, Donaldson JO. Neurologic abnormalities in Lyme disease without erythema chronicum migrans. Am J Med 1986; 81: 73–78.

87. Seidenberg KB, Leib M. Orbital myositis with Lyme disease. Am J Ophthalmol 1990; 109: 13–16.

88. Balcer LJ, Winterkorn JM, Galetta SL. Neuro-ophthalmic manifestations of Lyme disease. J Neuroophthalmol 1997; 17: 108–121.

89. Stanek G, Strle F. Lyme borreliosis. Lancet 2003; 362: 1639–1647.

90. Schwartz BS, Goldstein MD, Ribeiro JMC, et al. Antibody testing in Lyme disease: A comparison of results in four laboratories. JAMA 1989; 262: 3431–3434.

91. Luger SW, Krauss E. Serologic tests for Lyme disease: Interlaboratory variability. Arch Intern Med 1990; 150: 761–763.

92. Barbour AG. The diagnosis of Lyme disease: Rewards and perils. Ann Intern Med 1989; 110: 501–502.

93. Dattwyler RJ, Volkman DJ, Lugt BJ, et al. Seronegative Lyme disease dissociation of specific T- and B-lymphocyte responses to Borrelia burgdorferi. N Engl J Med 1988; 319: 1441–1446.

94. Russell H, Saampson JS, Schmid GP, et al. Enzyme-linked immunosorbent assay and indirect immunofluorescence assay for Lyme disease. J Infect Dis 1984; 149: 465–470.

95. Craft JE, Grodzicki RL, Steere AC. Antibody response in Lyme disease: Evaluation of diagnostic tests. J Infect Dis 1984; 149: 789–795.

96. Magnarelli LA, Anderson JF, Johnson RC. Cross-reactivity in serological tests of Lyme disease and other spirochetal infections. J Infect Dis 1987; 156: 183–188.

97. Hunter EF, Russell H, Farshy CE, et al. Evaluation of sera from patients with Lyme disease in the fluorescent treponemal antibody test for syphilis. Sex Transm Dis 1986; 13: 232–236.

98. Duffy J, Mertz LE, Wobig GH, et al. Diagnosing Lyme disease: The contribution of serologic testing. Mayo Clin Proc 1988; 63: 1116–1121.

99. Grodzicki RL, Steere AC. Comparison of immunoblotting and indirect enzyme-linked immunosorbent assay using different antigen preparations for diagnosing early Lyme disease. J Infect Dis 1988; 157: 790–797.

100. Mandell H, Steere AC, Reinhardt BN, et al. Lack of antibodies to Borrelia burgdorferi in patients with amyotrophic lateral sclerosis. N Engl J Med 1989; 320: 255–256.

101. Nocton JJ, Dressler F, Rutledge BJ, et al. Detection of Borrelia burgdorferi DNA by polymerase chain reaction in synovial fluid from patients with Lyme arthritis. N Engl J Med 1994; 330: 229–234.

102. Hilton E, Sood S. Ocular Lyme borreliosis diagnosed by polymerase chain reaction on vitreous fluid. Ann Intern Med 1996; 125: 424–425.

103. Steere AC, Grodzicki RL, Kornblatt AN, et al. The spirochetal etiology of Lyme disease. N Engl J Med 1983; 308: 733–740.

104. Guidelines Wormser GP, Nadelman, RB, Dattwyler RL, et al Practice guidelines for the treatment of Lyme disease. Clin Infect Dis 2000; 31(Suppl 1): S1–14.

105. Verdon ME, Sigal LH. Recognition and management of Lyme disease. Am Fam Phys 1997; 56: 427–436.

106. Steere AC, Taylor E, McHugh GL, et al. The overdiagnosis of Lyme disease. JAMA 1993; 269: 1812–1816.

107. Rosenbaum JT, Rahn DW. Prevalence of Lyme disease among patients with uveitis. Am J Ophthalmol 1991; 112: 462–463.

108. Breevald J, Kuiper H, Spanjaard L, et al. Uveitis and Lyme borreliosis. Br J Ophthalmol 1993; 77: 480–481.

109. Preac-Mursic V, Pfister HW, Spiegel H, et al. First isolation of Borrelia burgdorferi from an iris biopsy. J Clin Neuroophthalmol 1993; 13: 155–161.

110. Schubert HD, Greenebaum E, Neu HC. Cytologically proven seronegative Lyme choroiditis and vitritis. Retina 1994; 14: 39–42.

110a. Hilton E, Smith C. Sood S. Ocular Lyme borreliosis diagnosed by polymerase chain reaction on vitreous fluid. Ann Intern Med 1996; 125: 424–425.

111. Dattwyler RJ, Halperin JJ, Volkman DJ, et al. Treatment of late Lyme borreliosis – Randomised comparison of ceftriaxone and penicillin. Lancet 1988; 1: 1191–1194.

112. Bryceson ADM, Parry EHO, Perine PL, et al. Louse-borne relapsing fever: A clinical and laboratory study of 62 cases in Ethiopia and a reconstruction of the literature. QJ Med 1970; 39: 129–170.

113. Southern PM Jr, Sanford JP. Relapsing fever: A clinical and microbiological review. Medicine (Baltimore) 1969; 48: 129–149.

114. Rhee KY, Johnson WD Jr. Borrelia species (relapsing fever). In: Mandell GL, Bennett JE, Dolin R, eds. Mandell, Douglas and Bennett's Principles and Practice of Infectious Diseases, 6th edn. New York: Churchill Livingstone, 2005, pp 2795–2796.

115. Meader CN. Five cases of relapsing fever originating in Colorado, with positive blood findings in two. Colorado Med 1915; 12: 365–368.

116. Burgdorfer W. The enlarging spectrum of tick-borne spirochetoses: RR Parker memorial address. Rev Infect Dis 1986; 8: 932–940.

117. Horton JM, Blaser MJ. The spectrum of relapsing fever in the Rocky Mountains. Arch Intern Med 1985; 145: 871–875.

118. Perine PL, Parry EHO, Vukotich D, et al. Bleeding in louse-borne relapsing fever I. Clinical studies in 37 patients. Trans Roy Soc Trop Med Hyg 1971; 65: 776–781.

119. Quin CE, Perkins ES. Tick-borne relapsing fever in East Africa. J Trop Med 1946; 49: 30–32.

120. Hamilton JB. Ocular complications in relapsing fever. Br J Ophthalmol 1943; 27: 68–80.

121. Sciotto CG, Lauer BA, White WL, et al. Detection of Borrelia in acridine orange-stained blood smears by fluorescence microscopy. Arch Pathol Lab Med 1982; 107: 384–386.

122. Schwan TG, Schrumpf ME, Hinnebusch BJ, et al. GlpQ: an antigen for serological discrimination between relapsing fever and Lyme borreliosis. J Clin Microbiol 1996; 34: 2483–2492.

123. Kazragis RJ, Dever LL, Jorgensen JH, et al. In vivo activities of ceftriaxone and vancomycin against Borrelia spp. in the mouse brain and other sites. Antimicrob Agents Chemother 1996; 40: 2632–2636.

124. Warell DA, Perine PL, Krause DW, et al. Pathophysiology and immunology of the Jarisch–Herxheimer-like reaction in louse-borne relapsing fever: Comparison of tetracycline and slow-release penicillin. J Infect Dis 1983; 147: 898–908.

125. Weil A. Über eine Eigenümliche, mit Milztumor. Ikterus and Nephritis einhergehende, akute Infektionskrankheit. Deutsch Arch Klin Med 1886; 39: 209–232.

126. Barkay S, Garzozi H. Leptospirosis. In: Gold DH, Weingeist TA, eds. The Eye in Systemic Disease. Philadelphia, JB Lippincott, 1990, pp 226–228.

127. Palmer MF. Laboratory diagnosis of leptospirosis. Med Lab Sci 1988; 45: 174–178.

128. Waitkins SA. Update on leptospirosis. Br Med J 1985; 290: 1502–1503.

129. Graphs and maps for selected notifiable diseases in the United States. MMWR Morb Mortal Wkly Rep 1994; 42: 13–64.

130. Sasaki DM, Pang L, Minette HP, et al. Active surveillance and risk factors for leptospirosis in Hawaii. Am J Trop Med Hyg 1993; 48: 35–43.

130a. Priya CG, Rathinam SR, Muthukkaruppan V. Evidence for endotoxin as a causative factor for leptospiral uveitis in humans. Invest Ophthalmol Vis Sci 2008; 49: 5419–5424.

131. Bernard N, Moshe H. Human leptospirosis associated with eye

complications. Israel Med J 1963; 22: 182.

132. Barkay S, Garzozi H. Leptospirosis and uveitis. Ann Ophthalmol 1984; 16: 164–168.

133. Murdoch D. Leptospiral uveitis. Trans Ophthalmol Soc NZ 1980; 32: 73–75.

134. Duke-Elder S. System of Ophthalmology, vol VIII, Diseases of the Outer Eye. London: Henry Kimpton, 1965, pp 201–203.

135. Outbreak of acute febrile illness among athletes participating in triathlons – Wisconsin and Illinois, 1998. JAMA 1998; 280: 1473–1474.

136. Rathinam SR, Rathnam S, Slevaraj S, et al. Uveitis associated with an epidemic outbreak of leptospirosis. Am J Ophthalmol124: 71–79. 1997.

137. Dwyer AE, Crockett RS, Kalsow CM. Association of leptospiral seroreactivity and breed with uveitis and blindness in horses: 372 cases (1986–1993). J Am Vet Med Assoc 1995; 207: 1327–1331.

138. Rathinamsivakumar, Ratnam S, Sureshbabu L, et al. Leptospiral antibodies in patients with recurrent ophthalmic involvement. Indian J Med Res 1996; 103: 66–68.

139. Levin N, Nguyen-Khoa JL, Charpentier D, et al. Panuveitis with papillitis in leptospirosis. Am J Ophthalmol 1994; 117: 118–119.

140. Duke-Elder S. System of Ophthalmology, vol IX, Disease of the Uveal Tract. London: Henry Kimpton, 1966, pp 322–325.

141. Merien F, Perolat P, Manel E, et al. Detection of Leptospira DNA by polymerase chain reaction in aqueous humor of a patient with unilateral uveitis. J Infect Dis 1993; 168: 1335–1336.

142. Takafuji ET, Kirkpatrick JW, Miller RN, et al. An efficacy trial of doxycycline chemoprophylaxis against leptospirosis. N Engl J Med 1984; 310: 497–500.

143. Levett PN. Leptospirosis. In: Mandell GL, Bennett JE, Dolin R, eds. Mandell, Douglas and Bennett's Principles and Practice of Infectious Diseases, 6th ed. New York, Churchill Livingstone, 2005, pp 2789–2795.

144. Farr RW. Leptospirosis: State-of-the-art clinical article. Clin Infect Dis 1995; 21: 1–8.

145. Heath CW Jr, Alexander AD, Galton MM. Leptospirosis in the United States. N Engl J Med 1965; 273: 857–922.

146. Watt GW. Leptospirosis as a cause of uveitis. Arch Intern Med 1990; 150: 1130–1132.

Acquired Immunodeficiency Syndrome

Scott M. Whitcup

Key concepts

- Despite efforts at disease prevention there are still over 50 000 new HIV infections in the US every year, and HIV infection remains a global epidemic.
- HIV vasculopathy with cottonwool spots and retinal hemorrhage is the most common manifestation of the disease.
- HIV infection can be treated with highly active antiretroviral therapy (HAART), a combination of antiviral drugs. Despite therapy, HIV is has not been eradicated from any individual with our current medications.
- CMV retinitis is the most common opportunistic infection of the eye in patients with HIV infection.
- Treatment of CMV retinitis is based on location of the disease in the eye and time on HAART.
- Once the immune system improves on HAART and CD4+ T cell counts increase, specific anti-CMV therapy can be stopped without progression of the disease.
- An immune recovery uveitis (IRU) can occur in patients receiving HAART, and may require therapy.
- There are a number of opportunistic infections in HIV disease that can affect the eye. These should be looked for and treated appropriately.

Human immunodeficiency virus

The clinical course and disease manifestations of human immunodeficiency virus (HIV) infection have dramatically changed since the widespread use of potent antiretroviral therapy. It has been over 25 years since HIV was first established as the cause of the acquired immunodeficiency syndrome (AIDS). Although the use of combinations of antiviral drugs called highly active antiretroviral therapy (HAART) has led to greatly improved survival, a number of treatment challenges remain. First, nearly perfect adherence to complicated treatment regimens is required for sustained virologic suppression.[1] Adherence in the range of 50–70% is associated with poorer outcomes and development of drug resistance, and the goal should be greater than 90% adherence. Second, although patient outcomes have improved, eradication of the virus – the 'cure' – has remained elusive. Third, the initial hope of a vaccine for HIV has also proved problematic. Finally, access to therapy is limited for many, and as a result the incidence of HIV-1 infection continues to increase in many areas, including sub-Saharan Africa and parts of Asia.

HIV-1 is a retrovirus and therefore has only RNA copy in its genome. RNA viruses have both genetic diversity and latency, which makes control and eradication difficult. The virus can infect many types of human cell, but much of its pathologic effect is related to infection of the helper CD4+ T cell, which occurs within hours of entering the body.[2] Because this cell is crucial for the development of cell-mediated immune responses, infection of CD4+ T cells and subsequent cell death result in severe immunosuppression. The virion gp 120 Env protein binds to the CD4+ T cell, and once in the cell its RNA is translated into DNA by viral reverse transcriptase (**Fig. 11-1**). This DNA then enters the nucleus and incorporates into the cell genome with the assistance of integrase. The viral DNA is then capable of directing protein synthesis of new viral proteins using the infected cell's apparatus. Proteases are involved in processing HIV proteins into new viral particles, which are then shed from the cell. The infected cell eventually dies.

The earliest evidence of HIV-1 infection was obtained from a blood sample of a patient in the Congo. Clinical evidence of HIV-1 infection in the United States began in the late 1970s. Currently, HIV in humans is thought to originate from primate to human transmission. HIV-2 is classified as a separate virus, and although it causes effects that are clinically similar to those of HIV-1 infection, it is predominantly found in Western Africa.

Epidemiology

Infection is spread mostly through sexual transmission. Until the mid-1990s homosexual and bisexual activity was responsible for most of the transmission. Now, heterosexual activity is the major route of transmission in developed countries. Intravenous drug abuse is another common cause of disease transmission. Perinatal transmission from an infected mother to her offspring can occur in utero. Transmission can also occur during delivery or by breastfeeding. Finally, transmission to healthcare workers can also occur, usually as the result of a needlestick injury. Seroconversion to HIV after a needlestick injury is about 0.3% depending on viral load; this is about 10–100 times less than that with hepatitis C or B. Before the availability of a serologic test for HIV antibody, large numbers of patients, including those with hemophilia, were exposed to the virus through transfusion of blood products.

Although the number of patients with newly diagnosed HIV infection appears to be declining in the United States,

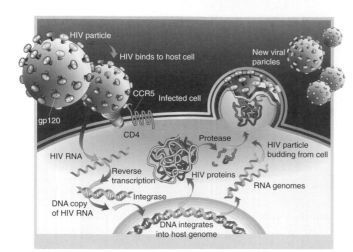

Figure 11-1. Diagram of the lifecycle of human immunodeficiency virus (HIV). *(From Weiss RA. Gulliver's travels in HIV land. Nature 2001; 410: 963–7.)*

HIV disproportionately affects certain segments of the population, including injection drug users, commercial sex workers, people living in poverty, and men who have sex with men. According to *Morbidity and Mortality Weekly Report* 2001, HIV infection has caused approximately 20 million deaths, and about 30 million people are infected.[3] In 2006, an estimated 39 400 persons were diagnosed with HIV in 22 states.[4] Extrapolation from these data suggests 56 300 new infections and an annual incidence rate of 22.8 per 100 000 population.

Diagnosis

HIV infection can be detected by the presence of antibody to viral antigens, 2–8 weeks after infection. The antibodies do not control the infection nor prevent its sequelae. Diagnosis of HIV infection is usually made by an enzyme-linked immunosorbent assay (ELISA) and is then confirmed by a Western blot test.[5,6] Some strains of HIV are not detected by some ELISA tests. Nevertheless, these tests are almost 100% sensitive, albeit not 100% specific, so false-positive results can occur. The virus can also be cultured from blood, semen, and solid tissues, but only rarely from saliva and tears. In the eye, the virus has been found in the cornea,[7] vitreous, and retina.[8] Rapid tests are now commercially available for HIV, although testing algorithms for these tests are still being assessed.

HIV disease

An acute retroviral syndrome usually occurs within 1–6 weeks after HIV infection. Patients typically develop fever, rash, myalgias, headache, or gastrointestinal symptoms. The CD4+ count is reduced, and many patients have elevated liver enzyme levels. Without treatment, CD4+ counts decline by about 75 cells/μL/year. The time from initial infection to the development of a disease that meets the definition of AIDS is about 10 years. AIDS is the most severe manifestation of HIV infection and occurs at a point at which the immune system is so damaged by the infection that opportunistic infections such as *Pneumocystis jiroveci*, *Cryptococcus neoformans*, cytomegalovirus (CMV), oral candidiasis, or unusual malignant processes such as Kaposi's sarcoma can

emerge.[5,6] There is also an encephalopathy caused by direct HIV infection of the brain.

Progression of HIV disease is related to the CD4+ lymphocyte count. The amount of HIV-1 viral RNA predicts the course of HIV disease, specifically, how rapidly the disease is likely to progress. Persons with HIV loads >30 000 copies/mL have an 80% likelihood of developing AIDS within 6 years. In contrast, those with HIV loads <500 copies/mL have a 5.4% chance of developing AIDS.[9] CD4+ lymphocyte counts are good predictors for the development of specific clinical manifestations of the disease, particularly opportunistic infections. For example, most cases of *P. jiroveci* pneumonia occur when CD4+ counts fall to <200 cells/μL. Typically, CMV retinitis occurs when CD4+ counts are <50 cells/μL.

HIV therapy

There is still some debate on when to start antiretroviral therapy for HIV disease. The decision regarding initiation of treatment should be individualized but can be based on symptoms, HIV-1 RNA level and CD4+ count. The potential benefit of antiretroviral therapy must be based on the risks of therapy and the impact on quality of life of adhering to a strict therapeutic regimen which is required to avoid drug resistance. Some clinicians start treatment as soon as HIV infection is diagnosed, although many begin treatment when the CD4+ count drops to <350 cells/μL or if symptoms are present. The rapidity of the decline in CD4+ count and HIV load are other factors in the decision of when to start therapy. Others wait until there is a significant risk of the patient developing HIV disease in the near future.

When therapy is started, a highly active regimen consisting of a combination of antiretroviral agents should be employed to minimize resistance. The goal of therapy is to suppress plasma HIV-1 RNA to below detectable limits using a sensitive assay. This highly active antiretroviral therapy (HAART) regimen has also been called the 'AIDS cocktail' or 'triple therapy,' because it usually consists of three medications. All regimens should combine drugs with synergistic antiviral activity. Regimens can include nucleoside or nucleotide analogue reverse transcriptase inhibitors with a protease inhibitor or combinations of two nucleoside reverse transcriptase inhibitors with a non-nucleoside reverse transcriptase inhibitor.[10] Other combinations have also been used successfully. Therapy is changed based on tolerability, HIV-1 RNA levels and CD4+ T-cell counts. **Box 11-1** lists currently available antiretroviral agents. HAART regimens involve multiple medications that need to be taken at specific times. Again, lack of adherence to these regimens can lead to resistance and failure of therapy, so this must be closely monitored.

Ocular manifestations of HIV infection

Ocular manifestations of HIV infection occur in every tissue of the eye, from the eyelids to the optic nerve (**Box 11-2**). The most common findings include dry eye, a retinal microvasculopathy, and CMV retinitis. Although direct HIV infection in the brain appears to produce a severe encephalopathy, there is still no definitive evidence that HIV infection of ocular tissue leads to clinically important pathologic effects. However, subclinical infection of retinal neural and

Box 11-1 Anti-HIV medications

Combination drugs

- Efavirenz/emtricitabine/Te... (Atripla)
- Lamivudine/zidovudine (Combivir)
- Abacavir/lamivudine (Epzicom)
- Abacavir/lamivudine/zidovudine (Trizivir)
- Embricitabine/tenofovir disoproxil... (Truvada)

Entry and fusion inhibitors

- Celsentri (Selzentry)
- DP 178 (Fuzeon)
- Enfuvirtide (Fuzeon)
- Fuzeon (Fuzeon)
- Maraviroc (Selzentry)
- MVC (Selzentry)
- Pentafuside (Fuzeon)
- Selzentry (Selzentry)
- T 20 (Fuzeon)
- UK-427,857 (Selzentry)

Integrase inhibitors

- Isentress (Isentress)
- MK-0518 (Isentress)
- RAL (Isentress)
- Raltegravir (T sentress)

Nonnucleoside reverse transcriptase inhibitors

- 136817–59–9 (Rescriptor)
- BI-RG-587 (Viramune)
- Delavirdine mesylate (Rescriptor)
- DLV (Rescriptor)
- DMP-266 (Sustiva)
- Efavirenz (Sustiva)
- EFV (Sustiva)
- ETR (Intelence)
- Etravirine (TMC125) (Intelence)
- ETV (Intelence)
- Intelence (Intelence)
- L 743726 (Sutiva)
- Nevirapine (Viramune)
- NVP (Viramune)
- Rescriptor (Rescriptor)
- Stocrin (Sustiva)
- Sustiva (Sustiva)
- TMC 125 (Intelence)
- U-90152S (Rescriptor)
- Viramune (Viramune)

Nucleoside reverse transcriptase inhibitors

- 3TC (Epivir)
- 524W91 (Emtriva)
- Abacavir (Ziagen)
- Abacavir/lamivudine (Epzicom)
- Abacavir/lamivudine/zidovudine (Trizivir)
- Abacavir sulfate (Ziagen)
- Abacavir sulfate/lamivudine (Epzicom)
- Abacavir sulfate/lamivudine... (Trizivir)
- ABC (Ziagen)

Taken from www.AIDSinfo.nih.gov

Box 11-2 Ocular manifestations of HIV infection

Eyelids

Molluscum contagiosum

Kaposi's sarcoma

Herpes zoster ophthalmicus

Herpes simplex virus cutaneous vesicles

Kaposi's sarcoma

Stevens–Johnson syndrome

Conjunctiva/sclera

Dry eye*

Kaposi's sarcoma

Microvasculopathy

Microsporidial conjunctivitis

Herpesvirus conjunctivitis

Scleritis

Cornea

Ulcerative keratitis

Dry eye*

Herpes simplex keratitis

Herpes zoster ophthalmicus

Microsporidiosis

Syphilitic keratitis

Tuberculosis

Gonorrhea

Lens

Cataract

Optic nerve

Optic neuropathy

Retina and choroid

Microvasculopathy (cotton-wool spots, retinal hemorrhages)*

CMV retinitis*

Acute retinal necrosis

Progressive outer retinal necrosis

Syphilis

Toxoplasmosis

Pneumocystis choroidopathy

Cryptococcosis

Mycobacterial infection

Intraocular lymphoma

Candidiasis

Histoplasmosis

*Occurs in >5% of patients.

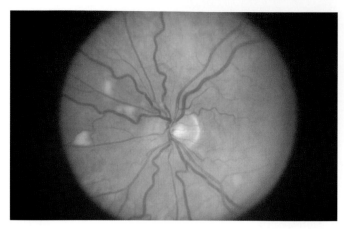

Figure 11-2. Multiple nerve fiber layer infarcts (cottonwool spots) in patient with AIDS.

endothelial cells has been reported.[8] The retinal microvasculopathy of HIV occurs in 25–92% of patients and includes small dot retinal hemorrhages and nerve fiber layer infarcts called cottonwool spots (**Fig. 11-2**).[11-14] This retinopathy may be caused by interactions between viral antigens and antibodies that circulate in the blood and then deposit in the eye, but this has not been clearly shown. The incidence of this retinal microvasculopathy increases with the degree of immunosuppression. The presence of the p24 antigen, a surface HIV antigen, in the blood also increases with more advanced disease, and it is possible that this antigenemia may be a cause of this retinopathy, with immune complex formation in the retinal vasculature. Superficial and deep retinal hemorrhages, retinal perivasculitis, and vascular occlusions also occur. Small peripheral blot hemorrhages are frequently noted on retinal examination and appear to be more common with decreasing CD4+ counts and anemia. Electron microscopic studies of these lesions reveal swollen endothelial cells and degenerating pericytes.[15] Inflammatory cell infiltrates and infectious organisms are not seen in cottonwool spots; however, the microvascular abnormalities are widespread throughout the retina and may provide an entrance for opportunistic viral infections of the retina.

Clinically, cottonwool spots are seen as superficial white fluffy lesions in the retina (Fig. 11-2). There may be small dilations of the microvasculature nearby. Visual symptoms are rarely associated with the presence of a cottonwool spot. A cottonwool spot cannot occur in the foveal avascular zone as there is no nerve fiber layer to become infarcted in this part of the retina. Perifoveal cottonwool spots may cause symptoms. Patients may notice a relative, but not absolute, scotoma. This can be useful in distinguishing a cottonwool spot from an early area of viral retinitis in which the scotoma is absolute. In patients with AIDS these lesions can sometimes be more than 0.5 disc diameter in size. They are distinguished from infectious retinitis by the fact that they do not enlarge over time. Although individual lesions will disappear over a period of several months, new lesions often appear. The retinal hemorrhages associated with HIV infection tend to be small dot hemorrhages and rarely cause visual symptoms. Occlusive vasculopathy, such as central retinal vein occlusions, may affect vision.

Dry eye is also a common finding in patients with HIV infection and may be due to reduced tear production associated with diminished lactoferrin and lysozyme.[16] In most patients the condition is mild to moderately severe and can be treated with artificial tears. More severe cases of dry eye can occur. Dry eye associated with Stevens–Johnson syndrome has also been reported in patients with AIDS.[17]

Even in the HAART era many patients with HIV infection have visual symptoms in the absence of active opportunistic infection.[18] Visual acuity, contrast sensitivity, and visual fields are worse than expected compared to a normal age-matched control group. Although the exact pathogenesis of this neuroretinopathy is unknown, causes may include HIV vasculopathy or a direct effect of HIV on the retina and optic nerve, undiagnosed coinfection, or effects from therapy.

Ocular infection

There are a number of other opportunistic infections associated with HIV infection (**Box 11-3**). CMV retinitis is the most common ocular infection in AIDS and is discussed in the next section. Other intraocular infections that more frequently occur in patients with AIDS include syphilis, toxoplasmosis, tuberculosis, *Candida* infection, and cryptococcosis.[19-23] These have been discussed in previous chapters and must be differentiated from CMV infection. Herpesvirus infections other than CMV infection can also cause a viral retinitis in patients with HIV infection. Herpes zoster ophthalmicus may be an early sign of HIV infection.[24] Herpes zoster retinitis accompanied by acute retinal necrosis (see Chapter 12) and herpes simplex retinitis have occasionally been seen in patients with AIDS.[15] These viral retinal infections are often difficult to differentiate clinically from CMV retinitis. Autopsy studies have shown that more than 95% of viral retinitis in patients with AIDS is due to CMV infection.[11,15] However, these studies were completed early in the history of the AIDS epidemic and the percentages may have changed.

Cytomegalovirus retinitis

CMV is a herpes class virus and contains double-stranded DNA. Systemic infection is a very common infection in the general population and causes a heterophil, antibody-negative mononucleosis syndrome. Therefore, many adults have CMV antibodies because of previous infection.

Approximately 50% of heterosexual men and 95% of homosexual men have evidence of a previous CMV infection. However, with the exception of a few unusual cases, CMV infection of the retina occurs as an opportunistic infection only in immunosuppressed persons or in infants with congenital CMV infection. The disease was first recognized as a congenital infection in 1947. In the past, immunosuppression associated with organ transplantation and chemotherapy was the most common cause of CMV retinitis.[25] It is interesting to note that CMV retinitis is much more frequent after renal transplantation than after bone marrow transplantation. In the current era, however, the increasing number of patients with AIDS has led to a marked increase in the number of occurrences of CMV retinitis. CMV retinitis tends to occur in patients whose immune systems are the most significantly suppressed by HIV infection,[11,26] rarely occurring if the CD4+ count is >100 cells/μL and typically occurring when CD4+ counts are <50 cells/μL. Before the widespread use of HAART, CMV retinitis was reported in 7–40% of patients with AIDS in several series, and probably occurred clinically in at least 15–20% of these patients at some time during the course of disease.[11,12,15,19]

CMV retinitis probably reaches the eye via the bloodstream, although the possibility of reactivation of latent virus has not been ruled out. Evidence of hematogenous spread includes the fact that one eye frequently develops retinitis several months before the other, and that new foci of retinitis can appear in an affected eye. It is unusual to see more than three separate areas of CMV retinitis in an eye, and most eyes contain one initial focus that then spreads across the retina.

CMV retinitis begins as small, white retinal infiltrates which, if seen early, may resemble a large cottonwool spot. Two types of clinical appearance may be seen. The first is a perivascular fluffy white lesion with many scattered hemorrhages (**Fig. 11-3**). Another manifestation is a more granular-appearing lesion that has few associated hemorrhages and often has a central area of clearing, with atrophic retina and stippled retinal pigment epithelium (**Fig. 11-4**). In autopsy studies CMV has been identified in both types of lesion in patients with AIDS. However, because we do not understand what factors predispose a person to one type of lesion, we cannot exclude the possibility that some of these lesions may be other viral retinal infections. It is possible that the underlying immune status of the patient influences the clinical appearance of the lesion. However, local factors also must be important, as an occasional patient will have different-appearing lesions. Both types of lesion respond to the therapeutic approach that will be discussed later, which is consistent with herpes class viral infections of the retina.

The diagnosis of CMV retinitis is based on clinical criteria. Although it is possible to confirm the diagnosis with a polymerase chain reaction (PCR) performed on a vitreous specimen or by culture of the virus from the vitreous or retina, this is rarely done in practice. As the number of treatment options grows and becomes more specific, accurate diagnosis will be increasingly important. Active CMV retinitis always has a faint granular border of intraretinal infiltrates that represent the new foci of viral activity in normal retina. In addition, the disease grows at approximately 250

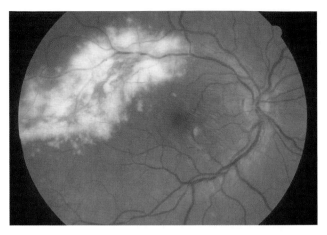

Figure 11-3. Cytomegalovirus retinitis in vascular distribution characterized by fluffy white retinal infiltration and small area of retinal hemorrhage.

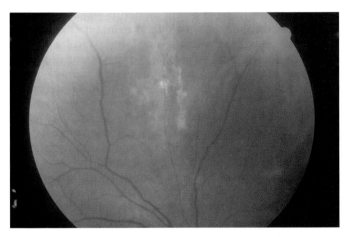

Figure 11-4. Cytomegalovirus retinitis may also have a granular appearance with mottling of retinal pigment epithelium and little associated retinal hemorrhage.

microns per week, and therefore there are usually areas that have begun to atrophy, as denoted by retinal pigment epithelial stippling. This is in contrast to acute retinal necrosis, in which the disease spreads rapidly, and one is less likely to find active retinitis surrounding an atrophic center. There is always a low-grade mild vitreous inflammation (vitritis) with CMV retinitis, frequently less than might be expected for the degree of retinal necrosis. Usually there are only trace vitreous cells with minimal vitreous haze. There may be fine anterior-chamber keratic precipitates (KPs), although most patients have no anterior chamber reaction. Vision is normal unless the optic disc or fovea is involved.

Patients with CMV retinitis may not complain of symptoms because the lesions begin in the periphery, or because the patient often does not notice an increase in floaters or a new scotoma. Therefore, it may make clinical sense to screen patients who are at risk with CD4+ counts <50–100 cells/μL. A reasonable screening frequency is every 3 or 4 months for this population, although this may need to be modified as use of oral prophylactic therapies becomes widespread. Because children more rarely complain of visual symptoms, ophthalmologic screening should be performed at least every 3 months when the CD4+ count is <50 cells/μL.

through the pars plana. The mean time to progression with this implant is 226 days, with about 50% of untreated contralateral eyes developing CMV retinitis during the study.[31] The efficacy of this device for treating local CMV retinitis is clear, but the implant does not treat systemic CMV infection or prevent occurrence in the contralateral eye; therefore, systemic treatment is often required in addition to the ganciclovir implant. Combinations of the ganciclovir implant with systemic therapy, such as oral ganciclovir, may treat both local and systemic infection while avoiding daily systemic infusions. In a multicenter clinical trial, 377 patients with unilateral CMV retinitis were randomly assigned to receive the ganciclovir implant with placebo, the ganciclovir implant with oral ganciclovir, or intravenous ganciclovir.[55] The primary endpoint was time to new CMV disease, defined as contralateral CMV retinitis or extraocular CMV disease proven on biopsy. At 6 months new CMV disease occurred in 44.3% of patients receiving the ganciclovir implant with placebo, 24.3% receiving the ganciclovir implant with oral ganciclovir, and 19.6% receiving intravenous ganciclovir. Interestingly, new CMV retinitis or extraocular CMV disease was rare in patients taking protease inhibitors, regardless of treatment group.

Historically, intravitreal injections of ganciclovir,[56] foscarnet,[57] or cidofovir were used to treat CMV retinitis.[58,59] We previously used injections of ganciclovir or foscarnet to treat recurrent CMV infection, especially in patients resistant to or intolerant of systemic therapy. However, in the era of HAART and the ganciclovir implant, this approach is rarely used.

Oral formulations of ganciclovir have been developed. A randomized controlled trial showed that once-daily oral valganciclovir was as clinically effective and well tolerated as oral ganciclovir three times daily for CMV prevention in high-risk sold organ transplant recipients.[60] Valganciclovir is an orally administered prodrug that is rapdily hydrolysed to ganciclovir and is now the formulation most commonly used. The recommended dose for newly diagnosed CMV retinitis is 900 mg twice daily for 2–3 weeks, followed by 900 mg once daily. If used in combination with a ganciclovir implant, the dose of valganciclovir is usually 900 mg once daily. Orally administered valganciclovir apears to be as effective as intravenous ganciclovir for induction treatment and effective for long-term maintentnace therapy for CMV retinitis in patients with AIDS.[61] As with intravenous ganciclovir, the major toxicity is bone marrow suppression with neutropenia and thrombocytopenia.

Current therapeutic approach to CMV retinitis in the era of HAART

How has HAART altered the treatment strategy for CMV retinitis? First, we now know that immune recovery following HAART has reduced the incidence of opportunistic infections and can also control pre-existing infections, including CMV retinitis. As a result, lifelong anti-CMV therapy is no longer required for most patients who have documented improvements in CD4+ T-cell counts following HAART. In fact, we currently consider stopping maintenance anti-CMV therapy in patients with stable CMV retinitis if CD4+ cell counts are stable or increasing and have been >100 cells/μL for at least 3 months. Freedom from anti-CMV therapy has

Table 11-1 Therapeutic approach for CMV retinitis

HAART Naïve or Receiving HAART for Less Than 3 Months	
Zone 1	**Zone 2 or 3**
Ganciclovir implant	Ganciclovir 900 mg po qd + valganciclovir 900 mg po qd
If patient refused intravitreal therapy:	
Valganciclovir 900 mg po bid	

HAART for more than 3 months	
Zone 1	**Zone 2 or 3**
Ganciclovir implant	Valganciclovir 900 mg po qd + ganciclovir implant Valganciclovir 900 mg po qd or Valganciclovir 900 mg po bid × 3 weeks then 900 mg po qd
If patient refused intravitreal therapy:	
Valganciclovir 900 mg po bid	

improved the quality of life of our patients. Nevertheless, they must be closely followed for reactivation of retinitis or the development of extraocular disease. If the CD4+ count falls to <50 cells/μL, the clinician should consider restarting anti-CMV therapy or, at least, plan to re-examine the patient more frequently.

The therapeutic approach to CMV retinitis is now based on the patient's immune status in relation to HAART, the location of CMV retinitis in the eye, and patient input (**Table 11-1**). Because we know that CMV can be effectively controlled with an improved immune status following HAART, if CMV retinitis occurs in a paitent who is HAART naïve, the goal is to control the CMV disease until the CD4+ counts rise. However, if a patient has failed to have a significant improvement in CD4+ counts despite HAART, one must assume that anti-CMV therapy will be required for longer than several months, and this will alter the therapeutic approach. Similarly, the approach to patients with CMV retinitis in zone 1, an area of the retina that extends 3000 μm from the center of the fovea or 1500 μm from the edge of the optic nerve, is different from that for patients who have more peripheral and less immediately sight-threatening disease.

Again, the main treatment goal for patients who are HAART naïve or who have started HAART within the last several months is to limit the CMV infection until the immune system improves and controls the infection on its own. For zone 1 disease, most clinicians still recommend a sustained-release ganciclvoir implant in combination with valganciclovir, regardless of whether patients are HAART naïve or HAART experienced.[62] This regimen provides the best ocular drug levels to control the CMV retinitis and prevent potentially sight-threatening disease progression, and also controls systemic CMV disease. Some patients refuse intravitreal therapy, and these patients are treated with higher induction doses of valganciclovir and watched very carefully for disease progression. For patients who have been receiving HAART for longer than 3 months we recommend a combination of a ganciclovir implant with valganciclovir for zone 1 disease; if they have zone 2 or 3 disease we will combine a ganciclovir implant with valganciclovir 900 mg once daily, or just valganciclovir 900 mg twice daily for 3 weeks followed by 900 mg once daily.

Previously, National Institutes of Health (NIH) guidelines on the therapy of HIV infection recommended that use of prophylactic medications be continued even if CD4+ cell counts increase above threshold levels.[63] Because of the clonal nature of the antigen-specific immune response, it is possible that the increased T-cell numbers after HAART may not restore adequate protection against opportunistic pathogens such as CMV. Current data now suggest that immune recovery after HAART is effective in controlling opportunistic infections, even in patients with a history of severe immunosuppression. Therefore, more recent NIH guidelines address discontinuation of maintenance anti-CMV therapy in patients receiving HAART who demonstrate immune recovery.[64]

Oral formulations of ganciclovir can be used for maintenance therapy for CMV retinitis but may be somewhat less effective than intravenous therapy. In an open-label study, after induction therapy with intravenous ganciclovir, patients were randomly assigned to receive maintenance intravenous ganciclovir or oral ganciclovir at a dose of 1000 mg three times a day.[65] Although the mean time to progression of retinitis was 62 days with intravenous therapy and 57 days with oral therapy, the median time to progression was 49 days with intravenous and 29 days with oral treatment. Valganciclovir, the orally administered prodrug of ganciclovir, appears to be as effective as intravenous ganciclovir for induction treatment and may be effective for the long-term management of CMV retinitis in patients with AIDS.[66] The usual dose is 900 mg once daily. An effective oral preparation of foscarnet is not available.

Retinal detachment

Retinal detachment develops in approximately 20% of patients with retinitis, 50% of these patients developing detachment in the second eye if it is involved with retinitis. Approximately 11% of patients with retinitis will experience a retinal detachment 6 months after diagnosis, and 24% will have detachment over the first year after diagnosis in the first eye.[67] The greater the amount of peripheral retinal involvement, the greater the risk of retinal detachment. Compared to eyes with 10% of the peripheral retina involved, eyes with more than 25% of involvement had a fivefold increase in detachment rate. This risk increased to 24-fold if active retinitis also was present.

Because the mechanism of retinal detachment in CMV retinitis is vitreous traction on the thinned, atrophic retina, multiple retinal breaks are usually present and large, relatively posterior breaks can occur. Tears can occur at the edge of the normal retina, but also throughout the atrophic areas. The risk of retinal detachment is increased if the patient with CMV retinitis is myopic. The posterior vitreous usually adheres to the retina, and the combination of low-grade vitritis with a thinned retina allows the vitreous to pull the retina forward, causing it to detach. The rate of growth of the detachment is variable and depends on the extent of traction and location within the eye.

The standard surgical approach for retinal detachment is not optimal for eyes with CMV retinitis. Scleral buckling is appropriate when retinal breaks are located near the vitreous base. The breaks in eyes with CMV retinitis often are more posterior and multiple. Scleral buckling may be successful in selected patients, but a more effective approach is vitrectomy, endolaser surgery, and the application of silicone oil tamponade. Head position can be more normal, although the patient still cannot lie on his or her back. Vision can be rehabilitated in a few days. The surgery can be performed as a local, outpatient procedure with minimal postoperative discomfort.

The major disadvantage of silicone oil is the induced hyperopia of 5 to 6 diopters, which, unless a contact lens is worn, will produce diplopia if surgery has been performed on only one eye. Both gas bubbles and silicone oil are associated with an increased risk of cataract formation. These cataracts commonly become visually significant 1 year after the surgery. Older patients may have a greater chance of cataract development than younger patients. As survival with CMV retinitis increases, more cataracts will need to be removed in this patient population. Of interest is the fact that the oil causes a hyperopic shift of approximately 1 to 2 diopters with a posterior chamber intraocular lens as opposed to the 5- to 6-diopter change in the phakic eye. One additional potential disadvantage of silicone oil is that intravitreal drug injections are more difficult and the therapeutic result is unpredictable.

The use of laser surgery to demarcate areas of retinitis and thereby prevent detachment has been suggested. A similar approach is often used in acute retinal necrosis due to herpes zoster infection. Although there is evidence in the literature to support this approach, it is not uniformly successful, and because CMV retinitis often continues to progress through a barrier of laser burns, this approach will not prevent either spread or detachment in all patients. It is unclear whether this approach should be widely utilized, but it may be possible to study this question and identify high-risk groups for whom prophylactic laser will be useful.

Prognosis

Advances in the drugs we use to treat both HIV and CMV disease have greatly improved the visual prognosis for patients with CMV retinitis. Reduced complications, including destruction of the macula from disease progression and retinal detachment, are a welcome outcome from improved treatment. Recent data suggest that patients with CMV retinitis have visual impairment at a rate of 0.10 case/eye-year and blindness at a rate of 0.06 case/eye-year.[68]

Immune recovery uveitis

Although HAART-associated improvements in immune function have improved the clinical course of CMV retinitis, immune restoration has also led to a change in the clinical manifestations of the disease. Vitritis was reported in immunocompromised patients with CMV retinitis before HAART.[69] However, more profound intraocular inflammation is occurring in patients with CMV retinitis receiving HAART.[38,42,70-73] Initially, this syndrome was referred to as immune recovery

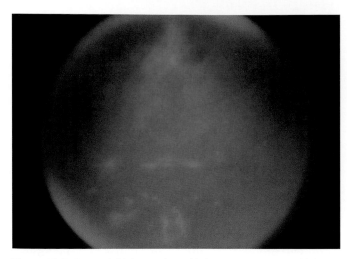

Figure 11-6. Dense vitritis in a patient with immune-recovery uveitis in the eye with inactive CMV retinitis.

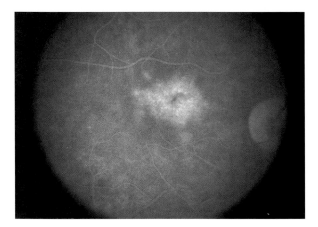

Figure 11-7. Cystoid macular edema in a patient with immune recovery uveitis and inactive CMV retinitis.

vitritis;[74] however, because the inflammation is characterized not only by a profound vitritis (**Fig. 11-6**) but also by anterior uveitis, cataract, macular edema (**Fig. 11-7**), epiretinal membranes, and optic disc edema, we referred to these findings as immune recovery uveitis (IRU).[39,75,76] In a prospective clinical trial in which specific anti-CMV therapy was discontinued in 14 patients with stable CMV retinitis and HIV infection during HAART, 12 (89.7%) of the 14 patients had IRU before they stopped their CMV therapy.[39] Three of these 12 patients had a profound increase in IRU during the course of the trial. Other investigators have reported high rates of IRU in patients with stable CMV retinitis receiving HAART;[77] however, there is large variability in the prevalence of this finding. High rates of IRU may be related to better immune responses in these patients due to strict compliance with aggressive HAART. The median CD4+ count at baseline in the study detailed above was >300 cells/μL. The amount of CMV antigen in the eye may also affect the development of IRU. The incidence of IRU may be lower in patients with CMV retinitis who have not received HAART before the control of retinal disease with anti-CMV therapy.[78]

Interestingly, in our prospective study of patients with CMV retinitis receiving HAART, no new retinal detachments occurred during the study.[39] This is surprising because the risk of retinal detachment in a similar population before the use of HAART was 19% at 6 months.[79] Intraocular inflammation and hypertrophy of the retinal pigment epithelium may lead to increased adherence of the retina and a reduced risk of retinal detachment.

Immune recovery uveitis may require treatment. Although the best therapy is unknown, we have treated anterior uveitis with topical prednisolone acetate. In addition, we have used periocular injections of triamcinolone or short courses of prednisone to treat vitritis and macular edema associated with decreased visual acuity. More recently, intravitreal triamcinolone has been used to treat macular edema associated with IRU.[80] The exact mechanism of immune recovery uveitis has not been elucidated. It does not occur in eyes without CMV retinitis; therefore, the inflammation appears to be related to the infection, but it is unclear whether IRU is related partly to subclinical viral replication in the eye. If this were true, therapy with specific anti-CMV therapy might limit the uveitis, but this has yet to be demonstrated. In any event, the severity of IRU appears to be related to the amount of infected retina. In our experience, eyes without IRU had very small areas of retinitis. This could be related either to the amount of CMV antigen in the eye or to the degree of the breakdown in the blood–retinal barrier as a result of the retinal necrosis. Finally, the type of anti-CMV therapy could also affect the amount of retinal involvement and CMV antigen in the eye. More effective treatment may reduce CMV involvement of the retina and limit the development of IRU.

Other inflammatory diseases have developed after immune recovery in patients receiving HAART. Patients with subclinical *Mycobacterium avium* complex infection develop fever, leukocytosis, and lymphadenitis after the initiation of HAART.[81] Meningitis has been reported in patients with latent cryptococcal central nervous system infection after initiation of HAART.[82] In developing countries tuberculosis is commonly noted after starting HAART, and is one of the major opportunistic infections seen in many parts of the world.

Herpes zoster

Herpes zoster ophthalmicus occurs more frequently in HIV-positive patients and may often be the presenting sign of the disease. Cutaneous zoster occurring in a severely immunosuppressed patient with AIDS is more likely to disseminate and may be more difficult to treat with aciclovir compared to its effectiveness in the immunocompetent patient. Intravenously administered aciclovir sometimes is required for cutaneous dermatomal zoster, and is certainly needed for disseminated zoster.

Varicella-zoster virus (VZV) retinitis in the HIV-positive patient has a somewhat more varied clinical spectrum than that seen in immunocompetent patients. Although the clinical picture in some patients is identical to that of acute retinal necrosis, other clinical appearances have been described. In one study 17% of HIV-positive patients with herpes zoster ophthalmicus subsequently developed acute retinal necrosis.[83] A form of retinitis termed progressive outer retinal necrosis (PORN) appears as multifocal areas of retinitis with good preservation of the inner retina and retinal vasculature in the early clinical stages[84] (discussed in detail in Chapter 12). The areas of necrosis occasionally appear similar to those in acute retinal necrosis. In progressive outer retinal necrosis the lesions are small, often multifocal, and consist of multiple punctate white retinal dots located in the outer retina (see Fig. 12-6). Still other patients may initially manifest multiple retinal vascular occlusions with areas of retinitis (see Fig. 12-5).

The response to systemic aciclovir in these immunosuppressed patients is inconsistent. Approximately half have a good response to intravenous aciclovir followed by oral aciclovir, with resultant quieting of the retinitis. Some of these patients can be weaned from the oral drug, but others have recurrences without maintenance therapy.[85] In contrast, other patients have progressive retinitis despite treatment with intravenous aciclovir. Also, because of the rapid progression of PORN and the difficulty of making a definitive diagnosis, many clinicians start therapy with aciclovir and foscarnet to cover CMV retinitis and provide 'double coverage' for the PORN. A combination of intravitreal and intravenous antiviral therapy has also been used to treat the disease.[86] Despite therapy the disease can be relentlessly progressive, and severe visual disability can result. The risk of retinal detachment appears similar for immunosuppressed and immunocompetent patients with VZV retinitis, and repair techniques are similar. With HAART, once the CD4+ T cell counts rise, antiviral therapy for zoster may be discontinued in some patients.

The major differential diagnosis in the HIV-positive patient is between CMV and VZV retinitis. This differentiation is important because aciclovir is considerably less toxic than either ganciclovir or foscarnet. CMV retinitis is at least 20 times more common than VZV retinitis, and the differential diagnosis is based primarily on clinical criteria, taking into account the rate of progression and the multifocality.

Pneumocystis jirovecii choroiditis

Pneumocystis carinii choroiditis was first reported by Macher et al.[87] Since that time it has been renamed *Pneumocystis jirovecii* and classified as a fungus. The choroiditis is characterized by multifocal white plaques in the choroid with little evidence of intraocular inflammation (**Fig. 11-8**).[88] It is an extrapulmonary form of pneumocystic disease usually seen in patients using a prophylactic inhalant for this condition, which prevents pulmonary involvement but does not provide systemic prophylaxis. This has become a less common problem as the use of aerosolized pentamidine has decreased. Histopathologic examination in these patients shows numerous cysts in the choroid (**Fig. 11-9**).

The lesions rarely cause visual loss because they are located beneath the retinal pigment epithelium (RPE) and have no associated inflammation. Trimethoprim-sulfamethoxazole is usually the first choice for therapy. Alternative therapy includes dapsone, aerosolized pentamidine, and atovaquone. Histologic examination has demonstrated large numbers of cysts with no host response. It is important to identify this disease so that the internist can be aware of the potential for extrapulmonary pneumocystic involvement. The ocular disease is associated with prophylactic aerosolized pentamidine and appears to be less common as aerosolized pentamidine use has decreased.

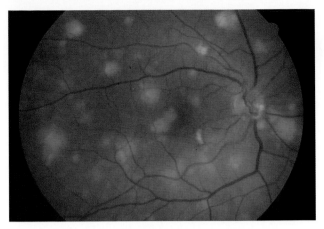

Figure 11-8. Fundus photograph of patient with AIDS and *Pneumocystis carinii* pneumonia shows multiple yellow deep choroidal lesions. Histopathologic examination revealed not only *P. carinii* cysts but also cytomegalovirus (see Fig. 11-9) and *Mycobacterium avium-intracellulare* (see Fig. 11-10). *(From Whitcup SM, Fenton RM, Pluda JM, et al.* Pneumocystis carinii *and* Mycobacterium avium-intracellulare *infection of the choroid.* Retina 1992; 12: 331–5.)

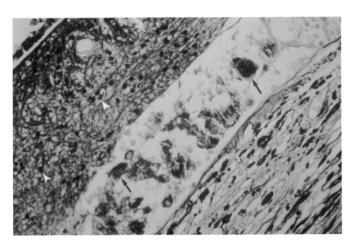

Figure 11-9. Photomicrograph of choroidal lesion in the right eye showing numerous *Pneumocystis carinii* cysts (white arrowheads) and cytomegalovirus cells in choroidal blood vessel (arrows). (Gomori's methenamine silver stain; ×400.) *(From Whitcup SM, Fenton RM, Pluda JM, et al.* Pneumocystis carinii *and* Mycobacterium avium-intracellulare *infection of the choroid.* Retina 1992; 12: 331–5.)

Mycobacterium avium-intracellulare choroiditis

M. avium-intracellulare manifests as infiltrates, usually 50–100 μm in size and scattered throughout the fundus.[89,90] It usually causes no visual symptoms, but, as in the case of pneumocystic disease, is evidence of disseminated systemic infection. *M. avium-intracellulare* is a common pathogen in patients with AIDS which often involves the bone marrow and leads to marrow failure.

Other diseases

Multiple infections in a single eye may be present in patients with AIDS. Choroidal lesions such as those caused by *Pneumocystis* can be seen concurrently with infections from other organisms such as CMV and *M. avium-intracellulare*

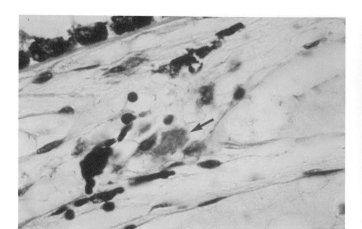

Figure 11-10. Photomicrograph of choroid adjacent to area infiltrated with *Pneumocystis carinii* shows cluster of acid-fast bacilli (arrow). (Ziehl-Neelsen stain; ×100.) *(From Whitcup SM, Fenton RM, Pluda JM, et al.* Pneumocystis carinii *and* Mycobacterium avium-intracellulare *infection of the choroid. Retina 1992; 12: 331–5.)*

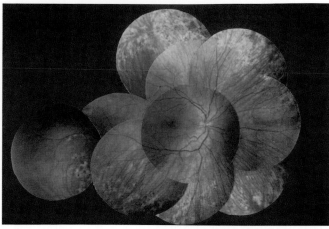

Figure 11-11. Photographic montage of patient with didanosine-related retinal lesions. Atrophic areas of RPE hypopigmentation and hyperpigmentation are seen in the midperiphery of the fundus.

(Figs 11-9 and 11-10), but the greatest concern is a CMV infection combined with herpes zoster or herpes simplex. In this situation the retinitis response can be atypical, and if the zoster infection is treated with aciclovir the CMV infection will continue to progress. Toxoplasmosis, which is discussed in Chapter 14, is also seen as a retinal infection with a vitritis and should be managed with an antitoxoplasmosis regimen.[90] In addition, B-cell lymphoma can occur in AIDS, manifesting as choroidal, retinal, or vitreous lesions.[91] A posterior ocular process that fails to respond to the therapy chosen on the basis of the clinical presentation may require a biopsy to ascertain the presence of lymphoma. Finally, syphilis is becoming increasingly common in HIV-infected patients and is discussed in detail in Chapter 10.[92]

Drug-related ocular inflammation

Several reports have identified both anterior and posterior uveitis in patients treated with rifabutin.[93] These inflammatory findings can occur months after the initiation of therapy. Rifabutin is used to treat *M. avium-intracellulare* infection. A severe uveitis that is often bilateral can result. The uveitis associated with rifabutin is most commonly seen in persons also receiving fluconazole or a macrolide drug, which raises serum levels of rifabutin. The inflammation responds to appropriate steroid therapy or to a reduction in the rifabutin dosage. The mechanism of this inflammation is unclear and may be either direct drug hypersensitivity or a response to mycobacterial death, with a subsequent inflammatory response. In addition, we have described retinal lesions in patients treated with the antiretroviral agent didanosine that appear to predominantly involve the RPE **(Fig. 11-11)**.[94] Uveitis has been reported in about one of four patients treated with fomivirsen. This uveitis appears to respond to topical corticosteroids. RPE changes have also been reported with fomivirsen.

Remarkable progress has been made in the treatment of HIV infection and the associated opportunistic infections, but of course we have far to go before we can claim victory over this disease. Nevertheless, there has been a dramatic change in the presentation and course of many of the ophthalmic manifestations of HIV infection, particularly CMV retinitis. Case 11-1 describes a typical case of CMV retinitis before HAART. Case 11-2 demonstrates the differences in the course of the disease after HAART.

Case 11-1

A 42-year-old man with a diagnosis of AIDS reported a 2-week history of reduced vision in the right eye. He had no light perception in this eye and 20/20 visual acuity in the left eye. The right eye contained 1+ vitreous cells and had a significant area of necrotic retinitis involving the optic disc. Blood cultures were positive for cytomegalovirus. The left eye had a small white infiltrate with an associated hemorrhage near the superior vascular arcade.

Over the next few weeks the area of involvement in the left eye increased in size. Treatment with ganciclovir was begun, with a marked improvement of the retinitis in both eyes. Vision did not return in the right eye. Ganciclovir therapy was discontinued after 3 weeks, and the vision in the left eye remained 20/20 for 2 weeks. It then decreased to 20/300 because of macular edema. The area of necrotic retinitis was larger. A second course of ganciclovir was begun, and the retinitis again resolved and the vision returned to 20/25. Maintenance therapy was begun, but because of neutropenia the patient could not tolerate a dose of 5 mg/kg 5 days/week. He lost all vision in the left eye approximately 2 months later and died several weeks after that.

Case 11-2

AIDS was diagnosed in a 37-year-old man who had a CD4+ cell count of 5/µL. A routine ophthalmologic examination revealed active CMV retinitis in both eyes. Highly active antiretroviral therapy was begun. The CMV retinitis was initially treated with intravenous ganciclovir, but the therapy was changed to intravenous foscarnet because of leukopenia.

The HIV load decreased to an undetectable level and the CMV retinitis remained quiescent with foscarnet therapy. On examination, visual acuity was 20/25 in the right eye and 20/40 in the left. Slit-lamp biomicroscopy revealed anterior chamber cells and flare and moderate vitritis in both eyes. Retinal examination revealed stable CMV retinitis involving the midperipheral retina bilaterally. Slight macular edema was noted, which was worse in the left eye. The CD4+ cell count increased and anti-CMV therapy was stopped. The CMV retinitis remained inactive when anticytomegalovirus therapy was stopped; however, over the next year vitritis and macular edema in both eyes worsened, with visual acuity dropping to 20/40 in the right eye and 20/63 in the left. The patient was offered treatment with periocular or systemic corticosteroids, but refused antiinflammatory drug therapy.

References

1. Achega JB, Hislop M, Dowdy DW, et al. Adherence to nonnucleoside reverse transcriptase inhibitor-based HIV therapy and virologic outcomes. Ann Intern Med 2007; 146: 564–573.

2. Gallo R. The AIDS virus. Sci Am 1987; 256: 46–56.

3. The global HIV and AIDS epidemic, 2001. MMWR Morb Mortal Wkly Rep 2001; 50: 434–439.

4. Hall HI, Song R, Rhodes P, et al. Estimation of HIV incidence in the United States. JAMA 2008; 300: 520–529.

5. Curran JW, Morgan WM, Hardy AM, et al. The epidemiology of AIDS: current status and future prospects. Science 1985; 229: 1352–1357.

6. Layon J, Warzynski M, Idus R. Acquired immunodeficiency syndrome in the United States – a selective review. Crit Care Med 1986; 14: 819–827.

7. Salahuddin SZ, Palestine AG, Heck E, et al. Isolation of the human T-cell leukemia/lymphotropic virus type III from the cornea. Am J Ophthalmol 1986; 101: 149–152.

8. Pomerantz RJ, Kuritzkes DR, de la Monte SM, et al. Infection of the retina by human immunodeficiency virus type I. N Engl J Med 1987; 317: 1643–1647.

9. Mellors JW, Munoz A, Giorgi JV, et al. Plasma viral load and CD4+ lymphocytes as prognostic markers of HIV-1 infection. Ann Intern Med 1997; 126: 946–954.

10. Hanna GJ, Hirsch MS. Antiretroviral therapy of human immunodeficiency virus infection. In Mandell GL, Bennett JE, Dolin R, editors: Principles and Practice of Infectious Diseases, ed 6, Philadelphia, 2005, Elsevier, pp 1655–1678.

11. Palestine AG, Rodrigues MM, Macher AM, et al. Ophthalmic involvement in the acquired immune deficiency syndrome. Ophthalmology 1984; 91: 1092–1099.

12. Freeman WR, Lerner CW, Mines JA, et al. A prospective study of the ophthalmologic findings in the acquired immune deficiency syndrome. Am J Ophthalmol 1984; 97: 133–142.

13. Newsome DA, Green WR, Miller ED, et al. Microvascular aspects of acquired immune deficiency syndrome retinopathy, Am J Ophthalmol 1984; 98: 590–601.

14. Kestelyn P, Van de Perre P, Rouvroy D, et al. A prospective study of the ophthalmologic findings in the acquired immune deficiency syndrome in Africa. Am J Ophthalmol 1985; 100: 230–238.

15. Pepose JS, Holland GN, Nestor MS, et al. Acquired immune deficiency syndrome: pathogenic mechanisms of ocular disease. Ophthalmology 1985; 92: 474–484.

16. Meillet D, Hoang PL, Unanue F, et al. Filtration and local synthesis of lacrimal proteins in acquired immunodeficiency syndrome. Eur J Clin Chem Clin Biochem 1992; 30: 319–323.

17. Belfort R Jr, de Smet M, Whitcup SM, et al. Ocular complications of Stevens–Johnson syndrome and toxic epidermal necrolysis in patients with AIDS. Cornea 1991; 10: 536–538.

18. Freeman WR, Van Natta ML, Jabs D, et al. Vision function in HIV-infected individuals without retinitis: report of the Studies of Ocular Complications of AIDS Research Group. Am J Ophthalmol 2008; 145: 453–462.

19. Schuman JS, Friedman AH. Retinal manifestations of the acquired immune deficiency syndrome. Trans Ophthalmol Soc UK 1983; 103: 177–189.

20. Weiss A, Margo CE, Ledford DK, et al. Toxoplasmic retinochoroiditis as an initial manifestation of the acquired immune deficiency syndrome. Am J Ophthalmol 1986; 101: 248–249.

21. Stoumbos VD, Klein ML. Syphilitic retinitis in a patient with acquired immunodeficiency syndrome-related complex. Am J Ophthalmol 1987; 103: 103–104.

22. Croxatto JO, Mestre C, Puente S, et al. Nonreactive tuberculosis in a patient with acquired immune deficiency syndrome. Am J Ophthalmol 1986; 102: 659–660.

23. Macher A, Rodrigue MM, Kaplan W, et al. Disseminated bilateral chorioretinitis due to Histoplasma capsulatum in a patient with the acquired immunodeficiency syndrome. Ophthalmology 1985; 92: 1159–1164.

24. Sandor EV, Millman A, Croxson TS, et al. Herpes zoster ophthalmicus in patients at risk for the acquired immune deficiency syndrome (AIDS). Am J Ophthalmol 1986; 101: 153–155.

25. Egbert PR, Pollard RB, Gallagher JG, et al. Cytomegalovirus retinitis in immunosuppressed hosts. II. Ocular manifestations. Ann Intern Med 1980; 93: 664–670.

26. Kupperman BD, Petty JG, Richman DD, et al. Correlation between CD4+ counts and the prevalence of cytomegalovirus retinitis and human immunodeficiency virus-related noninfectious retinal vasculopathy in patients with acquired immunodeficiency syndrome. Am J Ophthalmol 1993; 115: 575–582.

27. Studies of Ocular Complications of AIDS Research Group in collaboration with the AIDS Clinical Trials Group. Mortality in patients with the acquired immunodeficiency syndrome treated with either foscarnet or ganciclovir for cytomegalovirus retinitis. N Engl J Med 1992; 326: 213–220.

28. Jacobson MA, O'Donnell JJ, Porteous D, et al. Retinal and gastrointestinal disease due to cytomegalovirus in patients with the acquired immune deficiency syndrome: prevalence, natural history, and response to ganciclovir therapy. QJ Med 1988; 67: 473–486.

29. Lalezari JP, Stagg RJ, Kuppermann BD, et al. Intravenous cidofovir for peripheral cytomegalovirus retinitis in patients with AIDS: a randomized, controlled trial. Ann Intern Med 1997; 126: 257–263.

30. Studies of Ocular Complications of AIDS Research Group in collaboration with the AIDS Clinical Trials Group. Parenteral cidofovir for cytomegalovirus retinitis in patients with AIDS: the HPMPC peripheral cytomegalovirus retinitis trial: a randomized, controlled trial. Ann Intern Med 1997; 126: 264–274.

31. Martin DF, Parks DJ, Mellow SD, et al. Treatment of cytomegalovirus retinitis with an intraocular sustained-release ganciclovir implant. A randomized controlled clinical trial. Arch Ophthalmol 1994; 112: 1531–1539.

32. Cavert W, Notermans DW, Staskus K, et al. Kinetics of response in lymphoid tissues to antiretroviral therapy of HIV-1 infection. Science 1997; 276: 960–963.

33. Perelson AS, Essunger P, Cao Y, et al. Decay characteristics of HIV-1-infected compartments during combination therapy. Nature 1997; 387: 188–191.

34. Palella FJ, Delaney KM, Moorman AC, et al. Declining morbidity and mortality among patients with advanced human immunodeficiency virus infection. N Engl J Med 1998; 338: 853–860.

35. Holtzer CD, Jacobson MA, Hakley WK, et al. Decline in the rate of specific opportunistic infections at San Francisco General Hospital, 1994–1997. AIDS 1998; 12: 1931–1933.

36. Whitcup SM, Fortin E, Nussenblatt RB, et al. Therapeutic effect of combination antiretroviral therapy on cytomegalovirus retinitis. JAMA 1997; 277: 1519–1520.

37. Vrabec TR, Baldassano VF, Whitcup SM. Discontinuation of maintenance therapy in patients with quiescent cytomegalovirus retinitis and elevated CD4+ counts. Ophthalmology 1998; 105: 1259–1264.

38. Whitcup SM, Cunningham ET Jr, Polis MA, et al. Spontaneous and sustained resolution of CMV retinitis in patients receiving highly active antiretroviral therapy. Br J Ophthalmol 1998; 82: 845–846.

39. Whitcup SM, Fortin E, Lindblad AS, et al. Discontinuation of anticytomegalovirus therapy in patients with HIV infection and cytomegalovirus retinitis. JAMA 1999; 282: 1633–1637.

40. Reed JB, Schwab IR, Gordon J, et al. Regression of cytomegalovirus retinitis associated with protease inhibitor treatment in patients with AIDS. Am J Ophthalmol 1997; 124: 199–205.

41. Tural C, Romeu J, Siera G, et al. Long-lasting remission of cytomegalovirus retinitis without maintenance therapy in human immunodeficiency virus-infected patients. J Infect Dis 1998; 177: 1080–1083.

42. Macdonald JC, Torriani FJ, Morse LS, et al. Lack of reactivation of cytomegalovirus (CMV) retinitis after stopping maintenance therapy in AIDS patients with sustained elevations in CD4 T cells in response to highly active antiretroviral therapy. J Infect Dis 1998; 177: 1182–1187.

43. Jabs DA, Bolton SG, Dunn JP, et al. Discontinuing anticytomegalovirus therapy in patients with immune reconstitution after combination antiretroviral therapy. Am J Ophthalmol 1998; 126: 817–822.

44. Kirk O, Reiss P, Uberti-Foppa C, et al. Safe interruption of maintenance therapy against previous infection with four common HIV-associated opportunistic pathogens during potent antiretroviral therapy. Ann Intern Med 2002; 137: 239–250.

45. Komanduri KV, Viswanathan MN, Wieder ED, et al. Restoration of cytomegalovirus-specific CD4+ T-lymphocyte responses after ganciclovir and highly active antiretroviral therapy in individuals infected with HIV-1. Nature Med 1998; 4: 953–956.

46. Connors M, Kovacs JA, Krevat S, et al. HIV induces changes in CD4+ T-cell phenotype and depletions within the CD4+ T-cell repertoire that are not immediately restored by antiviral or immune-based therapies. Nature Med 1998; 3: 533–540.

47. Lederman MM, Connick E, Landay A, et al. Immunologic responses associated with 12 weeks of combination antiretroviral therapy consisting of zidovudine, lamivudine, and ritonavir: results of AIDS Clinical Trials Group protocol 315. J Infect Dis 1998; 178: 70–79.

48. Palestine AG, Stevens G, Lane HC, et al. Treatment of cytomegalovirus retinitis with dihydroxy propoxymethyl guanine. Am J Ophthalmol 1986; 101: 95–101.

49. Holland GN, Sakamoto MJ, Hardy D, et al. Treatment of cytomegalovirus retinopathy in patients with acquired immunodeficiency syndrome. Arch Ophthalmol 1986; 104: 1794–1800.

50. D'Amico DJ, Talamo JH, Felsenstein D, et al. Ophthalmoscopic and histologic findings in cytomegaovirus retinitis treated with BW-B759U. Arch Ophthalmol 1986; 104: 1788–1793.

51. Studies of Ocular Complications of Aids Research Group. Mortality in patients with the acquired immunodeficiency syndrome treated with either foscarnet or ganciclovir for cytomegalovirus retinitis. N Engl J Med 1992; 326: 213–220.

52. Palestine AG, Polis MA, De Smet MD, et al. A randomized controlled trial of foscarnet in the treatment of cytomegalovirus retinitis in patients with AIDS. Ann Intern Med 1991; 115: 665–673.

53. Studies of ocular complications of AIDS Research Group, in collaboration with the AIDS Clinical Trials Group. Morbidity and toxic effects associated with ganciclovir or foscarnet therapy in a randomized cytomegalovirus retinitis trial. Arch Intern Med 1995; 155: 65–74.

54. Perry CM, Balfour JA. Fomivirsen. Drugs 1999; 57: 375–380.

55. Martin DF, Kuppermann BD, Wolitz RA, et al. Oral ganciclovir for patients with cytomegalovirus retinitis treated with a ganciclovir implant. Roche Ganciclovir Study Group. N Engl J Med 1999; 340: 1063–1070.

56. Henry K, Cantrill H, Fletcher C, et al. Use of intravitreal ganciclovir (dihydroxy propoxymethyl guanine) for cytomegalovirus retinitis in a patient with AIDS. Am J Ophthalmol 1987; 103: 17–23.

57. Diaz-Llopis M, Chipont E, Sanchez S, et al. Intravitreal foscarnet of cytomegalovirus in a patient with acquired immunodeficiency syndrome. Am J Ophthalmol 1992; 114: 742–747.

58. Kirsch LS, Arevalo JF, De Clercq E, et al. Phase I/II study of intravitreal cidofovir for the treatment of cytomegalovirus retinitis in patients with the acquired immunodeficiency syndrome. Am J Ophthalmol 1995; 119: 466–476.

59. Kirsch L, Arevalo JF, Chavez de la Pax E, et al. Intravitreal cidofovir (HPMPC) treatment of cytomegalovirus retinitis in patients with acquired immune deficiency syndrome. Ophthalmology 1995; 102: 533–543.

60. Paya C, Humar A, Dominguez E, et al. Valganciclovir Solid Organ Transplant Study Group. Efficacy and safety of valganciclovir vs. oral ganciclovir for prevention of cytomegalovirus disease in solid organ transplant recipients. Am J Transplant 2004; 4: 611–620.

61. Martin DF, Sierra-Madero J, Walmsley S, et al. A controlled trial of valganciclovir as induction therapy for cytomegalovirus retinitis. N Engl J Med 2002; 346: 1119–1126.

62. Jabs DA. AIDS and Ophthalmology, 2008. Arch Ophthalmol 2008; 126: 113–1146.

63. Feinberg MB, Carpenter C, Fauci AS, et al. Report of the NIH panel to define principles of therapy of HIV infection. Ann Intern Med 1998; 128: 1057–1078.

64. Centers for Disease Control and Prevention. 1999 USPHS/IDSA guidelines for the prevention of opportunistic infections in persons infected with human immunodeficiency virus. MMWR Morb Mortal Wkly Rep 1999; 48: 1–66.

65. Drew WL, Ives D, Lalezari JP, et al. Oral ganciclovir as maintenance treatment for cytomegalovirus retinitis in patients with AIDS, N Engl J Med 1995; 333: 615–620.

66. Martin DF, Sierra-Madero J, Walmsley S, et al. A controlled trial of valganciclovir as induction therapy for cytomegalovirus retinitis. N Engl J Med 2002; 346: 1119–1126.

67. Freeman WR, Friedberg DN, Berry C, et al. Risk factors for the development of rhegmatogenous retinal detachment in patients with cytomegalovirus retinitis. Am J Ophthalmol 1993; 116: 713–720.

68. Thorne JE, Jabs DA, Kempen JH, et al. Incidence of and risk factors for visual acuity loss among patients with AIDS and cytomegalovirus retinitis in the era of highly active antiretroviral therapy. Ophthalmology 2006; 113: 1001–1008.

69. Palestine AG, Rodrigues MM, Macher AM, et al. Ophthalmic involvement in acquired immunodeficiency syndrome. Ophthalmology 1984; 91: 1092–1099.

70. Jabs DA, Bartlett JG. AIDS and ophthalmology: a period of transition. Am J Ophthalmol 1997; 124: 227–233.

71. Zegans ME, Walton RC, Holland GN, et al. Transient vitreous inflammatory reactions associated with combination antiretroviral therapy in patients with AIDS and cytomegalovirus retinitis. Am J Ophthalmol 1998; 125: 292–300.

72. Karavellas MP, Lowder CY, Macdonald JC, et al. Immune recovery vitritis

associated with inactive cytomegalovirus retinitis: a new syndrome. Arch Ophthalmol 1998; 116: 169–175.

73. Weinberg DV, Moorthy RS. Cystoid macular edema due to cytomegalovirus in a patient with acquired immunodeficiency virus. Retina 1996; 16: 1443–1445.

74. Zegans ME, Walton RC, Holland GN, et al. Transient vitreous inflammatory reactions associated with combination antiretroviral therapy in patients with AIDS and cytomegalovirus retinitis. Am J Ophthalmol 1998; 125: 292–300.

75. Whitcup SM. Cytomegalovirus retinitis in the era of highly active antiretroviral therapy. JAMA 2000; 283: 653–657.

76. Robinson MR, Reed G, Csaky KG, et al. Immune-recovery uveitis in patients with cytomegalovirus retinitis taking highly active antiretroviral therapy. Am J Ophthalmol 2000; 130: 49–56.

77. Karavellas MP, Plummer DJ, Macdonald JC, et al. Incidence of immune recovery vitritis in cytomegalovirus retinitis in patients following institution of successful highly active antiretroviral therapy. J Infect Dis 1999; 179: 697–700.

78. Ortega-Larrocea G, Espinosa E, Reyes-Teran G. Lower incidence and severity of cytomegalovirus-associated immune recovery uveitis in HIV-infected patients with delayed highly active antiretroviral therapy. Ophthalmology 2006; 19: 735–738.

79. The Studies of Ocular Complications of AIDS Research Group in collaboration with the AIDS Clinical Trials Group. Rhegmatogenous retinal detachment in patients with cytomegalovirus retinitis: the Foscarnet-Ganciclovir Cytomegalovirus Retinitis Trial. Am J Ophthalmol 1997; 121: 61–70.

80. Morrison VL, Kozak I, LaBree LD, et al. Intravitreal triamcinolone acetonide for the treatment of immune recovery uveitis macular edema. Ophthamology 2007; 114: 334–339.

81. Race EM, Adelson-Mitty J, Kriegel GR, et al. Focal mycobacterial lymphadenitis following initiation of protease-inhibitor therapy in patients with advanced HIV-1 disease. Lancet 1998; 351: 252–255.

82. Woods ML, MacGinley R, Eisen DP, et al. HIV combination therapy: partial immune restitution unmasking latent cryptococcal infection. AIDS 1998; 12: 1491–1494.

83. Sellitti TP, Huang AJ, Schiffman J, et al. Association of herpes zoster ophthalmicus with the acquired immunodeficiency syndrome and acute retinal necrosis. Am J Ophthalmol 1992; 116: 297–301.

84. Forster DJ, Dugel PU, Frangieh GT, et al. Rapidly progressive outer retinal necrosis in the acquired immunodeficiency syndrome. Am J Ophthalmol 1990; 110: 341–348.

85. Johnston WH, Holland GN, Engstrom RE, et al. Recurrence of presumed varicella zoster virus retinopathy in patients with the acquired immunodeficiency syndrome. Am J Ophthalmol 1993; 116: 42–50.

86. Yin PD, Kurup SK, Fischer SH, et al. Progressive outer retinal necrosis in the era of highly active antiretroviral therapy: successful management with intravitreal injections and monitoring with quantitative PCR. J Clin Virol 2007; 38: 254–259.

87. Macher AM, Bardenstein DS, Zimmerman LE, et al. *Pneumocystis carinii* choroiditis in a male homosexual with AIDS and disseminated pulmonary and extrapulmonary *P. carinii* infection. N Engl J Med 1987; 316: 1092.

88. Sha BE, Benson CA, Deutsch T, et al. *Pneumocystis carinii* choroiditis in patients with AIDS: clinical features, response to therapy and outcome. J AIDS 1992; 5: 1051–1058.

89. Whitcup SM, Fenton RM, Pluda JM, et al. *Pneumocystis carinii* and *Mycobacterium avium-intracellulare* infection of the choroid. Retina 1992; 12: 331–335.

90. Morinelli EN, Dugel PU, Riffenburgh R, et al. Infectious multifocal choroiditis in patients with acquired immune deficiency syndrome. Ophthalmology 1993; 100: 1014–1021.

91. Stanton CA, Sloan B III, Slusher MM, et al. Acquired immunodeficiency syndrome-related primary intraocular lymphoma. Arch Ophthalmol 1992; 110: 1614–1617.

92. Johns DR, Tierney M, Felsenstein D. Alteration in the natural history of neurosyphilis by concurrent infection with the human immunodeficiency virus. N Engl J Med 1987; 316: 1569–1572.

93. Shafran SD, Deschenes J, Miller M, et al. Uveitis and pseudojaundice during a regimen of clarithromycin, rifabutin and ethambutol. N Engl J Med 1994; 330: 438–439.

94. Whitcup SM, Butler KM, Caruso R, et al. Retinal toxicity in human immunodeficiency virus-infected children treated with 2′,3′-dideoxyinosine. Am J Ophthalmol 1992; 113: 1–7.

Acute Retinal Necrosis and Progressive Outer Retinal Necrosis

Scott M. Whitcup

Key concepts

- Despite effective antiviral therapies, herpes infection of the eye can lead to severe uveitis with substantial vision loss.
- Because acute retinal necrosis (ARN) can often begin as an anterior uveitis, examination of the peripheral retina is important in all patients with a new onset of anterior inflammation.
- Many patients with ARN benefit from antiviral therapy; oral aciclovir, valaciclovir, and famciclovir have all been used.
- Retinal detachment and optic nerve involvement remain important causes of vision loss in patients with ARN.
- Progressive outer retinal necrosis (PORN) is thought to be a variant of a necrotizing herpetic retinopathy in immunocompromised patients.
- Combination antiretrovial therapy in PORN may improve prognosis.

Despite many advances in the diagnosis and treatment of ocular disease, viral infections affecting the eye remain difficult to diagnose and difficult to treat. Many cases of uveitis, including multifocal choroiditis, acute posterior multifocal placoid pigment epitheliopathy (APMPPE), and multiple evanescent white-dot syndrome (MEWDS), are presumed to be caused by viral infection. Nevertheless, antiviral agents rarely are used in their treatment because the evidence supporting the viral etiology is anecdotal. For example, Epstein–Barr virus (EBV) infection has been associated with multifocal choroiditis and panuveitis;[1,2] however, because EBV infection is so ubiquitous it is difficult to prove a definite causal relationship between the virus and the choroidal disease. Many viral infections associated with uveitis are discussed in the chapter on white-dot syndromes (see Chapter 29). This chapter focuses on two disorders associated with herpes virus infections: acute retinal necrosis, and progressive outer retinal necrosis. Two other important viral infections causing uveitis – herpes simplex virus and herpes zoster virus – are discussed in Chapter 13.

Acute retinal necrosis

The evolution in our understanding of the etiology and pathophysiology of acute retinal necrosis (ARN) is an example of how scientific knowledge can improve our ability to accurately diagnose and treat inflammatory eye disease. ARN was initially described in 1971 in a report by Urayama and colleagues,[3] in which the authors documented the clinical findings of six patients with intraocular inflammation, retinal vascular sheathing, and large white confluent retinal infiltrates in one eye. The disease was called Kirisawa's uveitis, and these patients, in whom rhegmatogenous retinal detachments subsequently developed, were left with poor visual acuity. No etiologic agent was identified, and no therapy appeared to affect the outcome of the disease.

Additional cases of retinitis with rhegmatogenous retinal detachment were reported in the late 1970s,[4,5] and these retinal detachments were difficult to repair because of both tractional and rhegmatogenous components. Cases of bilateral acute retinal necrosis (BARN) were also described.[6] In 1982 the finding by Culbertson and colleagues[7] of herpes virus in the retina of patients with ARN paved the way for specific antiviral therapy for the disease. Nevertheless, late retinal detachment remains a serious complication despite the use of prophylactic laser photocoagulation and modern vitreoretinal surgical techniques.

Is ARN a new disease or just newly recognized? Few if any similar occurrences were reported before 1971, yet numerous reports on the topic have appeared in the literature since that time. Many investigators believe that ARN is a new disease, possibly due to mutations in the virus or changes in host susceptibility. Others believe that improved diagnostic techniques and awareness of the disease have led to increased recognition.

Epidemiology

Initially reported in Japan, ARN has now been widely reported throughout Europe and North America, with sporadic cases reported around the world. ARN can occur in patients of either sex and at any age, although there may be a slight male preponderance. Although the disease is typically thought to affect young adults, ARN has been reported in children[8,9] and in elderly patients as well. Although this disease was initially described in immunocompetent patients, ARN has now been documented in patients with immunosuppression, such as those with AIDS,[10,11] and in patients on immunosuppression or following bone marrow transplantation.[12]

Clinical features

The disease may affect one or both eyes; most cases begin with unilateral disease.[8] In almost one-third of patients the

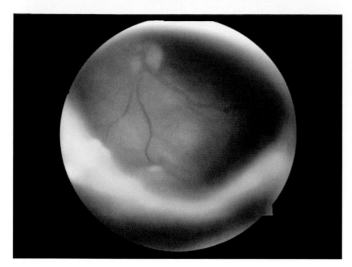

Figure 12-1. Acute retinal necrosis with dense white retinal infiltrate in retinal periphery.

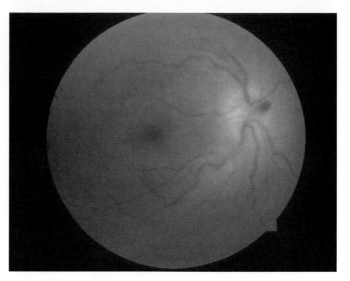

Figure 12-2. Posterior pole of the retina 1 week after the onset of symptoms of acute retinal necrosis and after vitrectomy had been performed demonstrating optic disc swelling and retinal perivascular sheathing.

second eye becomes involved, usually within 1–6 weeks; however, disease in the second eye has been reported to occur up to 20 years after that in the first eye.[13,14] Most patients have a history of pain, redness, floaters, and blurred vision. An anterior uveitis with or without keratic precipitates often occurs early in the disease, and although a plasmoid aqueous has been described in these patients, hypopyon is rare. Occasionally there is an associated herpes infection at another site,[4,15] but most patients are healthy, immunocompetent, and without systemic symptoms.

With the onset of vitritis, patients report floaters and diminished visual acuity. Vitritis tends to worsen as cellular immunity to the virus occurs, and the infiltrating inflammatory cells are predominantly lymphocytes and plasma cells.[7] The earliest retinal lesions are small, patchy, white-yellow areas that tend to enlarge, increase in number, and coalesce over time (**Fig. 12-1**). They usually start in the midperiphery; occasionally they occur in the posterior pole, but do not follow the architecture of the retinal vessels. After several weeks the lesions begin to resolve, with areas of clearing forming a Swiss cheese pattern. At this time perturbation of the retinal pigment epithelium (RPE) also develops. Retinal vasculitis is another manifestation of ARN (**Fig. 12-2**). Patients often have a severe retinal arteritis. Capillary nonperfusion can be documented on fluorescein angiography, and periphlebitis and venous occlusions have been described less commonly. Retinal hemorrhage can occur, especially in patients with venous occlusive disease. In contrast to findings with other venous occlusive diseases, neovascularization of the iris or retina is uncommon but reported.[16,17] The choroidal vasculature is also involved in this disease, and fluorescein angiography has shown areas of early hypofluorescence and late staining consistent with ischemia-induced inflammatory changes.

Optic neuropathy also occurs in patients with ARN. Disc edema is a common finding early in the course of the disease,[8] and Sergott and colleagues[18] described two patients with intraorbital optic nerve enlargement. Optic nerve involvement should be suspected in patients with an afferent pupillary defect and severe visual loss with few retinal findings. Visual field testing and color vision assessment can be instructive. Visual loss may be caused by vascular occlusive disease, viral infiltration of the nerve, or optic nerve distension. Optic nerve sheath fenestration has been proposed as a possible therapeutic intervention,[19] but its effect has been unproven in well-controlled clinical trials. ARN has also been reported in patients with clinical findings of viral meningitis.[20]

The acute inflammatory disease tends to resolve over several months with or without therapy. In untreated patients the acute phase usually resolves in 2–3 months. The course of the disease can also be predicted by the number of clock hours of initial retinal involvement. Unfortunately, within the next several months tractional and rhegmatogenous retinal detachments with many large breaks develop in up to 86% of patients.[8,21] Despite control of the active viral replication in the retina, cellular infiltration into the vitreous and the formation of vitreal membranes composed of RPE and fibroblasts develop and contribute to the tearing and detachment of an already thinned retina.[22]

The Executive Committee of the American Uveitis Society published a set of standard diagnostic criteria for the ARN syndrome,[23] stating that the designation of ARN syndrome should be based solely on clinical appearance and the course of infection. Clinical characteristics that must be seen include (1) one or more foci of retinal necrosis with discrete borders in the peripheral retina; (2) rapid progression of disease if antiviral therapy has not been given; (3) circumferential spread of disease; (4) evidence of occlusive vasculopathy with arteriolar involvement; and (5) a prominent inflammatory reaction in the vitreous and anterior chamber. Optic nerve involvement, scleritis, and pain support but are not required for the diagnosis, and macular lesions, although less common, do not preclude a diagnosis of ARN if peripheral lesions are present.

Etiology

ARN was initially believed to be an autoimmune disease.[22] In 1982 Culbertson and colleagues[7] described the first occurrence of an enucleated eye in a patient with ARN, in which

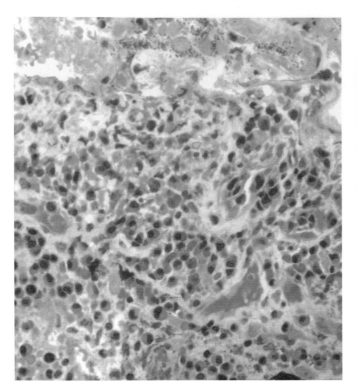

Figure 12-3. Histologic section of chorioretinal biopsy specimen from a patient with acute retinal necrosis showing lymphocytic infiltration and areas of necrosis. (Hematoxylin & eosin stain; ×400). *(Courtesy of Chi-Chao Chan, MD.)*

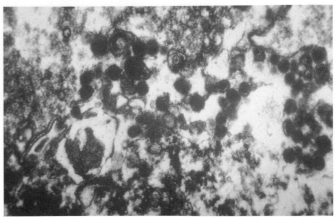

Figure 12-4. Electron micrograph demonstrating herpes class virions in retinal biopsy specimen from a patient with acute retinal necrosis.

herpes virus particles were noted in the retina on electron microscopy. However, virus was not cultured from the eye, and serum antibodies were found to herpes simplex, herpes zoster, cytomegalovirus (CMV), and EBV. Histologic examination showed prominent retinal arteritis and marked retinal necrosis with abrupt demarcation between normal and necrotic retina. Optic nerve inflammation was also noted. A similar histologic picture was seen in a retinal biopsy specimen we obtained from a patient with ARN in 1983, which revealed inflammatory cell infiltration and necrosis of the retina (**Fig. 12-3**). There was a predominance of T lymphocytes in the vitreous, but the retina contained many B lymphocytes, which suggested that antibody to the virus could be produced locally in the retina. Finally, the results of electron microscopy showed herpes class viral particles (**Fig. 12-4**), although virus was not cultured from the specimen. In 1986 Culbertson and colleagues[24] used immunohistochemical staining to reveal herpes zoster in two eyes with ARN, and also succeeded in culturing the virus from one of the two eyes. Varicella-zoster virus was initially thought to account for most of the typical cases of ARN; however, herpes simplex types 1 and 2, and rarely CMV were also implicated as a cause of the disease.[25–29] Herpes simplex virus was also implicated in ARN because of serially increasing serum and intraocular antibody levels; however, these may result from a nonspecific polyclonal activation of B cells in the inflammatory process rather than a humoral immune response against a specific virus involved in the current disease.

In a retrospective study of 28 patients, Ganatra and colleagues[30] used polymerase chain reaction (PCR) to show that varicella-zoster virus or herpes simplex virus type 1 caused ARN in patients older than 25 years, whereas herpes simplex virus type 2 caused ARN in patients younger than 25 years. Van Gelder and associates[31] also report that herpes simplex virus type 2 is an important cause of ARN, particularly in young patients. Sugita and colleagues more recently analyzed ocular fluid samples from 16 patients with ARN.[32] High copy numbers of HSV1, HSV2, or VZV were found in all the samples from the 16 patients, suggesting active viral replication.

Although data from PCR support the role of herpes virus infection in ARN, it is difficult to recommend the use of PCR for the diagnosis of ARN. First, vitreous specimens are probably needed for the analysis. Second, some caution in interpreting PCR data is warranted. PCR is so sensitive a test that viral DNA from a previous infection years earlier may yield confusing results, especially because viral infection with herpes simplex, CMV, and herpes zoster are quite common.

Other experimental data support the role of herpes virus infection in the pathogenesis of ARN. Injection of herpes simplex virus type 1 in BALB/c mice produces a necrotizing retinitis in the contralateral eye within about 10 days.[33] This animal model is similar to ARN in humans and has yielded interesting immunologic insights into the pathophysiologic course of the disease. The necrotizing retinitis develops only in immunocompetent animals. In addition, disease develops in the contralateral eye only if it is infected with virus via the optic nerve. Thus, as in other inflammatory eye diseases, retinal damage, initially induced by an infectious agent, leads to a secondary immune response against previously sequestered retinal antigens. This secondary immune response can then propagate the inflammatory damage to the retina.

Other factors may play a role in the pathogenesis of ARN. Holland and colleagues[34] showed an association between ARN and HLA-DQw7 and phenotype Bw62, DR4. These data suggest that some persons may have a genetically determined predisposition to mounting an immune response against certain infectious agents that promotes the development of ocular inflammatory disease. Some data provide evidence for antigen-specific immune deviation in patients with acute retinal necrosis. Varicella-zoster virus-associated ARN developed in patients in whom delayed hypersensitivity to viral antigens was absent.[35] In this study, delayed

Box 12-1 Differential diagnosis of acute retinal necrosis syndrome

Exogenous bacterial endophthalmitis
Fungal endophthalmitis
Behçet's disease
Pars planitis
Toxoplasmosis
Syphilis
Cytomegalovirus retinitis
Sarcoidosis
Intraocular lymphoma
Progressive outer retinal necrosis syndrome

hypersensitivity responses were restored in patients who recovered from the disease. In another study, Fas and Fas ligand expression were absent in a retinal biopsy from a patient with ARN.[36] Furthermore, apoptosis was noted on the specimen, suggesting a role in the disease. Finally, inflammatory cytokines may be involved in the development of ARN. Intraocular inoculation of herpes virus induced vascular endothelial growth factor, flk-1, transforming growth factor β_2, and interleukin (IL)-6 in the retina of injected and contralateral eyes in experimental animals.[37]

Differential diagnosis

Because ARN can often begin as an anterior uveitis, examination of the peripheral retina is important in all patients with a new onset of anterior inflammation. The differential diagnosis of ARN is listed in **Box 12-1**. In general, only Behçet's disease and endophthalmitis mimic the rapid progression and severity of ARN. The lesions of Behçet's disease rarely present with a uniform distribution in the periphery of the retina and are often associated with systemic symptoms and signs such as arthritis, mouth and genital ulcers, and skin lesions. Vitrectomy may be needed to rule out endophthalmitis. Toxoplasmic retinochoroiditis, syphilitic retinitis and intraocular lymphoma more rarely mimic ARN.[38]

Therapy

Many patients appear to benefit from treatment with aciclovir. Aciclovir has good activity against herpes simplex virus and, at slightly higher concentrations, is effective against herpes zoster. Although aciclovir is not as good a drug as ganciclovir or foscarnet for treating CMV infection, because CMV is rarely a cause of ARN and aciclovir is easier to administer and safer, it is the best initial therapy for the disease. Patients with newly diagnosed ARN can be treated with a 10–14-day course of intravenously administered aciclovir 500 mg/m^2 every 8 hours. Oral aciclovir 800 mg five times a day is then continued for an additional 6 weeks. The goal of therapy is to hasten the resolution of disease in the infected eye and to prevent contralateral spread. However, the therapeutic benefits of aciclovir for ARN have not been studied in well-controlled, randomized clinical trials. Severe side effects with aciclovir are relatively rare. A reversible rise in the serum creatinine level and elevation in liver function test results may occur. The most commonly reported side effects include nausea, vomiting, and headache, but most of these occur in fewer than 3% of patients.

Unfortunately, there have been no randomized prospective clinical trials of aciclovir specifically for the treatment of ARN. In a retrospective study by Palay and colleagues,[39] 87.1% of patients treated with aciclovir did not develop contralateral disease, compared to 35.1% of patients not receiving the drug. Other case series seem to show that retinal lesions resolve more quickly after initiation of aciclovir, but therapy does not appear to diminish vitritis or to prevent subsequent retinal detachment.[21,40] Patients with severe and progressive disease despite aciclovir therapy may be treated with ganciclovir or foscarnet. In addition, systemic corticosteroids such as prednisone 0.5–1.0 mg/kg can be added after the patient has received 24–48 hours of intravenous aciclovir. Steroids can be slowly tapered based on the amount of vitritis. Because of the extensive retinal arteritis and development of retinal vascular occlusions, some have suggested aspirin therapy,[41] but again this therapy has not been scrutinized in a clinical trial. Intravitreal injections with antiviral agents may be useful as adjunctive therapy in patients with ARN.[42]

Both valaciclovir and famciclovir offer more convenient dosage regimens. Famciclovir at a dose of 500 mg three times daily had efficacy similar to that of aciclovir in treating patients with ophthalmic zoster.[43] Valaciclovir is rapidly converted to aciclovir and the usual dose is 1 g orally three times daily, resulting in substantial vitreous penetration of aciclovir.[44] Importantly, in a 1-year prospective randomized clinical trial, recurrence of any type of ocular HSV disease was 23.1% in patients receiving valaciclovir compared to 23.1% in patients receiving aciclovir.[45] The use of either oral valaciclovir or famciclovir has resulted in regression of retinitis in patients in several case series.[46–48]

Retinal detachment and optic neuropathy remain the causes of severe visual loss in this disease. Laser photocoagulation to demarcate a zone between involved and uninvolved retina has been tried as a prophylactic therapy to prevent retinal detachment. Sternberg and colleagues[49] showed that retinal detachments occurred in two of 12 eyes receiving laser therapy and in four of six eyes not receiving laser therapy. However, this retrospective analysis may be biased because the condition of patients with the most severe disease and the worst vitritis may not have been amenable to laser therapy. Others have suggested prophylactic vitrectomy, scleral buckling, and endolaser treatment for eyes at high risk for retinal detachment, but there are few data to support this therapy.[50]

Clearly, surgery is warranted to repair retinal detachments in patients with ARN, although these detachments are difficult to repair and proliferative vitreoretinopathy is common.[21] Vitrectomy, fluid–gas exchange, and endolaser treatment have been suggested for complicated detachments.[51] Whether this therapy is better than vitrectomy with scleral buckling is unknown. Silicone oil has also been used successfully in some patients.

Less well studied is the effect of therapy on optic nerve disease. Optic nerve fenestration and corticosteroids have been used to treat optic neuropathy in ARN, but no well-controlled study data are available to support the effectiveness of these therapeutic interventions.

With the discovery of the viral etiology of ARN, specific therapy has been employed for the treatment of this disease. Nevertheless, many questions about ARN remain. We still do not know why certain individuals are more susceptible to developing the disease, because ARN is relatively rare but herpes virus infection is quite common. Finally, although aciclovir, valaciclovir, and famciclovir and corticosteroids are used to treat patients with ARN, there are still no randomized, masked, clinical trials definitively showing the benefits of therapy.

Progressive outer retinal necrosis

A syndrome characterized by rapidly progressive outer retinal necrosis (PORN) was initially described in immunocompromised patients. This syndrome seems to be different from ARN in immunocompromised patients and the prognosis is extremely poor. Unfortunately, it is thought to be the second most frequent opportunistic retinal infection in patients with AIDS in North America.[52]

Diagnosis

PORN is thought to be a variant of a necrotizing herpetic retinopathy in immunocompromised patients. The syndrome was described by Forster and colleagues in 1990[53] in two patients seropositive for human immunodeficiency virus (HIV). Margolis and coworkers[54] similarly described varicella-zoster virus retinitis in patients with AIDS, and also noted a rapidly progressive necrotizing retinitis with early patchy choroidal and deep retinal lesions which progressed relentlessly until patients were left with atrophic and necrotic retinas and pale optic nerves. Unlike typical ARN there is little or no vasculitis and less vitritis, and in many patients posterior pole involvement occurs early in the course of disease (**Fig. 12-5**).

Engstrom and colleagues[52] recently reviewed the cases of 38 AIDS patients with PORN. A definite history of cutaneous herpes zoster was documented in 22 of 33 patients (67%). The median CD4+ lymphocyte count in these patients was $21/mm^3$, with a range of $0–130/mm^3$. Most patients had a unilateral decrease in visual acuity, although about one-quarter of them had a presenting complaint of reduced peripheral vision or constriction of visual field. Asymptomatic disease was noted in seven of 65 eyes (11%). The median visual acuity at presentation was 20/30, but some patients had no light perception (NLP) vision at presentation. Anterior chamber and vitreous inflammation was minimal or absent in all patients. Multifocal, deep retinal lesions were typically found in the periphery; however, macular lesions were noted in 21 eyes (32%) at the time of diagnosis. Optic nerve involvement was present in 11 of 65 eyes (17%), and an afferent pupillary defect was noted in 11 of 29 patients (38%). Characteristic of this syndrome, the lesions rapidly progressed to confluence. Interestingly, although the syndrome is described as involving the outer retina, pathologic evidence suggests that the disease can cause substantial destruction of the inner retina late in its course.[53]

Differential diagnosis

The differential diagnosis for PORN is similar to that of ARN, and a comparison of their diagnostic criteria is noted in **Table 12-1**. It is important to differentiate these two disorders. Retinal lesions in PORN appear to predominantly involve the deep retina, whereas lesions in ARN appear to be full thickness. Posterior retinal lesions are more common in PORN, whereas anterior chamber inflammation and dense vitritis are characteristic of ARN but rare in PORN.

Table 12.1 Diagnostic criteria

Progressive Outer Retinal Necrosis Syndrome	Acute Retinal Necrosis Syndrome
Multifocal lesions characterized by deep retinal opacification without granular borders; there may be areas of confluent opacification	One or more foci of full-thickness retinal necrosis with discrete borders
Lesions located in the peripheral retina with or without macular involvement	Lesions located in the peripheral retina*
Extremely rapid progression of lesions No consistent direction of disease spread	Rapid progression of disease† Circumferential spread of disease around the peripheral retina
Absence of vascular inflammation	Evidence of occlusive vasculopathy, with arteriolar involvement
Minimal or absent intraocular inflammation	
Characteristics that support, but are not required, for diagnosis	Prominent inflammatory reaction in the vitreous and anterior chamber
Perivenular clearing of retinal opacification	Characteristics that support, but are not required, for diagnosis
	Scleritis
	Pain

From Engstrom RE Jr, Holland GN, Margolis TP, et al.: The progressive outer retinal necrosis syndrome: a variant of necrotizing herpetic retinopathy in patients with AIDS. Ophthalmology 1994; 101: 1488–1502.
*Involving the area adjacent to, or outside, the major temporal vascular arcades.
†Progression can be successfully halted in most patients with intravenous aciclovir therapy.

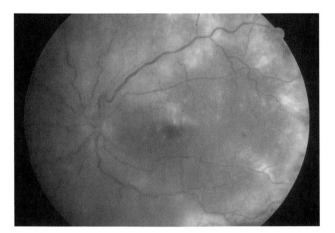

Figure 12-5. Diffuse retinitis involving posterior pole in patient with progressive outer retinal necrosis. Retinitis appears to involve the outer retina with little evidence of retinal vasculitis. *(Courtesy of Chris Walton, MD.)*

Similarly, vascular inflammation is also rare in PORN but common in ARN. Finally, lesions progress rapidly to confluence despite therapy in PORN, but are usually controlled with aciclovir therapy in ARN.

Etiology

Similar to ARN, varicella-zoster virus and herpes simplex virus have been implicated in the cause of PORN.[55] Most patients with PORN have had impaired immune status, due either to an underlying disease or to immunosuppressive therapy.

Therapy

We have tried various combinations of induction doses of intravenous ganciclovir and foscarnet, as well as intravitreal foscarnet, with little to no success. High-dose intravenous aciclovir at a dosage of 10 mg/kg every 8 hours for 2 weeks has also been used with inconsistent success. Others have reported that initial intravenous antiviral therapy appeared to reduce disease activity in 17 of 32 eyes (53%), but final visual outcome was not altered by therapy.[56] In this study, final visual acuity was NLP in 67% of eyes within 4 weeks after diagnosis. Some success has been reported with combination antiviral therapy, usually with intravenous foscarnet and either aciclovir or ganciclovir.[56] More recently, long-term preservation of vision has been reported using a combination of antiviral drugs with highly active antiretroviral therapy HAART).[57] Investigators treated patients with a ganciclovir implant, intravenous aciclovir (10 mg/kg every 8 hours, intravitreal foscarnet (2.4 mg), and HAART. Complications of the disorder included retinal detachment in 70% of eyes, despite prophylactic laser retinopexy in some.

Case 12-1

A 22-year-old woman developed sudden blurring of vision in the right eye, which was red and accompanied by a right-sided headache. One week later she saw an ophthalmologist, who diagnosed an anterior uveitis that was treated with topical corticosteroids. Three days later she developed a herpes simplex lesion on her lip, but an initial medical evaluation was uneventful. Two weeks after the initial symptoms, peripheral white lesions in the retina were noted. Vision in the right eye had decreased to 20/125. There were 3+ cells and 3+ flare in the anterior chamber and 4+ cells in the vitreous, and a diagnosis of acute retinal necrosis was made.

A vitrectomy was performed to improve visualization of the retinal lesions and for viral cultures. Viral culture results were negative; however, intravenous aciclovir was started after surgery. The white retinal lesions began to resolve. After 10 days the intravenous aciclovir was discontinued and the patient was treated with 200 mg of oral aciclovir five times daily. Laser photocoagulation was applied to the posterior edge of the white retinal lesions in an attempt to prevent retinal detachment. Two weeks later there was increased ocular inflammation and fibrin in the vitreous and the retina. Intravenous aciclovir was restarted and the inflammation slowly resolved. Vision 2 months later was 20/25 and remained stable without retinal detachment for more than 1 year.

Case 12-2

HIV infection was diagnosed in a 32-year-old African-American woman. Two years later she developed an immunoblastic B-cell non-Hodgkin's lymphoma involving the lung and nasopharynx. She was treated with six cycles of chemotherapy. After treatment, the patient reported a 3-day history of blurred vision in the left eye. Visual acuity was 20/16 in both eyes, and the results of slit-lamp biomicroscopy were normal. There were 1+ vitreous cells but no haze in the left eye, and funduscopic examination revealed multifocal lesions of the outer retina with no posterior pole involvement. The patient was immediately given induction doses of ganciclovir; however, the patches of retinitis continued to progress and coalesce. Induction doses of intravenous foscarnet were added to the regimen and seemed to halt progression of the retinitis. Nevertheless, 1 month later visual acuity had decreased to 5/125, with spread of the retinitis into the posterior pole (see Fig. 12-5), and a localized retinal detachment developed inferiorly. The CD4+ lymphocyte count at this time was <10 cells/mm^3. A diagnosis of PORN was made, and the patient was given maintenance doses of ganciclovir and foscarnet, with follow-up.

One week later the visual acuity had decreased to hand motions at a distance of 1 foot. The retinitis appeared to involve the deep retina; the retinal vessels were relatively spared. The patient was again treated with induction doses of foscarnet and maintenance doses of ganciclovir. The visual acuity remained limited to light perception in the left eye, but now multifocal lesions of the outer retina in the right eye developed (**Fig. 12-6**), which progressed rapidly. The patient was then treated with intravenous ganciclovir and intravitreal injections of foscarnet. Disease progression appeared to be halted in the right eye for the next 2 months, but she lost vision in that eye. At that time visual acuity was limited to light perception in the right eye and no light perception in the left. Retinal examination showed a cherry-red spot in the right macula with a diffuse area of retinitis and a large retinal detachment. The patient opted to stop therapy and died 2 years after the initial diagnosis of her ocular disease.

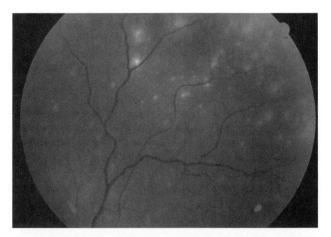

Figure 12-6. Multifocal punctate lesions involving outer retina early in the course of progressive outer retinal necrosis. These lesions quickly spread and coalesced despite therapy. *(Courtesy of Chris Walton, MD.)*

References

1. Tiedeman JS. Epstein–Barr viral antibodies in multifocal choroiditis and panuveitis. Am J Ophthalmol 1987; 103: 659–663.

2. Weber DJ, Hoffman KL, Thoft RA, et al. Endophthalmitis following intraocular lens implantation. Rev Infect Dis 1986; 8: 12–20.

3. Urayama A, Yamada N, Sasaki T, et al. Unilateral acute uveitis with periarteritis and detachment. Jpn J Clin Ophthalmol 1971; 25: 607–619.

4. Willerson D, Aaberg TM, Reeser FH. Necrotizing vaso-occlusive retinitis. Am J Ophthalmol 1977; 84: 209–219.

5. Young NJA, Bird AC. Bilateral acute retinal necrosis. Br J Ophthalmol 1978; 62: 581–590.

6. Price FW, Schlaegel TF. Bilateral acute retinal necrosis. Am J Ophthalmol 1980; 89: 419–424.

7. Culbertson WW, Blumenkranz MS, Haines H, et al. The acute retinal necrosis syndrome. II. Histopathology and etiology. Ophthalmology 1982; 89: 1317–1325.

8. Fisher JP, Lewis ML, Blumenkranz M, et al. The acute retinal necrosis syndrome. I. Clinical manifestations. Ophthalmology 1982; 89: 1309–1316.

9. Tan JCH, Byles D, Stanford MR, et al. Acute retinal necrosis in children caused by herpes simplex virus. Retina 2001; 21: 344–347.

10. Jabs DA, Schachat AP, Liss R, et al. Presumed varicella-zoster retinitis in immunocompromised patients. Retina 1987; 7: 9–13.

11. Friberg TR, Jost BF. Acute retinal necrosis in an immunosuppressed patient. Am J Ophthalmol 1984; 98: 515–517.

12. Kalpoe JS, van Dehn CE, Bollemeijer JG, et al. Varicella zoster virus (VZV)-related progressive outer retinal necrosis (PORN) after allogeneic stem cell transplantation. Bone Marrow Transplant 2005; 36: 467–469.

13. Saari KM, Boke W, Manthey KF, et al. Bilateral acute retinal necrosis. Am J Ophthalmol 1982; 93: 403–411.

14. Schlingemann RO, Bruininga M, Wertheim-van Dillen P, et al. Twenty years' delay of fellow eye involvement in herpes simplex virus type 2-associated bilateral acute retinal necrosis syndrome. Am J Ophthalmol 1996; 122: 891–892.

15. Ludwig IH, Zegarra H, Zakov ZN. The acute retinal necrosis syndrome: possible herpes simplex retinitis. Ophthalmology 1984; 91: 1659–1664.

16. Han DP, Abrams GW, Williams GA. Regression of disc neovascularization by photocoagulation in the acute retinal necrosis syndrome. Retina 1988; 8: 244–246.

17. Wang CL, Kaplan HJ, Waldrep JC, et al. Retinal neovascularization associated with acute retinal necrosis. Retina 1983; 3: 249–252.

18. Sergott RC, Belmont JB, Savino PJ, et al. Optic nerve involvement in the acute retinal necrosis syndrome. Arch Ophthalmol 1985; 103: 1160–1162.

19. Sergott RC, Anand R, Belmont JB, et al. Acute retinal necrosis neuropathy: clinical profile and surgical therapy. Arch Ophthalmol 1989; 107: 692–696.

20. Tada Y, Begoro K, Morimatsu M, et al. Findings in a patient with herpes simplex viral meningitis associated with acute retinal necrosis syndrome. Am J Neuroradiol 2001; 22: 1300–1302.

21. Blumenkranz MS, Culbertson WW, Clarkson JG, et al. Treatment of the acute retinal necrosis syndrome with intravenous acyclovir. Ophthalmology 1986; 93: 296–300.

22. Topilow HW, Nussbaum JJ, Freeman HM, et al. Bilateral acute retinal necrosis: clinical and ultrastructural study. Arch Ophthalmol 1982; 100: 1901–1908.

23. Holland GN, Executive Committee of the American Uveitis Society. Standard diagnostic criteria for the acute retinal necrosis syndrome. Am J Ophthalmol 1994; 117: 663–666.

24. Culbertson WW, Blumenkranz MS, Pepose JS, et al. Varicella zoster virus is a cause of the acute retinal necrosis syndrome. Ophthalmology 1986; 93: 559–569.

25. Matsuo T, Date S, Tsuji T, et al. Immune complex containing herpes virus antigen in a patient with acute retinal necrosis. Am J Ophthalmol 1986; 101: 368–371.

26. Sarkies M, Gregor Z, Forsey T, et al. Antibodies to herpes simplex type I in intraocular fluids of patients with acute retinal necrosis. Br J Ophthalmol 1986; 70: 81–84.

27. Lewis ML, Culbertson WW, Post JD, et al. Herpes simplex virus type I: a cause of the acute retinal necrosis syndrome. Ophthalmology 1989; 93: 875–878.

28. Margolis T, Irvine AR, Hoyt WF, et al. Acute retinal necrosis syndrome presenting with papillitis and arcuate neuroretinitis. Ophthalmology 1988; 95: 937–940.

29. Rungger-Brandle E, Roux L, Leuenberger PM. Bilateral acute retinal necrosis (BARN): identification of the presumed infectious agent. Ophthalmology 1984; 91: 1648–1658.

30. Ganatra JB, Chandler D, Santos C, et al. Viral causes of the acute retinal necrosis syndrome. Am J Ophthalmol 2000; 129: 166–172.

31. Van Gelder RN, Willig JL, Holland GN, et al. Herpes simplex virus type 2 as a cause of acute retinal necrosis syndrome in young patients. Ophthalmology 2001; 108: 8869–8876.

32. Sugita S, Shimizu N, Watanabe K, et al. Use of multiplex PCR and real-time PCR to detect human herpes virus genome in ocular fluids of patients with uveitis. Br J Ophthalmol 2008; 92: 928–932.

33. Whittum JW, McCulley JP, Niederkorn JT, et al. Ocular disease induced in mice by anterior chamber inoculation of herpes simplex virus. Invest Ophthalmol Vis Sci 1984; 25: 1065–1073.

34. Holland GN, Cornell PJ, Park MS, et al. An association between acute retinal necrosis syndrome and HLA-DQw7 and phenotype Bw62, DR4. Am J Ophthalmol 1989; 108: 370–374.

35. Kezuka T, Sakai J, Usui N, et al. Evidence for antigen-specific immune deviation in patients with acute retinal necrosis. Arch Ophthalmol 2001; 119: 1044–1049.

36. Chan CC, Matteson DM, Li Q, et al. Apoptosis in patients with posterior uveitis. Arch Ophthalmol 1997; 115: 1559–1567.

37. Vinores SA, Derevjanik NL, Shi A, et al. Vascular endothelial growth factor (VEGF), transforming growth factor-beta (TGFbeta), and interleukin-6 (IL-6) in experimental herpesvirus retinopathy: association with inflammation and viral infection. Histol Histopathol 2001; 16: 1061–1071.

38. Balansard B, Bodaghi B, Cassoux N, et al. Necrotising retinopathies simulating acute retinal necrosis syndrome. Br J Ophthalmol 2005; 89: 96–101.

39. Palay DA, Sternberg P, Davis J, et al. Decrease in the risk of bilateral acute retinal necrosis by acyclovir therapy. Am J Ophthalmol 1991; 112: 250–255.

40. Matsuo T, Nakayama T, Koyama T, et al. A proposed mild type of acute retinal necrosis syndrome. Am J Ophthalmol 1988; 112: 119–131.

41. Ando F, Kato M, Goto S, et al. Platelet function in bilateral acute retinal necrosis. Am J Ophthalmol 1983; 96: 27–32.

42. Luu KK, Scott IU, Chaudhry NA, et al. Intravitreal antiviral injections as adjunctive therapy in the management of immunocompetent patients with necrotizing herpetic retinopathy. Am J Ophthalmol 2000; 129: 811–813.

43. Tyring S, Engst R, Corriveau C, et al. The Collaborative Famciclovir Ophthalmic Zoster Research Group: Famciclovir for ophthalmic zoster: a randomised aciclovir controlled study. Br J Ophthalmol 2001; 85: 576–581.

44. Huynh TH, Johnson MW, Comer GM, et al. Vitreous penetration of orally administered valaciclovir. Am J Ophthalmol 2008; 145: 682–686.

45. Miserocchi E, Modorati G, Galli L, et al. Efficacy of valaciclovir vs aciclovir for the prevention of recurrent herpes simplex virus eye disease: a pilot study. Am J Ophthalmol 2007; 144: 547–551.

46. Aslanides IM, De Souza S, Wong DT, et al. Oral valaciclovir in the treatment of acute retinal necrosis syndrome. Retina 2002; 22: 352–354.

47. Emerson GG, Smith JR, Wilson DJ, et al. Primary treatment of acute retinal necrosis with oral antiviral therapy. Ophthalmology 2006; 113: 2259–2261.

48. Aizman A, Johnson MW, Elner SG. Treatment of acute retinal necrosis syndrome with oral antiviral medications. Ophthalmology 2007; 114: 307–312.

49. Sternberg P, Han DP, Yeo JH, et al. Photocoagulation to prevent retinal detachment in acute retinal necrosis. Ophthalmology 1988; 95: 1389–1393.

50. Blumenkranz M, Clarkson J, Culbertson WW, et al. Visual results and complications after retinal reattachment in the acute retinal necrosis syndrome: the influence of operative technique. Retina 1989; 9: 170–174.

51. Blumenkranz MS, Clarkson J, Culbertson WW, et al. Vitrectomy for retinal detachment associated with acute retinal necrosis. Am J Ophthalmol 1988; 106: 426–429.

52. Engstrom RE Jr, Holland GN, Margolis TP, et al. The progressive outer retinal necrosis syndrome: a variant of necrotizing herpetic retinopathy in patients with AIDS. Ophthalmology 1994; 101: 1488–1502.

53. Forster DJ, Dugel PU, Frangieh GT, et al. Rapidly progressive outer retinal necrosis in the acquired immunodeficiency syndrome. Am J Ophthalmol 1990; 110: 341–348.

54. Margolis TP, Iowder CY, Holland GN, et al. Varicella-zoster virus retinitis in patients with acquired immunodeficiency syndrome. Am J Ophthalmol 1991; 112: 119–131.

55. Kashiwase M, Sata T, Yamauchi Y, et al. Progressive outer retinal necrosis caused by herpes simplex virus type 1 in a patient with acquired immunodeficiency syndrome. Ophthalmology 2000; 107: 790–794.

56. Spaide RF, Martin DF, Teich SA, et al. Successful treatment of progressive outer retinal necrosis syndrome. Retina 1996; 16: 479–487.

57. Kim SJ, Equi R, Belair ML, et al. Long-term preservation of vision in progressive outer retinal necrosis treated with combination antiviral drugs and highly active antiretroviral therapy. Ocul Immunol Inflamm 2007; 15: 425–427.

Other Viral Diseases

Scott M. Whitcup

Key concepts

- Herpes simplex virus (HSV) is a common cause of inflammatory eye disease.
- Keratitis and anterior uveitis are frequent manifestations of HSV disease; secondary glaucoma is an important cause of vision loss.
- A number of randomized controlled trials help guide therapy for HSV ocular disease. Topical antiviral therapy is indicated for HSV keratitis. Although oral aciclovir did not improve outcome in patients with active epithelial keratitis receiving topical antiviral therapy, it did reduce recurrence and progression of HSV disease and appears to be beneficial for patients with HSV-associated uveitis.
- Varicella causes two distinct forms of disease: primary infection with varicella (chickenpox) and herpes zoster disease. Uveitis most commonly occurs with herpes zoster infection.
- Treatment with oral antiviral therapy appears to improve outcome in patients with herpes zoster infection.
- Viral infections associated with a transient mild uveitis during the acute stages of infection include measles (rubeola), mumps, influenza, dengue fever, Epstein–Barr virus (EBV), and human T-lymphotropic virus type I (HTLV-1).

Viruses are important causes of human disease and play a pathogenic role in a number of inflammatory eye diseases. Viruses were first identified in the late 1800s. The specific viral etiology of diseases such as foot-and-mouth disease and yellow fever soon followed. Viruses were first classified as a distinct group based on their small size. We now know that viral genomes are composed of either RNA or DNA, and can encode several to hundreds of proteins based on their size. By learning more about how viruses attach, infect, and replicate in cells has allowed new therapeutic approaches to fighting viral infection. Importantly, better detection of viruses has allowed us to determine a viral etiology for diseases previously thought to be idiopathic. For example, high-throughput sequencing of RNA obtained from the livers and kidneys of a cluster of patients with fatal transplant-associated diseases allowed the identification of a new arenavirus as the cause of the outbreak.[1]

Herpes simplex virus kerititis and keratouveitis

Although many viruses can induce intraocular inflammation, herpes simplex keratitis is probably the most common ocular disease associated with uveitis. Patients with stromal keratitis often have a concurrent anterior uveitis.[1] Although in some patients this uveitis develops during the initial onset of epithelial disease, most patients have uveitis with stromal involvement. Recurrent episodes are common and can severely damage the eye. Anterior uveitis may also occur in patients with a history of previous epithelial herpetic infection without currently active corneal disease. Herpetic keratouveitis manifests as a red, photophobic, and often very painful eye with decreased vision.[2] Secondary glaucoma frequently accompanies severe inflammatory episodes and can lead to vision loss.

Pathogenesis

It is difficult to know how much of the ocular inflammation is due to direct viral infection, an immune response against the virus, or induced autoimmunity as a result of molecular mimicry. Each may play a role and vary between patients. A similar disease to herpes stromal keratitis can be induced in experimental animals by infecting them with HSV type 1.[3,4] A herpes protein, UL6, has been identified as a viral protein resembling corneal progein. Interestingly, both tolerance and autoimmunity can be induced in the same model, depending on host susceptibility to keratitis (**Fig. 13-1**).[5]

Diagnosis

The diagnosis of herpes simplex keratouveitis is most easily made in patients with a known history of herpes simplex keratitis confirmed by typical dendritic epithelial defects (**Fig. 13-2**) or stromal disease confirmed by culture data. The disease should also be suspected in patients with a significant corneal opacity accompanied by synechiae and anterior chamber cells. Keratic precipitates in the area of corneal disease, hypopyon, and hyphema may be seen in some patients. In some patients the corneal disease may obscure the examination of the anterior chamber. Bacterial keratitis must be ruled out, as well as the possibility of secondary bacterial infection. The use of PCR is starting to help in identifying HSV as the causative agent in patients with uveitis of unknown etiology.[6]

It remains unclear whether the uveitis associated with herpes simplex keratitis is a secondary inflammatory response

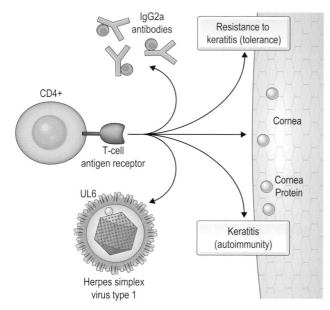

Figure 13-1. Experimentally induced herpes keratitis. Keratitis can be induced in mice by infecting them with herpes simplex virus type 1. Molecular mimicry may mediate both tolerance and autoimmunity in this animal model.[39,40] Mice that are resistant to keratitis after they have been infected with herpes simplex virus type 1 appear to be tolerant of the corneal protein because of similarities between a peptide sequence expressed in corneal cells and a sequence found within an IgG$_{2a}$-antibody variant that is unique to these animals. UL6, a protein expressed in herpes simplex virus type 1, is also similar to the corneal protein. In susceptible mice, this molecular mimicry is thought to be involved in the development of keratitis *(Albert LJ, Inman RD. Molecular mimicry and autoimmunity. N Engl J Med 1999;341:2068–74.)*

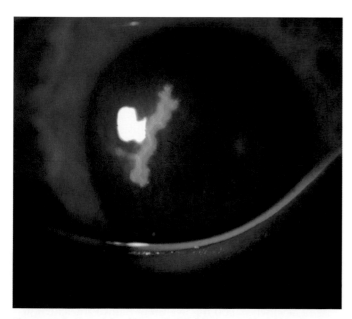

Figure 13-2. Typical dendritic epithelial defect caused by herpes simplex virus. *(Courtesy of Sue Lightman, MD.)*

to the corneal disease or whether it is induced by invasion of virus into the anterior uvea. Nevertheless, herpes simplex virus (HSV) has been isolated from the aqueous humor in some patients with the disorder.[2] In experimentally induced herpes simplex uveitis the combination of sensitized T lymphocytes, herpes-specific antibody, and herpes simplex

antigen is required to produce inflammation.[7] In addition, topical ciclosporin A was shown to effectively reduce stromal haze and inflammation in experimental herpes simplex keratitis.[8] If this situation applies to human disease, therapy that inhibits the cellular arm of the immune system could control the inflammation but enhance viral replication.

Experts differ on whether environmental factors can precipitate disease. Psychological stress has been cited as a potential trigger for recurrences of HSV ocular disease. However, when recall bias is controlled, a recent study failed to find an association between psychological stress and disease recurrence.[9]

Treatment

Herpetic eye disease is a disorder where numerous randomized clinical trials help guide clinicians on how to best care for patients. Herpes simplex keratitis is treated with topical antiviral therapy such as trifluridine solution (Viroptic) every 2 hours or vidarabine ointment (Vira A) every 3 hours. Cycloplegic agents are also employed to reduce pain and prevent synechiae. In addition, topical corticosteroids should be used in patients with associated uveitis, but their use is sometimes delayed until the corneal epithelial disease resolves. In a recent controlled trial of topical corticosteroids for herpes simplex stromal keratitis, Wilhelmus and colleagues[10] showed that prednisolone phosphate was significantly better than placebo in reducing persistence or progression of stromal keratitis, as well as the time to resolution of uveitis. In this study both groups received topical trifluridine. Although some episodes may resolve without therapy, inflammation may lead to severe ocular damage.

Oral aciclovir does not appear to be beneficial for patients with HSV epithelial keratitis treated with topical antiviral agents. In an initial study, Barron and colleagues for the Herpetic Eye Disease Study Group[11] reported no statistically or clinically significant beneficial effect of oral aciclovir in treating the stromal keratitis caused by HSV in patients receiving concomitant topical corticosteroids and trifluridine. The Herpetic Eye Disease Study Group also conducted a well-controlled, randomized clinical trial of oral aciclovir for the prevention of stromal keratitis or iritis in patients with herpes simplex virus epithelial keratitis.[12] Patients with HSV epithelial keratitis of 1 week or less duration were treated with topical trifluridine and then randomly assigned to receive a 3-week course of oral aciclovir 400 mg five times a day or placebo. The study showed that stromal keratitis or iritis developed in 17 of the 153 patients (11%) treated with aciclovir and in 14 of the 134 patients (10%) treated with placebo. In a second clinical trial the effect of oral aciclovir therapy for recurrences of HSV eye disease was investigated in 703 immunocompetent patients.[8] In this study the cumulative probability of a recurrence of any type of ocular HSV disease was 19% in the patients receiving aciclovir and 32% in patients receiving placebo. A benefit was seen for prevention of both epithelial and stromal keratitis.[9] There were only three patients with iritis; therefore the effect of treatment on uveitis could not be determined in this study. However, in another trial, The Herpetic Eye Disease Study Group assessed the benefit of adding oral aciclovir to a regimen of a topical corticosteroid and trifluridine for the treatment of HSV-associated iridocyclitis.[10] Patients with

HSV iridocyclitis were randomly assigned to receive a 10-week course of either oral aciclovir 400 mg five times daily or placebo in conjunction with topical trifluridine and a topical corticosteroid. The trial was stopped early because of slow recruitment after only 50 of the planned 104 patients were enrolled. Treatment failure, defined as persistence or worsening of ocular inflammation, withdrawal of medication because of toxicity, or withdrawal for any reason, occurred in 11 of 22 patients (50%) receiving aciclovir and in 19 of the 28 patients (68%) receiving placebo. Although the difference in failure rates was not statistically significant between the two groups, there was a trend toward a better outcome in the patients receiving oral aciclovir. Finally, oral aciclovir effectively prevents herpes-related recurrences after penetrating keratoplasty in herpetic eye disease, supporting the use of the drug.[13]

Valaciclovir and famciclovir are dosed less frequently than oral aciclovir and may be a useful alternative. In a small, prospective, randomized clinical trial of 52 immunocompetent patients oral valaciclovir (500 mg daily was as effective and well tolerated as aciclovir (400 mg twice daily) in reducing the rate of recurrent ocular herpes simplex virus disease.[14] In another small randomized clinical trial, oral valaciclovir had similar efficacy to topical aciclovir ointment in patients with herpes simplex keratitis.[15] Wilhelmus[16] compared the effects of various therapeutic interventions for dendritic or geographic HSV epithelial keratitis by searching the Cochrane Central Register of Controlled Trials. The conclusion of the review was that currently available antiviral agents are effective and nearly equivalent. The author also noted that the combination of a nucleoside antiviral with either debridement or with interferon seemed to speed healing.

Work to develop a vaccine for HSV infection is ongoing. In a small randomized clinical trial, the use of a vaccination with heat shock-inactivated herpes simplex virus type 1 (HSV-1) seemed to reduce the number and duration of relapses in HSV-1-related keratitis or keratouveitis.[17]

Secondary glaucoma is associated with herpetic keratouveitis and may be difficult to control, especially in patients with rubeosis. Glaucoma in these patients often requires surgical treatment with a drainage device. Nevertheless, vision loss related to glaucoma is common in these patients.

Herpes simplex retinitis is clearly caused by direct infection of the retina by the virus. As already stated, some cases of acute retinal necrosis may be caused by HSV infection (see Chapter 12). In addition, herpes simplex retinitis can occur in congenital HSV infection associated with herpes encephalitis.[18] This infection is usually caused by herpes simplex type 2 (HSV-2) and may be acquired in utero rather than during birth. Many patients with congenital herpes simplex retinitis have corneal and anterior chamber involvement as well, obscuring a clear view of the retina. When retinal lesions are seen clinically or pathologically, they appear as large, white retinal infiltrates associated with vitritis and retinal vascular sheathing. After the lesions heal, there are large areas of atrophic and scarred retina. The systemic infection with herpes simplex is often overwhelming and fatal.

Herpes simplex retinitis has also been reported in patients who have undergone chemotherapeutic immunosuppression, and again a viral encephalitis often accompanies this ocular condition. Large areas of white retinitis with retinal

necrosis result from the viral infection. The disorder may also occur in patients without immunosuppression, and diagnosis in some patients has been made after chorioretinal biopsy.[19] In some patients the disorder appears to respond to treatment with intravenous aciclovir.

Herpes zoster ophthalmicus

Varicella-zoster virus (VZV) causes two clinically distinct diseases. Primary infection causes varicella: chicken pox;[20] recurrent infection is known as herpes zoster infection. Although uveitis has been reported with varicella, most cases occur with herpes zoster infection. In fact, uveitis associated with herpes zoster infection often occurs with herpes zoster ophthalmicus. Ocular involvement is noted in two-thirds of patients with herpes zoster involving the ophthalmic division of the trigeminal nerve.[21] VZV is a DNA herpes class virus and remains latent in the ganglia after the patient has had chickenpox. Although reactivation occurs frequently in elderly patients, reactivation may also occur in young and healthy persons with no known immunosuppression. Cutaneous herpes zoster has been associated with defects in cellular immunity, and this disorder has been frequently seen with HIV infection.

Anterior uveitis can accompany herpes zoster ophthalmicus and probably results from vascular occlusion and secondary ischemia. Intraocular inflammation occurs in one-third to one-half of patients.[21,22] A severe glaucoma often arises in patients with severe inflammatory disease, and corneal disease manifested by dendritic keratitis, stromal keratitis, or exposure keratitis is a common finding. Large keratic precipitates and posterior synechiae accompany the anterior uveitis. Although the anterior uveitis may appear with the initial cutaneous lesions, it often develops 1–2 weeks after the onset of dermatologic disease. In a small number of patients, scleritis may be seen. The iris should be closely examined because it may be the key to correct diagnosis. Sector and patchy iris atrophy consistent with ischemic damage is characteristic of the disorder. Hyphema may occur, and some eyes develop phthisis because of severe ischemic destruction of the iris and ciliary body. Histologic study in severe disease reveals vascular inflammation and a granulomatous cellular infiltrate in the uvea.[23] Occasionally a retinal vascular occlusive disease or severe choroiditis with associated vitreal inflammation can be seen.

Treatment

Treatment with oral aciclovir early in the course of herpes zoster infection, when the cutaneous lesions are still active, appears to reduce viral proliferation and the complications of the infection, including anterior uveitis.[24–26] The usual dose of aciclovir is 800 mg five times daily. Famciclovir at a dose of 500 mg three times daily had efficacy similar to that of aciclovir for treating patients with ophthalmic zoster,[27] and valaciclovir has also been used effectively to treat the severity and duration of zoster infection. In contrast, aciclovir appears to have little effect on the development of postherpetic neuralgia. In addition, several weeks into the course of the disease the anterior uveitis is not caused by active viral replication but by ischemia. Therefore, antiviral therapy appears to be no longer useful. The anterior uveitis and glaucoma may persist for weeks to months and must be treated with topical corticosteroids, cycloplegics, and appropriate glaucoma therapy. It is not clear whether the prolonged inflammatory course is due solely to the residual ischemia or whether an immunologic response against retained viral antigen in the ocular tissue is also promoting persistent inflammation.

Although oral corticosteroids are sometimes necessary to treat postherpetic neuralgia, they should be used cautiously in the acute phase of ophthalmic zoster infection because of reports of associated ipsilateral cerebrovascular occlusion with contralateral hemiparesis.[21] Systemic corticosteroids should also be used cautiously in patients with herpes zoster infection associated with AIDS, because these agents may cause increased immunosuppression. A new topical inhibitor of substance P, capsaicin (Zostrix), may be effective in preventing postherpetic neuralgia of the skin, but a form for ocular use is not available.

Therapy requires a commitment to long-term management because even after the acute inflammation resolves, residual damage that limits acuity may be surgically repaired. Many patients are left with severe visual loss. A combination of dry eye, corneal disease, cataract, and posterior synechiae contributes to visual loss and often precludes a thorough evaluation of the posterior segment of the eye. Because the optic nerve and retina may also be involved in the disease process, it is often difficult to determine the exact cause of visual loss in any given patient. Nevertheless, it is important to try to ensure that the retina and optic nerve are not severely damaged before surgery for cataract, corneal disease, or glaucoma is performed.

In 2006, the US FDA approved a live attenuated vaccine for the prevention of herpes zoster and its sequelae. In a large, placebo-controlled clinical trial, the zoster vaccine reduced the overall incidence of zoster by 51.3%.[28] The Advisory Committee on Immunization Practices (ACIP) recommends routine vaccination of persons aged 60 years of age and older. Persons with a history of zoster can be vaccinated, although the safety and efficacy of zoster vaccine have not been assessed in this group. Zoster vaccine should not be administered to persons with primary or acquired immunodeficiency.

West Nile virus

West Nile virus is transmitted among birds by *Culex* mosquitoes in Africa, Asia, the Middle East and parts of Europe. Humans can acquire the disease through the bite of an infected mosquito. Originally identified in Africa in 1937, it was first detected in the western hemisphere in New York City in 1999 and has now spread across the United States. West Nile virus is an enveloped single-stranded RNA virus of the Flaviviridae family. Other flaviviruses cause yellow fever, dengue fever, Japanese encephalitis, St Louis encephalitis, and tick-borne encephalitis.

Epidemiology

Because West Nile virus is transmitted to humans by mosquitoes, in the US disease outbreaks occur during the summer season. In 2007, from 1 January through 13 November, 43 states reported 3304 cases of human WNV illness to the

Box 13-1 Ocular manifestations of West Nile virus infection

Multifocal chorioretinitis
Retinal hemorrhages
Vitritis
Chorioretinal linear streaks
Occlusive vascultis
Optic neuritis
Optic atrophy
Sixth-nerve palsy

Inflammation can be caused by direct infection, an immune response against the virus, or autoimmunity induced by molecular mimicry.

Centers for Disease Control and Prevention (CDC).[29] A total of 93 cases were fatal.

Diagnosis

A definitive diagnosis of West Nile virus infection is based on laboratory testing. Currently, there is an enzyme-linked immunosorbent assay (ELISA) to detect West Nile virus-specific IgM. However, clinicians must understand the presentations of the disease to know when to order the test, and both false positive and false negative results are possible.

Clinical description

Although most West Nile virus infections are asymptomatic, the virus can produce a flu-like illness with fever and chills, headache, arthralgia, myalgia, and retro-orbital pain.[30] A rash can be seen, and occasionally neurologic disease, including optic neuritis, has been reported.

Ophthalmic manifestations

Intraocular involvement with West Nile virus infection was first reported in 2003.[31] Multifocal choroiditis is the most common ocular finding in the disease. Other ophthalmic manifestations are listed in **Box 13-1** and include chorioretinitis and optic neuritis.[32]

Treatment

There is no proven treatment for West Nile virus infection. Supportive care should be provided to patients with severe manifestations of the disease, including neurologic complications. Fatalities occur mainly in older and compromised patients with underlying disease such as diabetes. Although antiviral agents have shown some activity against West Nile virus in vitro, these agents have not been effective against the virus clinically.[33] A number of researchers are working on vaccines for West Nile virus and other flaviviruses.[34] As with other mosquito-transmitted diseases, control of mosquito populations and the use of insect repellants are important in limiting the disease.

Prognosis

The symptoms and signs of West Nile virus infection can persist for months after disease presentation. In a longitudinal cohort study of 156 patients with West Nile virus infection, physical and mental function, as well as mood and fatigue, mostly returned to normal within 1 year of symptom onset.[35] Recovery was slightly longer in patients with neuroinvasive disease. Lack of comorbid conditions was associated with faster recovery of physical function.

Other viral infections

A number of other viral infections are associated with a transient mild anterior uveitis during the acute stages. These include measles (rubeola), mumps, influenza, Dengue fever, Epstein–Barr virus (EBV), and human T-lymphotropic virus type I (HTLV-1). The anterior uveitis rarely is accompanied by symptoms and is often undiagnosed because these patients do not undergo an ophthalmologic examination in the first week or two after the onset of disease. Retinitis and choroiditis caused by German measles (rubella) is rarely seen in the active stages of disease because rubella is a congenital infection. One other manifestation of measles virus infection is the rare, late presentation of subacute sclerosing panencephalitis. In addition to the progressive, fatal central nervous system disease characterized by dementia, ataxia, and myoclonus, an associated necrotizing retinitis involving the macula has developed in some patients.[36] Lesions have occasionally been mistaken for Vogt–Koyanagi–Harada syndrome, toxoplasmosis, or juvenile macular degeneration. Uveitis of varying severity has been associated with EBV infection.[37,38] One study reported positive antibody titers to early antigen (viral capsid antigen immunoglobulin M) in 10 patients with multifocal choroiditis;[39] however, subsequent studies have not confirmed this association.[40]

Human T-lymphotropic virus type I

Human T-lymphotropic virus type I (HTLV-1) is the first human retrovirus to be associated with malignancy, an adult T-cell leukemia/lymphoma.[41] HTLV-1 was initially associated with a chronic degenerative myelopathy also known as tropical spastic paraparesis.[42] Uveitis has also been associated with HTLV-1 infection. Interestingly, HTLV-I infection appears to be endemic to specific geographical areas, including Japan, central and equatorial regions of Africa, parts of Oceania, and South America.

HTLV-I associated uveitis is characterized by anterior uveitis, vitreous opacities, and retinal vasculitis.[43,44] The initial diagnosis in many patients was an idiopathic intermediate uveitis, and reduced visual acuity was often attributed to cataract and cystoid macular edema. Retinal degeneration, retinal hemorrhages, epiretinal membranes, and optic nerve atrophy can occur, and corneal involvement

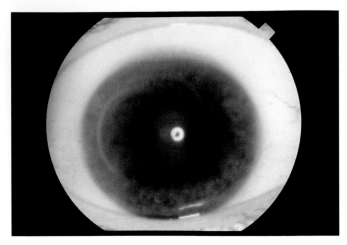

Figure 13-3. A 12-year-old girl with herpes simplex virus keratitis complicated by anterior uveitis, disciform stromal keratitis, and formation of a Wesseley immune ring. *(Courtesy of Roger George, MD.)*

with corneal haze, scarring, and neovascularization have been reported.[45] The uveitis can be treated with corticosteroids, but systemic immunosuppression is usually avoided, given the underlying viral infection.

As our ability to detect viral infection improves, and as new viral infections are described, a number of idiopathic forms of uveitis will very probably be attributed to a viral etiology. The section on West Nile virus uveitis was added to the fourth edition of this book, and as additional new viral causes of uveitis are identified, this chapter will undoubtedly become longer in future editions.

Case 13-1

Herpes simplex virus keratitis was diagnosed in a 12-year-old girl with dendritic keratitis. She was treated with topical trifluridine with resolution of the keratitis. Over the course of the next year she had several recurrences of the dendritic keratitis, but later developed a disciform stromal keratitis with an associated anterior uveitis. She was then treated with topical trifluridine and topical corticosteroids. On attempts to taper the topical corticosteroids there was an exacerbation of the stromal keratitis and anterior uveitis and the formation of a Wesseley immune ring (**Fig. 13-3**). Her clinical course was complicated by cataract and glaucoma, and she has required long-term therapy with topical trifluridine, corticosteroids, and betaxolol.

References

1. Palacios G, Druce J, Tran T, et al. A new arenavirus in a cluster of fatal transplant-associated diseases. N Engl J Med 2008; 358: 991–998.

2. O'Connor GR. Recurrent herpes simplex uveitis in humans. Surv Ophthalmol 1976; 21: 165–170.

3. Streilein JW, Dana MR, Ksander BR. Immunity causing blindness: five different paths to herpes stromal keratitis. Immunol Today 1997; 18: 443–449.

4. Zhao Z-S, Granucci F, Yeh L, et al. Molecular mimicry by herpes simplex virus type 1: autoimmune disease after viral infection. Science 1998; 279: 1344–1347.

5. Albert LJ, Inman RD. Molecular mimicry and autoimmunity. N Engl J Med 1999; 341: 2068–2074.

6. Sugita S, Shimizu N, Watanabe K, et al. Use of multiplex PCR and real-time PCR to detect human herpes virus genome in ocular fluids of patients with uveitis. Br J Ophthalmol 2008; (in press)

7. Oh JO, Minasi P. Role of lymphocyte and antibody in the pathogenesis of immune-mediated herpetic uveitis. Curr Eye Res 1985; 4: 685–691.

8. Yoon KC, Heo H, Is K, et al. Effect of topical cyclosproin A on herpectic stromal keratitis in a mouse model. Cornea 2008; 27: 454–460.

9. Herpetic Eye Disease Study Group. Psychological stress and other potential triggers for recurrences of herpes simplex virus eye infections. Arch Ophthalmol 2000; 118: 1617–1625.

10. Wilhelmus KR, Gee L, Hauck WW, et al. Herpetic eye disease study: a controlled trial of topical corticosteroids for herpes simplex stromal keratitis. Ophthalmology 1994; 101: 1883–1896.

11. Barron BA, Gee L, Hauck WW, et al. Herpetic eye disease study: a controlled trial of oral acyclovir for herpes simplex stromal keratitis. Ophthalmology 1994; 101: 1871–1882.

12. The Herpetic Eye Disease Study Group. A controlled trial of oral acyclovir for the prevention of stromal keratitis or iritis in patients with herpes simplex virus epithelial keratitis: the Epithelial Keratitis Trial. Arch Ophthalmol 1997; 115: 703–712.

13. van Rooij J, Rijneveld WJ, Remeijer L, et al. Effect of oral aciclovir after penetrating keratoplasty for herpetic keratitis: a placebo-controlled multicenter trial. Ophthalmology 2003; 110: 1916–1919.

14. Miserocchi E, Modorati G, Galli L, et al. Efficacy of valaciclovir vs aciclovir for the prevention of recurrent herpes simplex virus eye disease: a pilot study. Am J Ophthalmol 2007; 144: 547–551.

15. Sozen E, Avunduk AM, Akyol N. Comparison of efficacy of oral valaciclovir and topical aciclovir in the treatment of herpes simplex keratitis: a randomized clinical trial. Chemotherapy 2006; 52: 29–31.

16. Wilhelmus KR. Therapeutic interventions for herpes simplex virus epithelial keratitis. Cochrane Database Syst Rev 2008; Jan 23; (1): CD002898.

17. Pivetti-Pezzi P, Accoriniti M, Colabelli-Gisoldi RA, et al. Herpes simplex virus vaccine in recurrent herpetic ocular infection. Cornea 1999; 18: 47–51.

18. Reynolds JD, Griebel M, Mallory S, et al. Congenital herpes simplex retinitis. Am J Ophthalmol 1986; 102: 3336.

19. Grutzmacher RD, Henderson D, McDonald PJ, et al. Herpes simplex chorioretinitis in a healthy adult. Am J Ophthalmol 1983; 96: 788–796.

20. Strachman J. Uveitis associated with chicken pox. J Pediatr 1955; 46: 327–328.

21. Womack LW, Liesegang TJ. Complications of herpes zoster ophthalmicus. Arch Ophthalmol 1983; 101: 42–45.

22. Cobo M, Foulks GN, Liesegang T, et al. Observations on the natural history of herpes zoster ophthalmicus. Curr Eye Res 1987; 6: 195–199.

23. Hedges TR, Albert DM. The progression of the ocular abnormalities of herpes zoster: histopathologic observations of nine cases. Ophthalmology 1982; 89: 165–177.

24. Balfour HH Jr. Acyclovir therapy for herpes zoster: advantages and adverse effects. JAMA 1986; 255: 387–388.

25. Balfour HH Jr, Bean B, Laskin OL, et al. Acyclovir halts progression of herpes zoster in immunocompromised patients. N Engl J Med 1983; 308: 1448–1452.

26. Cobo LM, Foulks GN, Liesegang TJ, et al. Oral acyclovir in the treatment of acute herpes zoster ophthalmicus. Ophthalmology 1986; 93: 763–770.

27. Tyring S, Engst R, Corriveau C, et al. Famciclovir for ophthalmic zoster: a randomised aciclovir controlled study. Br J Ophthalmol 2001; 85: 576–581.

28. Oxman MN, Levin MJ, Johnson GR, et al. A vaccine to prevent herpes zoster and postherpetic neuralgia in older adults. N Engl J Med 2005; 352: 2271–2284.

29. Centers for Diseases Control and Prevention (CDC). West Nile virus update – United States, January 1–November 13, 2007. MMWR Morb Mortal Wkly Rep 2007; 16: 1191–1192.

30. Campbell GL, Marfin AA, Lanciotti RS, et al. West Nile virus. Lancet Infect Dis 2002; 9: 519–529.

31. Bains HS, Jampol LM, Caughron MC, et al. Vitritis and chorioretinitis in a patient with West Nile virus infection. Arch Ophthalmol 2003; 121: 205–207.

32. Chan CK, Limstrom SA, Tarasewicz DG, et al. Ocular features of West Nile virus infection in North America: a study of 14 eyes. Ophthalmology 2006; 113: 1539–1546.

33. Anderson JF, Rahal JJ. Efficacy of interferon alpha-2b and rabavirin against West Nile virus in vitro. Emerg Infect Dis 2002; 8: 107–108.

34. Chang DC, Liu WJ, Anraku I, et al. Single-round infectious particles enhance immunogenicity of a DNA vaccine against West Nile virus. Nature Biotechnol 2008; 26: 571–577.

35. Loeb M, Hanna S, Nicole L, et al. Prognosis after West Nile virus infection. Ann Intern Med 2008; 149: 232–241.

36. Otradovec J. Chorioretinitis centralis bei leuco-encephalitis subacuta sclerotisans. Van Bogaert Ophthalmol 1963; 146: 65–73.

37. Wilhelmus KR. Ocular involvement in infectious mononucleosis. Am J Ophthalmol 1981; 91: 117–118.

38. Wong KW, D'Amico DJ, Hedges III TR, et al. Ocular involvement associated with chronic Epstein–Barr virus infection. Br J Ophthalmol 1989; 73: 1002–1003.

39. Tiedman JS. Epstein–Barr viral antibodies in multifocal choroiditis and panuveitis. Am J Ophthalmol 1987; 103: 659–663.

40. Spaide RF, Sugin S, Yanuzzi LA, et al. Epstein–Barr virus antibodies in multifocal choroiditis and panuveitis. Am J Ophthalmol 1991; 112: 410–413.

41. Manns A, Hisada M, La Grenade L. Human T-lymphotropic virus type I infection, Lancet 1999; 353: 1951–1958.

42. Osame M, Usuku K, Izumo S, et al. HTLV-I associated myelopathy, a new clinical entity. Lancet 1986; 1: 1031–1032.

43. Mochizuki M, Watanabe T, Yamaguchi K, et al. HTLV-I uveitis: a distinct clinical entity caused by HTLV-I. Jpn J Cancer Res 1992; 83: 236–239.

44. Nakao K, Ohba N, Nakagawa M, et al. Clinical course of HTLF-I associated uveitis. Jpn J Ophthalmol 1999; 43: 404–409.

45. Buggage RR, Levy-Clarke GA, Smith JA. New corneal findings in human T-cell lymphotrophic virus type 1 infection. Am J Ophthalmol 2001; 132: 950–951.

Ocular Toxoplasmosis

Robert B. Nussenblatt

Key concepts

- Ocular disease can occur after both congenital and acquired disease.
- Recurrent disease frequently is seen as a satellite lesion.
- Immunodeficient patients are at risk for acquired disease and possibly reactivation of old disease.

Toxoplasmosis is a common disease in both mammals and birds. The disease is caused by the obligate intracellular protozoan *Toxoplasma gondii*. It is thought that this organism infects at least 500 million persons worldwide, and at least 50% of the adult population in the United States has the chronic symptomless form of the disease.[1] A survey of ophthalmologists in the US reported that 55% of those who responded saw one or more active ocular toxoplasmosis cases in last 2 years, and that 93% of those who responded had seen inactive cases in the last 2 years.[2] In the United Kingdom the estimated lifetime risk for ocular toxoplasmosis has been calculated to be 18 in 100 000.[3] In the developing world, its prevalence is probably underestimated.

A prospective study in Sierra Leone identified toxoplasmosis as the most common cause of uveitis. In Nepal, over 50% of those coming to hospital, not only for uveitis, but for other disorders such as malignancies and obstetric problems, had antibodies to toxoplasma, with over 5% being IgM positive, indicative of a recent infection.[4] The disease can cause a passing flu-like condition that has little consequence, but it can also cause lymphadenopathy, serious and sometimes fatal disease in immunocompromised hosts, spontaneous abortions, and congenital disease. For the ophthalmologist it is one of the most frequently encountered posterior uveitides, classically producing a necrotic retinitis. It is also one of the few uveitides for which we can potentially make a definitive diagnosis. In the past few years our understanding of the organism and its interrelationship with its host has brought into question several concepts that had been readily accepted in ophthalmology practice.

Organism

In 1908 *T. gondii* was first found in the brain of the North African rodent the gondi, by Nicolle and Manceaux[5] and then by Splendore[6] in a rabbit in Brazil. Janku[7] first described postmortem findings in a child who had died of disseminated toxoplasmosis. He noted what were probably *Toxoplasma* organisms in the eye, but inoculation of animals with infected tissue did not induce disease. The transmission of the organism to animals via inoculation of infected human tissue was accomplished by Wolf and coworkers.[8] Helenor Campbell Wilder identified the presence of the organism in the eye in 1952, confirming that it was the cause of uveitis.[9]

T. gondii is a 'cosmopolitan' parasite, being found all over the world. Members of the cat family are the definitive hosts. Oocysts of *Toxoplasma* are 10–12 μm in length and oval in shape. They are found uniquely in the intestinal mucosa of cats. Once they are released, they can be spread to humans or to other animals through a variety of vectors. Although invariably thought to be ingested, the organism may also enter the host through other mucosal surfaces.[10] Humans can also be infected secondarily by ingesting meat (pork and lamb particularly, as well as chicken in endemic areas, but probably not beef) contaminated with *Toxoplasma* cysts. The two forms of the organism that can be found in humans are cysts and tachyzoites (**Fig. 14-1**). The cysts are up to 200 μm in diameter, contain hundreds to thousands of organisms, and have a propensity for cardiac tissue, muscle, and neural tissue, including the retina. The cyst structure is complex and can include elements from the host. Cysts can remain intact outside of a host in soil for at least 1 year. Not all the factors that cause ultimate rupture of the cyst and the release of tachyzoites are totally clear. The tachyzoite is oval or arc shaped and about 6–7 mm in length. It is an obligate intracellular organism that actively proliferates and is the cause of the acute disease. The organism's entry into and residence within the host cell are clearly complex and dynamic events, and much is still not known. Joiner[11] found that the organism forms a parasitophorous vacuole that surrounds the parasite and that lacks plasma membrane markers from the host. It will not fuse with other compartments in the cell, and is sheltered from all cellular traffic.

Many of the antigens of the organism have been identified (**Table 14-1** and **Fig. 14-2**). Perhaps the most studied is SAG 1 or p30. This major surface antigen has a molecular mass between 27 and 30 kDa. It is useful in the serologic diagnosis of infection[12] and may play a role in the parasite's ability to invade a cell.[13] In animal models, immunization with this antigen or adoptive transfer of immune cells recognizing this antigen will confer a degree of protection against active infection. The p30 gene sequence has been deduced[14] and its mRNA appears to be 1500 nucleotides in length.

A second antigen that has been characterized is SAG 2 or p22. This cell surface antigen (molecular mass 22 kDa) can

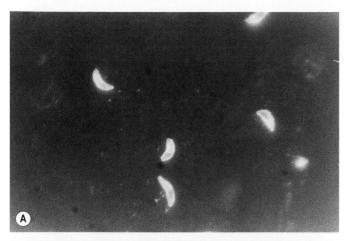

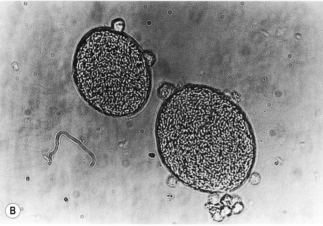

Figure 14-1. A, Tachyzoites in culture stained with immunofluorescent dye. **B,** *Toxoplasma* cysts containing large numbers of tachyzoites. *(Courtesy of Leon Jacobs, MD.)*

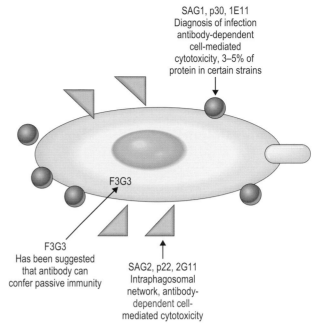

SAG1, p30, 1E11
Diagnosis of infection antibody-dependent cell-mediated cytotoxicity, 3–5% of protein in certain strains

F3G3

F3G3
Has been suggested that antibody can confer passive immunity

SAG2, p22, 2G11
Intraphagosomal network, antibody-dependent cell-mediated cytotoxicity

Figure 14-2. Cartoon showing anatomic areas from which purified *Toxoplasma* antigens have been isolated.

Table 14-1 *Toxoplasma gondii* antigens

Bradyzoite	Surface antigen (SAG) 2C,2D, and 4
	Bradyzoite specific recombinant (BSR) 4
	Matrix antigen (MAG) 1
	Lactate dehydrogenase (LDH) 2
	Enolase (ENO) 1
	Bradyzoite antigens (BAG) 1
	Phosphatidylinositol (Ptdins) b
	p-ATPase
Tachyzoite	SAG 1 (p30)
	SAG 2A and 2B (p22)
	LDH 1
	ENO 2
	Ptdins t
	SAG-related sequences (SRS) 1–3

participate in antibody-dependent, complement-mediated lysis of the tachyzoite.[15] It appears to be part of a complex phagosomal reticular network.[16] A third antigen that has been studied is known as the F3G3 antigen. This 58-kDa antigen is cytoplasmic and not expressed on the cell surface. Passive transfer of antibody that reacts to this antigen has been successful in protecting animals from a lethal challenge by the *Toxoplasma* organism.[17] The study of excreted/secreted antigens of toxoplasmosis continues[18] because it has been demonstrated that 90% of the circulating antigens detected during active infection are those that are actively excreted.[19] These antigens could be used as a basis for vaccine development, in that immunization against these antigens might abrogate rapid entry of the tachyzoite into the cell. Of interest have been attempts to classify the specific clonal lineages that may cause human toxoplasmosis. Howe and Sibley[20] determined the population genetic structure of *T. gondii* by using multiple restriction fragment length polymorphism analysis. They studied six loci in 106 independent *Toxoplasma* isolates from humans and animals. Although not separate strains, three distinct lineages seemed to be found, with only four of the isolates showing an extensively mixed genotype. In this study human isolates were found in all three lineages, although the majority of those had a type III genotype. However, one study performed in Europe reported that the cases evaluated were of the type I genotype.[21] This was also the type reported from Brazil.[22] However, the story is most probably more complicated than that. Grigg and colleagues[23] reported an abundance of atypical strains (i.e., lineages) that were associated with toxoplasmic disease. In the 12 samples they evaluated, three had typical type I lineage whereas five of 12 had recombinant genotypes typical of two lineages. Howe and colleagues[24] genotyped 68 of 72 samples isolated from human disease using the p22 (SAG2) antigen. They found that the vast majority of these 68 isolates (81%) were classified as type II, whereas only 10% were type I and 9% were type III. Khan et al.[25] evaluated other strains from various parts of Brazil and found that the genotypes were highly divergent compared to previous clonal lineages. They argued that limiting the genotyping to just the SAG 2 region will not fully recognize the diversity of this organism. This line of work is important in understanding the human disease and in devising ways to stop the strains that most commonly cause disease in humans.

Clinical manifestations

Systemic

The acquired disease in the nonimmunocompromised adult leads to lymphadenopathy in 90% of patients, with fever, malaise, and sore throat sometimes occurring. More severe disease can occur, affecting muscle, skin, brain, heart, and kidney, as well as other organs. Death due to toxoplasmosis rarely occurs in the immunocompetent. However, in the immunocompromised patient toxoplasmosis can be a fulminant central nervous system (CNS) disease that rapidly leads to death.

Ocular

The acquired disease in the immunocompetent person had been thought to cause ocular disease only rarely, but this appears not to be the case. In part, this concept stemmed from a report by Perkins,[26] discussed in some detail below (see Congenital versus Acquired disease). This is not to minimize the importance of pregnancy and the transmission of this parasite to the child. Pregnancy is the period during which acquisition of the disease causes the most concern. An older article suggests that in the United States up to six in 1000 women acquire the infection while pregnant,[1] with about a 40% risk of transmitting the infection to the fetus. In a report describing the national neonatal screening program for congenital toxoplasmosis in Denmark, there were 2.1 congenital toxoplasmosis cases per 10 000 newborns.[27] The congenital disease can lead to a wide range of symptoms, but most important to this discussion is that most cases of ocular toxoplasmosis are conjectured to be acquired congenitally, with late activation. In the Danish study 9.6% of those with congenital toxoplasmosis were born with retinal or macular lesions, with 15.6% manifesting these changes at 3 years of age.[27] In a European study reported by Koppe and Kloosterman in 1982,[28] 5% of the infants infected would either die or become severely affected by the disease. Further, about 70% of infants with congenital infections will show chorioretinal scars compatible with toxoplasmosis after a follow-up of 16 years, with 1–2% suffering severe visual impairment because of this infection. However, reports also support the notion that acquired infection may lead to ocular disease. In following up the results of an outbreak of systemic toxoplasmosis that occurred in Atlanta, Georgia, in October 1977, Wilson and Teutsch[29] reported that one patient of the original group who became ill or had serologic evidence of acute infection showed evidence of ocular disease.

A large atrophic scar, frequently in the macula – a result of congenital toxoplasmosis – is usually seen (**Fig. 14-3**). Although such lesions help in diagnosing an old problem, they do not present the ophthalmologist with a therapeutic

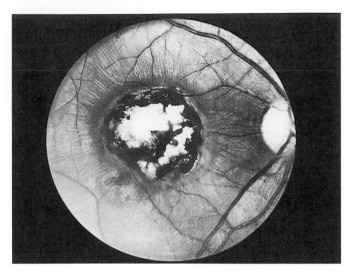

Figure 14-3. Large macular atrophic scar due to congenital toxoplasmosis.

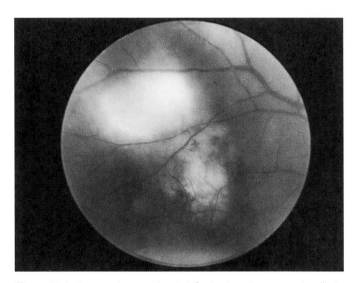

Figure 14-4. Large active toxoplasmic infection in retina; seen as 'satellite' to old healed atrophic lesion.

problem. Rather it is the reactivation or the recent acquisition of toxoplasmosis that poses the problem. In these instances, ocular toxoplasmosis manifests as a focal retinitis. The active lesion can vary greatly in size, but is usually oval or circular and rarely bullous. Frequently, reactivation sites will be 'satellite' lesions next to old atrophic lesions, indicative of previous toxoplasmic infections. The retina during the acute stage of infection appears thickened rather than transparent and is cream-colored (**Fig. 14-4**). Cells are found in the vitreous, particularly overlying the active lesion. Some eyes may have one or two small, old lesions, whereas others may have many, with some being very large and involving several clock hours of peripheral retina. In some large and particularly recalcitrant lesions the vitreal haze and cellular reaction can be so profound as to cause decreased vision. In the area surrounding the active retinitis one may see hemorrhage, as well as sheathing of the retinal blood vessels. Fluorescein angiography of the active lesion demonstrates early blockage with subsequent leakage of the lesion (**Fig. 14-5**). Indocyanine green angiography will show hypofluorescence of both active and inactive lesions.[30] ICG has shown areas

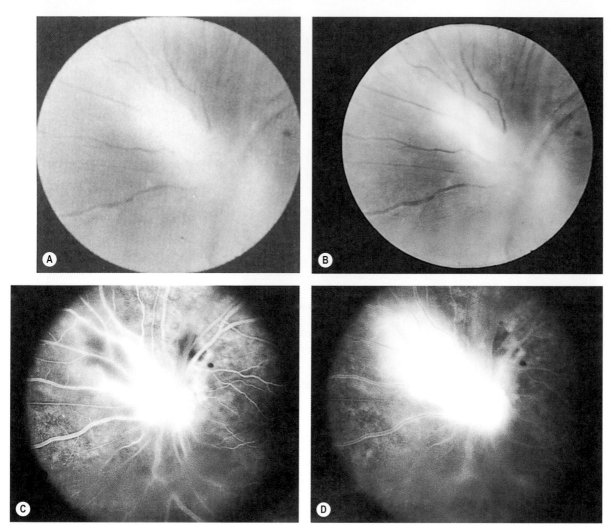

Figure 14-5. A, Fluorescein angiogram showing leakage around borders of macular lesion of toxoplasmosis. Note staining of retinal vein below lesion. *(Courtesy of JDM Gass, MD.)* **B,** Large toxoplasmosis lesion encroaching on optic disc. **C** and **D,** Fluorescein angiogram of lesion showing hyperfluorescence peripherally with later photograph showing leakage of dye from both lesion and disc.

of choroidal hypofluorescence that do not correspond to the defects seen on fluorescein angiography[31] (**Fig. 14-6**). Third-generation OCT has shown that the retinal layers are abnormally hyperflective at the active lesions, with thickening of the posterior hyaloids, which is often focally detached.[32] When lesions are close to the optic nerve, there can be considerable field loss;[33] one study reported that 94% of toxoplasmosis patients had visual field loss due to the disease.[34] As mentioned, there is a real risk of disease recurrence, hence the finding of 'satellite' lesions. It has been suggested that *Toxoplasma* cysts would be found in greater numbers near the site of a previous infection, which would seem reasonable. Holland and coworkers[35] reported that the risk of recurrence was greatest immediately after an episode, and Garweg et al.[36] found that younger ocular toxoplasmosis patients have a greater chance of recurrence than do older patients. In the questionnaire responses they received, two-thirds of the patients had a repeat attack.

Because the *Toxoplasma* organism has a propensity for neural tissue, it is important to bear in mind that the lesion classically begins in the retina, and only with ongoing inflammation will it involve not only multiple layers of the retina but also the choroid. Cells in the anterior

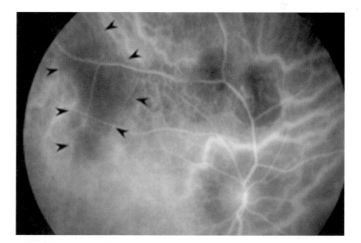

Figure 14-6. The ICG angiogram in the early phase can show hypofluorescent areas that do not correlate with that seen on fluorescein angiography (arrowheads). *(Reproduced with permission from Khairallah, Moncef, Acute Choroidal Ischemia Associated with Toxoplasmic Retinochoroiditis, 27(7):2007. Copyright 2007 Wolters Kluwer.)*

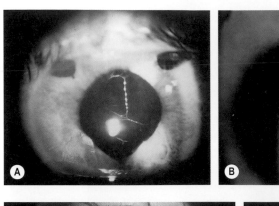
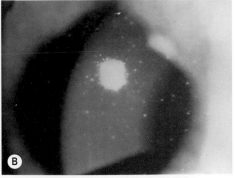

Figure 14-7. A, 'Scaffolding' seen in vitreous of patient with severe recurrent ocular toxoplasmosis. **B,** Keratic precipitates on cornea of same eye during inflammatory episode.

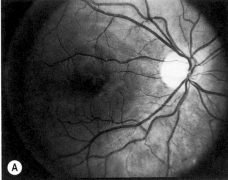
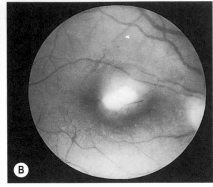

Figure 14-8. Punctate inner retinal layer toxoplasmosis. **A,** Lesion begins as subtle alteration in normal macular pattern. **B,** In a follow-up photograph lesion takes on appearance of more classic type of toxoplasmic infection. *(Courtesy of J.D.M. Gass, MD.)*

chamber may also be noted and may appear to be either a granulomatous or nongranulomatous uveitis. In the immunocompetent host, although evidence of old toxoplasmic activity may be present, the disease usually activates in only one eye at a time. With continuing inflammatory disease the lesion and overlying vitreous will undergo several changes. The vitreous may contract, and a posterior vitreal detachment is not uncommon. Further vitreal condensation leads to a 'scaffolding' of vitreal strands (**Fig. 14-7**). Roizenblatt and coauthors[37] refer to the development of vitreous cylinders in toxoplasmosis, a result of condensation of the collagen fibers. As the lesion becomes less acute, the area of retinal involvement takes on a less bright-yellow appearance, ultimately becoming atrophic, often with pigment heaping around its edges. Pigment clumping, however, does not surround all old lesions and should not be used as a diagnostic sign. The associated retinal disturbance will also begin to resolve. All patients will have visual field defects that correspond to the interruption of the retinal nerve fiber layer.[38] Although unusual, an unilateral toxoplasmic anterior optic neuropathy, presenting with sudden painless loss of vision, has been reported.[39]

Decreased Vision

The vision of the patient with toxoplasmosis is decreased for several reasons. As already mentioned, the vitreal inflammation by itself may be so great as to significantly reduce vision. Also, the lesion may be situated in the posterior pole (although not in the fovea per se), with edema and probable inflammatory byproducts of the reactions affecting central vision; however, the fovea may be relatively far from the center of the retinitis. This may be similar to the phenomenon seen in pars planitis. Another cause of decreased vision is infection involving the macula. Once the fovea is

involved in the actual infection itself, the potential for a significant return of good vision is poor, and all efforts must be made to prevent this from occurring. Schlaegel and Weber[40] noted that in 60 attacks of ocular toxoplasmosis seven patients (12%) had active retinitis within 5° of the umbo, and another seven (12%) demonstrated some evidence of mild macular edema. The observer should not forget that ocular toxoplasmosis patients often have elevated intraocular pressures. These need to be monitored, as clearly a loss of vision could be due to glaucoma.[41]

Ocular toxoplasmosis has been noted to present in a variety of ways besides the classic manifestation already described. Friedmann and Knox[42] and Doft and Gass[43] observed a subset of ocular toxoplasmosis that was characterized by gray-white fine punctate lesions of the deep retina and retinal pigment epithelium and, initially, with little or no overlying vitreal activity (**Fig. 14-8**). The resolution of these lesions may leave a typical toxoplasmosis scar. Another important presentation is papillitis. These patients may have severe papillitis even with a central retinal artery occlusion,[44] white centered retinal hemorrhages,[45] vitreal inflammation, and sector nerve, fiber-bundle defects, with no apparent retinal foci, as described by Folk and Lobes.[46] Other presentations that we are aware of are bullous-like inflammatory lesions in the midperiphery of the retina (**Fig. 14-9**), a wide ringlike lesion near the extreme periphery of the retina that resembles a severe uniocular pars planitis, and a scleritis due to the severe retinal inflammation caused by the *Toxoplasma* infection. The acute inflammation may be so severe that choroidal ischemia manifesting as retinal whitening[31] (**Fig. 14-10**) Numerous anecdotal reports concerning various presentations can be found in the literature. Although some may be without foundation, these reports emphasize the fact that one should suspect this disorder in a variety of clinical situations. Toxoplasmosis lesions can on occasion be

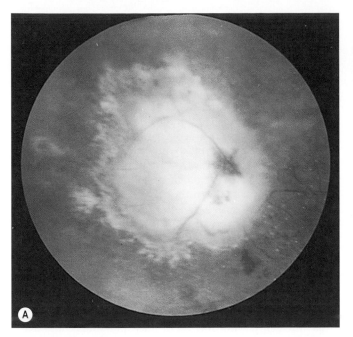

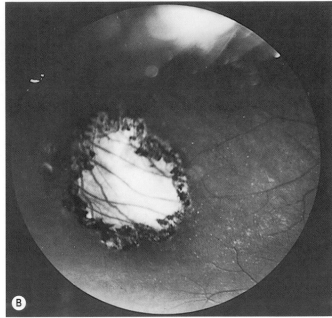

Figure 14-9. A, Large bullous lesion due to toxoplasmosis, with titer of 1 : 125. **B,** Lesion involuted only after anti-*Toxoplasma* medication.

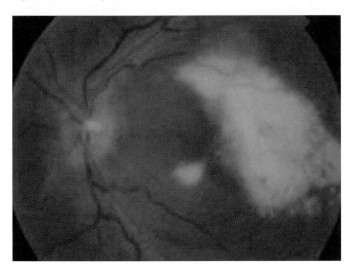

Figure 14-10. Toxoplasmosis lesion appearing as cytomegalovirus-like lesion which cleared with anti-toxoplasmosis medication. *(Reproduced with permission from Bilateral Toxoplasma Retinochoroiditis Simulating Cytomegalovirus Retinitis in an Allogeneic Bone Marrow Transplant Patient, Hyewon Chung, MD1, June-Gone Kim, MD1, Sang-Ho Choi, MD2, Sun Young Lee, MD1, Young Hee Yoon, MD1 Korean Journal of Ophthalmology 2008;22:197–200.)*

confused with other infectious disorders (see Case 14.4). In a patient who received an allogeneic bone marrow transplant for leukemia, ocular toxoplasmosis presented as a bilateral CMV retinitis with patient also found to have CNS lesions as well[47] (see Fig. 14-5). Friedmann and Knox[29] noted that the 63 patients whose cases they reviewed averaged 2.7 episodes each.

The involvement of the retinal vasculature needs to be emphasized. In one review of 64 patients[48] 59 had vascular changes in the quadrant of the active lesion. Five eyes had changes in all quadrants. Three of these patients also had retinal vascular occlusions. Frosted branch angiitis has been reported in ocular toxoplasmosis eyes even years after the acute event.[49]

In patients with ocular toxoplasmosis who are undergoing eye surgery there is a risk of reactivation of the disease. Bosch-Driessen and colleagues[50] reported that five of 15 eyes in patients with toxoplasmosis undergoing cataract extraction had a reactivation. They suggested that prophylactic anti-*Toxoplasma* therapy given perioperatively may be warranted.

Loss of Vision

The most important sequela of ocular toxoplasmosis is loss of vision due to direct involvement of the fovea by the infection. However, choroidal neovascularization can also occur as a late complication of the disease.[51, 52] Skorska and coworkers[52] found that subretinal neovascular lesions were present in seven of 36 patients studied. The new vessels were located either directly on the border of the scar or at a distance, with feeder vessels arising from the scar (**Fig. 14-11**). Retinochoroidal anastomoses have also been observed to occur in toxoplasmosis, with one study reporting an incidence of 2.7%[53] (**Fig. 14-12**). Other vascular complications have been reported. Rose[54] reported on a patient with ocular toxoplasmosis with a retinal vein occlusion, papillitis, and florid disc neovascularization. Pakalin and Arnaud[55] observed an occurrence that manifested with an arteriolar branch occlusion at a site passing through an area of necrosis. They emphasized the need to include toxoplasmosis in the differential diagnosis of even arterial inflammatory phenomena, something not usually done. Bosch-Driessen and associates[56] reported that nine of 150 patients (6%) with ocular toxoplasmosis had retinal detachments, and another seven (5%) had retinal breaks. Retinal detachment was seen more commonly in myopes, and the visual prognosis is guarded: five of nine eyes with retinal detachment were left with 20/200 visual acuity or worse. As with any disorder that disrupts Bruch's membrane, choroidal neovascularization, usually at the rim of an old lesion, needs to be looked for. One report describes multiple CNV lesions in one eye with punctate outer retinal *Toxoplasma* lesions.[57]

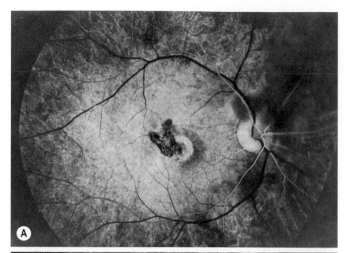

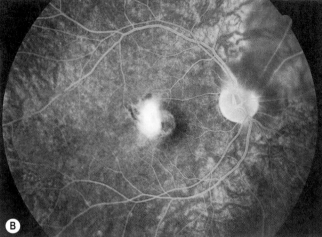

Figure 14-11. Subretinal neovascularization 8 months after acute attack of ocular toxoplasmosis. **A,** Nasal portion of lesion that stains corresponds to area of old scarred lesion. **B,** In the late-stage angiogram nasal hyperfluorescence has not increased in size; however, temporal subretinal neovascular lesion can be seen. *(Courtesy of Prof. G. Coscas. Reproduced with permission from Journal Francais d'Ophtalmologie 7: 211–218, 1984 © Masson.)*

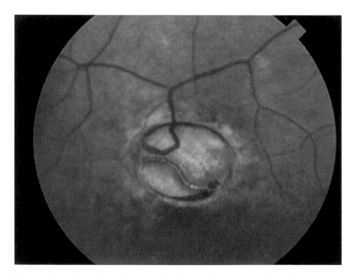

Figure 14-12. Fundus photograph of eye with congenital toxoplasmosis, with retinochoroidal shunt. *(Courtesy of J. Melamed, MD, Porto Alegre, Brazil.)*

A curious association between Fuchs' heterochromia and ocular toxoplasmosis was initially made by Toledo de Abreu and coworkers.[58] They studied 13 patients with Fuchs' syndrome who had focal necrotizing chorioretinal toxoplasmic lesions; none of these patients had ciliary injection or posterior synechiae but most had keratitic precipitates, anterior chamber reactions, and cataracts. Six of the 13 had iris transillumination. La Hey and colleagues[59] evaluated this possible association in a series of 88 patients with Fuchs' heterochromia, comparing them with control subjects and other patients with uveitis. Although nine of these patients (10.2%) with Fuchs' heterochromia had scars compatible with toxoplasmosis, the authors were unable to establish a special relationship between the two entities. Others have confirmed these observations[60]. Schwab,[61] in an interesting review, also looked for a relationship between toxoplasmosis and Fuchs' heterochromic iridocyclitis. In his review he found that 13 of 25 patients with Fuchs' heterochromic iridocyclitis had scars typical of toxoplasmosis and serologic evidence of the organism. This result was compared with results for 590 patients seen in the retina clinic at West Virginia University, with only 24 of these patients (4%) having retinal lesions typical of toxoplasmosis. Schwab concluded that a causal relationship between the two entities appears to exist, at least for a subgroup of patients with Fuchs' heterochromia.

Effects in immunocompromised host

Special mention seems appropriate for ocular toxoplasmosis in the immunocompromised host, particularly the patient with AIDS not being treated with HAART (see Chapter 11). In these patients the development of ocular toxoplasmosis does not meet the criteria for an opportunistic infection but can indicate to the clinician that a change in the patient's immune state has occurred. Indeed, we have seen active ocular toxoplasmosis in a patient with the AIDS-related complex in whom the full-blown picture of AIDS soon developed. In the patient with AIDS the degree of inflammatory disease associated with a toxoplasmic retinitis is usually far greater than that seen with cytomegalovirus (CMV) retinitis, perhaps indicating that reactivation (or acquisition) of the disease occurs earlier in the course of AIDS than in CMV retinitis, when the immune system is still capable of mustering a significant inflammatory response. In the United States, toxoplasmic retinitis is still a relatively uncommon disorder in patients with AIDS. Often in toxoplasmic retinitis numerous lesions will appear to be active at the same time, a most unusual finding in the immunocompetent patient.

The diagnosis of ocular toxoplasmosis in a patient with AIDS should initiate an evaluation of possible CNS disease as well. CNS toxoplasmosis has become a problem frequently seen in this patient population. The reason for the CNS and the eye incidence disparity is not known. The therapeutic management of these ocular lesions can be difficult. Despite therapy, disease can progress. Moorthy and colleagues[62] reported two patients in whom a severe necrotizing retinitis was seen, with one developing a panophthalmitis and orbital cellulitis despite sulfadiazine, pyrimethamine, and folinic acid therapy. Whether the ocular manifestations of this disease represent reactivation or acquired disease is not known. One could conjecture that both routes are possible. Gagliuso and coworkers[63] offer the observation that most ocular lesions in patients with AIDS are unassociated with a preexisting retinochoroidal scar and would therefore suggest acquired disease. This may be, but it is possible that cysts in the retina may remain dormant and become activated only in the immunosuppressed state. It is also possible that small lesions indicative of previous disease are simply engulfed in the large retinal necrotic lesion present in the patient with AIDS.

The patient who has undergone iatrogenic immunosuppression has a high risk of reactivation of ocular toxoplasmosis. As with patients with AIDS, if the immunosuppression cannot be reversed serious consequences may ensue, as reported by Yeo and colleagues.[64] Singer and coworkers[65] and Blanc-Jouvan and associates[66] have reported cases of ocular toxoplasmic retinochoroiditis occurring after liver transplantation. In the patient of Singer and coworkers, because of the difficulty of diagnosing the disorder, the eye was ultimately enucleated. These authors emphasize the fulminant nature of the disease, suggestive far more of the type of ocular disease seen in patients with AIDS.

We conclude with the interesting observation that immune recovery uveitis may be driven by *Toxoplasma* antigens and not only by CMV, as it is generally thought. Sendi and colleagues[67] reported the case of a 34-year-old HIV-positive man with a CD4 count of 11, who, after being placed on HAART therapy developed a uveitis after an increase in his CD4 count. Aqueous PCR for CMV was negative but positive for *Toxoplasma*, and his disease abated only after periocular steroid injections.

In summary, the diagnosis of ocular toxoplasmosis is primarily clinical. The typical lesions as described constitute the most important factor in our decision making. The one additional supportive test we believe to be very important is a positive toxoplasmosis titer at any dilution (see below). When the presentation is highly unusual, the diagnosis rests on a combination of multiple factors. In young children, infection with lymphochoriomeningitis virus, found in rodent feces, urine, and saliva, has been reported to mimic the ocular lesions associated with toxoplasmosis.[68] In these patients toxoplasmosis could be confused with the ocular histoplasmosis syndrome, although vitreal cells are not present in the latter entity and the peripapillary changes are rarely evident in toxoplasmosis. The deep retinal presentation of toxoplasmosis may be confused with the white-dot syndromes, such as an unusual case of acute posterior multifocal placoid pigment epitheliopathy (see Chapter 29). In the immunocompromised host a single toxoplasmosis lesion early on may be confused with CMV retinitis. One possible way to help discriminate between the two entities is the use of fluorescein angiography. In an active toxoplasmosis lesion the central area will block fluorescein early and stain late, because the central part is where the greatest inflammatory response is taking place. This is in contrast to CMV retinitis, in which the central area will be atrophic and more readily hyperfluorescent early in the angiogram (Phuc LeHoang, MD, personal communication, 1989). Indocyanine green angiography will show that the lesion extends beyond the visible area, with hypofluorescent foci at all phases.[69] A very good review of ocular disease can be found in Dr Gary Holland's Jackson Memorial lecture.[70,71]

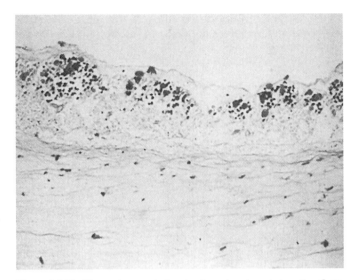

Figure 14-13. Photomicrograph showing toxoplasmic cysts in retina. Cysts are larger circular structures, located mainly in or close to the nerve fiber layer. *(Courtesy of D. Cogan, MD.)*

Histopathology and immune factors

In ocular toxoplasmosis, cysts and tachyzoites can be found in the retina (**Fig. 14-13**). The *Toxoplasma* organism most frequently is seen in the superficial portions of the retina. The lesion induced is necrotic, destroying the architecture of the retina. In many cases the underlying structures are destroyed as well, so that the disease at this point can certainly be classified as a chorioretinitis. Clinically, this destruction will permit the examiner to see underlying sclera quite clearly. Dutton and coworkers[72,73] were able to study these alterations more carefully using a murine model of congenital toxoplasmic retinochoroiditis. They noted that the inflammation ranged from a low-grade mononuclear infiltrate to total destruction of the outer retina, the retinal pigment epithelium, and choroid. Of great interest was the fact that photoreceptor outer segments were phagocytosed by macrophages, whereas the *Toxoplasma* cysts did not appear to be the center of the inflammatory attack. Roberts and colleagues[74] characterized histologically the eyes from 10 fetuses and two infants with congenital toxoplasmosis. Retinitis was present in 10 of 18 eyes, necrosis in four of 18, retinal pigment epithelial changes in 12 of 18, choroidal inflammation in 15 of 18, and optic neuritis in five of eight fetal eyes. Parasites were found on immunohistologic examination in 10 of 18 eyes. It appeared to the authors that the inflammatory response mounted by the host accounted for part of the damage seen.

Because of the selective photoreceptor destruction, one can speculate that autoimmune mechanisms may be important in the tissue destruction seen (see discussion of autoimmunity in Chapter 1). Indeed, when we had the opportunity to evaluate this issue, we found that in 16 of 40 patients (40%) with ocular toxoplasmosis an in vitro proliferative response to the retinal S-antigen was seen.[75] This finding could indicate that an autoimmune component to the inflammatory disease is initiated, with destruction of the retina by a parasite and subsequent sensitization to the uveitogenic antigen. We also found that proliferative responses to the p22 antigen approached those seen to crude toxoplasmosis antigen, whereas the response to the p30 membrane antigen was considerably less striking. Others have shown that *Toxoplasma* antigen stimulates CD25+ helper cells.[76]

Immune response

The host's immune response is exceptionally important in the ultimate expression of toxoplasmosis. In animal models, resistance, as measured by survival after challenge with the organism, has been reported to be regulated by at least five genes,[77] one of which is within the region of the H-2 antigen (the equivalent of the major histocompatibility complex [MHC] in humans).[78] Brown and McLeod[79] have found that class I MHC genes, as well as the CD8+ fraction of T cells, determine the cyst number in *Toxoplasma* infection. Jamieson et al.[80] reported polymorphism associations at the COL2A1 encoding type II collagen associated only with those who had ocular disease. Others have looked at the effect of cytokines on the multiplication of the *Toxoplasma* organism. Interferon (IFN)-γ, as well as tumor necrosis factor (TNF)-α and transforming growth factor-β all appear to play a role in inhibiting multiplication.[81, 82] Gazzinelli and colleagues[83] reported that a reactivation of *T. gondii*, at least in the experimental mouse model, is due to a downregulation of IFN-g and TNF-a, which leads to reduced macrophage (with a decrease in inducible nitric oxide synthase and macrophage activation gene 1) and glial activation, a release of parasite growth, and tissue damage. Shen and associates[84] found the presence of IFN in the eyes of *Toxoplasma*-infected mice, but that inflammatorily induced apoptosis was caused by several factors, not only Fas/FasL interactions. Beaman and colleagues[85] reported that interleukin (IL)-6 enhanced intracellular reproduction of *T. gondii* and actually reversed the effect of IFN-g-mediated killing, which contradicts the finding of Lyons and colleagues[86] who stated that IL-6 knockout mice in a chronic toxoplasmosis model had more severe disease and an increased parasite burden. This finding is particularly important in light of the fact that the retinal pigment epithelium produces large amounts of IL-6. An analysis of ocular fluids from uveitic eyes (including those with from patients with toxoplasmosis) demonstrated the presence of various cytokines, including IL-6, IFN, and IL-10. Recently, Zamora and coworkers showed that the *Toxoplasma* organism invades human retinal endothelial cells more efficiently than they do human dermal endothelial cells.[87] In another study, Feron and colleagues[88] characterized 10 T-cell specimens from the vitreous of patients with toxoplasmosis. Although the cell lines were initially generated by mitogenic stimulation, they were all CD4+ and appeared reactive to *Toxoplasma* antigens and not to any retinal antigens. The majority had a Th2 profile. It has also been suggested that CD8+ T cells directed against the *Toxoplasma* organism appear during the acute phase of the disease, whereas CD4+ parasite-specific T cells appear with chronicity of the disease.[89] Denkers and colleagues[90] reported that the *Toxoplasma* organism possesses a superantigen that expands murine Vβ5-expressing cells, most of which were CD8+. It may be that this superantigen-driven expansion of predominantly IFN-g-secreting CD8+ cells is partly why the early immune response is seen. Curiel and coworkers[91] reported the cloning of human CD3+, CD4+ T cells that lyzed autologous target cells

which had been pulsed with *Toxoplasma* antigen or infected with live tachyzoites. These results suggest that specific immunotherapy through the development of vaccine may be possible. Patients with acute toxoplasmosis have increased serum levels of CXCL8, part of the chemokines that control leukocyte infiltration and can even modulate angiogenesis.[92]

Although antibodies are usually readily made, it is the cellular component of the immune system that must be intact for a resolution of the disease process. However, antibody production may play an important role in establishing a state of premunition (immunity from infection) in *Toxoplasma* infection.[93] In an attempt to evaluate why newborn infants seem to have difficulty in fighting the *Toxoplasma* infection, Wilson and Haas[94] evaluated the cellular defenses against *T. gondii* in newborns. They noted that newborn and adult macrophages killed the organism equally well, but supernatants from cord blood-derived concanavalin A-stimulated mononuclear cells activated macrophages less effectively than supernatants produced from adult blood cells. This difference appeared to lie in the CD4+ fraction of T cells. The cord blood appeared to produce fewer lymphokines capable of activating macrophages, including IFN-g. The authors did not believe that enhanced generation of reactive oxygen intermediates was important in explaining the differences between the adult and newborn responses, although recent notions would suggest that nitrous oxide and its effects in macrophages may indeed play a very important role. Roberts and associates,[95] in a murine model, demonstrated that inhibition of nitric oxide by administration of Lω-*nitro*-L-arginine methyl ester made the disease worse. Of interest is the fact the organism replicates in the macrophage, and this reduced killing in the newborn may then lead to greater susceptibility.

Inflammatory response

What then is the cause of the focal, retinal inflammatory response? So far the data still support the notion that it is the release of actively proliferating tachyzoites, often from a long-dormant cyst. We know now of many immune components that can stimulate this tachyzoite–bradyzoite interconversion (**Fig. 14-14**) However, immune studies with patients with ocular toxoplasmosis suggest that other factors are involved. Wyler and coworkers[96] noted that lymphocytes from patients with ocular toxoplasmosis demonstrated in vitro responses not only to *Toxoplasma* antigens but also to a crude retinal preparation. As already mentioned, our patients with toxoplasmosis have demonstrated in vitro cellular responses to the retinal S-antigen, a purified antigen from the photoreceptor region, and the site of the most intense inflammatory response in Dutton and colleagues' murine model for toxoplasmosis.[73] Abrahams and Gregerson[97] detected circulating antibodies to various retinal antigens in patients with toxoplasmosis. Whittle and colleagues,[98] using indirect immunofluorescent techniques over normal human cadaver retina, determined the presence of human antiretinal antibodies in patients with ocular toxoplasmosis. Of the sera from 36 toxoplasmosis patients, 94% demonstrated photoreceptor layer reactivity. However, only 27 of these patients had anti-S-antigen antibodies as determined by an enzyme-linked immunosorbent assay (ELISA).

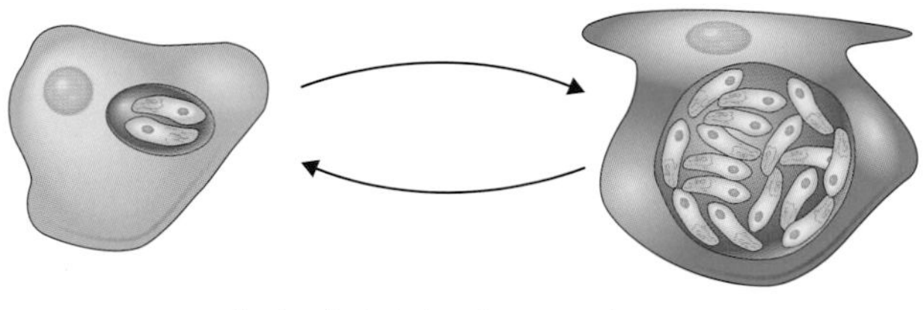

Tachyzoite to bradyzoite conversion

- High pH
- Low pH
- Heat shock
- Mitochondrial inhibition
- Presence of nitric oxide

Tachyzoite   Bradyzoite

Bradyzoite to tachyzoite conversion

- Lack of nitric oxide
- Lack of IFN-γ
- Lack of TNF-α
- Lack of T cells
- Lack of IL-12

Figure 14-14. Factors that affect conversion from tachyzoite to bradyzoite. *(From Lyons RE, McLeod R, Roberts CW. Toxoplasma gondii tachyzoite-bradyzoite interconversion. Trends Parasitol 18: 198, 2002, with permission.)*

The authors concluded that antiretinal activity can be accounted for by antibodies directed not only against S-antigen but also against other antigens. These observations raise the provocative argument that the inflammatory disease we see is at least partly, or at times, autoimmune driven. However, Vallochi et al.[99] reported that the peripheral blood from ocular toxoplasmosis patients also recognized retinal antigens. But their data suggest that such autoimmune responses were associated with less severe disease. We know that the *Toxoplasma* cyst may include tissue from the host, and perhaps S-antigen is sequestered there until the cyst breaks open. Alternatively, the initial destruction caused by the proliferating organism releases immunogenic antigens to the general circulation, thereby causing sensitization. This then results in a secondary autoimmune response, which can prolong the initial response or become the center of a recurrent inflammatory episode some time in the future.

The mechanism for the anterior uveitis and the Fuchs'-like syndrome seen in conjunction with the retinitis of ocular toxoplasmosis still is a subject of conjecture. In a rabbit model of experimental ocular toxoplasmosis, toxoplasmic antigen has been found in the vitreous.[100] In a feline model of ocular toxoplasmosis in which chorioretinal lesions form after injection of organisms into the carotid, an anterior uveitis can be seen in some of the animals.[101] It may be that in the human situation the antigen is also found in the anterior chamber, producing an inflammatory response there; alternatively, immune complexes formed more posteriorly in the eye may fix to the tissue in the anterior chamber, including the iris, giving the clinical findings described. However, an intact *Toxoplasma* organism has been found in only one immunocompromised person with AIDS.[102] Greven and Teot[103] reported recovering encysted bradyzoites from the cytospin of a vitrectomy specimen obtained in the course of a retinal detachment repair, which helped confirm the clinical impression and led to the initiation of therapy.

Methods of diagnosis

Serologic evidence of the *Toxoplasma* organism is of immense importance in helping the clinician make the diagnosis.

Research has suggested that there is a selective activation of a subset of B cells locally in nonlymphoid tissue, such as the eye.[104] Indeed, research evaluating serum and intraocular antibody responses has shown differences.[105] Antibody from the aqueous of patients with chronic toxoplasmosis stained more intensely to a 28-kDa antigen, believed to be the GRA-2 antigen, which is expressed in both tachyzoites and bradyzoites. We would accept seropositivity even in undiluted serum, although admittedly this can be problematic because the incidence of false-positive results is high. The presence of immunoglobulin (Ig) M titers to the organism suggests a recently acquired infection. Observations by Rubens Belfort Jr, MD, in Brazil (personal communication, 1993) suggested that at least in some cases the IgM peak may be highly ephemeral and thus easily missed. The type of serologic testing that is the most reliable is still being debated, although the ELISA technique has been recommended by many. Weiss and colleagues[106] reported their experience comparing the immunofluorescence antibody test, the Sabin–Feldman dye test, and the ELISA. They found that for three patients the immunofluorescence test result was negative (titer <1:16) whereas the Sabin–Feldman test result was positive for these three patients, as was the ELISA in the one patient tested. These data suggest that the Sabin–Feldman test or ELISA antibody test be performed before one excludes the diagnosis of ocular toxoplasmosis on the basis of a negative antibody test result.[106]

The polymerase chain reaction (PCR) is being used increasingly for diagnostic purposes and has become one of the mainstays for diagnosis but it does have its drawbacks.[107] Initial problems were raised about this methodology. In one early study comparing antibody determinations with the detection of *T. gondii* DNA,[108] intraocular IgG was more commonly found in recurrent ocular toxoplasmosis than in recently acquired disease (81% versus 41% of patients). However, DNA from *T. gondii* was found intraocularly in recently acquired disease compared with recurrent ocular toxoplasmosis (37% versus 4% of patients). Using the aqueous to diagnose posterior segment disorders is well accepted today.[109]

The diagnosis of this disease by serologic means alone may not always be reliable.[110] Rothova and coworkers noted that even though IgG antibody positivity was seen in 100% of their patients with clinically apparent ocular toxoplasmosis, 58% of the control subjects also showed positive results. Although seven of 25 patients (28%) with toxoplasmosis had detectable circulating immune complexes with IgG and *Toxoplasma* antigen, two of 12 control subjects (16%) did as well. In reviewing findings from normal control subjects and patients with suspected ocular toxoplasmosis, Phaik and coworkers[111] estimated that at least 77% of those with ocular toxoplasmosis had serotiters ≥1:256, somewhat higher than those found in control subjects. Nonetheless, we believe that the diagnosis is very much a clinical one, with serologic findings being supportive but not definitive.

The serologic examination of the aqueous is a technique reported by Desmonts.[112] In this classic paper, Desmonts postulated that in patients with purely an ocular recurrence of toxoplasmosis, local antibody formation against the organism will occur and therefore the local titer will be greater than that found in the circulation. His impressive demonstration of this phenomenon and the calculation of the C value is a result that the ophthalmologist should be aware of (see Chapter 5). This technique is not is widely used in the United States, although our European colleagues find it of value.[113] Although the clinical appearance of the disease is straightforward in most patients we have seen, this added technique can be helpful in the evaluation of those whose disease presents real diagnostic dilemmas (see Case 13-4). For example, consider the patient with an underlying malignant process, such as a lymphoma or leukemia, who manifests a focal inflammatory process in the retina, with overlying vitreal activity. Is this lesion a localized form of the neoplasm or an activation of toxoplasmosis because of a change in his or her immune status? The evaluation of the aqueous for anti-*Toxoplasma* antibodies may not be a perfect technique but could provide the clinician with important information. Turunen and colleagues[114] emphasized the reliability of this test and found that in both patients with toxoplasmosis and control subjects intraocular anti-mumps antibody formation was within the normal range, suggesting that the response may be specific.

So which test do you use, PCR or intraocular antibody? When comparing PCR and antibody levels in the eye, Westeneng et al.[115] found that antibody levels helped to diagnose toxoplasmosis in immunocompromised patients more often than did PCR, which often becomes negative in disease present for an extended period. Alternatively, PCR seemed better for the diagnosis of viral retinitis. This was the finding by Rothova et al. when comparing all patients regardless of their immune status.[109] In their report, they calculated that in 26/30 (87%) of those with toxoplasmosis the diagnosis would not have been made using PCR alone, and the majority of those would have been for toxoplasmosis. This is in contrast to the use of the Goldmann–Witmer quotient, where only two of the 30 patients with toxoplasmosis would not have been diagnosed if this were the only test performed. To make things a bit more confusing for the reader, Mahalakshmi et al.[116] compared local antibody production with a nested PCR method and found no difference in the sensitivity of the tests. They would prefer using PCR because of the amount of specimen needed, the rapidity of the test, and the cost. No perfect method of evaluation exists.

Using a different approach, Palkovacs et al.[117] reported the use of needle aspiration biopsy to diagnose acquired toxoplasmosis. It was performed in a 34-year-old woman who received a bone marrow transplantation for leukemia. The biopsy showed crescent-shaped intraretinal organisms and cysts. The patient was treated with anti-*Toxoplasma* medication.

Pregnancy

In pregnant women, testing for toxoplasmosis is routinely performed. It is generally believed that if the mother has anti-*Toxoplasma* antibodies before the beginning of the pregnancy, then the fetus is protected. If the disease is contracted during pregnancy, the highest number of children born with symptoms of *Toxoplasma* infection are those contracting the disease in the third trimester of the pregnancy. It is believed that if one child is born with signs of ocular toxoplasmosis, then succeeding siblings will be protected. Anecdotal reports have appeared that possibly disprove this concept, but in most instances extenuating circumstances have been present that could explain the unusual findings without disproving the concept. A recent case (see below) may in fact show that disease may be transmitted from a toxoplasmosis-positive mother. Pregnancy is a period of relative immunodepression: the body does not wish to reject the immunologically foreign object that is maturing in the uterus. For some autoimmune diseases this immune state may reduce the possibility of disease. However, with an infectious disorder the risk of disease may increase. There have been several cases reported of reactivation of ocular toxoplasmosis during pregnancy, and improvement of disease in some with delivery.[118,119] Although this supports the notion mentioned above, it is still a fairly unusual event, suggesting that immune surveillance still works in most people. However, it does need to be considered when following an ocular toxoplasmososis patient who becomes pregnant. What should one do with the woman who has a reactivation of her ocular disease during pregnancy? Many clinicians will try to follow the lesion if it appears not to be sight threatening. Martinez and colleagues[120] reported the successful management of ocular toxoplasmosis during pregnancy with intraocular injections of clindamycin and dexamethasone combined with systemic sulfadiazine.

Other methods

Other methods for diagnosis of toxoplasmosis have been developed. Western blot analysis[121] has been used to identify cytoplasmic and membrane antigens of *T. gondii*. Immunoblotting has also been shown to be useful.[122] Using recently identified genes believed to be specific to this organism as a template, and by means of the PCR, one can search for toxoplasmic DNA, even when it is present in minute quantities. PCR will permit adequate amplification of these DNA fragments to allow detection with standard laboratory techniques, such as Southern blot analysis. To date, two genes have been used. The gene for the p30 antigen encodes one of the major surface proteins of the organism.[12–14] The B1 gene,[123] which contains an intron but does not encode for a known protein, has been shown to be in the genome of many *Toxoplasma* strains, but not in the mammalian genome. The PCR technique has been applied to deparaffinized ocular sections from two patients. Although cysts could be identified by use of standard microscopic examination in one eye, PCR permitted the identification of the parasite in both patients.[107] This study demonstrated the feasibility of the PCR method even when paraffin slides are used. By means of this method, toxoplasmic DNA was identified in the aqueous of three patients with ocular toxoplasmosis.[124] The positive PCR response in these three patients was not related to the C coefficient, the analysis used to determine local production of specific antibody. Finally, tissue culturing using ocular tissue has been used to diagnose toxoplasmosis in HIV-positive patients.[125]

Another approach to diagnosis has been to develop in vivo tests. One method shown to work in rabbits is the use of in vivo immunofluorescence. Scheiffarth and associates[126] tagged specific anti-*Toxoplasma* antibodies with fluorescein, injected them intravenously, and found that samples from an experimentally induced chorioretinitis would stain with this technique. Much work is still needed before this technique can be used with the human form of the disease.

Congenital versus acquired disease

As discussed above, it was formerly an established 'given' in ophthalmology that most, if not all, of the ocular lesions ascribed to toxoplasmosis were due to a congenitally acquired infection. As mentioned earlier, Perkins,[26] in reviewing the literature, found that uveitis was described in 52 of 1669 cases (3.1%) of acquired toxoplasmosis, and was most commonly seen with toxoplasmic encephalitis.[26] In his treatise *Uveitis and Toxoplasmosis*,[127] Perkins states: 'It is probable that the vast majority of cases of toxoplasmic uveitis in adults and children are recurrences of a congenital infection.' It has therefore been assumed that acquired disease rarely manifests as a purely ocular disease.

The classic concepts were that subclinical infection would occur in most patients, resulting in overt clinical symptoms years later when the patient was a young adult. A corollary to this concept of congenital disease was that a mother, if infected before becoming pregnant, would not transmit the disease to her child. If she did become infected during pregnancy, then she would transmit the disease only to that one offspring; she would then be immunized and therefore any other children would be protected.

These ophthalmic 'givens' have been seriously questioned by the seminal observations of a family of ophthalmologists, the Silveiras, of Erechim, a small city located in the southernmost state (Rio Grande do Sul) of Brazil. These physicians had noted a very high rate of toxoplasmosis in the population of this region. In a survey of 100 normal children they found that 98% of those between the ages of 10 and 15 years had antibodies to toxoplasmosis. On the basis of their observations, the frequency of retinal scars in the population of this area was calculated to be 40 in 200, compared to 1 in 200 in the United States and 6 in 200 in São Paulo, Brazil. In a search for an explanation of this very high rate, it was noted that the residents of this region prepare sausage made of raw or poorly cooked pork. The preparation of the sausage is a family endeavor requiring much tasting, which custom could partly explain the high incidence of the disease.

Other observations regarding ocular toxoplasmosis in this region were most provocative. Ocular toxoplasmosis was observed in families in which the mother and several children (nontwins) had retinal lesions typical of toxoplasmosis; indeed, even three generations in one family were seen to have the disease.[128] The finding of toxoplasmic cysts, which provided a definitive diagnosis of this disorder, occurred in two siblings, each of whom required enucleation of an eye for intractable pain. Such findings could be better explained if the disease were acquired rather than congenital. Indeed, a rather typical systemic manifestation of this disease seen by one of us (RBN) when visiting Erechim was in a febrile child with rather marked lymphadenopathy. These children either have a necrotizing retinal lesion at the same time or will develop one some months later. Other studies showed that IgM antibodies could be found in patients, but the antibody titers do not stay elevated above baseline for very long.

To corroborate these earlier observations, a household survey was undertaken in the Erechim region. Of the 1042 persons examined, 184 (17.7%) were found to have ocular toxoplasmosis. On the basis of these observations, the prevalence of ocular toxoplasmosis was calculated to be 30 times higher than estimates for this disease in other parts of the world.[129] Also of interest was the finding that only 0.9% of young children tested had antibodies to *T. gondii*, further suggesting that the ocular disease seen was due to postnatal infection rather than congenital.

A prospective study investigating the incidence of congenital toxoplasmosis in this region was then undertaken.[130] During a 5-month period, serum was obtained from 283 of 599 newborns and 190 infants under 1 year of age. The study showed that 2.1% of the newborns and 0.5% of the infants had evidence of circulating antibodies to the *Toxoplasma* organism. For 21% of adults of this region of Brazil to have ocular toxoplasmosis due to a congenital infection, more than 20% of the mothers would have to be infected during pregnancy. Indeed, only 0.5–0.6% of the cord blood tested revealed anti-*Toxoplasma* antibodies. A questionnaire given to newly diagnosed ocular toxoplasmosis patients in the Erechim region showed that eating undercooked or raw meat, having a garden, and eating frozen lamb were associated with acquiring the disease.[131]

These studies clearly demonstrate that acquired disease is a major mode of transmission of this parasite that leads to the ocular form of the disease – at least for a corner of southern Brazil[132] – and perhaps in other areas as well.[133] In a recent study detailing results from the French program against congenital toxoplasmosis, Delair et al.[134] reported that in instances where the disease could be determined (100 cases), there were more cases of acquired disease than congenital cases. Only 4% of the acquired cases were bilateral, whereas 43.5% of the congenital cases were bilateral. A follow-up of the Erechim studies 7 years later provided further insight into this disorder.[135] In the 1990 study, 109 patients were seronegative, with 21 (19.3%) becoming seropositive by 1997 and two of them developing ocular lesions. In 1990, 131 individuals were only seropositive, with 11 (8.3%) developing ocular lesions of toxoplasmosis by 1997. Finally, in 1990 13 had small nonspecific ocular lesions, and by 1997 three of those (23%) had developed typical ocular toxoplasmosis. But do these observations have any relevance to the disease outside Brazil? The information now suggests that they do. However, the story is surely complex, because a recent survey in Rio Grande do Sul showed a marked difference in the prevalence rates between the region of Erechim and a more southern portion of the state.[136] The role of the environment is further emphasized by a report finding that residents of the United Kingdom born in West Africa had a 100 times higher incidence of ocular symptoms than those born in the United Kingdom.[3] The concept that acquired disease can lead to ocular lesions has now become accepted. These observations led to the speculation that the findings may be relevant to the North America population as well. Montoya and Remington[137] suggested that postnatally acquired disease was more common in the United States than previously thought. A recent report of a case series of acquired toxoplasmosis in British Columbia is a good example. An outbreak that lasted from October 1994 to March 1995 and appeared to be due to contaminated drinking water resulted in 100 patients with acquired disease and 12 with the congenital form.[138] Of the 100 patients with acquired disease, 20 presented with retinal findings; seven of these lesions were in the macular region. A similar epidemic was recently evaluated in Santa Isabel do Ivai in the Parana state of Brazil, where cat feces contaminated drinking water and led to over 600 occurrences of acquired toxoplasmosis (Cristina Muccioli, MD, Claudio Silveira, MD, and Rubens Belfort Jr, MD, personal communication 2005). In one study of 14 patients with postnatally acquired toxoplasmosis who were followed for 4.6 years, recurrent ocular disease occurred in 57%.[139] Another outbreak occurred in Coimbatore, India. This was first noted because of a sudden increase in September 2004 of seropositivity in patients coming to an eye clinic.[140] In this report by Palanisamy et al., 249 cases were tested and 178 had high titers of both IgG and IgM to the *Toxoplasma* organism. The majority of the cases came from an area with a single water reservoir, suggesting that contamination was through the municipal water system.

The notion that an unborn child may be 'protected' by the mother's being seropositive at the time of pregnancy has been questioned for years. The group in Brazil[141] has reported the case of a woman in whom toxoplasmosis had been diagnosed 20 years earlier and who then delivered a child with toxoplasmosis. Both reactivated and newly acquired disease with genetically different strains or lineages of *T. gondii* are possible explanations. An excellent review of this whole subject is available to those who read Portuguese.[142]

Therapy

An initial decision of whether the *Toxoplasma*-induced lesion needs to be treated must be made. We know that in the immunocompetent person the disease is ultimately self-limited. For us, the decision to treat generally would be based on the following criteria:

- A lesion within the temporal arcade;
- A lesion abutting the optic nerve or threatening a large retinal vessel;
- A lesion that has induced a large degree of hemorrhage;
- A lesion that has induced enough of a vitreal inflammatory response that the vision has dropped below 20/40 in a previously 20/20 eye, or at least has sustained a two-line drop from the visual acuity before the acute infection;
- A relative indication would be the case of multiple recurrences that develop marked vitreal condensation. Here one might be concerned that the continuation of this process might lead to retinal detachment.

Which drug or combination of drugs should one use? Few if any fully powered randomized studies have been published to answer this question completely. Results of a non-randomized study comparing three therapeutic regimens – pyrimethamine, sulfadiazine and steroid; clindamycin, sulfadiazine, and steroid; and trimethoprim and sulfamethoxazole – did not show a difference in the duration of the inflammation among therapy arms.[143] However, 52% of patients in the group receiving pyrimethamine had a reduction in the size of the retinal inflammatory focus, versus 25% of the untreated group (peripheral lesions). Stanford and colleagues,[144] after performing an evidence-based systematic

review of antibiotic therapy for toxoplasmosis, felt that there was lack of evidence to support routine antibiotic treatment for acute ocular disease. A single masked study in Iran compared trimethoprin/suflamethoxazole versus pyrimethamine/sulfadiazine (both groups received oral steroids): 59 patients were randomized and the authors reported no difference in the two groups in terms of retinal lesion quieting and visual acuity. A survey by Holland and Lewis[145] asked experts on uveitis how they manage this disease. The 97 respondents do treat, and reported using a total of nine drugs in 25 different regimens. As the first drug combination for the treatment of ocular toxoplasmosis we still use sulfadiazine (1 g orally four times daily) and pyrimethamine (50-mg loading dose and then 25 mg orally twice daily), always given concomitantly with folinic acid 3–5 mg three times per week; this is also the combination most commonly employed by the experts (28%) surveyed by Holland and Lewis. A baseline platelet count followed by weekly counts are obtained for the duration of the folinic acid therapy, which we continue for 1 week after stopping the pyrimethamine. We generally treat immunocompetent patients for 3–4 weeks with this regimen, and judiciously add prednisone to the regimen if the lesion is in the posterior pole or threatening the optic nerve head. Generally we use 20–40 mg/day of prednisone in the adult patient, beginning 12–24 hours after initiation of the specific antimicrobial therapy. If the macula or optic nerve is threatened we do not hesitate to see the patient frequently, trying to taper the prednisone in such a way that it is stopped before the anti-*Toxoplasma* therapy is discontinued. It is important to stress that immunosuppressive therapy (prednisone) should never be used alone, but only under the therapeutic cover of the specific antimicrobial therapy, nor do we give it at higher doses for any prolonged period. Periocular injections of corticosteroids are not to be used. Sabates and coworkers[146] reported the cases of seven patients in whom the disease was particularly destructive and disseminated, and all were initially treated with corticosteroids alone. We do not use intravitreal steroid injections to treat this disease, our concern being that such high levels in the eye will overcome the antimicrobial effect and lead to reactivation, echoing concerns raised by others.[147] Cytotoxic agents do not have a role in the treatment of this infection.

Clindamycin (150–300 mg orally three or four times daily) combined with sulfadiazine has also been shown to be effective in treating this disorder,[148,149] and as mentioned earlier has been used intravitreally in pregnant patients,[120] but also in those unable to tolerate systemic medication.[150] Because the two agents affect unrelated pathways, it may be that the combination could have synergistic effects, although not perhaps as effective as the combination of pyrimethamine and sulfadiazine.[151] Although it is a useful approach, the potential for diarrhea and the serious complication of pseudomembranous colitis at worst is problematic. In one study in Germany[152] 15 of 90 patients treated with clindamycin combined with fluorocortolone had side effects, including diarrhea, allergic exanthem, mild lymphopenia, hepatotoxicity, and gastrointestinal bleeding. The drug was withdrawn in eight patients. Clindamycin has also been given in 50-mg subconjunctival injections, with positive clinical results observed.[153] Kishore and associates[154] reported treating four patients with 1.0 mg of clindamycin (in 0.1 mL) and 1 mg of dexamethasone (in 0.1 mL) given intravitreally. In three of the patients systemic medications were continued. A favorable response was seen within 2 weeks. All patients needed three to four injections. As mentioned earlier, the question of which therapeutic combination is more effective in treating the acute disease and preventing recurrences has not been evaluated in a randomized study. It was initially thought that clindamycin might prevent recurrences, but this has not been the case (RJ Belfort, personal communication, 1992).

There is now evidence to suggest that treating congenitally acquired disease does have a positive therapeutic effect, though one could wish it were even more effective. In a cohort of 25 children diagnosed with congenital toxoplasmosis, who were not treated during their first year of life and who had an average followup of 5.7 years, 18 (72%) had at least one new lesion, with 13 of them having lesions in their macula.[155] Indeed, new lesions were noted after the first decade of life in some. This is in contrast to 132 children with congenital toxoplasmosis who were treated with anti-*Toxoplasma* medication (pyrimethamine, sulfadiazine, and leucovorin) during the first year: 34 (31%) developed new eye lesions, with 15 (14%) being in the macula.[156] McLeod and coworkers[157] have reported the overall neurologic long-term effects of therapy for 1 year (with sulfadiazine and pyrimethamine) in children with congenital toxoplasmosis. Those with no substantial neurologic damage all had normal cognitive, neurologic and auditory outcomes. For those with significant neurologic damage early in their life, the results are not as positive.

A trimethoprim/sulfamethoxazole combination has been used by some clinicians. In principle this would inhibit the synthesis of tetrahydrofolic acid, as does pyrimethamine. This combination of trimethoprim/sulfamethoxazole was evaluated in the treatment of toxoplasmosis by Opremcak and colleagues,[158] who found that in all 16 patients studied active retinochoroiditis resolved and vision improved. Two patients had drug allergies. In a recent study in Brazil[159] 124 patients with a history of ocular toxoplasmosis were randomly assigned either to receive intermittent trimethoprim/sulfamethoxazole (Bactrim) therapy or to be observed. Over a 20-month period of follow-up there was a significant reduction in ocular attacks in the trimethoprim/sulfamethoxazole-treated group.

Another drug used with positive results in the treatment of toxoplasmosis is atovaquone (Mepron). Of great potential interest is its ability to kill *Toxoplasma* cysts in vitro,[160] and others have shown that atovaquone reduced the number of cerebral cysts in a Syrian gold hamster model.[161] If this action were true in humans, it would be conceivable that one therapeutic course with this agent could prevent recurrences, assuming adequate levels of the drug were available to resolve the infection completely. Atovaquone is a quinolone derivative first developed because of its antimalarial properties. It has been used most extensively in the treatment of CNS toxoplasmosis, with reasonably good results.[162] We reported its use in the treatment of ocular toxoplasmosis in a patient with AIDS who was unable to continue more standard therapy, with a very good therapeutic response.[163] Anecdotal reports do not seem to support the notion that recurrences can be eliminated with atovaquone.[164] However, in a study of immunocompetent patients, therapy with atovaquone 750 mg four times daily for 3 months combined with 40 mg of prednisone in 17 patients resulted in a positive therapeutic outcome.[165]

Empiric observations in the immunoincompetent host (e.g., patients with AIDS) have shown that the disease will be arrested only with therapy and will reactivate once the therapy has been stopped. Allergies to drugs as well as other side effects always complicated the therapeutic approach. With the cellular response so important for host defense, before the availability of highly active antiretroviral therapy (HAART), long-term anti-*Toxoplasma* therapy was needed. However, it is not yet clear how HAART alters this treatment approach in patients with AIDS.

Additional therapeutic approaches

Cryotherapy of peripheral lesions that cause enough vitreal inflammatory activity to affect vision can also be considered. However, excessive cryotherapy applied to these 'hot' eyes could potentially induce unwanted and excessive vitreous condensation and membrane formation, ultimately pulling on the retina and causing retinal detachment. Photocoagulation has also been advocated by some as a means to treat toxoplasmosis. Ghartey and Brockhurst[166] described their experience in treating five eyes with toxoplasmic lesions unresponsive to antimicrobial therapy and corticosteroids. Photocoagulation treatment was thought to benefit four eyes, with healing of the lesion after a few weeks. Others have suggested that such treatment could reactivate dormant cysts, leading to a renewal of ocular disease.

Therapies addressing choroidal neovascularization have been evaluated in the treatment of this complication secondary to ocular toxoplasmosis. PDT[167, 168] and avastin injections[169,170] have been used by several, with the results (albeit in a small number of patients) that the CNV seems amenable to these therapies. There is one caveat: one report recounted a patient who received PDT and an intraocular steroid injection and returned 45 days later with a necrotizing retinitis and high IgG toxoplasmosis titers.[171] Laser therapy in the case reported above of multiple CNV lesions in one eye resulted in recurrence of the lesions.[57]

Vitrectomy and lensectomy can be performed on these eyes to remove vitreous and lens opacities that affect vision.[172] Significant vitreous condensations can form in eyes having a history of multiple episodes of inflammation due to toxoplasmosis. In patients with toxoplasmosis who are undergoing vitrectomy, we usually begin antimicrobial therapy before surgery and continue it postoperatively. Prophylaxis is also suggested for cataract extraction.[50] The rationale for this approach is the concern that the nonspecific inflammation induced by the vitrectomy might initiate an inflammatory episode of toxoplasmosis. We would not use periocular steroid injection after the procedure, but will give steroids by mouth if indicated.

Case 14-1

A 28-year-old white man was first seen at the National Eye Institute in March 1981. He was complaining of a reduction in vision with floaters in the left eye for over 1 week. The vision in his right eye was 20/20 and in the left 20/25. The anterior chambers were quiet. There was 1+ haze in the vitreous of the right eye, with a white retinal lesion, 1.5 disc diameters, encompassing the vessels of the superior temporal arcade and extending into the posterior pole. The more peripheral portion of the lesion seemed old – that is, less white and raised, with some pigment surrounding the edges – whereas the more active area seemed pointed toward the macula. The left eye also had an old inactive scar in the periphery of the superior portion of the retina. The clinical impression was that of ocular toxoplasmosis. The toxoplasmosis titer was positive at 1 : 128. The decision was made not to treat the patient.

The patient returned 1 week later with the same visual acuity. However, the lesion had progressed toward the macula. A decision was then made to initiate anti-*Toxoplasma* therapy: clindamycin 300 mg by mouth four times daily and sulfadiazine 0.5 g by mouth four times daily. No steroid was given. The patient was followed up weekly, and after 3 weeks of therapy the disease involuted. Therapy was stopped after 4 weeks. By late April 1981 the patient's visual acuity was 20/15 OU, and the lesion in the right eye was quiet. He had no problems until August 1985, when he noted an increase in floaters in the right eye. An examination at that time showed that there was a small area of active retinitis on the peripheral portion of the old lesion, on the side not facing the macula. It was elected not treat the patient, and the lesion regressed. He has been free of recurrence to date.

Comment 14-1. We elected to treat the patient despite good vision only after following the clinical course and noting its progression toward the macula. It did not seem reasonable to wait any longer. He has continued to have recurrences, even after clindamycin therapy, and needs to be seen regularly. In passing, it can be argued that a patient presenting today with his or her first attack of ocular toxoplasmosis deserves to be screened for HIV.

Case 14-2

This 43-year-old white man has congenital toxoplasmosis. He has never had good vision in the left eye because of a large atrophic scar in the macula. The right eye has multiple lesions, all compatible with the diagnosis of ocular toxoplasmosis. In the right eye there is a lesion that encroaches on the temporal side of the fovea, but his visual acuity was 20/25 in that eye when he was first seen at the National Eye Institute. Two years later he complained of a 'haziness' to his vision in the right eye. Examination of the parafoveal lesion could not detect an area of activity. Despite this, therapy with clindamycin, sulfadiazine, pyrimethamine (Daraprim), folinic acid, and prednisone was begun.

The haziness disappeared over the course of the 3-week therapy period. During the ensuing years his vision in the right eye has varied from 20/25 to 20/32. He has had one episode every 12 to 18 months when he feels there is a change in the quality of his vision. Examination of serial retinal photographs shows greater pigment around the atrophic scars but rarely evidence of activity.

Comment 14-2. The lack of observable activity on the edge of the old lesion abutting the fovea has not dissuaded us from

treating the patient each time he complains of a change in his vision. A small nidus of infection, enough to alter his vision but not enough for the observer to note, could very well be there. This patient always maintains a supply of his medication and begins the antimicrobial therapy (sulfadiazineand clindamycin) immediately when symptoms appear. He is seen within 24 hours and then pyrimethamine (after a baseline platelet count), folinic acid, and steroid are begun.

Case 14-3

This 36-year-old white man with AIDS-related complex had chronic granulomatous skin disease, chronic hepatitis, thrombocytopenia, and evidence of exposure to both the HIV and human T-cell leukemia/lymphoma-1 virus. We first saw him in November 1984, when he had had uveitis in the right eye for several months. He had active toxoplasmic retinitis in the right eye and an old pigmented lesion in the left eye, also compatible with ocular toxoplasmosis. The left eye also had a dense cataract. He was treated with clindamycin and sulfadiazine, with resolution of his inflammation after a 6-week course of sulfadiazine. The clindamycin was stopped after 3 weeks because of severe gastrointestinal problems, and pyrimethamine with folinic acid was begun for the next 3 weeks. A CT scan of the head showed no evidence of cerebral toxoplasmosis. Under this therapeutic regimen the patient underwent cataract surgery, with a good visual result.

The patient continued to have recurrences of his ocular toxoplasmosis as soon as the specific antimicrobial therapy was discontinued. It was therefore decided to maintain long-term sulfadiazine therapy, but this needed to be stopped because of hives. Pyrimethamine was then used. In August 1985 the cataract in the patient's right eye significantly reduced his vision and made it difficult to maintain close follow-up of his retinitis. There were now cottonwool spots in both eyes and cells in the left, but the lesion in the right eye seemed to be stable. He therefore underwent lensectomy and vitrectomy in the right eye. HIV was cultured out of the vitreous specimen, his Witmer quotient was markedly elevated, supporting the preoperative diagnosis, and after surgery his right eye revealed 4+ cells and 3+ haze. These responded only to the addition of sulfadiazine.

Comment 14-3. This man's ocular course emphasizes the rapidity of changes and the difficulty of treating them in the immunosuppressed host. The presence of HIV in the vitreous, in addition to his history of chronic hepatitis, emphasizes the great care needed in handling these samples. Further, without an intact cell-mediated immune arm, the disease simply recurred once therapy was discontinued. The only therapeutic option was to 'juggle' the available therapeutic agents. He ultimately succumbed to his underlying disease. HAART will certainly change this disease dynamic.

Case 14-4

A 67-year-old white man from Latin America underwent triple coronary artery bypass surgery in his home country. This surgery was complicated by renal failure and the need for acute hemodialysis and transfusions. He subsequently regained renal function and returned to his normal routine. Three months later he noted decreased visual acuity in his right eye (OD), followed a week later in the left eye (OS). He had cells in the anterior chamber and in the vitreous. There were deep retinal or subretinal whitish-yellow lesions in both eyes. Findings of a workup for a blood-borne infectious agent were negative, as were results of a CT scan of the head and a lumbar puncture. The clinical diagnosis was intraocular lymphoma. An OD vitrectomy showed no malignant cells. However, suspicion remained high and an OS vitrectomy and retinal biopsy were performed. Results of both were negative for a malignant process, and results of a CT scan of the abdomen and chest, as well as bone marrow biopsy, were all normal. The retinal biopsy showed a large number of mature plasma cells.

The patient was sent to the National Institutes of Health for further evaluation. Results of his physical examination were normal. A magnetic resonance image showed a few small areas of ischemia consistent with involutional change. The erythrocyte sedimentation rate was 34 mm/h, there were no antibodies to hepatitis B, and liver and thyroid test results were normal. Chest

X-rays showed no active disease. A repeat OS vitrectomy showed T cells and macrophages but no malignant cells; viral cultures for zoster, varicella, and CMV were negative but showed herpes simplex 1 and 2 antibodies that were higher in the cerebrospinal fluid. The patient's toxoplasmosis titer (IgG) was elevated at 1 : 1000. Analysis for Lyme disease and *Leptospira* organisms revealed seronegativity. Oral prednisone therapy was begun, and within 1 week new lesions developed in the fundus.

After the patient was seen by infectious disease specialists, an empirical regimen of pyrimethamine, sulfadiazine, and ganciclovir was begun. Rhegmatogenous retinal detachment developed, and during surgery the subretinal fluid was sent for toxoplasmosis titers and for culture. The C quotient for both vitreous and subretinal fluid was 300 compared to that for the serum. The ganciclovir was stopped, and the patient's inflammation resolved with the anti-*Toxoplasma* medication.

Comment 14-4. Although we evaluated the patient for toxoplasmosis, we did not consider this diagnosis as a high possibility. We would assume that the patient was infected via one of the transfusions he received after his coronary surgery. The C coefficient was the most helpful finding in this case.

References

1. Krick J, Remington J. Current concepts in parasitology. Toxoplasmosis in the adult – an overview. N Engl J Med 1978; 298: 550–553.

2. Lum F, Jones JL, Holland GN, et al. Survey of ophthalmologists about ocular toxoplasmosis. Am J Ophthalmol 2005; 140(4): 724–726.

3. Gilbert RE, Dunn DT, Lightman S, et al. Incidence of symptomatic toxoplasma eye disease: aetiology and public health implications. Epidemiol Infect 1999; 123: 283–289.

4. Rai SK, Upadhyay MP, Shrestha HG. Toxoplasma infection in selected patients in Kathmandu, Nepal. Nepal Med Coll J 2003; 5(2): 89–91.

5. Nicolle C, Manceaux L. Sur une infection a corps de Leishman (ou organismes voisins) du gondi. Compt Rend Acad Sci 1908; 147: 763–766.

6. Splendore A. Un nouvo protozoa parassita dei conigli: incontrato nell lesoni anatomiche d'une malattia che ricorda in molti punti il Kala-azar dell'uomo. Rev Soc Sci São Paulo 1908; 3: 109–112.

7. Janku J. Pathogenesis and pathologic anatomy of coloboma of macula lutea in eye of normal dimensions, and in microphthalmic eye, with parasites in retina. Cas Lek Cesk 1923; 62: 1021–1027, 154–1059, 1111–1115, 1138–1143.

8. Wolf A, Cowen D, Paige B. Human toxoplasmosis: Occurence in infants as an encephalomyelitis: Verification by transmission to animals. Science 1939; 89: 226–227.

9. Holland GN, Lewis KG, O'Connor GR. Ocular toxoplasmosis: a 50th anniversary tribute to the contribution of Helenor Campbell Wilder Foerster. Arch Ophthalmol 2002; 120: 1081–1084.

10. O'Connor, G. The mucosae as possible sites of entrance for Toxoplasma gondii. In: O'Connor G, ed. Immunologic Diseases of the Mucous Membranes, 1989, New York: Masson Publishing USA Inc. 71–78.

11. Joiner K. Cell entry by *Toxoplasma gondii*: All paths do not lead to success. Res Immunol 1993; 144(1): 34–38.

12. Santoro F, Afchain D, Pierce R, et al. Serodiagnosis of toxoplasma infection using a purified parasite protein. Clin Exp Immunol 1985; (62): 262–269.

13. Kasper L, Khan I. Role of p30 in host immunity and pathogenesis of *T. gondii* infection. Res Immunol 1993; 144(1): 45–48.

14. Burg J, Perelman D, Kasper LH, et al. Molecular analysis of the gene coding tha major surface antigen of *Toxoplasmosis gondii*. J Immunol 1988; (141): 3584–3591.

15. Kasper L, Crabb J, Pfefferkor E. Isolation and characterization of a monoclonal antibody-resistant antigenic mutant of Toxoplasma gondii. J Immunol 1982; 129: 1694–1699.

16. Sibley L, Krahenbuhl JL, Adams GM, et al. Toxoplasma modifies macrophage phagosomes by secretion of a vesicular network rich in surface proteins. J Cell Biol 1986; (103): 867–874.

17. Sharma S, Araujo F, Remington J. Toxoplasma antigen isolated by affinity chromatography with monoclonal antibody protects mice against lethal infection with *Toxoplasm gondii*. J Immunol 1984; 133: 2818–2820.

18. Cesbron-Delauw M, Capron A. Excreted/secreted antigens of *Toxoplasmosis gondii* – their origin and role in the host – parasite interaction. Res Immunol, 1993; 144(1): 41–44.

19. Hughes H, Van Knapen F. Characterization of a secretory antigen from *Toxoplasma gondii* and its role in circulating antigen production. Int J Parasit 1982; 12: 433–437.

20. Howe DK, Sibley LD. *Toxoplasma gondii* comprises three clonal lineages: correlation of parasite genotype with human disease. J Infect Dis 1995; 172: 1561–1566.

21. Switaj K, Master A, Borkowski PK, et al. Association of ocular toxoplasmosis with type I *Toxoplasma gondii* strains: direct genotyping from peripheral blood samples. J Clin Microbiol 2006; 44(11): 4262–4264.

22. Vallochi AL, Muccioli C, Martins MC, et al. The genotype of *Toxoplasma gondii* strains causing ocular toxoplasmosis in humans in Brazil. Am J Ophthalmol 2005; 139(2): 350–351.

23. Grigg ME, Ganatra J, Boothroyd JC, et al. Unusual abundance of atypical strains associated with human ocular toxoplasmosis. J Infect Dis 2001; 184: 633–639.

24. Howe DK, Honore S, Derouin F, et al. Determination of genotypes of

Toxoplasma gondii strains isolated from patients with toxoplasmosis. J Clin Microbiol 1997; 35: 1411–1414.

25. Khan A, Jordan C, Muccioli C, et al. Genetic divergence of *Toxoplasma gondii* strains associated with ocular toxoplasmosis, Brazil. Emerg Infect Dis 2006; 12(6): 942–949.

26. Perkins E. Ocular toxoplasmosis. Br J Ophthalmol 1973; 57: 7–17.

27. Schmidt DR, Hogh B, Andersen O, et al. The national neonatal screening programme for congenital toxoplasmosis in Denmark: results from the initial four years, 1999–2002. Arch Dis Child 2006; 91(8): 661–665.

28. Koppe J, Kloosterman G. Congenital toxoplasmosis: Long term follow up. Paediatr Padol 1982; 17: 171–179.

29. Wilson L, Teutsch S. Acquired toxoplasmosis. Ophthalmology 1982; 89: 1299–1302.

30. Atmaca LS, Simsek T, Atmaca SP, et al. Fluorescein and indocyanine green angiography in ocular toxoplasmosis. Graefes Arch Clin Exp Ophthalmol 2006; 244(12): 1688–1691.

31. Khairallah M, Yahia SB, Zaouali S, et al. Acute choroidal ischemia associated with toxoplasmic retinochoroiditis. Retina 2007; 27(7): 947–951.

32. Orefice JL, Costa RA, Campos W, et al. Third-generation optical coherence tomography findings in punctate retinal toxoplasmosis. Am J Ophthalmol 2006; 142(3): 503–505.

33. Stanford MR, Tomlin EA, Comyn O, et al. The visual field in toxoplasmic retinochoroiditis. Br J Ophthalmol 2005; 89(7): 812–814.

34. Scherrer J, Iliev ME, Halberstadt M, et al. Visual function in human ocular toxoplasmosis. Br J Ophthalmol 2007; 91(2): 233–236.

35. Holland GN, Crespi CM, ten Dam-van Loon N, et al. Analysis of recurrence patterns associated with toxoplasmic retinochoroiditis. Am J Ophthalmol 2008; 145(6): 1007–1013.

36. Garweg JG, Scherrer JN, Halberstadt M. Recurrence characteristics in European patients with ocular toxoplasmosis. Br J Ophthalmol 2008; 92(9): 1253–1256.

37. Roizenblatt J, Grant S, Foos R. Vitreous cylinders. Arch Ophthalmol 1980; 98: 734–739.

38. Benson W. Ocular toxoplasmosis and visual field defects. Am J Ophthalmol 1980; 90: 25–29.

39. Song J, Scott IU, Davis JL, et al. Atypical anterior optic neuropathy caused by toxoplasmosis. Am J Ophthalmol 2002; 133: 162–164.

40. Schlaegel TJ, Weber J. The macula in ocular toxoplasmosis. Arch Ophthalmol 1984; 102: 697–698.

41. Westfall AC, Lauer AK, Suhler EB, et al. Toxoplasmosis retinochoroiditis and elevated intraocular pressure: a retrospective study. J Glaucoma 2005; 14(1): 3–10.

42. Friedmann C, Knox D. Variations in recurrent active toxoplasmic retinochoroiditis. Arch Ophthalmol 1969; 81: 481–493.

43. Doft B, Gass J. Outer retinal layer toxoplasmosis. Graefes Arch Clin Exp Ophthalmol 1986; 224: 78–82.

44. Tandon R, Menon V, Das GK, et al. Toxplasmic papillitis with central retinal artery occlusion. Can J Ophthalmol 1995; 30(7): 374–376.

45. Hayashi S, Kim MK, Belfort RJ. White-centered retinal hemorrhages in ocular toxoplasmosis. Retina 1997; 17(4): 351–352.

46. Folk J, Lobes L. Presumed toxoplasmic papillitis. Ophthalmology 1984; 91: 64–67.

47. Chung H, Kim JG, Choi SH, et al. Bilateral toxoplasma retinochoroiditis simulating cytomegalovirus retinitis in an allogeneic bone marrow transplant patient. Korean J Ophthalmol 2008; 22(3): 197–200.

48. Theodossiadis P, Kokolakis S, Ladas I, et al. Retinal vascular involvement in acute toxoplasmic retinochoroiditis. Int Ophthalmol 1995; 19: 19–24.

49. Oh J, Huh K, Kim SW. Recurrent secondary frosted branch angiitis after toxoplasmosis vasculitis. Acta Ophthalmol Scand 2005; 83(1): 115–117.

50. Bosch-Driessen LH, Plaisier MB, Stilma JS, et al. Reactivations of ocular toxoplasmosis after cataract extraction. Ophthalmology 2002; 109: 41–45.

51. Fine S, Owens S, Haller J. Choroidal neovascularization as a late complication of ocular toxoplasmosis. Am J Ophthalmol 1981; 91: 318–322.

52. Skorska I, Soubrane G, Coscas G. Toxoplasmic choroiditis and subretinal neovessels. J Fr Ophthalmol 1984; 7: 211–218.

53. Potter J. Vascular anastomoses in ocular toxoplasmosis. J Am Optom Assoc 1982; 53: 549–552.

54. Rose G. Papillitis, retinal neovascularization and recurrent retinal vein occlusion in Toxoplasma retinochoroiditis: a case report with uncommon clinical signs. Aust NZ J Ophthalmol 1991; 19: 155–157.

55. Pakalin S, Arnaud B. Arterial occlusion associated with toxoplasmic chorioretinitis. J Fr Ophthalmol 1990; 13: 554–556.

56. Bosch-Driessen LH, Karimi S, Stilma JS, et al. Retinal detachment in ocular toxoplasmosis. Ophthalmology 2000; 107: 36–40.

57. Fujiwara T, Machida S, Hasegawa Y, et al. Punctate outer retinal toxoplasmosis with multiple choroidal neovascularizations. Retina 2006; 26(3): 360–362.

58. Toledo de Abreu M, Belfort RJ, Hirata P. Fuch's heterochromic cyclitis and ocular toxoplasmosis. Am J Ophthamol 1982; 93: 739–744.

59. La Hey E, et al. Fuch's heterochromia iridocyclitis is not associated with ocular toxoplasmosis. Arch Ophthalmol 1992; (110): 806–811.

60. Saraux H, Laroche L, Le Hoang P. Secondary Fuch's heterochromic cyclitis: a new approach to an old disease. Ophthalmologica 1985; 190: 193–198.

61. Schwab I. The epidemiologic association of Fuch's heterochromic iridocyclitis and ocular toxoplasmosis. Am J Ophthalmol 1991; 1: 356–362.

62. Moorthy R, Smith R, Rao N. Progressive ocular toxoplasmosis in patients with acquired immunodeficiency syndrome. Am J Ophthalmol 1993; 115: 742–747.

63. Gagliuso D, Teich SA, Friedman AH, et al. Ocular toxoplasmosis in AIDS patients. Trans Am Ophthalmol Soc 1990; (88): 63–86.

64. Yeo J, Jakobiec F, Iwamoto T. Opportunistic toxoplasmic retinochoroiditis following chemotherapy for systemic lymphoma. A light and electron microscopic study. Ophthalmology 1983; 90: 885–898.

65. Singer M, Hagler W, Grossniklaus H. *Toxoplasma gondii* retinochoroiditis after liver transplantation. Retina 1993; 13: 40–45.

66. Blanc-Jouvan M, Boibieux A, Fleury J, et al. Chorioretinitis following liver transplantation: Detection of *Toxoplasma gondii* in aqueous humor. Clin Infect Dis 1996; 22(1): 184–185.

67. Sendi P, Sachers F, Drechsler H, et al. Immune recovery vitritis in an HIV patient with isolated toxoplasmic retinochoroiditis. AIDS 2006; 20(17): 2237–2238.

68. Brezin AP, Thulliez P, Cisneros B, et al. Lymphocytic choriomeningitis virus chorioretinitis mimicking ocular toxoplasmosis in two otherwise normal children. Am J Ophthalmol 2000; 130: 245–247.

69. Auer C, Bornasconi O, Herbort CP. Indocyanine green angiography features in toxoplasmic retinochoroiditis. Retina 1999; 19(1): 22–29.

70. Holland GN. Ocular toxoplasmosis: a global reassessment. Part I: epidemiology and course of disease. Am J Ophthalmol 2003; 136(6): 973–988.

71. Holland GN. Ocular toxoplasmosis: a global reassessment. Part II: disease manifestations and management. Am J Ophthalmol 2004; 137(1): 1–17.

72. Dutton G, Hay J, Hair DM, et al. Clinicopathological features of a congenital murine model of ocular toxoplasmosis. Graefes Arch Clin Exp Ophthalmol 1986; (224): 256–264.

73. Dutton G, McMenamin PG, Hay J, et al. The ultrastructural pathology of congenital murine toxoplasmic retinochoroiditis. Part II: The morphology of the inflamatory changes. Exp Eye Res 1986; (43): 545–560.

74. Roberts F, Mets MB, Ferguson DJ, et al. Histopathological features of

ocular toxoplasmosis in the fetus and infant. Arch Ophthalmol 2001; 119(1): 51–58.

75. Nussenblatt R, Mittal KK, Fuhrman S, et al. Lymphocyte proliferative responses of patients with ocular toxoplasmosis to parasite and retinal antigens. Am J Ophthmol 1989; (107): 632–641.

76. Fatoohi F, Cozon GJ, Wallon M, et al. Systemic T cell response to *Toxoplasma gondii* antigen in patients with ocular toxoplasmosis. Jpn J Ophthalmol 2006; 50(2): 103–110.

77. McLeod R, Skamene E, Brown C, et al. Genetic regulation of early survival and cyst number after peroral *Toxoplasma gondii* infection of AXB/BXA recombinant inbred and B10 congenis mice. J Immunol 1989; (142): 3247–3255.

78. McLeod R, Brown C, Mack D. Immunogentics influence outcome of *Toxoplasma gondii* infection. Res Immunol 1993; 144(1): 61–65.

79. Brown C, McLeod R, Class I MHC genes and CD8+ T cells determine cyst number in toxoplasma infection. J Immunol 1990; 145: 3438–3441.

80. Jamieson SE, de Roubaix LA, Cortina-Borja M, et al. Genetic and epigenetic factors at COL2A1 and ABCA4 influence clinical outcome in congenital toxoplasmosis. PLoS ONE 2008; 3(6): e2285.

81. Chan C, Hu S, Gekker G, et al. Effects of cytokines on multiplication of *Toxoplasma gondii* in microglial cells. J Immunol 1993; (150): 3404–3410.

82. Nagineni CN, Pardhasaradhi K, Martins MC, et al. Mechanisms of interferon-induced inhibition of *Toxoplasma gondii* replication in human retinal pigment epithelial cells. Infect Immun 1996; 64(10): 4188–4196.

83. Gazzinelli R, Eltoum I, Wynn TA, et al. Acute cerebral toxoplasmosis is induced by in vivo neutralization of TNF-alpha and correlates with the down-regulated expression of inducible nitric oxide synthase and other markers of macrophage activation. J Immunol 1993; (151): 3672–3681.

84. Shen DF, Matteson DM, Tuaillon N, et al. Involvement of apoptosis and interferon-gamma in murine toxoplasmosis. Invest Ophthalmol Vis Sci 2001; 42: 2031–2036.

85. Beamon M, Hunter C, Remington J. Enhancement of intracellular replication of *Toxoplasma gondii* by IL-6. J Immunol 1994 153: 4583–4587.

86. Lyons RE, Anthony JP, Ferguson DJ, et al. Immunological studies of chronic ocular toxoplasmosis: up-regulation of major histocompatibility complex Class I and transforming growth factor β and a protective role for interleukin-6. Infect Immun 2001; 69(4): 2589–2595.

87. Zamora DO, Rosenbaum JT, Smith JR. Invasion of human retinal vascular endothelial cells by *Toxoplasma gondii* tachyzoites. Br J Ophthalmol 2008; 92(6): 852–855.

88. Feron EJ, Klaren VNA, Wierenga EA, et al. Characterization of *Toxoplasma gondii*-specific T cells recovered from vitreous fluid of patients with ocular toxoplasmosis. Invest Ophthalmol Vis Sci 2001; 42: 3228–3232.

89. Herion P, Saavedra R. human T-cell clones as tools for the characterization of the cell-mediated immune response to *Toxoplasma gondii*. Res Immunol 1993; 144(1): 48–51.

90. Denkers E, Caspar P, Sher A. *Toxoplasma gondii* possesses a superantigen activity that selectively expands murine T cell receptors Vbeta5-bearing CD8+ lymphocytes. J Exp Med 1994; 180: 985–994.

91. Curiel T, Krug ED, Purner MB, et al. Cloned Human CD4+ cytotoxic T lymphocytes specific for *Toxoplasma gondii* lysetachyzoite-infected target cells. J Immunol 1993; (151): 2024–2031.

92. Goncalves RM, Rodrigues DH, Camargos da Costa AM, et al. Increased serum levels of CXCL8 chemokine in acute toxoplasmic retinochoroiditis. Acta Ophthalmol Scand 2007; 85(8): 871–876.

93. Hafizi A, Modabber F. Effect of cyclophosphamide on *Toxoplasma gondii* infection: reversal of the effect by passive immunization. Clin Exp Immunol 1978; 33: 389–394.

94. Wilson C, Haas J. Cellular defense against *Toxoplasma gondii* in newborns. J Clin Invest 1984; 73: 1606–1616.

95. Roberts F, Roberts CW, Ferguson DJ, et al. Inhibition of nitric oxide production exacerbates chronic ocular toxoplasmosis. Parasite Immunol 2000; 22: 1–5.

96. Wyler D, Blackman J, Lunde M. Cellular hypersensitivity to toxoplasmal and retinal antigens in patients with toxoplasmal retinochoroiditis. Am J Trop Med Hyg 1980; 29: 1181–1186.

97. Abrahams IW, Gregerson DS. Longitudinal study of serum antibody responses to retinal antigens in acute ocular toxoplasmosis. Am J Ophthalmol 1982; 93(2): 224–231.

98. Whittle RM, Roberts CW, Ferguson DJ, et al. Human antiretinal antibodies in toxoplasma retinochoroiditis. Br J Ophthalmol 1998; 82: 1017–1021.

99. Vallochi AL, da Silva Rios L, Nakamura MV, et al. The involvement of autoimmunity against retinal antigens in determining disease severity in toxoplasmosis. J Autoimmun 2005; 24(1): 25–32.

100. Rollins D, Tabbara K, O'Connor G. Detection of toxoplasmal antigen and antibody in ocular fluids in experimental ocular toxoplasmosis. Arch Ophthalmol 1983; 101: 455.

101. Davidson MG, Lappin MR, English KV, et al. A feline model of ocular toxoplasmosis. Invest Ophthalmol Vis Sci 1993; (34): 3653–3660.

102. Rehder JR, Burnier MB Jr, Pavesio CE, et al. Acute unilateral toxoplasmic iridocyclitis in an AIDS patient. Am J Ophthalmol 1988; 106(6): 740–741.

103. Greven C, Teot L. Cytologic Identification of *Toxoplasma gondii* from Vitreous Fluid. Arch Ophthalmol 1994; 112: 1086–1088.

104. Klaren VNA, van Doornik CE, Ongkosuwito JV, et al. Differences between intraocular and serum antibody responses in patients with ocular toxoplasmosis. Am J Ophthalmol 1998; 126: 698–706.

105. Klaren VNA, Peek R. Evidence for a compartmentalized B cell response as a characterized by IgG epitope specifity in human ocular toxoplasmosis. J Immunol 2001; 167: 6263–6269.

106. Weiss M, Velazquez N, Hofeldt A. Serologic tests in the diagnosis of presumed toxoplasmic retinochoroiditis. Am J Ophthalmol 1990; 109: 407–411.

107. Brezin A, Egwuagu CE, Burnier M Jr, et al. Identification of *Toxoplasma gondii* in paraffin-embedded sections by the polymerase chain reaction. Am J Ophthalmol 1990; (110): 599–604.

108. Ongkosuwito JV, Bosch-Driessen EH, Kijlstra A, et al. Serologic evaluation of patients with primary and recurrent ocular toxoplasmosis for evidence of recent infection. Am J Ophthalmol 1999; 128: 407–412.

109. Rothova A, van Knapen F, Baarsma GS, et al. Usefulness of aqueous humor analysis for the diagnosis of posterior uveitis. Ophthalmology 2008; 115(2): 306–311.

110. Rothova A, van Knapen F, Baarsma G. Serology in ocular toxoplasmosis. Br J Ophthalmol 1986; 70: 615–622.

111. Phaik C, Seah S, Guan OS, et al. Anti-toxoplasma serotitres in ocular toxoplasmosis. Eye 1991; 5(5): 636–639.

112. Desmonts G. Definitive serological diagnosis of ocular toxoplasmosis. Arch Ophthalmol 1966; 76: 839–853.

113. Goichot E, Bloch-Michel E. Interet de l'etude detaillee de la serologie quantitative de l'humeur aqueuse pour le diagnostic de la toxoplasmose oculaire. A propos de 180 cas. J Fr Ophthalmol 1980; 3: 21–26.

114. Turunen H, Leinikki P, Saari K. Demonstration of intraocular synthesis of immunoglobulin G toxoplasma antibodies for specific diagnosis of toxoplasmic chorioretinitis by enzyme immunoassay. J Clin Microbiol 1983; 17: 988–992.

115. Westeneng AC, Rothova A, de Boer JH, et al. Infectious uveitis in immunocompromised patients and the diagnostic value of polymerase chain reaction and Goldmann – Witmer coefficient in aqueous

analysis. Am J Ophthalmol 2007; 144(5): 781–785.

116. Mahalakshmi B, Therese KL, Madhavan HN, et al. Diagnostic value of specific local antibody production and nucleic acid amplification technique-nested polymerase chain reaction (nPCR) in clinically suspected ocular toxoplasmosis. Ocul Immunol Inflamm 2006; 14(2): 105–112.

117. Palkovacs EM, Correa Z, Augsburger JJ, et al. Acquired toxoplasmic retinitis in an immunosuppressed patient: diagnosis by transvitreal fine-needle aspiration biopsy. Graefes Arch Clin Exp Ophthalmol 2008; 246(10): 1495–1497.

118. Kump LI, Androudi SN, Foster CS. Ocular toxoplasmosis in pregnancy. Clin Exp Ophthalmol 2005; 33(5): 455–460.

119. Garweg JG, Scherrer J, Wallon M, et al. Reactivation of ocular toxoplasmosis during pregnancy. Br J Obstet Gynaecol 2005; 112(2): 241–242.

120. Martinez CE, Zhang D, Conway MD, et al. Successful management of ocular toxoplasmosis during pregnancy using combined intraocular clindamycin and dexamethasone with systemic sulfadiazine. Int Ophthalmol 1999; 22: 85–88.

121. Ware P, Kasper L. Strain-specific antigens of Toxoplasma gondii. Infect Immun 1987; 55: 778–783.

122. Ho-Yen DO, Ashburn D. Immunoblotting can help the diagnosis of ocular toxoplasmosis. J Clin Pathol 2000; 53: 155–158.

123. Boothroyd J, Burg JL, Nagel S, et al. Antigen and tubulin genes Toxoplasma gondii. In:. Nogueria NAHGN, ed. Molecular Strategies of Parasitic Invasion. 1987, New York: A R Liss. 237–250.

124. Brezin A, Egwuagu CE, Silveira C, et al. Analysis of aqueous humor in ocular toxoplasmosis. N Engl J Med 1991; (324): 699.

125. Miller D, Davis J, Rosa R, et al. Utility of tissue culture for detection of Toxoplasma gondii in vitreous humor of patients diagnosed with toxoplasmic reitnochoroiditis. J Clin Microbiol 2000; 38: 3840–3842.

126. Scheiffarth O, Zrenner E, Disko R, et al. Intraocular in vivo immunofluorescence. Invest Ophthalmol Vis Sci 1990; (31): 272–276.

127. Perkins ES. Uveitis and Toxoplasmosis. 1961, Little, Brown: Boston.

128. Silveira C, Belfort R Jr, Burnier M, et al. Acquired toxoplasmosis infection as the cause of toxoplasmic retinochoroiditis in families. Am J Ophthalmol 1988; (106): 362–364.

129. Glasner P, Silveria C, Kruszon-Moran D, et al. An unusually high prevalence of ocular toxoplasmosis in southern Brazil. Am J Ophthalmol 1992; (114): 136–144.

130. Glasner P, Silveria CN, Camargo MG, et al. Low frequency of congenital Toxoplasmosis gondii (TG) infection in the Erechim region of Rio Grande do Sul, Brazil. Ophthalmology (suppl) 1992; (99): 150.

131. Jones JL, Muccioli C, Belfort R Jr, et al. Recently acquired Toxoplasma gondii infection, Brazil. Emerg Infect Dis 2006; 12(4): 582–587.

132. Nussenblatt R, Belfort RJ. Ocular toxoplasmosis, an old disease revisited. JAMA 1994; 271: 304–307.

133. Abreu MT, Boni D, Belfort R Jr. Toxoplasmose ocular em Venda Nova do Imagrante, ES, Brasil. Arq Bras Oftalmol 1998; 61: 541–545.

134. Delair E, Monnet D, Grabar S, et al. Respective roles of acquired and congenital infections in presumed ocular toxoplasmosis. Am J Ophthalmol 2008; 146(6): 851–855.

135. Silveira C, Belfort R Jr, Muccioli C, et al. A follow-up study of Toxoplasma gondii infection in southern Brazil. Am J Ophthalmol 2001; 131: 351–354.

136. Melamed J, Sebben JC, Maestri M, et al. Epidemiology of ocular toxoplasmosis in Rio Grande do Sul Brazil. Recent Advances in Uveitis, Proceedings of the Third International Symposium on Uveitis, Brussels, Belgium, ed. J.D.C.V.L. Caspers-Velu. 1993, Amsterdam: Tassignon Kugler Publications. 211–214.

137. Montoya JG, Remington JS. Toxoplasmic chorioretinitis in the setting of acute acquired toxoplasmosis. Clin Infect Dis 1996; 23(2): 277–282.

138. Burnett AJ, Shortt SG, Isaac-Renton J, et al. Multiple cases of acquired toxoplasmosis retinitis presenting in an outbreak. Ophthalmology 1998; 105(6): 1032–1037.

139. Bosch-Driessen EH, Rothova A. Recurrent ocular disease in postnatally acquired toxoplasmosis. Am J Ophthalmol 1999; 128: 421–425.

140. Palanisamy M, Madhavan B, Balasundaram MB, et al. Outbreak of ocular toxoplasmosis in Coimbatore, India. Indian J Ophthalmol 2006; 54(2): 129–131.

141. Silveira C, Ferreira R, Muccioli C, et al. Toxoplasmosis transmitted to a newborn from the mother infected 20 years earlier. Am J Ophthalmol 2003; 136(2): 370–371.

142. Silveira C. Toxoplasmose Duvidas e Controversias. 2002, Erechim, RS, Brazil: Edifapes.

143. Rothova A, Buitenhuis HJ, Meenken C, et al. Therapy of ocular toxoplasmosis. Int Ophthalmol 1989; 13: 415–419.

144. Stanford MR, See SE, Jones LV, et al. Antibiotics for toxoplasmic retinochoroiditis: an evidence-based systematic review. Ophthalmology 2003; 110(5): 926–931; quiz 931–932.

145. Holland GN, Lewis KG. An update on current practices in the management of ocular toxoplasmosis. Am J Ophthalmol 2002; 134(1): 102–114.

146. Sabates R, Pruett R, Brockhurst R. Fulminary ocular toxoplasmosis. Am J Ophthalmol 1981; 92: 497–503.

147. Aggio FB, Muccioli C, Belfort R Jr. Intravitreal triamcinolone acetonide as an adjunct in the treatment of severe ocular toxoplasmosis. Eye 2008; 22(9): 1200–1201.

148. Tabbara K, O'Connor G. Treatment of Ocular toxoplasmosis with clindamycin and sulfadiazine. Ophthalmology 1980; 87: 129–134.

149. Lakhanpal V, Schocket S, Nirankari V. Clindamycin in the treatment of toxoplasmic retinochoroiditis. Am J Ophthalmol 1983; 95: 605–613.

150. Sobrin L, Kump LI, Foster CS. Intravitreal clindamycin for toxoplasmic retinochoroiditis. Retina 2007; 27(7): 952–957.

151. Thiermann E, Apt W, Atias A. Comparative study of some combined treatment regimens in acute toxoplasmosis in mice. Am J Trop Med Hyg 1978; 27: 747–750.

152. Mittelviefhaus, H. Clindamycin therapy of suspected toxoplasmosis retinochoroiditis. Klin Monatsbl Augenheilkd 1992; 200: 123–127.

153. Ferguson JJ. Clindamycin therapy for toxoplasmosis. Ann Ophthalmol 1981; 13: 95–100.

154. Kishore K, Conway MD, Peyman GA. Intravitreal clindamycin and dexamethasone for toxoplasmic retinochoroiditis. Ophthalmic Surg Lasers 2001; 32(3): 183–192.

155. Phan L, Kasza K, Jalbrzikowski J, et al. Longitudinal study of new eye lesions in children with toxoplasmosis who were not treated during the first year of life. Am J Ophthalmol 2008; 146(3): 375–384.

156. Phan L, Kasza K, Jalbrzikowski J, et al. Longitudinal study of new eye lesions in treated congenital toxoplasmosis. Ophthalmology 2008; 115(3): 553–559 e8.

157. McLeod R, Boyer K, Karrison T, et al. Outcome of treatment for congenital toxoplasmosis, 1981–2004: the National Collaborative Chicago-Based, Congenital Toxoplasmosis Study. Clin Infect Dis 2006; 42(10): 1383–1394.

158. Opremcak EM, Scales, DK, Sharpe MR. Trimethoprim-sulfamethoxazole therapy for ocular toxoplasmosis. Ophthalmology 1992; 99: 920–925.

159. Silveira C, Belfort R Jr, Muccioli C, et al. The effect of long-term, intermittent trimethoprim/ sulfamethoxazole treatment on recurrencs of toxoplasmic retinochoroiditis. Am J Ophthalmol 2002; 134: 41–46.

160. Araujo F, Huskinson J, Remington J. Remarkable in vitro and in vivo activities of the hydroxynaphthoquinone 566C80 against tachyzoites and tissue cysts of Toxoplasma gondii. Antimicrob

Agents Chemother 1991; 35: 293–299.

161. Gormley PD, Pavesio CE, Minnasian D, et al. Effects of drug therapy on Toxoplasma cysts in an animal model of acute and chronic disease. Invest Ophthalmol Vis Sci 1998; 39: 1171–1175.

162. Lane H, Laughon Be, Falloon J, et al. NIH Conference: Recent advances in the management of AIDS-related opportunistic infections. Ann Intern Med 1994; (120): 945–955.

163. Lopez J, de Smet MD, Masur H, et al. Orally Administered 566C80 for treatment of ocular toxoplasmosis in a patient with the acquired immunodeficiency syndrone. Am J Ophthalmol 1992; (113): 331–333.

164. Baatz H, Mirshahi A, Puchta J, et al. Reactivation of toxoplasma retinochoroiditis under atovaquone therapy in an immunocompetent patient. Ocul Immunol Inflamm 2006; 14(3): 185–187.

165. Pearson PA, Piracha AR, Sen HA, et al. Atovaquone for the treatment of toxoplasma retinochoroiditis in immunocompetent patients. Ophthalmology 1999; 106: 148–153.

166. Ghartey K, Brockhurst R. Photocoagulation of active toxoplasmic retinochoroiditis. Am J Ophthalmol 1980; 89: 858–864.

167. Wirthlin R, Song A, Song J, et al. Verteporfin photodynamic therapy of choroidal neovascularization secondary to ocular toxoplasmosis. Arch Ophthalmol 2006; 124(5): 741–743.

168. Mauget-Faysse M, Mimoun G, Ruiz-Moreno JM, et al. Verteporfin photodynamic therapy for choroidal neovascularization associated with toxoplasmic retinochoroiditis. Retina 2006; 26(4): 396–403.

169. Benevento JD, Jager RD, Noble AG, et al. Toxoplasmosis-associated neovascular lesions treated successfully with ranibizumab and antiparasitic therapy. Arch Ophthalmol 2008; 126(8): 1152–1156.

170. Ben Yahia S, Herbort CP, Jenzeri S, et al. Intravitreal bevacizumab (Avastin) as primary and rescue treatment for choroidal neovascularization secondary to ocular toxoplasmosis. Int Ophthalmol 2008; 28(4): 311–316.

171. Nobrega MJ, Rosa EL. Toxoplasmosis retinochoroiditis after photodynamic therapy and intravitreal triamcinolone for a supposed choroidal neovascularization: a case report. Arq Bras Oftalmol 2007; 70(1): 157–160.

172. Fitzgerald C. Pars plana vitrectomy for vitreous opacity secondary to presumed toxoplasmosis. Arch Ophthalmol 1980; 98: 321–323.

Ocular Histoplasmosis

Robert B. Nussenblatt

Key concepts

- Amphotericin therapy does not help.
- Lesions have a high possibility of chorioretinal neovascularization.
- Laser therapy has been used to treat neovascularizations, as well as anti-VEGF therapies.
- Subretinal surgical removal of neovascular lesions is of minimal value.

Ocular histoplasmosis is the only syndrome in the spectrum of ocular inflammation in which 'presumed' has appeared in its name. Epidemiologic evidence supports the concept that an invading organism is the cause of this ocular disease. However, accruing evidence supports the notion that there is a complex interaction between the exogenous pathogen and the immune response. Also, the recent advances in submacular surgery have provided sufferers with this entity with a possible yet-to-be-fully-proven, alternative therapeutic approach to consider besides medical and laser therapy or simply observation.

Systemic findings

Histoplasma capsulatum, a fungus found worldwide in valleys with rivers, is endemic to the midwestern United States. Found in the soil, it is readily inhaled and phagocytosed. Although histoplasmosis may start in the lungs, it can spread to the liver and spleen, leaving small calcified lesions that can be seen on X-ray examination. The disease can take three major forms: a nonfatal acute pneumonitis with fever; an acute progressive form that can be fatal in 1–2 months; and a chronic form similar to tuberculosis.[1] These disease presentations rarely have ocular manifestations. The ocular histoplasmosis syndrome is rather a distinct entity found almost exclusively in the United States, and it usually occurs in symptom-free persons living in endemic regions. However, a similar clinical entity has been seen in nonendemic regions both in and outside the United States.

Ocular appearance

Probably Reid and coworkers[2] described the first ocular case that we now recognize as the ocular histoplasmosis syndrome, but Woods and Wahlen[3] were the first to describe the ocular syndrome in full detail. They believed that *H. capsulatum* might be the cause for both the typical atrophic spots in the retinal periphery and the disciform changes in the macula. Although the disorder is found most commonly in the midwestern United States, particularly in the Ohio–Mississippi River valleys, it also appears in the Middle Atlantic states such as Maryland. In these areas, skin tests for histoplasmosis show positive results in a high percentage of the population, indicating systemic sensitization by the immune system. The ocular histoplasmosis syndrome is a rare disease in other parts of the world, even in areas endemic for histoplasmosis.[4] From outside the United States there are reports of patients with symptoms that meet the criteria for the diagnosis; however, test results are negative for evidence of histoplasmosis infection and sensitization.[5, 6]

Studies in the United States have suggested that typical findings of ocular histoplasmosis will be found in 1.6%[1] to 12.9%[7] of the population in an endemic area. Further, Smith and Ganley[8] determined from the Walkersville, Maryland, study that maculopathy due to ocular histoplasmosis will develop in 1 of 1000 adults in an endemic area. The disease appears most commonly in the third to fourth decades of life, with men more likely to have involvement of both maculae.[4] It appears that the disease is considerably less common in African-Americans[9] (**Box 15-1**). *H. capsulatum* causes four major clinical manifestations of the ocular disease: 'histo' spots, maculopathy, peripapillary pigment changes, and clear vitreous.

'Histo' spots

A disseminated choroiditis produces the typical histo spots. Numbering on average four to eight per eye, these choroidal scars are circular, depigmented, and atrophic; they have a disc diameter of 0.2–0.7 and may have a pigment clump centrally[10] (**Fig. 15-1**). The peripheral lesions are not thought to be significant in terms of prognosis for the maintenance of good visual acuity. In a small number of patients these lesions occur in the equatorial ocular region as streaks running parallel to the ora serrata. They can become larger or smaller, and they may disappear.

Maculopathy

Maculopathy results in a macular lesion that is sight-threatening, causing a sudden, abrupt change in vision. During the initial stage the choroid may take on a ground-glass appearance and push the retina upward. In the macula a retinal pigment epithelial detachment can occur, and in 7% of patients a central serous choroidopathy is seen.[11] In a

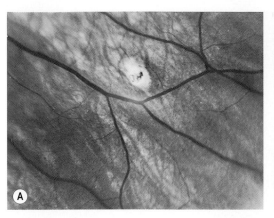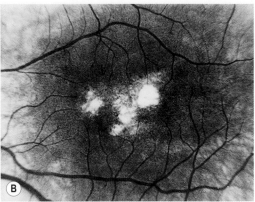

Figure 15-1. A, Peripheral 'histo' lesion. These lesions are round and deep to the retina. The media has no cells. **B,** Similar lesions in the macula.

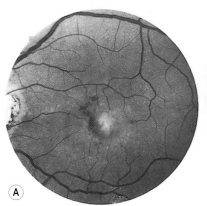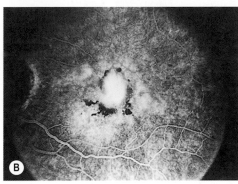

Figure 15-2. A, Patient with macular disciform lesion due to multiple recurrences of presumed ocular histoplasmosis. **B,** Late-stage fluorescein angiogram showing subretinal alterations.

Box 15-1 Characteristics of ocular histoplasmosis Syndrome

Resident of histoplasmosis belt of the US

White, 20–50 years of age

Multiple choroidal spots ('histo' spots)

Peripapillary changes

Disciform scar

No vitreous inflammatory disease

HLA-B7 positivity (macular disease)

---

large number of patients (63%) the lesion is hemorrhagic,[11] and in rare instances causes vitreous hemorrhage.[12] Intervals between macular attacks may vary from 1 month to years, leading to a disciform scar (**Fig. 15-2**). Schlaegel[4] informed his patients that if there were histo scars in the macula, then there was a 1 in 4 chance of recurrence in the macula over the ensuing 3 years. However, if no scars are noted, then the chances for ocular problems are about 1 in 50. About 60% of the time this process leads to severe visual impairment, and only 10–15% of patients will maintain 20/20 vision in the affected eye after a 2-year period. The development of a disciform lesion in the second eye depends on whether there are old atrophic histo scars in the macular region, because new lesions appear to arise at the edges of old ones.[9] At times these membranes can be difficult to diagnose because of the absence of hemorrhage or pigmentation.[13] Rarely, subretinal neovascularization leading to a disciform scar can appear in the absence of previous pigmentary changes, usually denoting a nidus of activity,[14] which supports the concept that there are invisible foci of choroidal inflammation in this disorder.[15] Indocyanine green angiography has shown areas of hypofluorescence in areas that can be mapped to points where patients were reporting visual disturbances.[16]

A point of great interest is the natural history of disciform lesions due to ocular histoplasmosis, particularly in light of new surgical techniques (see later discussion). In ocular histoplasmosis a spontaneous improvement of visual acuity is possible in patients with disciform changes due to this disorder. Jost and coworkers[17] found that 10 of 700 patients with ocular histoplasmosis had a spontaneous improvement. In a report by Kleiner and colleagues,[18] the visual outcome of 74 eyes having ocular histoplasmosis and active subretinal neovascular membranes was studied. Over a follow-up period that ranged from 12 to 109 months (median, 36.5 months) the authors found that 14% of eyes retained a visual acuity of 20/40 or better.

Some of the factors associated with the retention of good vision were the patient's age (<30 years), the small size of the membrane, and an absence of visual loss due to ocular histoplasmosis in the other eye. Campochiaro and colleagues[19] reported on five patients who maintained or spontaneously regained good visual acuity in the presence of a subfoveal neovascular membrane. They believed that a typical pattern emerged for all of these patients when the sequential photographs and angiograms were studied. A pigmented ring forms around the membrane, and the membrane begins to change character on the angiogram, going from one that leaks fluorescein to one that stains but does not leak. With time, there is resorption of subretinal fluid, with limitation of the hemorrhage and fibrosis (**Fig. 15-3**).

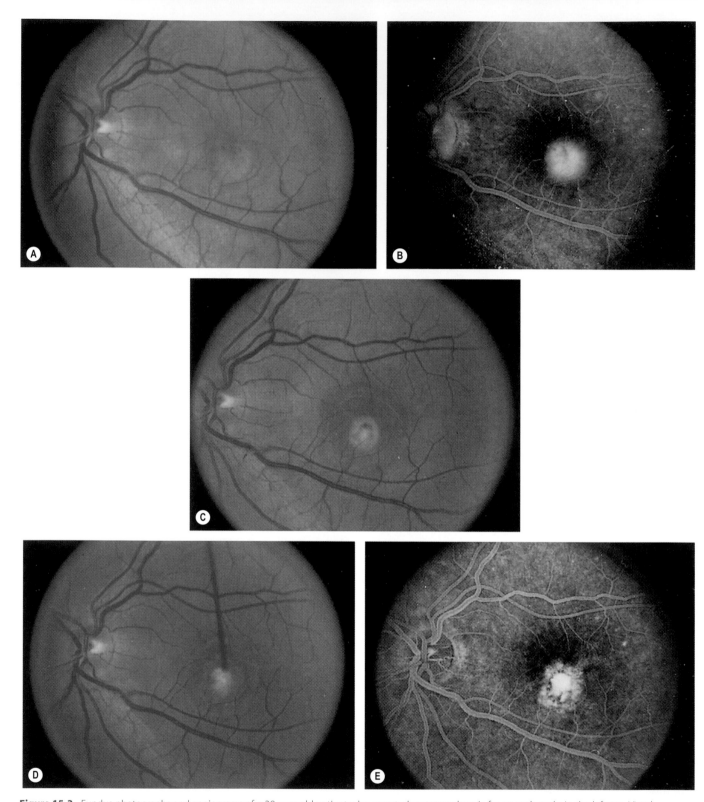

Figure 15-3. Fundus photographs and angiograms of a 30-year-old patient who reported metamorphopsia for several weeks in the left eye. Visual acuity was 20/40, with 20/20 vision in the right eye. **A,** Raised macular lesion. **B,** Angiogram shows hyperfluorescence compatible with subfoveal neovascularization. Vision in the left eye decreased to 20/100 at 3 months and was 20/80 at 6 months. However, a pigmented ring around the lesion (**C**) was noted. By 24 months vision had returned to 20/20, with an atrophic lesion in the macula (**D**), with staining but no leakage noted on angiography (**E**). *(Courtesy of Peter A. Campochiaro, MD.)*

Peripapillary pigment changes

Peripapillary pigment changes occur, presumably due to an underlying choroiditis. These changes are important because they can help the ophthalmologist diagnose the disease. A line of pigment is seen bordering the disc inside a depigmented area. Sometimes these lesions appear to be nodular and can harbor subretinal nets, with resultant hemorrhagic episodes. In a patient with documented disseminated histoplasmosis,[20] optic neuropathy and gaze palsy were also reported.

Clear vitreous

A clear vitreous is an important part of the clinical appearance of ocular histoplasmosis. The presence of cells must make the observer reconsider the diagnosis.

The differential diagnosis of this condition includes many granulomatous lesions that appear deep to the retina, including tuberculosis, coccidioidomycosis, cryptococcosis, multifocal choroiditis,[21] and sarcoidosis. The pseudohistoplasmosis entity reported by Nozik and Dorsch[22] has lesions in the posterior segment highly suggestive of ocular histoplasmosis. Deutsch and Tessler[23] found that sarcoidosis could be identified as the underlying cause of the histoplasmosis-like profile in many of the patients they observed. In the report of Parnell and coworkers[21] experienced observers felt (and showed) that they were able to differentiate between the histoplasmosis syndrome and multifocal choroiditis. In multifocal choroiditis symptoms wax and wane, and the patients (mostly female) will have an enlarged blind spot or other changes on visual field testing not explained by the clinical examination. Usually, patients with ocular histoplasmosis are asymptomatic unless the lesion affects their central vision. Most importantly, unlike the ocular histoplasmosis syndrome, all of these entities should have obvious inflammatory activity in the vitreous. Some noninflammatory conditions that simulate this condition include myopic degeneration, drusen of the optic disc, and angioid streaks. Again, it is important to keep in mind the fact that if vitreal cells are present, then the diagnosis of ocular histoplasmosis must be reconsidered.

Several reports describing ocular disease compatible with this diagnosis have appeared but in areas where H. capsulatum is not found.[24,25] In one study from The Netherlands, 51 patients were identified with the classic findings of the disease and another 31 with an incomplete form.[26] No evidence of Histoplasma could be found. Three patients from India with ocular disease suggestive of ocular histoplasmosis have been reported;[27] others in Brazil have reported five patients with classic findings but who had no antibodies to Histoplasma[28] These studies do not negate the reality of this syndrome but rather emphasize the fact that various insults to the eye may result in the same or similar clinical entities.

Etiology and immunology

Few clinically relevant tests are required to corroborate the clinical impression of ocular histoplasmosis. A skin test using histoplasmin antigen is most helpful, with this reactivity usually appearing early after exposure and persisting throughout the patient's life. However, there is a risk that ocular lesions may reactivate with this test, so that it is best not undertaken in patients with macular disease. One can argue that because 'invisible' lesions may be present in the macula, the test may pose a risk to all patients. The test is therefore not often performed. The complement fixation test for circulating antibodies is not a particularly effective way to evaluate exposure, with Schlaegel[4] finding seropositivity in only one-third of typical cases. A chest X-ray to detect any calcification can help establish whether the patient had been previously exposed to this pathogen.

The exact role that H. capsulatum plays in ocular histoplasmosis remains to be elucidated. Histoplasma organisms have been found in the eyes of patients who have been immunosuppressed.[29] Indeed, in one report of a patient with a 12-year history of relapsing disseminated histoplasmosis, the ocular lesion manifested was that of an endophthalmitis rather than the typical findings of the ocular histoplasmosis syndrome.[30] Specht and colleagues[31] reported the ocular findings in a patient with AIDS who had disseminated histoplasmosis. Creamy white intraretinal and subretinal lesions were noted, and postmortem examination of the globe showed the presence of Histoplasma yeast cells in the area of the retinitis, as well as in the optic nerve. Pulido and coworkers[32] reported a case of exogenous postoperative Histoplasma endophthalmitis. The enucleated specimen of this 60-year-old man (after intraocular lens surgery) showed Histoplasma organisms but seronegativity and an absence of systemic infection. However, other histopathologic correlations in which the presence of Histoplasma antigen has been suspected have occurred in cases thought to be compatible with the ocular histoplasmosis syndrome.[33–35]

Histoplasmosis has been seen to occur naturally in both cats and dogs, inducing a choroiditis and a retinitis, respectively.[36] Intracarotid inoculation of nonhuman primates with live H. capsulatum showed that acute lesions took on several clinical features seen in humans, including chorioretinal scarring and retinal pigment epithelial defects, as well as 'disappearing' lesions. However, organisms were not demonstrated by culture or special stains in lesions present for longer than 6 weeks.[37] Subretinal neovascularization was observed in one eye of a nonhuman primate 1 year after injection with the organism.[38] Of interest was the failure of fluorescein angiography to demonstrate the presence of this abnormality, presumably due to the presence of tight junctions and therefore no leakage.

Anderson and colleagues[39] have characterized the lesions of histoplasmic choroiditis in the nonhuman primate with the use of antihuman monoclonal antibodies. They found variability in the cellular components of typical histo spots, even in the same eye. Of interest was a chronic lesion with a B-cell focus having high numbers of mature B cells and helper/inducer T cells.

Immunologic monitoring has not been exceptionally helpful in understanding the basic mechanisms of this disease. Check and colleagues[40] believed that in vitro lymphocyte proliferation assays with Histoplasma organisms seemed to correlate with the severity of disease. Brahmi and coworkers[41] found similar lymphocyte transformation responses in patients with both presumed ocular disease and acute histoplasmosis syndrome, whereas other parameters, such as natural killer cell activity and helper/suppressor cell ratios, were different between these groups.

With use of HLA typing, a potential immunogenetic predisposition to the development of the macular lesions appears to have been identified. Godfrey and coworkers[42] and Braley and colleagues[43] found an association between HLA-B7 and the macular lesions of this syndrome, giving a calculated relative risk of 11.8. This association has not been noted with those patients manifesting only peripheral retinal lesions. Spaide and colleagues[44] found an absence of HLA-DR2 in 17 patients with multifocal choroiditis and panuveitis, whereas this antigen was found in 17 patients with subretinal neovascularization associated with the ocular histoplasmosis syndrome. The authors believed these data suggested that despite the ocular fundus similarities of these two entities, the disorders appear to have differing genetic dispositions. Ongkosuwito and colleagues,[45] analyzing DR sequencing, have suggested that isoleucine at amino acid 67 was most strongly associated with the ocular histoplasmosis syndrome.

Many questions remain concerning the underlying mechanism of this entity. Many years ago, Richard O'Connor, who at that time was at the University of California, San Francisco, studied patients in whom typical lesions of ocular histoplasmosis developed several decades after they left an endemic area. Several explanations for this can be given. It may be that genetically prone persons are unable to clear the organism and that they continuously 'shed' antigen from a site, such as the spleen. Once the organism has lodged in the eye, the low-grade inflammatory response in the choroid occurs again. Another possibility is that molecular mimicry may be the reason for repeated attacks (see Chapter 1). A third possibility is that in genetically prone persons the fungal antigen acts as an adjuvant to induce an inflammatory response wherever it lodges, for example in the choroid (**Fig. 15-4**). Ongkosuwito and colleagues[46] studied 23 patients in The Netherlands with peripapillary atrophy, punched-out retinal lesions, and macular disciform scars but no cells in the vitreous. None had antibodies to *H. capsulatum*, nor could any other risk factors be identified.

The subretinal membranes resulting from the ocular histoplasmosis syndrome have been studied. In one study reported by Grossniklaus and colleagues[47] 17 ocular histoplasmosis membranes were evaluated. All were fibrovascular, and some showed hemorrhage. The most common cellular elements were vascular endothelium and retinal pigment epithelium. It should be added that in one report, Mann and colleagues[48] reported a granulomatous inflammation. The membranes in this disorder were thinner and smaller in diameter, and photoreceptors were less likely to be found than in membranes removed from eyes with age-related macular degeneration.[47]

Nonsurgical therapies

Amphotericin B has no role in the treatment of ocular histoplasmosis. Not only is it ineffective, it also exposes the patient to a medication with serious secondary effects.

Corticosteroids can be given for the acute macular lesion that causes a sudden drop in visual acuity or in preparation for laser therapy. Patients with macular lesions, particularly

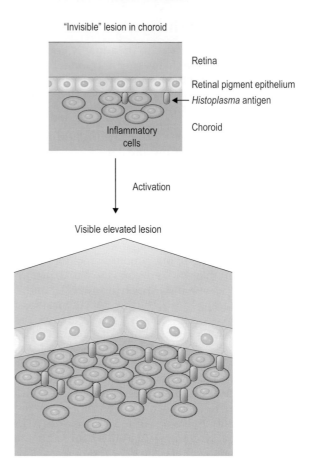

"Invisible" lesion in choroid

Retina

Retinal pigment epithelium

Histoplasma antigen

Inflammatory cells

Choroid

Activation

Visible elevated lesion

Figure 15-4. Scheme showing the presence of 'invisible' lesions in the choroid. Histoplasma antigen may be present, inducing a minimal inflammatory response, and therefore is not seen. If more antigen is released from distant site and lodges in the same area, or if *Histoplasma* antigen already there acts as adjuvant, more pronounced inflammatory response will occur, which now can be visualized as 'active' lesion.

those with one eye already visually handicapped because of the disease, may consider carrying prednisone with them and checking daily for any changes in vision or distortions that occur as noted on an Amsler grid. Short-term corticosteroid therapy should be given in high doses (60 mg daily, 50–120 mg every other day) to effect a change. The chronicity of the disorder (at least 2 years) suggests that a long-term therapeutic commitment must be made by both patient and physician. The final visual outcome when subretinal neovascular nets encroach on the foveal and juxtafoveal region is not affected by corticosteroid therapy;[49] with a follow-up of 39 months on average, 81% of eyes had visual acuities worse than 6/12, and almost 70% of these were 6/60 or worse using this form of therapy.

Steroids, given locally and systemically, have been used as antiangiogenic agents. In one study, 18 patients with ocular histoplasmosis were treated with either oral prednisone for 4–6 weeks (n = 10) or a single sub-Tenon's injection of triamcinolone (n = 8).[50] Oral prednisone resulted in short-term improvement in visual acuity and stabilization of the lesion. Intraocular steroid has also been used. Rechtman and colleagues[51] reported the use of intraocular triamcinolone injections for 10 ocular histoplasmosis patients with subfoveal or juxtafoveal choroidal neovascular lesions. They reported that three had an improvement in visual acuity, two

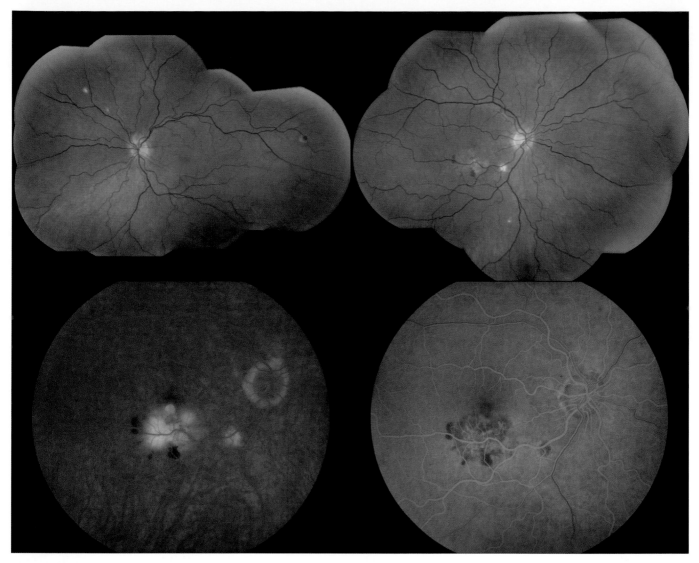

Figure 15-5. This Caucasian man had granulomatous nodules in the lung which upon work-up (lavage) were positive for histoplasmosis. He developed an active CNV in the right eye requiring avastin injections.

had a loss, and five had no change in visual acuity. This was with an average follow-up of 17 months (6–41 months). Increased intraocular pressure and 'mild' cataract development were noted as adverse effects. Continued intraocular injections of steroid would theoretically be necessary to effect a long-term result.

Holekamp and colleagues[52] reported the use of either a 2-mg or a 6-mg fluocinolone acetonide implant in 14 eyes with choroidal neovascularization not due to AMD, seven of them being due to ocular histoplasmosis. Ten of the 14 eyes saw an involution of the CNV, but interestingly four, all of whom were receiving the 2 mg implant, had recurrence of their lesions. The authors report 'significant' complications with the device.

Antiangiogenic therapies, particularly the intravitreal injection of anti-VEGF agents, have provided the practitioner with a new approach to ocular neovascular lesions. Adan and colleagues[53] reported a case of a juxtafoveal CNV responding well in the short term to an injection of bevacizumab. Schadlu et al.[54] performed a retrospective chart review of 28 eyes in 28 patients who received intravitreal injections of bevacizumab for CNV secondary to ocular

histoplasmosis. The follow-up was a mean of 22 weeks and patients received an average of almost two injections. Twenty of the eyes followed had an improvement in central visual acuity, four eyes stayed unchanged, and four had a decrease in vision. The real question is the long-term stability of these observations or whether continued injections of an anti-VEGF agent are needed (**Fig. 15-5**).

Laser therapy

Maumenee[35] first suggested the use of laser photocoagulation to treat the ocular histoplasmosis syndrome. The results of a randomized clinical trial evaluating the effectiveness of argon laser photocoagulation for choroidal neovascular membranes have shown this approach to be the treatment of choice until now.[55] After an 18-month follow-up, 34% (39 of 114) of untreated eyes versus 9.4% (11 of 117) of treated eyes lost six lines or more of visual acuity from baseline. In 1991 the Macular Photocoagulation Study Group[56] published their 5-year results of three randomized studies using argon laser photocoagulation in the treatment of extrafoveal choroidal neovascularization due to various disorders, including ocular histoplasmosis. In these studies, untreated eyes with extrafoveal choroidal neovascularization due to ocular histoplasmosis had a 3.6 times greater risk of losing six or more lines of visual acuity than did laser-treated eyes. However, recurrent neovascularization was noted in 26% of the treated eyes. In a multicenter, randomized controlled clinical trial the Canadian Ophthalmology Study Group[57] found that krypton red laser photocoagulation was no better for well-defined extrafoveal nets than was argon green laser photocoagulation.

A study was reported in which laser therapy treated subfoveal neovascular nets.[58] Only 25 patients were enrolled, and the follow-up period was fairly short. The observers could not conclude whether the approach was useful or not, but a marked decrease in vision did not appear to occur in the group treated with laser photocoagulation, nor was there a striking increase. One interesting aspect of this report was the difficulty of recruiting patients; the authors hypothesized that most patients' nets begin outside the fovea and therefore are treated before reaching the more advanced stage. Recurrence of subretinal neovascular nets is problematic. Green[59] reported a clinicopathologic study of treated choroidal neovascular membranes and noted that recurrences of choroidal neovascularization, some contiguous and some not contiguous to treated areas, occurred in nine of 12 lesions in the 10 eyes he studied. It is interesting to note that the scar induced by laser photocoagulation resembled that of the naturally occurring scar, portions of which consisted of hyperplastic retinal pigment epithelium.

Photodynamic therapy can be considered as a therapeutic approach for macular subretinal neovascular lesions associated with this disease.[60] Saperstein and colleagues[61] reported the results of a small (26-patient) open-label, three-center noncomparative case series using photodynamic therapy in the treatment of subfoveal neovascular lesions related to ocular histoplasmosis. By month 12 patients averaged 2.9 treatments, and there was a median improvement of seven letters from baseline for 14 patients, whereas four patients lost eight or more letters and two lost 15 or more. No serious systemic side effects or ocular adverse events were reported. More recently, Leslie and coworkers[62] retrospectively reviewed the cases of six patients with predominantly classic CNVs secondary to inflammatory disease and whose CNV apparently did not regress with immunosuppressive therapy. According to the report two of the six patients had ocular histoplasmosis. With a median follow-up of 10 months, an improvement in vision (median improvement 18 letters) occurred in all cases. Thus the authors felt that PDT was a useful consideration in such patients. Lim and colleagues[63] came to a different conclusion in their report, stating that PDT may stabilize but not improve the visual acuity of eyes with CNV secondary to inflammatory disease. Our experience, albeit based on few patients, has not been as positive, but certainly the literature seems to present a more nuanced picture.

Subretinal surgery

The removal of choroidal neovascular nets by means of subretinal surgery techniques has especially provocative implications. Although subretinal surgery reports appeared in the 1980s,[64,65] this type of surgery did not really develop until the 1990s, with the advent of new instruments and indications. Choroidal neovascularization due to ocular histoplasmosis has been one disease in which this approach has been explored in some depth. An initial paper by Thomas and Kaplan[66] reported on two patients with subfoveal neovascularization due to the ocular histoplasmosis syndrome whose visual acuities were 20/400. After surgery the visual acuity returned to 20/20 in one patient and to 20/40 in the other, with a short follow-up time. Subsequent reports have put the technique in perspective, albeit not definitively. Berger and Kaplan[67] reported that eight of 15 patients with subfoveal choroidal neovascularization due to ocular histoplasmosis had an improvement of two lines or better after subretinal surgery and removal of the membrane. They noted an improvement in vision even after 6 months of reduced vision. Recurrent neovascularization occurred in two of the 15 eyes. Thomas and coworkers[68] performed two types of procedure on patients with histoplasmosis who had subfoveal nets. After performing a vitrectomy, the authors either disconnected the choroidal circulation or extracted the net through their retinotomy site. Of 16 eyes that had membranes removed, six improved by at least two Snellen lines, whereas none of the eyes of four patients in which the membranes' choroidal circulation was disconnected showed such improvement. A large study of 117 patients with ocular histoplasmosis and subretinal neovascularization provided some insight into the long-term effects of subretinal surgery.[69,70] In a median 13-month follow-up, recurrence of disease was noted in 51 eyes (44%), the median time to recurrence being 3 months. Recurrences were extrafoveal (16%), juxtafoveal (18%), and subfoveal (66%). In this group of eyes with recurrent disease, 16 were treated with laser, 17 had repeat surgery, and 18 were observed. Visual outcome was better in the eyes treated with laser. During this median 13-month follow-up approximately 35% of eyes saw 20/40 or better, and 40% had improvement of three lines or better than before surgery. For those patients followed for at least 1 year, vision appeared to be stable or improved compared to the 3-month postoperative visual acuity measurements. Recently, Almony and colleagues[71] reported a retrospective review of patients with extensive peripapillary choroidal neovascularization, a different type of lesion than discussed before. They found that this approach yielded positive results with stabilization or improvement of visual acuity.

There was certainly enough information to support a randomized trial to evaluate the use of surgery for foveal or perifoveal choroidal neovascular lesions secondary to ocular histoplasmosis, or those that appear to be idiopathic. The results of this study were published in a series of papers and are important reading for those interested in the subject. The Submacular Surgery Trials (SST) Research Group randomized 225 patients to either observation (113) or subretinal surgery (112): 46% of the observation arm and 55% of those in the surgery arm had a successful outcome.[72] Five in the surgery arm had rhegmatogenous detachments. The conclusion overall was that there was no or a smaller benefit to surgery than the trial was designed to detect. One subgroup that may benefit more from surgery was a group with a visual acuity of 20/100 or worse and had other criteria mentioned in the report. To be fair, another report[73] of this study measured vision-targeted quality of life measures in these patients, and the surgical arm did show a larger improvement in the measure of this parameter than did the observation arm. The authors called it a 'possible small overall benefit.'

References

1. Asbury T. The status of presumed ocular histoplasmosis: including a report of a survey. Trans Am Ophthalmol Soc 1966; 64: 371–400.

2. Reid JD, Scherer JH, Herbut PA, et al. Systemic histoplasmosis diagnosed before death and produced experimentally in guinea pigs. J Lab Clin Med 1942; 27: 419–434.

3. Woods AC, Wahlen HE. The probable role of benign histoplasmosis in the etiology of granulomatous uveitis. Am J Ophthalmol 1960; 49: 205–220.

4. Schlaegel TFJ. Ocular histoplasmosis. 1977, New York: Grune & Stratton.

5. Saraux H, Pelosse B, Guigui A. Multifocal inner choroiditis: pseudohistoplasmosis – the European form of the presumed American histoplasmosis. J Fr Ophtalmol 1986; 9: 645–651.

6. Braunstein RA, Rosen DA, Bird AC. Ocular histoplasmosis syndrome in the United Kingdom. Br J Ophthalmol 1974; 58: 893–898.

7. Davidorff FH, Anderson JD. Ocular lesions in the Earth Day 1970 histoplasmosis epidemic. Int Ophthalmol Clin 1975; 15: 51–60.

8. Smith RE, Ganley JP. An epidemiologic study of presumed ocular histoplasmosis. Trans Am Acad Ophthalmol Otolaryngol 1971; 1971: 994–1005.

9. Gass JDM, Wilkinson CP. Follow-up study of presumed ocular histoplasmosis. Trans Am Acad Ophthalmol Otolaryngol 1972; 76: 672–694.

10. Smith RE, Ganley JP, Knox DL. Presumed ocular histoplasmosis. II. Patterns of peripheral scarring in persons with nonmacular disease. Arch Ophthalmol 1972; 87: 251–257.

11. Walma D, Schlaegel TFJ. Presumed ocular histoplasmosis. Am J Ophthalmol 1964; 57: 107–110.

12. Kranias G. Vitreous hemorrhage secondary to presumed ocular histoplasmosis syndrome. Ann Ophthalmol 1985; 17: 295–298.

13. Rivers MB, Pulido JS, Folk JC. Ill-defined choroidal neovascularization within ocular histoplasmosis scars. Retina 1992; 12: 90–95.

14. Ryan SJJ. De novo subretinal neovascularization in the histoplasmosis syndrome. Arch Ophthalmol 1976; 94: 321–327.

15. Schlaegel TFJ. The concept of invisible choroiditis in the ocular histoplasmosis syndrome. Int Ophthalmol Clin 1983; 23: 55–63.

16. Weinberger AWA, Kube T, Wolf S. Dark spots in late-phase indocyanine green angiographic studies in a patient with presumed histoplasmosis syndrome. Graefe's Arch Clin Exp Ophthalmol 1999; 237: 524–526.

17. Jost BF, Olk RJ, Burgess DB. Factors related to spontaneous visual recovery in the ocular histoplasmosis syndrome. Retina 1987; 7: 1–8.

18. Kleiner RC, Ratner CM, Enger C, et al. Subfoveal neovascularization in the ocular histoplasmosis syndrome: a natural history study. Retina 1988; 8: 225–227.

19. Campochiaro PA, Morgan KM, Conway BP, et al. Spontaneous involution of subfoveal neovascularization. Am J Ophthalmol 1990; 109: 668–675.

20. Perry JD, Girkin CA, Miller NR, et al. Disseminated histoplasmosis causing reversible gaze palsy and optic neuropathy. J Neuro-Ophthalmol 1999; 19: 140–143.

21. Parnell JR, Jampol LM, Yannuzzi LA, et al. Differentiation between presumed ocular histoplasmosis syndrome and multifocal choroiditis with panuveitis based on morphology of photographed fundus lesions and fluorescein angiography. Arch Ophthalmol 2001; 119: 208–212.

22. Nozik RA, Dorsch W. A new chorioretinopathy associated with anterior uveitis. Am J Ophthalmol 1973; 76: 758–762.

23. Deutsch TA. Tessler HH. Inflammatory pseudohistoplasmosis. Ann Ophthalmol 1985; 17: 461–465.

24. Suttorp-Schulten MSA. The etiology of the presumed ocular histoplasmosis syndrome. Ocul Immunol Inflamm 1997; 5: 71–72.

25. Watzke RC, Klein ML, Weiner MH. Histoplasmosis-like choroiditis in a nonendemic area. The Northwest United States. Retina 1998; 18: 204–212.

26. Suttorp-Schulten MSA, Bollemeijer JG, Bos PJ, et al. Presumed ocular histoplasmosis in the Netherlands – an area without histoplasmosis. Br J Ophthalmol 1997; 81: 7–11.

27. Sinha R, Raju S, Garg SP, et al. Presumed ocular histoplasmosis syndrome in India. Ocul Immunol Inflamm 2007; 15(4): 315–317.

28. Amaro MH, Muccioli C, Abreu MT. Ocular histoplasmosis-like syndrome: a report from a nonendemic area. Arq Bras Oftalmol 2007; 70(4): 577–580.

29. Scholz R, Green WR, Kutys R, et al. Histoplasma capsulatum in the eye. Ophthalmology 1984; 91: 1100–1104.

30. Goldstein BG, Buettner H. Histoplasmic endophthalmitis: a clinicopathologic correlation. Arch Ophthalmol 1983; 101: 774–777.

31. Specht CS, Mitchell KT, Bauman AE, et al. Ocular histoplasmosis with retinitis in a patient with acquired immune deficiency syndrome. Ophthalmology 1991; 98: 1356–1359.

32. Pulido JS, Folberg R, Carter KD, et al. Histoplasma capsulatum endophthalmitis after cataract extraction. Ophthalmology 1990; 97: 217–220.

33. Khalil MK. Histopathology of presumed ocular histoplasmosis. Am J Ophthalmol 1982; 94: 369–376.

34. Ryan SJJ. Histopathological correlates of presumed ocular histoplasmosis. Int Ophthalmol Clin 1975; 15: 125–137.

35. Maumenee AE. Clinical entities in 'uveitis': an approach to the study of intraocular inflammation. Am J Ophthalmol 1970; 69: 1–27.

36. Gwin RM, Makley TA Jr, Wyman M, et al. Multifocal ocular histoplasmosis in a dog and cat. J Am Vet Med Assoc 1980; 176: 638–642.

37. Smith RE, Dunn S, Jester JV. Natural history of experimental histoplasmic choroiditis in the primate. Invest Ophthalmol Vis Sci 1984; 25: 810–819.

38. Jester JV, Smith RE. Subretinal neovascularization after experimental ocular histoplasmosis in a subhuman primate. Am J Ophthalmol 1985; 100: 252–258.

39. Anderson A, Clifford W, Palvolgyi I, et al. Immunopathology of chronic experimental histoplasmic choroiditis in the primate. Invest Ophthalmol Vis Sci 1992; 33: 1637–1641.

40. Check IJ, Diddie KR, Jay WM, et al. Lymphocyte stimulation by yeast phase Histoplasma capsulatum in presumed ocular histoplasmosis syndrome. Am J Ophthalmol 1979; 87: 311–316.

41. Brahmi Z, Wheat J, Rubin RH, et al. Humoral and cellular immune response in ocular histoplasmosis. Ann Ophthalmol 1985; 17: 440–444.

42. Godfrey WA, Sabates R, Cross DE. Association of presumed ocular histoplasmosis with HLA-B7. Am J Ophthalmol 1978; 85: 854–858.

43. Braley RE, Meredith TA, Aaberg TM, et al. The prevalence of HLA-B7 in presumed ocular histoplasmosis. Am J Ophthalmol 1978; 85: 859–861.

44. Spaide RF, Skerry JE, Yannuzzi LA, et al. Lack of HLA-DR2 specificity in multifocal choroiditis and panuveitis. Br J Ophthalmol 1990; 74: 536–537.

45. Ongkosuwito JV, Tilanus MG, Van der Lelij A, et al. Amino acid residue 67 (isoleucine) of HLA-DRB is associated with POHS. Invest Ophthalmol Vis Sci 2002; 43: 1725–1729.

46. Ongkosuwito JV, Kortbeek LM, Van der Lelij A, et al. Aetiological study of the

presumed ocular histoplasmosis syndrome in the Netherlands. Br J Ophthalmol 1999; 83: 535–539.

47. Grossniklaus HE, Green WR, the Submacular Surgery Trials Research Group. Histopathologic and ultrastructural findings of surgically excised choroidal neovascularization. Arch Ophthalmol 1998; 116: 745–749.

48. Mann ES, Forgary SJ, Kincaid MC. Choroidal neovascularization with granulomatous inflammation in ocular histoplasmosis syndrome. Am J Ophthalmol 2000; 130: 247–250.

49. Olk RJ, Burgess DB, McCormick PA. Subfoveal and juxtafoveal subretinal neovascularization in the presumed ocular histoplasmosis syndrome. Ophthalmology 1984; 91: 1592–1602.

50. Martidis A, Miller DG, Ciulla TA, et al. Corticosteroids as an antiangiogenic agent for histoplasmosis-related subfoveal choroidal neovascularization. J Ocul Pharmacol Ther 1999; 15: 425–428.

51. Rechtman E, Allen VD, Danis RP, et al. Intravitreal triamcinolone for choroidal neovascularization in ocular histoplasmosis syndrome. Am J Ophthalmol 2003; 136(4): 739–741.

52. Holekamp NM, Thomas MA, Pearson A. The safety profile of long-term, high-dose intraocular corticosteroid delivery. Am J Ophthalmol 2005; 139(3): 421–428.

53. Adan A, Navarro M, Casaroli-Marano RP, et al. Intravitreal bevacizumab as initial treatment for choroidal neovascularization associated with presumed ocular histoplasmosis syndrome. Graefes Arch Clin Exp Ophthalmol 2007; 245(12): 1873–1875.

54. Schadlu R, Blinder KJ, Shah GK, et al. Intravitreal bevacizumab for choroidal neovascularization in ocular histoplasmosis. Am J Ophthalmol 2008; 145(5): 875–878.

55. Ocular Histoplasmosis Study. Argon laser photocoagulation for ocular histoplasmosis: results of a randomized clinical trial. Arch Ophthalmol 1983; 101: 1347–1357.

56. Macular Photocoagulation Study Group. Argon laser photocoagulation for neovascular maculopathy: five year results from randomized clinical trials. Arch Ophthalmol 1991; 109: 1109–1114.

57. Canadian Ophthalmology Study Group. Argon green vs krypton red laser photocoagulation for extrafoveal choroidal neovascularization. Arch Ophthalmol 1994; 112: 1166–1173.

58. Fine SL, Wood WJ, Isernhagen RD, et al. Laser treatment for subfoveal neovascular membranes in ocular histoplasmosis syndrome: results of a pilot randomized clinical trial. Arch Ophthalmol 1993; 111: 19–20.

59. Green WR. Clinicopathologic studies of treated choroidal neovascular membranes: a review and report of two cases. Retina 1991; 11: 328–356.

60. Sickenberg M, Schmidt-Erfurth U, Miller JW, et al. A preliminary study of photodynamic therapy using verteporfin for choroidal neovascularization in pathologic myopia, ocular histoplasmosis syndrome, angioid streaks, and idiopathic causes. Arch Ophthalmol 2000; 117: 327–336.

61. Saperstein DA, Rosenfeld PJ, Bressler NM, et al. Photodynamic therapy of subfoveal choroidal neovascularization with verteporfin in the ocular histoplasmosis syndrome. One-year results of an uncontrolled, prospective case series. Ophthalmology 2002; 109: 1499–1505.

62. Leslie T, Lois N, Christopoulou D, et al. Photodynamic therapy for inflammatory choroidal neovascularization unresponsive to immunosuppression. Br J Ophthalmol 2005; 89(2): 147–150.

63. Lim JI, Flaxel CJ, LaBree L. Photodynamic therapy for choroidal neovascularisation secondary to inflammatory chorioretinal disease. Ann Acad Med Singapore 2006; 35(3): 198–202.

64. Machemer R. Surgical approaches to subretinal strands. Am J Ophthalmol 1980; 90: 81–85.

65. de Juan EJ, Machemer R. Vitreous surgery for hemorrhage and fibrous complications of age-related macular degeneration. Am J Ophthalmol 1988; 105: 25–29.

66. Thomas MA, Kaplan HJ. Surgical removal of subfoveal neovascularization in the presumed ocular histoplasmosis syndrome. Am J Ophthalmol 1991; 111: 1–7.

67. Berger AS, Kaplan HJ. Clinical experience with the surgical removal of subfoveal neovascular membranes: short term postoperative results. Ophthalmology 1992; 99: 969–975.

68. Thomas MA, Grand MG, Williams DF, et al. Surgical management of subfoveal choroidal neovascularization. Ophthalmology 1992; 99: 952–968.

69. Melberg NS, Thomas MA, Dickinson JD, et al. Managing recurrent neovascularization after subfoveal surgery in presumed ocular histoplasmosis syndrome. Ophthalmology 1996; 103: 1064–1069.

70. Holekamp NM, Thomas MA, Dickinson JD, et al. Surgical removal of subfoveal choroidal neovascularization in presumed ocular histoplasmosis. Ophthalmology 1997; 104: 22–26.

71. Almony A, Thomas MA, Atebara NH, et al. Long-term follow-up of surgical removal of extensive peripapillary choroidal neovascularization in presumed ocular histoplasmosis syndrome. Ophthalmology 2008; 115(3): 540–545 e5.

72. Hawkins, BS, Bressler NM, Bressler SB, et al. Surgical removal vs observation for subfoveal choroidal neovascularization, either associated with the ocular histoplasmosis syndrome or idiopathic: I. Ophthalmic findings from a randomized clinical trial: Submacular Surgery Trials (SST) Group H Trial: SST Report No. 9. Arch Ophthalmol 2004; 122(11): 1597–1611.

73. Hawkins BS, Miskala PH, Bass EB, et al. Surgical removal vs observation for subfoveal choroidal neovascularization, either associated with the ocular histoplasmosis syndrome or idiopathic: II. Quality-of-life findings from a randomized clinical trial: SST Group H Trial: SST Report No. 10. Arch Ophthalmol 2004; 122(11): 1616–1628.

Toxocara canis

Robert B. Nussenblatt

Key concepts

- Toxocariasis is typically found in children, with the average age at diagnosis estimated to be 7.5 years.
- ELISA is the most reliable and readily available test for the evaluation of antibodies directed against this organism.
- If medical therapy is considered, anthelmintic drugs such as thiabendazole or diethylcarbamazine are frequently used, and prednisone can be used to reduce the secondary inflammatory response.

Nematode infections of the eye have been noted for some time; Calhoun,[1] in 1937, observed a larva in the anterior chamber of an 8-year-old boy that ultimately was resorbed. By its description it was thought to be an ascarid. In 1950, Wilder[2] reported on 24 patients in whom eyes enucleated for suspected retinoblastoma were found to have nematodes. Four of these lesions were later determined by Nichols[3] to be caused by *Toxocara canis*. Over the years, this entity has been recognized to cause a disorder with potentially serious consequences for vision.

T. canis is an ascarid (i.e., a member of the Ascariditae family) that can only complete its lifecycle in the dog. An adult dog can acquire the infection by ingesting eggs with stage I encapsulated larvae that are found in the soil; by ingesting second stage larvae from infected meat (mice, rabbits, etc.); or by ingesting advanced-stage larvae from the feces of prenatally infected pups.[4] In some parts of the United States toxocariasis is found in 100% of puppies less than 6 months of age.[5] Eggs in the intestine will ultimately hatch, and the larvae will migrate out of the intestine to all parts of the body. Most will encyst as stage II larvae and not develop further. However, pregnancy will reactivate some of these dormant larvae, allowing them to re-enter the bloodstream and pass through the placenta to infest the growing pups. At birth, the larvae will migrate to the lungs and become stage III. These can be coughed up and then swallowed, whereupon these larvae develop into stage IV and ultimately into the adult worm. These adult worms will lay massive numbers of eggs that pass out of the host in the feces. Humans enter the pathway when they ingest soil, food, or other materials contaminated with the eggs. A survey of sandpits in parks in Japan found *Toxocara* eggs in 12 of 13 surveyed. The eggs were present both on the surface and in the depths of the sand.[6] Once in the human intestine the stage II larva will enter the bloodstream, migrating throughout the body until the vascular lumen becomes small enough to block its progress. At this point the larva bores into the tissue and encysts. In addition to the eye, such cysts are frequently found in the brain, liver, and lungs. Because the larvae cannot migrate out of the human lungs, the life cycle ends at the stage II larval state, and *Toxocara* eggs will not be found in the feces of infected persons.

The encysted larvae may stay dormant without causing any clinically overt symptoms, although they are present in large numbers. However, one encysted larva in the eye can lead to serious visual disturbance. An acute systemic disease (visceral larval migrans [VLM]) is due to the migration of the stage II larva of *T. canis*.

T. canis infestation is associated with fever, pulmonary symptoms such as a dry, hacking cough or asthma-like attacks, splenomegaly and hepatomegaly, skin lesions, neurologic symptoms such as convulsions, and a meningitic picture.

T. canis is an ubiquitous parasite found worldwide. The incidence of infected puppies has been estimated to vary from 33% in London to 98% in Columbus, Ohio, to 100% in Brisbane, Australia.[7] In one case–control study comparing 24 age- and sex-matched patients with VLM with control subjects, 23 of the patients with VLM had had dogs in their homes some time before their illness, and an association with puppies in households of patients with VLM within 1 year of onset was statistically significant.[8]

The disease is thought to be fairly uncommon in the devleoped world. At the Francis I. Proctor Foundation at the University of California, San Francisco, over a 20-year period, there were 22 cases out of 22 185 seen (**Table 16-1**), In an article[9] estimating the prevalence of *T. canis* in Ireland, 120 00 participants were surveyed, and a prevalence of 6.6 cases/100 000 was calculated (**Table 16-2**). This rose to 9.7/100 000 if the cases thought to be highly suspect plus those diagnosed were included. The highest rate of seropositivity to *Toxocara* in adults seems to be on the island of Réunion, with a rate of 92.8%.[10] It should be mentioned here that another member of the Ascariditae family, *Toxocara cati*, also needs to be considered in the differential diagnosis.[11]

Ocular manifestations

Toxocariasis is typically found in children; the average age of diagnosis is estimated to be 7.5 years, with a range from 2 to 31 years,[12] and 80% of patients are under 16.[13] It is still a diagnosis that should be considered in adults, such as the case reported in a 36-year-old woman.[14] Yokoi and

Table 16-1 Demographics and other information on *Toxocara* patients seen at the Proctor Foundation, UCSF. (From Stewart JM, et al. Prevalence, clinical features, and causes of vision loss among patients with ocular toxocariasis. Retina 2005; 25: 1005–13, with permission.)

Variable	Finding
Gender	
Male	10 (45.5)
Female	12 (54.5)
Ethnicity	
Non-Hispanic, white	15 (68.1)
Hispanic	3 (13.6)
Asian	4 (18.1)
Residence	
United States	20 (90.9)
California	18 (81.8)
International	2 (9.1)
Opthalmologist referral	22 (100)
Puppy/kitten exposure	18 (81.8)
Mean/median age at presentation (range) (yrs)	
All patients	16.5/14 (1–37)
Male	15.3/11.5 (3–34)
Female	17.4/17.5 (1–37)
Mean/median age from onset to presentation (range) (months)	
All patients	18.8/5.5 (<1–212)
Male	7.9/6.3 (<1–22)
Female	28/5.5 (<1–212)

colleagues[15] reported this entity in 34 adults. Although exceptions have certainly been reported, this tends to be a uniocular disorder. The real prevalence of this disease may be underestimated because most reports dealing with blinding disorders chose patients with 6/60 or worse visual acuity in the best eye, and this disorder is typically unilateral.[16] However, Benitez del Castillo and associates[17] reported a bilateral occurrence of *T. canis* infestation in a patient who had a positive Witmer quotient for the parasite in both eyes.

Several 'typical' ocular presentations have been recognized. Probably the most common is a granuloma either in the posterior pole or in the periphery. This is presumed to arise after a stage II larva has been lodged in the choroid and becomes encysted.[18] The lesion itself will be raised and whitish in color, with a width of 0.75 to 2 or 3 disc diameters (**Fig. 16-1**). In the report[19] reviewing the 22 cases seen at the

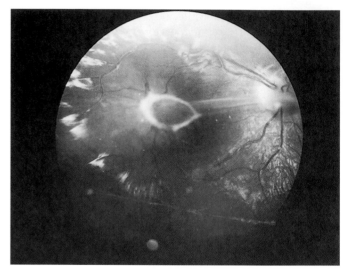

Figure 16-1. Toxocara lesion in the macula of a 6-year-old girl. The choroidal lesion is raised, pushing the overlying retina upward; note epiretinal changes.

Table 16-2 Risk factors for toxocariasis in a European population. (From Good B, et al. Ocular toxocariasis in schoolchildren. Clin Infect Dis 2004; 39(2): 173–8, with permission.)

Factor	Patients, n/N (%)*	Controls n/N (%)*	OR (95% CI)	p
Dog ownership ever	10/11 (90.9)	24/44 (54.5)	7.6 (0.97–394.4)	0.0552
Cat ownership ever	4/9 (44.4)	22/44 (50)	0.55 (0.05–4.2)	0.8214
Bird ownership ever	3/9 (33.3)	8/44 (18.2)	2.2 (0.31–12.7)	0.5248
Dog ownership in the past 2 years	9/11 (81.8)	18/44 (40.9)	5.5 (1.04–56.1)	0.0422
Cat ownership in the past 2 years	4/8 (50)	20/44 (45.5)	0.82 (0.08–6.7)	1
Bird ownership in the past 2 years	3/8 (37.5)	4/44 (9.1)	4.1 (0.54–28.1)	0.1884
Wheeze in the past 12 months	4/11 (36.4)	8/44 (18.2)	2.5 (0.43–13.3)	0.3687
Asthma	3/11 (27.3)	3/44 (6.8)	8.9 (0.62–498.4)	0.1312
Eczema	1/11 (9.1)	4/44 (9.1)	1 (0.02–14.1)	1
Hayfever	3/11 (27.3)	7/44 (15.9)	2.3 (0.25–20.0)	0.6149
Convulsion	4/10 (40)	1/44 (2.3)	16 (1.58–788)	0.0134
Geophagia	5/9 (55.6)	4.44 (9.1)	8.2 (1.4–62.2)	0.0183

Additional matching factors were age, gender, and urban/rural residence (patients, n = 11; controls n = 44).
*Number positive for the factor/replying to the question.

Proctor Foundation mentioned earlier, 50% presented with a peripheral retinal granuloma and 25% as macular lesions. This diagnosis must also be considered in the differential diagnosis of leukokoria because the lesion may become very large, encompassing a large portion of the vitreal cavity, and look suspiciously like a retinoblastoma. The disorder is frequently associated with a massive vitritis, probably the result of the release of highly immunogenic antigens from a dead worm.

Live larvae have been observed in the retinal vessels.[20] Another recognized presentation of this entity is a peripheral retinitis, which is thought to be the result of a larva lodging in the peripheral retinal vasculature.

A hypopyon uveitis can be seen with any of these posterior pole manifestations. Fuchs' heterochromia has been reported associated with this entity, just as has been noted in cases of ocular toxoplasmosis[21] (**Fig. 16-2**).

A less common presentation of *T. canis* infestation in the eye is optic nerve disease;[22,23] Brown and Tasman[24] reported an 11-year-old child with a presumed toxocaral neuroretinitis associated with a branch retinal artery obstruction. Karel and colleagues[25] reported a patient in whom the *Toxocara* larva observed in a choroidal granuloma migrated into the lens through the posterior capsule.

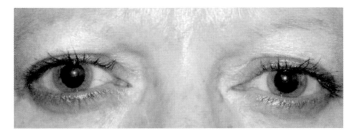

Figure 16-2. Right eye with heterochromia in a 20-year-old woman. The right eye fundus had a peripheral lesion compatible with *Toxocara*. *(Reproduced with permission from Teyssot, Cassoux, Lehoang, Bodaghi, Fuchs, Heterochromic Cyclitis and Ocular Toxocariasis. Am J Ophthalmol 2005;139:915–916.)*

Five cases of ocular toxocariasis in adults were reported by Steahly and Mader,[26] all with presentations similar to those seen in children. A recent report described a *Toxocara* lesion presenting as a vasoproliferative tumor in a 64-year-old man.[27]

As mentioned earlier, the most important alternative diagnosis to consider is retinoblastoma.[28] Shields[29] has written that *T. canis* endophthalmitis is the most common entity confused with retinoblastoma. Further, presumed ocular toxocariasis accounted for 26% of the pseudoretinoblastomas seen at the Oncology Service of the Wills Eye Hospital, Philadelphia. Children with retinoblastoma usually are younger than those with ocular toxocariasis, the vitreous is usually clear, and there may be a familial history of the disorder. Ultrasound,[30] radiographs, or other imaging methods will usually help distinguish this entity from retinoblastoma because calcification is found frequently in retinoblastoma, although it has also been reported in some patients with toxocariasis.[31] Using a standardized echographic approach, Wan and colleagues[32] studied the eyes of 11 patients with toxocariasis. In 10 of them the following characteristics were found: a solid highly reflective mass; vitreous bands or membranes that extended from the mass to the posterior pole; and a traction retinal detachment or fold from the mass to the posterior pole (**Fig. 16-3**). The migration of the *Toxocara* larva in the retina has been tracked by the use of OCT and fluorescein angiography.[33] OCT demonstrated larva to produce a highly reflective signature, moving in the nerve fiber layer (**Fig. 16-4**). Angiograms performed during this study showed severe inflammatory disease even before the presumed death of the organism.

The aqueous to serum lactate dehydrogenase ratio is >1 in patients with retinoblastoma, and the phosphoglucose to isomerase ratio should be >2 in eyes with retinoblastoma. Other diagnoses to consider include toxoplasmosis; primary hyperplastic primary vitreous; Coats' disease; focal choroiditis from another cause, such as sarcoid; and retrolental fibroplasia.

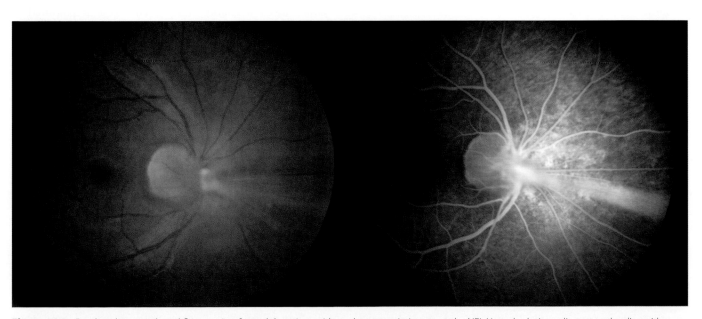

Figure 16-3. Fundus photograph and fluorescein of an adult patient with ocular toxocariasis seen at the NEI. Note the lesion adjacent to the disc with fibrotic stalk extending towards the periphery. This is perhaps better seen on the angiogram. *(Reproduced with permission from NEI.)*

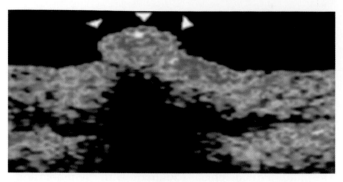

Figure 16-4. OCT of a *Toxocara* mass protruding into the vitreous. *(Reproduced with permission from Suzuki, T., et al., Following the migration of a Toxocara larva in the retina by optical coherence tomography and fluorescein angiography. Reprinted in part from Jpn J Ophthalmol 2005;49:159–161.)*

Histopathology and immune factors

The immune reaction to the *Toxocara* organism is similar to that seen for other parasites of this type. A profound eosinophilic response is initially noted histologically. Later, the immune response will change to include macrophages, lymphocytes, and epithelioid cells. A large granulomatous response to the organism is not unusual (see Fig. 16-1). In late lesions scarring may be prominent. The inflammatory response may be quite profound and cause more destruction than the offending organism. Therefore, a careful search of the lesion may be needed to discover the parasite. In addition, in severe inflammatory reactions the organism may be essentially destroyed, and therefore the diagnosis can only be suspected on the basis of the massive inflammatory response. In vitro work by Del Prete and colleagues[34] isolated clones of T cells from patients using the *T. canis* excretory/secretory antigen. They found that these clones secreted interleukin (IL)-4 and IL-5 but no or only minimal amounts of IL-2 and interferon-γ, the reverse of what was seen from clones that were specific to the purified protein derivative of *Mycobacterium tuberculosis*.

An eosinophilic amorphous material called the Splendore–Hoeppli phenomenon can be seen in the organs of children with VLM. Werner and colleagues[35] reported on the histopathologic examination of subretinal material removed from an eye with *T. canis* infection: eosinophilic amorphous material, possibly representing a Splendore–Hoeppli phenomenon was noted. This reaction is not specific to the *Toxocara* organism but rather is seen for several parasites that probably initiate a similar type of eosinophilic response. Experimentally induced disease will produce a marked eosinophilic response and a histologic picture not unlike that seen in humans.[36] Further, Rockey and colleagues[37] have noted that eosinophils adhere firmly to the larval sheath. However, the parasite is able to partially evade eosinophils in culture by shedding its sheath. This in vitro observation supports the notion that the larval sheath could act as an antigenic stimulus without the presence of the parasite itself. Kayes[38] has emphasized the important role of T cells in the host's immune response to this parasite.

Carter[39] used 35S-labeled *T. canis* to determine larval numbers in various tissues. It was found that although initially the larvae congregated in the liver, by day 14 after infection the majority of the isotope was found in the brain. Cuellar and colleagues[40] reported that measuring the level of immune complexes may be a good technique for monitoring treatment efficiency because they fell quickly and remained low with therapy. Various animal models have been used.[41] Hamsters and gerbils seem most susceptible to *Toxocara*. Gerbils may develop ocular lesions 55% of the time. Ollero et al.[42] studied the prevalence of eye disease in a mouse model of *Toxocara*. Eye disease occured after the larva reached the brain, but was not dependent on the inoculating dose.[42] Another animal model using Swiss mice[43] tested the administration of ciclosporin. Of interest was the fact that the medication increased the susceptibility of the mice to the *Toxocara* larvae, but the antiparasitic effect of the medication was great, leading to a diminution in the number of living larvae.

Laboratory tests can be important in the diagnosis of *T. canis* infection. Children with VLM will have an eosinophilia and hyperglobulinemia.[29] No eggs will be found in the stool because their lifecycle in humans would not reach this stage. Children with this condition tend to be 2–4 years of age. Those with ocular toxocariasis are generally older (7 years and older), and they may or may not have a history of VLM. Further, because there is no acute systemic illness, elevated immune parameters are rarely present.

Enzyme-linked immunoabsorbent assay

Many of the older methods used to evaluate antibody responses to *Toxocara* were not specific, cross-reacting with other ascarids. The enzyme-linked immunoabsorbent assay (ELISA) is the most reliable and readily available test for the evaluation of antibodies directed against this organism. This test has used at least two *Toxocara*-derived antigens: one from the embryonated egg and the excretory-secretory antigen or exoantigen. One report[44] suggested that the exoantigen may give more consistent findings. Gillespie and colleagues[45] found that a two-site antigen-capture ELISA that detects a carbohydrate epitope on the excretory–secretory antigens of *Toxocara* was reasonably efficient (in 50% of patients) in detecting antibodies in patients with acute toxocariasis, but not effective in detecting antibodies in those with inactive or ocular disease. One ELISA kit evaluated[46] had a calculated diagnostic sensitivity of 91%, but 14% of serum samples showed false-positive results because of cross-reactions with other protozoan or helminthic infections. This is why many feel that a negative serum test warrants testing ocular fluids if the clinical suspicion is high enough. De Visser and coworkers[47] paired fluid samples with serum samples. In their study, which found no adults with the disorder, two children with the ocular disease had low serum titers but significantly high antibody titers in the their ocular fluids, permitting the diagnosis.

Looking more closely at this test, a serum titer of 1 : 8 is usually taken as evidence of a positive test for ocular toxocariasis (**Table 16-3**). As with all tests, the ELISA is not foolproof. Albert and Marcus[48] reported a case of a 4-year-old boy with a serum ELISA titer of 1 : 4; examination of the enucleated eye revealed a second-stage larva of *Toxocara*. Kieler[49] reported the case of a 5-year-old with an ELISA titer of 1 : 2 in whom the *Toxocara* parasite was present in an eosinophilic granuloma in the vitreous cavity, whereas

Table 16-3 Sensitivity and specificity of ELISA for diagnosis of ocular toxocariasis. (From Hagler WS, Pollard ZF, Jarrett WH, et al. Results of surgery for ocular *Toxocara canis*. Ophthalmology 1981; 88: 1081–6, with permission)

Cutoff titer of Positive Test	Sensitivity (%)	Specificity (%)
1 : 2	95	72
1 : 4	93	86
1 : 8	90	91
1 : 16	85	94
1 : 32	73	95
1 : 64	51	97
1 : 128	24	99
1 : 256	15	100
1 : 512	5	100

Sharkey and McKay[50] reported a patient who had repeatedly negative ELISA test results. In a review of 383 Japanese patients with uveitis,[51] 55 had serum antibodies to *T. canis*, whereas 11 of 22 vitreous samples tested from these patients showed positive results. Interestingly, samples from eight patients had antibodies to *T. canis* in both serum and vitreous, but three had antibodies only in the vitreous. In another patient reported by Schneider and colleagues,[52] results from serum were negative but results from the polymerase chain reaction (PCR) performed on the aqueous were positive. A possible confounding factor is a cross-reactivity with *T. cati*. Sakai[53] and coauthors reported the case of a patient presumed to have *T. canis* infestation but observed that the titer for the ELISA directed against the second larval stage of *T. canis* was minimal. An ELISA using antigens from adult *canis* and *cati* showed very high antibody levels to *T. cati*.

Magnaval and colleagues[54] tested the value of Western blotting techniques against that of the standard ELISA. Using the same excretory/secretory antigens for both, results with the Western blotting technique correlated well with those for the ELISA technique. One advantage of the Western blotting technique was that banding patterns were such that problems of cross-reactivity with sera infected with other helminths were avoided.

A study of the aqueous or vitreous for local production of specific antibody or its cellular components has been done. Felberg and colleagues[55] found higher anti-*Toxocara* titers in the aqueous of patients with ocular toxocariasis than in those for serum, which suggests that local production of the antibody was taking place. Cytologic examination of the aspirate in ocular toxocariasis should demonstrate eosinophils and not lymphocytes as in other types of uveitides. Further, one may see tumor cells in the aspirate from an eye with retinoblastoma.

Treatment

Several treatment approaches have been suggested for this disorder, which suggests perhaps that the results for each therapy remain unclear or unsatisfactory. The medical therapy for *T. canis* infestation centers on two very different approaches. The first is treatment with anthelmintic drugs such as thiabendazole or diethylcarbamazine, and the second is treatment with prednisone to reduce the secondary inflammatory response. Rubin and colleagues[20] reported the use of systemic prednisone (40 mg/day) with thiabendazole (2 g daily for 5 days) which produced disappearance of the active larva 24 hours after the initiation of therapy but no change in the pre- and posttreatment visual acuity. Wilkinson and Welch[56] reported that thiabendazole and prednisone given to different patients were not successful in treating the disorder.

It has been always believed that the live larva may not induce a significant inflammatory response, but that on death the inflammation may be considerable, with serious sequelae to the eye. If that is the case, it would not be clear how helpful the addition of anthelmintics is. In most published studies successful treatment included the use of corticosteroids simultaneously with the anthelmintic. The use of corticosteroids seems justified when dealing with a severe intraocular infection, whereas the treatment of patients with an anthelmintic drug (thiabendazole), if used, should be accompanied by steroids, and the patients need to be followed up by either a pediatrician or an internist. Evidence reported by Suzuki[33] would suggest that mere movement of the larva through the retina induces an inflammatory response and justifies giving the anthelmintic. Dinning and colleagues[57] proposed a three-step approach for the ocular manifestations of toxocariasis. Initially, local, periocular, and systemic steroids combined with surgery, if appropriate, is suggested. If this approach is not successful, thiabendazole (50 mg/kg/day) should be considered. Finally, if the eye disease is associated with VLM or a high antibody titer, local and systemic steroid therapy combined with thiabendazole or albendazole (800 mg twice daily for adults or 400 mg twice daily for children, for 10 days to 2 weeks)[58] can be considered. In one study, Vermazol 300 mg was given for 1 week.[59] One concern we had was with a young patient with ocular toxocariasis who had a very high serum titer. Would systemic therapy induce a general immune response, similar to what is seen in onchocercisis (Mazzoti reaction) or in some cases of syphilis (Herxheimer reaction)? Upon discussion with infectious disease experts the feeling was that such a reaction would not occur, and it did not when we treated the child.

Vitreous surgery has also been suggested as an effective method by which the secondary effects of toxocariasis can be managed. Indeed, there is one report of the organism being recovered by vitrectomy.[59] Hagler and colleagues[60] operated on 17 patients with retinal complications of this disorder; three of them had active infection at the time of surgery. The authors were able to reattach the retina in 12 of these patients, and in 15 a stabilization or improvement of visual acuity was obtained. Belmont and colleagues[61] also reported a favorable outcome in patients with ocular toxocariasis who underwent pars plana vitrectomy. Gonvers and colleagues[62] reported the case of a 30-year-old patient with a traction detachment as a result of an inflammatory granuloma (see **Fig. 16-5**). The granuloma was removed in toto and showed a typical toxocariasis lesion. Results of the ELISA performed on the vitreous sample were strongly positive (see

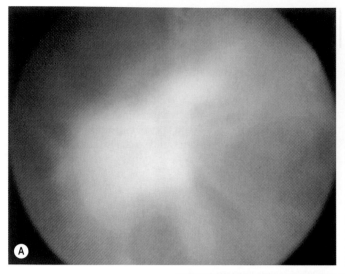

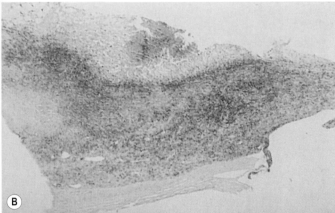

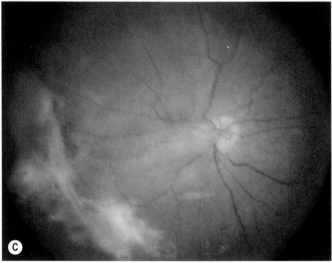

Figure 16-5. A, Posterior traction detachment caused by a large granuloma. After pars plana vitrectomy the lesion was removed in toto through the retinotomy site. **B,** The histologic findings of the lesion were characteristic of toxocariasis. Result of ELISA for *Toxocara canis* found the vitreous sample markedly positive. **C,** Posterior pole after surgery. Vision improved from hand motion to 15/200. *(Courtesy of Prof. M. Gonvers, Lausanne, Switzerland.)*

Fig. 16-2). Maguire and colleagues[63] performed a vitrectomy for vitreopapillary traction and extracted an intact *T. canis* organism. If the larva is visible and is at least 3 mm from the foveola, photocoagulation can be attempted to kill it.[24] This may induce inflammation that will require prednisone therapy. Amin and associates[64] reported an improvement in visual acuity in five of 10 eyes with *Toxocara* lesions having a traction retinal detachment needing repair, membrane removal, scleral buckle and fluid–gas exchange or silicone oil. Monshizadeh and colleagues[65] reported a choroidal neo-vascular membrane as a complication of an inactive *Toxocara* lesion in a 17-year-old woman. The lesion was treated with a laser, and vision went from 20/40 to 20/20. Cryopexy was used to treat the patient with a vasoproliferative tumor secondary to the organism.[27]

Case 16-1

A 5-year-old boy was referred for examination after having failed a routine eye-screening examination in his pediatrician's office. According to his parents, he had no visual complaints and his behavior, physical examination performed by the pediatrician and a complete blood cell count with a differential were normal. Although the family had no pets, several neighbors owned dogs. The visual acuity was 20/400 in the left eye, 20/20 in the right eye. There was a small-angle exotropia. The anterior segment was quiet. The intraocular pressure was normal. The lens was clear. The vitreous in the right eye had 1+ cells with trace haze. The vitreous of the left eye was quiet. In the macula of the right eye there was a gray-white subretinal granulomatous macular lesion, with preretinal gliosis extending from the disk to the macula associated with retinal wrinkling. The left eye was normal. Results of the ELISA for *T. canis* were positive, with a titer of 1 : 64, and the diagnosis of ocular toxocariasis was made. A course of systemic corticosteroids was started, but there was no improvement of visual acuity in the left eye, and the therapy was stopped. The posterior segment has remained unchanged for more than 3 years.

References

1. Calhoun FP. Intraocular lesion by the larva of ascaris. Arch Ophthalmol 1937; 18: 963–970.

2. Wilder HC. Nematode endophthalmitis. Trans Am Acad Ophthalmol Otolaryngol 1950; 55: 99–109.

3. Nichols RL. The etiology of visceral larva migrans. I. Diagnostic morphology of infective second stage Toxocara larvae. J Parasitol 1956; 42: 349–362.

4. Molk R. Ocular toxocariasis: a review of the literature. Ann Ophthalmol 1983; 15: 216–231.

5. Kazacos KR. Visceral and ocular larva migrans. Semin Vet Med Surg (small animal) 1991; 6: 227–235.

6. Uga S. Prevalence of Toxocara eggs and number of faecal deposits from dogs and cats in sandpits of public parks in Japan. J Helminthol 1993; 67: 78–82.

7. Mok CH. Visceral larva migrans. Clin Pediatr 1968; 7: 565–573.

8. Schantz PM, Weis PE, Pollard ZF, et al. Risk factors for toxocaral ocular larva migrans: a case-control study. Am J Public Health 1980; 12: 1269–1272.

9. Good B, Holland CV, Taylor MR, et al. Ocular toxocariasis in schoolchildren. Clin Infect Dis 2004; 39(2): 173–178.

10. Magnaval JF, Michault A, Calon N, et al. Epidemiology of human toxocariasis in La Reunion. Trans Roy Soc Trop Med Hyg 1994; 88: 531–533.

11. Sakai R, Kawashima H, Shibui H, et al. Toxocaria cati-induced ocular toxocariasis. Arch Ophthalmol 1998; 116: 1686–1687.

12. Brown DH. Ocular Toxocara canis. II. clinical review. J Pediatr Ophthalmol 1970; 7: 182–191.

13. Diallo JS, ed. Syndromes de larva migrans. Manifestations ophtalmologiques des parasitoses. 1985, Masson: Paris. 155–161.

14. Beerlandt N, Dralands L, Vanginderdeuren R, et al. Ocular toxocariasis in a 36 year old patient: a case report. Bull Soc Belge Ophtalmol 1995; 259: 177–181.

15. Yokoi K, Goto H, Sakai J, et al. Clinical features of ocular toxocariasis in Japan. Ocul Immunol Inflamm 2003; 11(4): 269–275.

16. Taylor MR. The epidemiology of ocular toxocariasis. J Helminthol 2001; 75: 109–118.

17. Benitez del Castillo JM, Herreros G, Guillen JL, et al. Bilateral ocular toxocariasis demonstrated by aqueous humor enzyme-linked immunosorbent assay. Am J Ophthalmol 1995; 119: 514–516.

18. Upadhyay M, Rai NC. Toxocara granuloma of the retina. Jpn J Ophthalmol 1980; 24: 278–281.

19. Stewart JM, Cubillan LD, Cunningham ET Jr. Prevalence, clinical features, and causes of vision loss among patients with ocular toxocariasis. Retina 2005; 25(8): 1005–1013.

20. Rubin ML, Kaufman HE, Tierney JP, et al. An intraretinal nematode. Trans Am Acad Ophthalmol Otolaryngol 1968; 72: 855–866.

21. Teyssot N, Cassoux N, Lehoang P, et al. Fuchs heterochromic cyclitis and ocular toxocariasis. Am J Ophthalmol 2005; 139(5): 915–916.

22. Bird AC, Smith JL, Curtin VT, Nematode optic neuritis. Am J Ophthalmol 1964; 69: 72–77.

23. Cox TA, Haskins GE, Gangitano JL, et al. Bilateral toxocara optic neuropathy. J Clin Neuro Ophthalmol 1983; 3: 267–274.

24. Brown GC, Tasman WS. Retinal arterial obstruction in association with presumed Toxocara canis neuroretinitis. Ann Ophthalmol 1981; 13: 1385–1387.

25. Karel I, Peleska M, Uhlíková M, et al. Larval migrans lentis. Ophthalmologia 1977; 174: 14–19.

26. Steahly LP, Mader T, Acute ocular toxocariasis in adults. J Ocul Ther Surg 1985; 4: 93–99.

27. Mori K, Ohta K, Murata T, Vasoproliferative tumors of the retina secondary to ocular toxocariasis. Can J Ophthalmol 2007; 42(5): 758–759.

28. Shields CL, Honavar S, Shields JA, et al. Vitrectomy in eyes with unsuspected retinoblastoma. Ophthalmology 2000; 107: 2250–2255.

29. Shields JA. Ocular toxocariasis: a review. Surv Ophthalmol 1984; 28: 361–381.

30. Kennedy JJ, Defeo E. Ocular toxocariasis demonstrated by ultrasound. Ann Ophthalmol 1981; 13: 1357–1358.

31. Howard GM, Ellsworth RM. Differential diagnosis of retinoblastoma. Am J Ophthalmol 1965; 60: 610–616.

32. Wan WL, Cano MR, Pince KJ, et al. Echographic characteristics of ocular toxocariasis. Ophthalmology 1991; 98: 28–31.

33. Suzuki T, Joko T, Akao N, et al. Following the migration of a Toxocara larva in the retina by optical coherence tomography and fluorescein angiography. Jpn J Ophthalmol 2005; 49(2): 159–161.

34. Del Prete GF, De Carli M, Mastromauro C, et al. Purified protein derivative of Mycobacterium tuberculosis and excretory-secretory antigen(s) of Toxocara canis expand in vitro human T cells with stable and opposite (type 1 T helper or type 2 T helper) profile of cytokine production. J Clin Invest 1991; 88: 346–350.

35. Werner JC, Ross RD, Green WR, et al. Pars plan vitrectomy and subretinal surgery for ocular toxocariasis. Arch Ophthalmol 1999; 117: 532–534.

36. Rockey JH, Donnelly JJ, Stromberg BE, et al. Immunopathology of Toxocara canis and Ascaris suum infections of the eye: the role of the eosinophil. Invest Ophthalmol Vis Sci 1979; 18: 1172–1184.

37. Rockey JH, John T, Donnelly JJ, et al. In vitro interaction of eosinophils from ascarid-infected eyes with Ascaris suum and Toxocara canis larvae. Invest Ophthalmol Vis Sci 1983; 24: 1346–1357.

38. Kayes SG. Human toxocariasis and the visceral larva migrans syndrome: correlative immunopathology. Chem Immunol 1997; 66: 99–124.

39. Carter KC. The use of 35S-labelled Toxocara canis to determine larval numbers in tissues. J Helminthol 1992; 66: 279–287.

40. Cuellar C, Fenoy S, Aguila C, et al. Evaluation of chemotherapy in experimental toxocariasis by determination of specific immune complexes. J Helminthol 1990; 64: 279–289.

41. Fenoy S, Ollero MD, Guillén JL, et al. Animal models in ocular toxocariasis. J Helminthol 2001; 75: 119–124.

42. Ollero MD, Fenoy S, Cuéllar C, et al. Experimental toxocariosis in BALB/c mice: effect of the inoculation dose on brain and eye involvement. Acta Trop 2008; 105(2): 124–130.

43. el-Ganayni GA, Handousa AE. The effect of cyclosporin A (CSA) on murine visceral toxocariasis canis. J Egypt Soc Parasitol 1992; 22: 487–494.

44. Glickman LT, Grieve RB, Lauria SS, et al. Serodiagnosis of ocular toxocariasis: a comparison of two antigens. J Clin Pathol 1985; 38: 103–107.

45. Gillespie SH, Bidwell D, Voller A, et al. Diagnosis of human toxocariasis by antigen capture enzyme linked immunosorbent assay. J Clin Pathol 1993; 46: 551–554.

46. Jacquier P, Gottstein B, Stingelin Y, et al. Immunodiagnosis of toxocariasis in humans: evaluation of a new enzyme-linked immunosorbent assay kit. J Clin Microbiol 1991; 29: 1831–1835.

47. de Visser L, Rothova A, de Boer JH, et al. Diagnosis of ocular toxocariasis by establishing intraocular antibody production. Am J Ophthalmol 2008; 145(2): 369–374.

48. Albert DM, Marcus L. Ocular toxocariasis presenting as leukocoria in a patient with low ELISA titer to Toxocara canis. Ophthalmology 1981; 88: 1302–1306.

49. Kieler RA. Toxocara canis endophthalmitis with low ELISA titer. Ann Ophthalmol 1983; 15: 447–449.

50. Sharkey JA, McKay PS. Ocular toxocariasis in a patient with repeatedly negative ELISA titre to Toxocara canis. Br J Ophthalmol 1993; 77: 253–254.

51. Yoshida M, Shirao Y, Asai H, et al. A retrospective study of ocular toxocariasis in Japan: correlation with antibody prevalence and ophthalmological findings of patients

with uveitis. J Helminthol 1999; 73: 357–361.

52. Schneider C, Arnaud B, Schmitt-Bernard CF. Toxocarose oculaire. Interet de l'immunodiagnostic local. J Fr Ophthalmol, 2000. 23.

53. Sakai R, Kawashima H, Shibui H, et al. *Toxocara cati*-induced ocular toxocariasis. Arch Ophthalmol 1998; 116: 1686–1687.

54. Magnaval JF, Fabre R, Maurières P, et al. Application of the western blotting procedure for the immunodiagnosis of human toxocariasis. Parasitol Res 1991; 77: 697–702.

55. Felberg NT, Shields JA, Federman JL. Antibody to *Toxocara canis* in the aqueous humor. Arch Ophthalmol 1981; 99: 1563–1564.

56. Wilkinson CP, Welch RB. Intraocular toxocara. Am J Ophthalmol 1971; 71: 921–930.

57. Dinning WJ, Gillespie SH, Cooling RJ, et al. Toxocariasis: a practical approach to management of ocular disease. Eye 1988; 2: 580–582.

58. Barisani-Asenbauer T, Maca SM, Hauff W, et al. Treatment of ocular toxocariasis with albendazole. J Ocul Pharmacol Ther 2001; 17: 287–294.

59. Acar N, Kapran Z, Utine CA, et al. Pars plana vitrectomy revealed *Toxocara canis* organism. Int Ophthalmol 2007; 27(4): 277–280.

60. Hagler WS, Pollard ZF, Jarrett WH, et al. Results of surgery for ocular *Toxocara canis*. Ophthalmology 1981; 88: 1081–1086.

61. Belmont JB, Irvine A, Benson W, et al. Vitrectomy in ocular toxocariasis. Arch Ophthalmol 1982; 100: 1912–1915.

62. Gonvers M, Mermoud A, Uffer S, et al. Ocular *Toxocara canis* in a 30-year-old adult. Klin Monatsbl Augenheilkd 1992; 200: 522–524.

63. Maguire AM, Green WR, Michels RG, et al. Recovery of intraocular *Toxocara canis* by pars plana vitrectomy. Ophthalmology 1990; 97: 675–680.

64. Amin HI, McDonald HR, Han DP, et al. Vitrectomy update for macular traction in ocular toxocariasis. Retina 2000; 20: 80–85.

65. Monshizadeh R, Ashrafzadeh MT, Rumelt S. Choroidal neovascular membrane: A late complication of inactive Toxocara chorioretinitis. Retina 2000; 20: 219–220.

Onchocerciasis and Other Parasitic Diseases

Robert B. Nussenblatt

Key concepts

- Onchocerciasis or river blindness is a disease that affects 17.7 million people worldwide, with some 123 million people living in its endemic regions; ivermectin is usually the drug of choice, but has not eradicated the disease.
- Worms of two sizes have been described in eyes with DUSN.
- The number of parasitic disorders affecting the eye is very large.

Onchocerciasis

Clinical appearance

Onchocerciasis or river blindness is a disease that affects 17.7 million people worldwide, with some 123 million people living in its endemic regions.[1] It is estimated that some 270 000 are blind and a half million are severely visually handicapped because of this disease. In developing countries, blindness occurs at 10 times the rate reported in the industrialized world.[2,3] Ocular onchocerciasis has been declared by the World Health Organization to be one of the five major preventable causes of blindness (the others include cataract, trachoma, glaucoma, and xerophthalmia). The disease is caused by a tissue-dwelling parasite, the nematode *Onchocerca volvulus*. It is spread by the blackflies of the Simulium species and is found in a broad belt across western and central Africa, as well as in Central America with small pockets in northern South America and the Arabian peninsula. Zoonotic infections have been reported in many countries, including Hungary.[4] The blackfly needs rapid running water to propagate, and therefore the endemic areas are usually the most fertile, which makes this disease of extraordinary importance for the Third World countries affected.

The infected blackfly bites humans, thereby introducing the infection. Polymerase chain reaction-mediated amplification methods and immunoblotting of the silk proteins permit the identification of sibling species of biting adult females.[5] Adult worms will ultimately develop and form into nodules found throughout the body, often subcutaneously. These adults will produce microfilariae that are released in extraordinary numbers. The diagnosis of the disease and the determination of the infestation rate is made by skin snips

and by counting the number of microfilariae found (**Fig. 17-1**) The microfilariae are the major cause of most of the ocular disease. **Table 17-1** describes other ocular manifestations involved in parasitic infections of the eye.

A major complication of *Onchocerca* infestation is corneal disease. Microfilarial infestation in the cornea is related to visual loss over time,[6] and the presence of a large number of microfilariae in the anterior segment is related to irreversible visual loss.[7] In the cornea there is a punctate keratitis; the presence of 'snowflake' opacities in the cornea is associated with a fairly mild infestation. With more intense infestation and over time, a sclerosing keratitis and loss of vision are seen (**Figs 17-2** and **17-3**).

An iridocyclitis can be seen in conjunction with other aspects of the disease, although the intensity of the reaction can vary considerably.[8] In addition to atrophy of the iris, more serious complications such as glaucoma and cataract can occur. Glaucoma has been recognized as a possibly important cause of irreversible visual loss in these patients.[9] In addition, even without the presence of the inflammatory response, microfilariae can be seen in the anterior chamber. However, the patient needs to be placed in a darkened room with his/her head down between the knees for a few minutes. With the use of a slit lamp the observer will note the presence of the swirling microfilariae in the anterior chamber.

Alterations of the posterior pole have been seen as well, and the degree of visual impairment caused by these changes has probably been underestimated in the past. Large areas of chorioretinitis as well as optic nerve disease leading to atrophy can be seen (**Fig. 17-4**). Newland and colleagues[10] examined 800 persons in a hyperendemic region of the rainforest in Liberia, West Africa. They found chorioretinal changes in 75% of those examined, which strongly suggests that the visual impairment in this region was due largely to chorioretinal disease and not to anterior segment changes. In a report describing recent Ethiopian immigrants to Israel, Enk et al[11] examined 1200 patients and found that 83 had cutaneous signs of onchocerciasis, with 48% having positive skin snips for microfilaria. Of the 65 patients who had an ocular examination, four eyes had evidence of active anterior segment inflammation and 11 had retinal or choroidal changes.

Relatively few eyes with this condition have been studied histologically. It is thought that the microfilariae may enter through the ciliary vessels, both the short and the long.[12,13] Another possibility is the passage of microfilariae through the cerebrospinal fluid into the optic nerve sheath[14] or direct

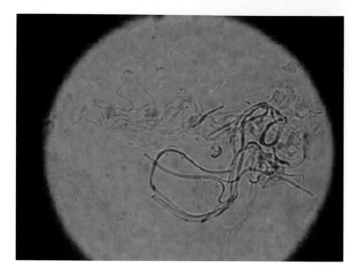

Figure 17-1. Microfilariae seen after immersion of skin snips in saline for 30 minutes. *(From Terranova, M. Padovese, V. Klaus, S. Morrone, A. Onchocerciasis in Tigray. Int J Dermatol 2007; 46 Suppl 2: 39-41.)*

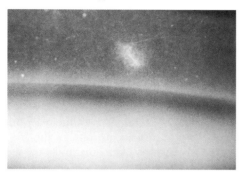

Figure 17-2. Dead microfilaria of *Onchocerca* in cornea inducing localized inflammatory response recognized clinically as snowflake opacity. *(Courtesy of Hugh Taylor, MD.)*

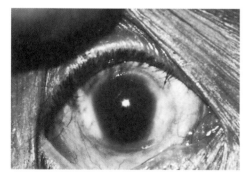

Figure 17-3. Sclerosing keratitis in a patient with onchocerciasis. *(Courtesy of Hugh Taylor, MD.)*

invasion through the sclera by the parasite's release of digestive enzymes.[15]

It should be noted that the ocular disease in most patients is thought to be a result of slow, chronic, and relatively insidious changes. However, acute episodes of glaucoma, uveitis, and optic nerve disease may be an important component to some patients' disease. Egbert and co-workers [16] examined patients in Ghana and found that 10.6% of those with glaucoma had concomitant onchocerchiasis, compared to 2.6% of those needing cataract extraction.

Laboratory studies have been attempted to better deduce the mechanism of systemic infestation, and to a lesser degree

Table 17-1 Parasitic infections of the eye

Ocular Manifestation	Disease
ANTERIOR CHAMBER	
Hyphema	Loiasis (Central and West Africa),[156–158] gnathostomiasis (Asia)[159–161]
Hypopyon	Amebiasis (worldwide),[162] cysticercosis (Latin America, India), gnathostomiasis, onchocerciasis (Africa, Latin America), toxocariasis
Anterior uveitis	Amebiasis, angiostrongyliasis (Pacific),[161] hookworm, ascariasis, schistosomiasis (tropics),[163] caterpillar hairs, cestodes (sparganosis),[164] cysticercosis, giardiasis, gnathostomiasis,[165] leishmania (Asia, Latin America), loiasis, myiasis, onchocerciasis, tapeworm trichinosis, toxocariasis, trypanosomiasis (Africa, Latin America), Kala-Azar (with HIV+)[166] Bancroft's filariasis (tropics)[167]
VITREOUS	
Hemorrhage	Ascariasis, schistosomiasis, loiasis, trichinosis
Vitreitis	Schistosomiasis,[168] caterpillar hairs, cysticercus, gnathostomiasis, onchocerciasis, toxocariasis, trichinosis
CHOROID/RETINA	
Degeneration, exudates, nodules, detachment	Angiostrongyliasis, amebiasis, babesiosis, caterpillar hairs, cysticercus, echinococcus (hydatid cyst),[169] leishmania, loiasis, myiasis, onchocerciasis, trichinosis,[170] toxocariasis
Hemorrhage	Amebiasis, hookworm, ascariasis, schistosomiasis, cysticercus, giardiasis, gnathostomiasis, leishmania, linguatulosis, loiasis, myiasis, malaria,[151] toxocariasis, trichinosis, trypanosomiasis
Arteriolar and venule occlusion	Toxocariasis, schistosomiasis, loiasis
Inflammation of retinal pigment epithelium and retinal vasculitis	Filariasis (*Wuchereria bancrofti*),[171] onchocerciasis, kala-azar (with HIV+)[172]

work has concentrated on ocular disease. The only known natural animal host besides the human is the gorilla,[17] although the disease has been induced in the chimpanzee[18] and the cynomolgus monkey, in which *Onchocerca lienalis* was used.[19] Using a rabbit model, Duke and Garner[20] placed *O. volvulus* into the vitreous or subretinally and observed chorioretinal alterations. The injection of *O. lienalis* subconjunctivally in guinea pigs produced a lesion resembling that seen in human onchocercal punctate keratitis.[21] A monkey model for this disease that was induced with the injection of 10 000 live *O. volvulus* microfilariae into the vitreous of monkeys has produced posterior segment lesions similar to those seen in the human disease.[22]

Immune characteristics

Laboratory studies suggest that the parasite induces a complex immune response, perhaps partly autoimmune.

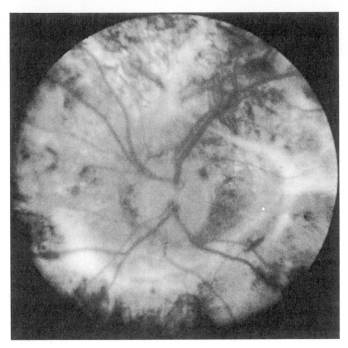

Figure 17-4. Montage of retina from a patient with ocular manifestations of onchocerciasis. Extensive chorioretinal alterations can be seen. This change is underrecognized as a cause of visual handicap in this disorder. *(Courtesy of David Cogan, MD.)*

Immunoglobulin (Ig) E production is a prominent feature of *Onchocerca* infestation, and circulating immune complexes that presumably contain parasite antigen can be detected.[23] Cell-mediated responsivity is reduced,[24] a phenomenon also noted in other helminth infections. Indeed, it appears that in addition to a predominantly B-cell (i.e., antibody) response, the immune system tries to minimize the bystander tissue damage after death of the microfilariae by producing blocking antibodies and downregulating cytokines.[25] Chan and colleagues[26] examined the ocular fluids and sera from patients with onchocerciasis for the presence of antiretinal autoantibodies, and found that these patients had antibodies directed toward the inner retina (nerve fiber, ganglion cell, and Müller cell) that could not be absorbed with the use of either S-antigen or the interphotoreceptor binding protein. These observations suggested that autoimmune mechanisms may play a role in the retinal degeneration and optic nerve disease seen so frequently in these patients. Van der Lelij and colleagues,[27] in finding high titers of anti-*Onchocerca* antibodies in the aqueous of patients with onchocerciasis and ocular disease, believed that retinal autoimmunity was an improbable factor in the pathogenesis of onchocercal chorioretinopathy.

However, an immunologic cross-reactivity between an antigen of *O. volvulus* and that found in the retinal pigment epithelium was identified. Antisera from patients with onchocerciasis identified a 22 kDa antigen from *Onchocerca*, whereas a 44 kDa antigen from cultured human retinal pigment epithelium immunoprecipitated with the same antiserum.[28] Klager and colleagues[29] used Western blots and showed that antibody reactions to this antigen were seen in all patients tested with onchocerciasis and posterior pole disease, but were not seen in controls. These provocative results suggest that molecular mimicry plays a role in the development of at least certain aspects of the ocular complications noted in this disorder. It further strengthens the notion that as with ocular toxoplasmosis our notions of inflammatory systems can no longer be restricted to only one mechanism but rather to many, and in some ways intellectually contradictory routes may have been stimulated. Autoantibody responses are not restricted to the eye. Such cross-reactivity has been reported against five major autoantigens, anticalreticulin activity, and the 65-kDa arthritis-associated mycobacterial heat shock protein.[30]

The corneal lesions of onchocerciasis have been studied using animal models. There is an infiltration of granulocytes and eosinophils into the clear structures. Kaifi and co-workers[31] found that vascular adhesion molecules are important in this process. They demonstrated a regulatory role for platelet endothelial cell adhesion molecule 1 and intercell adhesion molecule in their recruiting neutrophils and eosinophils to the cornea as does P-selectin.[32] Because antibodies exist that are directed against these molecules, it raises the possibility of their use in immune therapy to the cornea. Work by the same group[33,34] demonstrated the importance of CD4+ T cells in the development of corneal opacification but not in the early stages of the disease. Saint Andre and colleagues[35] proposed that the predominant inflammatory response seen in the cornea of *Onchocerca*-infected animals is really directed against the endosymbiont of *Onchocerca*, *Wolbachia*. Indeed, it may be the essential player in the pathogenesis of river blindness.[36] This endosymbiont is so essential to the nematode that embryogenesis of the *Onchocerca* is completely dependent on the presence of *Wolbachia*. The *O.volvulus/Wolbachia* combination initiates activation of many immune indicators[37] (**Table 17-2**). Indeed this may open a new avenue for therapy (see below).

With the study of the specialized mechanisms of the parasite, a provocative concept has recently emerged.[38] Lipid-binding proteins in the nematode, with no known counterpart in mammalian systems, exist. One of these, Ov-FAR-1, has a high affinity for retinal and fatty acids and is present in all life stages of the parasite.[39] Retinol is believed to be important for the growth and differentiation as well as for the embryogenesis and glycoprotein synthesis of the organism.[40] The concentration of retinol is eight times higher in the *Onchocerca* nodule than in the surrounding tissue.[41] It is possible that Ov-FAR-1 causes a relative local or systemic depletion of vitamin A in patients with onchocerciasis and may also be a trigger for the production of collagen, which is found in large quantity in *Onchocerca* nodules. These could explain why ivermectin therapy may not be effective for retinal disease in this disorder, because microfilaria already in the retina would continue to produce this lipid-binding protein (see later discussion on ivermectin).

The regulation of interleukin (IL)-5 production in onchocerciasis has been evaluated. It has been suggested that in some helminthic infections the production of IL-5 may be associated with an immune or resistant state. It appears that in patients who are 'immune' to the effects of *Onchocerca*, both IL-2 and IL-5 are produced in significantly higher levels than in those with acute infection. IL-2 production is required to induce IL-5.[42] Toll-like receptor 2 (TLR2) appears to regulate chemokine production and neutrophil recruitment to the cornea in experimentally induced *Onchocerca/*

Table 17-2 Filarial and endobacterial molecules capable of inducing an inflammatory response. Pathogenesis and host responses in human onchocerciasis: impact of *Onchocerca filariae* and *Wolbachia endobacteria*. (Reproduced with permission from Pathogenesis and host responses in human onchocerciasis: Impact of *Onchocerca filariae* and *Wolbachia endobacteria* N.W. Brattig Microbes and Infection 6(2004) 113–128)

Response	Mechanisms Operative in Immunopathogenesis of Onchocerciasis	
	Proinflammatory	Antiinflammatory
Regulatory cells	Th2, Th1[a]	Th3
	Macrophage	Alternatively activated macrophage
	Mast cell	
Regulatory molecules	IL-5, IL-4, IL-13[b]	IL-10, TGF-β[c]
	IFN-γ[d]	IL-4
	TNF-α[e], IL-8, IL-12	
Effector cells	B cell	B cell
	Eosinophil, neutrophil	Alternatively activated macrophage
	Macrophage, mast cell	
Effector molecules	IgG1, IgG3, IgE[f]	IgG4, polyclonal IgE
	MBP, EDN, ECP	
	Peroxidases (EPO, MPO)	
	Defensins	
	Oxygen, nitrogen radicals	
	Proteases	

[a]Th, T helper cells.
[b]IL, interleukin.
[c]TGF, transforming growth factor.
[d]IFN, interferon.
[e]TNF, tumor necrosis factor.
[f]IG, immunoglobulin.

Wolbachia keratitis.[43] Interferon (IFN)-γ responses from TLR2 knockout mice are also deficient.[44]

Therapy

Therapeutic strategies have been varied. A long-term approach has been to attempt to rid the endemic regions of the vector, the blackfly. This approach has been moderately successful in a large area of West Africa, but it has been expensive, needs constant monitoring to prevent encroachment of blackflies from non-insecticide-treated regions, and is officially coming to an end. Three modalities were traditionally available to treat the patient. The first was nodulectomy, i.e., removing the adult worms that produce the microfilariae. Nodulectomy was reported by Rodolfo Robles in Central America in 1915 to improve the ophthalmic disease, and this approach has been practiced in Guatemala since 1935. Indeed, although hard evidence concerning its

effectiveness is lacking, the rate of blindness in the endemic regions has decreased from 1935 to 1979, during which time 1.5 million people have been examined and 257 883 nodules excised.[45] Nodulectomy has not significantly altered the number of microfilariae in skin snips from patients in West Africa.

Other modalities available are specific therapies against the *Onchocerca* organism. For many years these were limited to diethylcarbamazine citrate (DEC-C) and suramin. DEC-C is microfilaricidal, and with the massive killing of these organisms a severe systemic reaction occurs (Mazzotti reaction). An aggravation of the ocular condition, with limbitis, an increase in corneal opacities, and advancement of sclerosing keratitis, can also occur. Further, Bird and colleagues[46] observed that DEC-C administration induced transient pigment epithelial lesions, optic disc leakage, and visual field loss. Its administration sometimes necessitates corticosteroid treatment. Although suramin is more toxic to adult worms than to microfilariae, killing of the microfilariae still leads to secondary reactions. Further, this drug has an intrinsic toxicity that may be fatal. For these reasons, suramin is best given in progressive doses over 6–8 weeks until a total dosage of 60–67 mg/kg is reached. Both of these drugs were used with great care, and patients needed to be followed up closely by physicians with experience in their use. They are not used much today.

Other drugs that have been evaluated include the benzimidazoles, and a quantification of ocular reactions as a result of the therapy has been published.[47] These compounds have an effect on the embryogenesis of various *Onchocerca* species, thereby sterilizing the adult worms. Testing of these compounds suggested that embryogenesis was interrupted in adult worms in the nodules of patients with onchocerciasis 2 months after therapy.[48] However, these drugs are poorly absorbed orally, and standard dosages may not be particularly effective.

The agent ivermectin was shown to be successful for treatment of onchocerciasis in 1982.[49] Given as a single oral dose of 150 µg/kg, the belief was that it would control or curtail the disease if given on a wide scale in endemic areas.[2,57] Ivermectin is not thought to kill adult worms, nor does it effect embryogenesis or spermatogenesis, but rather it prevents the release of the microfilariae from the adult female worm, resulting in their in utero degeneration. Ivermectin was compared to DEC-C in a randomized, double-masked study in the treatment of the ocular changes caused by onchocerciasis.[50] It was found that although DEC-C caused a marked increase in both living and dead microfilariae in the cornea, inducing a limbitis and punctate keratitis, ivermectin did not. Further, ivermectin resulted in a long-term reduction in intraocular microfilariae when given in a single oral dose of 200 µg/kg. Other studies have demonstrated similar results.[51,52] Diallo and colleagues[51] noted that microfilarial densities reached 4% of pretherapy levels 1 year after a single 12-mg dose of ivermectin, but one of 10 ivermectin-treated patients needed systemic steroid therapy to deal with adverse systemic reactions. In this study, adult worms taken from patients treated with ivermectin were examined; they contained deformed and degenerated intrauterine forms of the microfilariae. In one report outlining preliminary findings for the distribution of ivermectin to 118 925 persons in Nigeria, Ogunba and Gemade[53] found that the drug was extremely well tolerated: only 0.7% of recipients reported adverse reactions within 3 days of treatment. Whitworth and colleagues[54] reported the results of a randomized, double-masked study in Sierra Leone that compared the effects of ivermectin with those of placebo on ocular disease. They found that the 296 persons who received ivermectin had less anterior segment disease, a lower prevalence of microfilariae in the anterior chamber and cornea, and less punctate keratitis and iritis than that seen in the 272 patients who received placebo. No difference was found between the two groups for optic atrophy or chorioretinitis, and the visual acuities in the two groups were not statistically significantly different, although the results for the ivermectin group were more favorable. Dadzie and colleagues[55] found very low ocular microfilariae loads in 334 patients in Ghana who were treated twice with the medication. Blindness did occur in three patients in the ivermectin group; these patients were thought to have advanced disease. Because of these and other reports, between March 1992 and February 1993 an estimated 1.5 million people were treated in the Onchocerciasis Control Programme (OCP) area.[56] The OCP has covered 11 countries in West Africa, and by 2002 10 million people had received ivermectin;[57] by 2006 nongovernmental development organizations had helped to treat 62 million people[58] (**Fig. 17-5**). Will this therapeutic program eradicate this disease? In some smaller endemic regions, such as Ecuador, it has the potential to do so.[59] However, in the vast area of West Africa the challenge is enormous. Because of the characteristics of ivermentin, it has been estimated that 90 million at-risk individuals would need to be treated for

25 years, a daunting task.[60] Reports such as those by Semba and co-workers[61] and Njoo and colleagues[62] are not heartening. In the study reported by Njoo and colleagues of a fairly small number of patients with onchocerciasis from an hyperendemic area with no vector control, 44% of 25 patients who received three doses of ivermectin still had positive results for skin snips, but the number of adverse reactions did decrease with repeated administration. In one long-term follow-up study performed in Sierra Leone and reported by Mabey and colleagues,[63] ivermectin-treated patients had full ocular examinations in 1989 and again in 1994. These authors concluded that annual treatment with ivermectin controlled all aspects of ocular disease except chorioretinal lesions. Changing the dosing interval to every 6 months did not seem to help either. Chippaux and colleagues[64] found that repeated ivermectin doses failed to prevent the appearance of initial retinal lesions or the worsening of preexisting ones. Awadzi and coinvestigators[65] treated patients with doses of ivermectin varying from 150 µg/kg to 1600 µg/kg of body weight. Their findings suggested that administration of larger doses of the medication was probably no better than giving repeated lower doses. It appears that ivermectin therapy needs to be given regularly to produce any long-term benefit.[66] A controlled study using ivermectin every 3 months showed that this regimen greatly reduced the number of female worms as well as acute itching and skin lesions.[67] Studies in the past with at least a 1-year follow-up did not show a statistically significant better visual outcome between ivermectin and placebo.[68] Awadzi et al.[69] reported that over a 30-month period they were able to confirm the existence of a population of female *O. volvulus* that respond poorly to ivermectin. A randomized study[70] giving patients high doses (800 µg/kg) annually, or the normal dose at 3-month intervals, did show a greater effect than the standard dose (150 µg/kg) annually. However, in this particular study transitory ocular complaints were noted, suggesting that the higher-dose approach should be considered only with caution. Studies suggest that therapy alone without vector control may not control disease in endemic areas, and models[71,72] suggest that therapy alone (without vector control) will not control disease in the next quarter-century. These projections once again point to the need to find new drugs to treat this disorder. There have been recent new therapeutic considerations. As mentioned earlier, *Wolbachia* appears to be one of the major sources of antigenic stimulation for the corneal disease, and in its symbiotic relationship with *Onchocerca* appears to be essential for the fertility of *O. volvulus*. Treatment with doxycycline, 100mg/day for 6 weeks, will deplete *Wolbachia* in the *Onchocerca* after several months and inhibit embryogenesis.[3] Further, even if a medication that safely kills adults appears, there is an interest in other medications such as moxidectin. This inhibits embryogenesis and may last longer than ivermectin.[3]

Giardiasis

Giardia lamblia is a flagellated binucleate protozoan about 12–14 µm in length. It can be in a motile form (trophozoite) or in a cystic state. The organism was first seen microscopically by van Leeuwenhoeck in 1681.[73] Ingestion of

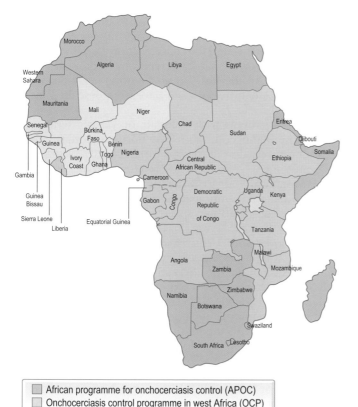

African programme for onchocerciasis control (APOC)
Onchocerciasis control programme in west Africa (OCP)

Figure 17-5. The geographical distribution of African programs for onchocerciasis control. *(Reproduced with permission from Onchocerciasis – is it all solved? AD Hopkins, Eye (2005) 19:1057–1066.)*

contaminated food or drinking water is the usual mode of spread. *Giardia* has a propensity to inhabit the jejunum of humans, where it will multiply and cause swelling of the microvilli of the intestinal epithelial cells. Gastrointestinal symptoms include epigastric burning, cramps, diarrhea, constipation, and weight loss. Although extraintestinal spread of the organism has not been documented to date, there have been reports of patients with extraintestinal manifestations attributed to *Giardia*.[74,75] These include nervousness, headache, and emotional instability. To our knowledge, Barraquer[76] was the first to make the association between giardiasis and ocular inflammatory disease, noting choroiditis, hemorrhagic retinopathy, and iridocyclitis. Knox and King[77] reported finding *Giardia* in the stools of three patients with retinal arteritis, which was associated with an iridocyclitis in two of them. It was felt that antiparasitic therapy improved their ocular state. Pettoello Mantovani and colleagues[78] examined 90 children with intestinal *Giardia* for ocular disease. They noted that eight of them (9%) had 'salt and pepper' alterations at the level of the retinal pigmented epithelium in all quadrants of the midperiphery. Some of these patients also had atrophic regions and hard exudates associated with the lesions. In addition, one other patient was noted to have temporal 'discoloration' of the optic disk, and another had a chorioretinitis that resolved with steroid therapy. These patients were treated, and after 1 year of follow-up no alteration in the salt and pepper changes were noted. In two control groups, one of 200 children with gastrointestinal symptoms not due to *Giardia* and 200 healthy children did not have salt and pepper changes. In a similar study reported by Corsi and colleagues,[79] 141 children with *Giardia* were examined and 28 (19.9%) were noted to have salt and pepper changes in their fundus.

The underlying cause of the ocular inflammatory disease is unknown, although the most plausible explanation at this point is that the inflammation results from a hypersensitivity reaction. The organism has never been isolated from lesions (besides the gut) associated with the parasite (such as urticarial lesions). Immune complexes have been reported in patients with *Giardia*,[80] and it has been suggested that the ocular lesions are a hypersensitivity reaction. HLA studies have been performed, with a higher expected frequency seen for HLA-A1 (46.7% vs 32%) and HLA-B12 (47.8% vs 25.3%).[81]

The diagnosis is based on finding the organism in the stool, which is not always easy to do. Multiple examinations or even biopsy of jejunal tissue are needed. In the past the disease was treated with quinacrine hydrochloride (Atabrine) (100 mg) given three times a day for 10 days, but a single dose of tinidazole (50 mg/kg) has been used more recently.[79] In one report, oral corticosteroids and metronidazole (250 mg tid) were used.[82]

Ophthalmomyiasis

The term ophthalmomyiasis refers to the infestation of the eye by the larval forms of flies (maggots) of the order Diptera. Ophthalmomyiasis externa indicates infestation of the conjunctiva, whereas ophthalmomyiasis interna (posterior or anterior) means infestation inside the globe.[83] Usually, these larval forms are obligate tissue parasites that require the

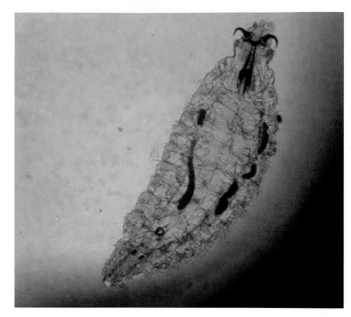

Figure 17-6. First instar larva from *Oestrus ova*. Note oral hooks. Removed from the conjunctiva of a patient. *(Reproduced with permission from An Outbreak of Human External Ophthalmomyiasis Due to Oestrus ovis in Southern Afghanistan, James Dunbar et al Clinical Infectious Diseases 2008;46:e124–6. University of Chicago Press.)*

host's tissue to complete their developmental cycle. In addition to humans, the usual hosts for these larvae include cattle, deer, sheep, horses, and reindeer. The larvae may get to the eye via a vector such as an adult fly that carries the larvae or eggs to the region, or by touching of the ocular region with hands contaminated with the larvae. Most patients do not give a history of being 'bitten.' The larva is thought to bore through the coats of the eye until they come to rest within. However, an early report by DeBoe[84] described the emergence of the larva from the optic nerve head into the vitreous. A handful of cases have been described in the literature.

Seventeen patients with ophthalmomyiasis externa were seen by Amr and colleagues[85] in northern Jordan. These occurrences were due to the sheep nasal botfly, *Oestrus ovis*; the symptoms were mild to severe conjunctivitis, cellulitis, and lacrimation. Four cases due to *O. ovis* in Kuwait both before and after Operations Desert Shield and Desert Storm were reported.[86] Another species involved is *Cochliomyia hominivorax*,[87] whose larvae can lie over the conjunctiva and can be removed with a cotton swab[88] (**Fig. 17-6**).

With ophthalmomyiasis interna the invading larva may initially cause little or no pain, but discomfort and an intraocular inflammatory reaction can certainly occur,[89] particularly after its death.[90] The characteristic features of ophthalmomyiasis interna include the presence of subretinal tracks[91,92] along with the finding of an encysted larva either subretinally or even free floating in the vitreous. Without finding the maggot in the eye, a definitive diagnosis cannot be made; the maggot is white or semitranslucent, segmented, and tapered at both ends.[91] Vision may be lost because of macular hemorrhage, optic nerve invasion by the maggot, or retinal detachment. Jakobs and colleagues[93] reported a patient with a larva that appeared to enter the eye via the optic nerve, migrated subretinally yielding tracts, and then apparently entered the optic nerve again. Billi and co-workers[94] reported such a case after cataract extraction, conjecturing that the site of entry into the eye was the surgical wound. The organism was removed from the eye by vitrectomy and thought to be of the Sarcophagidae family of flies. Interestingly, no retinal pigment epithelium tracking was noted. Campbell and colleagues[95] reported that an interesting retinopathy that resembled ophthalmomyiasis interna was seen in 10% of a sample Chamorro population examined on the island of Guam. In addition, this retinopathy was found in 50% of a population with amyotrophic lateral sclerosis–parkinsonism–dementia complex. Although the retinopathy appears to be similar to the changes seen with parasitic infestation, they were not able to establish a definitive diagnosis despite obtaining eyes for histologic study.

The treatment of ophthalmomyiasis must be tailored to the ocular findings. If the worm is situated in the anterior chamber it should be removed as quickly as possible, as it may migrate elswehere in the eye.[96] A Fuchs' heterochromic iridocyclitis has been been described after a case of ophthalmomyiasis interna posterior.[97] Saraiva and colleagues[98] reported a case of the removal of a worm from the anterior segment, and histology showed the larva to be covered with macrophages and foreign body giant cells (**Fig. 17-7**). The granulomatous reaction cleared with removal of the worm. In the case of an immobile subretinal worm, with no inflammatory disease and good vision, the ophthalmologist may elect to follow the patient. However, if there is a severe inflammatory reaction, antiinflammatory therapy should be instituted. Hemorrhage may require a vitrectomy because it may indicate that the larva is alive and migrating. If the larva can be visualized in the subretinal space, and if the decision is made to treat it, Gass and Lewis[91] have recommended the use of photocoagulation over removal of the organism by sclerotomy. Others have suggested either laser or vitrectomy.[99] Forman and colleagues[100] described a case of a 16-year-old patient with a subretinal fly larva in which the larva was killed with argon laser therapy. The patient's visual acuity improved from 20/200 to 20/20. Syrdalen and colleagues[101] reported that removal of a reindeer warble fly larva through a pars plana opening after vitrectomy freed the surrounding vitreous attachments. Others have reported a caribou botfly infecting an eye.[99] The patient retained good vision. However, the visual result varies, depending on whether the macula and the optic nerve were involved in the process.[93]

Cysticercosis

Cysticercosis is more common in areas with poor hygiene. It is usually seen in the first four decades of life and is rare in the United States, but is frequently seen in Central and South America and is the most common parasitic infection affecting the nervous system.[102] This disease is caused by the ingestion of the eggs of *Taenia solium*. The larva migrates to the eye, where it encysts (**Fig. 17-8**). The cyst can appear in any part of the eye. In the anterior chamber it can induce an anterior uveitis with fibrous changes and a secondar glaucoma. Excision of the cyst containing the worm has been reported to be therapeutic[103,104] (**Fig. 17-9**). Often the scolex of the larva can be seen moving slowly in the vitreous.[105] An anterior chamber tap will reveal a large number of

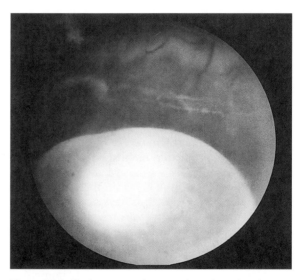

Figure 17-8. Cysticerca organism seen through cystic retina. *(Courtesy Miguel Burnier, Jr., M.D.)*

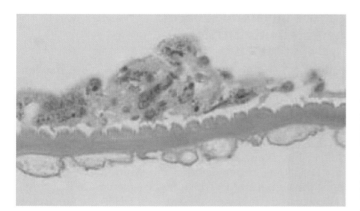

Figure 17-7. Macrophages and foreign body giant cells on the surface (cuticle) of the larva (H&E, original magnification ×600). *(Reproduced with permission from A case of anterior internal ophthalmomyiasis: case report Arq Bras Ofthalmol. 2006:69. Vinicius da Silveira Saraiva, Miguel Hage Amaro, Rubens Belfort Jr. Miguel Noel Burnier Jr.)*

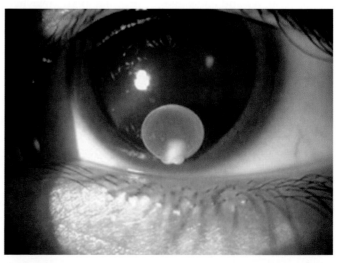

Figure 17-9. A 6-year-old girl with discomfort and drop in vision in one eye. Scolex exiting the cyst. *(From Cortez MA, Giuliari GP, Escaf L, et al. Ocular cysticercosis of the anterior segment. J AAPOS 2007; 11: 628–62, with permission.)*

eosinophils. The presence of the parasite can be disastrous for the eye, particularly if it is located in the subretinal space. Vitrectomy can be used to remove the larva if it is in the vitreous,[106] with the potential for good vision postoperatively. However, the removal of subretinal lesions may not lead to a good visual outcome.[107] The larva can be removed via a sclerotomy site, and repair of the detachment caused by the presence of the parasite with a scleral buckling procedure can be tried.[106] Others have removed the organism through a retinotomy at the apex of the induced serous retinal detachment using a soft silicone-tipped extrusion cannula.[108] There are usually no overt systemic findings in this disorder. However, cysticercosis has been identified as the cause of severe medial rectus muscle myositis.[109] In one recent report an optic nerve lesion ascribed to cysticerci (no confirmatory biopsy could be obtained) was seen using high-resolution CT.[110] Albendazole has been used to treat neurocysticercosis, with regression of the cyst in some patients.[111]

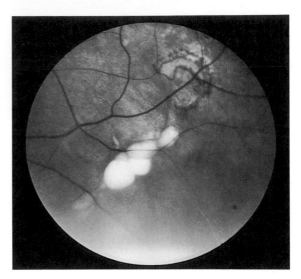

Figure 17-10. Presumed caterpillar hairs causing track anteroposteriorly in temporal retina.

Caterpillar hairs

Caterpillar hairs have been known since ancient times to be toxic to humans. Ocular disease was first associated with the caterpillar in the last century when reported by Schon in 1861. Several species of caterpillar have hairs forming a row on their dorsal surface and containing histamine-liberating substances[112] that are released only if the hair is broken. It is theorized that these hairs reach the eye by being airborne, or when a person prunes a tree or bush containing these caterpillars. Once the hair reaches the eye, the movement of the globe and lids may force the hair into the eye itself and cause the disease described here. If it stays on the surface of the globe, then a small granulomatous reaction in the conjunctiva will ensue. A caterpillar hair keratitis has also been reported.[113] A seasonal epidemic was reported in the Kangra district of India, with over 136 affected individuals.[114]

The initial entry into the eye may cause an immediate inflammatory reaction with pain, photophobia, and anterior uveitis. Later findings include chorioretinal lesions. According to Raspiller and colleagues,[115] this may occur anywhere from 0.5 to 16 years after the initial insult. They stress two characteristics of these chorioretinal lesions. The first is the presence of a track or tracks that align in the anteroposterior direction and reflect the hairs' migration from the anterior to the posterior portion of the globe. The second aspect is the formation of white nodules or outpouchings along the track (**Fig. 17-10**).

Treatment lies in trying to prevent situations in which caterpillar hairs can be released. Certainly if a caterpillar hair can be seen sticking out of the ocular surface, one should attempt to remove it at the slit lamp. It has been suggested that setae subconjunctivally and intracorneally positioned can be asypmtomatic.[114] If the hair is noted in the anterior chamber or vitreous, then its surgical removal may be considered. Only about 10% of cases will have vitreoretinal involvment. Fraser and David[116] performed a vitrectomy to remove the hairs. Raspiller and colleagues[115] have suggested placing a barrier of laser photocoagulation in front of the progressing track to prevent it from extending into the macular region. The use of antiinflammatory agents is certainly indicated to reduce the inflammatory response and to make the patient more comfortable.

Amebiasis

It is estimated that 10% of the world population is infested with amebae, and at least half of the population of Central and South America as well as Asia. Most of the symptoms are gastrointestinal. However, intraocular inflammatory disease has on occasion been associated with the parasite. Rodger and colleagues[117] reported that intermediate uveitis was common in patients with amebic dysentery. Several researchers have reported that various entamoebae[118] as well as *Acanthamoeba*[119] species cause a chorioretinal lesion. The disease is characterized by a subretinal whitish exudative lesion, most commonly in the macular region. Associated with this lesion will be hemorrhage and disturbances of the retinal pigment epithelium. In patients with dysentery the amoeba can be found in stool samples, but this is not always the case in hepatic amebiasis.

Diffuse unilateral subacute neuroretinitis (DUSN)

Although *Toxocara canis* involvement of the eye has long been recognized, there is certainly a possibility that other heretofore unrecognized nematodes may also cause ocular disease. An example of this is diffuse unilateral subacute neuroretinitis. This was first described by Gass in 1977,[120] who called it the unilateral wipe-out syndrome. In 1978 he changed the name to diffuse unilateral subacute neuroretinitis (DUSN) to better describe the syndrome.[121] Gass later published an article in which he observed a motile subretinal nematode in two patients with DUSN.[122] On further searching of the literature, Gass was able to identify previously reported cases of similar nematodes that produced the same clinical picture appearing as early as 1952. Hence a syndrome of initially unknown cause that was classified only by clinical description was later found to be related to a

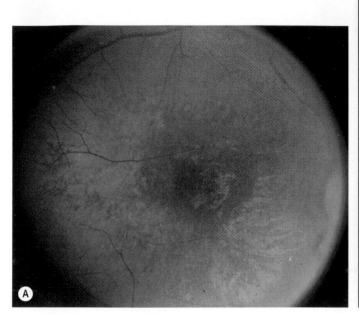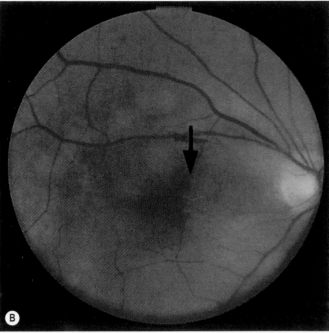

Figure 17-11. Fundus photographs of worms causing DUSN from (**A**) the southern part of the United States and (**B**) the northern part of United States. *(Courtesy of J. Donald Gass, MD.)*

nematode in the subretinal space. The understanding of the cause suggested possible therapies that were not considered when the disease was thought to be idiopathic.[123]

DUSN begins as scattered recurrent deep gray-white retinal lesions with marked loss of central acuity. There is often moderate vitreal inflammation, but in some patients there may be no observable inflammation. Optic disc swelling may be present. As the disease advances there is progressive optic atrophy, narrowing of the retinal vessels, pigment epithelial stippling, and further visual field loss. The electroretinogram response is significantly reduced. Careful examination with a contact lens may disclose a motile worm moving in the subretinal space. The details of the worm's size will be discussed below. Occasionally the worm may be seen in the vitreous. In some patients subretinal tracks that correspond to previous movement of the worm can be seen. The examination light may cause the worm to move. Granulomatous masses, such as those that are seen in classic *T. canis* infestation, are not observed in DUSN. There have been reports of unusual presentations of the disease, including a worm that appeared to be below the retinal pigment epithelium[124] and a large worm that produced a macular cyst.[125] Fluorescein angiography has demonstrated no fluorescence of the gray-white lesions in the early angiogram stages with late staining of these lesions.[83] Perivascular staining and mottled retinal pigment epithelial window defects are also seen. ICG has demonstrated choroidal areas of hypofluorescence suggesting involvement of the choroid in addition to the subretinal space.[126] Before the worm has been identified, several disorders can be considered in the differential diagnosis. These include acute multifocal posterior placoid epitheliopathy, toxoplasmosis, and optic neuritis, as well as posttraumatic retinal and choroidal ischemia.

Because the movement of the worm is thought to cause destruction of the retinal outer segments, visual loss is rarely reversible. Visual acuity of less than 20/200 is seen in about one-half of patients.[122] Occasional patients have retained good vision without treatment. An associated creeping skin eruption suggestive of systemic nematode infection is seen in some patients.

Worms of two sizes have been described in eyes with DUSN. A smaller worm between 400 and 700 μm in length was seen in most patients who lived in southeastern United States and was reported in the Caribbean and South America (Brazil).[127] A larger (1500–2000 μm) worm has been seen in patients residing in the northern and midwestern states (**Fig. 17-11**) and in Germany,[128,129] China,[130] and Brazil.[131] However, this geographic relationship does not always hold up to careful scrutiny. The worms have been described as being about 1/20th their length in diameter (**Fig. 17-12**).

The identification of the type of nematode that causes DUSN is still unsettled. *Toxocara* organisms rarely exceed 400 μm in length. Titers for *T. canis* have been looked for in patients with DUSN, and results are invariably negative.[132] Eosinophilia is occasionally seen. In 1984 it was suggested that the larger worms in patients living in more northern climates were *Baylisascaris procyonis*, a nematode found in raccoons.[133] Experimental infection of subhuman primates and other experimental animals by *B. procyonis* eggs orally has produced a clinical picture similar to that of DUSN.[134] Goldberg and co-workers[135] reported a patient from the western United States with unilateral DUSN whose evaluation implicated *Baylisascaris* as the causative agent. However, no patient with DUSN has had the neurologic complications that have been associated with infection by this nematode. It is likely that the clinical picture of DUSN can be produced by a variety of nematodes that find their way by chance to the eye and destroy the retina. These may include *Toxocara* in some patients despite the very low levels of *Toxocara* antibodies that are found, because the smaller worms seen in

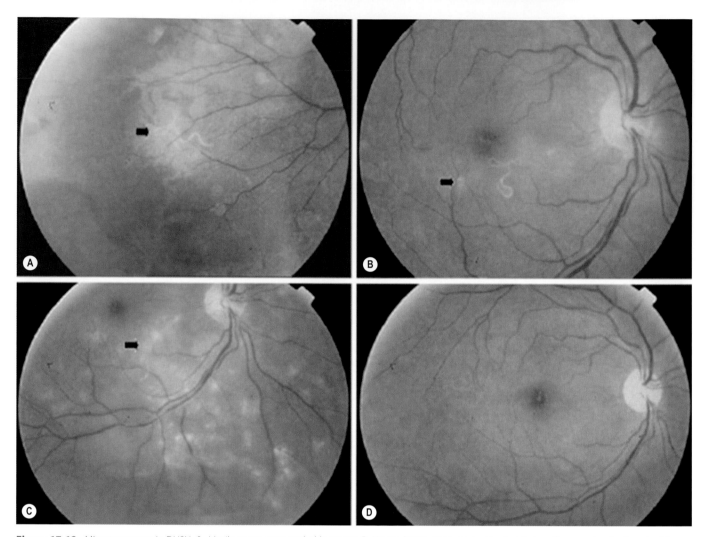

Figure 17-12. Migratory worm in DUSN. **A,** Motile worm surrounded by tracts. **B,** Worm (1500–2000 mm) migrating below the macula after laser had been applied (arrow). **C,** Dead worm with multiple white dots. **D,** Resolution 3 weeks post laser. *(Reproduced from K Myint, R Sahay, S Mon, V R Saravanan, V Narendran, B Dhillon, "Worm in the eye": the rationale treatment of DUSN in South India. 90:1125–1127. Copyright 2006, with permission of the BMJ Publishing Group.)*

DUSN are of the correct size for *Toxocara.* Indeed, in one report in which the organism was removed from the eye transvitreally, the larva was thought to be a third-stage *Toxocara.*[136]

Therapy with thiabendazole, an anthelmintic agent, or corticosteroids had not been successful in the treatment of DUSN. However, more recently, Souza et al.[137] treated 12 DUSN patients in Brazil with albendazole, 400 mg/day for 30 days, and saw an improvement in visual acuity and and a reduction in inflammation. The worm had been successfully destroyed by photocoagulation.[123,138] The need to treat with laser as rapidly as possible is emphasized by several. Venkatesh et al.[139] reported a case in India which was photographed but not initially lasered, and although laser therapy was applied later it resulted in only a partial improvement in visual acuity. In a series of two papers, Garcia and colleagues[140,141] emphasize the need to treat with laser as early as possible. Their results suggest that early therapy resulted in an improvement in vision, whereas late therapy helped few. It has been shown that nerve fiber layer thickness is decreased in DUSN, and it would make sense that early treatment would minimize this.[142] In this disease, death of the worm is usually not associated with an increased inflammatory response. However, as reported by Muccioli and Belfort,[143] a patient with DUSN did develop an acute iridocyclitis and hypopyon uveitis, presumably related to the death of the organism. Therefore, most practitioners will add oral steroids to the therapeutic regimen after laser therapy is initiated.[144] In addition, if the worm can be localized in the periphery of the retina, it can be surrounded by photocoagulation and then excised. Destruction of the worm by photocoagulation appears to halt the progression of DUSN (**Fig. 17-13**). Although the risk factors for the development of this type of ocular larval migrans are uncertain and the exact type of nematode in each case is still not specified, the recognition of the cause of this disease has led to the beginnings of a logical therapeutic approach. There may be a resultant epiretinal membrane needing surgical removal that could cause a persistent traction detachment even after adequate photocoagulation has been administered.[145]

Although nematodes have been reported in the eye, there are few reports of trematodes. McDonald and colleagues[146] reported finding *Alaria mesocercaria,* a trematode, in the eyes of two unrelated Asian men who presumably were exposed to the organism while eating poorly cooked frogs' legs. They both presented with unilateral disease,

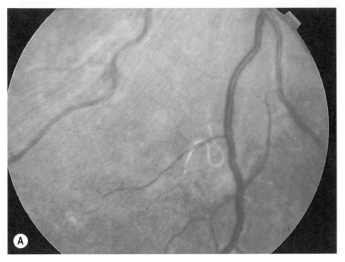
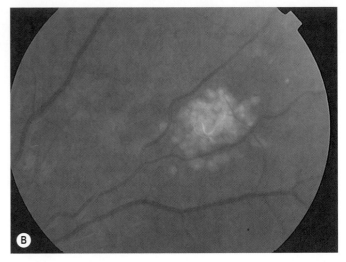

Figure 17-13. Fundus photo of a subretinal worm (**A**), which was successfully photocoagulated (**B**). *(Courtesy of Rubens Belfort, MD and Marcelo Casela, MD.)*

choroidal tracks, and other findings similar to those of DUSN. In one patient the organism was killed with laser therapy, and in the other the trematode was removed surgically from the vitreous.

Finally, it is fitting to finish this segment with a footnote from Gass and his associates. In a report from Brazil, Cunha de Souza and colleagues[147] described the first patient with the documented presence of nematodes in both eyes. Based on this bilaterality, the paper's discussion ends with the proposal that a more appropriate term for this entity is diffuse subacute neuroretinitis.

Malaria

Some mention of malaria must be made here. This is a disorder that is spreading and its incidence is increasing even in nonendemic areas because of increased international travel. Malaria is caused by a protozoon, most commonly *Plasmodium falciparum* and *Plasmodium vivax*. It is estimated that approximately 300 million people in the world harbor the parasite, and it has been suggested that malaria was the underlying problem of Jefferson Davis' (President of the Confederacy during the American Civil War) chronic ocular problems.[148] Of patients with malaria, 10–20% have been reported to have ocular manifestations,[149] which range from subconjunctival hemorrhages to optic neuritis and retinal hemorrhages. In a report[150] generated from the Blantyre (Malawi) Malaria Project, 1000 children with cerebral malaria were examined ophthalmologically. These children ranged in age from 2 to 14 years; 5% had cottonwool spots. There were retinal vessel abnormalities and retinal hemorrhages with white centers, resembling Roth spots. Retinal whitening was seen very frequently, perhaps due to retinal edema. Although papilledema was not seen very frequently, it was a poor prognosic sign. Biswas and colleagues[151] reported a clinical and histopathologic study of three patients, one with multiple, blotchy retinal hemorrhages, a second with bilateral panuveitis, perivasculitis, retinal hemorrhages and glaucoma, and a third with cerebral malaria having retinal hemorrhages as well.[151] Histopathologic examination showed cytoadherence of

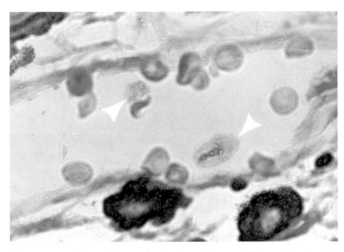

Figure 17-14. Photomicrograph showing schizonts of *Plasmodium vivax* in the choroid. (Hematoxylin & eosin, ×1000.) *(Courtesy of Professor Jyotirmay Biswas. Reproduced from Ophthalmology 1996; 103: 1471–5, with permission.)*

parasitized erythrocytes as well as schizonts and gametocytes of *P. vivax* with the retinal and choroidal blood vessels (**Fig. 17-14**).

Seasonal hyperacute panuveitis (SHAPU)

A curious entity has been reported by Malla[152] and by Upadhyay and colleagues[153] in Nepal. This severe and usually unilateral disease has been noted to occur principally in children, with sporadic cases in adults. The oldest reported patient was 44 years old. About one-third to one-half of patients revealed a history of contact with a moth in the few days preceding the onset of ocular symptoms. In 249 patients with newly diagnosed uveitis seen at the Eye Department of Tribhuvan University's Teaching Hospital from October 1997 to September 1999, 13 patients with seasonal hyperacute panuveitis were seen. All racial groups in Nepal seem to be affected. (Dr Dev Shah, personal communication).

It has occurred in 2-year cycles, the first having been recognized soon after the monsoon season of 1975. The disease begins very acutely with a red eye and leukocoria with little

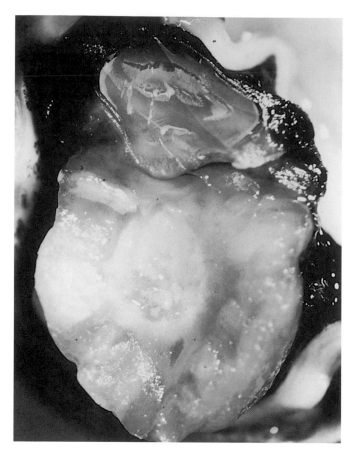

Figure 17-15. Sectioned eye with seasonal hyperacute panuveitis. The eye has intraocular hemorrhage and cataract. The dense white structure in the center of the vitreous is a totally detached retina.

pain. There may be a fibrinoid reaction in the anterior chamber, and often there is also a hypopyon. This is followed by hypotony and a very sudden decrease in vision. Examination of the posterior segment is obscured by the leukocoria. The anterior chamber ultimately becomes flat and the eye becomes phthisical (**Fig. 17-15**). Ultrasound may show remarkable choroidal thickening. Therapy has so far been unable to reverse the course of the disease.

Examination of these children has revealed no systemic abnormalities. Patients' sedimentation rates are normal or minimally elevated, and results of tests for rheumatoid factor and antinuclear antibodies are negative. The levels of circulating immune complexes were not elevated. Anti-*Toxoplasma* antibodies have not been present in the majority of patients, and anti-*Toxocara* antibodies have been found only in a few. Evidence of S-antigen sensitization could not be demonstrated.[154] Several children were noted to have been exposed to moths, but laboratory experiments attempting to define whether antigens from the moth-induced uveitis were not successful.[85] Histologic examination revealed a severe inflammatory response, with lymphocytes and plasma cells noted and with the retina drawn up into the retrolenticular mass. Eosinophils did not comprise a significant proportion of the cell population. Scanning electron microscopic examination has shown prominent Russel bodies and plasma cells. Neither worms nor virus particles could be identified. The underlying cause of this disorder remains unknown, and therapy has been problematic. In a study performed in Pokhara, Nepal, 14 patients underwent vitrectomy and half of them had a final vision of 6/60, which appears to be an improvement over the phthisis which is frequently seen as the end result.[155]

References

1. World HO. Onchocerciasis and its control. WHO Tech Rep Ser 1995; 852: 1–103.

2. Narita AS, Taylor HR. Blindness in the tropics. Med J Aust 1993; (159): 416–420.

3. Boatin BA, Richards FO Jr. Control of onchocerciasis. Adv Parasitol 2006; 61: 349–394.

4. Sallo F, Eberhard ML, Fok E, et al. Zoonotic intravitreal Onchocerca in Hungary. Ophthalmology 2005; 112(3): 502–504.

5. Brockhouse CL, Vajime CG, Marin R, et al. Molecular identification of onchocerciasis vector sibling species in black flies (Diptera: Simuliidae). Biochem Biophys Res Commun 1993; (194): 628–634.

6. Anderson J, Fuglsang H, Marshall TF. Effects of diethylcarbamazine on ocular onchocerciasis. Tropenmed Parasit 1976; (27): 263–275.

7. Thylefors B, Brinkman UK. The microfilarial load in the anterior segment of the eye. A parameter of intensity of onchocerciasis. Bull Org Mond Santé 1977; (5): 731–737.

8. Maertens K. Tonography in onchocerciasis. Bull Soc Panafr Ophthalmol 1982; (5): 23–27.

9. Thylefors B, Duppenthaler JL. Epidemiological aspects of intra-ocular pressure in an onchocerciasis endemic area. Bull Org Mond Santé 1979; (57): 963–969.

10. Newland HS, White AT, Greene BM, et al. Ocular manifestations of onchocerciasis in a rain forest area of West Africa. Br J Ophthalmol 1991; (75): 163–169.

11. Enk CD, Anteby I, Abramson N, et al. Onchocerciasis among Ethiopian immigrants in Israel. Isr Med Assoc J 2003; 5(7): 485–488.

12. Neumann E, Gunders AE. Pathogenesis of the posterior segments lesion of ocular onchocerciasis. Am J Ophthalmol 1973; (75): 82.

13. Budden FH. The natural history of ocular onchocerciasis over a period of 14–15 years and the effect on this of a single course of suramin. Trans Roy Soc Med Hyg 1976; (70): 484–491.

14. Duke BOL, Vincelette J, Moore PJ. Microfilariae in the cerebrospinal fluid, and neurological complications during treatment of onchocerciasis with diethylcarbamazine. Tropenmed Parasit 1976; (27): 123–132.

15. Tonjum AM, Thylefors B. Aspects of corneal changes in onchocerciasis. Br J Ophthalmol 1978; (62): 458–461.

16. Egbert PR, Jacobson DW, Fiadoyor S, et al. Onchocerciasis: a potential risk factor for glaucoma. Br J Ophthalmol 2005; 89(7): 796–798.

17. Van den Berghe L, Chardome M, Peel E. The filiarial parastites of the eastern gorilla in the Congo. J Helminthol 1964; (38): 349–368.

18. Duke BOL. Experimental transmission of *Onchocerca volvulus* from man to chimpanzee. Trans Roy Soc Trop Med Hyg 1962; (56): 271.

19. Donnelly JJ, Taylor HR, Young E, et al. Experimental ocular onchocerciasis in Cynomolgus monkeys. Invest Ophthalmol Vis Sci 1986; (27): 492–499.

20. Duke BOL, Garner A. Fundus lesions in the rabbit eye following inoculation of *Onchocerca volvulus* microfilariae into the posterior segment. II. Pathology. Tropenmed Parasit 1976; (27): 19–29.

21. Sakla AA, Donnelly JJ, Lok JB, et al. Punctate keratitis induced by subconjunctivally injected microfilariae of *Onchocera lienalis*. Arch Ophthalmol 1986; (104): 894–898.

22. Semba RD, Donnelly JJ, Young E, et al. Experimental ocular onchocerciasis in Cynomolgus monkeys. IV. Chorioretinitis elicited by *Onchcerca volvus* microfilariae. Invest Ophthalmol Vis Sci 1991; (32): 1499–1507.

23. Somorin AO, Hewer DC, Ajugwo RE. Immunoglobulin in Nigerian onchocerciasis. Ann J trop Med Hyg 1977; (26): 872–876.

24. Ngu JL, Blackett K. Immunological studies in onchocerciasis in Cameroon. Trop Geog Med 1976; (28): 111–120.

25. Ottesen EA. Immune responsiveness and the pathogenesis of human onchocerciasis. J Infect Dis 1995; 171: 659–671.

26. Chan CC, Nussenblatt RB, Kim MK, et al. Immunopathology of ocular onchocerciasis. 2. Anti-retinal autoantibodies in serum and ocular fluids. Ophthalmology 1987; (94): 439–443.

27. Van der Lelij A, Rothova A, De Vries JP, et al. Analysis of aqueous humour in ocular onchocerciasis. Curr Eye Res 1991; (10): 169–176.

28. Braun G, McKechnie NM, Connor V, et al. Immunological crossreactivity between a cloned antigen of *Onchocerca volvulus* and a component of the retinal pigment epithelium. J Exp Med 1991; (174): 169–177.

29. Klager S, McKechnie NM, Braun G, et al. Immunologic crossreactivity in the pathogenesis of ocular onchocerciasis. Invest Ophthalmol Vis Sci 1993; (34): 2888–2902.

30. Meilof JF, Van der Lelij A, Rokeach LA, et al. Autoimmunity and filariasis: Autoantibodies against cytoplasmic cellular proteins in sera of patients with onchocerciasis. J Immunol 1993; (151): 5800–5809.

31. Kaifi JT, Diaconu E, Pearlman E, Distinct roles for PECAM-1, ICAM-1, and VCAM-1 in recruitment of neutrophils and eosinophils to the cornea in ocular onchocerciasis (river blindness). J Immunol 2001; 166: 6795–6801.

32. Kaifi JT, Hall LR, Diaz C, et al. Impaired eosinophil recruitment to the cornea in P-selectin-deficient mice in *Onchocerca volvulus* keratitis (river blindness). Invest Ophthalmol Vis Sci 2000; 41(12): 3856–3861.

33. Hall LR, Pearlman E, Pathogenesis of onchocercal keratitis (river blindness). Clin Microbiol Rev 1999; 12: 445–443.

34. Hall LR, Kaifi JT, Diaconu E, et al. CD4+ depletion selectively inhibits eosinophil recruitment to the cornea and abrogates *Onchocerca volvulus* keratitis (river blindness).

Infect Immun 2000; 68(9): 5459–5461.

35. Saint Andre AV, Blackwell NM, Hall LR, et al. The role of endosymbiotic *Wolbachia* bacteria in the pathogenesis of river blindness. Science 2002; 295: 1892–1895.

36. Gillette-Ferguson I, Hise AG, Sun Y, et al. *Wolbachia*- and *Onchocerca volvulus*-induced keratitis (river blindness) is dependent on myeloid differentiation factor 88. Infect Immun 2006; 74(4): 2442–2445.

37. Brattig NW. Pathogenesis and host responses in human onchocerciasis: impact of *Onchocerca filariae* and *Wolbachia* endobacteria. Microbes Infect 2004; 6(1): 113–128.

38. Bradley JE, Nirmalan N, Kläger SL, et al. River blindness: a role for parasite retinoid-binding proteins in the generation of pathology? Trends Parasitol 2001; 17(10): 471–475.

39. Tree TI, Gillespie AJ, Shepley KJ, et al. Characterization of an immunodominant glycoprotein antigen of *Onchocerca volvulus* with homologues in other filarial nematodes and *Caenorhabditis elegans*. Mol Biochem Parasitol 1995; 69: 185–195.

40. Gudes LJ, Sporn MB. Roberts AB. Cellular biology and biochemistry of retinoids, In: The Retinoids, Sporn MB, et al. eds. 1994, Raven Press. 443–520.

41. Sturcheler D, Wyss F, Hanck A, et al. Retinol, onchocerciasis, and *Onchocerca volvulus*. Trans Roy Soc Trop Med Hyg 1981; 75: 617.

42. Steel C, Nutman TB. Regulation of IL-5 in onchocerciasis. a critical role for IL-2. J Immunol 1993; (150): 5511–5518.

43. Gillette-Ferguson I, Daehnel K, Hise AG, et al. Toll-like receptor 2 regulates CXC chemokine production and neutrophil recruitment to the cornea in *Onchocerca volvulus*/*Wolbachia*-induced keratitis. Infect Immun 2007; 75(12): 5908–5915.

44. Daehnel K, Gillette-Ferguson I, Hise AG, et al. *Filaria*/*Wolbachia* activation of dendritic cells and development of Th1-associated responses is dependent on toll-like receptor 2 in a mouse model of ocular onchocerciasis (river blindness). Parasite Immunol 2007; 29(9): 455–465.

45. UNDP, W. Bank, and WHO. Special Programme for research and training in tropical disease: The pathogenesis and treatment of ocular onchocerciasis: report of the eighth meeting on the scientific working grop on filariasis in collaboration with the programme for the preventon of blindness. in Special Programme for research and training in tropical disease: The pathogenesis and treatment of ocular onchocerciasis: report of the eighth meeting on the scientific working grop on filariasis in collaboration with the programme for the preventon of blindness. 1982. Geneva, Switzerland.

46. Bird AC, el-Sheikh H, Anderson J, et al. Changes in visal function and i the posterior segment of the eye during treatment of onchocerciasis with diethylcarbamazine citrate. Br J Ophthalmol 1980; (64): 191–200.

47. Hero M, Bird AC, Awadzi K. Quantifcation of the ocular reactions to microfilaricides in the chemotherapy of onchocerciasis. Eye 1992; (6 (pt 1)): 93–96.

48. Rivas-Alcala AR, Greene BM, Taylor HR, et al. Chemotherapy of onchocerciasis: A controlled comparison of mebendazole, levamisole, and diethylcarbamazine. Lancet, 1981(ii): 485–492.

49. Aziz MA, Diallo S, Diop IM, et al. Efficacy and tolerance of ivermectin in human onchocerciasis. Lancet 1982; 2: 171–173.

50. Taylor HR, Murphy RP, Newland HS, et al. Treatment of onchocerciasis. The ocular effects of ivermectin and diethylcarbamazine. Arch Ophthalmol 1986; (104): 863–870.

51. Diallo S, Aziz MA, Lariviere M, et al. A double-blind comparison of the efficacy and safety of ivermectin and diethylcarbamazine in a placebo controled study of Senegalese patients with onchocerciasis. Trans Roy Soc Trop Med Hyg 1986; (80): 927–934.

52. Dadzie KY, Bird AC, Awadzi K, et al. Ocular findings in a double-blind study of ivermectin versus diethylcarbazine versus placebo in the treatment of onchocerciasis. Br J Ophthalmol 1987; (71): 78–85.

53. Ogunba EO, Gemade EL. Preliminary observations on the distribution of ivermectin in Nigeria for control of river blindness. Ann Trop Med Parasitol 1992; (86): 649–655.

54. Whitworth JA, Gilbert CE, Mabey DM, et al. Effects of repeated doses of ivermectin on ocular onchocerciasis: community-based trial in Sierra Leone. Lancet 1991; (338): 1100–1103.

55. Dadzie KY, Remme J, De Sole G. Changes in ocular onchocerciasis after two rounds of community-based ivermectin treatment in a holo-endemic onchocerciasis. Doc Ophthalmol 1991; (79): 261–267.

56. OCP/EAC, OCP Expert Advisory Committee on Onchocerciasis. 1993.

57. Boatin B. The Onchocerciasis Control Programme in West Africa (OCP). Ann Trop Med Parasitol 2008; 102(Suppl 1): 13–17.

58. Haddad D. The NGDO Co-ordination Group for Onchocerciasis Control. Ann Trop Med Parasitol 2008; 102(Suppl 1): 35–38.

59. Vieira JC, Cooper PJ, Lovato R, et al. Impact of long-term treatment of onchocerciasis with ivermectin in Ecuador: potential for elimination of infection. BMC Med 2007; 5: 9.

60. Hopkins AD. Ivermectin and onchocerciasis: is it all solved? Eye 2005; 19(10): 1057–1066.

61. Semba RD, Murphy RP, Newland HS, et al. Longitudinal study of lesions of the posterior segment in onchocerciasis. Ophthalmology 1990; 97: 1334–1341.

62. Njoo FL, Stilma JS, van der Lelij A. Effects of repeated ivermectin treatment in onchocerciasis. Doc Ophthalmol 1992; (79): 261–267.

63. Mabey D, Whitworth JA, Eckstein M, et al. The effects of multiple doses of ivermectin on ocular onchocerciasis. Ophthalmology 1996; 103: 1001–1008.

64. Chippaux JP, Boussinesq M, Fobi G, et al. Effect of repeated ivermectin treatments on ocular onchocerciasis: evaluation after six to eight dosings. Ophthalmic Epidemiol 1999; 6(4): 229–246.

65. Awadzi K, Attah SK, Addy ET, et al. The effects of high-dose ivermectin regimens on *Onchocerca volvulus* in onchocerciasis patients. Trans Roy Soc Trop Med Hyg 1999; 93: 189–194.

66. Gardon J, Boussinesq M, Kamgno J, et al. Effects of standard and high doses of ivermectin on adult worms on *Onchocerca volvulus*: a randomised controlled trial. Lancet 2002; 360: 203–210.

67. Klager SL, Whitworth JA, Downham M. Viability and fertility of adult *Onchocerca volvulus* after 6 years of treatment with ivermectin. Trop Med Int Health 1996; 1(5): 581–589.

68. Ejere H, Schwartz E, Wormald R. Ivermectin for onchocercal eye disease (river blindness) (Cochrane Review), in The Cochrane Library. 2001, Oxford: update software.

69. Awadzi K, Attah SK, Addy ET, et al. Thirty-month follow-up of sub-optimal responders to multiple treatments with ivermectin, in two onchocerciasis-endemic foci in Ghana. Ann Trop Med Parasitol 2004; 98(4): 359–370.

70. Fobi G, Gardon J, Kamgno J, et al. A randomized, double-blind, controlled trial of the effects of ivermectin at normal and high doses, given annually or three-monthly, against *Onchocerca volvulus*: ophthalmological results. Trans Roy Soc Trop Med Hyg 2005; 99(4): 279–289.

71. Plaisier AP, van Oortmarssen GJ, Remme J, et al. The risk and dynamics of onchocerciasis recrudescence after cessation of vector control. Bull WHO 1991; 69: 169–178.

72. Davies JB. Description of a computer model of forest onchocerciasis transmission and its application to field scenarios of vector control and chemotherapy. Ann Trop Med Parasitol 1993; 87: 41–63.

73. Sucs FE, Zanen A. Ocular manifestations secondary to giardiasis. Bull Soc Belge Ophtalmol 1986; 219: 63–69.

74. Welch PB. Giardiasis with unsual clinical findings. Am J Digest Dis 1943; 1943: 10.

75. Webster BH. Human infection with *Giardia lamblia*. Am J Dig Dis (New Series) 1958; (3): 64–71.

76. Barraquer I. Sur la coincidence de la lambliase et de certaines lesions du fond de l'oeil. Bull Soc Pathol Exot (Paris) 1938; (31): 55–58.

77. Knox DL, King JJ. Retinal arteritis, iridocyclitis, and giardiasis. Ophthalmology 1982; (89): 1303–1308.

78. Pettoello Mantovani M, Giardino I, Magli A, et al. Intestinal giardiasis associated with ophthalmologic changes. J Pediatr Gastroenterol 1990; 11: 196–200.

79. Corsi A, Nucci C, Knafelz D, et al. Ocular changes associated with *Giardia lamblia* infection in children. Br J Ophthalmol 1998; (82): 59–62.

80. Wania J. De Ocampo Lecture. The eye and intestinal parasitic diseases, In: Current aspects of ophthalmology, Shimizu K, ed. 1992, Elsevier Science: Amsterdam. 1–7.

81. Roberts-Thornson IC, Mitchel GI. Genetic studies in human and murine giardiasis. Gut 1980; 21: 397–401.

82. Anderson ML, Griffith DG. Intestinal giardiasis associated with ocular inflammation. J Clin Gastroenterol 1985; 7(2): 169–172.

83. Behr C. Ophthalmomyiasis interna and externa. Klin Mbl Augenheilkd 1920; 64: 161–180.

84. DeBoe MP. Dipterous larva passing from the optic nerve into the vitreous chamber. Arch Ophthalmol 1933; (10): 824–825.

85. Amr ZS, Amr BS, Abo-Shehada MN. Ophthalmomyiasis externa caused by *Oestrus ovis* L. in the Ajloun area of northern Jordan. Ann Trop Med Parasitol 1993; (87): 259–262.

86. Hira PR, Hajj B, al-Ali F, et al. Ophthalmomyiasis in Kuwait: first report of *Oestrus ovis* before and after the Gulf conflict. J Trop Med Hyg 1993; (96): 241–244.

87. Chodosh J, Clarridge J. Ophthalmomyiasis: A review with special reference to *Cochliomyia hominivorax*. Clin Infect Dis 1992; (14): 444–449.

88. Dunbar J, Cooper B, Hodgetts T, et al. An outbreak of human external ophthalmomyiasis due to *Oestrus ovis* in southern Afghanistan. Clin Infect Dis 2008; 46(11): e124–6.

89. Dixon JM, Winkler CH, Nelson JH. Ophthalmomyiasis interna caused by *Cuterebra* larva. Trans Am Ophthalmol Soc 1969; (67): 110–115.

90. Godde-Jolly D, Brumpt ML, Stofft P. Un cas d'ophthalmomyase 'hypoderma boris' de la chambre anterieure. Bull Soc Ophthal Fr 1966; (2): 48–56.

91. Gass JDM, Lewis RA. Subretinal tracks in ophthalmomyiasis. Arch Ophthalmol 1976; (94): 1500–1505.

92. Slusher MM, Holland WD, Weaver RG, et al. Ophthalmomyiasis interna posterior. Subretinal tracks and intraocular larvae. Arch Ophthalmol 1979; (97): 885–887.

93. Jakobs EM, Adelberg DA, Lewis JM, et al. Ophthalmomyiasis interna posterior. Report of a case with optic atrophy. Retina 1997; 17: 310–317.

94. Billi B, Lesnoni G, Audisio P, et al. Pars plana vitrectomy for retinal detachment due to internal posterior ophthalmomyiasis after cataract extraction. Graefe's Arch Clin Exp Ophthalmol 1997; 235: 255–258.

95. Campbell RJ, Steele JC, Cox TA, et al. Pathologic findings in the retinal pigment epitheliopathy associated with the amyotrophic lateral sclerosis/Parkinsonism-dementia complex of Guam. Ophthalmology 1993; (100): 37–42.

96. Sharifipour F, Feghhi M. Anterior ophthalmomyiasis interna: an ophthalmic emergency. Arch Ophthalmol 2008; 126(10): 1466–1467.

97. Spirn MJ, Hubbard GB, Bergstrom C, et al. Ophthalmomyiasis associated with Fuchs heterochromic iridocyclitis. Retina 2006; 26(8): 973–974.

98. Saraiva Vda S, Amaro MH, Belfort R, et al. A case of anterior internal ophthalmomyiasis: case report. Arq Bras Oftalmol 2006; 69(5): 741–743.

99. Lagace-Wiens PR, Dookeran R, Skinner S, et al. Human ophthalmomyiasis interna caused by *Hypoderma tarandi*, Northern Canada. Emerg Infect Dis 2008; 14(1): 64–66.

100. Forman AR, Cruess AF, Benson WE. Ophthalmomyiasis treated by argon-laser photocoagulation. Retina 1984; (4): 163–165.

101. Syrdalen P, Nitter T, Mehl R. Opthalmomyiasis interna posterior: report of case caused by reindeer warble fly larva and review of previous reported cases. Br J Ophthalmol 1982; (66): 589–593.

102. Barry M, Kaldiian LC, Neurocysticercosis. Semin Neurol 1993; 13: 131–143.

103. Cortez MA, Giuliari GP, Escaf L, et al. Ocular cysticercosis of the anterior segment. J Am Assoc Pediatr Ophthalmol Strabismus 2007; 11(6): 628–629.

104. Mahendradas P, Biswas J, Khetan V, Fibrinous anterior uveitis due to cysticercus cellulosae. Ocul Immunol Inflamm 2007; 15(6): 451–454.

105. Meyerson L, Pienaar BT. Intraocular cysticercus. Br J Ophthalmol 1961; (45): 148–153.

106. Topilow HW, Yimoyines DJ, Freeman HM, et al. Bilateral multifocal intraocular cysticercosis. Ophthalmology 1981; (88): 1166–1172.

107. Segal P, Mrzyglod S, Dudarewiex JS. Subretinal cysticercosis in the macular region. Am J Ophthalmol 1964; (57): 655–664.

108. Chuck RS, Olk RJ, Weil GJ, et al. Surgical removal of a subretinal proliferating cysticercus of

Taeniaeformis crassiceps. Arch Ophthalmol 1997; 115(4): 562–563.

109. Stewart CR, Salmon JF, Murray AD, et al. Cysticercosis as a cause of severe medical rectus muscle myositis. Am J Ophthalmol 1993; (116): 510–511.

110. Menon V, Tandon R, Khanna S, et al. Cysticercosis of the optic nerve. J Neuro-Ophthalmol 2000; 20(1): 59–60.

111. Takayanagui OM, Jardim E. Therapy for neurocysticercosis: comparison between albendazole and praziquantel. Arch Neurol 1992; 49: 290–294.

112. Diallo JS. Manifestations Ophtalmologiques des Parasitoses. 1985. Masson, Paris.

113. Teske SA, Hirst LW, Gibson BH, et al. Caterpillar induced keratitis. Cornea 1991; (10): 317-321.

114. Sood P, Tuli R, Puri R, et al. Seasonal epidemic of ocular caterpillar hair injuries in the Kangra District of India. Ophthalmic Epidemiol 2004; 11(1): 3–8.

115. Raspiller A, Lepori JC, George JL. Chorioretinopathie par migration de poils de chenilles. Bull Mem Soc Fr Ophtalmol 1984; (95): 153–156.

116. Fraser SG, Dowd TC, Bosanquet RC. Intraocular caterpillar hairs (setae): clinical course and management. Eye 1994; 8(Pt 5): 596–598.

117. Rodger FC, Chir PK, Hosain ATMM. Night blindness in the tropics. Arch Ophthalmol 1960; (63): 927–935.

118. Braley AE, Hamilton HE. Central serous choroiditis associated with amebiasis. Arch Ophthalmol 1957; (58): 1–14.

119. Schlaegel TFJ, Culbertson C, Experimental *Hartmanella* optic neuritis and uveitis. Ann Ophthalmol 1972; (4): 103–112.

120. Gass JDM. Some problems in the diagnosis of macular disease. in Symposium on Retinal Disease. 1977. St Louis.

121. Gass JDM, Scelfo R. Diffuse unilateral subacute neuroretinitis. J Roy Soc Med 1978; (71): 95–111.

122. Gass JDM, Braunstein RA. Further observations concerning the diffuse unilateral subacute neuroretinitis syndrome. Arch Ophthalmol 1983; (101): 1689–1697.

123. Parson HE. Nematode chorioretinitis: report of a case with photographs of a viable worm. Arch Ophthalmol 1952; (47): 799–800.

124. Anshu A. Chee SP, Diffuse unilateral subacute neuroretinitis. Int Ophthalmol 2008; 28(2): 127–129.

125. Vedantham V, Vats MM, Kakade SJ, et al. Diffuse unilateral subacute neuroretinitis with unusual findings. Am J Ophthalmol 2006; 142(5): 880–883.

126. Vianna RN, Onofre G, Ecard V, et al. Indocyanine green angiography in diffuse unilateral subacute neuroretinitis. Eye 2006; 20(9): 1113–1116.

127. Küchle M, Knorr HL, Medenblik-Frysch S, et al. Diffuse unilateral subacute neuroretinitis syndrome in a German most likely caused by the raccoon roundworm, *Baylisascaris procyonis*. Graefe's Arch Clin Exp Ophthalmol 1993; 231: 48–51.

128. Naumann GOH, Knorr HLJ. DUSN occurs in Europe. Letter to the Editor. Ophthalmology 1994; 101(6): 971–972.

129. Cunha de Souza E, Lustosa da Cunha S, Gass JDM. Diffuse unilateral subacute neuroretinitis in South America. Arch Ophthalmol 1992; 110: 1261–1263.

130. Cai J, Wei R, Zhu L, et al. Diffuse unilateral subacute neuroretinitis in China. Arch Ophthalmol 2000; 118: 721–722.

131. Cialdini AP, Cunha de Souza E, Avila MP. The first South American case of diffuse unilateral subacute neuroretinitis caused by a large nematode. Arch Ophthalmol 1999; 117: 1431–1432.

132. Garcia CA, Sabrosa NA, Gomes AB, et al. Diffuse unilateral subacute neuroretinitis – DUSN. Int Ophthalmol Clin 2008; 48(3): 119–129.

133. Kazacos KR, Vestre WA, Kazacos EA, et al. Diffuse unilateral subacute neuroretinitis syndrome: a probable cause. Arch Ophthalmol 1984; 102: 967–968.

134. Kazacos KR, Raymond LA, Kazacos EA, et al. The racoon ascarid: a probable cause of human ocular larva migrans. Ophthalmology 1985; (92): 1735–1744.

135. Goldberg MA, Kazacos KR, Boyce WM, et al. Diffuse unilateral subacute neuroretinitis. Morphologic, serologic, and epidemiologic support for *Baylisascaris* as a causative agent. Ophthalmology 1993; 100: 1695–1701.

136. Cunha de Souza E, Nakashima Y. Diffuse unilateral subacute neuroretinitis. Report of transvitreal surgical removal of a subretinal nematode. Ophthalmology 1995; 102: 1183–1186.

137. Souza EC, Casella AM, Nakashima Y, et al. Clinical features and outcomes of patients with diffuse unilateral subacute neuroretinitis treated with oral albendazole. Am J Ophthalmol 2005; 140(3): 437–445.

138. Raymond LA, Gutierrez Y, Strong LE, et al. Living retinal nematode destroyed by photocoagulation. Ophthalmology 1978; (85): 944–949.

139. Venkatesh P, Sarkar S, Garg S. Diffuse unilateral subacute neuroretinitis: report of a case from the Indian subcontinent and the importance of immediate photocoagulation. Int Ophthalmol 2005; 26(6): 251–254.

140. Garcia CA, Gomes AH, Garcia Filho CA, et al. Early-stage diffuse unilateral subacute neuroretinitis: improvement of vision after photocoagulation of the worm. Eye 2004; 18(6): 624–627.

141. Garcia CA, Gomes AH, Vianna RN, et al. Late-stage diffuse unilateral subacute neuroretinitis: photocoagulation of the worm does not improve the visual acuity of affected patients. Int Ophthalmol 2005; 26(1–2): 39–42.

142. Garcia CA, de Oliveira AG, de Lima CE, et al. Retinal nerve fiber layer analysis using GDx in 49 patients with chronic phase DUSN. Arq Bras Oftalmol 2006; 69(5): 631–635.

143. Muccioli C, Belfort RJ. Hypopyon in a patient with presumptive diffuse unilateral subacute neuroretinitis. Ocul Immunol Inflamm 2000; 8(2): 119–121.

144. Myint K, Sahay R, Mon S, et al. 'Worm in the eye': the rationale for treatment of DUSN in south India. Br J Ophthalmol 2006; 90(9): 1125–1127.

145. Matsumoto BT, Adelberg DA, Del Priore LV. Transretinal membrane formation in diffuse unilateral subacute neuroretinitis. Retina 1995; 15: 146–149.

146. McDonald HR, Kazacos KR, Schatz H, et al. Two cases of intraocular infection with *Alaria mesocercaria* (Trematoda). Am J Ophthalmol 1994; 177(4): 447–455.

147. Cunha de Souza E, Abujamra, Nakashima S, Gass Y. JDM Diffuse bilateral subacute neuroretinitis. Arch Ophthalmol 1999; 117: 1349–1351.

148. Hertle RW, Spellman R. The eye disease of Jefferson Davis (1808–1889). Surv Ophthalmol 2006; 51(6): 596–600.

149. Hidayet AA, Nalbandian RM, Sammons DW et al. The diagnostic histopathologic features of ocular malaria. Ophthalmology 1993; 100: 1183–1186.

150. Hirneiss C, Klauss V, Wilke M, et al. [Ocular changes in tropical malaria with cerebral involvement–results from the Blantyre Malaria Project]. Klin Monatsbl Augenheilkd 2005; 222(9): 704–708.

151. Biswas J, Fogla R, Srinivasan P, et al. Ocular malaria. A clinical and histopathologic study. Ophthalmology 1996; 103: 1471–1475.

152. Malla OK. Endophthalmitis probably caused by Tussock moth, in Report of the Proceedings of the first National Seminar on Prevention of Blindness. 1978: Kathmandu. 44.

153. Upadhyay MP, Rai NC, Ogg JE, et al. Seasonal hyperacute panuveitis of unknown etiology. Ann Ophthalmol 1984; (16): 38–44.

154. Upadhyay MP, Rai NC, Ogg JE, et al. Seasonal hyperacute panuveitits., In: Uveitis Update, Saari K, ed. 1984, Excerpta Medica: Amsterdam. 257–262.

155. Byanju RN, Pradhan E, Rai SC, et al. Visual outcome of vitrectomy in seasonal hyperacute panuveitis. Kathmandu Univ Med J 2003; 1(2): 121–123.

156. Botero D, Aguledo LM, Uribe FJ, et al. Intraocular filaria, a Loaina species, from a man in Columbia. Am J Trop Med Hyg 1984; (33): 578–582.

157. Lee BY, McMillian R. Loa loa: ocular filariasis in an African student in Missouri. Ann Ophthalmol 1984; (16): 456–458.

158. Padgett JJ, Jacobsen KH. Loiasis: African eye worm. Trans Roy Soc Trop Med Hyg 2008; 102(10): 983–989.

159. Tuder RC, Blair E. Gnathostoma spingerum: an unsual cause of ocular nematodiasis in the western hemisphere. Am J Ophthalmol 1971; (72): 185–190.

160. Bathrick ME, Mango CA, Mueller JF. Intraocular gnathostomiasis. Ophthalmology 1981; (88): 1293–1295.

161. Singalavanija A, Wangspa S, Teschareon S. Intravitreal angostrongyliasis. Aust NZ J Ophthalmol 1986; (14): 381–384.

162. Matsuo T, Notohara K, Shiraga F, et al. Endogenous amoebic endophthalmitis. Arch Ophthalmol 2001; 119: 125–128.

163. Newton JC, Kanchanaranya C, Previte LR. Intraocular Schistosoma mansoni. Am J Ophthalmol 1968; (65): 774–778.

164. Mougeot G, Cambon M, Menerath JM, et al. Human eye anterior chamber sparganosis. Parasite 1999; 6: 365–366.

165. Kannan KA, Vasantha K, Venugopal M. Intraocular gnathostomiasis. Indian J Ophthalmol 1999; 47(4): 252–253.

166. Blanche P, Gombert B, Rivoal O, et al. Uveitis due to Leishmania major as part of HAART-induced immune restitution syndrome in a patient with AIDS. Clin Infect Dis 2002; 34(9): 1279–1280.

167. Mathai E, David S. Intraocular filariasis due to Wuchereria bancrofti. Trans Roy Soc Trop Med Hyg 2000; 94: 317-318.

168. Vedy J, Carrica A, Rivaud C, et al. A propos d'un cas de retinite chez un bilharzien. Med Trop 1979; 39: 603–609.

169. Behrens-Baumann W, Freissler G. Retinochoroidopathy in a patient with seropositive trichinosis. Klin Monatsbl Augenheilkd 1991; 119: 114–117.

170. Muftuoglu G, Cicik E, Ozdamar A, et al. Vitreoretinal surgery for a subretinal hydatid cyst. Am J Ophthalmol 2001; 132: 435–437.

171. Gupta A, Agarwal A, Dogra MR. Retinal involvement in Wucheria bancrofti filariasis. Acta Ophthalmol (Copenh), 1992; (70): 832–835.

172. Ramos A, Cruz I, Muñez E, et al. Post-kala-azar dermal leishmaniasis and uveitis in an HIV-positive patient. Infection 2008; 36(2): 184–186.

Postsurgical Uveitis

Robert B. Nussenblatt

Key concepts

- The causes of postoperative inflammation need to be divided into those occurring acutely and those occurring after the passage of time.
- Fungal endophthalmitis may occur sometime after surgery.
- Lens-induced uveitis may occur spontaneously in an eye with a hypermature lens or may follow ocular trauma or cataract surgery.

Intraocular inflammation can occur after any ocular surgical procedure. It is especially important in the postoperative patient to differentiate infectious causes of uveitis from other causes of intraocular inflammation because bacterial and fungal endophthalmitis require prompt treatment with specific antimicrobial therapy. The major causes of postsurgical uveitis are listed in **Box 18-1**.

Patients with a preexisting uveitis often have an exacerbation of intraocular inflammation after surgery. The flare-up usually occurs 3 days to a week postoperatively in patients who receive subconjunctival corticosteroids at the end of the surgical procedure. In patients who do not receive steroids the inflammation may occur earlier. Occasionally, the uveitis can be severe enough to be confused with an infectious endophthalmitis, although hypopyon and severe pain are rare in patients with noninfectious postsurgical uveitis. In contrast, low-grade intraocular inflammation is common after many ocular procedures, especially after cataract extraction. This inflammation appears to be mediated by prostaglandins and can be inhibited by prostaglandin inhibitors.[1] In contrast, a rat model of bacterial endophthalmitis showed that a wide range of proinflammatory cytokines are released, including tumor necrosis factor (TNF)-α, interleukin-1β, and the rat equivalent of interleukin-8.[2] During these severe infections, a better idea is emerging of the host/pathogen interactions;[3] the eye upregulates αB crystallin in an attempt to prevent apoptosis of the retinal cells.[4] However, some infectious agents, such as *Propionibacterium acnes*, may produce a low-grade postsurgical endophthalmitis that may take months to develop.

Acute bacterial endophthalmitis

Most cases of bacterial endophthalmitis occur after intraocular surgery and are a surgical emergency. Fortunately, postoperative endophthalmitis is a rare condition. Allen and Mangiaracine[5] reported 22 occurrences of endophthalmitis in a series of 20 000 ocular operations (0.11%), and nine occurrences in a second series of 16 000 operations (0.056%).[6] The overall prevalence has been estimated to be 0.07%.[7] Post-keratoplasty endophthalmitis is associated with grafts from those who die in hospital from cancer.[8] The rate for endophthalmitis after pars plana vitrectomy is low, reported at 0.039%,[9] with a recent publication reporting the incidence of infection after 20 and 25 gauge vitrectomies to be the same (0.03%).[10] However, the visual outcome of these cases is usually not good. For cataract extraction older studies suggested a rate between 0.07% and 0.12%5;[11,12] 75% of patients present within 11 days of cataract surgery or a secondary implant.[13] West et al.[14] suggested that the rate has been increasing over the years, from 0.1% in the 1990s to 0.2% for 2000–2003. Ng and co-workers[15] reported that in their series of endophthalmitis secondary to cataract surgery 48% occurred after phacoemulsification and 39% after planned extracapsular extraction. In Sweden, the rate was calculated to be 0.048%, with a higher rate seen with a clear cornea approach (0.053%) versus a sclerocorneal incision (0.036%); the difference was statistically significantly different.[16] Thoms and coworkers[17] reviewed 815 clear cornea cataract extraction cases, almost equally divided between sutured and unsutured, and found that there were five cases of culture-positive endophthalmitis in the unsutured group and none in the sutured group (p = 0.022). In addition, those who did not receive topical antibiotics until the day after surgery and those who did not receive 5% povidone-iodine drops immediately after wound closure were at greater risk. In a survey sent to 4000 American Society of Cataract and Refractive Surgery (ASCRS) members, of the 1312 who responded, 30% said that they used intracameral antibiotics either via injection or in the irrigating solution.[18] Wound problems appear to be an important contributing factor in about 25% of occurrences of endophthalmitis,[19] and infectious endophthalmitis may be a more common problem after glaucoma surgery, with late-onset endophthalmitis after trabeculectomy and antimetabolites seen in 2.7–8% of patients.[20–22] Others[23] have reported endophthalmitis associated with glaucoma drainage implants, usually due to exposure of the drainage tube. Kuang et al.[24] evaluated 988 trabeculectomy procedures performed over a 5-year period. In their experience there was one case of early endophthalmitis, but six cases (0.6%) that had a late onset. Mitomycin use increased the risk of late onset infection. It has been reported after Ahmad valve placement. Endophthalmitis was noted in one study in nine

---

Box 18-1 Causes of postoperative intraocular inflammation

DAY 1 to DAY 30
Acute aerobic bacterial endophthalmitis
Sterile endophthalmitis
Increased activity of previous uveitis
Phacogenic (lens-related) uveitis
Toxic reaction to intraocular lens

DAY 15 to 2 YEARS
Fungal endophthalmitis
Propionibacterium acnes or other anaerobic endophthalmitis
Low virulence aerobic bacterial endophthalmitis
Phacogenic (lens-related) uveitis
Sympathetic ophthalmia
Toxic reaction to intraocular lens
Iris–ciliary body irritation related to physical contact with
  intraocular lens
Glaucoma drainage device
New onset of idiopathic uveitis

---

of 542 eyes (1.7%), and the rate was five times higher in children.[25]

The interval between surgery and the onset of inflammation is sometimes helpful in distinguishing bacterial endophthalmitis from other causes of postoperative inflammation. Most aerobic bacterial infections occur within 11 days after surgery. Pain and diminished vision are accompanied by conjunctival hyperemia, chemosis, and lid edema. Anterior uveitis with fibrin, hypopyon, and vitritis is also characteristic of a bacterial endophthalmitis. These symptoms and signs should prompt a diagnostic evaluation that includes culture of intraocular fluids, usually obtained during vitrectomy surgery. Even in patients with endophthalmitis after anterior segment surgery, cultures of the vitreous yield positive cultures more frequently than those of the aqueous.[26] The most common organisms are the Gram-positives, particularly coagulase-negative staphylococcus.[27] Methicillin-resistant *Staphylococcus aureus* (MRSA) needs to be considered in the diagnosis. Deramo and colleagues[28] reported that in 64 cases of acute endophthalmitis secondary to cataract extraction, 33/164 were culture positive, and 6/33 (18.2%) were MRSA. All were sensitive to gentamicin and vancomycin.

The management of bacterial endophthalmitis in the past included vitrectomy, intravitreal, systemic, subconjunctival and topical antibiotics, and corticosteroids.[19,29] The approach to postoperative endophthalmitis has been helped by the results of the Endophthalitis Vitrectomy Study,[30] in which all patients received intravitreal amikacin and vancomycin. One group was randomized to pars plana vitrectomy and the other group received a vitreous tap. Each of these larger groups was further subdivided into those receiving systemic antibiotics and those who did not. In general, patients did reasonably well in terms of visual results. It was noted that vitrectomy was of help in patients presenting with poor vision. Systemic antibiotics did not seem to help the outcome. Therefore, the approach today is usually a vitrectomy and the use of broad-spectrum antibiotics given intravitreally, such as vancomycin and ceftazidime or vancomycin and amikacin.[31] However, only 75% of eyes with a clinical picture consistent with bacterial endophthalmitis will have positive bacterial culture results.[19] The polymerase chain reaction is being used more and more in these situations, often with panbacterial 16S rDNA gene primers or cytochrome P-450L primers for fungus.[32] PCR techniques have developed rapidly and have real clinical importance. Chiquet and coworkers[33] used eubacterial PCR primers for bacterial detection in 100 acute post-cataract endophthalmitis cases. When they evaluated the detection rate of culture versus PCR when using aqueous there was little difference (38.2% vs 34.6%) from when a vitreous tap was used. However, with vitrectomy the PCR positivity rate was 70% for PCR versus 9% for culture. When PCR and culture were combined, the detection rate was 68% from a vitreous tap, 72% from a vitrectomy specimen, and 47% from an aqueous sample.

These patients should, however, initially be treated as though they have bacterial endophthalmitis until their condition has improved or until other clinical information suggests an alternative diagnosis. Although sterile endophthalmitis can occur in the early postoperative period and may mimic a bacterial infection, the consequences of untreated bacterial endophthalmitis are so severe that culturing and antibiotic therapy should not be delayed.

What about patients with intraocular foreign bodies? Clearly this subject is too complex to discuss fully here. However, in a retrospective study of 589 eyes with an intraocular foreign body seen over a 12-year period at the King Khaled Eye Hospital,[34] 44 (7.5%) developed clinical evidence of endophthalmitis. A positive culture, however, was obtained on 17 eyes. The issue of whether prophylactic use of antibiotics in cases of intraocular foreign bodies will diminish the risk of infection was addressed by Soheilian and coworkers,[35] who performed a randomized study on 346 eyes with intraocular foreign bodies. In addition to the surgery (repair of the globe and removal of the object) the eyes were randomized to receiving either 40 µg of gentamicin sulfate and 45 µg of clindamycin intravitreally, or BSS injected intravitreally; 8/167 of those receiving BSS developed endophthalmitis, compared to 1/179 in the antibiotic group. Some have questioned the specifics of the study,[36] but the larger issue regarding the value of antibiotics in these circumstances is strengthened.

It is useful to add a comment about intravitreal injections, which are being used more and more frequently. Contamination from the ocular surface is a real possibility. De Caro et al.[37] cultured sites and needles from patients undergoing intravitreal injections and found that 2% (2/114) of needles were contaminated with bacteria. Injection site prophylaxis does make a big difference, with positive cultures found in 43% of the sites tested without prophylaxis and 13% positive after prophylaxis. This is still a relatively rare occurrence clinically. Although endophthalmitis hase been reported after bevacizumab intravitreal injections,[38] in one study of 5233 consecutive injections only one case of acute endophthalmitis was found.[39]

Chronic bacterial endophthalmitis

Although most patients with postoperative bacterial endophthalmitis present with the acute onset of severe inflammation, loss of vision and pain, some bacteria can

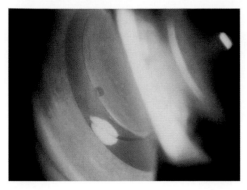

Figure 18-1. Infiltrate on lens haptic in patient with late-onset postoperative endophthalmitis caused by *Propionibacterium acnes*. *(From Murase KH, et al. A case of lens induced uveitis following metastatic endophthalmitis. Jpn J Ophthalmol 2007;51(4):304–6, with permission.)*

cause a chronic indolent intraocular infection. These organisms are more difficult to culture and grow more slowly.

Propionibacterium acnes has been recognized as an organism that can cause a chronic postoperative uveitis, especially after cataract extraction with intraocular lens placement.[40–42] It has also been reported after a cataract extraction and Molteno placement in a 7-year-old with congenital glaucoma.[43] The typical patient with *P. acnes* endophthalmitis presents with chronic low-grade anterior segment inflammation that starts from 2 months to 2 years after cataract surgery. Topical corticosteroids often suppress the inflammation early in the course of the disease, but do not prevent the protracted low-grade inflammatory response. White plaques composed of bacteria are often seen between the intraocular lens and the posterior capsule or on the intraocular lens haptics (**Fig. 18-1**). The clinical course of *P. acnes* endophthalmitis may resemble that of pseudophakic phacoanaphylaxis,[44,45] and it is not clear whether some of these patients actually had undiagnosed *P. acnes* infections.

In addition to the predominance of polymorphonuclear cells, the inflammatory infiltrate in eyes with *P. acnes* endophthalmitis includes a large number of macrophages (10–15%).[46] The presence of residual lens material in some patients suggests that lens-induced uveitis may be contributing to the inflammation.[41,45] Others have suggested that *P. acnes* immunopotentiation may be the result of inhibition of suppressor T cells caused by stimulated macrophages.[47]

Diagnosis of *P. acnes* endophthalmitis is based on culture data. It is important to instruct the microbiology laboratory not to discard the cultures after the normal 3–4 days, because the organism is slow growing and cultures should be maintained by the laboratory for 14 days before they are read as negative. Therapy for *P. acnes* endophthalmitis usually involves a combination of vitrectomy with posterior capsulectomy, intravitreal vancomycin, and sometimes systemic cephalosporins. Although the intraocular lens does not need to be removed at the time of initial therapy, recurrent disease is managed with repeat courses of intravitreal antibiotics and removal of the residual posterior capsule and the intraocular lens. Clark and coworkers[48] reported the following results in their study of eyes with *P. acnes*: 100% of eyes treated with intraocular antibiotics only had persistent disease; 50% of eyes treated with pars plana vitrectomy and antibiotics had persistent disease; and 14% of eyes treated with pars plana vitrectomy, antibiotics, and subtotal

capsulotomy had persistent disease. None of the eyes receiving a total capsulotomy and removal of the intraocular lens had recurrent disease.

Despite the delay in diagnosis and therapy of this chronic endophthalmitis, the visual prognosis is usually good. *P. acnes* infection has been reported after Ahmed valve placement.[49] Other organisms, including *Propionibacterium granulosum*, *Achromobacter*, *Pseudomonas oryzihabitans*,[50] *Mycobacterium*,[51] and *Staphylococcus epidermidis* may also cause a chronic bacterial endophthalmitis.[52] However, in addition to these bacteria, fungal endophthalmitis may also cause chronic smoldering postoperative intraocular inflammation.

Fungal endophthalmitis

Fungal endophthalmitis is a relatively rare condition; however, as our diagnostic abilities improve, the incidence of this condition appears to be increasing. Recent studies show that fungus accounts for 8–13% of culture-positive isolates; in some reports the *Candida* species predominate,[19,26] in others *Aspergillus*.[53] Fungal infections may not become symptomatic until months after surgery. They often start with low-grade iridocyclitis or vitritis, and some may have corneal involvement.[53] Symptoms of blurred vision, redness, and pain gradually increase. Corticosteroid therapy can temporarily ameliorate the symptoms but should be avoided. With time the infection progresses, and 'fluff balls' may form in the vitreous in addition to anterior uveitis and vitritis. A discrete fungal mass may be present in the vitreous or anterior chamber in some eyes.[54] There may be a 'string of pearls' in the posterior segment, a mass in the iris, a corneal infiltrate, or a necrotizing scleritis.[55] The risk factors for and ocular characteristics of postoperative and endogenous fungal infections are listed in **Table 18-1**.

Untreated fungal endophthalmitis leads to blindness. Even after the correct diagnosis is made, treatment initiated late in the course of the disease may not successfully restore vision. In a recent study only 42% of eyes had a visual acuity of 20/400 or better after treatment for fungal endophthalmitis.[54] Patients who present early with good acuity (better than 20/60) have a more favorable visual prognosis.[54] Infections with *Acremonium* or *Fusarium* are associated with a poorer prognosis.

The diagnosis of fungal endophthalmitis should be suspected in all patients with postoperative inflammation that occurs weeks to months after surgery. Rarely, fungal infection may occur within 1 week after the surgical procedure. If fungal infection is suspected, it is helpful to pass part of the vitreous specimen through a Millipore filter and to culture the filter as a method of concentrating the organisms. Fungal organisms do not stain well on Gram stain. One needs to search for fungus using either a Giemsa or Gomori methenamine silver stain. It takes days for the cultures to grow, and *Candida*, *Fusarium*, and *Aspergillus* are the most common causes of the disorder. The use of Calcofluor or Calcofluor white staining techniques on vitreous samples allows the rapid identification of fungal elements and has improved diagnostic speed and accuracy.[56] As with bacterial conditions PCR is being employed more and more often, but with as much usefulness as has been shown in bacterial

Table 18-1 Characteristics of fungal infections (postsurgical and endogenous)

Organism	Risk Factors	Ocular Characteristics
Candida sp.	IV drug use, chronic IV therapy, surgery	Yellow-white chorioretinal lesions, vitreous fluff balls
Aspergillus sp.	IV drug use, immunosuppression, surgery	Yellow-white chorioretinal lesions, vitreous fluff balls
Coccidioides immitis	Southwestern United States	Multiple yellow-white chorioretinal lesions, punched-out choroidal lesions; often associated with pulmonary *C. immitis* infection
Cryptococcus neoformans	Immunosuppression, lymphoma	Small or large yellow-white chorioretinal lesions; often associated with meningitis
Histoplasma capsulatum	Immunosuppression	Panuveitis with iris involvement
Sporotrichum schenckii	Horticulturists	Panuveitis
Blastomyces dermatitidis	Systemic North American blastomycosis	Panuveitis or multiple small chorioretinal lesions

disease. In one study of 50 cases of nonbacterial endophthalmitis, six cases were detected using panfungal primers (ITS1 and ITS4).[57]

Antifungal therapy combined with vitrectomy and removal of an intraocular lens offers the best chance of a favorable outcome. Some patients have been successfully managed without intraocular lens removal, especially those with *Candida* endophthalmitis.[54,58] Intravitreal and intravenous amphotericin B, oral fluconazole, and oral flucytosine are used to treat the infection. Ten micrograms of amphotericin B are instilled into the vitreous; this dose can be repeated once if needed. Intraocular miconazole (25–50 µg) can be used in patients not responding to treatment with amphotericin B. Topical and subconjunctival antifungal agents may be used in infections that involve the cornea. Oral flucytosine is useful in candidal infections that are not resistant to this drug.

Endogenous endophthalmitis

This disorder increasingly needs to be considered as we see more patients with altered immune states. At present it accounts for a small number, 5–7%, of documented cases.[59] Most series have shown that the majority of these cases are fungal, but a large minority of cases are bacterial in origin.[60–63] Scheidler et al.[62] reviewed 21 eyes with culture-proven endogenous endophthalmitis and fungal isolates were found in 13. Six of these patients died within 2 months of the diagnosis. Perhaps a harbinger of the future, Agarwal et al.[64] reported the case of a 65-year-old woman who developed gradual loss of vision in the right eye that occurred during treatment with infliximab (3 mg/kg). Gram-positive cocci were cultured from the eye. Some of the factors predisposing to endogenous endophthalmitis include immunosuppressive therapy, AIDS, systemic autoimmune disease, intravenous hyperalimentation, malignancy, diabetes, intravenous drug use, and hematologic disorders[60] (**Box 18-2**).

Lens-induced uveitis

Phacoanaphylactic (phacoantigenic) uveitis is a granulomatous inflammatory response that is thought to represent an immunologic reaction against lens proteins released after surgical or traumatic disruption of the lens capsule. The term phacoanaphylactic uveitis is somewhat of a misnomer

---

Box 18-2 Factors putting patients at higher risk for endogenous endophthalmitis

AIDS
Intravenous drug use
Intravenous hyperalimentation
Indwelling catheters
Diabetes mellitus
Cancer
Hemodialysis
Immunosuppression for autoimmune disease and transplant
Bone marrow suppression
Hepatic disease
Postpartum
Underlying systemic autoimmune disease

---

because the reaction is not an anaphylactoid or type I hypersensitivity reaction. This form of lens-induced uveitis is differentiated from the nongranulomatous phacogenic (phacotoxic) uveitis, although there is no evidence to support the theory that lens degradation products are directly toxic to the eye.[65,66] It now appears that all these entities may represent varying severities of the same immunologic process that is better termed lens-induced uveitis.

Lens-induced uveitis may occur spontaneously in an eye with a hypermature lens or may follow ocular trauma or cataract surgery. It may occur under rather unusual circumstances. One such example is a case of lens induced uveitis which followed metastatic endophthalmitis secondary to a septic pneumonia. Six months after the event the patient developed a drop in vision and pain which resulted in an enucleation, which demonstrated changes compatible with this disease[67] (**Fig. 18-2**). A number of researchers have reported a high incidence of lens-induced uveitis after sympathetic ophthalmia.[65,66] However, isolated lens-induced uveitis is usually uniocular, occurring in the eye most recently treated with surgery; sympathetic ophthalmia is a bilateral disease.[68] The inflammation may occur hours or months after disruption of the lens capsule. Granulomatous keratic precipitates, anterior chamber cells and flare, and occasionally a hypopyon may be seen.

The inflammation can be severe and associated with both anterior uveitis and vitritis. Removal of all residual lens material is usually curative. Response to the administration of corticosteroids is poor. If some lens material is mixed with

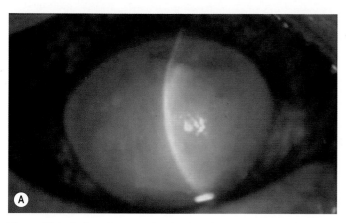

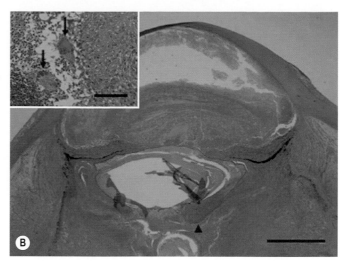

Figure 18-2. A, Eye of patient who developed a severe anterior chamber immune response 6 months after suffering from metastatic endophthalmitis secondary to a septic pneumonia. The eye was enucleated. **B,** Histopathology of eye showing phacoanaphylaxis. *(From Murase KH, et al. A case of lens-induced uveitis following metastatic endophthalmitis. Jpn J Ophthalmol 2007; 51(4): 304–6, with permission.)*

vitreous, a vitrectomy may be indicated. Lens-induced uveitis was rare in the 1960s when intracapsular cataract surgery was performed, but it is much more common with extracapsular cataract extraction. Lens-induced uveitis may be difficult to distinguish clinically from chronic endophthalmitis such as *P. acnes* infection;[40,41] therefore, cultures should be obtained from most eyes with chronic postoperative intraocular inflammation. Some have proposed the use of modified Papanicolaou or May–Grunwald–Giemsa staining of the aqueous cytospin or thin prep to help with the diagnosis.[69]

Toxic anterior segment syndrome (TASS)

This entity is a sterile postoperative inflammatory response to noninfectious agents entering the anterior chamber.[70] It is usually seen early – up to 2 days – after anterior segment manipulation. Initially, the entity was seen with early intraocular lenses. These lenses were associated with a variety of toxic reactions caused by problems with lens design material. Some causes of intraocular lens-related uveitis included reactions against metal haptics,[45] impurities on the lens from the manufacturer,[68] certain methods of sterilization,[71] and degradation of lens haptics.[72] Although these reactions are usually not immunologically driven, the resultant tissue damage can then lead to prostaglandin and cytokine release and the recruitment of lymphocytes and other inflammatory cells into the eye. This secondary immune-mediated inflammation can often be more damaging than the initial toxic reaction to the intraocular lens. Some old models of anterior chamber intraocular lenses were associated with the development of a syndrome characterized by uveitis, glaucoma, and hyphema (the UGH syndrome).[73] Fortunately, the UGH syndrome is uncommon with current anterior chamber intraocular lenses with flexible haptics.

Intraocular lenses sometimes cause mild inflammation that leads to the accumulation of cellular deposits on the anterior surface of the lens.[9,13,74] These deposits are often composed of macrophages and giant cells, but may be acellular,[51] and membranes are often associated with them. Clearly, most eyes tolerate a posterior chamber intraocular

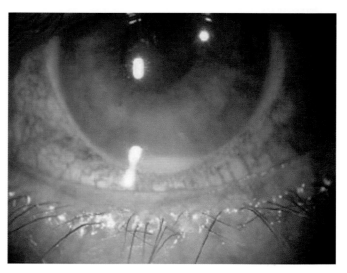

Figure 18-3. Example of toxic anterior segment syndrome. *(From Mamalis N, et al. Toxic anterior segment syndrome. J Cataract Refract Surg 2006; 32(2): 324–33, with permission.)*

lens with little inflammation.[75] However, some patients have a mild iridocyclitis that can be seen histologically, even if the lens was clinically well tolerated.[76] Indeed, over the years there have been many known causes of the toxic anterior segment syndrome. These include the irrigating solutions or viscosurgical devices not at the correct pH or osmolality; incorrect chemical composition or residual preventatives; instrument contaminants; and IOL contaminants such as polishing, cleaning and sterilizing materials (**Fig. 18-3**).

Laser-induced uveitis

Yttrium–aluminum–garnet (YAG) laser capsulotomy has been associated with low-grade inflammation.[77] The shock wave created by the laser is capable of causing a physical alteration in the blood–eye barrier. We have observed several cases of patients with a history of ongoing intraocular inflammation in which YAG laser capsulotomy caused a significant increase in inflammation. In some patients increased amounts of topical, periocular, or even systemic corticosteroids may be required at the time of the laser procedure. We saw an unusual case of endophthalmitis that appeared to be induced by a YAG laser iridectomy. The iridectomy was performed in a patient with closed-angle glaucoma with minimal bleeding from an iris vessel. Two days after the procedure the patient developed a hypopyon. Sepsis was diagnosed, and the same organism grew from cultures of both the eye and blood.

Case 18-1

A 66-year-old woman underwent bilateral extracapsular cataract surgery with posterior chamber intraocular lens implantation. The two surgical procedures were performed 6 weeks apart. After surgery the visual acuity was 20/20 in each eye. Two months after surgery an anterior uveitis developed in the right eye, and white material was noted on the polypropylene lens haptic (see Fig. 18-1).

The anterior uveitis initially resolved with administration of topical and periocular corticosteroids. However, the patient had recurrent episodes of uveitis and eventually developed a hypopyon and vitritis. The intraocular lens was removed and replaced with a new one. Bacterial and fungal culture results were reported as negative. The intraocular inflammation persisted despite therapy with oral corticosteroids. Repeat aqueous and vitreous cultures were obtained, and both results were positive for *P. acnes* 5 days after inoculation. Cytologic examination of the specimens showed macrophages and neutrophils with few lymphocytes. The patient received intravitreal cefazolin and intravenous cephalexin. Two weeks later there was a moderate amount of persistent inflammation and a second intravitreal injection of cefazolin was given. The inflammation resolved, and the patient's vision improved to 20/20.

References

1. Huang K, Peyman GA, McGetrick J, et al. Indomethacin inhibition of prostaglandin mediated inflammation following intraocular surgery. Invest Ophthalmol Vis Sci 1977; 16: 1760–1762.

2. Giese MJ, Sumner HL, Berliner JA, et al. Cytokine expression in a rat model of *Staphylococcus aureus* endophthalmitis. Invest Ophthalmol Vis Sci 1998; 39(13): 2785–2790.

3. Callegan MC, Gilmore MS, Gregory M, et al. Bacterial endophthalmitis: therapeutic challenges and host-pathogen interactions. Prog Retin Eye Res 2007; 26(2): 189–203.

4. Whiston EA, Sugi N, Kamradt MC, et al. alphaB-crystallin protects retinal tissue during *Staphylococcus aureus*-induced endophthalmitis. Infect Immun 2008; 76(4): 1781–1790.

5. Allen HF, Mangiaracine AB. A study of 22 infections in 20,000 operations. Arch Ophthalmol 1964; 72: 454–462.

6. Allen HF, Mangiaracine AB. Bacterial endophthalmitis after cataract extraction. II. Incidence in 36,000 consecutive operations with special reference to preoperative topical antibiotics. Arch Ophthalmol 1974; 91: 3–7.

7. Kattan HM, Flynn HW Jr, Pflugfelder SC, et al. Nosocomial endophthalmitis survey. Ophthalmology 1991; 98: 227–238.

8. Hassan SS, Wilhelmus KR, Dahl P, et al. Infectious disease risk factors of corneal graft donors. Arch Ophthalmol 2008; 126(2): 235–239.

9. Eifrig DE. Deposits on the surface of intraocular lenses. South Med J 1980; 73: 6–8.

10. Shimada H, Nakashizuka H, Hattori T, et al. Incidence of endophthalmitis after 20- and 25-gauge vitrectomy: causes and prevention.

11. Ophthalmology, 2008;115(12): 2215-2220.

11. Results of the Endophthalmitis Vitrectomy Study. A randomized trial of immediate vitrectomy and of intravenous antibiotics for the treatment of postoperative bacterial endophthalmitis. Endophthalmitis Vitrectomy Study Group. Arch Ophthalmol 1995; 113(12): 1479–1496.

12. Javitt JC, Vitale S, Canner JK, et al. National outcome of cataract extraction. Arch Ophthalmol 1991; 109: 1085–1089.

13. Berrocal AM, Davis JL. Uveitis following intraocular surgery. Opthalmol Clin North Am 2002; 15: 357–364.

14. West ES, Behrens A, McDonnell PJ, et al. The incidence of endophthalmitis after cataract surgery among the U.S. Medicare population increased between 1994 and 2001. Ophthalmology 2005; 112(8): 1388–1394.

15. Ng JQ, Morlet N, Pearman JW, et al. Management and outcomes of postoperative endophthalmitis since the endophthalmitis vitrectomy study: the Endophthalmitis Population Study of Western Australia (EPSWA)'s fifth report. Ophthalmology 2005; 112(7): 1199–1206.

16. Lundstrom M, Wejde G, Stenevi U, et al. Endophthalmitis after cataract surgery: a nationwide prospective study evaluating incidence in relation to incision type and location. Ophthalmology 2007; 114(5): 866–870.

17. Thoms SS, Musch DC, Soong HK. Postoperative endophthalmitis associated with sutured versus unsutured clear corneal cataract incisions. Br J Ophthalmol 2007; 91(6): 728–730.

18. Chang DF, Braga-Mele R, Mamalis N, et al. Prophylaxis of postoperative endophthalmitis after cataract surgery: results of the 2007 ASCRS member survey. J Cataract Refract Surg 2007; 33(10): 1801–1805.

19. Driebe WT, Mandelbaum S, Forster RK, et al. Pseudophakic endophthalmitis: diagnosis and management. Ophthalmology 1986; 93: 442–448.

20. Higgenbotham EJ, Stevens RK, Musch DC. Bleb-related endophthalmitis after trabeculectomy with mitomycin C. Ophthalmology 1996; 103: 650–656.

21. Wolner B, Liebmann JM, Sassani JW, et al. Late bleb-related endophthalmitis after trabeculectomy with adjunctive 5-fluorouracil. Ophthalmology 1991; 98: 1053–1060.

22. Katz IJ, Cantor LB, Spaeth GL. Complications of surgery in glaucoma: early and late bacterial endophthalmitis following glaucoma filtering surgery. Ophthalmology 1985; 92: 959–963.

23. Gedde SJ, Scott IU, Tabandeh H, et al. Late endophthalmitis associated with glaucoma drainage implants. Ophthalmology 2001; 108: 1323–1327.

24. Kuang TM, Lin YC, Liu CJ, et al. Early and late endophthalmitis following trabeculectomy in a Chinese population. Eur J Ophthalmol 2008; 18(1): 66–70.

25. Al-Torbak AA, Al-Shahwan S, Al-Jadaan I, et al. Endophthalmitis associated with the Ahmed glaucoma valve implant. Br J Ophthalmol 2005; 89(4): 454–458.

26. Forster RK, Zachary IG, Cottingham AJ Jr, et al. Further observation on the diagnosis, cause, and treatment of endophthalmitis. Am J Ophthalmol 1976; 81: 52–56.

27. Han DP, Wisniewski SR, Kelsey SF, et al. Microbiologic yields and complication rates of vitreous needle aspiration versus mechanized vitreous biopsy in the Endophthalmitis Vitrectomy Study. Retina 1999; 19: 98–102.

28. Deramo VA, Lai JC, Winokur J, et al. Visual outcome and bacterial sensitivity after methicillin-resistant *Staphylococcus aureus*-associated acute endophthalmitis. Am J Ophthalmol 2008; 145(3): 413–417.

29. Weber DJ, Hoffman KL, Thoft RA, et al. Endophthalmitis following intraocular lens implantation. Rev Infect Dis 1986; 8: 12–20.

30. Doft BH. Treatment of postcataract extraction endophthalmitis: a summary of the results from the Endophthalmitis Vitrectomy Study. Arch Ophthalmol 2008; 126(4): 554–556.

31. Bron A. Le traitement curatif des endophtalmies aigues post chirurgicales. J Fr Ophtalmol 1999; 22: 1076–1083.

32. Okhravi N, Adamson P, Lightman S. Use of PCR in endophthalmitis. Ocul Immunol Inflamm 2000; 8: 189–200.

33. Chiquet C, Cornut PL, Benito Y, et al. Eubacterial PCR for bacterial detection and identification in 100 acute postcataract surgery endophthalmitis. Invest Ophthalmol Vis Sci 2008; 49(5): 1971–1978.

34. Chaudhry IA, Shamsi FA, Al-Harthi E, et al. Incidence and visual outcome of endophthalmitis associated with intraocular foreign bodies. Graefes Arch Clin Exp Ophthalmol 2008; 246(2): 181–186.

35. Soheilian M, Rafati N, Mohebbi MR, et al. Prophylaxis of acute posttraumatic bacterial endophthalmitis: a multicenter, randomized clinical trial of intraocular antibiotic injection, report 2. Arch Ophthalmol 2007; 125(4): 460–465.

36. Essex RW, Lamoureux E, Charles PG, et al. Prophylaxis for posttraumatic endophthalmitis. Arch Ophthalmol 2008; 126(5): 742–743; author reply 743–4.

37. de Caro JJ, Ta CN, Ho HK, et al. Bacterial contamination of ocular surface and needles in patients undergoing intravitreal injections. Retina 2008; 28(6): 877–883.

38. Yenerel NM, Dinc UA, Gorgun E. A case of sterile endophthalmitis after repeated intravitreal bevacizumab injection. J Ocul Pharmacol Ther 2008; 24(3): 362–363.

39. Mason JO 3rd, White MF, Feist RM, et al. Incidence of acute onset endophthalmitis following intravitreal bevacizumab (Avastin) injection. Retina 2008; 28(4): 564–567.

40. Meisler DM, Palestine AG, Vastine DW, et al. Chronic *Propionibacterium* endophthalmitis after extracapular cataract and intraocular lens implantation. Am J Ophthalmol 1986; 102: 733–739.

41. Roussel TJ, Culbertson WW, Jaffe NS. Chronic postoperative endophthalmitis associated with *Propionibacterium acnes*. Arch Ophthalmol 1987; 105(9): 1199–1201.

42. Jaffe NS. *Propionibacterium acnes* and endophthalmitis seven months after extracapsular cataract extraction and intraocular lens implantation. Ophthalmic Surg 1986; 17: 791–793.

43. Hollander DA, Dodds EM, Rossetti SB, et al. *Propionibacterium acnes* endophthalmitis with bacterial sequestration in a Molteno's implant after cataract extraction. Am J Ophthalmol 2004; 138(5): 878–879.

44. Apple DJ, Mamalis N, Steinmetz RL, et al. Phacoanaphylactic endophthalmitis associated with extracapsular cataract extraction and posterior chamber intraocular lens. Arch Ophthalmol 1984; 102: 1528–1532.

45. McMahon MS, Weiss JS, Riedel KG, et al. Clinically unsuspected phacoanaphylaxis after extracapsular cataract extraction with intraocular lens. Br J Ophthalmol 1985; 69: 836–840.

46. Whitcup SM, Belfort R Jr, de Smet MD, et al. Immunohistochemistry of the inflammatory response in *Propionibacterium acnes* endophthalmitis. Arch Ophthalmol 1991; 109: 978.

47. Maguire HCJ, Cipriano D. Immunopotentiation of cell-mediated hypersensitivity by *Corynebacterium parvum* (*Propionibacterium acnes*). Int Arch Allergy Appl Immun 1983; 70: 34–39.

48. Clark WL, Kaiser PK, Flynn HW Jr, et al. Treatment strategies and visual acuity outcomes in chronic postoperative *Propionibacterium acnes* endophthalmitis. Ophthalmology 1999; 106: 1665–1670.

49. Gutierrez-Diaz E, Montero-Rodríguez M, Mencía-Gutiérrez E, et al. *Propionibacterium acnes* endophthalmitis in Ahmed glaucoma valve. Eur J Ophthalmol 2001; 11: 383–385.

50. Yu EN, Foster CS, Chronic postoperative endophthalmitis due to *Pseudomonas oryzihabitans*. Am J Ophthalmol 2002; 134: 613–614.

51. Abu El-Asrar A, Tabbara K. Chronic endophthalmitis after extracapsular cataract extraction caused by *Mycobacterium chelonae* subspecies *absecessus*. Eye 1995; 9(pt. 6): 798–801.

52. Flicker L, Meredith TA, Wilson LA, et al. Chronic bacterial endophthalmitis. Am J Ophthalmol 1987; 103: 745–748.

53. Narang S, Gupta A, Gupta V, et al. Fungal endophthalmitis following cataract surgery: clinical presentation, microbiological spectrum, and outcome. Am J Ophthalmol 2001; 132(5): 609–617.

54. Pflugfelder SC, Flynn HW Jr, Zwickey TA, et al. Exogenous fungal endophthalmitis. Ophthalmology 1988; 95: 19–30.

55. Samson CM, Foster CS. Chronic postoperative endophthalmitis. Int Ophthalmol Clin 2000; 40: 57–67.

56. Sutphin JE, Robinson NM, Wilhelmus KR, et al. Improved detection of oculomycoses using induced fluorescence with Cellufluor. Ophthalmology 1986; 93: 416–417.

57. Tarai B, Gupta A, Ray P, et al. Polymerase chain reaction for early diagnosis of post-operative fungal endophthalmitis. Indian J Med Res 2006; 123(5): 671–678.

58. Gilbert CM, Novak MA. Successful treatment of postoperative *Candida* endophthalmitis in an eye with an intraocular lens implant. Am J Ophthalmol 1984; 97: 593–595.

59. Smith SR, Kroll AJ, Lou PL, et al. Endogenous bacterial and fungal endophthalmitis. Int Ophthalmol Clin 2007; 47(2): 173–183.

60. Jackson TL, Eykyn SJ, Graham EM, et al. Endogenous bacterial endophthalmitis: a 17-year prospective series and review of 267 reported cases. Surv Ophthalmol 2003; 48(4): 403–423.

61. Romero CF, Rai MK, Lowder CY, et al. Endogenous endophthalmitis: case report and brief review. Am Fam Phys 1999; 60(2): 510–514.

62. Schiedler V, Scott IU, Flynn HW Jr, et al. Culture-proven endogenous endophthalmitis: clinical features and visual acuity outcomes. Am J Ophthalmol 2004; 137(4): 725–731.

63. Zhang YQ, Wang WJ. Treatment outcomes after pars plana vitrectomy for endogenous endophthalmitis. Retina 2005; 25(6): 746–750.

64. Agarwal PK, Gallaghar M, Murphy E, et al. Endogenous endophthalmitis in a rheumatoid patient on tumor necrosis factor alpha blocker. Indian J Ophthalmol 2007; 55(3): 230–232.

65. Blodi FC. Sympathetic uveitis as an allergic phenomenon. Trans Am Acad Ophthalmol Otolaryngol 1959; 63: 642–656.

66. Easom HA, Zimmerman LE. Sympathetic ophthalmia and bilateral phacoanaphylaxis. Arch Ophthalmol 1964; 72: 9–15.

67. Murase KH, Goto H, Kezuka T et al. A case of lens-induced uveitis following metastatic endophthalmitis. Jpn J Ophthalmol 2007; 51(4): 304–306.

68. Meltzer DW. Sterile hypopyon following intraocular lens surgery. Arch Ophthalmol 1980; 98: 100–104.

69. Kalogeropoulos CD, Malamou-Mitsi VD, Asproudis I, et al. The contribution of aqueous humor cytology in the differential diagnosis of anterior uvea inflammations. Ocul Immunol Inflamm 2004; 12(3): 215–225.

70. Mamalis N, Edelhauser HF, Dawson DG, et al. Toxic anterior segment syndrome. J Cataract Refract Surg 2006; 32(2): 324–333.

71. Stark WJ, Rosenblum P, Maumenee AE, et al. Postoperative inflammatory reactions to intraocular lens sterilized

with ethylene oxide. Ophthalmology 1980; 87: 385–389.

72. Krause U, Alanko HI. Dislocated intraocular lens after biodegradation of fixation loops. Acta Ophthalmol 1986; 64: 338–343.

73. Ellington FT. The uveitis–glaucoma–hyphema syndrome associated with the Mark VIII anterior-chamber lens implant. J Am Intraocul Implant Soc 1978; 4: 50–53.

74. Wolter JR, Sugar A, Meyer RF. Reactive membranes on posterior chamber lens implants. Ophthalmic Surg 1985; 16: 699–702.

75. Crawford JB. A histopathologic study of the position of the Shearing intraocular lens in the posterior chamber. Am J Ophthalmol 1981; 91: 458–461.

76. McDonnell PJ, Green WR, Maumenee AE, et al. Pathology of intraocular lenses in 33 eyes examined postmortem. Ophthalmology 1983; 90: 386–403.

77. Flohr MJ, Robin A, Kelley JS. Early complications following Q-switched neodymium YAG laser posterior capsulotomy. Ophthalmology 1985; 92: 360–363.

Anterior Uveitis

Scott M. Whitcup

Anterior uveitis is the most common form of uveitis and the least likely to be referred to a uveitis specialist. The diagnosis of anterior uveitis is based on inflammation limited to the anterior chamber. Because many patients have only a single episode of disease without recurrence or complications, there is a debate on how to evaluate and treat patients with newly diagnosed anterior uveitis. Although anterior uveitis is usually the most easily managed form, associated complications such as glaucoma may result in severe visual loss. In addition, many disorders that can cause a panuveitis, such as sarcoidosis, Behçet's disease, bacterial endophthalmitis, and ocular malignancies may start as an anterior uveitis. Therefore, the approach to patients with anterior uveitis requires careful thought and planning.

As we learn more about the pathophysiology of uveitis, it is becoming increasingly clear that many forms of uveitis may be triggered by a microbial agent. There are a number of conditions where the line between infectious and noninfectious causes becomes blurred. Therefore, this section is now titled Uveitic Conditions not Caused by Active Infection.

Epidemiology

Anterior uveitis accounts for approximately three-quarters of cases of uveitis, with an annual incidence rate of about eight per 100 000 population.[1–3] Most cases have no identifiable cause and are classified as idiopathic; however, in some series HLA-B27 is associated with the disease in up to a third of patients.[4]

Clinical description

Anterior uveitis includes diseases previously categorized as both iritis (inflammation of the iris) and iridocyclitis (inflammation of the iris and ciliary body). Patients with anterior uveitis often complain of redness, pain, and photophobia; some are relatively asymptomatic. Tearing may occur, but ocular discharge is rare. Some patients with severe anterior uveitis may also complain of blurred vision. Conjunctival injection is frequently noted on examination. Ciliary flush – conjunctival injection in the perilimbal area, is characteristic of many forms of the disease. Pupillary miosis, posterior synechiae, and dilated iris vessels are common findings in all forms of anterior uveitis. However, sector abnormalities of the iris may suggest herpes zoster ophthalmicus as an underlying cause. The iris may also adhere to the trabecular meshwork, forming peripheral anterior synechiae (PAS). These PAS should be looked for on gonioscopic examination because patients with severe PAS are at increased risk for secondary glaucoma. In addition, patients with severe posterior synechiae – iris adhesions to the lens – can develop pupillary block and may require prophylactic iridectomy.

The major indicators of anterior uveitis are the presence of cells and flare in the anterior chamber. Anterior chamber inflammation is assessed on slit-lamp biomicroscopic examination and is discussed in detail in Chapter 3. These cells and flare represent extravasated inflammatory cells and protein as a result of a breakdown of the blood–aqueous barrier. A device has been developed that uses laser photometry to objectively assess anterior chamber cells and flare. Guex-Crosier and colleagues[5] used laser flare-cell photometry to demonstrate that blood–aqueous barrier disruption was very pronounced in idiopathic anterior uveitis and acute retinal necrosis, but minimal in patients with toxoplasmosis or Fuchs' heterochromic cyclitis. These authors suggested that laser flare-cell photometry provides a quantitative and sensitive assessment of anterior segment inflammation and may be useful for the management of patients with uveitis.

Fibrin may accumulate in the anterior chamber and may cause the once-mobile cells that circulate in the aqueous to become frozen. This plasmoid aqueous is a sign of severe anterior uveitis that requires aggressive therapy. Another sign of severe anterior uveitis is a hypopyon composed of layered leukocytes. A hypopyon can be seen in a number of forms of anterior uveitis, but it is frequently associated with Behçet's

Table 19-1 Syndromes of Anterior Uveitis

Disease	Age (yr)	Sex	Ocular Redness	HLA-B27	Systemic Findings	Steroid Response
Idiopathic	Any	Either	Yes	No	None	Yes
HLA-B27, ocular only	15–40	M > F	Yes	Yes	None	Yes
Ankylosing spondylitis	15–40	M > F	Yes	Yes	Spondylitis, sacroiliitis	Yes
Reactive arthritis	15–40	M > F	Yes	Yes	Arthritis, urethritis, mucocutaneous lesions	Yes
Juvenile rheumatoid arthritis	3–16	F > M	No	No	Pauciarticular arthritis, ANA-positive, RF-negative	Yes
Fuchs' iridocyclitis	Any	Either	No	No	None	Yes/no
Posner–Schlossman syndrome	Adult	Either	No	No	None	Yes
Schwartz syndrome	Adult	Either	No	No	None	No
Ocular ischemia	>50	Either	Yes	No	Carotid insufficiency	No
Kawasaki disease	1–18	Either	Yes	No	Skin rash, lymphadenopathy fever, cardiac lesions	Yes

ANA, antinuclear antibody; RF, rheumatoid factor.

disease or infectious endophthalmitis. Anterior uveitis, including some cases with hypopyons, has been described in patients with AIDS who are receiving the drug rifabutin as treatment or prophylaxis for mycobacterial infection.[6–8] Also, hyphema may occur in patients with anterior uveitis, but it usually resolves without permanent damage.[9]

Inflammatory cells may also collect and adhere to the corneal endothelium and form keratic precipitates. The mechanism appears to involve the expression of cell adhesion molecules that are upregulated in the presence of inflammatory cytokines such as interleukin-1.[10–12] Large, greasy-appearing keratic precipitates are suggestive of a granulomatous inflammation and may help in determining the cause of the uveitis (see Chapter 4). In vivo confocal microscopy of keratic precipitates showed heterogeneous features of KP and may have diagnostic relevance.[13]

During the acute inflammatory episode, the intraocular pressure is often reduced because of ciliary body shutdown and reduced aqueous production. As the inflammation subsides, however, the intraocular pressure may rapidly increase, especially in patients with severe PAS. In some patients it is difficult to determine whether the increased intraocular pressure is a result of underlying inflammation or a steroid response to the corticosteroids used to control the disease. In secondary glaucoma caused by active inflammatory disease, increased corticosteroid therapy will lead to a reduction in intraocular pressure.

Although some of the clinical symptoms and signs of anterior uveitis are specific for certain diseases, most disorders are differentiated by their associated systemic findings. The clinical findings of the common disorders that cause anterior uveitis are summarized in **Table 19-1**. Some disorders, such as postsurgical inflammation, infectious uveitis, Behçet's disease, sarcoidosis, and the masquerade syndromes, are discussed in separate chapters.

Idiopathic anterior uveitis

After a thorough medical history and an ocular and general physical examination, almost 50% of patients are found to have an anterior segment inflammation that is not associated with other defined clinical syndromes. This form of anterior uveitis is referred to as idiopathic anterior uveitis. Patients with idiopathic anterior uveitis must not only lack systemic disease associations but also cannot have the HLA-B27 haplotype, which is associated with anterior segment inflammatory disease. In one study, 47% of patients with anterior uveitis had HLA-B27-associated anterior uveitis;[1] however, about one-quarter of these patients also had underlying systemic disorders, including ankylosing spondylitis and Reiter's syndrome. Nevertheless, the diagnosis of idiopathic anterior uveitis depends greatly on the extent of the evaluation for an underlying condition. Many of the conditions initially diagnosed as idiopathic anterior uveitis are later found to be a specific disorder.

Importantly, one should rule out masquerade syndromes that present with an anterior uveitis (see Chapter 30). Conditions, including the presence of intraocular foreign bodies, malignancies including leukemia and lymphoma, and pigment dispersion syndrome, can be misdiagnosed as an idiopathic anterior uveitis. Medications including rifabutin, sulfonamides, topical prostaglandin analogs for glaucoma and ocular hypertension, and vaccines have been associated with anterior uveitis.[14,15] Nevertheless, a specific etiology for anterior uveitis cannot be determined in many patients. It has been hypothesized that these patients may have an immune responsiveness that may explain the development of anterior segment inflammation. Patients with a history of acute anterior uveitis but no signs of ocular inflammation at the time of recruitment showed a high innate immune responsiveness compared with control subjects.[16] In a whole blood culture assay, levels of tumor necrosis factor-α and C-reactive protein were significantly higher in patients with a history of anterior uveitis than in control subjects.

Diagnostic workup

A controversial topic in uveitis concerns the diagnostic evaluation of patients with a first episode of anterior uveitis. Some suggest that no evaluation is needed. Others state that a long list of laboratory tests and diagnostic procedures should be ordered. The prudent approach probably lies somewhere in the middle, and, as discussed in Chapter 4, a complete medical history and thorough examination can help target the workup. For example, if the patient complains of lower back pain, a diagnosis of ankylosing spondylitis is suggested and the evaluation might consist solely of sacroiliac joint films and HLA-B27 testing. Similarly, for a child with anterior uveitis with band keratopathy and a history of arthritis a diagnosis of juvenile rheumatoid arthritis is suggested, and a targeted evaluation consisting of tests for antinuclear antibody (ANA) and rheumatoid factor may suffice.

However, when a thorough history and examination fail to suggest specific diagnoses, what tests should be ordered? We tend to do a limited workup of all patients with anterior uveitis even if it is their first episode. If the uveitis is non-granulomatous, we order a fluorescent treponemal antibody absorption test to rule out syphilis, because this test is both highly sensitive and specific for the disease and because syphilis is treatable, and early treatment can prevent long-term complications. Similarly, we obtain results of a complete blood cell count and urinalysis to rule out an underlying systemic disorder such as connective tissue disease, because the associated renal disease or anemia may be asymptomatic yet warrant therapy. If the inflammation is granulomatous, a number of other disorders are suggested (see Chapter 4). For granulomatous anterior uveitis we will also require a purified protein derivative test, a chest X-ray, and a serum and urine calcium test and a serum angiotensin-converting enzyme level to rule out asymptomatic tuberculosis or sarcoidosis.

Treatment

The breakthrough in the treatment of ocular inflammation came with the discovery of corticosteroids. In 1949, Hench and colleagues[17] reported the beneficial effect of 17-hydroxy-11-dehydrocorticosterone and pituitary adrenocorticotropic hormone in patients with rheumatoid arthritis. During the following year, two papers were published in the *Journal of the American Medical Association* showing effects on ocular inflammatory disease.[18,19] This was a vast improvement from previous therapy. Earlier in the 20th century, patients with ocular inflammation were treated by inducing hyperpyrexia. Early on, patients were placed in steam baths in which their temperature was raised to 40–41°C for 4–6 hours. In some patients the inflammation improved, but many developed severe complications. Later, patients were injected with milk protein or typhoid toxin to induce fever. Despite complications with their use, corticosteroids were a welcome advance in our treatment of inflammation.

Patients with idiopathic anterior uveitis tend to have non-granulomatous inflammation that responds well to topical corticosteroid therapy. Acetate preparations of topical corticosteroids tend to penetrate the cornea better than other preparations especially if the epithelium is intact, and we tend to use prednisolone acetate 1%. To prevent the development of posterior synechiae and to moderate symptoms of pain and photophobia caused by inflammation of the ciliary muscle, mydriasis and cycloplegia are indicated. Scopolamine 0.25% given twice daily is usually sufficient. For resistant disease, periocular injections of corticosteroids may be useful. Systemic corticosteroids are rarely needed to treat anterior uveitis. However, patients with anterior uveitis may develop posterior segment disease. These patients frequently require more aggressive antiinflammatory therapy including periocular or systemic corticosteroids or other immunosuppressive therapy.

HLA-B27–associated anterior uveitis

HLA-B27-associated anterior uveitis appears to be a distinct clinical disorder. This form of the disease has frequent associations with systemic diseases, including ankylosing spondylitis, Reiter's syndrome, inflammatory bowel disease, Whipple's disease, and psoriatic arthritis.[20] Nevertheless, as stated earlier, many patients with the HLA-B27 haplotype and anterior uveitis have no associated systemic illness.

Epidemiology

Some studies suggest that as many as 50% of patients with acute anterior uveitis are HLA-B27 positive, and half of these have spondyloarthropathies.[21] In a systematic review of 126 articles describing 29 877 patients with spondyloarthropathy, Zeboulon and colleagues[22] reported a uveitis prevalence of 32.7%. This prevalence increased with the duration of disease.

Demographics and clinical findings

Patients with HLA-B27-associated anterior uveitis are more often male and tend to develop uveitis at a younger age than those who are HLA-B27 negative.[3] However, some studies indicate that the long-term visual prognosis is similar for both groups.[3]

In a retrospective cohort study of 177 HLA-B27 patients with uveitis, the average age at onset of acute anterior uveitis was 36 years with no difference between males and females.[23] HLA-B27-associated systemic disease developed earlier in males and bilateral uveitis developed more frequently in females.

Should HLA typing be performed in all patients with anterior uveitis? We obtain HLA typing for patients with their first episode of acute anterior uveitis, especially if they have back pain or other systemic symptoms or signs. In addition, if patients develop severe chronic anterior uveitis, we will obtain HLA typing for the patient because the finding of the HLA-B27 haplotype often obviates the need for an extensive laboratory evaluation to rule out infectious or other treatable causes of the disease.

Etiology

The finding of the HLA-B27 haplotype is also of interest as a clue to the possible pathogenesis of the disease. Of particular interest is the potential role of Gram-negative bacteria and their interaction with major histocompatibility complex (MHC) class I antigens in triggering the anterior uveitis.[20,24] More recently, *Helicobacter pylori* has also been associated with anterior uveitis.[21] Unfortunately, this possible link between microbial antigens, HLA-B27, and anterior uveitis has not lead to improved therapy for the disorder because antimicrobial agents have not been proved to affect the course of disease. This may be due to a lack of efficacy or the dearth of trials investigating this therapeutic approach. A possible explanation for the lack of efficacy of antimicrobial agents is that the infection induces inflammation through toll-like receptors (TLR) and the process becomes separate from the active infection.[25]

Other immunologic studies have been performed in an attempt to determine the pathogenesis of anterior uveitis. Increased levels of complement and immunoglobulin (Ig) G compatible with breakdown of the blood–aqueous barrier can be detected in the aqueous of patients with anterior uveitis.[26] There is also evidence of complement activation in the aqueous of patients with anterior uveitis, measured by the presence of C3a, C4a, and C5a.[27] Evidence of increased serum fibrin degradation products has suggested a pathogenic role of the clotting pathways.[28] Increased expression of cell adhesion molecules has been associated with the development of intraocular inflammation. Increased expression of intercellular adhesion molecule-1 (ICAM-1) in the irides of patients with uveitis has been reported,[29] and expression of cell adhesion molecules in the anterior uvea has been shown to precede the infiltration of inflammatory cells in animal models of acute anterior uveitis.[10,11] Finally, polymorphisms within the tumor necrosis factor (TNF)-α promoter region have been identified, and individuals with these single-nuleotide polymoprhisms (SNPs) show a higher susceptibility towards developing uveitis.[30]

HLA-B27–associated anterior uveitis with systemic disease

Ankylosing spondylitis

Ankylosing spondylitis is a chronic, inflammatory arthritis that primarily affects the spine and sacroiliac joints. The disease was previously known as Bechterew's disease and Marie Strumpell disease, and is now discussed as a spondlyoarthropathy. Without treatment, the disease can progress and result in fusion and rigidity of the spine known as bamboo spine.

Ocular involvement occurs in 25% of patients with ankylosing spondylitis.[31] In 80% of patients both eyes are involved, but they are rarely inflamed simultaneously. Although the ocular findings associated with ankylosing spondylitis include both iritis and conjunctivitis, the iritis is the more significant manifestation. The disease course is quite variable. Recurrence of the ocular inflammation may occur as frequently as every 2–3 weeks. Some patients have fewer than one exacerbation per year. Interestingly, recurrence may be seasonal, although this variation appears to be more frequent in patients with idiopathic anterior uveitis.[32]

The anterior uveitis associated with ankylosing spondylitis usually has a presentation similar to that of idiopathic disease, occurring as a unilateral acute iritis with pain, photophobia, and redness (**Fig. 19-1A**). Patients often complain of the onset of an attack 1–2 days before anterior chamber cell and flare are evident on slit-lamp biomicroscopy. The use of laser photometry may help determine when initial breakdown of the blood–aqueous barrier occurs in relation to the development of symptoms and clinical signs of inflammation. Vision may decrease transiently during an acute episode as a result of anterior chamber inflammation, or less often because of associated cystoid macular edema. A fibrin clot may form in the anterior chamber (Fig. 19-1B). Posterior synechiae commonly develop unless attacks are treated promptly with corticosteroids and cycloplegic agents (**Fig. 19-2**).

Ankylosing spondylitis has been reported to affect men 2.5–3 times more frequently than women. Women may have a milder disease that may present with more peripheral joint manifestations. It is a common disorder that affects 0.1% of white adults.[33] Because HLA-B27 antigen is dominantly inherited and expressed, 50% of offspring will carry the gene, but the disease will be manifest in only 10% of them. Approximately 96% of patients with ankylosing spondylitis have the HLA-B27 antigen, compared to 6–14% of a control white population without ankylosing spondylitis. HLA-B27 is found in 0–4% of African-Americans. Thus the relative risk for ankylosing spondylitis in patients with the HLA-B27 antigen is as high as 100. Nevertheless, only 1.3% of all HLA-B27-positive patients will have the disease.

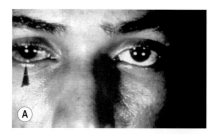

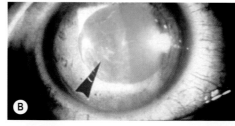

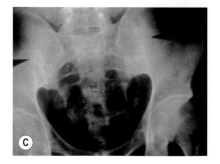

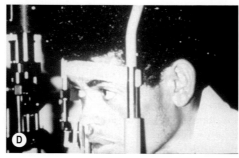

Figure 19-1. A, Unilateral redness caused by iritis associated with ankylosing spondylitis. **B,** Fibrin clot in the anterior chamber in iritis associated with ankylosing spondylitis. **C,** X-ray of the sacroiliac joints demonstrating increased radiodensity caused by ankylosing spondylitis. **D,** Flexed neck caused by ankylosis of the cervical spine in ankylosing spondylitis. (*Courtesy of Fernando Orefice, MD, and Rubens Belfort Jr, MD.*)

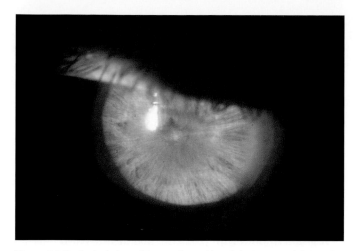

Figure 19-2. Occluded pupil in a patient with ankylosing spondylitis and recurrent iritis.

Sacroiliitis may be asymptomatic early in the course of disease, but can be associated with severe lower back pain and debilitating stiffness and decreased range of motion. X-rays of the sacroiliac joints show blurring of the joints followed by sclerotic changes and eventually obliteration as the disease progresses (see Fig. 19-1C). A common mistake in the initial evaluation of patients with possible ankylosing spondylitis is to order lumbosacral spine films instead of radiographs of the sacroiliac joints. In severe disease, however, patients develop a fusion of the spine that begins in the lumbar region but can involve all parts of the spine. This leads to back pain and stiffness, and in severe disease may cause pulmonary restriction and a stiff, flexed neck, making positioning for slit-lamp biomicroscopic examination difficult (see Fig. 19-1D). Interestingly, the associated uveitis does not appear to correlate with the severity of the underlying spondylitis. Aortic insufficiency, cardiomegaly, and conduction defects are also associated with this disease.

Etiology

The reason for the association between HLA-B27 and ankylosing spondylitis remains unknown. As mentioned above, some data suggest that environmental triggers such as infection with Gram-negative bacteria are important for the development of the disease. This information has led to several theories. One hypothesis suggests that HLA-B27 is a receptor for the infectious agent. A second suggests that HLA-B27 may cross-react with foreign antigens and induce tolerance. Others have suggested that HLA-B27 is a marker for an immune response gene that determines susceptibility to an environmental stimulus, or that microbial agents activate toll-like receptors and induce inflammation.

Treatment

It is important to make the diagnosis of ankylosing spondylitis in patients with uveitis because if the disease is recognized and treated early, spinal deformity can be prevented. Treatment usually involves physical therapy and antiinflammatory drugs, including nonsteroidal antiinflammatory drugs (NSAIDs). Sulfasalazine is used in patients who fail to respond to NSAIDs or who have contraindications to NSAID therapy. Cytotoxic therapy such as methotrexate is reserved

for severe cases, but can reduce rates of recurrence.[34] More recently, anti-TNF drugs have been used to treat ankylosing spondylitis. NSAIDs may have some role in treating the uveitis associated with this disorder; however, data from large controlled trials are lacking. A meta-analysis of four placebo-controlled studies with anti-TNF agents in ankylosing spondylitis reviewed the effect on anterior uveitis. The frequency of flares of anterior uveitis was significantly less in patients receiving anti-TNF therapy than in patients receiving placebo (6.8 anterior uveitis flares per 100 patient-years vs 15.6 uveitis flares per 100 patient-years).[35]

Reactive arthritis (Reiter's syndrome)

Reactive arthritis is a systemic disorder characterized by arthritis, conjunctivitis, and urethritis. It was first described in 1818, but is named after Reiter, who described the entity in 1916.[36] Reiter's syndrome is now more commonly referred to as reactive arthritis, a form of seronegative spondyloarthropathy that includes ankylosing spondylitis, psoriatic arthritis, juvenile chronic arthritis, and the arthropathy associated with inflammatory bowel disease. This change is due in part to the desire to use names that are more clinically descriptive, and because of Reiter's activities with the Nazis during WWII. Reactive arthritis is the most common cause of inflammatory oligoarthropathy in young males and, like ankylosing spondylitis, is related to both HLA-B27 and a specific infection that may trigger the disease. The disease develops in at least 1% of patients with nonspecific urethritis and occurs in about 2% of patients after dysentery caused by *Shigella* spp.

Many patients do not manifest the classic triad of arthritis, conjunctivitis, and urethritis. In addition, many of the findings of reactive arthritis are easily missed. For example, urethritis may be mild and missed. Other systemic associations include a scaling skin eruption called keratoderma blennorrhagicum, balanitis, and an aphthous stomatitis. Rheumatologic features of the disease include arthralgias, plantar fasciitis, and tenosynovitis. About 20% of patients with reactive arthritis develop sacroiliitis and ascending spinal disease similar to ankylosing spondylitis. Hyperkeratotic skin lesions occur and may be indistinguishable from psoriasis. A number of classification systems have been proposed for reactive arthritis (**Box 19-1**),[37] but none are used uniformly in clinical practice.

In one review, arthritis was the presenting symptom in 25% of patients and genitourinary symptoms in 19%.[37]As the syndrome progresses, 94% of patients developed arthritis at some point, mostly in the joints of the hands, wrists, feet, and knees. Sacroiliitis occurred in 19% of patients, and almost any joint can be involved. Urethritis occurred in 75% of patients, with cystitis, orchitis, vaginitis, and epididymitis occurring in occasional patients. Oral ulcers occurred in 19% of patients and external genital lesions in 39%. Skin lesions are common in reactive arthritis: they are seen in about 20% of patients but occur rarely in patients with ankylosing spondylitis.

Conjunctivitis is the most common ocular finding in patients with reactive arthritis and occurs in 30–60% of patients. Some patients develop a mucoid discharge, but the conjunctivitis is usually not chronic. Iritis and keratitis are less common. Iritis occurs in 3–12% of patients and is

---

Box 19-1 Reactive arthritis

MAJOR CRITERIA

Polyarthritis

Conjunctivitis, iridocyclitis

Urethritis

Keratoderma blennorrhagica, balanitis circinata

MINOR CRITERIA

Fasciitis, tendonitis, sacroiliitis, spondylitis

Keratitis

Cystitis, prostatitis

Oral mucosal lesions, psoriasis-like rash, nail changes

Diarrhea, leukocytosis, increased serum globulins, inflammation in the synovial fluid

Reactive arthritis is:

    Definite if three major criteria or two major and three minor

    Probable if two major and two minor

Modified from Lee DA, Barker SM, Su WPD et al.: The clinical diagnosis of Reiter's syndrome, Ophthalmology 1986; 93: 350–6.

---

nongranulomatous and mild. The keratitis is characterized by multifocal punctate subepithelial and anterior stroma infiltrates. A small pannus may also develop.

As stated previously, reactive arthritis may occur after dysentery caused by Gram-negative bacteria or after non-gonococcal urethritis caused by *Chlamydia trachomatis* and *Ureaplasma urealyticum*.[38] Nevertheless, treatment of the dysentery does not appear to alter the development or course of the syndrome. Most patients have signs of this syndrome 2–4 weeks after the onset of dysentery, but the full syndrome may take years to develop.[37]

The diagnosis of reactive arthritis is based on clinical findings in association with the HLA-B27 haplotype. Rheumatoid factor and autoantibodies are usually absent. The ocular disease associated with reactive arthritis is usually mild and can be treated with topical corticosteroids and mydriatic agents. However, the joint involvement may lead to significant long-term dysfunction and require treatment with NSAIDs. Immunosuppressive therapy with agents such as azathioprine and methotrexate may be required for systemic sequelae. Anti-TNF agents have also been used to treat the disease.

Juvenile idiopathic arthritis

Juvenile idiopathic uveitis (JIA) is a chronic arthritis that was previously called juvenile rheumatoid arthritis (JRA). Until recently, the term juvenile rheumatoid arthritis was used inappropriately to describe all forms of childhood arthritis. As in adults, arthritis in children may be associated with infections such as Lyme disease, psoriasis, inflammatory bowel disease, and other systemic diseases. The diagnosis is based on the presence of arthritis in a child under 16 and is usually with a negative rheumatoid factor test result and no other known cause for the joint disease.[39] The joint inflammation may be polyarticular or pauciarticular, and the majority of patients have negative rheumatoid factor test results. A systemic form of JIA is characterized by a symmetric polyarthritis with an associated fever, rash, hepatosplenomegaly, and leukocytosis.

Diagnosis

Identifying the subclassification of JIA is important to determine the risk for developing uveitis. Children with uveitis are often asymptomatic and rarely complain of ocular symptoms, especially if the disease is uniocular. Uveitis is rare in children with systemic JIA.[40,41] Patients with polyarticular arthritis only occasionally develop uveitis. In contrast, patients with the pauciarticular form of JIA have a much higher risk for developing ocular inflammation. Girls with pauciarticular arthritis and a positive ANA test result have the highest risk for developing chronic iridocyclitis.[39] A higher risk of uveitis is also associated with arthritis sparing the wrists but involving a lower-extremity joint: 14% of girls in this high-risk group will develop chronic anterior uveitis.

A group of boys with pauciarticular arthritis also have an increased risk for developing anterior uveitis:[42] 75% of boys with pauciarticular arthritis are HLA-B27 positive, and the ocular inflammation they develop is similar in appearance to that of ankylosing spondylitis. The uveitis is characterized by an acute, episodic, nongranulomatous anterior uveitis, and some of these boys develop ankylosing spondylitis later in life.[42]

Unlike males who develop uveitis, girls with JIA tend to have chronic indolent disease, which can cause permanent ocular damage before it is recognized. In fact, the inflammation is clinically silent in more than 50% of patients. Therefore, girls with pauciarticular arthritis with test results that are positive for ANA and negative for rheumatoid factor should be screened every 3–4 months for the development of chronic smoldering uveitis. Parents should be told that a red eye should not be dismissed as conjunctivitis. Frequently, the first sign of uveitis in these girls is an irregular pupil as a result of posterior synechiae.

The chronic uveitis in JIA is characterized by anterior chamber cells and flare. Usually, patients only have 1 to 2+ cells, and once the uveitis has developed, chronic flare is typical. Anterior chamber cells and not flare should be used to determine the severity of disease and the need for therapy. The number of cells will fluctuate with the severity of inflammation and diminish with corticosteroid therapy. Similar to the uveitis associated with other arthropathies, the severity of the uveitis is unrelated to the severity of the underlying joint disease. Although the joint disease often diminishes with age, ocular disease frequently persists into adulthood. Chronic inflammation may lead to band keratopathy, posterior synechiae, cataract, hypotony, and glaucoma. Glaucoma has been reported in up to 20% of eyes and may be caused by pupillary block or chronic inflammatory disease, with presumed damage to the trabecular meshwork.[43] Band keratopathy occurs in more than half of patients and can cause significant visual disturbance (**Fig. 19-3**).[42] Cataract occurs in at least 60% of eyes and in young patients may lead to amblyopia. Chronic inflammation in the presence of posterior synechiae and a small pupil can lead to the development of a fibrin membrane over the pupil. Finally, although the ocular inflammatory disease associated with JIA primarily involves the anterior segment, vitritis, macular edema, and macular folds may occur. Therefore, visual loss may be caused by multiple factors in patients with JIA, and a thorough evaluation is necessary to develop an appropriate therapeutic approach.

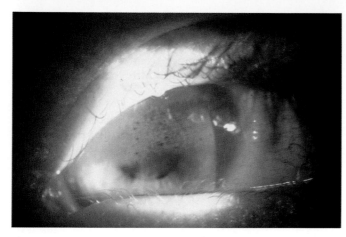

Figure 19-3. Band keratopathy in a patient with long-standing pauciarticular juvenile rheumatoid arthritis and chronic iritis.

The joint disease in patients who develop acute uveitis has an average age of onset of 7.5–9 years.[39,42] In contrast, patients with chronic uveitis develop joint symptoms earlier in life, with an average age of onset of 4–6.3 years. In one study, half of the patients had chronic uveitis by age 6.[43] Joint inflammation usually precedes ocular disease by several years, but iritis can precede the joint symptoms by months to years.[42]

Pathology

Pathologic studies have been performed only on a few eyes of patients with JIA.[44,45] Histologic findings show that the inflammation predominantly involves the iris and ciliary body. Plasma cells and lymphocytes are the most common inflammatory cells, and scattered giant cells have been noted. A similar histologic picture is seen in the involved joints of these patients. In view of the association between ANAs and other autoantibodies with JIA, some have hypothesized that infiltrating plasma cells are responsible for local synthesis of autoantibodies against ocular antigens.[45] However, these proposed autoantibodies or ocular antigens have not been identified.

Differential diagnosis

Ocular sarcoidosis in children is the disease that most closely mimics JIA. Children with sarcoidosis develop arthritis and skin lesions and often lack radiographic evidence of pulmonary disease. JIA can be distinguished from sarcoidosis by the presence of a positive ANA test result, the characteristic distribution of involved joints, the nongranulomatous inflammation limited primarily to the anterior segment of the eye, and the absence of systemic symptoms and signs. Nevertheless, early in the course of JIA children may have no history of joint disease and present only with chronic uveitis and band keratopathy. Other diseases to consider include Lyme disease, psoriatic arthritis, juvenile Reiter's syndrome, ankylosing spondylitis, inflammatory bowel disease-associated anterior uveitis, Kawasaki disease, trauma, and keratouveitis caused by herpes simplex or herpes zoster infection.

Treatment and prognosis

Patients with chronic anterior uveitis associated with JIA need to be seen regularly – no less than every 3 months. Topical corticosteroids remain the mainstay of therapy.[46,47] Corticosteroid therapy should be used to reduce the number of anterior chamber cells, but chronic flare in the absence of cells should not be treated. Glaucoma and cataract are frequent side effects of topical steroid therapy in children with JIA. Especially in young patients, cataracts may lead to the development of amblyopia and require prompt surgical removal.

Chylack[47] studied 210 patients with JIA and found that in 39% of patients the uveitis responded to short courses of topical corticosteroids. However, in 61% of patients JIA did not respond to corticosteroids or required prolonged treatment. Repeated periocular injections of depot preparations of corticosteroids are needed to manage some occurrences of chronic active inflammation that cannot be controlled with topical corticosteroids alone. For most children this requires general anesthesia for each injection. Short courses of oral corticosteroids can be tried, but we do not favor the long-term use of oral corticosteroids in children because of the overwhelming side effects on growth and bone formation. Alternate-day therapy may reduce the side effects and may be tried for unusually severe ocular disease requiring prolonged therapy.

The use of NSAIDs may allow a reduction in the dosage of corticosteroids required to treat chronic uveitis.[48] Tolmetin and naproxen are the NSAIDs most commonly used in children. A number of other immunosuppressive agents, including azathioprine, chlorambucil, cyclophosphamide, and methotrexate have been used to treat severe uveitis associated with JIA. We are hesitant to use many of the cytotoxic agents in children for fear of inducing a secondary malignancy. A double-masked trial of methotrexate versus placebo in the treatment of resistant JIA showed that joint disease improved with methotrexate therapy; however, the study did not address the response of the uveitis.[49] We have found ciclosporin to be useful for the treatment of many forms of childhood uveitis but have rarely treated children with JIA using this agent.

More recently, anti-TNF agents have been used to treat JIA. In a retrospective case series, the use of the anti-TNF agents led to a prompt reduction in intraocular inflammation.[50] However, not all patients respond to anti-TNF therapy, and children need to be following closely to monitor for therapeutic response and potential relapse.[51]

Surgery is often needed in the management of JIA-associated uveitis. Cataracts are common in children with JIA and require surgical removal, but only in eyes that have been 'quiet' for at least 3 months. Cataract extraction may be performed by either phacoemulsification or as a pars plana lensectomy.[52,53] The need for a secondary surgical procedure appears to be reduced in patients undergoing a pars plana lensectomy with vitrectomy.[53] Many uveitis specialists also recommend removal of the posterior capsule at the time of surgery because a secondary laser posterior capsulotomy may be difficult to perform in children. Foster and Barrett[54] reported their surgical experience in patients with JIA. Cataracts were common in their patients and developed in 13 of 72 patients (18%) during follow-up. The authors performed phacoemulsification extracapsular cataract extraction followed by a pars plana vitrectomy, and emphasized the need for aggressive antiinflammatory therapy both before and after surgery. The average postoperative visual acuity in this study was 20/40.

Medical management of glaucoma in patients with JIA is problematic. Aggressive use of topical IOP-lowering agents is warranted. Surgery is required for a number of patients for whom medical management has failed. Laser iridectomy is indicated for glaucoma caused by pupillary block with iris bombé. In patients with secondary glaucoma caused by chronic intraocular inflammation the success of traditional surgery with trabeculectomy is poor.[55] Filtering devices such as Molteno implants may improve the prognosis. Cyclocryotherapy should only be used when other surgical procedures have failed to control the pressure.

Band keratopathy is seen in 77% of patients with severe JIA-associated iridocyclitis.[41] This band keratopathy can be treated with chemical chelation with topical application of 0.37 M ethylenediamine tetraacetic acid solution after debridement of the epithelium with 70% isopropyl alcohol and scraping. The excimer laser may have a role in the management of this complication in the future. Keratoconjunctivitis sicca can also occur in JIA. In a study of 64 patients with JIA, 12.5% complained of dry eye with lower Schirmer test results and tear break-up times than age- and gender-matched controls.[56]

Prognosis is related to early diagnosis and meticulous treatment of ocular inflammation and management of secondary complications. Because ocular inflammation does not always mirror joint disease, routine ophthalmologic examinations at least every 3 months are recommended.[57] This makes sense, as complications and vision loss are common. In a retrospective cohort study of 75 patients with JIA, the incidence of any ocular complication was 0.33 per eye-year.[58] Rates of vision loss to 20/50 or worse and 20/200 or worse were 0.10 per eye-year and 0.08 per eye-year, respectively. Risk factors included anterior chamber flare 1+ or greater and elevated IOP. Immunosuppressive drug therapy reduced the rates of complications, including hypotony and blindness.

Psoriatic arthropathy

Psoriasis is a skin disease caused by hyperproliferation of the epidermis with resultant scaling. Uveitis occurs predominantly in patients who develop arthropathy. About 20% of patients with psoriasis develop psoriatic arthropathy, and about 20% of these patients develop uveitis, sacroiliitis, and ascending spine disease.[59] The arthropathy usually involves the distal joints of the hands and feet as well as the sacroiliac joints. The uveitis predominantly involves the anterior segment of the eye and is similar to HLA-B27-associated disease. Because psoriasis is a common disorder, not all anterior uveitis that occurs in patients with psoriasis will be causally related, especially if the patient does not have arthritis. The psoriasis and arthropathy in these patients have been treated separately. Anti-TNF agents have also been used to treat both components of the disease.[60] The uveitis tends to respond well to standard therapy with topical corticosteroids and a drop to induce cycloplegia and mydriasis.

Inflammatory bowel disease

Patients with both ulcerative colitis and Crohn's disease can develop uveitis.[61,62] About 5% of patients with ulcerative colitis will develop ocular disease. Conjunctivitis, episcleritis, and anterior uveitis are most commonly described;

however, posterior uveitis may also occur. Similar ocular inflammatory disease has been associated with Crohn's disease. The ophthalmologist should ask patients with anterior uveitis whether they have recurrent diarrhea, bloody diarrhea, or abdominal cramping. Although the uveitis often responds to therapy with topical corticosteroids, early diagnosis of inflammatory bowel disease will lead to prompt treatment for the gastrointestinal complications that frequently occur. Similar to other spondyloarthropathies, anti-TNF agents are now used in the management of the disease. The effect on uveitis is less well documented in clinical trials.

Whipple's disease

Whipple's disease is a chronic infectious disease caused by *Tropheryma whipplei* that has been associated with uveitis.[63] Now that the causative organism has been identified, the description of this disease has been moved to the chapter on bacterial and fungal disease (Chapter 9).

Disease associations

Fuchs' heterochromic iridocyclitis

The association of iris heterochromia and cataract was initially described by Lawrence in 1843.[64] In 1906, Fuchs[65] described seven patients with heterochromic iridocyclitis, and later described 38 patients with the disease and reported on the pathologic features of six eyes. The classic hallmark of Fuchs' heterochromic iridocyclitis is, as the name suggests, iris heterochromia (**Fig. 19-4A and B**). However, this classic finding may be difficult to perceive. It is easiest to see in blue-eyed patients, in whom the affected eye appears more intensely blue.[66] In addition, 7–15% of patients have bilateral involvement and no obvious heterochromia. A more consistent finding appears to be blurring of the iris stroma and loss of detail and density of the iris surface that can only be seen on careful slit-lamp biomicroscopic examination.[66,67] Fuchs observed that most patients with this disorder develop cataracts.

The typical patient is young and presents with iris heterochromia and a mild disturbance of vision. Pain and redness are rare. Slit-lamp examination shows small stellate keratic precipitates (KPs) with fine filaments that are uniformly scattered over the endothelium, unlike most other occurrences of anterior uveitis in which the precipitates occur predominantly on the lower half of the cornea. Anterior chamber inflammation is mild, and low-grade vitritis may be seen. The posterior segment of the eye is usually unaffected, although cystoid macular edema has been reported in a few patients. Abnormal vessels bridging the anterior chamber angle are frequently described, but iris neovascularization and neovascular glaucoma are rare.[68] It is well documented that hyphema is likely to occur after intraocular surgery. Amsler[69] first noted the occurrence of hyphema after paracentesis. Anterior chamber paracentesis was initially proposed as a diagnostic test for Fuchs' heterochromic iridocyclitis, but appears unwarranted for this purpose.[68]

Many patients with Fuchs' heterochromic iridocyclitis are unaware of their disease until their vision decreases because of cataract or progressive glaucoma. Rarely, vitreous

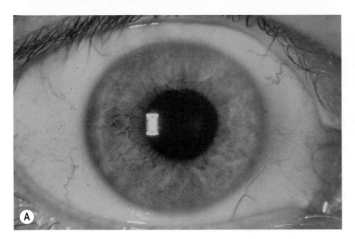
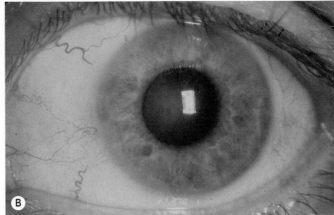

Figure 19-4. Photograph of irides of a patient with Fuchs' heterochromic iridocyclitis demonstrating heterochromia. **A,** The unaffected right eye. **B,** The affected left eye has the lighter colored iris.

inflammation is severe enough to cause floaters. The presence of fine, evenly distributed KPs in a white eye with mild anterior chamber cells and flare, cataract, and increased intraocular pressure should suggest the diagnosis. Patients often note that one iris has been lighter in color for many years. Brown eyes become less brown and blue eyes appear more blue with this disorder, because the heterochromia is due to a loss of anterior iris pigment. Gray eyes may appear green.

The differential diagnosis of Fuchs' heterochromic iridocyclitis includes disorders that produce iris heterochromia. Malignant melanoma of the iris, Horner's syndrome, and chronic anterior uveitis with iris atrophy caused by infections such as herpes zoster should all be considered. In addition, Posner–Schlossman syndrome and neovascular glaucoma may cause ocular disease that looks like Fuchs' heterochromic iridocyclitis.

Etiology

A number of researchers have hypothesized an infectious cause for Fuchs' heterochromic iridocyclitis. Fuchs described peripheral chorioretinal scars in some patients with this disease. Several authors have associated Fuchs' heterochromic iridocyclitis with toxoplasmosis (**Fig. 19-5**). Ocular toxoplasmosis may cause fine KPs and anterior uveitis and mimic Fuchs' heterochromic iridocyclitis. This would explain why many patients with Fuchs' heterochromic iridocyclitis lack findings of toxoplasmosis. Others suggest that infection with *Toxoplasma* may be causally related to the development of the disorder. Chorioretinal scars consistent with ocular histoplasmosis have also been noted, but a causal relationship between infectious agents and Fuchs' heterochromic iridocyclitis is unproven. Others have proposed that a lack of normal sympathetic innervation and neurogenic factors cause the findings associated with the disease, but again these associations are unproven.[68]

Recently, investigators have suggested an association of rubella virus with Fuchs' heterochromic iridocyclitis. In one study, rubella virus – but not herpes simplex virus, varicella zoster virus, or toxoplasmosis – was associated with the disease.[70] Antibody against rubella was identified in the aqueous humor of 13 of 14 patients studied; antibody against the other infectious agents was not found. In another study, antibody against rubella virus using nested PCR was found in all 52 eyes with Fuchs' heterochromic cyclitis.[71]

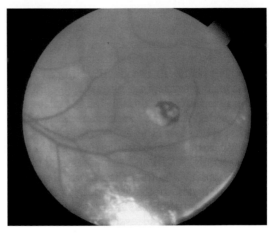

Figure 19-5. Chorioretinal scar consistent with toxoplasmosis observed in the patient shown in Figure 19-4. *(Courtesy of Rubens Belfort Jr, MD.)*

The finding of infiltrating plasma cells and lymphocytes on pathologic examination of ocular specimens from patients with Fuchs' iridocyclitis confirms an inflammatory cause for the disease.[72] Electron microscopic examination of iris biopsy specimens showed both a reduction in the number of stromal melanocytes and a decrease in melanosome size.[73] Plasma cells, mast cells, and lymphocytes were present in the tissue, but no infectious organisms were seen. Although Fuchs' heterochromic iridocyclitis may be a single pathologic entity with a single cause, much of the evidence suggests that many occurrences represent a common ocular response that can develop from a variety of etiologic insults.

Treatment and prognosis

Fuchs' heterochromic iridocyclitis is generally chronic. Although therapy with topical corticosteroids can reduce the clinical signs of inflammation, long-term topical therapy is often unnecessary and may serve only to hasten cataract formation and induce glaucoma in steroid responders. Cataracts can be safely removed in patients with Fuchs' heterochromic iridocyclitis; however, the glaucoma associated with the disease may not be easily controlled and can result in significant and permanent visual loss. Uveitis in these patients must be controlled. Although medications can control the glaucoma, surgery is often required but is fraught

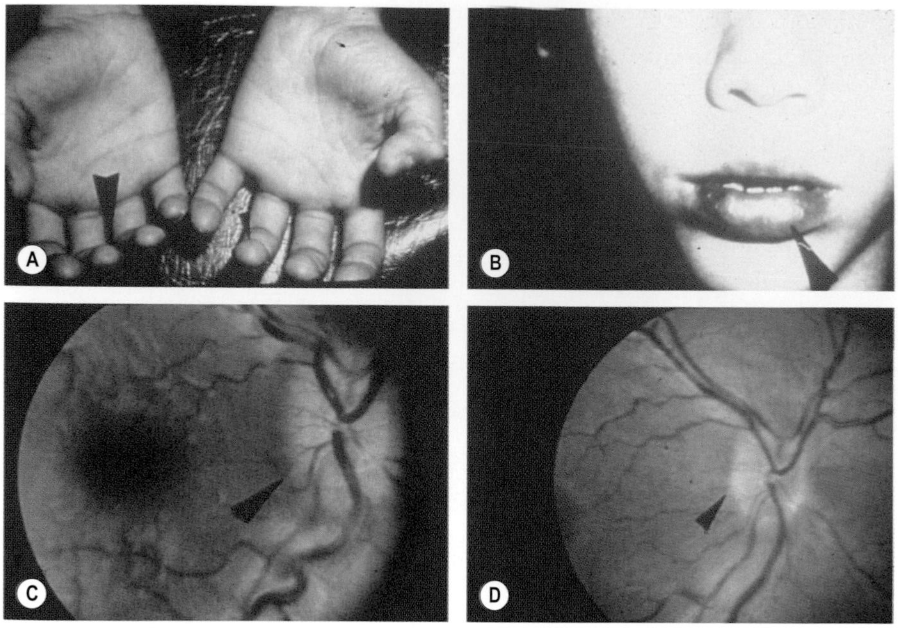

Figure 19-6. A, Distal cutaneous erythematous lesions seen in patient with Kawasaki disease. **B,** Oral mucocutaneous lesions in a patient with the disease. **C,** Papilledema and dilated retinal veins in a patient with Kawasaki disease that **(D)** resolved after the acute phase. *(Courtesy of Fernando Orefice, MD, and Rubens Belfort Jr, MD.)*

with the complications and difficulties associated with glaucoma surgery in other patients with uveitis.[67,68]

Kawasaki disease

Kawasaki disease, also called mucocutaneous lymph node syndrome, is a disease of children and young adults characterized by an erythematous and desquamative exanthem **(Fig. 19-6A)**, oral mucosal erythema (Fig. 19-6B), conjunctivitis, fever, and an asymmetric cervical adenopathy.[74] Anterior uveitis has also been noted in many patients with this disorder. Although the cause is unknown, patients with active Kawasaki disease have an antibody to α-interferon-activated endothelial cells from the umbilical vein that express MHC class II antigens.[75] In one study 66% of patients had evidence of anterior uveitis that occurred most commonly during the first week of illness.[76] The uveitis does not appear to be severe or chronic, and usually resolves without therapy. Optic disc edema and dilated retinal veins may also be seen (Fig. 19-6C and D).

Tubulointerstitial nephritis and uveitis syndrome (TINU)

Anterior uveitis has been associated with acute interstitial nephritis. In 1975 two publications each reported two patients with interstitial nephritis and anterior uveitis.[77,78] This syndrome is now called tubulointerstitial nephritis and uveitis syndrome (TINU).[79] Patients usually present with an acute uveitis and later develop manifestations of acute interstitial nephritis with cellular casts in the urine.[80] Renal biopsy results show infiltration with eosinophils and mononuclear cells. The nephritis usually responds to corticosteroid therapy. Anterior uveitis has also been reported in patients with IgA nephropathy.[81] This disease often occurs in children and is associated with an upper respiratory tract infection. The uveitis appears to occur with the pulmonary disease and responds to standard therapy with topical corticosteroids and mydriatic and cycloplegic drops.

Pathogenesis

The pathogenesis of TINU appears to involve an immune response mediated by a number of possible insults, including infection and medication. There appears to be a genetic component, and the disease has been described in monozygotic twins.[82] Seroreactivity against renal and retinal antigens has been reported.[83]

Glaucomatous cyclitic crisis

Glaucomatous cyclitic crisis, also known as Posner–Schlossman syndrome, is an inflammatory glaucoma manifested by fine KPs, mydriasis, and elevated intraocular pressure.[84] Conglomerates of inflammatory cells are occasionally noted in the anterior chamber angle, and an accompanying reduction in aqueous outflow has been documented. Episodes are treated with topical corticosteroids, β-blockers, and carbonic anhydrase inhibitors.

Schwartz syndrome

Rhegmatogenous retinal detachment is frequently associated with a mild reduction in intraocular pressure. In some patients, intraocular pressure is elevated and associated with anterior uveitis. This syndrome of increased intraocular pressure, an open anterior chamber angle, and anterior segment inflammation is termed Schwartz syndrome.[85] It remains unclear whether the increased intraocular pressure is secondary to the anterior uveitis, concomitant damage to the trabecular meshwork, or blockage of the trabecular meshwork from retinal pigment epithelium or components of the photoreceptors.[86] It should also be noted that anterior uveitis is a frequent finding in blunt ocular trauma and usually resolves with topical corticosteroid therapy.

Anterior segment ischemia

Anterior segment ischemia caused by carotid artery insufficiency may simulate an anterior uveitis in older patients with the presence of cells and flare. The amount of flare is often out of proportion to the number of cells in the anterior chamber compared to other types of anterior uveitis. The pupil is poorly reactive, and patients often complain of dull, deep, and chronic pain. Anterior segment ischemia is often associated with other signs of ischemia, such as venous stasis and neovascularization.[87] Therapy should be focused on improving the ischemia rather than treating the secondary ocular findings.

Lens-induced uveitis

Anterior uveitis occurs in association with several forms of lens-induced glaucoma. Phacolytic glaucoma occurs when a hypermature cataract leaks liquefied cortical material into the anterior chamber. Macrophages are found in the aqueous humor, although KPs are rare.[88] Treatment involves suppressing the inflammation with topical corticosteroids and removing the cataract. Phacoantigenic glaucoma occurs after rupture of the lens capsule and is characterized by conjunctival chemosis and anterior segment inflammation that develops within days to weeks after the capsular disruption. A phacotoxic glaucoma may also occur after recent cataract extraction or traumatic rupture of the lens capsule.[89] In these patients inflammation is treated with topical, periocular, or systemic corticosteroids in addition to antiglaucoma medications. These conditions must be distinguished from endophthalmitis, especially in the context of recent trauma or ocular surgery.

Anterior uveitis associated with AIDS

Anterior uveitis is found in a number of patients with AIDS.[90] The anterior uveitis is often associated with other infectious diseases such as syphilis, cytomegalovirus retinitis, toxoplasmosis, herpes simplex, or herpes zoster.[91] A mild anterior uveitis may be associated with human immunodeficiency virus (HIV) infection in the absence of coinfection. In addition, anterior uveitis may result as an adverse reaction to one of the many medications that patients with AIDS receive. As stated earlier, anterior uveitis, occasionally with hypopyon, has been associated with rifabutin use in patients with AIDS.[6-8,92]

The ocular manifestations of AIDS have changed dramatically with the advent of highly active antiretroviral therapy (HAART). The use of HAART has lead to reduced HIV viral loads and increased CD4+ T-cell counts. This has had an especially profound effect on cytomegalovirus (CMV) retinitis. Patients previously requiring persistent anti-CMV therapy are able to stop treatment without progression of the retinitis. However, an immune recovery uveitis has been described in some eyes with quiescent CMV retinitis in patients with elevated CD4+ counts.[93] In addition to an anterior uveitis, the immune recovery uveitis can include cataract, vitritis, and cystoid macular edema.

Other disease associations

In addition to the disorders described here, anterior uveitis can occur in many forms of uveitis. Infectious causes of uveitis such as syphilis, herpes simplex virus keratitis, herpes zoster infection, and toxoplasmosis are frequently accompanied by an anterior uveitis. Noninfectious causes of uveitis, such as Behçet's disease, sarcoidosis, and multiple sclerosis are also associated with anterior segment inflammation. Anterior uveitis may also be caused by postoperative infection. Acute bacterial endophthalmitis may present with a hypopyon. *Propionibacterium acnes* infection has been associated with an indolent smoldering anterior uveitis after cataract surgery. Anterior uveitis may also be a sign of corneal allograft rejection, especially when seen in conjunction with corneal inflammation such as a Koudadoust line. Anterior uveitis can occur after immunization or vaccination and may develop as a toxic effect of certain medications.[6,92,94] Finally, a number of malignancies such as leukemia, retinoblastoma, and intraocular lymphoma may masquerade as an idiopathic anterior uveitis.[95,96] These entities are discussed in detail in Chapter 30.

References

1. Wakefield D, Dunlop I, McClusky PJ, et al. Uveitis: aetiology and disease associations in an Australian population, Aust NZ J Ophthalmol 1986; 14: 181–187.

2. Vedot E, Barth E, Billet P. Epidemiology of uveitis: preliminary results of a prospective study in Savoy. In: Sarri KM, ed. Uveitis update. Amsterdam, 1984, Elsevier, pp 13–16.

3. Rothova A, Veenedaal WG, Linssen A, et al. Clinical features of acute anterior uveitis. Am J Ophthalmol 1987; 103: 137–145.

4. Wakefield D, Montanaro A, McCluskey P. Acute anterior uveitis and HLA-B27. Surv Ophthalmol 1991; 36: 223–232.

5. Guex-Crosier Y, Pittet N, Herbort CP. Evaluation of laser flare-cell photometry in the appraisal and management of intraocular inflammation in uveitis. Ophthalmology 1994; 101: 728–735.

6. Frank MO, Graham MB, Wispelway B. Rifabutin and uveitis [letter]. N Engl J Med 1994; 330: 868.

7. Jacobs DS, Piliero PJ, Kuperwaser MG, et al. Acute uveitis associated with rifabutin use in patients with human immunodeficiency virus infection. Am J Ophthalmol 1994; 118: 716–722.

8. Saran BR, Maguire AM, Nichols C, et al. Hypopyon uveitis in patients with acquired immunodeficiency syndrome treated for systemic *Mycobacterium avium* complex infection with rifabutin. Am J Ophthalmol 1994; 112: 1159–1165.

9. Fong DS, Raizman MB. Spontaneous hyphema associated with anterior uveitis. Br J Ophthalmol 1993; 77: 635–638.

10. Whitcup SM, Wakefield D, Li Q, et al. Endothelial leukocyte adhesion molecule-1 in endotoxin-induced uveitis. Invest Ophthalmol Vis Sci 1992; 33: 2626–2630.

11. Whitcup SM, DeBarge LR, Rosen H, et al. Monoclonal antibody against CD11b/CD18 inhibits endotoxin-induced uveitis. Invest Ophthalmol Vis Sci 1993; 34: 673–681.

12. Elner VM, Elner SG, Pavilack MA, et al. Intercellular adhesion molecule-1 in human corneal endothelium: modulation and function. Am J Pathol 1991; 138: 525–536.

13. Wertheim MS, Mathers WD, Planck SJ, et al. In vivo confocal microscopy of keratic precipitates. Arch Ophthalmol 2004; 122: 1773–1781.

14. Moorthy RS, Valluri S, Jampol LM. Drug-induced uveitis. Surv Ophthalmol 1998; 42: 557–570.

15. Fraunfelder FW, Rosenbaum JT. Drug-induced uveitis. Incidence, prevention and treatment. Drug Safety 1997; 17: 197–207.

16. Huhtinen M, Repo H, Laasila K, et al. Systemic inflammation and innate immune response in patients with

previous anterior uveitis. Br J Ophthalmol 2002; 86: 412–417.

17. Hench PS, Kendall EC, Slocumb CH, et al. The effect of a hormone of the adrenal cortex (17-hydroxy-11-dehydrocorticosterone: compound E) and of pituitary adrenocorticotropic hormone on rheumatoid arthritis. Proc Staff Meet Mayo Clin 1949; 24: 181–197.

18. Gordon DM, McLean JM. Effects of pituitary adrenocorticotropic hormone (ACTH) therapy in ophthalmologic conditions. JAMA 1950; 142: 1271–1276.

19. Olson JA, Steffensen EH, Margulis RR, et al. Effect of ACTH on certain inflammatory diseases of the eye. JAMA 1950; 142: 1276–1278.

20. Wakefield D, Montanaro A, McCluskey P. Acute anterior uveitis and HLA-B27. Surv Ophthalmol 1991; 36(3): 223–232.

21. Otasevic L, Zlatanovic G, Stanojevic-Paovic A, et al. *Helicobacter pylori*: an underestimated factor in acute anterior uveitis and spondyloarthropathies? Ophthalmologica 2007; 221: 6–13.

22. Zeboulon N, Dougados M, Gossec L. Prevalence and characteristics of uveitis in the spondyloarthropathies: a systematic literature review. Ann Rheum Dis 2008; 67: 955–959.

23. Braakenburg AM, de Valk HW, de Boer J, et al. Human leukocyte antigen-B27-associated uveitis: long-term follow-up and gender differences. Am J Ophthalmol 2008; 145: 472–479.

24. Wakefield D, Abi-Hanna D. HLA antigens and their significance in the pathogenesis of anterior uveitis: a mini review. Curr Eye Res 1986; 5: 465–473.

25. Chang JH, McCluskey PJ, Wakefield D. Toll-like receptors in ocular immunity and the immunopathogenesis of inflammatory eye disease. Br J Ophthalmol 2006; 90: 103–108.

26. Mondino BJ, Rao H. Hemolytic complement activity in aqueous humor. Arch Ophthalmol 1983; 101: 465–468.

27. Mondino BJ, Sumner H. Anaphylatoxin levels in human aqueous humor. Invest Ophthalmol Vis Sci 1986; 27: 1288–1292.

28. Sen DK, Sarin GS, Mathur MD. Serum fibrin degradation products in acute idiopathic anterior uveitis. Acta Ophthalmol 1986; 64: 632–636.

29. Wakefield D, McCluskey P, Palladinetti P. Distribution of lymphocytes and cell adhesion molecules in iris biopsy specimens from patients with uveitis. Arch Ophthalmol 1992; 110: 121–125.

30. El-Shabrawi Y, Wegscheider BJ, Weger M, et al. Polymorphisms within the tumor necrosis factor-alpha promoter region in patients with HLA-B27-associated uveitis: association with susceptibility and clinical manifestations. Ophthalmology 2006; 113: 695–700.

31. Brewerton DA, Caffrey M, Hart FD, et al. Ankylosing spondylitis and HLA-B27. Lancet 1973; 1: 904–907.

32. Ebringer R, White L, McCoy R, et al. Seasonal variation in acute anterior uveitis: differences between HLA-B27 positive and HLA-B27 negative disease. Br J Ophthalmol 1985; 69: 202–204.

33. Masi AT. Epidemiology of B27 associated disease. Ann Rheum Dis 1979; 38: 131–134.

34. Munoz-Fernandez S, Garcia-Aparicio AM, Hidalgo MV, et al. Methotrexate: an option for preventing the recurrence of acute anterior uveitis. Eye 2009; 23: 1130–1133.

35. Braun J, Baraliakos X, Listing J, et al. Decreased incidence of anterior uveitis in patients with ankylosing spondylitis treated with the anti-tumor necrosis factor agents infliximab and etanercept. Arthritis Rheum 2005; 52: 2447–2451.

36. Reiter H. Uber eine bisher unerkannte Spirochateninfektion. Dtsch Med Wochenschr 1916; 42: 1535–1536.

37. Lee DA, Barker SM, Su WPD, et al. The clinical diagnosis of Reiter's syndrome. Ophthalmology 1986; 93: 350–356.

38. Keat A. Reiter's syndrome and reactive arthritis in perspective. N Engl J Med 1983; 39: 1606–1615.

39. Cassidy JT, Levinson JE, Bass JC, et al. A study of classification criteria for a diagnosis of juvenile rheumatoid arthritis. Arthritis Rheum 1986; 29: 274–281.

40. Rosenberg AM. Uveitis associated with juvenile rheumatoid arthritis. Semin Arthritis Rheum 1987; 16: 158–173.

41. Wolf MD, Lichter PR, Ragsdale CG. Prognostic factors in the uveitis of juvenile rheumatoid arthritis. Ophthalmology 1987; 94: 1242–1247.

42. Smiley WK. The eye in juvenile rheumatoid arthritis. Trans Ophthalmol Soc UK 1974; 94: 817–829.

43. Key SW III, Kimura SJ. Iridocyclitis associated with juvenile rheumatoid arthritis. Am J Ophthalmol 1975; 80: 425–429.

44. Merriam JC, Chylack LT, Albert DM. Early onset pauciarticular juvenile rheumatoid arthritis: a histopathologic study. Arch Ophthalmol 1983; 101: 1085–1092.

45. Sabates R, Smith T, Apple D. Ocular histopathology in juvenile rheumatoid arthritis. Ann Ophthalmol 1979; 1979: 733–737.

46. Kanski JJ. Anterior uveitis in juvenile rheumatoid arthritis. Arch Ophthalmol 1977; 95: 1794–1797.

47. Chylack LT. The ocular manifestations of juvenile rheumatoid arthritis. Arthritis Rheum 1977; 20: 217–223.

48. Olson NY, Lindsley CB, Godfrey WA. Nonsteroidal antiinflammatory drug therapy in chronic childhood iridocyclitis. Am J Dis Child 1988; 142: 1289–1292.

49. Giannini EH, Brower EJ, Kuzmind N, et al. Methotrexate in resistant juvenile rheumatoid arthritis. Results of the

USA–USSR double-blind, placebo-controlled trial. N Engl J Med 1992; 326: 1043–1049.

50. Kahn P, Weiss M, Imundo LF, et al. Favorable response to high-dose infliximab for refractory childhood uveitis. Ophthalmology 2006; 113: 860–864.

51. Sauremann RK, Levin AV, Rose JB, et al. Tumour necrosis factor alpha inhibitors in the treatment of childhood uveitis. Rheumatology (Oxford) 2006; 45: 92–99.

52. Diamond JG, Kaplan HG. Lensectomy and vitrectomy for complicated cataract secondary to uveitis. Arch Ophthalmol 1978; 96: 1798–1804.

53. Praeger DL, Schneider HA, Sakowski AD, et al. Kelman procedure in the treatment of complicated cataract of the uveitis of Still's disease. Trans Ophthalmol Soc UK 1976; 96: 168–171.

54. Foster CS, Barrett F. Cataract development and cataract surgery in patients with juvenile rheumatoid arthritis-associated iridocyclitis. Ophthalmology 1993; 100: 809–817.

55. O'Brien JM, Albert DM. Therapeutic approaches for ophthalmic problems in juvenile rheumatoid arthritis. Rheum Dis Clin North Am 1989; 15: 413–437.

56. Akinci A, Cakar N, Uncu N, et al. Keratoconjunctivitis sicca in juvenile rheumatoid arthritis. Cornea 2007; 26: 941–944.

57. Reininga JK, Los LI, Wulffraat NM, et al. The evaluation of uveitis in juvenile idiopathic arthritis (JIA) patients: are current ophthalmologic screening guidelines adequate? Clin Exp Rheumatol 2008; 26: 367–372.

58. Thorne JE, Woreta F, Kedhar SR, et al. Juvenile idiopathic arthritis-associated uveitis: incidence of ocular complications and visual acuity loss. Am J Ophthalmol 2007; 143: 840–846.

59. Calin A. The spondyloarthropathies. In: Wyngaarden JB, Smith LH Jr, Bennett JC, eds. Cecil textbook of medicine, ed 19, Philadelphia, 1992, WB Saunders, pp 1515–1521.

60. Tobin AM, Kirby B. TNF alpha inhibitors in the treatment of psoriasis and psoriatic arthritis. BioDrugs 2005; 19: 47–57.

61. Ellis PP, Gentry JH. Ocular complications of ulcerative colitis. Am J Ophthalmol 1964; 58: 779–784.

62. Duker JS, Brown GC, Brooks L. Retinovasculitis in Crohn's disease. Am J Ophthalmol 1987; 103: 654–668.

63. Selsky EJ, Knox DL, Maumanee AE, et al. Ocular involvement in Whipple's disease. Retina 1984; 4: 103–106.

64. Lawrence W. Changes in colour in the iris. In: Hays I, ed. A treatise on diseases of the eye. Philadelphia, 1843, Lea & Blanchard, pp 411–416.

65. Fuchs E. Über Komplicaationen der Heterochromie. Z Augenheilkd 1906; 15: 191–212.

66. Kimura SJ, Hogan MJ, Thygeson P. Fuchs' syndrome of heterochromic cyclitis. Arch Ophthalmol 1955; 54: 179–186.

67. Liesegang TJ. Clinical features and prognosis in Fuchs' uveitis syndrome. Arch Ophthalmol 1982; 100: 1622–1626.

68. Jones NP. Fuchs' heterochromic uveitis: an update. Surv Ophthalmol 1993; 37: 253–272.

69. Amsler M. New clinical aspects of the vegetative eye. Trans Ophthalmol Soc UK 1948; 68: 45–74.

70. de Groot-Mijnes JD, de Visser L, Rothova A, et al. Rubella virus is associated with Fuchs' heterochromic iridocyclitis. Am J Ophthalmol 2006; 141: 212–214.

71. Quentin CD, Reiber H. Fuchs' heterochromic cyclitis: rubella virus antibodies and genome in aqueous humor. Am J Ophthalmol 2004; 138: 46–54.

72. Goldberg MF, Erozan YS, Duke JR, et al. Cytopathologic and histopathologic aspects of Fuchs' heterochromic iridocyclitis. Arch Ophthalmol 1965; 74: 604–609.

73. McCartney AC, Bull TB, Spalton DJ. Fuchs' heterochromic cyclitis: an electron microscopy study. Trans Ophthalmol Soc UK 1986; 105: 324–329.

74. Bligard CA. Kawasaki disease and its diagnosis. Pediatr Dermatol 1987; 4: 75–84.

75. Leung DY, Collins T, Lapierre LA, et al. Immunoglobulin M antibodies present in the acute phase of Kawasaki syndrome lyse cultured vascular endothelial cells stimulated by gamma interferon. J Clin Invest 1986; 77: 1428–1435.

76. Burns JC, Joffe L, Sargent RA, et al. Anterior uveitis associated with Kawasaki syndrome. Pediatr Infect Dis 1985; 4: 258–261.

77. Kikkawa Y, Sakurai M, Mano T, et al. Interstitial nephritis with concomitant uveitis. Report of two cases. Contrib Nephrol 1975; 4: 1–11.

78. Dobrin RS, Venier RL, Fish AL. Acute eosinophilic interstitial nephritis and renal failure with bone marrow-lymph node granulomas and anterior uveitis. A new syndrome. Am J Med 1975; 59: 325–333.

79. Vanhaesebrouck P, Carton D, De Bel C, et al. Acute tubulo-interstitial nephritis and uveitis syndrome (TINU syndrome). Nephron 1985; 40: 418–422.

80. Gafter U, Ben-Basat M, Zevin D, et al. Anterior uveitis, a presenting symptom in acute interstitial nephritis. Nephron 1986; 42: 249–251.

81. Moller-Jensen J, Marthinsen L, Linne T. Anterior uveitis in IgA nephropathy. Am J Ophthalmol 1989; 108: 604–605.

82. Howarth L, Gilbert RD, Bass P, et al. Tubulointerstitial nephritis and uveitis in monozygotic twin boys. Pediatr Nephrol 2004; 19: 917–919.

83. Shimazaki K, Jirawuthiworavong GV, Nguyen EV, et al. Tubulointerstitial nephritis and uveitis syndrome: a case with an autoimmune reactivity against retinal and renal antigens. Ocul Immunol Inflamm 2008; 16: 51–53.

84. Posner A, Schlossman A. Syndrome of unilateral recurrent attacks of glaucoma with cyclitic symptoms. Arch Ophthalmol 1948; 39: 517–528.

85. Schwartz A. Chronic open-angle glaucoma secondary to rhegmatogenous retinal detachment. Am J Ophthalmol 1973; 75: 205–211.

86. Matsuo N, Takabatake M, Ueno H, et al. Photoreceptor outer segments in the aqueous humor in rhegmatogenous retinal detachment. Am J Ophthalmol 1986; 101: 673–679.

87. Jacobs NA, Ridgway AE. Syndrome of ischaemic ocular inflammation: six cases and a review. Br J Ophthalmol 1985; 69: 682–687.

88. Epstein DL, Jedziniak JA, Grant WM. Identification of heavy molecular weight protein in aqueous humor in human phacolytic glaucoma. Invest Ophthalmol 1978; 17: 398–402.

89. Irvine SR, Irvine AR Jr: Lens-induced uveitis and glaucoma. II. The 'phacotoxic' reaction. Am J Ophthalmol 1952; 35: 370–375.

90. Shuler JD, Engstrom RE, Holland GN. External ocular disease and anterior segment disorders associated with AIDS. Int Ophthalmol Clin 1989; 29: 98–104.

91. Verma S, Hughes JD, Mabey D, et al. Symptomatic anterior uveitis in HIV-positive patients. Int J STD AIDS 1999; 10: 268–274.

92. Fuller JD, Stanfield LE, Craven DE. Rifabutin prophylaxis and uveitis [letter, comment]. N Engl J Med 1994; 330: 1315–1316.

93. Robinson MR, Reed G, Csaky KG, et al. Immune-recovery uveitis in patients with cytomegalovirus retinitis taking highly active antiretroviral therapy. Am J Ophthalmol 2000; 130: 49–56.

94. Yeomans SM, Knox DL, Green WR, et al. Ocular inflammatory pseudotumor associated with propranolol therapy. Ophthalmology 1983; 90: 1422–1425.

95. Woog JJ, Chess J, Albert DM, et al. Metastatic carcinoma of the iris simulating iridocyclitis. Br J Ophthalmol 1984; 68: 167–173.

96. Hertler AA, Rosenwasser GO, Gluck WL. Isolated anterior chamber relapse in acute monoblastic leukemia. Am J Hematol 1986; 23: 401–403.

Scleritis

Scott M. Whitcup

Scleritis is a painful and potentially sight-threatening disorder. From a strict anatomical viewpoint, scleritis is not a form of uveitis but rather an inflammatory disorder that is similar in pathogenesis to many forms of uveitis. When severe, scleritis is often associated with inflammation in the underlying uveal tissue. Entire books have been written on scleritis, and some of its key features are discussed in this chapter. Like uveitis, scleritis is often associated with underlying systemic disease. Additionally, the therapeutic approaches to scleritis and uveitis share many similarities. In contrast to scleritis, episcleritis is a disorder involving the more superficial episclera and tends to be more acute and less severe than scleritis. Importantly, episcleritis is rarely, if ever, vision threatening and may resolve without therapy. Episcleritis is also discussed in this chapter.

Episcleritis

Episcleritis is an inflammatory disorder involving the episcleral tissue that lies superficial to the sclera, just beneath Tenon's capsule. Although it occurs in both sexes and at all ages, it is seen more frequently in young to middle-aged women. Episcleritis is usually mild, characterized by slight conjunctival injection and the presence of a foreign body sensation. The episodes often resolve without treatment, but can recur. Occasionally patients may experience more severe redness and pain. Inflamed episcleral blood vessels tend to have a salmon color in natural light, radiate from the limbus, and can be moved over the sclera with a cotton-tipped applicator. In addition, these more superficial vessels will blanch after administration of topical phenylephrine. A nodular episcleritis has been described.

In 50% or more of patients episcleritis is idiopathic; however, many of the diseases associated with scleritis have also been associated with episcleritis. In a review of 100 patients with episcleritis, an associated systemic disease was found in 36 (36%).[1] Although often self-limited, episcleritis can be associated with corneal involvement, uveitis, and glaucoma.

Extensive evaluation for underlying disease may not be warranted for mild forms of the disease, especially if it is not recurrent. When treatment is required, the disease often responds to topical or oral nonsteroidal antiinflammatory drugs (NSAIDs) or to topical corticosteroids. Although topical vasoconstrictors can reduce the redness, they should be used sparingly. In patients with episcleritis that fails to respond to initial therapy one should suspect the possibility of a masquerade syndrome, such as a conjunctival malignancy or the presence of an underlying systemic disease.

The differential diagnosis of episcleritis includes conjunctivitis, a conjunctival malignancy such as lymphoma, medications, and scleritis. Conjunctivitis, whether allergic or infectious, can frequently be distinguished from episcleritis based on symptoms and examination. Infectious conjunctivitis is usually associated with a discharge and allergic conjunctivitis with itching and chemosis. Scleritis is anatomically deeper and has a distinct appearance. Malignant conjunctival lesions also tend to have a specific appearance and are rarely mistaken for episcleritis. A number of medications have been associated with both episcleritis and scleritis and are listed in **Box 20–1**.

The visual prognosis for patients with episcleritis is usually good. Some patients have a single episode, and in those with recurrent disease the frequency tends to diminish over time. As up to a third of patients can have an associated systemic disease, and because episcleritis can be associated with ocular complications usch as uveitis and glaucoma, patients with more severe or recurrent episcleritis should be carefully assessed and treated. **Table 20-1** compares the features of episcleritis and scleritis.

Scleritis

The severity of scleritis varies greatly, but the disease can result in loss of vision and be difficult to treat. Scleritis is characterized by eye pain and redness of the sclera and episclera. The pain is usually gradual in onset but can become excruciating, with the feeling of something boring into the eye, and can wake the patient from sleep. The pain may radiate to the forehead or to other parts of the face, and may be associated with photophobia and tearing. Corneal involvement, anterior uveitis, and exudative retinal detachments can occur and cause decreased vision. The inflamed sclera is deep to the episclera, typically with a violaceous hue, and the inflamed vessels cannot be moved with a cotton-tipped applicator (**Fig. 20-1**). The disease is most common in the fourth to sixth decades of life and more common in women. Scleritis is bilateral in more than 50% of patients, but frequently starts in one eye. It can be divided into anterior and posterior disease (Table 20-1). Anterior scleritis has been classified into four additional categories (**Table 20-2**): diffuse, nodular, necrotizing with inflammation, and necrotizing without inflammation.[2] Necrotizing scleritis without inflammation is also called scleromalacia perforans.

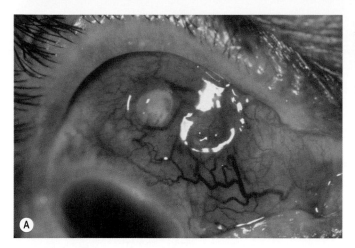
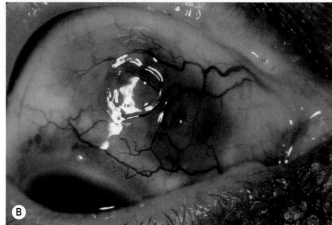

Figure 20-1. A, Nodular anterior scleritis in patient with rheumatoid arthritis. Inflammation of the deep scleral vessels is characterized by violaceous hue. **B,** After 2 months of systemic corticosteroids the scleral vessels are less inflamed; however, signs of scleral thinning can be noted.

Table 20-1 Characteristics of episcleritis and scleritis

Feature	Episcleritis	Scleritis
Anatomy	Episclera (deep to Tenon's capsule)	Sclera
Age (years)	20s–40s	20s–60s
Gender	Predominantly women	Predominantly women
Clinical features	Mild pain, transient	Painful
Underlying systemic disease	Occasional	Common
Complications	Rare	Frequent
Treatment	May not be needed	Needed
Prognosis	Excellent	Variable

Table 20-2 Classification of scleritis with approximate disease prevalence

Classification	Prevalence (%)
Anterior scleritis	40
Diffuse scleritis	
Nodular scleritis	40–45
Necrotizing scleritis with inflammation	10
Necrotizing scleritis without inflammation (scleromalacia perforans)	1–5
Posterior scleritis	1–5

Box 20-1 Medications associated with episcleritis and scleritis

Bisphosphonates
Erlotinib
Procainamide

Necrotizing scleritis is a severe form of the disorder, frequently associated with both blinding ocular disease and life-threatening systemic disease. An underlying systemic disease was found in approximately one-half of patients with necrotizing scleritis.[2] Necrotizing scleritis with inflammation is almost always painful. The sclera is edematous, and inflammation leads to scleral thinning, which allows the underlying choroid to become visible. Intraocular inflammation is often seen in severe cases of scleritis. Fluorescein angiography shows hypoperfusion or nonperfusion of the scleral vessels. Other complications of scleritis include cataract and glaucoma.

Posterior scleritis is defined as inflammation of the sclera posterior to the ora serrata. Symptoms of posterior scleritis can be subtle, and the disease is frequently misdiagnosed. As with other forms of scleritis, pain is the most common symptom; however, vision is more frequently affected. Unlike other forms of scleritis, redness can be subtle and missed on examination. Other findings include retinal and or choroidal folds, exudative retinal detachments, or choroidal masses. As with anterior scleritis, masquerade syndromes should be suspected in atypical cases of posterior scleritis, especially when the disease does not respond to treatment. Some of the malignant diseases masquerading as posterior scleritis include lymphoma, metastatic carcinoma, and choroidal melanoma. We have also seen occurrences of benign lymphoid hyperplasia involving the choroid and juvenile xanthogranuloma misdiagnosed as posterior scleritis. Nonmalignant disorders, including retinal detachments and central serous retinopathy, can also masquerade as posterior scleritis.

Disease associations

An underlying systemic disease is diagnosed in about one-half of patients with scleritis. **Box 20-2** lists some of the diseases associated with scleritis. Rheumatoid arthritis is probably the most common disease of these. Scleritis has been associated with several forms of systemic vasculitis, including Wegener's granulomatosis (**Fig. 20-2**), polyarteritis nodosa, and relapsing polychondritis. The presence of necrotizing scleritis is thought to be associated with increased severity of disease in patients with rheumatoid arthritis[3] and is an indication for systemic immunosuppression; however, this association may not hold true for other autoimmune diseases. Wegener's granulomatosis is a multiorgan disease

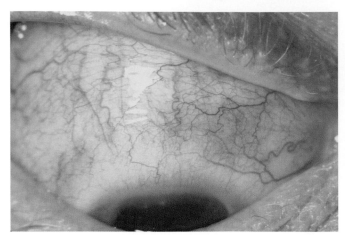

Figure 20-2. Diffuse anterior scleritis in a patient with Wegener's granulomatosis.

Box 20-2 Diseases associated with scleritis

Rheumatoid arthritis
Juvenile rheumatoid arthritis
Reiter's syndrome
Crohn's disease
Ankylosing spondylitis
Ulcerative colitis
Polymyositis
Relapsing polychondritis
Systemic lupus erythematosus
Wegener's disease
Polyarteritis nodosa
Cogan's syndrome
Sarcoidosis
Lyme disease
Bartonellosis
Syphilis
Tuberculosis
Herpes zoster infection
Acanthamoeba keratitis

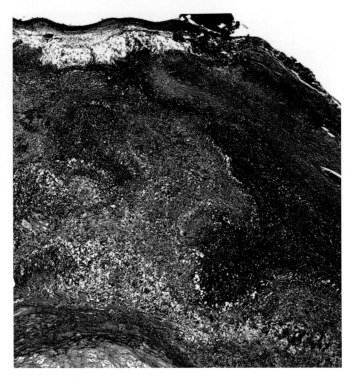

Figure 20-3 Photomicrograph showing diffuse replacement of the collagen fibers of the sclera with inflammatory infiltrates. The inflammation consists of focal granulomas, vasculitis, hemorrhage, and necrosis. (Hematoxylin & eosin, original magnification ×50.) *(Courtesy of Chi-Chao Chan, MD.)*

characterized by a necrotizing granulomatous vasculitis. The disease frequently involves the kidneys and respiratory tract; the eye is involved in more than half of patients. Polyarteritis nodosa is another systemic vasculitis that affects multiple organs. It involves small- and medium-sized arteries and is associated with abdominal pain, myalgias, peripheral neuritis, and renal disease. Eye involvement can also occur. Cogan's syndrome is a form of systemic vasculitis associated with interstitial keratitis and hearing loss. Arthritis, aortitis, or a vasculitis resembling polyarteritis nodosa have also been described.

A number of infectious diseases have been associated with scleritis. Historically, tuberculosis and syphilis were common causes. More recently, scleritis has been described in patients with Lyme disease and other diseases such as bartonellosis.

Other causes of scleritis

Scleritis has been associated with a number of surgical procedures, including cyclodestructive procedures, pterygium surgery, vitreretinal surgery, and other corneal and anterior segment operations. Medications have been associated with both episcleritis and scleritis, including the bisphosphonates.[4,5]

Diagnostic testing

Although the diagnosis of scleritis is based on medical history and clinical examination, diagnostic testing is often indicated as many patients have an associated systemic disease. Posterior scleritis is more difiicult to diagnose based on clinical signs and symptoms, and B-scan ultrasonography can be useful in demonstrating thickening of the posterior sclera. In complicated cases a CT scan may be useful in identifying associated orbital disease. If an underlying rheumatologic disease is suspected, a laboratory assessment should be based on the history and physical examination of the patient. An FTA-ABS should be obtained to rule out a treatable cause of scleritis. The antineurotrophic cytoplasmic antibody test (ANCA) may be useful in predicting the presence of an underlying systemic disease in patients with scleritis.[6] ANCA-positive scleritis patients in this series were also more likely to have ocular complications and thus warrant more aggressive antiinflammatory therapy.

Pathogenesis

Most of the pathologic data suggest that scleritis is an immune-mediated disease.[7] Pathologic examination shows both granulomatous and nongranulomatous inflammation and an associated vasculitis.[8] Histologic examination reveals diffuse infiltration with inflamatory cells that eventually replaces the collagen, leading to scleral thinning (**Fig. 20-3**).

Deposition of circulating immune complexes has been thought to be the cause of the disorder; however, the disease may also be caused by a T-cell-mediated response to antigens in the sclera, such as type II collagen, or to antigens in the scleral blood vessels. Increased expression of cell adhesion molecules such as ICAM-1 on the sclera may play a role in the pathogenesis of the disease.[9] Sporadic case reports discuss possible infectious causes of scleritis.[10]

Differential diagnosis

Episcleritis is the most challenging condition to differentiate from scleritis, and because the severity and treatment of episcleritis differ greatly from those of scleritis, it is important to distinguish the two diseases. Severe uveitis can be associated with overlying scleral inflammation, but the diagnosis of underlying uveitis is obvious on ophthalmic examination. Malignancies such as melanoma or metastatic disease can mimic a scleritis and should be considered.

Treatment

Use of topical corticosteroids or oral NSAIDs usually controls inflammation in patients with mild scleritis. For more severe forms of the disease, treatment with oral corticosteroids or other systemic immunosuppressive agents is often required.[11-13] Methotrexate is commonly used to treat moderately severe scleritis. Recently, mycopheonlate mofetil was shown to have efficacy in treating patients with scleritis, some who had failed or were intolerant to other therapies.[14,15]

The scleritis associated with necrotizing systemic vasculitis may be diffuse, nodular, or necrotizing. Necrotizing scleritis in these diseases is especially difficult to treat and almost always requires systemic immunosuppressive therapy.[16] Importantly, immunosuppression is required to control the underlying necrotizing systemic vasculitis, because in untreated patients mortality is high. Treatment recommendations are therefore based to a large degree on trials examining the effect of immunosuppression on mortality and disease severity in patients with Wegener's granulomatosis and polyarteritis nodosa. Treatment with cyclophosphamide produced complete remission in 93% of patients.[17] Deaths occurred in only 7% of patients over a mean follow-up of 51 months. Similarly, cyclophosphamide reduced the 5-year mortality for patients with polyarteritis nodosa from 53% to 20%.[18]

Although there have been no randomized, controlled clinical trials, several studies have evaluated the treatment of scleritis associated with necrotizing systemic vasculitis. Cyclophosphamide was the only effective immunosuppressive drug used in three patients with necrotizing scleritis associated with relapsing polychondritis in whom treatment with high-dose systemic corticosteroids, penicillamine, methotrexate, and azathioprine had failed.[16] Treatment of scleritis in patients with necrotizing systemic vasculitis should be guided both by the ophthalmic response and control of the underlying disease. The antineutrophil cytoplasmic antibody test, for example, is a useful laboratory measure of the therapeutic response in patients with Wegener's granulomatosis. Cyclophosphamide, starting at a dose of 2 mg/kg/day, may be the drug of choice for scleritis associated with necrotizing systemic vasculitis. Concomitant administration of prednisone at a dose of 1 mg/kg/day may be needed for disease uncontrolled by a maximally tolerated dose of cyclophosphamide. Oral corticosteroids can usually be tapered and often discontinued over the first 6–12 weeks of cytotoxic therapy.

Other immunosuppressive agents, including methotrexate, azathioprine, ciclosporin, and chlorambucil, have been successfully used for the treatment of necrotizing systemic vasculitis, but reports are based on small case series. Because of its widespread use in the treatment of rheumatologic disease, methotrexate is probably more commonly used to treat scleritis than some of the other agents. Inflammation control was achived in 11 of 18 patients with chronic, noninfectious, nonnecrotizing scleritis treated with methotrexate at a dose of 7.5–35 mg weekly.[19] Complete corticosteroid sparing was achieved in 10 of these 11 patients.

Periocular injections of corticosteroids have not been widely used for the treatment of scleritis, mainly for fear of exacerbating scleral thinning or precipitating scleral perforation. Subconjunctival corticosteroid injections for nonnecrotizing anterior scleritis resistant to topical or systemic therapy was evaluated in 38 eyes of 35 patients.[20] Thirty-six of the 38 eyes had complete resolution of signs and symptoms within 6 weeks of therapy. However, 15 had perforation, and other adverse events included cataract and glaucoma. No scleral necrosis or scleral meltine was observed over a median follow-up of 29 months. Although preliminary, these data suggest that there may be a role for local corticosteroid therapy in some patients with anterior scleritis; however, additional data are needed to fully assess the safety and efficacy of this therapeutic approach. Other therapeutic approaches have included the use of rituximab[21] and topical ciclosporin A.[22]

Although there has been success in treating rheumatologic diseases such as rheumatoid arthritis with inhibitors of tumor necrosis factor (TNF), the clinical experience in treating ocular inflammatory diseases is more variable. A recent case series reported nine patients with uveitis and seven with scleritis treated with etanercept or infliximab.[23] Only six of the 16 patients experienced improvement in their eye disease, and five developed inflammatory eye disease for the first time while taking a TNF inhibitor. There are a number of other reports of patients successfully treated with a TNF inhibitor, but larger randomized trials are needed to more definitely assess this therapeutic approach.[24,25]

Scleral perforation and severe glaucoma are two of the more devastating complications of scleritis. Surgical treatment of scleral perforation can be successfully performed, but it is critical that inflammation be well controlled with systemic immunosuppressive medications. Glaucoma can also lead to blindness in patients with scleritis. The glaucoma can usually be controlled with topical medications; however, surgical treatment may be warranted in rare cases where intraocular pressure cannot be controlled with drops.

References

1. Akpek EK, Uy HS, Christen W, et al. Severity of episcleritis and systemic disease association. Ophthalmology 1999; 106: 729–731.
2. Watson PG, Hayreh SS. Scleritis and episcleritis. Br J Ophthalmol 1976; 60: 163–191.
3. Foster CS, Forstot L, Wilson LA. Mortality rate in rheumatoid arthritis patients with destructive ocular lesions: effect of systemic immunosuppression. Ophthalmology 1984; 91: 1253–1263.
4. Fraunfelder FW. Ocular side effects associated with bisphosphonates. Drugs Today (Barc) 2003; 39: 829–835.
5. Turgeon PW, Slamovits TL. Scleritis as the presenting manifestation of procainamide-induced lupus. Ophthalmology 1989; 96: 68–71.
6. Hoang LT, Lim LL, Vaillant B, et al. Antineutrophil cytoplasmic antibody-associated active scleritis. Arch Ophthalmol 2008; 126: 651–655.
7. Watson PG. Doyne Memorial Lecture, 1982. The nature and the treatment of scleral inflammation. Trans Ophthalmol Soc UK 1986; 102: 257–281.
8. Sevel D. Necrogranulomatous scleritis. Clinical and histologic features. Am J Ophthalmol 1967; 64: 1125–1134.
9. Sangwan VS, Merchant A, Sainz de la Maza M, et al. Leukocyte adhesion molecule expression in scleritis. Arch Ophthalmol 1998; 116: 1476–1480.
10. Krist D, Wenkel H. Posterior scleritis associated with *Borrelia burgdorferi* (Lyme disease) infection. Ophthalmology 2002; 109: 143–145.
11. Foster CS, Sainz de la Maza M. The sclera. New York, 1994, Springer-Verlag.
12. Jabs DA, Mudun A, Dunn JP, et al. Episcleritis and scleritis: clinical features and treatment results. Am J Ophthalmol 2000; 130: 469–476.
13. Okhravi N, Odufuwa B, McCluskey P, et al. Scleritis. Surv Ophthalmol 2006; 51: 351–363.
14. Thorne JE, Jabs DA, Qazi FA, et al. Mycophenolate mofetil therapy for inflammatory eye disease. Ophthalmology 2005; 112: 1472–1477.
15. Sobrin L, Christen W, Foster CS. Mycophenolate mofetil after methotrexate failure or intolerance in the treatment of scleritis and uveitis. Ophthalmology 2008; 115: 1416–1421.
16. Hoang Xuan T, Foster CS, Rice BA. Scleritis in relapsing polychondritis. Ophthalmology 1990; 97: 892–898.
17. Fauci AS, Haynes BF, Katz P, et al. Wegener's granulomatosis: prospective clinical and therapeutic experience with 85 patients for 21 years. Ann Intern Med 1983; 98: 76–85.
18. Leib ES, Restivo C, Paulus HE. Immunosuppression and corticosteroid therapy of polyarteritis nodosa. Am J Med 1979; 67: 941–947.
19. Jachens AW, Chu DS. Retrospective review of methotrexate therapy in the treatment of chronic, noninfectious, nonnecrotizing scleritis. Am J Ophthalmol 2008; 145: 487–492.
20. Albini TA, Zamir E, Read RW, et al. Evaluation of subconjunctival triamcinolone for nonnecrotizing anterior scleritis. Ophthalmology 2005; 112: 1814–1820.
21. Ahmadi-Simab K, Lamprecht P, Nolle B, et al. Successful treatment of refractory anterior scleritis in primary Sjogren's syndrome with rituximab. Ann Rheum Dis 2005; 64: 1087–1088.
22. Shimura M, Yasuda K, Fuse N, et al. Effective treatment with topical cyclosporin A of a patient with Cogan syndrome. Ophthalmologica 2000; 214: 429–432.
23. Smith JR, Levinson RD, Holland GN, et al. Differential efficacy of tumor necrosis factor inhibition in the management of inflammatory eye disease and associated rheumatic disease. Arthritis Rheum 2001; 45: 252–257.
24. Murphy CC, Ayliffe WH, Booth A, et al. Tumor necrosis factor alpha blockage with infliximab for refractory uveitis and scleritis. Ophthalmology 2004; 111: 352–356.
25. Sobrin L, Kim EC, Christen W, et al. Infliximab therapy for the treatment of refractory ocular inflammatory disease. Arch Ophthalmol 2007; 125: 895–900.

Intermediate Uveitis

Scott M. Whitcup

Key concepts

- Diagnosis is based on the anatomic location of ocular inflammation: vitreous and peripheral retina with macular edema.
- Frequently associated with a systemic or infectious disease.
- Pars planitis is a subtype of intermediate uveitis.
- Complications include macular edema, epiretinal membrane, vitreous hemorrhage, retinal detachment, and glaucoma.
- Treatment involves corticosteroids, immunosuppressive agents, or biologics.
- Cryoretinopexy and vitrectomy my be beneficial for some patients.

Intermediate uveitis is a diagnosis based on the anatomic location of ocular inflammation; it is not a distinct clinicopathologic condition. The diagnosis of intermediate uveitis is made when ocular inflammation primarily involves the vitreous and peripheral retina. Intermediate uveitis was first described as chronic cyclitis by Fuchs in 1908.[1] The clinical description of intermediate uveitis was further elucidated by Schepens in 1950,[2] when he described patients with a peripheral uveitis characterized by inflammation centered around the vasculature and exudative changes in the retinal periphery. In 1960, Brockhurst and colleagues[3] described additional patients with peripheral vascular abnormalities and an exudate along the ora serrata and pars plana, and Welch and colleagues[4] used the term pars planitis to describe an inflammation characterized by the white accumulation on the pars plana. Other terms used in the literature to describe patients with intermediate uveitis include vitreitis, peripheral exudative retinitis, cyclochorioretinitis, chronic posterior cyclitis, and peripheral uveoretinitis. Unfortunately, there is still confusion and controversy, even among uveitis specialists, on how to classify patients with this anatomic distribution of intraocular inflammation. Grouping conditions with the anatomic features of intermediate uveitis does provide value as it helps with developing a differential diagnosis and in determining response to therapy and long-term prognosis.

We use the term intermediate uveitis, as suggested by the International Uveitis Study Group, to classify patients with intraocular inflammation predominantly involving the vitreous and peripheral retina. Some specialists use this diagnosis only if a more specific diagnosis cannot be made. Specific diseases such as sarcoidosis and multiple sclerosis are known to cause an intermediate uveitis, and we will often classify patients as having an intermediate uveitis associated with sarcoidosis or associated with multiple sclerosis, when an underlying disease can be identified. The reason for this is that diseases like sarcoidosis can also present with other manifestations, such as a predominant retinitis, and these patients will respond differently to therapy. We also use the term pars planitis to describe a subset of patients with intermediate uveitis when a white opacity (commonly called a snowbank) occurs over the pars plana and ora serrata. Although pars planitis probably does not represent a clinical entity distinct from intermediate uveitis, patients with pars planitis often have worse vitreitis, more severe macular edema, and a worse prognosis than patients with intermediate uveitis who do not have a pars plana exudate.[5]

Epidemiology

Intermediate uveitis accounts for approximately 4–8% of cases of uveitis in a referral practice.[6-8] In approximately 15% of patients with uveitis referred to us at the National Institutes of Health (NIH), intermediate uveitis is diagnosed. In a retrospective, population-based cohort study the incidence of pars planitis was 2.077 per 100 000 persons (95% confidence interval, 1.43–2.62).[9] Although the incidence of uveitis in children is low, intermediate uveitis may account for up to 25% of cases.[10] Intermediate uveitis has been reported in both young children and the elderly, but it tends to mostly affect people in their teens to their 40s.[7] There appears to be no gender or race predilection.

There have been occasional reports of intermediate uveitis occurring in families, suggesting that either hereditary or environmental factors may predispose one to develop the disease. HLA associations have been identified in patients with multiple sclerosis and intermediate uveitis, but there is debate about whether there are other HLA haplotypes associated with intermediate uveitis.[11] In 1963, Kimura and Hogan[12] first reported multiple family members with intermediate uveitis. There are only about 20 instances of familial intermediate uveitis of which we are aware, and a number of these have been reported.[10,13-16] In one instance of familial pars planitis, the two affected brothers were not twins but had identical HLA haplotypes.[13] There have also been cases of intermediate uveitis of the pars planitis subtype in identical twins.[17] Some of the familial occurrences of intermediate uveitis are associated with demyelinating disease.[18,19] Studies have indicated a possible association of intermediate uveitis with HLA-A28, HLA-DR15, HLA-DR51, and HLA-DR17 haplotypes.[20-22]

Clinical manifestations

Most patients present with blurred vision and/or floaters. Pain and photophobia are rare. Early in the course of the disease, visual acuity is often reduced to the 20/40 range as a result of a moderate vitritis and cystoid macular edema. However, if inflammation is not well controlled severe visual loss can ensue, associated with chronic cystoid macular edema, glaucoma, inflammatory changes in the retina, and retinal detachment. We have seen sudden loss of vision in several patients after vitreous hemorrhage. Bilateral involvement is seen in 70–80% of patients at the time of presentation, and approximately one-third of patients who have unilateral disease initially will later develop bilateral involvement.[5,7]

Most adults with intermediate uveitis have minimal anterior segment inflammation;[23] the exception is patients with intermediate uveitis associated with multiple sclerosis, who typically develop a granulomatous anterior uveitis with formation of mutton-fat keratic precipitates. Anterior segment inflammation is more common in children with uveitis, when there may be a moderate degree of anterior chamber cells with posterior synechiae. Brockhurst and colleagues[3] noted peripheral anterior synechiae in 24% of patients and posterior synechiae in 18%. Band keratopathy may be seen in children. Occasionally patients may present with significant anterior segment inflammation with pain and photophobia and only later develop signs typical of an intermediate uveitis.

Autoimmune endotheliopathy is a rare finding associated with pars planitis. Khodadoust and colleagues[24] reported four of 10 patients with pars planitis who demonstrated areas of peripheral corneal edema with keratic precipitates arranged linearly on the border between edematous and normal cornea. This morphologic finding was reminiscent of a corneal graft endothelial rejection line. Although other investigators have not observed this finding as frequently as Khodadoust and associates, the possible association of an autoimmune phenomenon is intriguing.

Glaucoma has been described as a cause of severe visual loss in patients with intermediate uveitis. In a study of 182 eyes with intermediate uveitis, glaucoma was diagnosed in 15 (8%).[25] However, 11 of the 15 cases were thought to be related to corticosteroid use, and only four of the 182 eyes (2%) had disease-induced glaucoma. Cataract is a more common finding in these patients; it develops as a result of the ocular inflammatory disease and corticosteroid therapy. Similar to other cataracts in patients with uveitis, posterior subcapsular cataract is the most common lenticular opacity found in patients with intermediate uveitis.

The most characteristic findings in this disease are in the vitreous and peripheral retina. Cells are always present in the vitreous in active intermediate uveitis. Some patients may only have 1+ vitreous cells, but the absence of cellular activity in the vitreous precludes a diagnosis of an active intermediate uveitis. White and yellow-colored aggregates of inflammatory cells called vitreous snowballs tend to accumulate in the inferior vitreous. Occasionally, the vitreitis is dense enough to obscure the retina entirely. This dense vitreitis must be differentiated from vitreous hemorrhage that may also occur as a result of neovascularization, usually in the vitreous base or peripheral retina.

Brockhurst and colleagues[3] described the early stages of peripheral uveitis as the accumulation of yellow-gray exudates at the ora serrata. Although this clinical finding is not required for a diagnosis of intermediate uveitis, it is the major clinical feature in the subset of intermediate uveitis that we call pars planitis. Not all patients with intermediate uveitis have a snowbank, and because some patients may have it in one eye only, the inferior white snowbank is an important finding but not an absolute requirement. As the disease progresses, Brockhurst and colleagues note that these exudates coalesce to form the material commonly referred to as a snowbank. This is usually located inferiorly only, but in rare patients it can extend for 360°. The snowbank may be discontinuous. It may form a fine band along the ora serrata or be broad and extend onto both the peripheral retina and the pars plana. It can be dense and extend several millimeters into the vitreous, and is usually best seen with scleral depression (see Fig. 3-16). However, a high dense snowbank on the pars plana can often be better seen with the indirect ophthalmoscope without using the 20-diopter lens while the patient looks down. Although this material has been termed an exudate, it is probably a fibroglial mass and not a true protein exudate, as will be discussed later. When a snowbank is observed, the area should be carefully examined for the presence of neovascularization because these areas are a source of potential vitreous hemorrhage.

The peripheral retinal vascular abnormalities may be obscured by the dense vitreal inflammation in some patients. When the vitreous is fairly clear, sheathing or obliteration of the small peripheral venules can be seen. Periarteritis of the small arteries is found less commonly. The perivasculitis is often associated with whitish infiltrates of the peripheral retina. In rare patients the peripheral neovascularization can evolve into a vascular cyclitic membrane (**Fig. 21-1**).

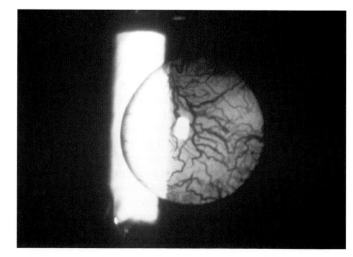

Figure 21-1. Retroillumination photograph demonstrates a vascular cyclitic membrane in a patient with intermediate uveitis of pars planitis subtype. *(Courtesy of Rubens Belfort Jr, MD.)*

Many patients have a mild course of intermediate uveitis or pars planitis and have no loss of visual acuity and may not require treatment. However, when visual acuity does decrease early in the disease process, cystoid macular edema is the most common cause; these patients usually warrant therapy. Fluorescein angiography or clinical examination frequently reveals cystoid macular edema. In addition, there is often diffuse retinal vascular leakage and optic disc edema when the disease is active. Interestingly, optic disc edema occurs in 50% of children with this entity.[26]

Vitreous hemorrhage from peripheral neovascularization may occur in a small percentage of patients.[3] It occurs more frequently in intermediate uveitis of the pars planitis subtype, and appears to be more common in children, occurring in 28% of children compared to 6% of adults in one case series.[27] Vitreous hemorrhage has also been reported as a characteristic finding of intermediate uveitis associated with multiple sclerosis.[28] In many eyes the hemorrhage will resolve, but some will require surgical intervention to remove a persistent vitreous hemorrhage. We have observed one patient in whom the neovascularization extended well into the posterior pole, leading to recurrent vitreous hemorrhages (**Fig. 21-2**). Rhegmatogenous retinal detachment can occur from vitreoretinal traction; it is seen in 3.7–22% of patients, depending on the published series.[3,7] In our experience, rhegmatogenous retinal detachment is an uncommon complication of intermediate uveitis that occurs in less than 3% of patients. Retinal detachments, when they occur, tend to develop later in the disease process, because persistent vitreal inflammation leads to vitreal contraction and retinal traction. In addition to rhegmatogenous retinal detachments, Brockhurst and colleagues[3] described nonrhegmatogenous retinal detachments associated with choroidal detachments.

Although macular edema is the most common cause of visual loss in patients with intermediate uveitis and is present in most of the patients who are referred to us, other series have reported an incidence of macular edema ranging from 28% to 50%.[5,7,29] Epiretinal membranes have been reported in 36% of eyes with intermediate uveitis.[30] Long-standing macular edema can lead to the development of retinal pigment epithelial stippling in the macula and may be a subtle sign of previous edema in patients with chronic intermediate uveitis. Unfortunately, this postcystoid macular degeneration can be a cause of severe visual loss in these patients.

Disc edema, optic atrophy, and optic disc neovascularization have been reported in patients with intermediate uveitis. Neovascularization of the disc is associated with severe retinal ischemia but responds to panretinal laser photocoagulation.[31] Phthisis bulbi may be the final outcome for an eye with chronic poorly controlled intermediate uveitis. Oftentimes these eyes have had total retinal detachments, proliferative vitreoretinopathy, or a cyclitic membrane leading to ciliary body traction and hypotony.[32]

Prognosis

Brockhurst and colleagues[3] originally described five possible types of intermediate uveitis; 28% of their patients had a benign course during which the inflammation subsided with good visual outcome. In fact, Schlaegel[6] stated that 80% of patients with intermediate uveitis of the pars planitis subtype need no therapy, and we have seen a number of patients with intermediate uveitis with or without pars plana exudates who have low-grade inflammation but never develop macular edema or decreased visual acuity. However, patients in the second group of Brockhurst and colleagues developed choroidal and serous retinal detachments. Patients in the third group developed vascularized high snowbanks that eventually formed cyclitic membranes that led to retinal detachments or glaucoma. Patients in the fourth group had significant vascular obliteration that led to visual field loss and optic atrophy. The fifth group, accounting for 46% of his patients, developed chronic smoldering inflammation.

In a later article, Brockhurst and Schepens[33] condensed the classification into four groups: benign (31%), mild chronic (49%), severe chronic (15%), and relentlessly progressive (10%). In an article published 5 years later, Smith and colleagues[7] found that 19% of patients with intermediate uveitis had mild disease, 42% had moderate inflammation, and 39% had severe inflammation. Clearly, the exact percentage of patients in any given category depends on the patient populations of the institutions in which the studies are performed. Tertiary referral centers will have more severe disease than primary care institutions. For example, Brockhurst and Schepens[33] reported retinal detachments in 50% of their patients; however, patients with intermediate uveitis and retinal detachments were probably preferentially referred to their retina practice. We have found retinal detachment to occur rarely in patients with intermediate uveitis, but this may reflect the positive effect of therapy with corticosteroids.

Long-term prognosis varies greatly based on treatment and development of complications including epiretinal membrane and glaucoma. At the time of presentation, one half of patients have a visual acuity of 20/30 or better.[5] Nevertheless, the disease can produce long-term visual disability in more than one third of patients.[7] Schlaegel and Weber[34] found that two-thirds of eyes in patients treated with corticosteroids maintained visual acuity of 20/40 or better, and

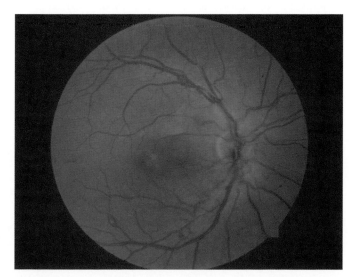

Figure 21-2. Retinal photograph demonstrates small areas of neovascularization in the posterior pole in a patient with pars planitis and recurrent vitreous hemorrhages.

other studies have noted that long-term prognosis for vision is often good with strict control of inflammation and proper management of complications.[35] In a 20-year cohort study, mean visual acuity after 10 years of follow-up was 20/30, with 75% of patients maintaining a visual acuity of 20/40 or better.[36] One-third of patients in this study maintained normal visual acuity without treatment. The presence of pars plana exudation or snowbanks may be of some prognostic value. Henderly and colleagues[5] observed that eyes with pars plana exudates had more vitreitis and macular edema, although the difference was not statistically significant. In addition, severity of disease appears to be more related to visual outcome than duration of disease.[7,37]

Although inflammatory disease does remit in some patients, Smith and colleagues[7] found only a 5% remission rate in patients followed from 4 to 26 years. Similarly, Hogan and colleagues[1] reported only one remission in 56 patients followed from 1 to 9 years. Patients with intermediate uveitis are often told that their disease will 'burn out' after a number of years, and although many patients may maintain useful vision, the disease is usually characterized by either a chronically active course or a course of exacerbations interrupted by apparent remissions. In fact, Aaberg[26] stated that ophthalmologists rarely observe a permanent spontaneous resolution of the disease.

Differential diagnosis

Although intermediate uveitis may exist as an isolated idiopathic disorder, a number of underlying diseases are associated with this condition. Evidence of systemic disorders can be found in up to one-third of patients with intermediate uveitis, depending on the study.[38] In one study of 83 patients, 10 had presumed sarcoidosis, six had multiple sclerosis, two had optic neuritis, two had inflammatory bowel disease, four had thyroid abnormalities, and two had histories consistent with Epstein–Barr virus infection.[38] Recently, infectious diseases have been associated with intermediate uveitis. It has been reported in patients with Lyme disease,[39,40] human T-cell lymphoma virus type 1 (HTLV-1) infection,[41] cat scratch disease,[42] and hepatitis C.[43] The diagnoses associated with intermediate uveitis are listed in **Box 21-1**. Many of these disorders are discussed in detail elsewhere in this book. Sarcoidosis is discussed in Chapter 22, Lyme disease in Chapter 10, toxocariasis in Chapter 16, intraocular lymphoma in Chapter 30, and iridocyclitis with Irvine–Gass syndrome in Chapter 18. Intermediate uveitis associated with multiple sclerosis is discussed later in this chapter. Other autoimmune disorders can cause an intermediate uveitis in the eye, including Crohn's disease.[44] Although specific diseases associated with intermediate uveitis can be identified in many patients, clinical investigation often fails to yield an exact diagnosis despite clinical findings that may suggest a unique condition. We reported 19 phakic patients with vitreitis, cystoid macular edema, retinal periphlebitis, and good visual outcome in whom no specific disease could be discerned.[45]

Our diagnostic evaluation of patients with intermediate uveitis includes a thorough evaluation for sarcoidosis, including a chest X-ray, a serum angiotensin-converting enzyme (ACE) level, serum calcium level, pulmonary

Box 21-1 Differential diagnosis of intermediate uveitis

Sarcoidosis
Multiple sclerosis
Inflammatory bowel disease
Lyme disease
Toxocariasis
Intraocular lymphoma
Retinoblastoma
Whipple's disease
Iridocyclitis
Multifocal choroiditis
Irvine–Gass syndrome
Amyloidosis
Interstitial nephritis and uveitis syndrome
HTLV-1 infection
Cat scratch disease
Hepatitis C
Crohn's disease

function testing, and a gallium scan. Patients with a history of chronic or bloody diarrhea are referred to a gastroenterologist for evaluation for inflammatory bowel disease. A neurologic history and examination are performed and a magnetic resonance imaging (MRI) scan is performed in patients suspected of having multiple sclerosis. For patients with a history of a rash who live in an area endemic for Lyme disease, and especially those with a history of chronic arthritis, a serologic test for Lyme disease is performed. If the inflammation is unilateral, a serologic test for *Toxocara* is performed especially in younger patients. Intraocular lymphoma is suspected in older patients, who undergo a MRI scan of the brain, a lumbar puncture for cytologic evaluation of the cerebral spinal fluid, and a diagnostic vitrectomy. Other tests are ordered on the basis of a clinical suspicion of a specific disorder.

We usually obtain a fluorescein angiogram for these patients for two reasons: to assess the presence and extent of cystoid macular edema, and to examine the retinal vasculature for signs of perivasculitis, including staining of the vessel wall and vascular leakage of dye (**Fig. 21-3**). Ultrasonography can demonstrate cyclitic membranes or the extent of vitreous debris when the view of the posterior pole is obscured by cataract. Ultrasound biomicroscopy may reveal vitreoretinal adhesions that are not observed clinically.[46]

Multiple sclerosis

Intermediate uveitis may occur in patients with multiple sclerosis. Although some authors classify multiple sclerosis in a list of masquerade syndromes, the author prefers to consider it as a cause of uveitis, like other uveitides with both CNS and ocular manifestations, such as Vogt–Koyanagi–Harada syndrome. Optic neuritis is a frequent finding in patients with multiple sclerosis, and Rizzo and Lessell[47] showed that within 15 years multiple sclerosis develops in more than 50% of patients with optic neuritis. Multiple

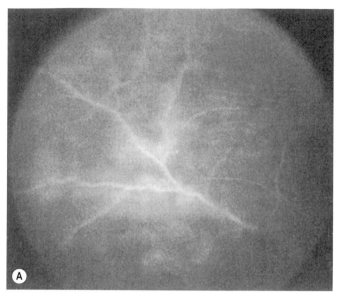
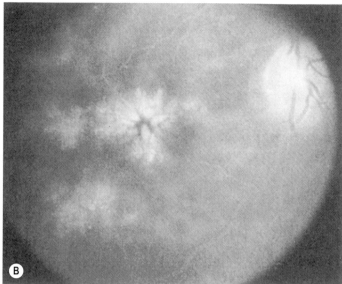

Figure 21-3. A, Late phase of fluorescein angiogram from a patient with intermediate uveitis shows substantial leakage of dye from peripheral retinal vessels. **B,** Late phase of fluorescein angiogram from a patient with pars planitis shows vascular leakage and prominent cystoid macular edema.

sclerosis was first associated with inflammatory eye disease in the early 1900s, and Breger and Leopold[48] found uveitis in 14 of 52 patients with multiple sclerosis. The most common ocular findings in patients with multiple sclerosis include intermediate uveitis, anterior uveitis, and periphlebitis, and the uveitis may precede or follow the development of multiple sclerosis. In one study, the diagnosis of MS preceded the onset of uveitis in 56% of patients, followed it in 25%, and was made concurrently in 19% of cases.[49]

Ohguro and colleagues[50] showed that eight of 14 patients with multiple sclerosis had serum antibodies to arrestin (retinal S-antigen), although none of them had uveitis. In addition, antibody titers were higher during relapses than during remissions. These findings suggest that antibodies reactive with arrestin may be related to the clinical course of multiple sclerosis. Also, because arrestin is found in the eye, antiarrestin antibodies may explain the development of uveitis in some patients with multiple sclerosis.

The uveitis associated with multiple sclerosis has been treated with corticosteroids and immunosuppressive agents similar to other causes of intermediate uveitis. Interferon is used to treat multiple sclerosis and may have a beneficial effect on the uveitis associated with this disease.[51]

Etiology

The cause of intermediate uveitis and pars planitis has not been elucidated. Evidence suggests that patients with intermediate uveitis probably do not all have the same disease. Although intermediate uveitis is a fairly common condition in uveitis clinics, the limited amount of pathologic material that has been studied has prevented a thorough clinicopathologic classification of the disease process.

The exudate deposited in eyes with intermediate uveitis of the pars planitis subtype typically localizes to a broad area of the inferior pars plana (see Fig. 3-16). The inferior location of the exudate is attributed to gravity. A diffuse phlebitis leads to breakdown of the blood–ocular barrier and release

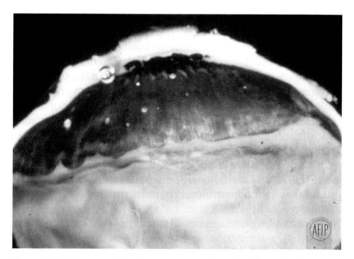

Figure 21-4. Gross pathologic appearance of peripheral snowbank in patient with intermediate uveitis of pars planitis subtype. *(Courtesy of Lorenz Zimmerman, MD.)*

of inflammatory cells, cytokines, and other inflammatory mediators that settle inferiorly.[52] Gross pathologic examination of the peripheral snowbank in pars planitis shows exudate deposited on the peripheral retina and pars plana (**Fig. 21-4**). Histologic examination of this snowbank reveals a collapsed vitreous, blood vessels, fibroglial cells including fibrous astrocytes, and scattered inflammatory cells, predominantly lymphocytes (**Fig. 21-5**).[32] Peripheral veins show lymphocytic cuffing and infiltration. The vascular component of the snowbank is continuous with the retina in some cases; this suggests that the neovascularization associated with pars planitis may be the result of retinal vessels extending through breaks in the inner limiting membrane of the vitreous base.[32] Only mild inflammation is noted in the choroid and ciliary body, suggesting that the inflammatory process in intermediate uveitis primarily involves the vitreous base and peripheral retina and not the uvea.

Case 21-1

An 8-year-old boy presented with a 1-year history of progressive unilateral visual loss. Examination revealed a visual acuity of 20/100, 2+ vitreous cells and haze, and a pars plana exudate (snowbank); the diagnosis was intermediate uveitis of the pars planitis subtype. He received cryopexy to the snowbank and a periocular injection of 40 mg methylprednisolone acetate (Depo-Medrol). Over the next 2 weeks his visual acuity improved from 20/100 to 20/30, with a concurrent reduction in inflammation. Visual acuity remained stable for the next 9 months, but intraocular inflammation began to recur. One year after the first cryopexy and periocular injection with corticosteroids, vision decreased to 20/80. The patient was treated with a second cryopexy and periocular injection of corticosteroids. Vision again improved to 20/30, but 1 year later the vision again decreased to 20/80. A third cryopexy procedure and periocular corticosteroid injection had no effect. However, two additional periocular injections led to decreased ocular inflammation and improvement of vision to 20/30.

Case 21-2

An 11-year-old girl developed bilateral intermediate uveitis with pars plana exudates that resulted in reduced vision in both eyes. She was treated with systemic prednisone, and visual acuity improved. The patient, however, developed intolerable weight gain, mood changes, and gastroitestinal distress, and the prednisone therapy was discontinued. She received three periocular injections of corticosteroids without improvement in vision. Cryotherapy to one eye similarly had no effect. Two years after the start of the disease, the patient was left with bilateral cystoid macular edema, moderate vitreitis, and visual acuity of 20/50 in the right eye and 20/80 in the left eye.

Therapy was begun with ciclosporin at a dose of 4 mg/kg daily and bromocriptine at 10 mg/day. Over the next 2 months the vitreal inflammation and cystoid macular edema resolved, and the visual acuity improved to 20/20 in the right eye and 20/32 in the left. The patient tolerated these medications without problems, and this therapeutic regimen has been continued.

References

1. Hogan MJ, Kimura SJ, O'Connor GR, et al. Peripheral retinitis and chronic cyclitis in children. Trans Ophthalmol Soc UK 1965; 85: 39–52.
2. Schepens CL. L'inflammation de la region de l'ora serrata et ses sequelles. Bull Soc Ophthalmol Fr 1950; 73: 113–124.
3. Brockhurst RJ, Schepens CL, Okamura ID. Uveitis II. Peripheral uveitis: clinical description, complications and differential diagnosis. Am J Ophthalmol 1960; 49: 1257–1266.
4. Welch RB, Maumenee AE, Wahlen HE. Peripheral posterior segment inflammation, vitreous opacities, and edema of the posterior pole. Arch Ophthalmol 1960; 64: 540–549.
5. Henderly DE, Haymond RS, Rao NS, et al. The significance of the pars plana exudate in pars planitis. Am J Ophthalmol 1987; 103: 669–671.
6. Schlaegel TF Jr. Differential diagnosis of uveitis. Ophthalmol Digest 1973; 35: 34.
7. Smith RE, Godfrey WA, Kimura SJ. Chronic cyclitis. I. Course and visual prognosis. Trans Am Acad Ophthalmol Otolaryngol 1973; 77: 760–768.
8. Van Metre TE. Role of the allergist in diagnosis and management of patients with uveitis, JAMA 1966; 195: 167–172.
9. Donaldson MJ, Pulido JS, Herman DC, et al. Pars planitis: a 20-year study of incidence, clinical features, and outcomes. Am J Ophthalmol 2007; 144: 812–817.
10. Giles CL. Uveitis in childhood. In: Tasman W, Jaeger EA, eds. Duane's clinical ophthalmology. Philadelphia, 1981, JB Lippincott, pp 1–8.

11. Arocker-Mettinger E, Mayr WR, Huber SV, et al. Do HLA antigens play a role in intermediate uveitis? Vox Sang 1992; 63: 282–284.
12. Kimura SJ, Hogan MJ. Chronic cyclitis. Arch Ophthalmol 1964; 71: 193–201.
13. Wetzig RP, Chan CC, Nussenblatt RB, et al. Clinical and immunopathological studies of pars planitis in a family. Br J Ophthalmol 1988; 72: 5–10.
14. Culbertson WW, Giles CL, West CW, et al. Familial pars planitis. Retina 1983; 3: 179–181.
15. Augsburger JJ, Annesley WH, Sergott RC, et al. Familial pars planitis. Ann Ophthalmol 1981; 13: 553–557.
16. Fitt A, Harrison RJ. Familial intermediate uveitis: a case report of two brothers. Eye 1999; 13: 808–809.
17. Biswas J, Raghavendran SR, Vijaya R. Intermediate uveitis of pars planitis type in identical twins: report of a case. Int Ophthalmol 1998; 22: 275–277.
18. Haimovici R, Lightman SL, Bird AC. Familial pars planitis and dominant optic atrophy. Ophthalmic Genet 1997; 18: 43–45.
19. Lee AG. Familial pars planitis. Ophthalmic Genet 1995; 16: 17–19.
20. Martin T, Weber M, Schmitt C, et al. Association of intermediate uveitis with HLA-A28: definition of a new systemic syndrome? Graefes Arch Clin Exp Ophthalmol 1995; 233: 269–274.
21. Tang WM, Pulido JS, Eckels DD, et al. The association of HLA-DR15 and intermediate uveitis. Am J Ophthalmol 1997; 123: 70–75.
22. Oruc S, Duffy BF, Mohanakumar T, et al. The association of HLA class II

with pars planitis. Am J Ophthalmol 2001; 131: 657–659.
23. Capone A Jr, Aaberg TM. Intermediate uveitis. In: Albert DM, Jacobiec FA, eds. Principles and practice of ophthalmology. Philadelphia, 1994, WB Saunders, pp 423–442.
24. Khodadoust AA, Karnama Y, Stoessel KM, et al. Pars planitis, an autoimmune endotheliopathy. Am J Ophthalmol 1986; 102: 633–639.
25. Smith RE, Godfrey WA, Kimura SJ. Complications of chronic cyclitis. Am J Ophthalmol 1976; 82: 277–282.
26. Aaberg TM. The enigma of pars planitis. Am J Ophthalmol 1987; 103: 828–830.
27. Lauer AK, Smith JR, Robertson JE, et al. Vitreous hemorrhage is a common complication of pediatric pars planitis. Ophthalmology 2002; 109: 95–98.
28. Valentincic NV, Kraut A, Rothova A. Vitreous hemorrhage in multiple sclerosis-associated uveitis. Ocul Immunol Inflamm 2007; 15: 19–25.
29. Hogan MJ, Kimura SJ, O'Connor GR. Peripheral retinitis and chronic cyclitis in children. Trans Ophthalmol Soc UK 1965; 85: 39–52.
30. Donaldson MJ, Pulido JS, Herman DC, et al. Pars planitis: a 20-year study of incidence, clinical features, and outcomes. Am J Ophthalmol 2007; 144: 812–817.
31. Felder KS, Brockhurst RJ. Neovascular fundus abnormalities in peripheral uveitis. Arch Ophthalmol 1982; 100: 750–754.
32. Pederson JE, Kenyon KR, Green WR, et al. Pathology of pars planitis. Am J Ophthalmol 1978; 86: 762–774.

33. Brockhurst RJ, Schepens CL. Uveitis IV. Peripheral uveitis: the complications of retinal detachment. Arch Ophthalmol 1968; 80: 747–753.

34. Schlaegel TF, Weber JC. Corticosteroids for pars planitis. Surv Ophthalmol 1977; 22: 120–130.

35. Bonfioli AA, Damico FM, Curi AL, Orefice F. Intermediate uveitis. Semin Ophthalmol 2005; 20: 147–154.

36. Donaldson MJ, Pulido JS, Herman DC, et al. Pars planitis: a 20-year study of incidence, clinical features, and outcomes. Am J Ophthalmol 2007; 144: 812–817.

37. Chester GH, Blach RK, Cleary PE. Inflammation in the region of the vitreous base: pars planitis. Trans Ophthalmol Soc UK 1976; 96: 151–157.

38. Boskovich SA, Lowder CY, Meisler DM, et al. Systemic diseases associated with intermediate uveitis. Cleve Clin J Med 1993; 60: 460–465.

39. Breeveld J, Rothova A, Kuiper H. Intermediate uveitis and Lyme borreliosis. Br J Ophthalmol 1992; 76: 181–182.

40. Guex CY, Herbort CP. Lyme disease in Switzerland: ocular involvement. Klin Monatsbl Augenheilkd 1992; 200: 545–546.

41. Mochizuki M, Watanabe T, Yamaguchi K, et al. Uveitis associated with human T-cell lymphotropic virus type I. Am J Ophthalmol 1992; 114: 123–129.

42. Soheilian M, Markomichelakis N, Foster CS. Intermediate uveitis and retinal vasculitis as manifestations of cat scratch disease. Am J Ophthalmol 1996; 122: 582–584.

43. Perez-Alvarez AF, Jimenez-Alonso J, Reche-Molina I, et al. Retinal vasculitis and vitreitis in a patient with chronic hepatitis C virus. Arch Intern Med 2001; 161: 2262.

44. Rosenbaum JT, Kurz D. An old crone finds a new home: Crohn's disease and pars planitis. Ocul Immunol Inflamm 2002; 10: 157–160.

45. Park DW, Folk JC, Whitcup SM, et al. Phakic patients with cystoid macular edema, retinal periphlebitis, and vitreous inflammation. Arch Ophthalmol 1998; 116: 1025–1029.

46. Haring G, Nolle B, Wiechens B. Ultrasound biomicroscopic imaging in intermediate uveitis. Br J Ophthalmol 1998; 82: 625–629.

47. Rizzo JF, Lessell S. Risk of developing multiple sclerosis after uncomplicated optic neuritis. Neurology 1988; 38: 185–190.

48. Breger BC, Leopold IH. The incidence of uveitis in multiple sclerosis. Am J Ophthalmol 1966; 62: 540–545.

49. Zein G, Berta A, Foster CS. Multiple sclerosis-associated uveitis. Ocul Immunol Inflamm 2004; 12: 137–142.

50. Ohguro H, Chiba S, Igarashi Y, et al. â-Arrestin and arrestin are recognized by autoantibodies in sera from multiple sclerosis patients. Proc Natl Acad Sci USA 1993; 90: 3241–3245.

51. Becker MD, Heiligenjaus A, Hudde T, et al. Interferon as a treatment for uveitis associated with multiple sclerosis. Br J Ophthalmol 2005; 89: 1254–1257.

52. Deschenes J, Freeman W, Char DH, et al. Lymphocyte subpopulations in uveitis. Arch Ophthalmol 1986; 104: 233–236.

53. Green WR, Kincaid MC, Michels GG, et al. Pars planitis. Trans Ophthalmol Soc UK 1981; 101: 361–367.

54. Thorne JE, Daniel E, Jabs DA, et al. Smoking as a risk factor for cystoid macular edema complicating intermediate uveitis. Am J Ophthalmol 2008; 145: 841–846.

55. Hultsch E. Peripheral uveitis in the owl monkey. Mod Probl Ophthalmol 1977; 18: 247–251.

56. Gartner J. The vitreous base of the human eye and 'pars planitis': electron microscopic observations. Mod Probl Ophthalmol 1972; 10: 250–255.

57. Bora NS, Bora PS, Tandhasetti MT, et al. Molecular cloning, sequencing, and expression of the 36 kDa protein present in pars planitis: sequence homology with yeast nucleopore complex protein. Invest Ophthalmol Vis Sci 1996; 37: 1877–1883.

58. Bora NS, Bora PS, Tandhasetti MT, et al. Molecular cloning, sequencing, and expression of the 36 kDa protein present in pars planitis. Sequence homology with yeast nucleopore complex protein. Invest Ophthalmol Vis Sci 1996; 37: 2363–2364.

59. Murray PI, Young DW. Soluble interleukin-2 receptors in retinal vasculitis. Curr Eye Res 1992; 11(suppl): 193–195.

60. Arocker-Mettinger E, Steurer-Georgiew L, Steurer M, et al. Circulating ICAM-1 levels in serum of uveitis patients. Curr Eye Res 1992; 11(suppl): 161–166.

61. Perez VL, Papaliodis GN, Chu D, et al. Elevated levels of interleukin 6 in the vitreous of patients with pars planitis and posterior uveitis: the Massachusetts Eye & Ear experience and review of previous studies. Ocul Immunol Inflamm 2004; 12: 193–201.

62. Kaplan HJ. Intermediate uveitis (pars planitis, chronic cyclitis) – a four step approach to treatment. In: Saari KM, ed. Uveitis update, Amsterdam, 1984, Excerpta Medica, pp 169–172.

63. Young S, Larkin G, Branley M, et al. Safety and efficacy of intravitreal triamcinolone for cystoid macular oedema in uveitis. Clin Exp Ophthalmol 2001; 29: 2–6.

64. Devenyi RG, Mieler WF, Lambrou FH, et al. Cryopexy of the vitreous base in the management of peripheral uveitis. Am J Ophthalmol 1988; 106: 135–138.

65. Pulido JS, Mieler WF, Walton D, et al. Results of peripheral laser photocoagulation in pars planitis. Trans Am Ophthalmol Soc 1998; 96: 127–137.

66. Kaplan HJ. Surgical treatment of intermediate uveitis. Dev Ophthalmol 1992; 23: 185–189.

67. Bacskulin A, Eckardt C. Results of pars plana vitrectomy in chronic uveitis in childhood. Ophthalmologe 1993; 90: 434–439.

68. Miller WF, Will BR, Lewis H, et al. Vitrectomy in the management of peripheral uveitis. Ophthalmology 1988; 95: 859–864.

69. Wiechens B, Nolle B, Reichelt JA. Pars-plana vitrectomy in cystoid macular edema associated with intermediate uveitis. Graefes Arch Clin Exp Ophthalmol 2001; 239: 474–481.

70. Stavrou P, Baltatzis S, Letko E, et al. Pars plana vitrectomy in patients with intermediate uveitis. Ocul Immunol Inflamm 2001; 9: 141–151.

71. Foster CS. Vitrectomy in the management of uveitis. Ophthalmology 1988; 95: 1011–1012.

72. Michelson JB, Friedlander MH, Nozik RA. Lens implant surgery in pars planitis. Ophthalmology 1990; 97: 1023–1026.

Sarcoidosis

Scott M. Whitcup

Key concepts

- Sarcoidosis is a multisystem granulomatous disease that can affect almost every organ in the body in people of all racial and ethnic groups.
- The cause of sarcoidosis remains unknown, but a number of recent studies have elucidated the immunologic basis for the disease pathogenesis with the macrophage playing a central role.
- Most patients with sarcoidosis present with respiratory symptoms, although some have generalized symptoms such as fever, fatigue, or weight loss.
- Many patients with sarcoidosis are asymptomatic at the time of diagnosis, and it is only recognized after an abnormal chest X-ray or laboratory test result. Uveitis may be the initial manifestation of the disease.
- Definitive diagnosis is made on biopsy; however, diagnosis if frequently based on clinical findings and chext X-ray or CT scan.
- Ophthalmic findings occur in as many as 50% of patients including anterior and posterior uveitis, retinal vasculitis, and optic nerve disease.
- Secondary glaucoma is a common cause of vision loss.
- Systemic corticosteroids and immunosuppressive agents, including the biologics, are used to treat the disease.

Sarcoidosis is a multisystem granulomatous disease that can affect almost every organ in the body in people of all racial and ethnic groups. The organs most commonly involved are the lungs, thoracic lymph nodes, and skin. The adrenal glands, which produce corticosteroids, are the only organs consistently spared by this disease. Sarcoidosis was initially described as a dermatologic disease by Hutchinson in 1869, and Boeck used the term sarkoid to describe the skin biopsies that had a histologic appearance similar to that of sarcomas.[1] Uveitis was described in patients with sarcoidosis in the early 1900s, and in 1936 sarcoid uveitis associated with a facial nerve palsy and uveoparotid fever was termed Heerfordt's syndrome.[2] Although the cause of sarcoidosis remains unknown, it is important to make the diagnosis of sarcoidosis in patients with uveitis not only to allow appropriate therapy for the eye disease, but also to alert the physician to the possible systemic manifestations that may also require treatment.

Epidemiology

Epidemiologic studies of sarcoidosis are prone to considerable error because of variability in the criteria for diagnosis. Nevertheless, there are substantial differences in the yearly incidence rate in different parts of the world, from 0.2 per 100 000 in Japan and Spain to 64 per 100 000 in Sweden.[3,4] In one study, the age-adjusted annual incidence in African-Americans was 82 per 100 000 and in whites was eight per 100 000.[5] More recently, the adjusted annual incidence of sarcoidosis among black Americans was 35.5 per 100 000, compared to 10.9 per 100 000 in white Americans.[6] In addition, African-Americans with chronic sarcoidosis are more likely to develop ocular manifestations than are whites.[7] There are conflicting data in the literature on whether sarcoidosis is more common in females.[7,8]

Etiology

Although the cause of sarcoidosis remains unknown, a number of recent studies have elucidated the immunologic basis for the disease pathogenesis (**Fig. 22-1**).[9] The macrophage, acting as an antigen-presenting cell, is hypothesized to initiate the inflammatory response in sarcoidosis.[10-13] Possibly in response to presentation of an unknown antigen, macrophages are thought to release cytokines such as TNF-α and interleukin (IL)-12 that cause the infiltration of T-helper lymphocytes. These lymphocytes will also release cytokines and recruit other inflammatory cells to the site of inflammation. In response to these events, granulomas are formed and immunoglobulins produced in large quantities by stimulated B lymphocytes and released into the circulation. The immunohistochemical staining of one eye with sarcoidosis showed granulomas in the choroid and anterior uvea composed of macrophages and T-helper cells.[14]

The primary involvement of the lung in sarcoidosis suggests sensitization and a resultant immune response to an endogenous lung antigen or an inhaled infectious agent or other antigen. Frequent involvement of the eye and skin also supports this hypothesis. A number of epidemiologic studies have now reported associations between environmental exposure and sarcoidosis. Early studies suggested associations of sarcoidosis with exposure to tree pollen and smoke from wood-burning stoves in rural areas.[15] Other environmental associations with sarcoidosis include mold and insecticides.[16] Microbial triggers have also been described in sarcoidosis.[17] The development of sarcoidosis has been

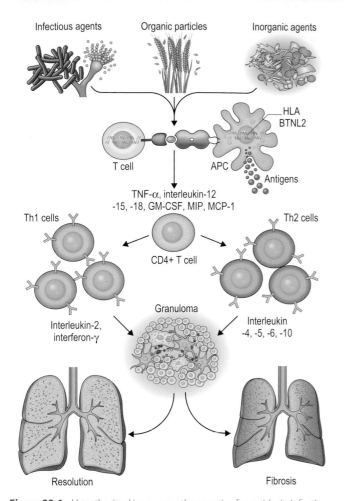

Table 22-1 Uveitis associated with sarcoidosis

DIAGNOSTIC CRITERIA	
Suspected sarcoidosis	Hilar adenopathy, erythema nodosum, increased serum ACE level, positive lung or lacrimal or salivary gland gallium scan results, increased serum globulin level, increased serum or urinary calcium level, lymphadenopathy, decreased lung diffusing capacity
Definite sarcoidosis	Histologic confirmation of noncaseating granulomas
Associated findings	Uveitis, arthritis, neurologic signs and symptoms, anemia, decreased pulmonary function, lymphadenopathy
OCULAR FINDINGS	
Common	Acute nongranulomatous or chronic granulomatous iridocyclitis, vitritis, vitreal snowballs, macular edema, perivenous sheathing, small yellow choroidal, and retinal pigment epithelial patches of inflammation, optic disc swelling, retinal neovascularization
Rare	Large choroidal granulomas, subretinal neovascularization, optic neuropathy

Figure 22-1. Hypothesized immunopathogenesis of sarcoidosis. Infectious, organic, and inorganic agents are possible antigens in sarcoidosis. Any causative microbe, if present, is probably cleared, leaving behind an undegradable product or initiating a cross-reacting immune response to self-antigen. Antigen-presenting cells (APC), in addition to producing high levels of tumor necrosis factor-α (TNF-α), secrete IL-12, IL-15, and IL-18, macrophage inflammatory protein 1 (MIP-1), monocyte chemotactic protein 1 (MCP-1), and granulocyte–macrophage colony-stimulating factor (GM-CSF).[57] A cardinal feature of sarcoidosis is the presence of CD4+ T cells that interact with APCs to initiate the formation and maintenance of granulomas. CD4+ T cells release IL-2 and IFN-γ. Activated CD4+ cells differentiate into type 1 helper (Th1)-like cells and secrete predominantly IL-2 and IFN-γ. The efficiency of antigen processing, antigen presentation, and cytokine release is probably under genetic control; evidence strongly supports a role for macrophage HLA and BTNL2 alleles in sarcoidosis susceptibility and phenotype.[48,49] However, T-cell genes that may confer a predisposition to sarcoidosis or affect the phenotype have not yet been identified. Sarcoidal granulomas are organized, structured masses composed of macrophages and their derivatives, epithelioid cells, giant cells, and T cells. Sarcoidal granulomas may persist, resolve, or lead to fibrosis. Alveolar macrophages activated in the context of a predominant type 2 helper (Th2) T-cell response appear to stimulate fibroblast proliferation and collagen production, leading to progressive fibrosis. *(From Iannuzzi M et al. Sarcoidosis N Engl J Med 2007;357:2153–2165. Copyright 2007 Massachusetts Medical Society. All rights reserved)*

associated with IFN-α treatment for hepatitis, although the association may be related to the underlying hepatitis C infection.[18]

Additional data suggest that sarcoidosis is an abnormal immune response directed against one of many different antigens in a patient with a hereditary or acquired abnormality of the immune system. There does appear to be some genetic predilection to the disease. Sarcoidosis has been reported more commonly in monozygotic than in dizygotic twins.[19] Furthermore, there have been associations between both class I antigens (HLA-B8)[20] and class II antigens (HFA-DRB1).[21] There are a number of immune defects in patients with sarcoidosis. Despite the inflammatory response seen in multiple tissues, delayed-type hypersensitivity is depressed, causing anergy on skin testing, and a generally depressed cellular immunity has been reported.

Clinical manifestations

Most patients with sarcoidosis present with respiratory symptoms, although some have generalized symptoms such as fever, fatigue, or weight loss. Many are asymptomatic at the time of diagnosis, and sarcoidosis is only recognized after an abnormal chest X-ray or laboratory test result. Sarcoid uveitis is diagnosed when ocular inflammation is found in a patient with extraocular findings diagnostic of sarcoidosis. The definitive diagnosis of sarcoidosis requires the demonstration of a noncaseating, granulomatous, non-infectious inflammatory process on biopsy; however, a number of laboratory and other diagnostic tests can strongly support the diagnosis. Two-thirds of patients with sarcoidosis have a remission within a decade after diagnosis with minimal health consequences; however, one-third have recurrent, progressive disease leading to significant organ damage.[9]

Ophthalmic involvement occurred in 50% of patients with sarcoidosis in one report,[17a] but most series report eye findings in about 25% of patients.[7,22,23] The common ocular findings in patients with sarcoidosis are listed in **Table 22-1**. Of patients with chronic systemic sarcoidosis, 26% have ophthalmic involvement at some point during the course of their disease.[7] Ocular disease is usually bilateral, but may be unilateral or markedly asymmetric. It is important to examine both the conjunctiva and the lacrimal gland in patients with possible sarcoidosis. The palpebral conjunctiva should be carefully scrutinized for sarcoid granulomas (**Fig. 22-2**),

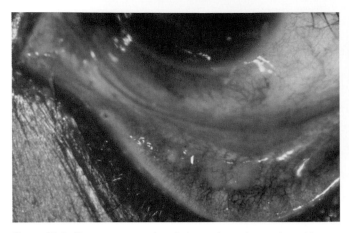

Figure 22-2. Biopsy-proven conjunctival granulomas in a patient with sarcoidosis.

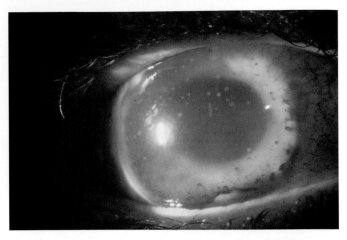

Figure 22-3. Large granulomatous mutton-fat keratic precipitates in a patient with chronic uveitis and sarcoidosis.

which are seen in 7–17% of patients with ophthalmic involvement.[7,22,23] The lacrimal gland, which is clinically involved in 7–26% of patients with ocular sarcoidosis,[7,22,23] should also be examined for possible enlargement as a result of the disease. Although a positive conjunctival biopsy for sarcoidosis does not correlate with the presence of anterior uveitis in sarcoidosis,[24] the demonstration of a noncaseating granuloma in the conjunctiva can be diagnostic.

Anterior uveitis

Anterior uveitis is the most common ocular manifestation and occurs in almost two-thirds of patients with ocular sarcoidosis. From 53% to 60% of patients with ocular sarcoidosis will have a chronic granulomatous uveitis.[7,22,23] Most of these patients will have mutton-fat keratic precipitates (KPs) that may be extremely large and dense, as shown in **Figure 22-3**. Iris nodules, albeit characteristic for granulomatous inflammation, occur in only 11% of all patients with ocular sarcoidosis (**Fig. 22-4**).[13] Occasionally, an iris nodule can enlarge to the point where it resembles a tumor. Although the presence of other signs of inflammation and the yellow color of the lesion may be reassuring, only a reduction in the size of the lesion after corticosteroid therapy can prove that the nodule is inflammatory and not malignant.

This chronic form of anterior inflammation generally occurs in patients with sarcoidosis in the fourth to sixth decades[23] and results in secondary damage to the eye, including cataract and glaucoma. The incidence of both of these complications is difficult to estimate from the literature because there is an increasing incidence of both cataracts and glaucoma with increased duration of the chronic inflammation. The prevalence of cataracts in patients with chronic sarcoid uveitis is 8–17%, and the prevalence of glaucoma varies from 11% to 23%.[7,22,23] Both pupillary block and trabecular meshwork damage can cause glaucoma in these patients and may exist simultaneously. In contrast, chronic inflammation will occasionally lead to hypotony and phthisis.[14,25]

Acute iridocyclitis of limited duration associated with small fine KPs occurs in 15–45% of patients with ocular sarcoidosis.[7,22,23] Even among patients with chronic systemic sarcoidosis, those with anterior iridocyclitis frequently have one attack early in the course of their disease and no further recurrences. Some will develop a pattern of acute recurrent

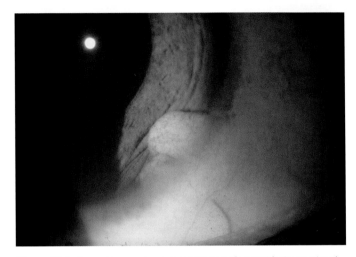

Figure 22-4. Large iris granuloma in a patient with sarcoidosis associated with chronic anterior and posterior uveitis.

uveitis without granulomatous signs. Therefore, although granulomatous uveitis is the more common presentation of ocular sarcoidosis, even a patient with recurrent anterior iritis may have sarcoidosis as an underlying cause. We have followed several patients with recurrent anterior uveitis who developed mild vitritis years later, along with systemic manifestations of sarcoidosis. As will be discussed later, there is currently little proof that the lesions of acute iritis in patients with sarcoidosis are due to the same pathologic process that is responsible for the noncaseating granulomas of the thorax.

Posterior segment findings

Inflammation of the vitreous, retina, and choroid is less common but more visually disabling than inflammation in the anterior segment, and occurs in 6–33% of patients with sarcoidosis.[7,22,23] Many of these patients will also have anterior inflammation. The presence of clumps of cells and proteinaceous debris called snowballs in the vitreous should suggest the diagnosis of sarcoidosis. Often these snowballs are located inferiorly and lie on the retinal surface anterior to the equator. The classic 'candle wax dripping' (*en taches de bougie*) along the retinal veins is not frequently seen (**Fig. 22-5**), but many patients with posterior inflammation will have perivenous sheathing.[22,26] In contrast, periarterial

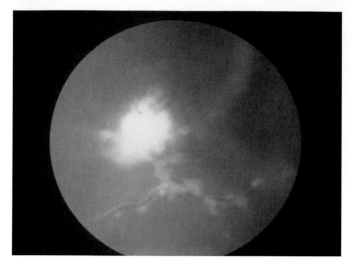

Figure 22-5. Peripheral perivenous sheathing (candle wax drippings) and peripheral retinal exudate in sarcoidosis.

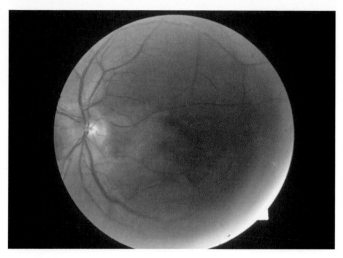

Figure 22-7. Choroidal granuloma with associated serous retinal detachment in a patient with sarcoidosis.

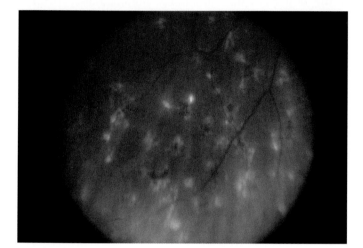

Figure 22-6. Multiple Dalen–Fuchs nodules in patient with sarcoidosis.

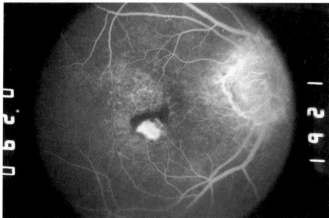

Figure 22-8. Fluorescein angiogram of subretinal neovascular membrane in patient with sarcoidosis.

sheathing is rarely observed. Small areas of peripheral venous occlusion have been reported, but large vein occlusions are uncommon. Deep yellow choroidal lesions consistent with Dalen–Fuchs nodules and mottling of the pigment epithelium occur in 36% of these patients (**Fig. 22-6**) and are more common than true elevated choroidal granulomas.[26] These smaller lesions are probably small choroidal granulomas that evolve and lead to secondary pigment epithelial alterations. They are similar in appearance and histologic findings to the Dalen–Fuchs nodules of sympathetic ophthalmia, although the lesions may be somewhat larger in sarcoidosis than in sympathetic ophthalmia. Large granulomas of the choroid can also occur and may resemble choroidal tumors.[27,28] These appear as yellow-white or yellow-gray discrete elevated masses. Large granulomas can have overlying serous retinal detachments and will cause decreased acuity if they involve the fovea (**Fig. 22-7**). These lesions will block fluorescence in the early stages of a fluorescein angiogram and will stain in the late phase. If the lesions occur under the macula, one needs to be concerned about the development of a submacular neovascular net extending from the granuloma.

Chronic cystoid macular edema is usually the cause of decreased acuity in patients with posterior uveitis and sarcoidosis. However, the vitreous opacities can occasionally be sufficiently dense in this disease to contribute to a decrease in visual acuity. Nevertheless, we have been surprised that visual acuity is only minimally affected in most uveitis patients with even dense vitreous opacity as long as the macula and optic nerve are uninvolved. Neovascularization of the optic disc occurs in approximately 15% of patients with posterior uveitis related to sarcoidosis.[26] In our experience, prompt steroid therapy will frequently lead to an involution of these vessels, which implies that the ischemic stimulus that promoted the neovascularization is reversible and related to the inflammation. If there is significant peripheral vascular ischemia or neovascularization, therapy with antiinflammatory drugs may not be adequate and photocoagulation may be indicated.

In contrast to retinal neovascularization, subretinal neovascularization in sarcoidosis is much less common and does not respond to medical therapy.[25,29,30] Case reports usually describe a peripapillary or macular subretinal neovascular membrane (**Fig. 22-8**). It is likely that choroidal inflammation with secondary retinal pigment epithelial damage leads to breaks in Bruch's membrane that permit the development of the neovascular net. The natural course of these vascular abnormalities is not well defined, but they

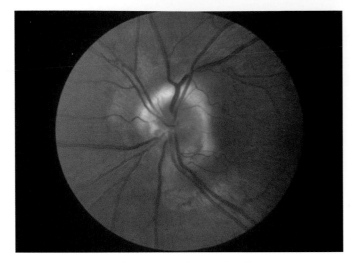

Figure 22-9. Optic disc hyperemia and peripapillary fibrous ring in a patient with sarcoidosis and a history of optic disc swelling.

Table 22-2 Systemic involvement of sarcoidosis (Modified from Siltzbach LE, James DG, Neville E et al. Course and prognosis of sarcoidosis around the world. Am J Med 1974; 57: 847–52.)

Locus	Occurrence (%)
Hilar adenopathy	74
Lung parenchyma	46
Lymphadenopathy	28
Skin lesions (excluding erythema nodosum)	18
Erythema nodosum	15
Splenomegaly	10
Bone	4
Parotid	6
Central nervous system	5

probably have a prognosis similar to that for subretinal membranes as a result of other causes.

Optic disc swelling occurs in 39% of patients with posterior uveitis, but is usually mild and not associated with visual dysfunction.[26] The optic disc may also be hyperemic. Papilledema can occur due to sarcoid granulomas that invade the optic nerve, but it is probably not the common cause of disc swelling as the swelling follows a course that parallels the severity of the posterior uveitis.[26] After the disc edema resolves, a peripapillary fibrous ring may remain (**Fig. 22-9**). Retrobulbar neuritis without intraocular signs of inflammation has also been reported and is presumably related to direct involvement of the optic nerve by granulomatous inflammation.[31]

Systemic involvement

Sarcoidosis is a systemic disease, and the other organ systems involved in this disease are listed in **Table 22-2**. Skin lesions are common (**Fig. 22-10**), and a biopsy of granulomatous lesions can be diagnostic. Both erythema nodosum and granulomatous sarcoid nodules of the skin have been described. Erythema nodosum is a nodular subcutaneous inflammation that presents on the lower extremities and occasionally on the upper extremities or face. The nodules are elevated, red, and tender. It is a hypersensitivity reaction and occurs in drug allergies and in diseases such as streptococcal infection, colitis, and Behçet's disease as well as in sarcoidosis. The lesions of erythema nodosum are not granulomatous, and the condition is generally self-limited. It usually occurs in women with sarcoidosis in the second and third decades, and is frequently associated with an acute presentation of sarcoidosis that also includes fever, arthralgia, hilar adenopathy, and iritis.[5] The granulomatous nodules of sarcoidosis in the skin appear as movable nontender subcutaneous nodules, usually on the lower extremities. Biopsy of these lesions often reveals noncaseating granulomas diagnostic of sarcoidosis.

The arthritis of sarcoidosis can be either acute or chronic in nature. Of North American whites with sarcoidosis 21% have joint symptoms,[32] and the percentage in African-Americans may be somewhat higher. Arthritis is most common during acute sarcoidosis, but in these patients it rarely becomes chronic. Although granulomas may be seen in the joint synovium, mild nongranulomatous synovitis is more common. Arthritis occurs less frequently in patients with chronic sarcoidosis, but these patients are more likely to have synovial granulomas.

A wide range of neurologic signs and symptoms, including cranial nerve palsies, neuropathy, myopathy, and aseptic meningitis, can result from the meningoencephalitis of sarcoidosis. Overall, the CNS is involved in up to 25% of patients.[9] A lumbar puncture and central nervous system imaging studies are important to define the nature of the neurologic involvement that occurs in these patients.[5] Sarcoidosis that involves the base of the brain and chiasm may be clinically difficult to prove without a biopsy. The facial nerve is the cranial nerve most commonly involved in patients with sarcoidosis. Because Lyme disease is also a cause of facial nerve paresis, arthralgias, rash, and uveitis, it should be considered in the differential diagnosis of patients with these findings.

Other organs are frequently involved in sarcoidosis. Although hilar adenopathy is a more frequent finding in sarcoidosis, splenomegaly and lymphadenopathy occur in respectively 10% and 28% of patients with sarcoidosis.[5] These findings are detectable by physical examination and should be looked for in patients with possible sarcoidosis. Enlarged lymphoid organs are unusual in most types of endogenous uveitis and point to a clinical diagnosis of sarcoidosis. Liver involvement is also common. Approximately 10% of patients have elevated liver enzymes, and hepatic lesions can be detected on CT scans in about 5% of patients.[33] Renal involvement can occur as a result of hypercalciuria. Importantly, cardiac granulomas are found in about 25% of patients with sarcoidosis at autopsy, but are clinically apparent in only about 5% of all patients.[9] Furthermore, mortality from sarcoidosis frequently occurs as a result of end-stage pulmonary disease, neurologic disease, or cardiac complications, including arrhythmias or cardiomyopthy. The arrhythmias may present as sudden death.

Although less common in the pediatric population, sarcoidosis is a cause of uveitis in children under 5 years of age. The disease in these cases is typically characterized by a granulomatous anterior uveitis, polyarticular arthritis, rash, and lymphadenopathy.[34] Posterior uveitis and orbital disease can also occur. Pulmonary disease occurs in only

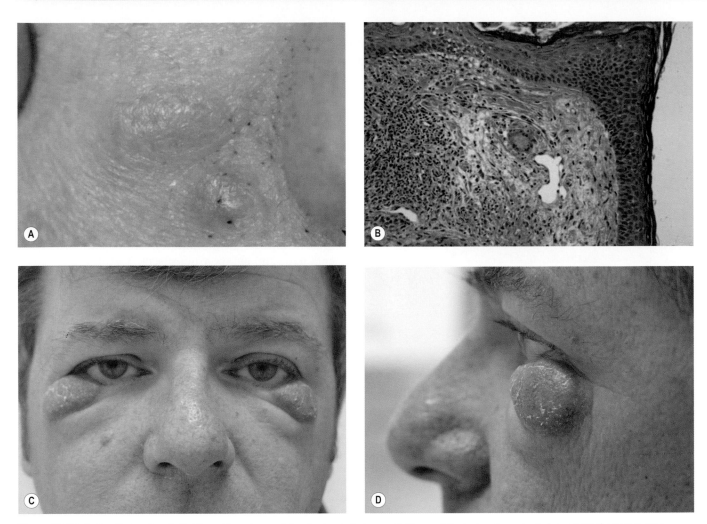

Figure 22-10 A. Two flesh-colored, slightly eyrthematous, minimally elevated plaques. **B**. Biopsy of the lesion shown in **A** shows typical noncaseating granuloma consistent with the diagnosis of sarcoidosis. **C**. and **D**. show thick, erythematous, scaling plaques in the inferior periorbital area in a patient with sarcoidosis. *(A and B Courtesy of Chi-Chao Chan, MD; C and D Courtesy of Teresa Soriano, MD.)*

one-third of younger patients, but these children often have skin and joint disease.[35] Finding an anterior uveitis and arthritis in a young child with a normal chest X-ray often leads to the misdiagnosis of juvenile rheumatoid arthritis. Intermittent fever and synovial swelling can delay the diagnosis of sarcoidosis in young children.[36] In infants, sarcoidosis may present as a more multisystem illness.[37] Nevertheless, like that seen in patients with juvenile rheumatoid arthritis, the anterior uveitis may lead to permanent loss of vision, especially in young children susceptible to the development of amblyopia. In these children especially, aggressive therapy is often warranted. In older children the presentation and course of sarcoidosis more closely parallels those of adults.

One genetic disease that occurs in children that can mimic sarcoidosis is Blau syndrome, a disorder characterized by familial granulomatosis, arthritis, uveitis, and skin rash.[38] Although some of these patients may have elevated serum ACE levels, the disorder is otherwise clinically distinct. Patients with Blau syndrome may have camptodactyly and do not have pulmonary disease, hypercalcemia, or positive reactions to Kveim skin testing. The disease has been associated with CARD15 gene mutations.[39] Blau syndrome may be misdiagnosed as early-infantile sarcoidosis.[40]

Although many patients with sarcoid uveitis maintain good visual acuity, permanent visual loss can occur despite appropriate therapy. In our patients with biopsy-proven ocular sarcoidosis, 14 of 21 (67%) had a visual acuity of 20/40 or worse in at least one eye. Visual acuity worse than 20/200 was most often caused by secondary glaucoma, and aggressive treatment of this complication is therefore warranted.

Pathology

The definitive diagnosis of sarcoidosis requires the finding of noncaseating epithelioid cell granulomas on biopsy. The typical sarcoid granuloma consists of whorls of epithelioid cells surrounding multinucleated giant cells (**Fig. 22-11**). Mononuclear cells, fibroblasts, and lymphocytes may be found at the periphery of these nodules, and surrounding areas of fibrosis are common. True caseation, however, is absent. Although suggestive of sarcoidosis, these pathologic findings are nonspecific, and the presence of infectious agents or foreign bodies should be excluded. This may be accomplished with the use of cultures, special stains, and microscopic examination for foreign bodies under polarized

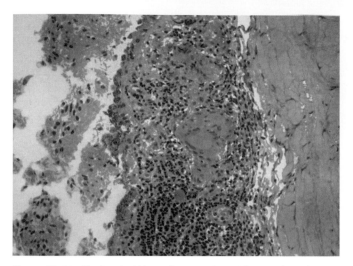

Figure 22-11. Chorioretinal biopsy from a patient with sarcoidosis shows inflammatory cell infiltration into retina with noncaseating granuloma. (Hematoxylin & eosin; original magnification ×400.) *(Courtesy of Chi-Chao Chan, MD.)*

light. Several types of inclusion bodies have been noted in biopsies of sarcoid granulomas. Asteroid bodies composed of vimentin intermediate filaments, Schaumann's bodies composed of aggregates of basophilic material, and crystalline inclusions containing calcium carbonate crystals have all been described.

Sarcoidosis is thought to be a Th1-driven inflammatory process. Activated Th1-type CD4+ T lymphocytes are fundamental to the development of the disease, including granuloma formation.[41] A number of Th1 cytokines have also been associated with disease activity. A reduced expression of regulatory T cell-associated forkhead box P3 (FoxP3) genes in CD4+ T cells obtained from bronchoalveolar lavage fluid of patients with sarcoidosis suggests a possible defect in regulatory T cells with disease pathogenesis.[42]

Most histologic specimens from enucleated eyes have shown granulomas of the retina, choroid, or the region of the retinal pigment epithelium.[14,43] Histologic examination of the vitreous and perivascular and retinal infiltrates revealed epithelioid cells.[43] The deeper lesions at the level of the retinal pigment epithelium are granulomas like the Dalen–Fuchs nodules of sympathetic ophthalmia. Choroidal involvement is infrequent, and Gass and Olson[43] wrote that many lesions that have been called focal choroiditis in sarcoidosis may be granulomas below the pigment epithelium and not discretely involving the choroid. However, large choroidal granulomas do occur (see Fig. 22-7).

The pathologic findings of the acute iritis of sarcoidosis can resemble erythema nodosum rather than the pulmonary granulomas that are prominent and diagnostic of sarcoidosis. Some suggest that iritis may be a hypersensitivity reaction of the eye that occurs in a number of diseases of diverse cause in a manner similar to the occurrence of erythema nodosum in association with a variety of unrelated diseases. It is clear that the granulomatous reaction that is characteristic of sarcoidosis is not necessarily the cause of some of the clinical pathologic conditions but rather a secondary response to an underlying immune sensitization.

Diagnosis

Although the definitive diagnosis of sarcoidosis requires biopsy confirmation, sarcoidosis can sometimes be diagnosed in patients with a characteristic clinical presentation. Asymptomatic patients between the ages of 20 and 40 years with bilateral symmetric hilar and paratracheal lymphadenopathy are likely to have sarcoidosis. This likelihood is increased in patients who also have arthralgias, erythema nodosum, or an associated uveitis. However, in most patients a biopsy is needed to make the diagnosis.

Our diagnostic approach is to closely examine the skin, conjunctiva, and lacrimal glands for nodular lesions to biopsy. Biopsy of nodular skin lesions can show granulomas diagnostic for sarcoidosis; however, biopsy of lesions of erythema nodosum shows a nonspecific vasculitis and is not useful. The incidence of positive conjunctival biopsy results in patients with biopsy-proven sarcoidosis is 27–55% in patients without a discrete conjunctival lesion but falls to 12% in patients in whom sarcoidosis is suspected.[24] Granulomas were found on biopsy of the lacrimal gland in 22% of patients with presumed ocular sarcoidosis.[44] The diagnostic yield of lacrimal gland biopsy is improved if there is increased uptake on a gallium scan or if the gland is clinically enlarged. The presence of specific inflammatory markers on biopsies of the conjunctiva and lacrimal gland may also improve the sensitivity and specificity of these biopsies. We studied lacrimal gland biopsy specimens from 14 patients with sarcoidosis.[45] Although few biopsies showed classic histopathologic findings of noncaseating granuloma, immunohistochemical staining showed a consistent preponderance of infiltrating activated CD4+ T cells and macrophages. In addition to the presence of tumor necrosis factor (TNF)-α, we noted increased expression of the major histocompatibility complex antigens, HLA-DR and HLA-DQ, and the cell adhesion molecules, intercellular adhesion molecule-1 (ICAM-1) and lymphocyte function antigen-1 (LFA-1).

Of patients with sarcoidosis 90% will have an abnormal chest X-ray (**Fig. 22-12**), and transbronchial biopsy is often a sensitive and specific diagnostic test. Approximately 60% of patients with sarcoidosis have granulomas on a transbronchial lung biopsy, even those with a normal chest radiograph (stage 0 disease).[3] When there is a parenchymal abnormality on the chest film, almost 90% of patients will have granulomas on transbronchial lung biopsy. However, some patients do require multiple biopsies to make the correct diagnosis. Some data suggest that a CT scan of the chest may be useful in diagnosing sarcoidosis because it is more sensitive than conventional chest roentgenography. Kosmorsky and co-workers[46] reported on two elderly patients with uveitis for whom chest CT scans showed mediastinal lymphadenopathy. Subsequent lymph node biopsy by mediastinoscopy demonstrated sterile noncaseating granulomas consistent with the diagnosis of sarcoidosis. Endoscopic ultrasound-guided fine needle aspiration of intrathoracic lymph nodes was reported to have a diagnostic yield of 82% in one series.[47]

Laboratory testing may be useful in the diagnosis of sarcoidosis. Transbronchial lung biopsy cannot be performed on all patients with a uveitis compatible with ocular sarcoidosis, and diagnostic tests can help determine which

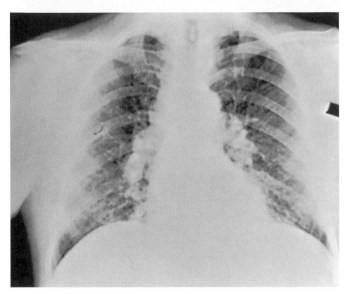

Figure 22-12. Chest radiograph showing the characteristic features of stage II sarcoidosis. Bilateral hilar adenopathy and diffuse interstitial lung disease are seen. *(From Weinberger SE: Principles of Pulmonary Medicine, p 164. Copyright 2003 Elsevier.)*

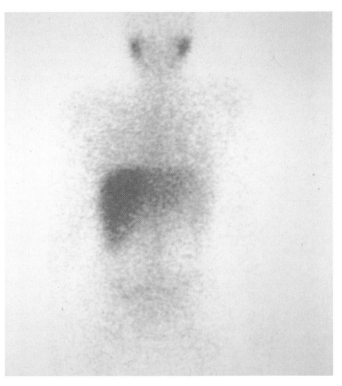

Figure 22-13. Gallium scan of the upper torso and head of a patient with active systemic sarcoidosis demonstrates uptake in the parotid gland.

should undergo more invasive diagnostic procedures. ACE is predominantly produced in pulmonary macrophages and vascular endothelium, and serum ACE levels are elevated in 60–90% of patients with sarcoidosis in whom the disease is active.[48] Unfortunately, serum ACE levels may be normal in patients with quiescent or isolated disease. In addition, ACE is produced by epithelioid cells present in granulomas associated with a number of diseases, including tuberculosis, leprosy, silicosis, primary biliary cirrhosis, asbestosis, and histoplasmosis. ACE levels may be elevated in the aqueous humor of patients with ocular sarcoidosis[49] or in the cerebrospinal fluid of patients with neurosarcoidosis. ACE levels may be high in normal children and are more difficult to interpret as a diagnostic test.

Serum lysozyme levels may also be elevated in patients with sarcoidosis but are less specific than ACE and hence rarely obtained. Hypercalcemia and hypercalciuria occur in some patients as a result of increased calcium absorption after increased production of 1,25-dihydroxycholecalciferol; they can be detected on routine laboratory tests. Lymphopenia and elevated liver enzymes, particularly alkaline phosphatase, may also occur.

The Kveim skin test used to be an accepted method to diagnose sarcoidosis. Kveim antigen is prepared from the spleens of patients with proven sarcoidosis and is then injected intradermally into a patient with suspected sarcoidosis.[32] The presence of granulomatous inflammation in a skin biopsy performed 6 weeks after the injection was considered to be diagnostic for sarcoidosis. Although Kveim test results are positive in about 80% of patients with sarcoidosis, negative test results can occur in those with more limited disease.[50] In addition, the fear of transmitting infectious agents has led to reduced use of the test, and there is still no commercial preparation of Kveim antigen for clinical use. Anergy on skin testing is also seen in about one-half of patients with sarcoidosis and may help support the diagnosis.

The gallium scan, which detects concentrated radioactive gallium in areas of inflammation, can be useful for showing involvement of organs such as the lungs, lacrimal glands, and parotid glands (**Fig. 22-13**).[25,51] Bronchoalveolar lavage may show a lymphocytosis in patients with sarcoidosis. However, because bronchoalveolar lavage findings are not diagnostic for sarcoidosis, it is not commonly performed in the evaluation of patients with sarcoidosis. Pulmonary function tests can be useful in evaluating patients with suspected sarcoidosis. Limited diffusing capacity, noted as a diminished carbon monoxide diffusion in the lung, can occur before radiographic abnormalities are seen on a chest X-ray. Diminished lung volumes are later seen with the development of restrictive lung disease and reduced forced expiratory volume in 1 second (FEV_1) are also noted. We retrospectively reviewed the records of 46 patients with biopsy-proven sarcoidosis at the National Institutes of Health; 21 had uveitis. Only 61% of the patients with sarcoid uveitis had an abnormal chest X-ray, and only 36% had an elevated serum ACE level. The most sensitive diagnostic test in our patients was the pulmonary diffusing capacity, which was diminished in 78% of the patients we tested. Interestingly, there was no statistical difference in test results between patients with sarcoidosis with or without uveitis. Our current diagnostic approach is to obtain pulmonary consultation for transbronchial biopsy in patients with suspected ocular sarcoidosis who have a reduced diffusing capacity, especially if other diagnostic tests support the diagnosis.

Treatment

Asymptomatic patients with hilar adenopathy do not require therapy and can be followed. Treatment is usually reserved to prevent organ damage. Two main indications for therapy in patients with sarcoidosis are symptomatic pulmonary

285

disease and uveitis. The mainstay of therapy for both systemic and ocular sarcoidosis is administration of corticosteroids.[5,25] Internists must rely on a number of indicators of disease activity to guide their therapy. Doses of corticosteroids are adjusted, depending on clinical symptoms and signs as well as pulmonary function tests, chest X-rays, serum ACE levels, and occasionally the results of bronchoalveolar lavage. In a Cochrane Review of nine randomized clinical trials examining the use of corticosteroids for pulmonary sarcoidosis, the reviewers concluded that oral steroids improved the chest X-ray, symptoms, and spirometry over 6–24 months.[52] However, they noted that there is little evidence of an improving lung function.

The ophthalmologist is fortunate in being able to judge the severity of disease by clinical examination, and as described in Chapter 7, therapy must be tailored to the severity of the ocular disease. Acute anterior inflammation is best managed by topical corticosteroids, but frequently periocular injections of corticosteroids are needed to control severe anterior uveitis complicated by iris nodules and glaucoma.

The treatment of chronic anterior or posterior uveitis is more difficult. Systemic therapy is often required for bilateral chronic uveitis, and patients with chronic ocular inflammatory disease frequently require higher daily doses of oral corticosteroid than those with chronic sarcoid pulmonary disease. However, sarcoidosis is often responsive to corticosteroids, and the use of high initial doses with slow tapering is effective in managing most patients. Two or three high doses of intravenous pulse corticosteroids (1 g methylprednisolone) on consecutive days may induce a more rapid remission. In patients with chronic sarcoidosis who require prolonged corticosteroid therapy, side effects often require the addition of a steroid-sparing drug. Ciclosporin and other immunosuppressive agents have had therapeutic effects in patients with sarcoidosis, although most of the data are anecdotal, coming from case series. A Cochrane Review of immunosuppressive and cytotoxic therapy for pulmonary sarcoidosis concluded that the evidence supporting the use of these therapies is limited and that side effects with some of the therapies were severe.[53] We have observed improvement of both the ocular and systemic manifestations of sarcoidosis after ciclosporin therapy,[25] but there is still no optimal safe long-term approach for the use of this drug. Supplementation with periocular steroids and pulse systemic steroids can assist in keeping the dose of ciclosporin low. Local intravitreal administration of corticosteroids as an injection or in a sustained-release implant may be useful, especially for patient with active disease limited to the eye.

Methotrexate is being used more frequently as an effective corticosteroid-sparing agent in the treatment of sarcoidosis. In a small randomized, double-masked trial of methotrexate versus placebo, patients receiving methotrexate appeared to require less prednisone to control their disease.[54] Low-dose methotrexate also appeared to be an effective and safe adjunctive therapy in patients with sarcoid-associated panuveitis.[55] In this retrospective case series, 100% of patients requiring oral corticosteroids were able to reduce their corticosteroids from a mean initial dose of 26.6 mg/day to 1.5 mg/day, and 86% completely discontinued oral corticosteroids after receiving methotrexate. However, one must remember that up to 6 months may be required for methotrexate to take effect.

Other treatments are needed for some patients with resistant disease. Hydroxychloroquine can be an effective treatment for skin disease, CNS involvement, and some cases of pulmonary sarcoidosis.[56] Gallium nitrate, approved by the Food and Drug Administration for the treatment of hypercalcemia of malignancy, also has immunosuppressive properties. We previously showed that gallium nitrate inhibits experimental autoimmune uveitis.[57] Clinical trials studying the safety and efficacy of gallium nitrate for treating sarcoidosis and rheumatoid arthritis are in progress.[58] Recently, treatments targeting TNF have been shown to be effective in treating some patients with chronic sarcoidosis. TNF-α appears to be important in the pathogenesis of sarcoidosis. The administration of infliximab, a chimeric monoclonal antibody that inhibits TNF-α, led to a significant improvement in chronic pulmonary sarcoidosis in three patients.[59] However, a randomized, controlled clinical trial in 138 patients reported only a small increase in forced vital capacity in patients treated with infliximab compared to placebo.[60] Sarcoidosis involving the central nervous system may be resistant to treatment, and radiotherapy has been tried for unresponsive disease. Gelwan and colleagues[61] have reported the use of radiotherapy for cases of sarcoidosis involving the anterior visual pathway. Lung, heart, and liver transplantations have been performed in patients with sarcoidosis, with results similar to those seen in other diseases.[9]

Sarcoidosis produces a high incidence of glaucoma and cataract, and surgical intervention is frequently required. Because of the changes in the anterior segment and the substantial vitreous opacities that often occur in sarcoidosis, some uveitis specialists prefer to use a pars plana lensectomy to remove the cataract. However, there are no data on the relative benefits of this procedure compared to those of extracapsular cataract extraction in patients with sarcoidosis. Patients with sarcoidosis frequently have severe exacerbations of their ocular inflammation in the immediate postoperative period, and the optic disc may not be seen for the first few days. This occurs with both pars plana lensectomy and extracapsular cataract extraction. This inflammatory response peaks about 48 hours after surgery and lasts for 5 or 6 days, and patients with sarcoidosis should therefore be treated with high doses of systemic corticosteroids for the first week. The patient's immediate postoperative vision may be greatly reduced because of the vitreous haze, but it will improve as the vitritis resolves. The retinal and optic disc neovascularization that occurs in sarcoidosis frequently responds to oral corticosteroid therapy.[26] However, the subretinal neovascularization requires laser photocoagulation if it is in a treatable location.[25]

Fortunately, many patients with sarcoidosis show complete remission of their disease after several years. If sarcoidosis regresses spontaneously, it rarely recurs. In all patients with ocular manifestations of sarcoidosis the goal is to control the inflammatory disease and thereby prevent permanent visually impairing changes such as photoreceptor damage caused by chronic cystoid macular edema. The ideal therapy for all forms of sarcoidosis awaits discovery, but advances in the therapy of ocular sarcoidosis should follow both an improved understanding of the cause of systemic sarcoidosis and an insight into the relationship between the ocular manifestations and the systemic inflammatory disease.

Case 22-1

A 25-year-old white woman with sarcoidosis developed floaters and blurred vision in one eye. Examination revealed granulomatous KPs, vitreous cells, fluff balls, and a choroidal granuloma in the posterior pole temporal to the macula. Vision was 20/200, primarily because of macular edema. The patient received a periocular depot steroid injection that resulted in a partial reduction in the inflammation but no visual improvement. Four additional injections given 3 weeks apart resulted in total resolution of the inflammation and an improvement in visual acuity to 20/25. The disease remained quiet for 6 months, at which time the inflammation began to increase and vision dropped to 20/50. One periocular depot steroid injection resulted in resolution of the inflammation and a return of vision to 20/25. The patient has required one or two injections of periocular steroid every 6 months to maintain good vision in the affected eye. The other eye has remained normal.

References

1. Hunter DG, Foster CS. Systemic manifestations of sarcoidosis. In: Albert DA, Jakobiec FA, eds. Principles and practice of ophthalmology. Philadelphia, 1994, WB Saunders, pp 3132–3142.
2. Bruins Slot WJ. Ziekte van Besnier-Boeck en Febris uveoparotidea (Heerfordt). Ned Tijdshr Geneeskd 1936; 80: 2859–2870.
3. Fanburg BL. Sarcoidosis. In: Wyngaarden JB, Smith LH Jr, Bennett JC, eds. Cecil textbook of medicine. ed 19, Philadelphia, 1992, WB Saunders, pp 430–435.
4. Bresnitz EA, Strom BL. Epidemiology of sarcoidosis. Epidemiol Rev 1983; 5: 124–156.
5. Siltzbach LE, James DG, Neville E, et al. Course and prognosis of sarcoidosis around the world. Am J Med 1974; 57: 847–852.
6. Rybicke BA, Major M, Popovich J Jr, et al. Racial differences in sarcoidosis incidence: a 5-year study in a health maintenance organization. Am J Epidemiol 1997; 145: 234–241.
7. Jabs DA, Johns CJ. Ocular involvement in chronic sarcoidosis. Am J Ophthalmol 1986; 102: 297–301.
8. Milman N, Selroos O. Pulmanory sarcoidosis in the Nordic countries 1950–1982: epidemiology and clinical picture. Sarcoidosis 1990; 7: 50–57.
9. Iannuzzi MC, Rybicki BA, Teirstein AS. Sarcoidosis. N Engl J Med 2007; 357: 2153–2165.
10. Thomas PD, Hunninghake GW. Current concepts of the pathogenesis of sarcoidosis. Am Rev Respir Dis 1987; 135: 747.
11. Crystal RG, Roberts WC, Hunninghake GW, et al. Pulmonary sarcoidosis: a disease characterized and perpetuated by activated lung T-lymphocytes. Ann Intern Med 1981; 94: 73–94.
12. Hunninghake GW, Crystal RG. Pulmonary sarcoidosis: a disorder mediated by excess helper T-lymphocyte activity at sites of disease activity. N Engl J Med 1981; 305: 429–434.
13. Sememzato G, Pezzutto A, Pizzolo G. Immunohistological study in sarcoidosis: evaluation at different sites of disease activity. Clin Immunol Immunopathol 1984; 30: 29–40.
14. Chan CC, Wetzig RP, Palestine AG, et al. Immunohistopathology of ocular sarcoidosis: report of a case and discussion of immunopathogenesis. Arch Ophthalmol 1987; 105: 1398–1402.
15. Bresnitz EA, Strom BL. Epidemiology of sarcoidosis. Epidemiol Rev 1983; 5: 124–156.
16. Newman LS, Rose CS, Bresnitz EA, et al. A case control etiologic study of sarcoidosis: environmental and occupational risk factors. Am J Respir Crit Care Med 2004; 170: 1324–1330.
17. Haijzadeh R, Sato H, Carlisle J, et al. Mycobacterium tuberculosis antigen 85A induces Th-1 immune responses in systemic sarcoidosis. J Clin Immunol 2007; 27: 445–454.
17a. Crick RP, Hoyle C, Smellie H. The eyes in sarcoidosis. Br J Ophthalmol 1961; 45: 461–481.
18. Hwang CJ, Gausas RE. Sarcoid-like granulomatous orbital inflammation induced by interferon-alpha treatment. Ophthalm Plast Reconstruct Surg 2008; 24: 311–313.
19. Familial associations in sarcoidosis: a report to the Research Committee of the British Thoracic and Tuberculosis Association. Tubercle 1973; 54: 87–98.
20. Brewerton DA, Cockburn C, James DC, et al. HLA antigens in sarcoidosis. Clin Exp Immunol 1977; 27: 227–229.
21. Rossman MD, Thompson B, Ferderick M, et al. HLA-DRB1*1101: a significant risk factor for sarcoidosis in blacks and whites. Am J Hum Genet 2003; 73: 720–735.
22. Obenauf CD, Shaw HE, Sydnor CF, et al. Sarcoidosis and its ophthalmic manifestations. Am J Ophthalmol 1978; 86: 648–655.
23. James DG, Neville E, Langley DA. Ocular sarcoidosis. Trans Ophthalmol Soc UK 1976; 96: 133–139.
24. Nichols CW, Eagle RC, Yanoff M, et al. Conjunctival biopsy as an aid in the evaluation of the patient with suspected sarcoidosis. Ophthalmology 1980; 87: 287–291.
25. Palestine AG, Nussenblatt RB, Chan CC. Treatment of intraocular complications of sarcoidosis. Ann NY Acad Med 1986; 465: 564–573.
26. Spalton DJ, Sanders MD. Fundus changes in histologically confirmed sarcoidosis. Br J Ophthalmol 1981; 65: 348–358.
27. Marcus DF, Bovino JA, Burton TC. Sarcoid granuloma of the choroid. Ophthalmology 1982; 89: 1326–1330.
28. Campo RV, Aaberg TM. Choroidal granuloma in sarcoidosis. Am J Ophthalmol 1984; 97: 419–427.
29. Frank KW, Weiss H. Unusual clinical and histopathologic findings in ocular sarcoidosis. Br J Ophthalmol 1983; 67: 8–16.
30. Gragoudas ES, Regan CDJ. Peripapillary subretinal neovascularization in presumed sarcoidosis. Arch Ophthalmol 1981; 99: 1194–1197.
31. Rush JA. Retrobulbar optic neuropathy in sarcoidosis. Ann Ophthalmol 1980; 12: 390–394.
32. Mitchell DN, Scadding JG, Heard BE, et al. Sarcoidosis: histopathological definition and clinical diagnosis. J Clin Pathol 1977; 30: 395–408.
33. Scott GC, Berman JM, Higgins JL Jr. CT patterns of nodular hepatic and splenic sarcoidosis: a review of the literature. J Comput Assist Tomogr 1997; 21: 369–372.
34. Hoover DL, Khan JA, Giangiacomo J. Pediatric ocular sarcoidosis. Surv Ophthalmol 1986; 30: 215.
35. Perruquet JL, Harrington TM, Davis DE, et al. Sarcoid arthritis in a North American Caucasian population. J Rheumatol 1984; 11: 521–525.
36. Yotsumoto S, Takahashi Y, Takei S, et al. Early onset sarcoidosis masquerading as juvenile rheumatoid arthritis. J Am Acad Dermatol 2000; 43: 969–971.
37. Roy M, Sharma OP, Chan K. Sarcoidosis presenting in infancy: a rare occurrence. Sarcoidosis Vasc Diffuse Lung Dis 1999; 16: 224–227.
38. Raphael SA, Blau EB, Zhang WH, et al. Analysis of a large kindred with Blau syndrome for HLA, autoimmunity, and sarcoidosis. Am J Dis Child 1993; 147: 842–848.
39. Schurmann M, Valentonyte R, Hampe J, et al. CARD15 gene mutations in sarcoidosis. Eur Respir J 2003; 22: 748–754.

40. Manouvrier-Hanu S, Puech B, Piette F, et al. Blau syndrome of granulomatous arthritis, iritis, and skin rash: a new family and review of the literature. Am J Med Genet 1998; 76: 217–221.

41. Grunewald J, Eklund A. Role of CD4+ T cells in sarcoidosis. Proc Am Thorac Soc 2007; 4: 461–464.

42. Idali F, Wahlström J, Müller-Suur C, et al. Analysis of regulatory T cell associated forkhead box P3 expression in the lungs of patients with sarcoidosis. Clin Exp Immunol 2008; 152(1): 127–137. Epub 2008 Feb 14.

43. Gass JDM, Olson CL. Sarcoidosis with optic nerve and retinal involvement. Arch Ophthalmol 1976; 94: 945–950.

44. Cohen KL, Peiffer RL, Powell DA. Sarcoidosis and ocular disease in a young child. Arch Ophthalmol 1981; 99: 422–424.

45. Smith JA, Chan CC, Egwuagu CE, et al. Immunohistochemical examination of lacrimal gland tissue from patients with ocular sarcoidosis. Adv Exp Med Biol 1998; 438: 599–602.

46. Kosmorsky GS, Meisler DM, Rice TW, et al. Chest computed tomography and mediastinoscopy in the diagnosis of sarcoidosis-associated uveitis. Am J Ophthalmol 1998; 126: 132–134.

47. Annema JT, Veselic M, Rabe KF. Endoscopic ultrasound-guided fine-needle aspiration for the diagnosis of sarcoidosis. Eur Respir J 2005; 25: 405–409.

48. Lieberman J. Enzymes in sarcoidosis: angiotensin converting enzyme (ACE). Clin Lab Med 1989; 9: 745.

49. Weinreb RN, Sandman R, Ryder MI, et al. Angiotensin converting enzyme activity in human aqueous humor. Arch Ophthalmol 1985; 34: 103.

50. Munro CS, Mitchell DN. The Kveim response: still useful, still a puzzle. Thorax 1987; 42: 321.

51. Weinreb RN. Diagnosing sarcoidosis by transconjunctival biopsy of the lacrimal gland. Am J Ophthalmol 1984; 97: 573–576.

52. Paramothayan NS, Jones PW. Corticosteroids for pulmonary sarcoidosis. Cochrane Database Syst Rev 2005; 2: CD001114.

53. Paramothayan S, Lasserson TJ, Walters EH. Immunosuppressive and cytotoxic therapy for pulmonary sarcoidosis. Cochrane Database Syst Rev 2006; 3: CD003536.

54. Baughman RP, Winget DB, Lower EE. Methotrexate is steroid sparing in acute sarcoidosis: results of a double blind, randomized trial. Sarcoidosis Vasc Diffuse Lung Dis 2000; 17: 60–66.

55. Dev S, McCallum RM, Jaffe GJ. Methotrexate treatment for sarcoid-associated panuveitis. Ophthalmology 1999; 106: 111–118.

56. Baltzan M, Mehta S, Kirkham TH, et al. Randomized trial of prolonged chloroquine therapy in advanced pulmonary sarcoidosis. Am J Respir Crit Care Med 1999; 160: 192–197.

57. Lobanoff MC, Kozhich AT, Mullet DI, et al. Effect of gallium nitrate on experimental autoimmune uveitis. Exp Eye Res 1997; 65: 797–801.

58. Apseloff G. Therapeutic uses of gallium nitrate: past, present, and future. Am J Ther 1999; 6: 327–329.

59. Baughman RP, Lower EE. Infliximab for refractory sarcoidosis. Sarcoidosis Vasc Diffuse Lung Dis 2001; 18: 70–74.

60. Baughman RP, Drent M, Kavuru M, et al. Infliximab therapy in patients with chronic sarcoidosis and pulmonary involvement. Am J Respir Crit Care Med 2006; 174: 795–802.

61. Gelwan MJ, Kellen RI, Burde RM, et al. Sarcoidosis of the anterior visual pathway: successes and failures. J Neurol Neurosurg 1988; 51: 1473.

Sympathetic Ophthalmia

Robert B. Nussenblatt

Key concepts

- This is a bilateral condition.
- Some reports suggest that this entity is more commonly seen after vitrectomy than is endophthalmitis.
- Dalen–Fuchs nodules are commonly seen in the retinal periphery of eyes with this entity but they are not pathognomonic for the disease.

Sympathetic ophthalmia probably is the intraocular inflammatory condition best known to practitioners outside of ophthalmology. Albeit not yet defined at that time, it has been suggested that JS Bach's poor vision after couching for cataracts may have been due to this disorder.[1] It has also stimulated enormous interest within our field since its clinical description by MacKenzie[2] early in the 19th century. The number of patients having this problem each year is relatively small, but the dread of losing not only the involved eye but the contralateral, untouched eye as well in a potentially sight-threatening process is indeed great, and justifiably so. Further, the potential mechanisms to explain such a process are many, which has provided the more intellectually (and imaginatively) inclined with ample material for thought. Newer observations have certainly helped place this disorder in perspective.

Clinical appearance and prevalence

Sympathetic ophthalmia is a bilateral granulomatous uveitis that occurs after either intentional or unintentional penetrating trauma to one eye. Thereby trauma to one eye (the exciting eye) will result in an inflammatory response not only in that eye but also in the contralateral eye (the sympathizing eye). It is a disease that was known to the ancient Greeks and was referred to in the teachings of Hippocrates.[3] It was recognized also during the early and late Middle Ages and into the 18th and 19th centuries with MacKenzie's full clinical description. Fuchs[4] published the classic description of the disease in 1905, establishing it as a separate entity. The disease can begin as early as several days after the penetrating insult up to decades later, with the clinical diagnosis becoming apparent in 80% of patients some 3 months after injury to the exciting eye[5] and in 90% within 1 year of trauma.[6,7] Sympathetic ophthalmia occurs more often after nonsurgical trauma. Liddy and Stuart[8] reported that the disorder occurred in 0.2% of eyes with nonsurgical wounds, and Holland[9]

found the disorder in 0.5% of eyes with nonsurgical trauma. Marak[5] estimated the incidence of this disease to be fewer than 10 cases in 100 000 surgical penetrating wounds. In a review by Gass,[10] in which 26 eye pathology laboratories were surveyed for a 5-year period from 1975 through 1980, sympathetic ophthalmia was diagnosed in 53 eyes (two of every 1000 eyes examined); 55% of these occurrences were posttraumatic. In the same report a survey of 34 retinal surgeons who had performed 14 915 vitrectomies disclosed that sympathetic ophthalmia occurred in nine eyes (incidence of 0.06%), with one eye having vitrectomy as the only operative procedure performed (incidence of 0.01%). Recent studies suggested a change in the major initiating factor of sympathetic ophthalmia, with ocular surgery, particularly vitreoretinal surgery, now being the major risk for this disorder.[11,12] This trend is being seen worldwide. In a review of 10 cases of sympathetic ophthalmia in Singapore from 1993 to 2003,[13] the authors report that the disease occurred in three after trauma, and after surgery in seven. Of those seven, four cases were seen after vitreoretinal surgery, but two after diode laser cyclophotoablation and one after Nd:YAG laser cyclotherapy. In their commentary, Kilmartin and colleagues[11] calculated the risk of sympathetic ophthalmia to be 1 : 1152 retinal surgical procedures and perhaps as much as 1 : 800.[14] If this calculation reflects a true trend, the risk would be twice that reported previously for vitrectomy (0.06%).[10] The authors raise the issue as to whether patients should be informed of this risk in the consent form, because the calculated risk is more than twice the 0.05% risk of infectious endophthalmitis after vitrectomy (**Table 23-1**).

It is interesting to note that no cases of sympathetic ophthalmia were reported in the 467 perforated globes observed by the US military during World War II, the Korean War, and the Vietnam War.[15] However, there was one recent case of a soldier injured in the Iraq conflict.[16] These findings are in contrast to the older literature of the last century, which suggested an incidence of about 2%,[7] and it was believed that 16% of ocular injuries during the American Civil War resulted in sympathetic ophthalmia. In a recent prospective surveillance study in the UK and the Republic of Ireland[12] drawn from a surveillance of 59 million citizens, 17 patients with newly diagnosed sympathetic ophthalmia were reported in a 12-month period, and a minimum estimated incidence of 0.03 in 100 000 was calculated.

Sympathetic ophthalmia is thought to be more common in males – almost certainly because of their higher incidence of ocular trauma – but this demographic is changing as the causes of sympathetic ophthalmia change (see below). Also, it is thought to be more common in lighter-skinned ethnic

Table 23-1 Changes in SO trends worth taking into consideration. (From Vote BJ, et al. Changing trends in sympathetic ophthalmia. Clin Exp Ophthalmol 2004; 32: 542–5.)

Trend	Historical	Current
Cause	Post trauma	Post surgery (especially vitreoretinal)
Patients	Males and children (reflecting trauma peaks)	No sex preference (reflects positive impact of injury prevention programs) and increasingly elderly patients (reflects impact of ocular surgery)
Incidence	Considered disappearing 30 years ago	Probably increasing (underdiagnosed?)
Onset	For 65% within 2–8 weeks (for 90%, onset <1 year from trauma or most recent surgery)	Many delayed presentations (for significant percentage onset >1 year from trauma or most recent surgery)
Presentation	Granulomatous panuveitis	Any clinical uveitis
Outcome	Enucleation within 2 weeks for prevention of SO	Enucleation solely of SO prevention questionable
Visual prognosis	Poor	Reasonable due to moden immunosuppression

groups, but this may be because of better reporting and recognition of the disease.

We reviewed 32 patients with sympathetic ophthalmia seen at the National Eye Institute during a 10-year period.[17] They represented 1.4% of the 2287 patients with uveitis seen by us during that period. There was no sex preponderance (16 males and 16 females) and 23 of the 32 patients had their disease develop after accidental injury. The patients' ages spanned from 3 years to 80 years. In our group of patients, sympathetic ophthalmia developed within 1 year of injury in 56%, with approximately 31% of them developing disease between 2 weeks and 3 months after the ocular insult, whereas one patient's disease developed some 46 years later. Hakin and associates[18] reported their experience with 18 patients: 15 of their cases followed trauma, 11 of which occurred after a known penetrating wound, and the other four occurred after a posterior scleral rupture. Three cases occurred after retinal detachment, with patients having on average three surgical interventions. Surgical trauma, particularly vitrectomy,[19] is well recognized as an antecedent event to sympathetic ophthalmia and, as mentioned above, appears to be more common than accidental trauma as the initiating event[10,20–22] (**Fig. 23-1**).

Classic presentation

In the classic presentation the inflammatory response seen in the anterior chamber is granulomatous, with mutton-fat keratic precipitates on the corneal endothelium and findings of an acute anterior uveitis. However, the anterior chamber inflammatory response can be relatively mild, with the inflammation taking on a nongranulomatous appearance as well. There is generally a moderate to severe vitritis accompanied by changes in the posterior segment. Of particular note are multiple white-yellow lesions in the periphery, which sometimes become confluent (**Fig. 23-2**). These represent the clinical appearance of a Dalen–Fuchs nodule, a histologic finding. Swelling of the disc (papillitis) can be prominent, and circumpapillary choroidal lesions can also occur. Retinal involvement is not an uncommon finding in sympathetic ophthalmia, although this involvement, classically thought of as a choroidal disease, has been amply corroborated by histologic findings (see following discussion). Although rare, subretinal neovascularization has been reported to occur in sympathetic ophthalmia,[23] as it has been

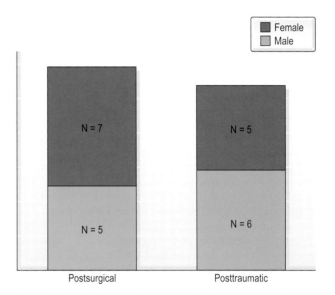

Figure 23-1. Distribution of patients at the National Eye Institute in whom sympathetic ophthalmia developed after surgery and after trauma. Although these data were collected in the early 1990s, the number of postsurgical occurrences is interesting. *(From Arch Ophthalmol 113: 597–600, 1995. Copyright © 1995, American Medical Association. All rights reserved.)*

in the Vogt–Koyanagi–Harada syndrome (VKH) (see Chapter 24) (see Fig. 24-2).

A small number of patients with sympathetic ophthalmia report or demonstrate extraocular findings not dissimilar from those seen in VKH (see Chapter 24), such as cells in the cerebrospinal fluid, hearing disturbances such as high-frequency deafness,[24] and hair and skin changes. These extraocular findings are rare in sympathetic ophthalmia compared to VKH, in which they are fairly common symptoms that are important indicators in making the diagnosis. They are also important in the conceptualization of autoimmune disease, because sympathetic ophthalmia is the only disease for which we know when a specific event leading to autosensitization has occurred. The development of extraocular signs must be secondary to ocular immunization.

It should be noted that the clinical appearance of sympathetic ophthalmia comprises a spectrum that ranges from the very mild to the severe. Lewis and coworkers[25] reported a patient with sympathetic ophthalmia after trauma and vitrectomy that was confined to the posterior segment in such

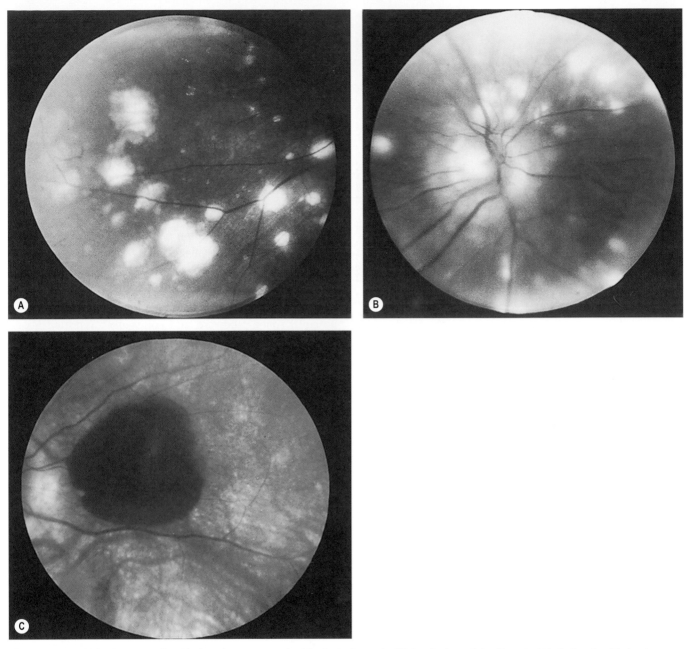

Figure 23-2. A, Multiple cream-colored lesions that correspond to histologic diagnosis of Dalen–Fuchs nodules. Characteristically they tend to be strewn throughout the periphery and can extend to the disc and at times into the posterior pole (**B**). Initially they appear to have 'substance' to them, raising the overlying retina. With time they appear atrophic. Although considerably less common in sympathetic ophthalmia than in VKH (see Chapter 24), subretinal neovascularization with resultant hemorrhage (**C**) can occur, in this case nasal to the disc in a one-eyed patient and not affecting vision.

a way that it resembled focal lesions of acute posterior multi-focal placoid pigment epitheliopathy (APMPPE) (see Chapter 29). A mild anterior uveitis has also been reported, but this has not been our experience. Carrying the concept to the extreme, some have proposed the notion of a unilateral sympathetic ophthalmia. It is quite possible that the sympathizing response may be so mild as to disappear with minimal or no sequelae, and the spectrum of the histologic response seen would support this concept. However, if no inflammatory disease is noted, or if none is seen on a histologic specimen, it seems inappropriate to use the term sympathetic ophthalmia to describe the disease under observation. Marak[5] describes a phenomenon he has called sympathetic irritation, which occurs in the fellow eye after

injury to or disease in one eye. About one-third of these patients may have cells and flare in the anterior chamber, with 67% of patients complaining of photophobia and a smaller number having perilimbal or conjunctival injection or both. The distinction between this entity and 'mild' sympathetic ophthalmia seems to us quite unclear. There has been a suggested variant of sympathetic ophthalmia with diffuse subretinal fibrotic changes. In one report of a patient who developed the disease after multiple operations for the repair of a retinal detachment, there was fast detererioration of vision with the fibrotic changes becoming more extensive (**Fig. 23-3**). This eye had many CD20+ cells (B cells) along with CD3+ (T cells) and CD68+ cells (macrophages).[26] In another report of a multifocal granuloma and fibrosis, PCR

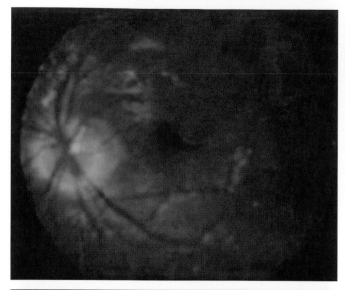

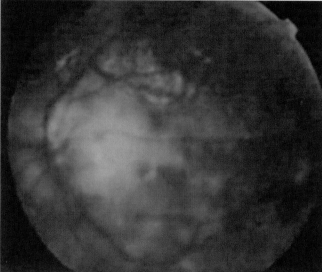

Figure 23-3. Sympathetic ophthalmia developed in this eye after successful retinal detachment surgery and vitrectomy. Note that the OCT shows areas of exudative detachment and hyperreflectivity at the level of the RPE, probably scarring. *(From Abu El-Asrar AM, Al Kuraya H, and Al-Ghamdi A, Sympathetic ophthalmia after successful retinal reattachment surgery with vitrectomy. Eur J Ophthalmol 2006; 16(6): 891–4.)*

was negative for herpes viruses, and types III, IV, V, and VI collagens were noted in the fibrosis; antibodies to photoreceptors were also seen.[27]

Several ocular entities have been associated with sympathetic ophthalmia. Phacoanaphylaxis has been observed,[28] and Blodi[29] noted its occurrence in 23% of eyes with sympathetic ophthalmia. He believed that the presence of the two entities in the same eye reflected the fact that these patients have a predisposition for autoimmune phenomena. In their excellent review of 105 cases, Lubin and coworkers[6] found an incidence of 46%. It should be noted that both entities can be found in the sympathizing (noninjured) eye as well,[30] and the phacoanaphylaxis can be a confounding element in attempting to make the diagnosis of sympathetic ophthalmia (see later discussion). It had been suggested in the past that infection would 'protect' from sympathetic ophthalmia. However, this disorder has been reported after

a central corneal perforation secondary to an *Aspergillosis fumigatus* keratitis.[31]

Malignant melanoma has also been associated with sympathetic ophthalmia.[32–34] In 400 cases of sympathetic ophthalmia evaluated by Easom and Zimmerman[35] at the Armed Forces Institute of Pathology, seven were found to involve a malignant melanoma. Fries and colleagues[36] reported sympathetic ophthalmia after helium ion irradiation of a choroidal melanoma, whereas Margo and Pautler[37] reported the development of a granulomatous bilateral uveitis after therapy with proton-beam irradiation. In the latter case the authors stressed the fact that the sutures securing the four tantalum rings to the sclera did not penetrate the uvea.

Sympathetic ophthalmia has been reported to occur after cyclocryotherapy.[38] Harrison[39] discussed the development of sympathetic ophthalmia in a patient who underwent cyclocryotherapy for neovascular glaucoma. No penetration of the sclera was noted in that patient. However, in one case of sympathetic ophthalmia after cyclocryotherapy it was felt that the procedure resulted in microperforations with inflammatory cells as well as uveal pigment found in the subconjunctival space.[40] Edward and colleagues[41] reported a case after noncontact neodymium yttrium–aluminum–garnet (Nd:YAG) laser cyclotherapy. Lam and coworkers[42] reported three others, and the problem was discussed by Tessler and colleagues.[43] There may still be the rare case of no obvious clinical penetration into the globe, such as the case of penetrating trauma resulting in hyphema.[44] Of course it is possible that a micropentatrating wound did occur.

Cataract surgery has been mentioned rarely as a cause of this entity.[45] In one report[46] the disease occurred 3 months after an intracapsular cataract extraction and anterior chamber lens placement in which the immediate postoperative problems of flat chamber, pupillary block, and wound dehiscence occurred, with one of the haptics protruding into the subconjunctival space. Vitrectomy and removal of the lens resulted in control of the disease and improvement of vision. A similar case was reported by El-Asrar and Al-Obeidan.[47] We saw a patient who had a history of retinal detachment repair but whose sympathetic ophthalmia was diagnosed weeks after having received laser therapy for a retinal tear in the other eye,[17] as did El-Asrar et al.[48] reporting a case after retinal detachment surgery and vitrectomy.

There is an ongoing debate as to whether an evisceration or enucleation should be performed. Many have claimed that evisceration carries a risk of sympathetic ophthalmia. Du Toit[49] et al. reviewed 1392 patients who had penetrating eye trauma at the Groote Schuur Hospital in South Africa: 491 (35.5%) had a primary evisceration and no cases of sympathetic ophthalmia were seen in this group. However, we do see sporadic cases develop after this procedure, as with the patient from the Iraq conflict who had an evisceration.[16]

Sequelae

The sequelae of the inflammation noted in sympathetic ophthalmia are quite variable, depending on the severity of the ocular inflammation and whether therapy has been instituted (see later discussion of therapy). Secondary glaucoma and cataract can result from the inflammatory process, as well as retinal and optic atrophy in association with retinal detachment and/or subretinal alterations such as fibrosis and underlying choroidal atrophy. Disc neovascularization has been reported, which initially regressed with steroid therapy but was finally stabilized only with the addition of methotrexate.[50]

Tests and immunologic characteristics

Clinical testing of patients will help to put into perspective the amount and severity of sympathetic ophthalmia but will not help make the diagnosis. Fluorescein angiography is useful in evaluating the degree of posterior segment disease. Spitznas[51] noted that the fluorescein angiogram obtained during the acute stage of sympathetic ophthalmia reflects an exudative process, with multiple subretinal enlarging hyperfluorescent spots and pooling of dye (**Fig. 23-4**). This observation is further emphasized by OCT. Abu Azar et al.[48] reported the presence of multiple exudative retinal detachments and areas of hyperreflectivity at the level of the RPE (**Fig. 23-5**). Although Spitznas thought that the retinal vasculature was not involved, we have seen evidence of late staining of the retinal vessels. During the cicatricial phase there is a coarsening of the pigment pattern in the fundus. The areas that are believed to correspond to Dalen–Fuchs nodules will, in the later stages of the disease, become atrophic and appear on the angiogram as window defects.

Sympathetic ophthalmia has been studied using indocyanine green angiography.[52] Two patterns of fluorescence were observed. The first was a pattern of hypofluorescence in the intermediate phase of the angiogram, followed by a fading, and the second was a hypofluorescent pattern that persisted throughout the course of the study. The first was interpreted as showing active lesions, whereas the persistent pattern was that of a cicatricial or atrophic lesion. Saatci and colleagues[53] used ICG to follow the therapeutic response of a patient who developed sympathetic ophthalmia after a perforated anterior staphyloma. During active disease there were multiple hyperflourescent dots which coalesced and then with adequate therapy there was a minimal residual noted[53] (**Fig. 23-6**).

As might be expected, findings on both electroretinography and electrooculography can be affected by the disease.

Dreyer and associates[54] observed changes in the photopic cone b-wave amplitudes and scotopic rod b-wave amplitudes during acute disease, with improvement in these functions after successful therapy.

The immunogenetics of the disease have been studied and appear to be identical to those of the Vogt–Koyanagi–Harada syndrome. Davis and coworkers[55] reported HLA typing results in a small series of patients with sympathetic ophthalmia that appeared to be the same as that of the larger VKH group. Haplotypes HLA-DR4, DRw53, and DQw3 were found more often in both groups than in control subjects. Further work using high-resolution DNA-based HLA typing has been done. In a study reported by Kilmartin and coworkers[56] the highest relative risk was found for the haplotype HLA-DRB1*0404-DQA1*0301. Patients with that haplotype were more prone to develop sympathetic ophthalmia earlier and needed more immunosuppressive therapy to control the disease. It is significant that this association appears to be the same in both Japanese patients[57] and those of European origin. Further work suggests that there was a significant association between the IL-10–1082 SNP and disease recurrence, whereas the GCC IL-10 promoter haplotype (IL-10-1082G, -819C, and -592C) was seen to be protective against disease recurrence.[58] Of interest, yet another single nucleotide polymorphism (SNP) of IL-10 (-1082A) was found to be associated with unremitting sympathetic ophthalmia.[59]

The histologic features of sympathetic ophthalmia, which are rather distinctive, were first described by Fuchs in 1905.[4] In the full-blown picture the choroid is markedly thickened by a sea of lymphocytes, with a granulomatous nonnecrotizing reaction as the predominant feature (**Fig. 23-7**). In general, the choriocapillaris tends to be spared, although this is not always the case. The infiltrate in the choroid can also have large numbers of eosinophils. Although plasma cell infiltration into the choroid was not thought to be a part of the disease, these cells were noted in 85.7% of the cases reviewed by Lubin and coworkers.[6] Marak and colleagues[60] reported the presence of more choroidal granulomas and eosinophils in African-American than in white patients, but no differences have been noted between Chinese patients and those from the United States.[61] As already noted, retinal changes are not rare. Croxatto and coworkers[62] described retinal detachment and retinal perivasculitis in 50% of the 100 eyes with sympathetic ophthalmia they examined, whereas 18% had mild inflammatory infiltrates into the retina.

Dalen–Fuchs nodules

A typical but by no means pathognomonic finding in sympathetic ophthalmia is Dalen–Fuchs nodules (**Fig. 23-8**), which occur in about one-third of eyes with sympathetic ophthalmia.[2,6] On fluorescein angiography the lesion may block early (i.e., become hypofluorescent) and then stain late (i.e., hyperfluorescence).[63] As the lesions mature, with ultimate disruption of the retinal pigment epithelium (RPE) and probably a decrease in the inflammatory process, these lesions may simply appear as window defects. These lesions were thought by Fuchs[4] to represent RPE cells that had migrated and transformed. Although early Dalen–Fuchs nodules may represent such a phenomenon,[64] Jakobiec and coworkers[65] and Chan and colleagues[66,67] used monoclonal

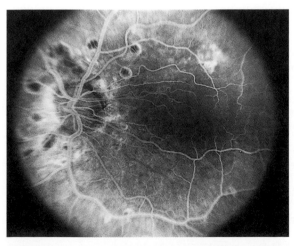

Figure 23-4. Fluorescein angiogram showing initial blockage of Dalen–Fuchs nodules, with ultimate hyperfluorescence of the lesion.

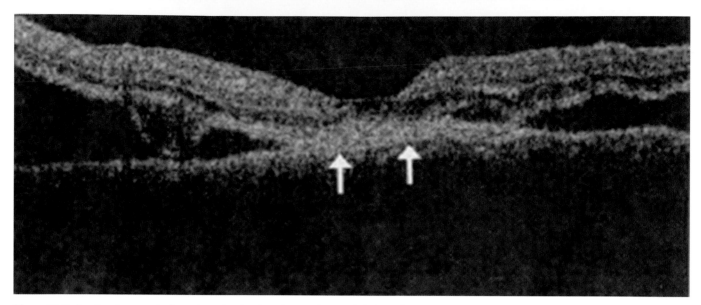

Figure 23-5. Fundus photograph of a patient who developed sympathetic ophthalmia after retinal surgery. Peripapillary subretinal fibrosis was seen initially, involving the macula 3 months later. *(Reproduced with permission from Immunopathology of Progressive Subretinal Fibrosis: A Variant of Sympathetic Ophthalmia, Wee-Kiak Lim, FRCOphth, FRCS (Ed), Soon-Phaik Chee, FRCOphth, FRCS(G), Ivy Sng, FRCPA, Robert Burton Nussenblatt, MD, and Chi-Chao Chan, MD Am J Ophthalmol 2004;138:475–477)*

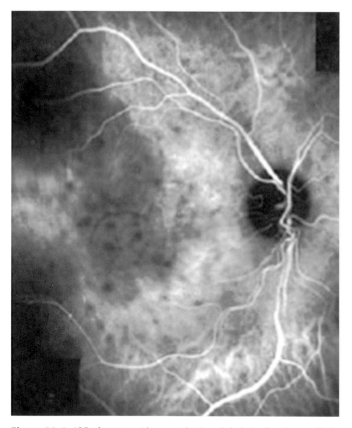

Figure 23-6. ICG of an eye with sympathetic ophthalmia showing multiple hypocyanescent dots during the intermediate phase of the study.

(Reproduced with permission from A Osman Sattci, Eser Pasa, Meltem Söylev, Nilüfer Koçak, Ismet Durak, Süleyman Kaynak, Sympathetic Ophthalmia and Indocyanine Green Angiography, Arch Opthalmol. Vol 122, Oct 2004 www.archophthalmol.com)

antibodies and structural analysis to demonstrate that Dalen–Fuchs nodules were made up of a mixture of Ia+, OKM1+ cells (presumably histiocytes), and depigmented RPE cells, which were Ia⁻ and OKM1⁻. These authors' conclusions, which were similar for the epithelioid cells seen in the choroid itself, were corroborated by Rao and coworkers.[68] The subsets of infiltrating lymphocytes into the choroid have been identified with the use of immunohistochemical techniques. Jakobiec and colleagues[65] noted that the predominant T cell was of the CD8+ subset (suppressor/cytotoxic cell) in the choroid of an eye removed 1.5 years after the initial surgical trauma. Chan and coworkers[69] evaluated an eye enucleated for the disease only several months after the initial nonsurgical trauma and found that the predominant T cell was the CD4 (Leu-3a) subset, the helper/inducer subset. The sympathizing eye of the same patients was eventually studied,[69] and in this eye the predominant T-cell subset had changed to the suppressor/cytotoxic (CD8+) subset, as had been seen in the study of Jakobiec and coworkers. The interpretation of these observations is that the human eye's inflammatory response in this disease parallels that seen in the experimentally induced uveitis model in lower mammals (see Chapter 1), that is, there is a dynamic, changing cellular immune response initiated by the helper T cell. As the disease progresses the body attempts to downregulate the immune response, and this is done by an influx of large numbers of the suppressor subset of T cells. Others have emphasized the presence of B cells in the infiltrate, found in more chronic conditions.

Chemokines that have been found in sympathetic ophthalmia include matrix metalloproteinase-9, stromal cell-derived factor-1, and monocytic chemotactic protein-1.[70] None of these is surprising, all being found in the context of an inflammatory response.

Preservation of the choriocapillaris

One of the classic findings in both sympathetic ophthalmia and the Vogt–Koyanagi–Harada syndrome is the preservation of the choriocapillaris. This is seen even with the choroid filled with inflammatory cells. It has been suggested that the RPE can play both a pro- and an antiinflammatory role in the eye.[71] Although RPE cells in culture may generate proinflammatory cytokines such as interleukin (IL)-1 and IL-6,

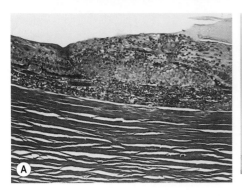
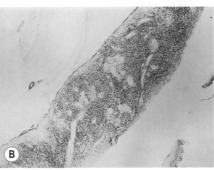

Figure 23-7. A, Markedly thickened choroid with nonnecrotizing granulomatous inflammation surrounded by lymphocytes, which is typical of sympathetic ophthalmia. **B,** Immunohistochemical techniques reveal dark areas of cells that bear OKT3 marking, indicating that they are mature T cells. Central areas that have no black staining represent areas of granulomatous reaction. Retina can be seen above the choroid.

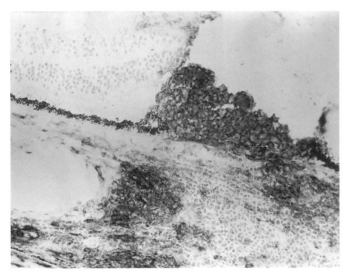

Figure 23-8. Immunohistochemical staining of a Dalen–Fuchs nodule with monoclonal antibody OKM1, which is specific for macrophages. Note that most cells in this particular nodule are of that lineage, with smaller area of macrophages in the choroid.

they may suppress the inflammatory response by releasing factors such as retinal pigment epithelial protective protein, which is believed to suppress neutrophil superoxide generation.[72,73]

The foregoing scenario, however, may not explain all cases. Several authors[62,67,74,75] have stressed the fact that the classic findings just outlined represent one point in a spectrum of disease recognized clinically as sympathetic ophthalmia. An immunohistochemical study was completed in 29 patients with sympathetic ophthalmia.[76] In 20 eyes, T cells predominated in the choroidal infiltration, whereas in four eyes – all from male patients – B cells were predominantly found. The presence of B cells was correlated to long-term disease (more than 9 months) and phthisical changes. It has classically been taught that the presence of B cells in the choroid of an eye with sympathetic ophthalmia is extremely rare. The authors of this study suggested that these findings may reflect a secondary pathologic process. They further speculated on these findings from a therapeutic point of view. It could be argued that in light of these observations, cytotoxic agents rather than more T-cell-specific drugs (e.g., ciclosporin, tacrolimus (FK506), or perhaps daclizumab) may be a more logical choice for patients whose disease does not respond to steroid therapy.

There is no established and accepted laboratory test for sympathetic ophthalmia. Sen and coworkers[77] measured the level of serum β_2-microglobulin levels in the blood of patients with sympathetic ophthalmia. They found levels to be high in these patients compared to those with traumatic uveitis and in control subjects. The levels appeared to be higher in the initial stages and reflected the severity of the disease. These results need to be corroborated. Immunohistochemistry of eight eyes with sympathetic ophthalmia showed an increased expression of TNF-α in the photoreceptor layer, whereas iNOS was found in the mitochondria, suggesting that photoreceptor oxidative stress occurs in the absence of a leukocyte infiltrate and that this may lead to vison loss.[78] A recent report by Chan's group has shown the presence of IL-17 in the macrophages and granuloma of sympathetic ophthalmia eyes. This is in agreement with the concept that the IL-17 is a major player in propagating chronic inflammatory disease.[79]

Sympathetic ophthalmia and Vogt–Koyanagi–Harada syndrome

The question arises whether sympathetic ophthalmia can be distinguished histologically from VKH because it may be the same from an immunogenetic perspective. It would appear that the two entities represent the spectrum of very similar inflammatory responses.[7] It is thought that 'classic' sympathetic ophthalmia neither involves the choriocapillaris nor has chorioretinal scarring, both of which are common in VKH. Although these changes can be seen in sympathetic ophthalmia,[5] they probably occur in fewer patients. In addition, the lack of chorioretinal scarring and obliteration of the choriocapillaris in eyes with sympathetic ophthalmia (a phenomenon seen late) may reflect the fact that eyes with sympathetic ophthalmia are usually removed early in the course of the inflammatory disease. In contrast, the eyes with VKH that have been studied were removed late in the course of the disease. Is the inflammatory response seen in sympathetic ophthalmia unique to this entity? Chan and coinvestigators[67] evaluated the cellular composition of granulomas of sympathetic ophthalmia and sarcoidosis. Most of the cells within the lesions were found to be identical and were mainly cells from bone-derived monocytes (**Table 23-2**). It has been suggested that Dalen–Fuchs nodules in sarcoidosis are larger.

A complicating factor is the presence of phacoanaphylaxis. Easom and Zimmerman[35] reported cases in which the clinical diagnosis in the exciting eye was thought to be sympathetic ophthalmia, but histologic confirmation could not be obtained; the so-called sympathizing eye showed evidence only of phacoanaphylaxis, rather than the alterations

Table 23-2 Sympathetic ophthalmia versus sarcoidosis

Disease	Uveitis	Dalen–Fuchs Nodules	Other		
HISTOPATHOLOGY					
Sarcoidosis	Focal or diffuse granulomatous	Some larger	'Snowbanking' conjunctival and iris nodules		
Sympathetic ophthalmia	Diffuse granulomatous	Many	Sparing of choriocapillaris; retina may not be involved		
Disease	T cells	T-helper cells	T-suppressor cells	B cells	Macrophages
IMMUNOPATHOLOGY					
Sarcoidosis	Majority	Many	Some	A few	In granuloma and Dalen–Fuchs nodules
Sympathetic ophthalmia	Majority	Early – more; late – less	Early – less; late – more	Some	In granuloma and Dalen–Fuchs nodules

typical of the suspected disorder. Although it is not always true, de Veer[28] emphasized that in phacoanaphylaxis disease in the first eye involved has already become quiescent by the time the second eye is involved. This is in contrast to sympathetic ophthalmia, in which both eyes are inflamed at the same time. A history of penetrating trauma is imperative. If this is not available, or if it is not clear whether ocular penetration occurred, then the diagnosis becomes even more difficult. VKH and sarcoidosis perhaps most resemble the disorder, but the diagnosis of localized posterior segment disorders such as APMPPE (see Chapter 29) must also be considered.

The concept that an autoimmune inflammatory response is the basis of sympathetic ophthalmia is not new, having been proposed by Elschnig in 1910.[80] For years the notion was that uveal pigment was the antigenic stimulus for this disease. A report by Woods[81] in 1921 outlined the interesting observation that patients who had sustained ocular trauma without resultant sympathetic ophthalmia had circulating antibodies to uveal pigment, but that in all patients with sympathetic ophthalmia circulating antibodies were absent. Furthermore, in one of these latter patients a cellular immune response to uveal pigment was seen, as measured with an intradermal skin test. These observations are striking, considering our knowledge of the predominant T-cell response in the eye. In vitro cell-culturing techniques have been used to evaluate cell-mediated anamnestic responses of lymphocytes from patients with sympathetic ophthalmia, and in these patients a positive response to uveal or uveoretinal preparations was seen.[82,83]

Of interest were the observations of Marak and coworkers[84] that blastogenic activity of lymphocytes from a small group of patients with sympathetic ophthalmia could be elicited only with RPE and retinal antigens, but not with antigens from the choroid. De Smet and colleagues[85] tested two patient populations, one from the National Eye Institute's clinic and the other from a uveitis clinic in Japan. Patients with sympathetic ophthalmia were tested for their cellular immune response to both S-antigen and interphotoreceptor retinoid-binding protein (IRBP). Patients' lymphocytes were found to respond to several autoantigens and to several fragments. Chan and colleagues,[86] using an enzyme-linked immunoabsorbent assay, found no circulating antiretinal S-antigen antibodies. However, when serum

from patients with sympathetic ophthalmia was placed over normal human retinal tissue, a few showed antiretinal antibodies directed against the outer segments of the photoreceptors and against Müller cells. However, the titers of the antiretinal antibodies and the number of patients with these circulating antibodies were considerably higher in the VKH group than in the sympathetic ophthalmia group. An association between HLA-A11 and sympathetic ophthalmia has been suggested.[87] However, this study reports the results in a population that is multiethnic and multiracial, making the validity of the results difficult to evaluate. As mentioned before, Davis and colleagues[55] found a strong association between HLA-DR4, DRw53, and Bw54 haplotypes and both VKH and sympathetic ophthalmia, but in the latter disease the small number of patients precluded statistical analysis.

No exact experimental model for sympathetic ophthalmia exists. The induction of uveitis with the ocular antigens IRBP and S-antigen will produce a disease in monkeys and mice that has many characteristics of sympathetic ophthalmia, including Dalen–Fuchs nodules (see Fig. 23-8 and Chapter 1). However, although there may some choroidal involvement, the disease induced in these animals is essentially retinal in nature. Another important factor in the development of the human disorder is the fact that penetrating trauma may permit the development of intraocular lymphatics and the presentation of ocular antigens to the systemic immune system in an unusual manner.[75]

Is it then possible to develop a working hypothesis to explain the development of sympathetic ophthalmia? The dominant T-cell response certainly seems clear. But what of the precipitating factors leading to the disease? The possibility of an autoimmune role still seems quite attractive, based on the type of disease in the monkey that is induced with retinal antigens. It is possible to hypothesize that the perforating injury permits several events to take place (**Fig. 23-9**). The first is that drainage of antigen from the eye can occur via the lymphatics, an event that does not occur under normal conditions. The second is that small amounts of adjuvant, such as bacterial cell wall or other immunostimulators, might now enter the eye. These products may come from already killed bacteria on the skin (such as *Propionibacterium acnes*), and therefore active proliferation of the organism is not significant to the hypothesis. Rather, these products may profoundly 'upgrade' the local immune response,

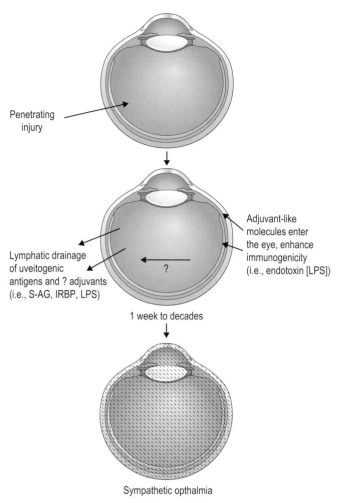

Penetrating injury

Lymphatic drainage of uveitogenic antigens and ? adjuvants (i.e., S-AG, IRBP, LPS)

Adjuvant-like molecules enter the eye, enhance immunogenicity (i.e., endotoxin [LPS])

1 week to decades

Sympathetic opthalmia

Figure 23-9. Hypothesis explaining the development of sympathetic ophthalmia.

Table 23-3 Relationship between clinical treatment and visual outcome

	Visual Outcome in No. (%) of Patients	
	Visual Acuity >0.5	Visual Acuity <0.1
Adequate and rapid medication	16/16 (100)	4/10 (40)
Enucleation	9/16 (56)	7/10 (70)
Time interval of diagnosis made		
<2 months	10/16 (62)	4/10 (40)
>1 year	6/16 (38)	6/10 (60)

From Chan C, Roberge F, Whitcup S, et al. Thirty two cases of sympathetic ophthalmia examined at the National Eye Institute: a retrospective study at the National Eye Institute, Bethesda, MD, from 1982–1992. Arch Ophthalmol 1995; 113: 597–600.

causing it to bypass certain inherent suppressor mechanisms in genetically prone persons. This then leads to the inflammatory kinetic process that we ultimately recognize as sympathetic ophthalmia.

Therapy

Enucleation of an injured eye before the sympathizing eye becomes involved is the only known way to prevent sympathetic ophthalmia. Enucleation has classically been thought to have no effect on the course of the sympathizing eye once the disease has begun. However, on rare occasions this may not be true. Bellan[88] reported the case of a patient who suffered penetrating trauma to one eye and who had enucleation of the nonseeing eye 5 days after his injury. At the time his remaining eye was reported to be normal. Three months later he developed presumed sympathetic ophthalmia (it was not histologically proven) in his remaining eye. Indeed, experience from the era before steroids suggested that enucleation did not help to improve the patient's ultimate visual outcome.[89] However, the review by Lubin and coworkers[6] suggested that enucleation within 2 weeks of the initiation of the inflammatory response may beneficially affect the visual outcome of the remaining eye. Reynard and associates,[90] in their retrospective clinicopathologic study, also noted that enucleation within 2 weeks of the beginning of symptoms resulted in a fairly benign course. However, in our retrospective study[17] and the prospective study reported by Kilmartin and coauthors,[12] enucleation was not seen to correlate with a better visual outcome. Indeed, in our experience it appears that adequate and rapid immunosuppressive therapy was the most important factor in achieving good vision (**Table 23-3**). Bellan[88] questioned the need for prophylactic enucleation, given the high treatment to benefit ratio in this disorder.[88] Therefore, we would hesitate to suggest early enucleation of an eye with any prognosis for useful vision. It may be that the exciting eye's visual acuity could be superior to that obtained in the sympathizing eye. Brackup and coworkers[91] evaluated 50 eyes that had global rupture and were not removed within 2 weeks of injury with visual acuities of no better than hand motion. Seventeen of the eyes were later removed, nine of them being painful. The other 33 eyes were not removed and remained comfortable for a mean follow-up of 66 months. Of interest was the fact that there were no cases of sympathetic ophthalmia. An interesting question has been raised by Hollander et al.[92] In their discussion of penetrating injuries to an already blind eye, it could be argued that enucleation instead of a primary repair could have a role.

The decision as to when to treat a patient with sympathetic ophthalmia with immunosuppressive therapy usually is not problematic. The patient is first seen with a marked, bilateral inflammation and decrease in vision. On rare occasions, although an inflammatory response can be observed, the patient's vision remains good, and the practitioner may need to follow other parameters, such as changing visual fields, to decide whether a therapeutic intervention is indicated.

Corticosteroids

If the decision has been made to intervene with antiinflammatory therapy, the initial approach, in most cases, should be the use of systemic corticosteroids. They should be given at a dose of at least 1–1.5 mg/kg of prednisone or equivalent on a daily basis. Some practitioners recommend even higher doses, from 100 to 200 mg/day of prednisone.[5] To deal with a particularly severe inflammatory process intravenous pulse steroid therapy can be employed,[93] but this needs invariably

patient's condition. Baseline visual fields and electroretinogram were obtained. Although her vision remained 20/20, the visual field was noted to become increasingly more constricted and the electroretinogram showed a change from baseline as well. The patient also noted subjective changes in her vision. Despite the good visual acuity, it was elected to treat these alterations with steroids. The subjective alterations disappeared, but no improvement in the visual field changes was seen, although there was no further progression.

In summary, we have seen a changes in trends when we consider sympathetic ophthalmia, as suggested by Vote et al.[14] Although in the past the disease was more commonly seen after penetrating trauma, we are seeing it more often after surgery, particularly vitreoretinal and ciliary body ablation, and the incidence may be increasing. It remains questionable as to whether the risk of this disease is greater with evisceration than with enucleation. Whereas once we saw more men with the disease, there probably is no gender preference, and it is being noted in more elderly patients. The disease may present with any type of uveitis, and the concept that enucleation soon after the onset of disease ameliorates the course is now in question. Although once the outcome often resulted in a very poor visual outcome, we can now be guardedly optimistic about the outcome.

References

1. Zegers RH. The eyes of Johann Sebastian Bach. Arch Ophthalmol 2005; 123(10): 1427–1430.
2. MacKenzie W. A practical treatise on disease of the eye. 1830, London: Longmans.
3. Albert D, Diaz-Rohena R. A historical review of sympathetic ophthalmia and its epidemiology. Surv Ophthalmol 1989; 34: 1–14.
4. Fuchs E. Über sympathislerende Entzündung zuerst Bemerkungeen über seröse traumatische Iritis. Albrect Von Graefes Arch Ophthalmol 1905; 61: 365–456.
5. Marak GJ. Recent advances in sympathetic opthalmia. Surv Ophthalmol 1979; 24: 141–156.
6. Lubin J, Albert D, Weinstein M. Sixty-five years of sympathetic ophthalmia. A clinicopathologic review of 105 cases (1913–1978). Ophthalmology 1980; 87: 109–121.
7. Goto H, Rao N. Sympathetic ophthalmia and Vogt–Koyanagi–Harada syndrome. Int Ophthalmol Clin 1990; 30: 279–285.
8. Liddy N, Stuart J. Sympathetic ophthalmia in Canada. Can J Ophthalmol 1972; 7: 157–159.
9. Holland G. About the indication and time for surgical removal of an injured eye. Klin Monatsbl Augenheilkd 1964; 145: 732–740.
10. Gass J. Sympathetic ophthalmia following vitrectomy. Am J Ophthalmol 1982; 93: 552–558.
11. Kilmartin D, Dick A, Forrester J. Commentary. Sympathetic ophthalmia risk following vitrectomy: should we counsel patients? Br J Ophthalmol 2000; 84: 448–449.
12. Kilmartin D, Dick A, Forrester J. Prospective surveillance of sympathetic ophthalmia in the UK and Republic of Ireland. Br J Ophthalmol 2000; 84: 259–263.
13. Su DH, Chee SP. Sympathetic ophthalmia in Singapore: new trends in an old disease. Graefes Arch Clin Exp Ophthalmol 2006; 244(2): 243–247.
14. Vote BJ, Hall A, Cairns J, et al. Changing trends in sympathetic ophthalmia. Clin Exp Ophthalmol 2004; 32(5): 542–545.
15. Hoefle F. Initial treatment of eye injuries. Arch Ophthalmol 1968; 79: 33–35.
16. Freidlin J, Pak J, Tessler HH, et al. Sympathetic ophthalmia after injury in the Iraq war. Ophthalm Plast Reconstruct Surg 2006; 22(2): 133–134.
17. Chan C, Roberge RG, Whitcup SM, et al. Thirty two cases of sympathetic ophthalmia examined at the National Eye Institute. A retrospective study at the National Eye Institute, Bethesda, MD, from 1982–1992. Arch Ophthalmol 1995; 113: 597–600.
18. Hakin K, Pearson R, Lightman S. Sympathetic ophthalmia: Visual results with modern immunosuppressive therapy. Eye 1992; 6: 453–455.
19. Pollack A, McDonald HR, Ai E, et al. Sympathetic ophthalmia associated with pars plana vitrectomy without antecedent penetrating trauma. Retina 2001; 21: 146–154.
20. Smith R, Webb R, van Heusen W. Sympathetic ophthalmia as a complication of pars plana vitrectomy. Perspect Ohthalmol 1978; 2: 117–120.
21. Green W, Maumene A, Sanders T. Sympathetic uveitis following evisceration. Trans Am Acad Ophthalmol Otolaryngol 1972; 76: 625–644.
22. Awan K. Sympathetic uveitis in intraocular implant surgery. J Ocul Ther Surg 1984; 3: 134–135.
23. Carney M, Tessler HH, Peyman GA, et al. Sympathetic ophthalmia and subretinal neovascularization. Ann Ophthalmol 1990; 22: 184–186.
24. Comer M, Taylor C, Chen S, et al. Sympathetic ophthalmia associated with high frequency deafness. Br J Ophthalmol 2001; 85: 496–503.
25. Lewis M, Gass J, Spencer W. Sympathetic uveitis after trauma and vitrectomy. Arch Ophthalmol 1978; 96: 263–267.
26. Lim WK, Chee SP, Sng I, et al. Immunopathology of progressive subretinal fibrosis: a variant of sympathetic ophthalmia. Am J Ophthalmol 2004; 138(3): 475–477.
27. Wang RC, Zamir E, Dugel PU, et al. Ophthalmology 2002; 109(8): 1527–1531.
28. de Veer J. Bilateral endophthalmitis phacoanaphylactica. Arch Ophthalmol 1953; 49: 607–632.
29. Blodi F. Sympathetic uveitis as an allergic phenomenon. Trans Am Acad Ophthalmol Otolaryngol 1959; 63: 642–649.
30. Allen J. Sympathetic uveitis and phacoanaphylaxis. Am J Ophthalmol 1967; 63: 280–283.
31. Buller AJ, Doris JP, Bonshek R, et al. Sympathetic ophthalmia following severe fungal keratitis. Eye 2006; 20(11): 1306–1307.
32. Romaine H. Malignant melanoma of the choroid with sympathetic ophthalmia. Arch Ophthalmol 1949; 42: 102–103.
33. Melanowski W. Contribution to the pathogenesis of sympathetic ophthalmia: a case of sympathetic ophthalmia due to intraocular melanosarcoma. Klin Monatsbl Augenheilkd 1936; 97: 52–59.
34. Garcia-Arumi J, Gil MM, Palau MM, et al. Sympathetic ophthalmia after surgical resection of iridociliary melanoma. A case report. Graefe's Arch Clin Exp Ophthalmol 2006; 244: 1353–1356.
35. Easom H, Zimmerman L. Sympathetic ophthalmia and bilateral phacoanaphylaxis. A clinicopathologic correlation of the sympathogenic and sympathizing eyes. Arch Ophthalmol 1964; 72: 9–15.
36. Fries P, Char DH, Crawford JB, et al. Sympathetic ophthalmia complicating helium ion irradiation of a choroidal melanoma. Arch Ophthalmol 1987; 105: 1561–1564.
37. Margo C, Pautler S. Granulomatous uveitis after treatment of a choroidal melanoma with proton-beam irradiation. Retina 1990; 10: 140–143.
38. Sabates R. Choroiditis compatible with the histopathological diagnosis

of sympathetic ophthalmia following cyclocryotherapy of neovasuclar glaucoma. Ophthalmic Surg 1988; 19: 176–182.

39. Harrison T. Sympathetic ophthalmia after cyclocryotherapy of neovascular glaucoma without ocular penetration. Ophthalmic Surg 1993; 24: 44–46.

40. Biswas J, Fogla R. Sympathetic ophthalmia following cyclocryotherapy with histopathologic correlation. Ophthalmic Surg Lasers 1996; 27: 1035–1038.

41. Edward D, Brown SV, Higginbotham E. et al. Sympathetic ophthalmia following neodymium:YAG cyclotherapy. Ophthalmic Surg 1989; 20: 544–546.

42. Lam S, Tessler HH, Lam BL, et al. High incidence of sympathetic ophthalmia after contact and non-contact neodymium:YAG cyclotherapy. Ophthalmology 1992; 99: 1818–1822.

43. Tessler H, Lam S, Wilensky J, et al. Sympathetic ophthalmia after non-contact neodymium:YAG cyclotherapy., In: Dernouchamps J, et al, eds. Recent advances in Uveitis, Proceeding of the Third International Symposium on Uveitis, 1993, Kugler Publications: Amsterdam. p. 201–202.

44. Bakri SJ, Peters GB, 3rd. Sympathetic ophthalmia after a hyphema due to nonpenetrating trauma. Ocul Immunol Inflamm 2005; 13(1): 85–86.

45. Glavici M. Sympathetic ophthalmia after a cataract operation. Oftalmolgia 1992; 36: 397–401.

46. Lakhanpal V, Dogra M, Jacobson M. Sympathetic ophthalmia associated with anterior chamber intraocular lens implantation. Ann Ophthalmol 1991; 23: 139–143.

47. Abu El-Asrar A, Al-Obeidan S. Sympathetic ophthalmia after complicated cataract surgery and intraocular lens implantation. Eur J Ophthalmol 2001; 11: 193–196.

48. Abu El-Asrar AM, Al Kuraya H, Al-Ghamdi A. Sympathetic ophthalmia after successful retinal reattachment surgery with vitrectomy. Eur J Ophthalmol 2006; 16(6): 891–894.

49. du Toit N, Motala MI, Richards J, et al. The risk of sympathetic ophthalmia following evisceration for penetrating eye injuries at Groote Schuur Hospital. Br J Ophthalmol 2008; 92(1): 61–63.

50. Sampangi R, Venkatesh P, Mandal S, et al. Recurrent neovascularization of the disc in sympathetic ophthalmia. Indian J Ophthalmol 2008; 56(3): 237–239.

51. Spitznas M. Fluorescein angiography of sympathetic ophthalmia. Klin Monatsbl Augenheilkd 1976; 169: 195–200.

52. Bernasconi O, Auer C, Zografos L, et al. Indocyanine green angiographic findings in sympathetic ophthalmia. Graefe's Arch Clin Exp Ophthalmol 1998; 236: 635–638.

53. Saatci AO, Paşa E, Söylev MF, et al. Sympathetic ophthalmia and indocyanine green angiography. Arch Ophthalmol 2004; 122(10): 1568–1569.

54. Dreyer WJ, Zegarra H, Zakov ZN, et al. Sympathetic ophthalmia. Am J Ophthalmol 1981; 92: 816–823.

55. Davis J, Mittal KK, Freidlin V, et al. HLA Associations and ancestry in Vogt–Koyanagi–Harada disease and sympathetic ophthalmia. Ophthalmology 1990; 97: 1137–1142.

56. Kilmartin D, Wilson D, Liversidge J, et al. Immunogenetics and clinical phenotype of sympathetic ophthalmia in British and Irish patients. Br J Ophthalmol 2001; 85: 281–286.

57. Shindo Y, Ohno S, Usui M, et al. Immunogenetic study of sympathetic ophthalmia. Tissue Antigens 1997; 49(2): 111–115.

58. Atan D, Turner SJ, Kilmartin DJ, et al. Cytokine gene polymorphism in sympathetic ophthalmia. Invest Ophthalmol Vis Sci 2005; 46(11): 4245–4250.

59. Glover N, Ah-Chan JJ, Frith P, et al. Unremitting sympathetic ophthalmia associated with homozygous interleukin-10-1082A single nucleotide polymorphism. Br J Ophthalmol 2008; 92(1): 155–156.

60. Marak G, Font R, Zimmerman L. Histologic variations related to race in sympathetic ophthalmia. Am J Ophthalmol 1974; 78: 935–938.

61. Kuo P, Lubin JR, Ni C, et al. Sympathetic ophthalmia: A comparison of the histopatholgical features from a Chinese and American series. Int Ophthalmol Clin 1982; 22: 125–139.

62. Croxato J, Rao NA, McLean IW, et al. Atypical histopathologic features in sympathetic ophthalmia. A study of a hundred cases. Int Ophthalmol 1981; 3: 129–135.

63. Allinson R, Le TD, Kramer TR, et al. Fluorescein angiographic appearance of Dalen–Fuchs nodules in sympathetic ophthalmia. Ann Ophthalmol 1993; 25: 152–156.

64. Font R, Fine BS, Messmer E, et al. Light and electron microscopic study of Dalen–Fuchs nodules in sympathetic ophthalmia. Ophthalmology 1983; 90: 66–75.

65. Jakobeic F, Marboe CC, Knowles DM, et al. Human sympathetic ophthalmia. An analysis of the inflammatory infiltrate by hybridoma-monoclonal antibodies, immunochemistry, and correlative electron microscopy. Ophthalmology 1983; 90: 76–95.

66. Chan C, BenEzra D, Hsu SM, et al. Granulomas in sympathetic opthalmia and sarcoidosis.

Immunohistochemical study. Arch Ophthalmol 1985; 103: 198–202.

67. Chan C, Nussenblatt RB, Fujikawa LS, et al. Sympathetic ophthalmia Immunohistochemical study of epithelioid and giant cells. Ophthalmology 1986; 93: 690–695.

68. Rao N, Xu S, Font R. Sympathetic ophthalmia. An immunohistochemical study of epithelioid and giant cells. Ophthalmology 1985; 92: 1660–1662.

69. Chan C, Benezra D, Rodrigues MM, et al. Immunohistochemistry and electron microscopy of choroidal infiltrates and Dalen–Fuchs nodules in sympathetic ophthalmia. Ophthalmology 1985; 92: 580–590.

70. Abu El-Asrar AM, Struyf S, Van den Broeck C, et al. Expression of chemokines and gelatinase B in sympathetic ophthalmia. Eye 2007; 21(5): 649–657.

71. Rao N. Mechanisms of inflammatory response in sympathetic ophthalmia and VKH syndrome. Eye 1997; 11: 213–216.

72. Wu G, Rao N. A novel retinal pigment epithelial protein suppresses neutrophil superoxide generation. I. Characterization of the suppressive factor. Exp Eye Res 1996; 63: 713–725.

73. Wu G, Swiderek K, Rao N. A novel retinal pigment epithelial protein suppresses neutrophil superoxide generation. II. Purification and microsequencing analysis. Exp Eye Res 1996; 63: 727–737.

74. Kaplan H, Waldrep JC, Chan WC, et al. Human sympathetic ophthalmia. Immunologic analysis of the vitreous and uvea. Arch Ophthalmol 1986; 104: 240–244.

75. Rao N, Robin J, Hartmann D, et al. The role of the penetrating wound in the development of sympathetic ophthalmia. Experimental observations. Arch Ophthalmol 1983; 101: 102–104.

76. Shah D, Piacentini MA, Burnier MN Jr, et al. Inflammatory cellular kinetics in sympathetic ophthalmia. A study of 29 traumatized (exciting) eyes. Ocul Immunol Inflamm 1993; 1: 255–262.

77. Sen D, Sarin G, Mathur M. Serum beta-2 microglobulin level in sympathetic ophthalmitis. Acta Ophthalmol (Copenh) 1990; 68: 200–204.

78. Parikh JG, Saraswathy S, Rao NA. Photoreceptor oxidative damage in sympathetic ophthalmia. Am J Ophthalmol, 2008; 146: 866–875.

79. Chan CC, et al. Th1 cells made IFN gamma, M1 macrophages made CCL19/CXCL11 and IL-17/IL-18 in sympathetic ophthalmia. ARVO abstract 2009.

80. Elschnig A. Studies in sympathetic ophthalmia. II. The antigenic effect of

eye pigments. Albrecht von Graefes Arch Ophthalmol 1910; 76: 509–546.

81. Woods A. Immune reactions following injuries to the uveal tract. JAMA 1921; 77: 1317–1322.

82. Wong V, Anderson R, O'Brien P. Sympathetic ophthalmia and lymphocyte transformation. Am J Ophthalmol 1971; 72: 960–965.

83. Hammer H. Cellular hypersensitivity to uveal pigment confirmed by leucocyte migration tests in sympathetic ophthalmitis and the Vogt–Koyanagi–Harada syndrome. Br J Ophthalmol 1974; 58: 773–776.

84. Marak GJ, Font RL, Johnson MC, et al. Lymphocyte-stimulating activity of ocular tissues in sympathetic ophthalmia. Invest Ophthalmol Vis Sci 1971; 10: 770–774.

85. de Smet M, Yamamoto JH, Mochizuki M, et al. Cellular immune responses of patients with uveitis to retinal antigens and their fragments. Am J Ophthalmol 1990; 110: 135–142.

86. Chan C, Palestine AG, Nussenblatt RB, et al. Anti-retinal auto-antibodies in Vogt–Koyanagi–Harada syndrome, Behçet's disease, and sympathetic ophthalmia. Ophthalmology 1985; 92: 1025–1028.

87. Reynard M, Shulman IA, Azen SP, et al. Histocompatibility antigens in sympathetic ophthalmia. Am J Ophthalmol 1983; 95: 216–221.

88. Bellan L. Sympathetic ophthalmia: a case report and review of the need for prophylactic enucleation. Can J Ophthalmol 1999; 34: 95–98.

89. Winter F. Sympathetic uveitis. A clinical and pathologic study of the visual result. Am J Ophthalmol 1955; 101: 102–104.

90. Reynard M, Riffenburgh R, Maes E. Effect of corticosteroid treatment and enucleation on the visual prognosis of sympathetic ophthalmia. Am J Ophthalmol 1983; 96: 290–294.

91. Brackup A, Carter KD, Nerad JA, et al. Long-term follow-up of severely injured eyes following globe rupture. Ophthalmol Plast Reconstruct Surg 1991; 7: 194–197.

92. Hollander DA, Jeng BH, Stewart JM. Penetrating ocular injuries in previously injured blind eyes: should we consider primary enucleation? Br J Ophthalmol 2004; 88(3): 438.

93. Hebestreit H, Huppertz HI, Sold JE, et al. Steroid-pulse therapy may suppress inflammation in severe sympathetic ophthalmia. J Pediatr Ophthalmol Strabismus 1997; 34: 124–126.

94. Makley T, Azar A. Sympathetic ophthalmia. A long term follow up. Arch Ophthalmol 1978; 96: 257–262.

95. Jonas JB, Spandau UH. Repeated intravitreal triamcinolone acetonide for chronic sympathetic ophthalmia. Acta Ophthalmol Scand 2006; 84(3): 436.

96. Jonas JB, Rensch F. Intravitreal steroid slow-release device replacing repeated intravitreal triamcinolone injections for sympathetic ophthalmia. Eur J Ophthalmol 2008; 18(5): 834–836.

97. Schaelgel T, Azar A. Uveitis of suspected viral origin, in Clinical Ophthalmology, T. Duane, ed. 1978, Harper and Row: Hagerstown, MD.

98. Tessler H, Jennings T. High-dose short-term chlorambucil for intractable sympathetic ophtahlmia and Behçet's disease. Br J Ophthalmol 1990; 74: 353–357.

99. Kilmartin D, Forrester J, Dick A. Cyclosporine-induced resolution of choroidal neovascularization associated with sympathetic ophthalmia. Arch Ophthalmol 1998; 116: 249–250.

100. Gupta V, Gupta A, Dogra MR. Posterior sympathetic ophthalmia: a single centre long-term study of 40 patients from North India. Eye, 2007; 22: 1459–1464.

101. DeAngelis D, Gupta N, Howcroft M, et al. Cataract extraction by phacoemulsification in a sympathizing eye. Can J Ophthalmol 2000; 35: 26–28.

102. Ganesh SK, Sundaram PM, Biswas J, et al. Cataract surgery in sympathetic ophthalmia. J Cataract Refract Surg 2004; 30(11): 2371–2376.

103. Kinge B, Syrdalen P, Bjornsson OM. Photodynamic therapy for choroidal neovascularization secondary to sympathetic ophthalmia. Retina 2005; 25(3): 375–377.

104. Bom S, Young S, Gregor Z, et al. Surgery for choroidal neovascularization in sympathetic opthalmia. Retina 2002; 22(1): 109–111.

Vogt–Koyanagi–Harada Syndrome

Robert B. Nussenblatt

Key concepts

- Diagnostic criteria for both the complete and incomplete forms of the disease are becoming better defined.
- Personality changes because of the CNS involvement may be seen in this entity.
- Posterior pole disease should be treated very aggressively as the drop in vision may be very marked.

The Vogt–Koyanagi–Harada syndrome (VKH) is a systemic disorder involving many organ systems, including the eyes, ears, skin, and meninges. It includes a constellation of clinical signs and symptoms, and no definitive confirmatory diagnostic tests are yet available. In the 12th century a physician from the Arab world, Mohammad-al-Ghafiqi, described a disease with poliosis, neuralgias, and hearing changes.[1] In more modern times, in 1906 Alfred Vogt[2] presented one case, and Koyanagi in 1929[3] described in detail six patients with bilateral nontraumatic chronic iridocyclitis associated with poliosis, vitiligo, and dysacousia. Harada, in 1926,[4] described an essentially posterior uveitis with an exudative retinal detachment associated with a pleocytosis in the cerebrospinal fluid (CSF). As more of these cases were recognized, it became clear that many of the features seen in each of these entities overlapped. Babel[5] suggested that these symptoms were manifestations of the same underlying disorder, and that only intensity and distribution varied from one patient to the next; it therefore seemed appropriate to call the entity the Vog–Koyanagi–Harada syndrome, although it sometimes appears in the literature under other names, for example uveomeningitis.

Clinical aspects

Although VKH has been reported throughout the world, its appearance seems to be concentrated in certain racial and ethnic groups. Recently diagnostic criteria have been discussed and published (**Table 24-1**). It is a common type of endogenous uveitis in Japan, constituting at least 8% of these cases.[6] The same holds true for certain parts of Latin America, particularly Brazil. It is, however, relatively uncommon in the United States and seems to be an exceedingly unusual diagnosis in persons of northern European extraction. VKH patients seen in France were all of Mediterranean origin.[7] Some years ago, when we reviewed our examinations of 75 patients with VKH, we noted that most (79%) were female (Table 24-1). A similar observation has been made of patients in Latin America (Rubens Belfort Jr, personal communication, 1995). However, Ohno and coworkers,[8] in their series of 186 patients, reported that more males than females had the disease. In our series, 44% of the patients were African-American, 37% were white, 11% were Hispanic, and 6% were Oriental. Of interest is the fact that a very high percentage of the patients with VKH whom we have seen have American-Indian heritage, albeit sometimes distant. This observation is a most provocative one, because certainly this may be the unifying genetic bond between patients in the United States and those in the Orient. VKH is commonly seen in the Hispanic population of Southern California, an ethnic group often with Native American ancestry as well.[9] VKH is generally a disease of persons in the second to fourth decades of life, although the disease has been reported in children.[10] Lacerda[11] reported a case in a 7-year-old child. Tabbara and coworkers[12] reported that 13 of 97 patients with VKH seen at the King Khaled Eye Hospital in Saudi Arabia were children, whereas Berker et al.[13] reported that 15% of Turkish VKH patients were under 16 years of age. Rathinam and associates[14] found that only three of their 98 patients with VKH were children. This latter number is closer to our experience. The visual prognosis is generally favorable.[15]

Systemic findings

VKH is a systemic disorder, and the extraocular findings are most important in securing the diagnosis. Perry and Font[16] stressed that in patients with the Harada form of the disease some extraocular findings, such as hair and skin alterations, are uncommon. However, in our opinion, even patients with ocular lesions typical of this disorder cannot definitively be said to have VKH without these extraocular findings. A 'revised' guideline for diagnosis has been developed that reflects these concerns (see below).

The disease may be preceded by a prodromal stage, in which the patient may complain of headache, orbital pain, stiff neck, and vertigo. There may also be a fever. In the group of mostly Hispanic patients of Beniz and coworkers,[17] headache was by far the most common neurologic complaint. Others[18,19] have reported presentation with a mild facial weakness, migraine-like headaches with a sensorimotor hemisyndrome, and cognitive brain dysfunction.

The patient complaining of central nervous system symptoms needs to be evaluated rapidly. A lumbar puncture will reveal a pleocytosis in 84%,[8] with mostly lymphocytes and

Table 24-1 Characteristics of patients with VKH seen at the NEI. (From Lertsumitkul S, Whitcup SM, Chan CC, et al. Subretinal fibrosis and choroidal neovascularization in Vogt–Koyanagi–Harada syndrome. Graefes Arch Clin Exp Ophthalmol 1999; 237: 1039–1045.)

Characteristics	No. (%)	Range
Gender		
Male	16 (21.3)	
Female	59 (78.7)	
Race		
White/Native American ancestry	17 (22.7) /3	
African-American/Native American ancestry	39 (52.0) /16	
Hispanic	9 (12.0)	
Oriental	9 (12.0)	
Asian Indian	1 (1.3)	
Age (mean, yr)	32.8 ±12.6	11–72
Duration of disease (mean, mo)	29.0 ± 50.7	1–240
Systemic manifestations		
Ocular only	12 (16.9)	
Ocular + cutaneous	10 (14.1)	
Ocular + neurologic	30 (42.3)	
Ocular + cutaneous + neurologic	19 (26.7)	
Glaucoma	16 (21.3)	
Cataract	12 (16.0)	
Visual acuity mean (ETDRS letters read)	41.7 ± 29.3	1–85
Subretinal fibrosis	30 (40)	
Choroidal neovascularization	11 (14.7)	

monocytes present. The CSF glucose level should show a normal relationship to the serum glucose level. A lumbar puncture should be performed early in the course of the disease because the pleocytosis will ultimately disappear, even though the inflammatory disease in the eye may continue. These CSF findings were central to the diagnosis criteria as proposed by Sugiura,[20] and not to the revised criteria (see below). The CSF pleocytosis and the number of cells noted are significantly higher in those patients who develop a sunset glow fundus (see below). Further, it is occasionally very helpful in terms of determining the severity of the disease. If we see a pleocytosis we know we need to be very aggressive in our therapeutic approach. On occasion it can help with the diagnosis, as in a case where melanin-laden macrophages in the CSF specimen helped to make the diagnosis in a patient with titers positive for syphilis.[21]

The auditory difficulties associated with this disorder are central and will often occur concurrently with the ocular disease. The auditory disorder may be the presenting problem, however. The hearing loss usually involves the higher frequencies and may affect more than three-quarters of patients with the disorder. Dysacousia, which was observed in 74% of patients in one study,[8] may resolve after several months; however, we and others have noted that it may persist for years. Some patients will have tinnitus without an objective decrease in hearing. When we reviewed 24 patients, we noted that some may indeed present with tinnitus and even sudden hearing loss. However, audiology revealed many more with hearing alterations.[22] Detailed auditory testing, carried out by competent professionals, is important to rule out a noncentral reason for a reduction in hearing.

Skin lesions may also be a prominent part of the disease complex. Approximately 72% of patients[8] report sensitivity to touch of both hair and skin during the active phase of their disease. Vitiligo and poliosis occur in a large number of patients (63% and 90%, respectively) during the convalescent stage, whereas alopecia was reported in 70–73% of one group with VKH[23,24] (**Fig. 24-1**). It should be noted that ethnic groups may manifest varying systemic symptoms, as suggested by the study of Beniz and colleagues,[17] in which the authors found dermatologic involvement only rarely in the group of mostly Hispanic patients with VKH whose cases they followed. One area frequently overlooked during an examination for such changes is the axilla.

Ocular findings

VKH is a bilateral ocular condition. Although only one eye may be inflamed initially, in 94% of patients the disease involves the second eye within 2 weeks. There is a tendency for the ocular disease to occur in spring and autumn.[8] The inflammatory disease is granulomatous in nature, with mutton-fat keratic precipitates on the corneal endothelium. Perilimbal vitiligo (Sugiura's sign) may be a striking feature, occurring in 85% of Oriental patients.[8] The inflammatory activity can be quite severe and involves both the anterior chamber and the anterior vitreous in about 56% of patients. Nodules may be noted on the pupillary margin, as well as in the iris stroma (**Fig. 24-2**). An early finding in the disease is the shallowing of the anterior chamber and a moderate increase in intraocular pressure.[25] This appears to be related to a swelling of the ciliary processes, which has been noted to occur early in this disease.[26] This finding is apparent only with careful gonioscopic evaluation. Other patients, however, may have hypotony, probably as a result of the edema of the ciliary body. A high incidence of neovascularization of the angle has been reported by one group of Japanese investigators,[27] but this has not been our personal experience. The severity of the inflammatory response is reflected by the fact that pupillary membranes often develop, and cataract formation occurs. The glaucoma associated with VKH can be difficult to control. In a series reported by Forster and coworkers,[28] 16 of 42 patients with VKH required either surgical or medical therapy for their glaucoma, with nine having open-angle glaucoma and seven having angle closure due to pupillary block. A thickened iris is commonly noted in this disease. This is important for at least two reasons. The first is that laser iridotomy is very difficult to perform and the hole created by the laser often closes quickly. The second is that the patient may experience angle closure with a plateau iris, which often adheres completely to the lens, making it impossible to bow forward as one would expect in a more typical case of iris bombé. A rare presentation in dark-skinned persons is scleral perforation, presumably at the site of emergence of the scleral nerves, which are involved as innocent bystanders in the immune response directed against the melanocytes surrounding them[29] (**Fig. 24-3**).

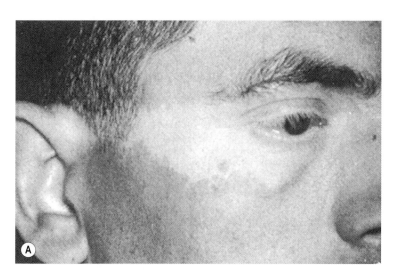

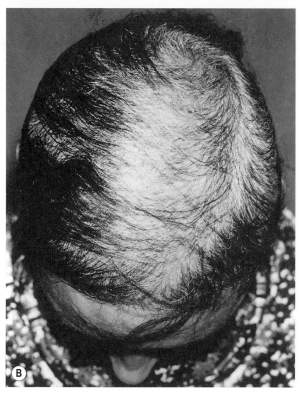

Figure 24-1. A, Area of vitiligo and poliosis of the cilia in a patient with VKH. *(Courtesy of D. Cogan, MD.)* **B,** Alopecia in a patient with VKH. The hair ultimately regrew.

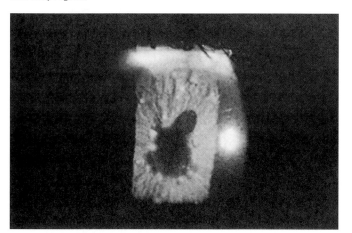

Figure 24-2. Iris nodules and mutton-fat keratitic precipitates in a patient with VKH.

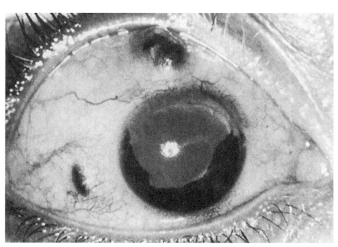

Figure 24-3. VKH with areas of focal scleritis and thinning of sclera anterior to insertion of rectus muscles. There is a large sector iridectomy superiorly. *(Reproduced with permission from Tabbara KF: Scleromalacia associated with Vogt-Koyanagi-Harada syndrome. Am J Ophthalmol 105:694–695, 1988)*

Severe and rather characteristic changes are noted to occur in the posterior portion of the eye as this disorder evolves. A swelling of the optic nerve head is seen early in 87% of patients;[8] this usually occurs concurrently with a severe vitreous inflammatory response. In addition, retinal edema may be one of the first signs of the disease and may be seen in the posterior pole. As the disease process continues, an exudative nonrhegmatogenous retinal detachment may occur, which is an important diagnostic finding. The inferior portion of the retina is most frequently involved. In the periphery of the retina, yellow-white, well-circumscribed lesions may appear, similar to those seen in sympathetic ophthalmia (see Chapter 23). It had been thought that these were the clinical equivalent of Dalen–Fuchs nodules; however new findings would suggest that

perhaps that is not always the case (see below). Macular edema, although relatively rare, is seen in eyes with a more protracted inflammation or those that have epiretinal membranes.[30]

Several fundus alterations occur as the disease process continues. Neovascularization of the retina and optic nerve can be seen, with subsequent recurrent and clinically significant vitreous hemorrhages. Subretinal neovascularization of the macula can also occur. Also, extramacular disciform lesions have been reported,[31] presumably in areas of reactive proliferation of the retinal pigment epithelium (RPE) and perturbation of Bruch's membrane. Moorthy and coworkers[32] reported that subretinal neovascular membranes developed in seven of 58 patients with VKH they were following. They found that these seven affected patients showed more anterior and vitreous inflammation as well as more pigmentary disturbances in the fundus. As expected, the visual outcomes for these patients were also significantly poorer than those for patients with less severe alterations.

The nonrhegmatogenous detachments frequently do not persist after the initial presentation, although the other signs of inflammation continue to be present – for example 'demarcation lines' representing the extent of previous detachments. Rhegmatogenous detachments may also occur in these eyes, and constant surveillance for such changes is vital.

Diagnostic criteria for both the complete and incomplete forms of the disease have been published (**Box 24-1**). There have been mixed reviews concerning the use of the criteria. A report by Gaspar et al.[33] from Brazil reported a 100% concordance in a retrospective review of 67 patients, 46 of whom were in the early phase of the disease. Rao et al.[34] reported a very good concordance rate as well when the criteria were applied retrospectively. However, Yamaki et al.[35] found that the criteria were effective for the final diagnosis but not for the early stage of the disease. They felt it better to include criteria suggested by Sugiura, namely pleocytosis in the CSF and HLA typing. Retrospective studies are helpful as starting points, but prospective studies are very much needed to effectively evaluate the usefulness of any criteria.

As the disease process begins to wane, a characteristic depigmentation of the posterior portion of the globe occurs. This 'sunset glow' appearance to the fundus, which reflects the changes occurring at the level of the RPE or choroid, is seen commonly in Oriental patients. Keino and colleagues[36] found that the sunset glow fundus was more commonly seen in eyes with a chronic inflammation that persisted for months. In the United States, the fundus of a white person with this disease has a more mottled appearance as well as a profound loss of pigment, causing what is known as a 'blond' fundus. At times profound subretinal changes, such as subretinal fibrosis, disciform scars, and RPE migration, can be quite striking (**Figs 24-4 to 24-6**).

Mondkar and colleagues[37] reported their experience with VKH in India, which represented only 2.2% of referrals. Extraocular manifestations were seen in 64% of patients at the time of presentation. More than 95% of these patients had a meningismus. In the 78 patients with VKH we reviewed, the disease manifested predominantly as posterior pole changes. We have not seen patients with only anterior segment disorders. In our experience there can be a wide distribution of visual acuities in patients with VKH. However, the acuities appear to be 'bunched' at the extremes of the vision chart. A large number of the eyes will demonstrate visual acuities that are 20/200 or worse, whereas a large proportion have a visual acuity of 20/40 or better. This reflects the observations of Ohno and coworkers.[8] We have noted that our patients have had a far more persistent ocular inflammatory disease than is generally described in the literature. Rubsamen and Gass[38] found in their series of 26 patients that the disease recurred in nine of 21 patients in the first 3 months, sometimes associated with a rapid taper of therapy. This may reflect referral patterns.

Box 24-1 Revised criteria for diagnosis of VKH (Modified from Read et al. Vogt–Koyanagi–Harada disease diagnostic criteria. Int Ophthalmol 2007; 27:195–199)

Complete VKH: Criteria 1–5 must be present
Incomplete VKH: Criteria 1–3 and either 4 or 5 must be present
Probable VKH (isolated ocular disease): Criteria 1–3 must be present

1. No history of penetrating ocular trauma or surgery preceding the initial onset of uveitis
2. No clinical or laboratory evidence suggestive of other ocular disease entities
3. Bilateral ocular involvement (a or b must be met, depending on the stage of disease when the patient is examined)
   a) Early manifestations of disease
      (1) Evidence of diffuse choroiditis (with or without anterior uveitis, vitreous inflammatory reaction or optic disc hypermia) which may manifest as (a) focal areas of subretinal fluid or (b) bullous serous retinal detachments
   b) Late manifestations of disease
      (1) History suggestive of prior presence of early findings noted in 3a and either (2) or (3) below, or multiple signs from 3.
      (2) Ocular depigmentation: either (a) nummular chorioretinal depigmented scars or (b) retinal pigment epithelium clumping and/or migration or (c) recurrent or chronic anterior uveitis
4. Neurological/auditory findings (may resolve by time of evaluation)
   (a) Meningismus (malaise, fever, headache, nausea, abdominal pains, stiffness of the neck and back or a combination of these factors); Note that headache alone is not sufficient to meet the definition of meningismus
   (b) Tinnitus
   (c) Cerebrospinal fluid plenocytosis
5. Integumentory finding (not preceding onset of central nevous system or ocular disease)
   (a) Alopecia, or
   (b) Poliosis, or
   (c) Vitiligo

Course of disease

The clinical course of VKH is quite varied. The ideal patient is the one with severe acute finding, followed by a period of quiescence during which there is a depigmentation of tissue, with a later stage of recurrent anterior segment inflammation disease. Some patients may have a limited period of severe ocular inflammatory activity, followed by rapid depigmentation and no further episodes. Other patients, however, continue to have ongoing, chronic disease. It is this group that requires constant vigilance. Anterior segment alterations, such as cataract and secondary glaucoma, occur in about one-third of patients. Peripapillary atrophy >2 disc diopters was associated with greater visual dysfunction, and interestingly the use of a multivariate analysis steroid was the main determinant for peripapillary atrophy.[39,40] With aggressive therapy, one can assume that the nonrhegmatogenous detachment will reattach. Reattachment usually results

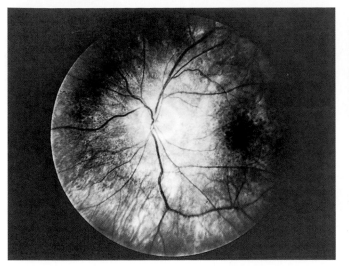

Figure 24-4. Sunset glow fundus in Asian patient after inflammatory disease of the posterior segment due to VKH. Note 'blond' appearance of fundus. *(Courtesy of K. Masuda, MD, and M. Mochizuki, MD.)*

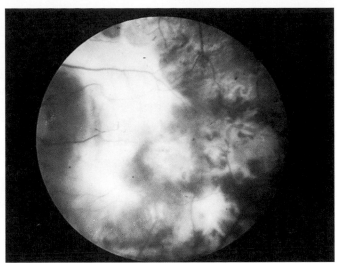

Figure 24-5. Dramatic subretinal alterations with subretinal fibrosis can occur in severe posterior pole inflammatory attacks.

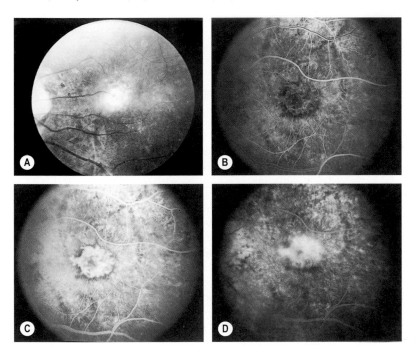

Figure 24-6. A–D, A Hispanic woman with poor vision in the left eye after having uveitis due to VKH. Fluorescein angiography findings demonstrated a subretinal neovascular net.

in reasonably good vision. However, a close evaluation of the retina will demonstrate changes, such as preretinal membranes, RPE stippling, extensive posterior pole atrophy,[41] and subtle folds in the retina precluding a return to previous levels of vision and subretinal fibrosis.[42] In a report of 75 patients seen at the National Eye Institute (NEI)[43] (**Table 24-2**), 30 (40%) had subretinal fibrosis, and 14.7% of eyes had choroidal neovascularization. The subretinal fibrosis was associated with longer duration of disease and a worse visual acuity. The disease in children appears to be aggressive. Tabbara and colleagues[12] reported that 61% of children with VKH versus 17% of adults needed cataract surgery, and that the final visual acuity in those children needing surgery was worse than that seen in adults. Rathinam and associates[14] found that all of their small number of pediatric patients with VKH had cataracts. Clinical findings at presentation, the duration of the disease, as well as the develop-

ment of extraocular manifestations all are prognostic factors relating to final visual acuity and recurrent inflammation.[44]

When patients manifest the classic findings of acute VKH, there is little difficulty in making the diagnosis. However, when the patient is examined at a later stage, the sequelae of the inflammatory disease cannot reliably help one to decide what the original problem had been, particularly if the nonocular findings are absent. The problems faced in diagnosing this condition were considered by Kayazawa and Takahashi,[45] who described two patients, both of whom had multiple yellow-white placoid lesions and a decrease in vision. On the basis of fluorescein angiographic findings, one patient was believed to have acute posterior multifocal placoid pigment epitheliopathy. However, the fluorescein angiographic findings in the other patient showed multiple pinpoint leaks, and later the fundus developed a sunset glow appearance. Rao and Marak[46] reported four patients with

Table 24-2 Clinical features of patients with subretinal fibrosis, choroidal neovascularization, history of glaucoma, cataract, and treatment with immunosuppressive agents. (From Lertsumitkul S, Whitcup SM, Chan CC, et al. Subretinal fibrosis and choroidal neovascularization in Vogt–Koyanagi–Harada syndrome. Graefes Arch Clin Exp Ophthalmol 1999; 237: 1039–1045.)

Clinical Features	Yes (%)	No (%)	p Value
Subretinal fibrosis			
Visual acuity (ETDRS letters read)	26.2	52.0	0.0001
Duration of disease (mo)	42.6	19.1	0.074
Age (yr)	31.5	33.6	0.48
Vitreous haze (0.5–4)	0.50	0.43	0.65
Choroidal neovascularization			
Visual acuity (ETDRS letters read)	27.8	44.0	0.074
Duration of disease (mo)	44.5	26.5	0.43
Age (yr)	30.3	33.2	0.52
Vitreous haze (0.5–4)	0.44	0.46	0.91
Glaucoma			
Visual acuity (ETDRS letters read)	35.2	43.4	0.32
Duration of disease (mo)	32.9	27.9	0.68
Age (yr)	30.3	33.5	0.28
Vitreous haze (0.5–4)	0.65	0.42	0.21
Cataract			
Visual acuity (ETDRS letters read)	28.3	44.2	0.10
Duration of disease (mo)	66.0	21.5	0.10
Age (yr)	37.1	32.0	0.30
Vitreous haze (0.5–4)	0.68	0.42	0.20
Use of immunosuppressive agent			
Visual acuity (ETDRS letters read)	46.2	39.8	0.33
Duration of disease (mo)	21.8	31.7	0.31
Age (yr)	28.5	34.6	0.07
Vitreous haze (0.5–4)	0.53	0.44	0.61

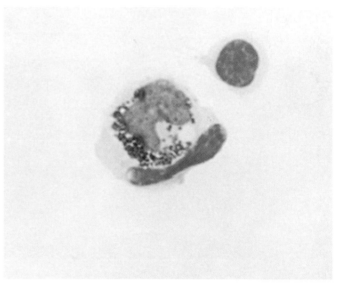

Figure 24-7. Basophilic granules in a melanin-laden macrophage taken from the cerebrospinal fluid of the patient described in reference 46. *(Reproduced with permission from Kamondi A, Szegedi A, Papp A et al: Vogt-Koyanagi-Harada disease presenting initially as aseptic meningoencephalitis, Eur J Neurol 7:719–722, 2000.)*

indications (such as hepatitis) can induce a serous detachment simulating VKH.[51] While recognizing this possible complication, some have argued that the positive therapeutic value of interferon outweighs any possible negative adverse events.[52]

The observer should set minimal ocular criteria for the diagnosis of this condition, because diagnosis is mainly a clinical decision. Our minimal criteria include a bilateral acute inflammatory response, with retinal edema and typical pinpoint leakage at the level of the RPE early on, as noted on examination with fluorescein angiography (see next section). Disc edema (and leakage seen on the fluorescein angiogram) is an important confirmatory sign, and many patients will have a central nervous system pleocytosis early in the disease. The presence of other extraocular findings already enumerated is helpful but these may be missed late in the disease. A history of Native American heritage is helpful information. We have no knowledge of the presence of Sugiura's sign in white patients with this disease.

Laboratory tests, etiology, and histopathology

Several tests can be performed to evaluate alterations occurring in the eye as a result of the inflammatory disease. The use of fluorescein angiography is helpful in evaluating the extent of the disease in the posterior segment of the globe. Early in the disease, multiple pinpoint areas of leakage are noted at the level of the RPE. The later frames of the angiogram may show a large confluent area of leakage (**Fig. 24-8**), and late leakage of the disc usually occurs. Subretinal neovascularization can be evaluated best with fluorescein angiography (see Fig. 24-6). Manger and Ober[53] reported the presence of retinal arteriovenous anastomoses in a young woman with VKH. By using fluorescein angiography, they noted that these vessels were collaterals that had developed in areas of damaged RPE. Both fluorescein angiographic changes and ICG findings have been well described. Herbort

sympathetic ophthalmia, all of whom had penetrating wounds, and in whom two or more extraocular manifestations usually associated with VKH developed, that is, vitiligo, poliosis, dysacousia, and meningitis (see Chapter 23). Other disorders that can mimic VKH include sarcoidosis (see Chapter 22) (particularly if there is choroidal involvement and subretinal changes) and some of the white-dot syndromes (see Chapter 29). One patient was reported as presenting with an aseptic meningitis (**Fig. 24-7**) and only manifesting ocular findings typical of VKH many months later.[47] Kouda and associates[48] reported a patient with VKH who first presented with a unilateral posterior scleritis and 12 months later was found to have a bilateral, severe granulomatous uveitis. Other diseases may rarely mimic the fundus picture seen in VKH. *Bartonella* has been reported to present as an unilateral VKH.[49] In addition, another patient, who had an ICG and IVFA compatible with VKH ultimately was diagnosed as having an intravascular lymphoma.[50] Admittedly, these are rare occurrences. A short note to alert the treating physician that interferon therapy given for other

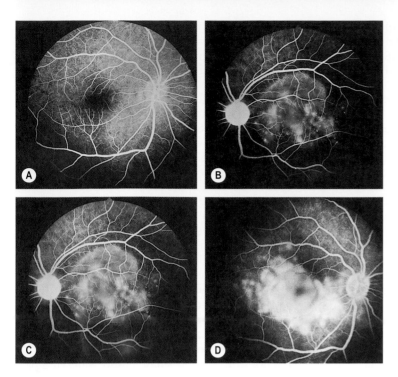

Figure 24-8. Fluorescein angiograms of the right eye (**A and D**) and left eye (**B and C**) of a patient with VKH, demonstrating pinpoint subretinal leakage, which later coalesced into a large area of leakage.

and coworkers[54] describe four general findings in VKH. First there is an early choroidal stromal vessel hyperfluorescence and hypofluorescent dark dots. In addition, one sees a fuzzy vascular pattern to the large stromal vessels and disc hyperfluorescence. With adequate immunosuppressive therapy the dark dots will resolve. Others have used ICG to examine the peripheral lesions usually identified as Dalen–Fuchs nodules.[55] They found one group of patients whose nodules, which were more common inferiorly and temporally, to be hyperfluorescent in the early phase and then becoming hypofluorescent in the later frames. They felt that these patients had shorter disease. Those with nodules that showed small round hypofluorescent lesions early had longer disease.

The electroretinogram and electrooculogram findings show varying degrees of abnormality, depending on the ocular disease. Studies have shown that multifocal electrongraphic responses in patients can be severely altered, and that with therapy there is a delayed but limited recovery of macular function over several months.[56] It is important to note that improvement in the results of both tests may occur during certain time points of the clinical course, with worsening associated with a recurrence.[57] Although electrophysiologic testing and fluorescein angiography are helpful adjuncts, we have seen patients with dramatic alterations of the posterior pole who maintain very good vision despite poor test results. However, macular function appears to be altered. During the convalescent stage foveal cone photoreceptor regeneration and recovery is delayed in VKH.[58] An image analyzer, measuring the number of red pixels to the total number of pixels, has been used to determine sunset glow changes early in the disease.[59]

Optical coherence tomography (OCT) has permitted the clinician to observe changes in this disorder more precisely.[60] It has been used to document anterior segment changes in the acute glaucoma that can be seen in VKH.[61] Using the cirrus OCT,[62] during the acute stage of VKH one can visualize troughs of RPE undulations which on clinical examination appears to be choroidal striations. Choroidal folds are not unusual in the eyes of patients with VKH, with one study reporting the finding in 12% of patients, often with hypofluorescent bands radiating from the optic disc.[63]

An interesting report evaluated glucose tolerance testing in patients with VKH.[64] These authors studied 20 patients during their acute and convalescent period and found that 55% of them showed glucose intolerance but not an insulin secretion deficiency. Four of seven patients tested during the convalescent period of their disease showed an improvement in glucose tolerance test results.

Antigen-specific and immune responses

Much attention has been focused on defining the immunoregulatory alteration that leads to VKH. Monoclonal antibodies directed to cell surface markers of various components of the immune system and to markers of cellular activation that appear at times have been utilized to study this disorder. In early studies, Okubo and coworkers[65] evaluated the various cellular immune components of seven patients with VKH who had active uveitis compared with those of 98 control subjects. They noted that the numbers of total T cells (OKT3+), helper T cells (OKT4+), and putative suppressor cells (OKT11+) were lower in patients than in control subjects. Liu and Sun[65] reported that the CD4/CD8 ratio was increased in patients whose disease recurred, an observation seen previously by us when patients with uveitis were evaluated in the United States. However, in the study by Okubo and coworkers[66] the number of cells bearing the antigen defined by the OK1a antibody was elevated. Ia or DR expression can be taken as a sign of immune system activation. DR expression can be enhanced by T-cell products released during the lymphokine cascade. In particular, interferon-γ (IFN-γ) is a powerful stimulus for DR activation on cell-surface membranes and does not have antiviral activity. The presence of circulating IFN-γ was evaluated in VKH patients.

Significantly increased IFN levels were detected in the blood of patients with VKH 1 and 2 months after the initiation of ocular symptoms; further evaluation of the IFN present revealed it to be IFN-γ. IFN-γ could not be detected in the CSF in those patients whose blood samples showed positivity.[67] Similar observations have been made in diseases of putative autoimmune origin, such as systemic lupus erythematosus, rheumatoid arthritis, and Sjögren's syndrome.[68] Sakaguchi and coworkers[69] established nine T-cell clones from patients with VKH and found that all of them spontaneously produced greater amounts of IFN-γ, interleukin (IL)-6, and IL-8 than were produced by cells from control subjects. Imai and associates[70] repeatedly saw high IFN-γ levels produced by T-cell clones obtained from patients with VKH. The evaluation of cell-surface markers on lymphocytes in VKH has shown that CD3+ T cells were more commonly seen in the aqueous and CSF than in peripheral blood.[71] CD45+Ro+ (i.e., memory cells) cells were seen in a higher percentage in the aqueous and CSF than in the peripheral blood, with Fas+ cells seen more in the aqueous than in the CSF. The CSF in VKH patients has been reported to have high amounts of the chemokine CXCL10 and lower amounts of CXCL17 than in the serum, whereas CCL2/MCP-1 is lower in VKH CSF than in controls.[72] These findings are similar to those seen in the CSF of patients with multiple sclerosis. More recent studies have tried to evaluate the presence of other markers of immune activation or immunoregulation. Li et al.[73] reported the upregulation of t-bet RNA expression in the peripheral blood of patients with VKH. T-bet is involved in the differentiation of T cells into Th1 cells. They also found that these cells, when stimulated, produced large amounts of IFN-γ, which is not surprising if they are Th1 cells. It has been suggested at least one source of immunoregulatory cells (i.e., those that can suppress or 'modulate' the immune response) is found in a subgroup of CD4+ cells that bear large numbers of receptors for IL-2 (the receptor is called CD25), and therefore they are labeled at CD4+ CD25^{high} cells. Chen et al.[74] reported there was a reduced frequency of these cells in the peripheral blood of VKH patients, and that another marker for immunoregulatory cells, FoxP3, was also low. In our experience the decrease of these markers of immunoregulation is not as consistently seen in human peripheral blood as in mouse models. Another cell that has received much attention is the Th17 cell. It has been proposed that Th1 cells initiate, and Th17 cells potentiate, inflammatory responses (see Chapter 1). Chi et al.[75] reported that higher IL-23 levels were seen in VKH patients, a lymphokine associated with IL-17, and that there was an increased production of IL-17 in peripheral blood cells of VKH patients, when stimulated polyclonally. This finding is not surprising. Along those lines, leptin, which is structurally similar to IL-6, IL-12, and IL-15, was seen to be elevated in the serum of VKH patients.[76] Further when peripheral blood mononuclear cells are cultured in the presence of leptin, there was proliferation of the cells and an increase in secretion of IL-17 and IFN.

The notion that a specific antigen-driven immune response is occurring in this disorder remains an intriguing possibility. Initial hypotheses centered on the role of pigment as the antigen driving the immune response. Several reports observed positive in vitro immune phenomena when patients' lymphocytes were placed in an environment containing uveal extracts or pigment.[77] Most of these reports used a nonhuman – usually bovine – source for antigen, thereby raising the possibility that the positive test results were due to a sensitization against bovine antigens in meat-eating humans. Yuasa and coworkers,[78] however, used human uveal preparations. They observed that 13 of 30 patients tested had positive macrophage migration inhibition test results, evidence that the immune system is capable of a memory response to the antigen(s). Maezawa and colleagues[79] evaluated the role of cytotoxic T cells in this disorder and how they may react against melanocyte-associated antigens. They noted that in the six patients with VKH they studied, the cytotoxic T-cell component of the immune repertoire appeared to demonstrate specific killing against a P-36 melanoma cell line, which bears cross-reactive antigens with normal melanocytes. Further, they demonstrated that the monoclonal antibody Leu-2a, specifically directed against the cytotoxic T-cell subset, blocked this reaction. They observed that the cytotoxic activity depended on the presence of DR+-adherent cells, and the activity could be augmented by the addition of interleukins into the in vitro system.[80] More recent work has centered on tyrosinase family proteins. Yamaki and colleagues[81] demonstrated that a 30-mer sequence from the tyrosinase family induced a proliferative response in lymphocytes taken from patients with VKH. Sugita et al.[82] reported that that CD4+ cells infiltrating the eye responded to tyrinosinase and gp100 peptide, producing RANTES and IFN-g. Additionally, when injected into Lewis rats these antigens induce both ocular and extraocular disease (skin and meninges) approximately 12 days after immunization.[83] Gocho and coworkers[84] were able to establish 28 T-cell clones directed against tyrosinase and another 34 directed against tyrosinase-related protein 1. Yamada and associates[85] reported a higher prevalence of immunoglobulin G antilens epithelium-derived growth factor in patients with VKH. A rather interesting example of the power these autoaggressive immune cells can be seen in a report by Yeh et al.[86] in which a patient with systemic melanoma received tumor infiltrating cells (TIL) with IL-2 therapy. The patient developed a Vogt–Koyanagi–Harada syndrome affecting the eye. This suggests the fine balance between autoaggressive cells being therapeutically positive in preventing tumor spread as opposed to the induction of an autoimmune response.

Immune responses directed against the retina can also be seen. Patients with VKH have circulating lymphocytes that have been noted to have in vitro proliferative responses to the retinal S-antigen,[87] although this finding is by no means unique to this disorder. Chan and coworkers,[88] however, noted that sera from these patients had particularly unique properties. Using the avidin–biotin–peroxidase technique for the detection of retinal antibodies, they found particularly large titers of antiretinal antibodies in these patients' sera directed against the outer segments of photoreceptors and Müller cells. Considerably lower titers were found in some patients with Behçet's disease and in a few with sympathetic ophthalmia. Whether this observation is reflective of a primary immune process or a result of the severe posterior pole disease seen in these patients still remains to be evaluated. It is also of interest that nonspecific triggering mechanisms can lead to the full disease. Several years ago we followed a patient in whom typical VKH developed after the placement of a purified protein derivative (PPD) skin test (see Case 24-2). Rathinam and coworkers[89] reported three patients who developed VKH after cutaneous injury, with the skin initially becoming vitiliginous. It is thought-provoking to speculate on the role of other exogenous triggering factors.

Because of the increased prevalence of this disorder in certain ethnic groups, it is logical to hypothesize an immunogenetic basis for this disease. Cases of siblings with this disorder have been reported,[90] as have those of monozygotic twins.[91] Ohno[67] evaluated the frequency of HLA antigens in Japanese patients with this disease compared with that in control subjects. HLA-DR4 was present in 88% of patients but in only 32% of controls, with a calculated relative risk of 15.2. All the patients had the supertypical DR antigen MT3 (HLA-B53), compared to 53% of the control subjects, with a resultant relative risk of 74.5. Kunikane[92] reported an association with HLA-DQWa and Harada's disease in Japanese patients (relative risk 5.17), confirming Ohno's previous work with the same antigen. However, using two-dimensional electrophoresis and restriction fragment length polymorphism analysis, Kunikane noted that these antigen molecules differed in Japanese and white subjects tested. In typing 25 Han Chinese with VKH, Zhao and coworkers[93] found an association with HLA-DR4 (relative risk 16.0) and HLA-Dw53 (relative risk 34.2), similar to that seen in Japan. Zhang and coworkers[94] reported a strong association between VKH and HLA-DR4, with a calculated relative risk of 10.0, whereas a reduced frequency of HLA-DQw1 was seen in fewer patients. Numaga and colleagues,[95] using a polymerase chain reaction technique, demonstrated that the HLA-DR β1 in 19 of 20 patients had a specific amino acid sequence in positions 70 and 71. However, Yu and colleagues[96] found an association with HLA-B22, with a relative risk calculated at 8.69. In Korean patients with VKH, Kim and colleagues[97] reported an association with HLA-DRB1*0405 or the HLA-DRB1*0405-DQA1*0302-DQB1*0401 haplotype.

Davis and colleagues[98] evaluated the HLA associations of 23 American patients with VKH. A strong association was found with HLA-DR4 and HLA-DRw53. HLA-DQw3 was strongly associated with this disease, because this antigen was in linkage disequilibrium with DR4. An interesting report by Rutzen and coworkers[99] described the development of VKH in monozygotic twins of Vietnamese ancestry. HLA typing disclosed HLA-DR4 positivity. In addition, the anecdotal association of VKH with Native American ancestry was confirmed. In the report by Martinez and colleagues[100] of North American patients of Cherokee Indian ancestry with VKH, assay results in seven patients showed the HLA-DRw52 haplotype. Five of these patients were homozygous for this allele, whereas patients in Mexico of Mestizo background had DRB1*04 on their cells.[101] Levinson et al.[102] also reported an increase in combined DR4 alleles in Mestizo VKH patients in Southern California, and he and coworkers[103] reported a trend towards B KIR haplotypes, a finding similar to those in other autoimmune disorders.

Others have examined whether other specific gene alleles or single nucleotide polymorphism might be associated with VKH. Horie and coworkers[104] investigated any relationship between the tyronsinase gene family TYR and dopachrome tantomerase. Although a very strong association was noted between VKH and HLA-DRB1*0405, no risk was sign

identified with the tyrosinase gene family; nor did the group identify a genetic susceptibility with VKH and the IFN-g gene.[105] Du et al.[106] reported an association with the cytotoxic lymphocyte-associated antigen-4 (CTLA-4), a negative regulator of T-cell responses, and VKH; however the odds ratio was not very impressive.

The concept that this disorder is of viral origin has been an attractive one for many, and numerous attempts have been made to substantiate this theory. However, studies aimed at isolating virus from either the eye[107] or the CSF[108] have not been successful. Sunakawa and Okinami[109] determined anti-Epstein–Barr virus antibody levels in control subjects and in patients with panuveitis, including patients with VHK, and found that the frequency of elevated titers was lower in the patients than in the controls. In work mentioned above in which Sugita et al.[82] found CD+ ocular infiltrating cells recognizing tyrinosinase, they also recognized the cytomegalovirus envelope glycoprotein H- which has a high amino acid homology to tyrinosinase.

Vogt–Koyanagi–Harada syndrome versus sympathetic ophthalmia

The histologic evaluation of VKH in several patients has appeared in the literature.[6] A major discussion point has been how this disorder differs from sympathetic ophthalmia (see Chapter 23). As in the latter condition, in VKH there is a marked thickening of the choroid, with macrophages and lymphocytes, as well as epithelioid cells that contain melanin. Unlike sympathetic ophthalmia, in VKH plasma cells are readily observed. Dalen–Fuchs nodules are present, and involvement of the choriocapillaris is more common, unlike the classic 'sparing' of this portion of the choroid in sympathetic ophthalmia. Although much has been said about the histologic differences between sympathetic ophthalmia and VKH, it is clear that both represent a spectrum of disease, and that most of the time standard histologic evaluation of the posterior globe cannot definitively differentiate one from the other. An interesting note about sparing of the choriocapillaris is that, as suggested by Rao,[110] this sparing is due to the production of antiinflammatory molecules by the RPE, which produces both transforming growth factor-β and retinal pigment epithelial protective protein, which would suppress the generation of superoxides by phagocytes. A more recent report by Rao[111] challenges another thought about VKH. In chronic VKH, the peripheral fundus scars were not Dalen–Fuchs nodules but areas of focal chorioretinal atrophy with loss of the retinal pigment epithelium (**Fig. 24-9**). In the chronic stage of the disease the histology takes on a nongranulomatous appearance and there is involvement of the choriocapillaris; finally, in the chronic recurrent stage the disease appears to become granulomatous again. This may indicate different mechanisms of immune response during different stages of the disease course.

Kahn and colleagues[112] used immunohistochemical techniques to study enucleated eyes from a patient with active VKH. They found that the uveal infiltrates were composed predominantly of T cells and HLA-DR+ macrophages. Nondendritic CD1 (Leu-6)-positive cells were also seen. Emulsified chorioretinal tissue was processed for viral isolation and other tissue for isolation of *Treponema pallidum*, with no

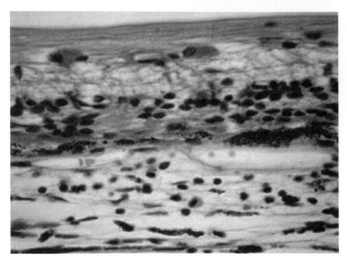

Figure 24-9. Chronic stage of VKH with atrophic lesion that was thought in the past to have been a Dalen–Fuchs nodule. *(With kind permission of Springer Science & Business Media: Rao, N.A. Pathology of vogt-koyanagi-harada's disease. International Ophthalmology. 2007 27:81.)*

microorganisms identified. Sakamoto and colleagues[113] studied the eyes from autopsies performed on two Japanese patients with this disease. They found that the choroidal infiltrate was made up mostly of T cells, with more helper/ inducer (CD4+) than suppressor/cytotoxic (CD8+) cells. They also noted that major histocompatibility complex (MHC) class II molecules were expressed on both the choroidal melanocytes and the endothelium of the choriocapillaris. Skin biopsies performed 1 month after the onset of ocular disease has shown infiltrating cells that are primarily HLA-DR+ T cells, with a CD4+ to CD8+ ratio of 3 : 1.[114]

Experimentally induced autoimmune uveoretinitis in monkeys bears a resemblance to VKH.[115] After immunization with S-antigen, eyes showed both CD3– and CD19/ CD22+ lymphocytes. Class II MHC proteins and adhesion molecules were expressed on the surface of resident ocular cells. In addition to T cells, there is an influx of B cells and the development of subretinal fibrosis. Another model of human disease, melanin protein-induced uveitis,[116] is a disease characterized by an anterior uveitis and bilateral uveal infiltrations with mainly CD4+ lymphocytes as well as monocytes.[117] Rats, Akita dogs, and monkeys immunized with tyrosinase-related protein develop inflammation ocular disease suggestive of VKH, with the rat manifesting extraocular changes as well.[118] Of interest is the fact that Cheung and coworkers[119] at the NEI tested eight patients with VKH for serum antimelanin antibodies, all of whom had such antibodies. Studies with tyrosinase demonstrate similar immune findings.[81]

Therapy

Medical management is the main therapeutic approach to VKH. The initial drug of choice remains a corticosteroid. Usually given systemically (but sometimes now given intraocularly) for this bilateral condition, the dosage needed to effect a positive therapeutic result may be high. Oral steroid administrataion has been associated with reducing the loss of vision associated with this disorder.[120] In patients with severe disease, with bilateral retinal detachments and a dramatic drop in visual acuity, a starting dose of 100–120 mg or higher (e.g., 2 mg/kg) of prednisone can be used. It is clear that when such high doses are used the patient should preferably be hospitalized, with careful follow-up. Hayasaka and colleagues[121] reported using drip infusions of 200 mg of prednisolone per day. They have seen resolution of both intraocular and extraocular symptoms in most patients treated in this fashion. Their suggestion is that less steroid may be needed for the Harada type of the disease than for the Vogt–Koyanagi component, although this has not been our own experience. In patients with particularly severe ocular disease some practitioners use intravenous high-dose pulse steroid therapy (up to 1 g/day of methylprednisolone given for 3 days) followed by oral prednisone at levels of about 1 mg/kg/day (**Fig. 24-10**). Pregnancy, a state of immunotolerance, should theoretically make the inflammatory disease less severe, which is what we have usually seen. However, Doi and coworkers[122] reported the need for high-dose steroid treatment in a pregnant 26-year-old Japanese woman with VKH just after the 18th week of gestation, whereas others have reported both mild and severe disease.[123] We are seeing the use of intracameral triamcinolone therapy, either to treat particularly severe acute retinal disease or frequently as an adjunct to systemic therapy[124,125] (**Fig. 24-11**). Although one can certainly conceive of instances where such local therapy may be useful, repeated injections are problematic, particularly with large detachments. Some may be rhegamatogenous, or the injection may create a hole, compounding the problem. Aggressive therapy does seem to make a difference in the long-term outcome of these patients.[126] Miyanaga et al.[127] examined the visual outcome of patients referred to them long after the disease had begun and treated with low-dose steroid or only topical agents, and compared them to those who had had a CSF examination and early pulse steroid therapy. They found that those with early and aggressive therapy had less integumentary involvement and less recurrent uveitis. That group all had a vision of 0.8 or better, whereas 55% of those in the delayed group did not. Read and coworkers[128] collected the results of nine clinics where they compared the results of VKH patients who either received oral steroid alone versus those receiving oral steroids plus intravenous pulse steroid therapy. No difference was seen in change in visual acuity nor fundus changes.

The duration of treatment and the rate of therapy taper must be individualized for each patient. Rubsamen and Gass[38] treated patients with steroid for 6 months on average, and longer if the disease became chronic. In our experience in patients with severe disease, one needs to continue immunosuppressive therapy for at least 1 year, with a slow, gradual taper during this time. Whereas in the past steroids were given as the sole agent for extended periods (1 year), we now would add a second or even a third immunosuppressive agent to reduce the steroid dose or stop it if possible. Paredes et al.[129] reported that those VKH patients receiving early immunosuppressive therapy did better long term with their vision than did those receiving steroid alone. This may reflect the fact that steroids cannot be maintained at an adequate dose to treat the inflammation effectively.[130] Recurrences are possible, and patients need to be monitored. The presence of new inflammatory cells in the vitreous or extraocular complaints such as headache should arouse the physician's suspicion that the

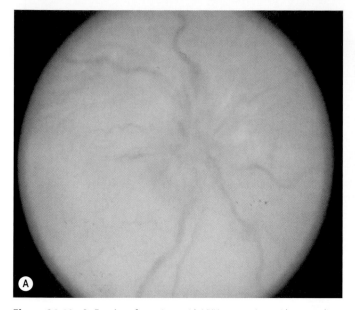
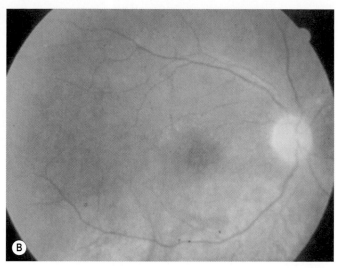

Figure 24-10. A, Fundus of a patient with VKH presenting with acute disease and visual acuity of hand motions. **B,** Appearance of fundus 10 weeks after methylprednisolone, 1 g intravenously, given every day for 3 days. The patient was then given lower doses of prednisone with a steroid-sparing agent added.

disorder may be recurring. However, continued RPE perturbation or increased prominence of peripheral white spots may or may not represent true disease activity. Visual field testing can be helpful in such cases. Some patients regain and keep good vision only at doses of prednisone that are unacceptably high for long-term use. It is at this point, in our mind set arbitrarily at about 3 months, that we would consider other therapeutic alternatives. Although other immunosuppressive agents have been used, the number of patients thus treated is relatively small.[131] Cytotoxic agents have not been used widely in the treatment of this disorder, but a positive therapeutic response to their administration has been reported.[132] We have noted that ciclosporin has been effective in the treatment of patients with VKH who had posterior pole involvement and who were not able to continue systemic corticosteroid therapy because of side effects or the extremely high doses needed to maintain good vision (see Case 24-1).[133] Using ciclosporin, we have been able to reduce dramatically the amount of steroid needed for treatment of the disease. Wakatsuki and coworkers[134] reported that the combination of ciclosporin and prednisone was effective in a patient who required 200 mg or more of prednisone to control his disease, paralleling our experience. Others used prednisone and ciclosporin combined with azathioprine,[135] and Kim et al.[136] suggested the use of low-dose azathioprine, which in our hands has not been very effective. Others have also reported its therapeutic efficacy but stressed the secondary effects and the possibility of disease relapse with drug withdrawal.[137] Tacrolimus (FK506)[138] has been used in a small number of patients with VKH with a positive therapeutic response, but with the induction of a variety of adverse side effects. Recently, a patient was treated using adalimumab (Humira) who received 40 mg every other week for 8 months, permitting discontinuance of his steroids and ciclosporin.[139]

Subretinal neovascular membranes can occur in this disorder and need to be treated. PDT was used in a report of six eyes, with five demonstrating recent and classic lesions, and five having active inflammation.[140] The results appeared

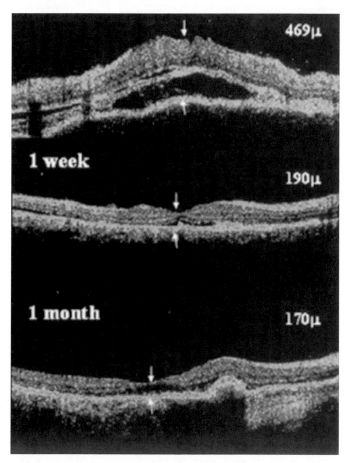

Figure 24-11. Results of an intravitreal injection of triamcinolone in a patient with acute VKH. *(From Andrade RE, Muccioli C, Farah ME, et al. Intravitreal triamcinolone in the treatment of serous retinal detachment in Vogt–Koyanagi–Harada syndrome. Am J Ophthalmol 2004;137:752–4.)*

to be mixed. Although it appeared to control the membrane, subretinal fibrosis developed. We would rather use anti-VEGF therapies today, or possibly add rapamycin to the patient's therapeutic regimen (see Therapy).

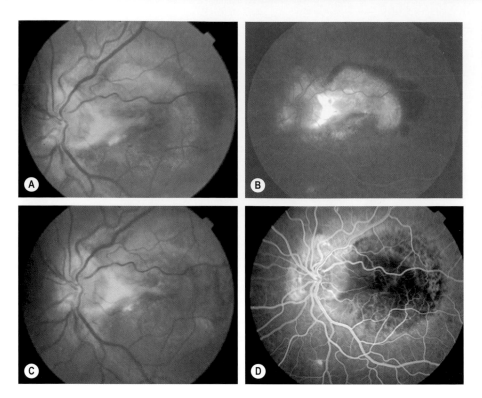

Figure 24-12. A and B, A 10-year-old girl with VKH and a large subretinal neovascular membrane involving her whole posterior pole. Vision was 20/800. **C and D,** Photodynamic therapy was given, and vision stabilized at 20/320. *(Courtesy of Rubens Belfort Jr, MD, and Cristina Muccioli, MD, São Paulo, Brazil.)*

Nonmedical treatment methods have been employed in a small number of patients. Although usually not a primary therapeutic approach, drainage of the nonrhegmatogenous detachment might be beneficial in some patients whose disease did not resolve with medical therapy (R. Nozik, personal communication).[141] It should be kept in mind that rhegmatogenous detachments can occur and need to be re-attached as quickly as permitted by the inflammatory condition. Laser therapy for the neovascular lesions that arise as a result of the inflammatory disease is an important adjunct. Photodynamic therapy had been employed for patients with VKH that manifest subretinal neovascular membranes (**Fig. 24-12**). However, anti-VEGF therapy would nowadays probably be employed first. Plasmapheresis has been used in a limited number of patients with initially good responses in some, but it is not clear whether this therapy will have a long-term beneficial response.

Cataract extraction

Cataract extraction in patients with VKH is a complicated issue. Moorthy and colleagues[142] found that cataracts developed over the course of therapy in 26 of 65 consecutive patients with VKH. One can find reports in the literature suggesting that intraocular lens (IOL) placement after a planned extracapsular cataract extraction resulted in no exacerbation of the patient's disease and an improvement of visual acuity from vision preoperatively.[143] Although this clinical result certainly can happen, the treating physician must be very careful in the evaluation of the patient with VKH. Extensive synechiae may belie a tendency that will manifest after the surgery, with resultant lens capture by the iris, as well as collection of myriad keratic precipitates on the anterior and posterior surfaces of the lens or the development of retrolental membranes necessitating repeated YAG laser procedures. Many patients who have undergone pars plana vitrectomy along with their cataract extraction adapt well to aphakic correction. This approach almost always prevents the bound-down small pupil that makes it essentially impossible to visualize the posterior pole. With the bound-down pupil changes in visual acuity become difficult to assess, and one must deal with the question of whether it is due to ongoing posterior segment inflammation, neovascular membrane, unrecognized glaucoma, or even a low-lying retinal detachment. Despite these concerns, certain well-chosen patients have shown benefit from IOL placement, but in our experience they comprise only a small number. However, cataract extraction may result in a marked improvement in visual acuity and should be considered strongly in these patients.[142]

Case 24-1

A 39-year-old white woman with Native American ancestry developed bilateral posterior uveitis with serous retinal detachments. Her vision fell to 20/400 in both eyes (OU). She began to have severe headaches. A lumbar puncture was performed, and 25/mm³ mononuclear cells were noted. Soon after, a profound hearing loss developed in both ears, which was documented on an audiogram. She was given 120 mg/day of prednisone for 1 month, with no improvement in her condition. At this point the oral prednisone dose was tapered as quickly as was medically permissible, and the patient was given ciclosporin. The response in both eyes was slow, but a constant reduction in inflammatory disease was followed by a gradual improvement in visual acuity OU. Her vision reached 20/40 OU. Some months after her vision was stabilized, an attempt was made to reduce and then stop the ciclosporin. Renewed intraocular inflammatory disease was observed. The patient's condition was stabilized with a dose of 10 mg of prednisone coupled with 2–3 mg/kg day of ciclosporin.

Case 24-2

A 17-year-old African-American woman with no Native American ancestry was known to have a positive PPD test reaction (but no radiologic evidence of tuberculosis), for which she was treated with isoniazid and p-aminosalicylic acid for 1 year. The patient had no history of ocular disease. She underwent a repeat PPD test for a physical examination, and 5 days later her vision decreased to hand-motion vision in the

right eye and counting-fingers vision in the left. She had bilateral serous retinal detachments with creamy deep spots throughout the fundus. She complained of intermittent tinnitus. In addition, the site of the PPD test developed vitiligo, and a skin biopsy revealed a marked decrease in melanocytes in this region. A spinal tap was not performed. She was given a dose of 120 mg prednisone daily. Her visual acuity began to improve rapidly, and after 4–6 weeks it had returned to the 20/30–20/40 range. An audiologic evaluation failed to demonstrate a hearing loss. Results of the ocular examination showed that the retinal detachments had resolved. However, striae in the macular region were seen in both eyes. She has maintained this good vision, with no recurrences, for over 5 years after stopping all medication.

References

1. Herbort CP, Mochizuki M. Vogt–Koyanagi–Harada disease: inquiry into the genesis of a disease name in the historical context of Switzerland and Japan. Int Ophthalmol 2007; 27(2–3): 67–79.
2. Vogt A. Frühzeitiges Ergrauen der Zilien und Bemerkungen üben den sogannten plözlichen Eintritt dieser Veränderung. Klin Monatsbl Augenheilkd 1906; 44: 228–242.
3. Koyanagi Y. Dysakusis, Alopecia un Poliosis bei schwerer Uveitis nicht traumatischen Ursprungs. Klin Monatsbl Augenheilkd 1929; 82: 194–211.
4. Harada E. Clinical observations of nonsuppurative choroiditis. Acta Soc Ophthalmol Jpn 1926; 30: 356.
5. Babel J. Syndrome de Vogt–Koyanagi. Schweiz Med Wochenschr 1932; 44: 1136–1140.
6. Sugiura S. Vogt–Koyanagi–Harada disease. Jpn J Ohthalmol 1978; 22: 9–35.
7. Abad S, Monnet D, Caillat-Zucman S, et al. Characteristics of Vogt–Koyanagi–Harada disease in a French cohort: ethnicity, systemic manifestations, and HLA genotype data. Ocul Immunol Inflamm 2008; 16(1): 3–8.
8. Ohno S, Minakawa R, Matsuda H. Clinical studies on Vogt–Koyanagi–Harada's disease. Jpn J Ophthalmol 1988; 32: 334–343.
9. Sukavatcharin S, Tsai JH, Rao NA. Vogt–Koyanagi–Harada disease in Hispanic patients. Int Ophthalmol 2007; 27(2–3): 143–148.
10. Garcia LA, Carroll MO, Garza Leon MA. Vogt–Koyanagi–Harada syndrome in childhood. Int Ophthalmol Clin 2008; 48(3): 107–117.
11. Lacerda R. Sindrome de Vogt–Koyanagi–Harada: Descrição de um caso especial em criança de sete anos de idade. Arq Bras Oftal 1994; 57: 46–48.
12. Tabbara KF, Chavis PS, Freeman WR. Vogt–Koyanagi–Harada syndrome in children compared to adults. Acta Ophthalmol Scand 1998; 76: 723–726.
13. Berker N, Ozdamar Y, Soykan E, et al. Vogt–Koyanagi–Harada syndrome in children: report of a case and review of the literature. Ocul Immunol Inflamm 2007; 15(4): 351–357.
14. Rathinam SR, Vijayalakshmi P, Namperumalsamy P, et al. Vogt–Koyanagi–Harada syndrome in children. Ocul Immunol Inflamm 1998; 6: 155–161.
15. Abu El-Asrar AM, Al-Kharashi AS, Aldibhi H, et al. Vogt–Koyanagi–Harada disease in children. Eye 2008; 22(9): 1124–1131.
16. Perry H, Font R. Clinical and histopathologic observations in severe Vogt–Koyanagi–Harada syndrome. Am J Ophthalmol 1977; 83: 242–254.
17. Beniz J, Forster DJ, Lean JS, et al. Variations in clinical features of the Vogt–Koyanagi–Harada syndrome. Retina 1991; 11: 275–280.
18. Ikeda M, Tsukagoshi H. Vogt–Koyanagi–Harada disease presenting meningoencephalitis. Report of a case with magnetic resonance imaging. Eur Neurol 1992; 32: 83–85.
19. Katterer C, Kaeser H, Steiger U. Rare form of uveitis with neurological symptoms: the Vogt–Koyanagi–Harada uveomeningoencephalitic syndrome. Schweiz Med Wochenschr 1992; 33: 281–292.
20. Sugiura S. Some observations on uveitis in Japan, with special reference to Vogt–Koyanagi–Harada and Behçet diseases (author's transl). Nippon Ganka Gakkai Zasshi 1976; 80(11): 1285–1326.
21. Kim LA, Khurana RN, Parikh JG, et al. Melanin-laden macrophages in the CSF to diagnose Vogt–Koyanagi–Harada simulating ocular syphilis. Ocul Immunol Inflamm 2008; 16(1): 59–61.
22. Ondrey FG, Moldestad E, Mastroianni MA, et al. Sensorineural hearing loss in Vogt–Koyanagi–Harada syndrome. Laryngoscope, 2006; 116(10): 1873–1876.
23. Rosen E, Uveitis, with poliosis, vitiligo, alopecia and dysacousia, (Vogt–Koyanagi syndrome). Arch Ophthalmol 1945; 33: 281–292.
24. Igawa K, Endo H, Yokozeki H, et al. Alopecia in Vogt–Koyanagi–Harada syndrome. J Eur Acad Dermatol Venereol 2006; 20(2): 236–238.
25. Kimura R, Sakai M, Okabe H. Transient shallow anterior chamber as initial symptom in Harada's syndrome. Arch Ophthalmol 1981; 99: 1604–1606.
26. Kimura R, Kasai M, Shoji K, et al. Swollen ciliary processes as an initial symptom in Vogt–Koyanagi–Harada syndrome. Am J Ophthalmol 1983; 95: 402–403.
27. Okinami S, Ogino N, Matsumura M, et al. Neovascularization at the angle of anterior chamber in cases of uveitis – high incidence in Vogt–Koyanagi–Harada disease. Nippon Ganka Gakkai Zasshi 1982; 86: 2186–2189.
28. Forster DJ, Rao NA, Hill RA, et al. Incidence and management of glaucoma in Vogt–Koyanagi–Harada syndrome. Am J Ophthalmol 1993; 100: 613–618.
29. Tabbara KF. Scleromalacia associated with Vogt–Koyanagi–Harada syndrome. Am J Ophthalmol 1988; 105: 694–695.
30. Rutzen AR, Ortega-Larrocea G, Frambach DA, et al. Macular edema in chronic Vogt–Koyanagi–Harada syndrome. Retina 1995; 15: 475–479.
31. Ober, R, Smith R, Ryan S. Subretinal neovascularization in the Vogt–Koyanagi–Harada syndrome. Int Ophthalmol 1983; 6: 225–234.
32. Moorthy R, Chong LP, Smith RE, et al. Subretinal neovascular membranes in Vogt–Koyanagi–Harada Syndrome. Am J Ophthalmol 1993; 116: 164–170.
33. Gaspar FT, Da Silva C, Damico FM, et al. Revised diagnostic criteria for Vogt–Koyanagi–Harada Disease:

Considerations on the different disease categories. Am J Ophthalmol, 2009; 147(2): 339–345.

34. Rao NA, Sukavatcharin S, Tsai JH. Vogt–Koyanagi–Harada disease diagnostic criteria. Int Ophthalmol, 2007; 27(2–3): 195–199.

35. Yamaki K, Hara K, Sakuragi S. Application of revised diagnostic criteria for Vogt–Koyanagi–Harada disease in Japanese patients. Jpn J Ophthalmol 2005; 49(2): 143–148.

36. Keino H, Goto H, Usui M. Sunset glow fundus in Vogt–Koyanagi–Harada disease with or without chronic ocular inflammation. Graefe's Arch Clin Exp Ophthalmol 2002; 240: 878–882.

37. Mondkar SV, Biswas J, Ganesh SK. Analysis of 87 cases with Vogt–Koyanagi–Harada Disease. Jpn J Ophthalmol 2000; 44: 296–301.

38. Rubsamen P, Gass D. Vogt–Koyanagi–Harada Syndrome. Clinical course, therapy, and long-term visual outcome. Arch Ophthalmol 1991; 109: 682–687.

39. Chee SP, Luu CD, Cheng CL, et al. Visual function in Vogt–Koyanagi–Harada patients. Graefes Arch Clin Exp Ophthalmol 2005; 243(8): 785–790.

40. Jap A, Luu CD, Yeo I, et al. Correlation between peripapillary atrophy and corticosteroid therapy in patients with Vogt–Koyanagi–Harada disease. Eye 2008; 22(2): 240–245.

41. Sonoda S, Nakao K, Ohbo N. Extensive chorioretinal atrophy in Vogt–Koyanagi–Harada disease. Jpn J Ophthalmol 1999; 43: 113–119.

42. Kuo IC, Rechdouni A, Rao NA, et al. Subretinal fibrosis in patients with Vogt–Koyanagi–Harada disease. Ophthalmology 2000; 107: 1721–1728.

43. Lertsumitkul S, Whitcup SM, Nussenblatt RB, et al. Subretinal fibrosis and choroidal neovascularization in Vogt–Koyanagi–Harada syndrome. Graefe's Arch Clin Exp Ophthalmol 1999; 237: 1039–1045.

44. Al-Kharashi AS, Aldibhi H, Al-Fraykh H, et al. Prognostic factors in Vogt–Koyanagi–Harada disease. Int Ophthalmol 2007; 27(2–3): 201–210.

45. Kayazawa F, Takahashi H. Acute posterior multifocal placoid pigment epitheliopathy and Harada's disease. Ann Opthalmol 1983; 15: 58–62.

46. Rao N, Marak G. Sympathetic ophthalmia simulating Vogt–Koyanagi–Harada's disease: a clinico-pathologic study of four cases. Jpn J Ophthalmol 1983; 27: 506–511.

47. Kamondi A, Szegedi A, Papp A, et al. Vogt–Koyanagi–Harada disease presenting initially as aseptic meningoencephalitis. Eur J Neurol 2000; 7: 719–722.

48. Kouda N, Sasaki H, Harada S, et al. Early Manifestation of Vogt–Koyanagi–Harada Disease as

unilateral posterior scleritis. Jpn J Ophthalmol 2002; 46: 590–593.

49. Khurana RN, Albini T, Green RL, et al. *Bartonella henselae* infection presenting as a unilateral panuveitis simulating Vogt–Koyanagi–Harada syndrome. Am J Ophthalmol 2004; 138(6): 1063–1065.

50. Pahk PJ, Todd DJ, Blaha GR, et al. Intravascular lymphoma masquerading as Vogt–Koyanagi–Harada syndrome. Ocul Immunol Inflamm 2008; 16(3): 123–126.

51. Papastathopoulos K, Bouzas E, Naoum G, et al. Vogt–Koyanagi–Harada disease associated with interferon-A and ribavirin therapy for chronic hepatitis C infection. J Infect 2006; 52(2): e59–e61.

52. Touitou V, Sene D, Fardeau C, et al. Interferon-alpha2a and Vogt–Koyanagi–Harada disease: a double-edged sword? Int Ophthalmol 2007; 27(2–3): 211–215.

53. Manger CI, Ober R. Retinal arteriovenous anastomoses in the Vogt–Koyanagi–Harada syndrome. Am J Ophthalmol 1980; 89: 186–191.

54. Herbort CP, Mantovani A, Bouchenaki N. Indocyanine green angiography in Vogt–Koyanagi–Harada disease: angiographic signs and utility in patient follow-up. Int Ophthalmol 2007; 27(2–3): 173–182.

55. Wu W, Wen F, Huang S, et al. Indocyanine green angiographic findings of Dalen–Fuchs nodules in Vogt–Koyanagi–Harada disease. Graefes Arch Clin Exp Ophthalmol 2007; 245(7): 937–940.

56. Yang P, Fang W, Wang L, et al. Study of macular function by multifocal electroretinography in patients with Vogt–Koyanagi–Harada syndrome. Am J Ophthalmol 2008; 146(5): 767–771.

57. Nagaya T. Use of the electro-oculogram for diagnosing and following the development of Harada's disease. Am J Ophthalmol 1972; 74: 99–109.

58. Okamoto Y, Miyake Y, Horio N, et al. Delayed regeneration of foveal cone photopigments in Vogt–Koyanagi–Harada disease at the convalescent stage. Invest Ophthalmol Vis Sci 2004; 45(1): 318–322.

59. Suzuki S. Quantitative evaluation of 'sunset glow' fundus in Vogt–Koyanagi–Harada disease. Jpn J Ophthalmol 1999; 43: 327–333.

60. Gallagher MJ, Yilmaz T, Cervantes-Castañeda RA, et al. The characteristic features of optical coherence tomography in posterior uveitis. Br J Ophthalmol 2007; 91(12): 1680–1685.

61. Yamamura K, Mori K, Hieda O, et al. Anterior segment optical coherence tomography findings of acute angle-closure glaucoma in Vogt–Koyanagi–Harada disease. Jpn J Ophthalmol 2008; 52(3): 231–232.

62. Gupta V, Gupta A, Gupta P, et al. Spectral-domain cirrus optical coherence tomography of choroidal striations seen in the acute stage of Vogt–Koyanagi–Harada disease. Am J Ophthalmol 2009; 147(1): 148–153.

63. Wu W, Wen F, Huang S, et al. Choroidal folds in Vogt–Koyanagi–Harada disease. Am J Ophthalmol 2007; 143(5): 900–901.

64. Yawata N, Nakamura S, Kijima M, et al. High incidence of glucose intolerance in Vogt–Koyanagi–Harada disease. Br J Ophthalmol 1999; 83: 39–42.

65. Liu T, Sun S. Peripheral lymphocyte subsets in patients with Vogt–Koyanagi–Harada syndrome (VKH). Chung Hua Yen Ko Tsa Chih 1993; 29: 138–140.

66. Okubo K, Kurimoto S, Okubo K, et al. Surface markers of peripheral blood lymphocytes in Vogt–Koyanagi–Harada disease. J Clin Lab Immunol 1985; 17: 49–52.

67. Ohno S. Immunological aspects of Behçet's and Vogt-Koyanagi-Harada's diseases. Trans Ophthalmol Soc UK 1981; 101: 335–341.

68. Hooks J, Moutsopoulos HM, Geis SA, et al. Immune interferon in the circulation of patients with autoimmune disease. N Engl J Med 1979; 301: 5–8.

69. Sakaguchi M, Sugita S, Sagawa K, et al. Cytokine production by T cells infiltrating in the eye of uveitis patients. Jpn J Ophthalmol 1998; 42: 262–268.

70. Imai Y, Sugita M, Nakamura S, et al. Cytokine production and helper T cell subsets in Vogt–Koyanagi–Harada's disease. Curr Eye Res 2001; 22: 312–318.

71. Ohta K, Yoshimura N. Expression of Fas antigen on helper T lymphocytes in Vogt–Koyanagi–Harada disease. Graefe's Arch Clin Exp Ophthalmol 1998; 236: 434–439.

72. Miyazawa I, Abe T, Narikawa K, et al. Chemokine profile in the cerebrospinal fluid and serum of Vogt–Koyanagi–Harada disease. J Neuroimmunol 2005; 158(1–2): 240–244.

73. Li B, Yang P, Zhou H, et al. Upregulation of T-bet expression in peripheral blood mononuclear cells during Vogt–Koyanagi–Harada disease. Br J Ophthalmol 2005; 89(11): 1410–1412.

74. Chen L, Yang P, Zhou H, et al. Diminished frequency and function of CD4+CD25[high] regulatory T cells associated with active uveitis in Vogt–Koyanagi–Harada syndrome. Invest Ophthalmol Vis Sci 2008; 49(8): 3475–3482.

75. Chi W, Yang P, Li B, et al. IL-23 promotes CD4+ T cells to produce IL-17 in Vogt–Koyanagi–Harada disease. J Allergy Clin Immunol 2007; 119(5): 1218–1224.

76. Liu L, Yang P, He H, et al. Leptin increases in Vogt–Koyanagi–Harada (VKH) disease and promotes cell proliferation and inflammatory cytokine secretion. Br J Ophthalmol 2008; 92(4): 557–561.

77. Momoeda S. Lymphocyte transformation test in Vogt–Koyanagi–Harada syndrome. Acta Soc Ophthalmol Jpn 1976; 80: 491–495.

78. Yuasa T, Murai Y, Hoki T, et al. Lymphocyte transformation test and migration inhibition test of macrophages in Vogt–Koyanagi–Harada's syndrome. Acta Soc Ophthalmol Jpn 1973; 77: 1652–1657.

79. Maezawa N, Yano A, Taniguchi M, et al. The role of cytotoxic T lymphocytes in the pathogenesis of Vogt–Koyanagi–Harada disease. Ophthalmologica 1982; 185: 179–186.

80. Maezawa N, Yano A. Requirement of Ia-positive nylon wool adherent cells for the activation of cytotoxic T lymphocytes specific for melanocyte-associated antigens in patients with Vogt–Koyanagi–Harada's disease. Jpn J Opthalmol 1988; 32: 348–357.

81. Yamaki K, Gocho K, Hayakawa K, et al. Tyrosinase family proteins are antigens specific to Vogt–Koyanagi–Harada disease. J Immunol 2000; 165: 7323–7329.

82. Sugita S, Takase H, Taguchi C, et al. Ocular infiltrating CD4+ T cells from patients with Vogt–Koyanagi–Harada disease recognize human melanocyte antigens. Invest Ophthalmol Vis Sci 2006; 47(6): 2547–2554.

83. Yamaki K, Kondo I, Nakamura H, et al. Ocular and extraocular inflammation induced by immunization of tyrosinase related protein 1 and 2 in Lewis rats. Exp Eye Res 2000; 71: 361–369.

84. Gocho K, Kondo I, Yamaki K. identification of autoreactive T cells in Vogt–Koyanagi–Harada disease. Invest Ophthalmol Vis Sci 2001; 42: 2004–2009.

85. Yamada K, Senju S, Shinohara T, et al. Humoral immune response directed against LEDGF in patients with VKH. Immunol Lett 2001; 78: 161–168.

86. Yeh S, Karne NK, Kerkar SP, et al. Ocular and systemic autoimmunity after successful tumor-infiltrating lymphocyte immunotherapy for recurrent, metastatic melanoma. Ophthalmology 2009; 116(5): 981–989.

87. Nussenblatt R, Gery I, Ballintine EJ, et al Cellular immune responsiveness of uveitis patients to retinal S-antigen. Am J Ophthalmol 1980.

88. Chan C, Palestine AG, Nussenblatt RB, et al. Anti-retinal auto-antibodies in Vogt–Koyanagi–Harada syndrome, Behçet's disease, and sympathetic ophthalmia. Ophthalmology 1985; 92: 1025–1028.

89. Rathinam SR, Namperumalsamy P, Nozik RA, et al. Vogt–Koyanagi–Harada syndrome after cutaneous injury. Ophthalmology 1999; 106: 635–638.

90. Ashkenazi I, Gutman I, Melamed S, et al. Vogt–Koyanagi–Harada syndrome in two siblings. Metab Pediatr Syst Ophthalmol 1991; 14: 64–67.

91. Itho S, Kurimoto S, Kouno T. Vogt–Koyanagi–Harada disease in monozygotic twins. Int Ophthalmol 1992; 16: 49–54.

92. Kunikane H. Analysis of HLA-DQWa antigen ethnic polymorphism among a Japanese and Caucasian population and an association with Harada's disease. Hokkaido Igaku Zasshi 1986; 61: 672–681.

93. Zhao M, Yougin J, Abrahams I. Association of HLA antigens with Vogt–Koyanagi–Harada syndrome in a Han Chinese population. Arch Ophthalmol 1991; 109: 368–370.

94. Zhang X, Wang X, Hu T. Profiling human leukocyte antigens in Vogt–Koyanagi–Harada syndrome. Am J Ophthalmol 1992; 113: 567–572.

95. Numaga J, Matsuki K, Tokunaga K, et al. Analysis of human leukocyte antigen HLA-DR beta amino acid sequence in Vogt–Koyanagi–Harada syndrome. Invest Ophthalmol Vis Sci 1991; 32: 1958–1961.

96. Yu Q, Mao W, Xie C, et al. HLA antigens and Vogt–Koyanagi–Harada's disease. Yen Ko Hsueh Pao 1991; 7: 3–5.

97. Kim MH, Seong MC, Kwak NH, et al. Association of HLA with Vogt–Koyanagi–Harada syndrome in Koreans. Am J Ophthalmol 2000; 129: 173–177.

98. Davis J, Mittal KK, Freidlin V, et al. HLA associations and ancestry in Vogt–Koyanagi–Harada disease and sympathetic ophthalmia. Ophthalmology 1990; 97: 1137–1142.

99. Rutzen A, Ortega-Larrocea G, Schwab IR, et al. Simultaneous onset of Vogt–Koyanagi–Harada syndrome in monozygotic twins. Am J Opthalmol 1995; 119: 239–240.

100. Martinez J, Lopez PF, Sternberg P Jr, et al. Vogt–Koyanagi–Harada syndrome in patients with Cherokee Indian ancestry. Am J Opthalmol 1992; 144: 615–620.

101. Alaez C, del Pilar Mora M, Arellanes L, et al. Strong association of HLA class II sequences in Mexicans with Vogt–Koyanagi–Harada's disease. Hum Immunol 1999; 60: 875–882.

102. Levinson RD, See RF, Rajalingam R, et al. HLA-DRB1 and -DQB1 alleles in Mestizo patients with Vogt–Koyanagi–Harada's disease in Southern California. Hum Immunol 2004; 65(12): 1477–1482.

103. Levinson RD, Du Z, Luo L, et al. KIR and HLA gene combinations in Vogt–Koyanagi–Harada disease. Hum Immunol 2008; 69(6): 349–353.

104. Horie Y, Takemoto Y, Miyazaki A, et al. Tyrosinase gene family and Vogt–Koyanagi–Harada disease in Japanese patients. Mol Vis 2006; 12: 1601–1605.

105. Horie Y, Kitaichi N, Takemoto Y, et al. Polymorphism of IFN-gamma gene and Vogt–Koyanagi–Harada disease. Mol Vis 2007; 13: 2334–2338.

106. Du L, Yang P, Hou S, et al. Association of the CTLA-4 gene with Vogt–Koyanagi–Harada syndrome. Clin Immunol 2008; 127(1): 43–48.

107. Morris W, Schlaegel TJ. Virus-like inclusion bodies in subretinal fluid in uveo-encephalitis. Am J Opthalmol 1964; 58: 940–945.

108. Moreira M, Moreira C. Virus search in cerebrospinal fluid in Vogt–Koyanagi syndrome: report of a case. Arq Neuropsiquiatr 1984; 42: 408–410.

109. Sunakawa M, Okinami S. Epstein–Barr virus-related antibody pattern in uveitis. Jpn J Opthalmol 1985; 29: 423–428.

110. Rao NA. Mechanisms of inflammatory response in sympathetic ophthalmia and VKH syndrome. Eye 1997; 11: 213–216.

111. Rao NA. Pathology of Vogt–Koyanagi–Harada disease. Int Ophthalmol 2007; 27(2–3): 81–85.

112. Kahn M, Pepose JS, Green WR, et al. Immunocytologic findings in a case of Vogt–Koyanagi–Harada syndrome. Ophthalmology 1993; 100: 1191–1198.

113. Sakamoto T, Murata T, Inomata H. Class II major histocompatibility complex on melanocytes of Vogt–Koyanagi–Harada disease. Arch Opthalmol 1991; 109: 1270–1274.

114. Okada T, Sakamoto T, Ishibashi T, et al. Vitiligo in Vogt–Koyanagi–Harada disease: immunohistological analysis of inflammatory site. Graefe's Arch Clin Exp Ophthalmol 1996; 234: 359–363.

115. Fujino Y, Li Q, Chung H, et al. Immunopathology of experimental autoimmune uveoretinitis in primates. Autoimmunity 1992; 13: 303–309 (beta).

116. Broekhuyse R, Kuhlmann ED, Winkens HJ, et al. Experimental autoimmune anterior uveitis (EAAU), a new form of experimental uveitis. I. Induction by a detergent-insoluble, intrinsic protein fraction of the retina pigment epithelium. Exp Eye Res 1991; 52: 465–474.

117. Chan C, Hikita N, Dastgheib K, et al. Experimental melanin-protein induced uveitis in the Lewis rat: Immunopathological processes. Opthalmology 1994; 101: 1275–1280.

118. Yamaki K, Ohono S. Animal models of Vogt–Koyanagi–Harada disease (sympathetic ophthalmia). Ophthalmic Res 2008; 40(3–4): 129–135.

119. Cheung M, Walton C, Chan CC, et al. Subretinal fibrosis in Vogt–Koyanagi–Harada disease. Invest Ophthalmol Vis Sci 1995; 36: 5782.

120. Bykhovskaya I, Thorne JE, Kempen JH, et al. Vogt–Koyanagi–Harada disease: clinical outcomes. Am J Ophthalmol 2005; 140(4): 674–678.

121. Hayasaka S, Okabe H, Takahashi J. Systemic corticosteroid treatment in Vogt–Koyanagi–Harada disease. Graefes Arch Clin Exp Ophthalmol 1982; 218: 9–13.

122. Doi M, Matsubara H, Uji Y. Vogt–Koyanagi–Harada syndrome in a pregnant patient treated with high-dose systemic corticostoids. Acta Ophthalmol Scand 2000; 78: 93–96.

123. Miyata N, Sugita M, Nakamura S, et al. Treatment of Vogt-Koyanagi-Harada's disease during pregnancy. Jpn J Ophthalmol 2001; 45: 177–180.

124. Andrade RE, Muccioli C, Farah ME, et al. Intravitreal triamcinolone in the treatment of serous retinal detachment in Vogt–Koyanagi–Harada syndrome. Am J Ophthalmol 2004; 137(3): 572–574.

125. Moreker MR, Lodhi SA, Pathengay A. Role of intravitreal triamcinolone as an adjuvant in the management of Vogt–Koyanagi–Harada disease. Indian J Ophthalmol 2007; 55(6): 479–480.

126. Yang P, Ren Y, Li B, et al. Clinical characteristics of Vogt–Koyanagi–Harada syndrome in Chinese patients. Ophthalmology 2007; 114(3): 606–614.

127. Miyanaga M, Kawaguchi T, Shimizu K, et al. Influence of early cerebrospinal fluid-guided diagnosis and early high-dose corticosteroid therapy on ocular outcomes of Vogt–Koyanagi–Harada disease. Int Ophthalmol 2007; 27(2–3): 183–188.

128. Read RW, Yu F, Accorinti M, et al. Evaluation of the effect on outcomes of the route of administration of corticosteroids in acute Vogt–Koyanagi–Harada disease. Am J Ophthalmol 2006; 142(1): 119–124.

129. Paredes I, Ahmed M, Foster CS. Immunomodulatory therapy for Vogt–Koyanagi–Harada patients as first-line therapy. Ocul Immunol Inflamm 2006; 14(2): 87–90.

130. Andreoli CM, Foster CS. Vogt–Koyanagi–Harada disease. Int Ophthalmol Clin 2006; 46(2): 111–122.

131. Fang W, Yang P. Vogt–Koyanagi–Harada syndrome. Curr Eye Res 2008; 33(7): 517–523.

132. Limon S, Girard R, Bloch-Michel E, et al. Les aspects actuels du syndrome du Vogt–Koyanagi–Harada. Apropos de 9 cas. J Fr Opthalmol 1985; 8: 29–35.

133. Nussenblatt R, Palestine A, Chan C. Cyclosporin A therapy in the treatment of intraocular inflammatory disease resistant to systemic corticosteroids and cytotoxic agents. Am J Ophthalmol 1983; 96: 275–282.

134. Wakatsuki Y, Kogure M, Takahashi Y, et al. Combination therapy of cyclosporin A and steroid in the severe case of Vogt–Koyanagi–Harada's disease. Jpn J Ophthalmol 1988; 32: 358–360.

135. Agarwal M, Ganesh SK, Biswas J. Triple agent immunosuppressive therapy in Vogt–Koyanagi–Harada syndrome. Ocul Immunol Inflamm 2006; 14(6): 333–339.

136. Kim SJ, Yu HG. The use of low-dose azathioprine in patients with Vogt–Koyanagi–Harada disease. Ocul Immunol Inflamm 2007; 15(5): 381–387.

137. Wakefield D, McCluckey P. Cyclosporine: a therapy in inflammatory eye disease. J Ocul Pharmacol 1991; 7: 221–226.

138. Mochizuki M, Masuda K, Sakane T, et al. A clinical trial of FK506 in refractory uveitis. Am J Ophthalmol 1993; 115: 763–769.

139. Diaz Llopis M, Amselem L, Romero FJ, et al. [Adalimumab therapy for Vogt–Koyanagi–Harada syndrome]. Arch Soc Esp Oftalmol 2007. 82(3): 131–132.

140. Nowilaty SR, Bouhaimed M. Photodynamic therapy for subfoveal choroidal neovascularisation in Vogt–Koyanagi–Harada disease. Br J Ophthalmol 2006; 90(8): 982–986.

141. Gaun S, Kurimoto Y, Komurasaki Y, et al. Vitreous surgery for bilateral bullous retinal detachment in Vogt–Koyanagi–Harada syndrome. Ophthalmic Surg Lasers 2002; 33: 508–510.

142. Moorthy R, Rajeev B, Smith RE, et al. Incidence and management of cataracts in Vogt–Koyanagi–Harada Syndrome. Am J Ophthalmol 1994; 118: 197–204.

143. Chung Y, Yeh T. Intracular lens implantation following extracapsular cataract extraction in uveitis. Ophthalmic Surg 1990; 21: 272–276.

Birdshot Retinochoroidopathy

Robert B. Nussenblatt

Key concepts

- HLA-A29 is very strongly associated with this entity.
- Long term the disorder can lead to severe visual handicap.
- Long-term therapy is often needed to control this disease.

The spectrum of posterior uveitic entities is quite broad, with similar or identical entities known by various names in the literature. Better definition of these entities is obviously a constant goal. Birdshot retinochoroidopathy fits the aforementioned spectrum, and fits into the broad scheme of 'white-dot (perhaps 'splotch' is a better word!) syndromes.' However, this disorder seems to have better-defined boundaries than some of the others in the white-dot group. Laboratory tests, albeit not definitive, appear to help the clinician in making this diagnosis. The entity appears to have distinct characteristics; it occurs more frequently in whites of northern European extraction and has a strong genetic association. Several reviews have described it.[1–4] As this is a chronic, ongoing disease, we need to be very cognizant of the fact that it has a significant impact on the non-visual aspects of patients' quality of life.[5]

Clinical manifestations

Birdshot retinochoroidopathy was first described by Ryan and Maumenee[6] in 1980 and soon after by Gass in 1981,[7] who called it vitiliginous chorioretinitis. According to Gass – and this has been our experience as well – it is seen in healthy persons, more commonly women, with an onset somewhat later than that of other uveitic entities in the third to the sixth decades. One recent report described a patient with birdshot retinochoroidopathy as also having psoriasis;[8] another reported a patient with birdshot retinochoroidopathy as also having an autoimmune sensorineural hearing loss;[9] these may be chance occurrences. This disorder affects a small percentage of the patients with uveitis whom we see at the National Eye Institute. In our experience, 58% of these patients are women, whose average age is 48 years.[10] Patients report an increased number of floaters and often have difficulty with night vision or color distinctions. In the original description by Ryan and Maumenee,[6] the key elements of the clinical presentation are as outlined in **Box 25-1**; see also **Figure 25-1**. For research purposes, the following criteria

have been assembled, not really different in any major way from the clinical presentation outlined (**Box 25-2**).

Fuerst and colleagues[11] believed they could distinguish four patterns of birdshot-spot distribution in the nine patients they evaluated: those with (1) macular sparing or (2) macular predominance; those that were (3) asymmetric with a concentration of spots, particularly inferiorly; and those that were (4) diffuse. In our experience the lesions tend to be present in the posterior pole and extend to the equator, but not generally beyond that. The lesions themselves appear deep in the fundus, are circular or oval, and are fairly large (at times 0.75 disc diameter in area). The edges of the lesions are usually not sharply defined, and frequently do not stand out as being sharply demarcated, particularly in a 'blond' fundus. Often they are best observed with the indirect ophthalmoscope. The lesions themselves may have 'substance' to them; we have interpreted this appearance as evidence of an active lesion, whereas with time they may flatten out, giving a more atrophic appearance (**Fig. 25-2**). The lesions can disappear. Usually the lesions in the posterior pole do not have a significant amount of pigment surrounding them and those in the periphery perhaps have even less. The overlying retina may be quite normal, although in more advanced disease an edematous or thinned retina can be perceived. In the late stages, examination of the posterior segment reveals a strikingly blond fundus, suggestive in our minds of the involvement of the outer retina and the retinal pigment epithelium. Rothova and von Schooneveld[12] reported end-stage findings in one patient who did not receive immunosuppressive therapy. The patient's electroretinograms (ERGs) ultimately were flat, and the retina resembled a tapetoretinal dystrophy. Using fundus autofluorescence, the hypopigmented lesions did not correspond to the white-cream colored lesions[13] (**Fig. 25-3**). They are however, reflective of retinal pigment epithelial damage or death and could explain the poor vision seen in some patients.

Ocular examination and ancillary clinical tests

Examination of the macula is imperative, as cystoid edema is a significant sequela to this disease. We noted it in 41% of the eyes with birdshot retinochoroidopathy we followed.[10] Its presence is important in establishing the diagnosis and in deciding on a correct therapeutic approach. Monnet and coworkers[14] reported that cystoid macular edema was the most common casue of a drop in visual acuity in the 80 patients they reported. Thorne et al.[15] reported cystoid macular edema in 20% of their patient group, noting that

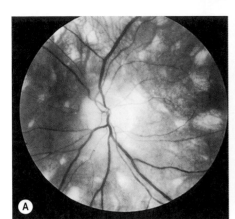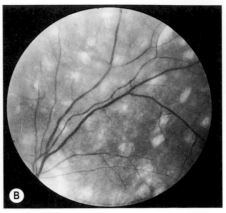

Figure 25-1. Multiple cream-colored lesions, circular or oval, deep to the retina, are seen in birdshot retinopathy. They tend to be clustered in the posterior pole **(A)** out to the midperiphery **(B)**.

Box 25-1 Findings supporting diagnosis of birdshot retinochoroidopathy

PATIENT

White

Female

Late 40s to 50s

OCULAR EXAMINATION FINDINGS

Quiet anterior chamber

Vitreal inflammation but no snowbanking

Retinal vascular leakage and cystoid macular edema

Deep circular cream-colored lesions, mostly in the posterior pole and surrounding areas

Bilateral

Low to moderate risk of subretinal neovascularization

ADDITIONAL TESTS

Abnormal electroretinogram and electrooculogram findings

Evidence of retinal autoimmunity

HLA-A29+

Box 25-2 Birdshot chorioretinopathy: diagnostic criteria for research purposes[81]

Required characteristics

1. Bilateral disease
2. Presence of at least three peripapillary 'birdshot lesions'* inferior or nasal to the optic disc in one eye
3. Low-grade anterior segment Intraocular inflammation (defined as ≤1 + cells in the anterior chamber†)
4. Low grade vitreous inflammatory reaction (defined as ≤2 + vitreous haze‡)

Supportive findings

1. HLA-A29 positivity
2. Retinal vasculitis
3. Cystoid macular edema

Exclusion criteria

1. Keratic precipitates
2. Posterior synechiae
3. Presence of infectious, neoplastic, or other inflammatory diseases that can cause multifocal choroidal lesions§

---

*Cream-colored, irregular or elongated, choroidal lesions with indistinct borders, the long axis of which is radial to the optic disc. Typical lesions are illustrated in the Figure 25-1.
†As defined by the Standardization of Uveitis Nomenclature (SUN) Working Group.[12]
‡As defined by Nussenblatt and associates.[13]
§Patient should be evaluated for the following disorders by appropriate history taking, physical examination, or laboratory tests: sarcoidosis with panuveitis or posterior uveitis; intraocular lymphoma; acute posterior multifocal placoid pigment epitheliopathy (APMPPE); multifocal choroiditis and panuveitis; punctate inner choroidopathy (PIC); multifocal evanescent white dot syndrome (MEWDS); pars planitis syndrome; posterior scleritis; sympathetic ophthalmia; Vogt–Koyanagi–Harada disease (chronic stage); syphilis; tuberculosis.

---

the longer the patient had had the disease the greater the chance of developing cystoid macular edema and the greater the chance of a decrease in vision. Patients with birdshot retinochoroidopathy have a vitreal reaction, although if cystoid edema is not present visual acuity will often be quite good despite the opacities. The disease may initially be low grade, and patients may not be aware of visual alterations, with lesions being noted because of a routine examination or after cataract surgery.[16,17]

The use of fluorescein angiography is helpful in delineating the degree of retinal vascular leakage and the severity of the macular edema. This technique very dramatically underscores the rather marked retinal vascular component of this disease, as well as inflammatory disease affecting the optic nerve head (**Fig. 25-4**). However, as Gass first noted – as have all the investigators reporting their findings concerning this disease – the cream-colored lesions are far more prominent ophthalmoscopically than with fluorescein angiography. Although mild hyperfluorescence may be noted in the later stage of the angiogram, early photographs in the angiogram may not demonstrate either hypo- or hyperfluorescence (**Fig. 25-5**). Optical coherence tomography (OCT) has been a useful way to determine the presence of macular edema and also to monitor for its disappearance. Ultrahigh-resolution OCT has provided us with a new and important

view of the damage that can occur with the inflammatory disease of birdshot.[18] Monnet et al.[19] have corroborated what we showed years ago: that a drop in visual acuity is associated with macular thickness rather than the area of fluorescein leakage. They did report that the loss of the third highly reflective band (HRB) seen on OCT is associated with poorer visual acuity[19] (**Fig. 25-6**). Forooghian et al.,[20] using high-definition OCT, showed that foveal atrophy was a complication of many uveitic syndromes, including birdshot retinochoroidopathy.

Indocyanine green (ICG) has been used to study this disorder (**Fig. 25-7**). Although the use of ICG will elucidate more lesions than are seen clinically, early on in its use it was suggested that it was not particularly useful in following

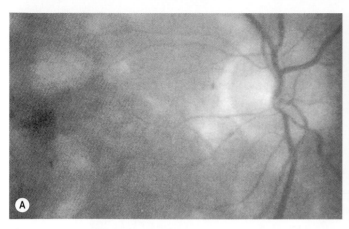
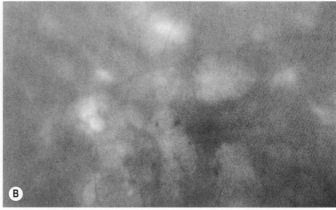

Figure 25-2. A and B, High-magnification fundus photographs of lesions in long-standing disease. There is loss of retinal pigment epithelium in some areas, and choroidal vessels are apparent.

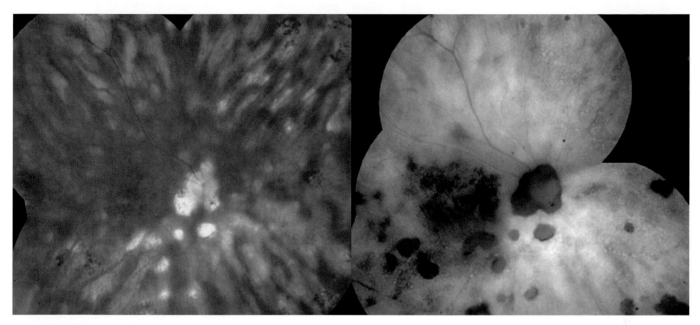

Figure 25-3. Fundus autofluorescence in a patient with birdshot retinochoroidopathy. Note that the area of presumed RPE death or damage does not correlate with the fundus lesions. *(From Koizumi H, Pozzoni MC, Spaide RF. Fundus autofluorescence in birdshot chorioretinopathy. Ophthalmology 2008; 115: e15–e20.)*

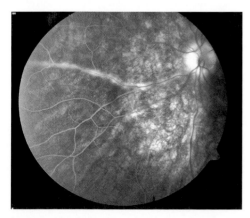

Figure 25-4. Fluorescein angiogram of birdshot fundus showing late staining of the retinal vasculature, emphasizing the vascular component of this disease.

the disease course.[21] More recently, Herbort et al.[22] have shown that choroidal lesions evolve differently than do the retinal lesions, with the former seeming more responsive to immunusuppressive therapy. Lommatzsch and coworkers[23] studied choroidal blood flow using perfusion-pressure videoangiography in a patient with birdshot retinochoroidopathy. They found that in this patient fluorescein dye penetrated through the vessel walls of the large choroidal arterioles close to the short posterior ciliary arteries. These investigators thought that this leakage was the cause of the typical birdshot pattern seen in this disorder. It does not explain, however, why most patients initially may not have dramatic angiographic evidence of disease.

Many of these patients will show altered retinal function in spite of good visual acuity. The visual field and electroretinographic results are two good ways to follow the course of these patients. Visual field testing will often reveal scotomata, even in patients with good vision and minimal ocular complaints.[24,25] In a report by Thorne et al.,[26] 75% of 48 eyes had abnormal I-4 changes. Of the 28 eyes from

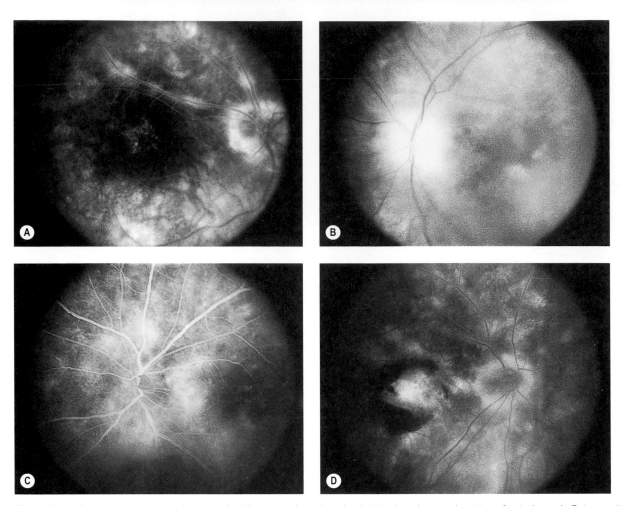

Figure 25-5. Fluorescein angiogram changes in birdshot retinochoroidopathy. **A,** Macular edema and staining of retinal vessels. **B,** Late staining of disc. **C,** Areas of hyperfluorescence corresponding to birdshot lesions can sometimes be seen, but not usually. **D,** Subretinal neovascular net in macula of a patient with birdshot retinochoroidopathy.

patients receiving immunosupprssion, the rate of visual field loss prior to therapy was 107° per year for the I-4 isopter. After therapy was initiated, there was a rate of gain of 53° per year for the isopter. Therefore therapy may reverse visual field loss. Problems with night vision and color discrimination are not uncommon in patients with this disorder, sometimes despite excellent central visual acuity. They should not be taken lightly, because alterations in retinal functions other than visual acuity can be demonstrated.

In reports investigating psychophysical and electrophysiologic testing of patients with this entity, disturbances in both the electroretinogram and the electrooculogram have been noted. Fuerst and colleagues[11] reported a b-wave amplitude reduction and an implicit time prolongation. We have seen abnormal ERGs in the majority of patients we have tested, results similar to those reported by others[10] (**Fig. 25-8**). Several electrophysiologic changes have reported. Holder et al.[27] reported that the cone-mediated flicker ERG responses are delayed before therapy initiation. Sobrin and coworkers[28] also saw the cone b-wave flicker implicit time alterations and that they seemed to improve with therapy. Zacks et al.[29] suggested that the bright scotoptic response amplitudes and the 30 Hz flicker implicit times were associated with recurrence of disease as immunosuppressive therapy is tapered. Robson et al.[30] suggest that post-

phototransduction involvement of the optic nerve pathway may be seen as well. Color-vision alterations can be found, and some patients complain of colors being 'washed out' or faded. Others may note a difference in color discrimination between their two eyes. Holland et al,[31] using the desaturated Lanthony 15-Hue Test, showed that 49 of 80 patients tested (61.3%) had abnormal color confusion scores, and this included patients with normal vision. Dark adaptation thresholds are invariably abnormal. Indeed, Kappel and coworkers[32] evaluated birdshot patients with contrast sensitivity testing. Reduced contrast sensitivity is a common finding in these eyes, being abnormal in 92% of 126 eyes tested. Although they are often related to poor vision, these authors also found that of the 38 eyes tested with normal vision, 31 (82%) had abnormal contrast sensitivity. A meta-analysis of several studies describing the clinical features of the disease can be seen in **Table 25-1**.

Because the retinal lesions can be very striking, the diagnosis would appear to be relatively easy to make. However, as with all diseases, some occurrences fall within the 'gray' zone. One should consider other diagnoses, such as multifocal choroiditis and panuveitis, described by Nozik and Dorsch[33] and also discussed by Dreyer and Gass.[34] The patients with the condition described by Nozik and Dorsch tend to be younger, to have unilateral disease more often,

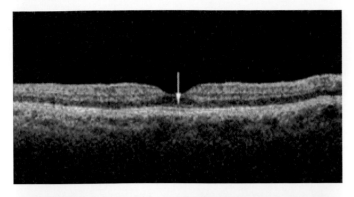

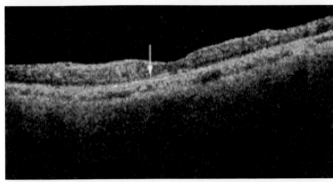

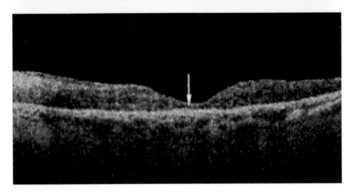

Figure 25-6. OCT showing changes in the third highly reflective band (HRB) in birdshot retinochoroidopathy. The top panel shows an intact HRB; the middle panel an HRB partially present; the lower panel absent HRB. *(From Monnet D, Levinson RD, Holland GN, et al. Longitudinal cohort study of patients with birdshot chorioretinopathy. III. Macular imaging at baseline. Am J Ophthalmol 2007; 144: 818–828.)*

have a greater degree of vitreous inflammation, and are less likely to have night blindness or abnormal ERG findings.[33] Further, the lesions in this entity tend to become pigmented, smaller, and better defined than those seen in birdshot retinochoroidopathy. Sarcoidosis has been often considered as an alternative diagnosis in the patients we have seen and evaluated.[35] Brinkman and Rothova[36] reported on six patients with neurosarcoidosis who demonstrated multifocal chorioretinal lesions, as well as optic nerve disease and a periphlebitis. In addition, the multiple evanescent white-dot syndrome, described by Jampol and colleagues,[37] and primary intraocular lymphoma (referred to as reticulum cell sarcoma in the old literature) need to be considered (see Chapter 30). Noble and Greenberg[38] reported a patient with myelodysplasia syndrome and fundus lesions resembling the appearance of birdshot retinochoroidopathy. Cases of posterior scleritis with fundus lesions reminiscent of

birdshot have been reported.[39] In a report of 11 patients with birdshot retinochoroidopathy, three had antibodies against *Borrelia burgdorferi*.[40] It is not known whether these were examples of false-positive reactions or whether in some patients the organism causing Lyme disease may play a role. Cunningham and colleagues[41] described two patients with posterior scleritis associated with choroidal thickening who, upon resolution, had posterior segment lesions resembling those of birdshot retinochoroidopathy. Neither patient was HLA-A29 positive (see below). Sommer et al.[42] reported the fundus appearance similar to birdshot that was associated with tamoxifen toxicity.

The physician should consider an alternative diagnosis to birdshot retinochoroidopathy, particularly in nonwhite patients, because this condition appears rarely, if at all, in nonwhites. It was not reported in a survey of uveitis cases from a center in China, and in Japan it is very rare (see below).[43] We have seen an African-American patient in whom birdshot retinochoroidopathy had been diagnosed but who, after an extensive evaluation, was found to have benign choroidal lymphoid hyperplasia (see Chapter 30).

Tests, histology and etiology

The exact cause of birdshot retinochoroidopathy is unknown. However, observations have provided provocative hypotheses. We have found a strong correlation between birdshot retinochoroidopathy and HLA-A29 in white patients.[44] Of the patients tested, 80% showed HLA-A29 within their genetic makeup, whereas only 7% of control subjects had this antigen. This unusually high correlation yielded a relative risk of almost 50 (see discussion on HLA in Chapter 1). This finding suggests a strong genetic predisposition for this disease. Several other studies have demonstrated the same strong association with HLA-A29[45–47] (**Table 25-2**). Le Hoang and coworkers[48] reported that 54 of 58 French patients with birdshot retinochoroidopathy showed HLA-A29 positivity (93.1%, relative risk 157.3), and that subtyping results for 33 of these patients showed the HLA-A29.2 subtype in all. HLA-A29.2 is considerably more common than HLA-A29.1. In the initial patient evaluation the absence of the HLA-A29.1 subtype raised questions about a possible 'resistance motif' in the HLA-A29.1 molecule. A single difference was found in the extracellular domain between the two HLA-A29 subtypes (i.e., A29.1 versus A29.2). Because the HLA-A29.1 subtype contains a unique mutation, it was conjectured by these authors that the ancestral type was HLA-A29.2 and that the HLA-A29.1 mutation came later and conferred resistance to birdshot retinochoroidopathy. Work by Tabary and coworkers[49] showed that the sequence of HLA-A29.2 was identical in both patients and healthy controls. The position of the HLA-A29.1 mutation would not permit it to interact with the T-cell receptor, but rather it interacted with an accessory molecule, such as CD8.

De Waal and colleagues[50] examined the question of HLA-A29 subtypes and found that in a white population from The Netherlands and Belgium, HLA-A29.2 was the more common, found in 90% of control subjects. They found that the distribution of HLA-A29.2 versus that of HLA-A29.1 did not differ among the patients with birdshot retinochoroidopathy whom they examined. Both subtypes

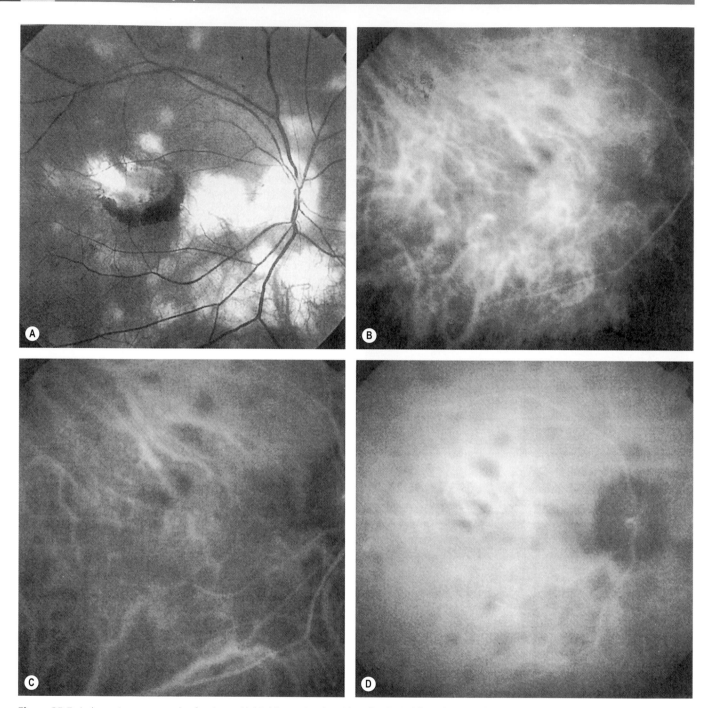

Figure 25-7. Indocyanine green study of patient with birdshot retinochoroidopathy. **A,** Red-free photograph shows blood in the macula. **B to D,** Areas of hypofluorescence in the choroid remain late into the study, whereas ICG staining also demonstrates a macular area that suggests a subfoveal net.

were found, but HLA-A29.2 predominated simply because it is almost 10 times more commonly seen, at least in this population. Others have reported the same findings.[51,52] In contrast to the northern European and American experience, some Japanese and Brazilian observers are not sure that they have seen a classic case (M. Mochizuki and R. Belfort, personal communication, 1990). Saito and colleagues[53] reported a case in Japan, but neither the patient nor 10 other Japanese patients reported were HLA-A29 negative. All of our patients have been European, apart from one who was Hispanic. HLA-B12 has been found in 68% of birdshot patients and has a relative risk of 6.15 (which is small compared to the calculated A29 relative risk).[54] This antigen is in linkage

disequilibrium with HLA-A29. Levinson and coworkers[55] have evaluated the association between this entity and HLA class I specific killer cell immunoglobulin-like receptors (KIR). KIR are important receptors of human NK cells, as well on CD8+ and CD4+ CD28 null cells. An association was noted with birdshot and the genes KIR2DS2/S3/S4, genes associated with autoimmunity. It may be that these genes activate natural killer cells and T cells, perhaps to respond to intraocular self antigens.

Additional information to support the notion that endogenous immune mechanisms play a role is the finding that patients' lymphocytes demonstrate an in vitro cell-mediated response to retinal antigens, most notably the retinal S-

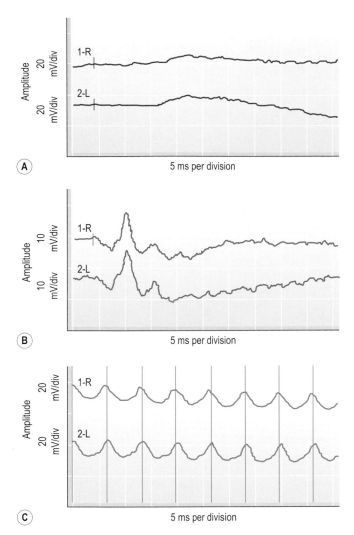

Figure 25-8 Examples of rod- and cone-mediated electroretinogram, and flicker responses from the eye of a patient with birdshot retinochoroidopathy. Rod responses (**A**) demonstrate markedly reduced amplitude, but cone responses (**B**) less so. Flicker responses (**C**), produced by cones, also have reduction of amplitude. *(From Smith JA, Whitcup SM. Birdshot retinochoroidopathy. Br J Ophthalmol 83: 241–249, 1999, with permission from the BMJ Publishing Group.)*

antigen[40] (**Fig. 25-9** and Table 25-2). Jobin and coworkers,[56] using either a lymphocyte proliferation assay or basophil degranulation, found that in vitro positivity to S-antigen appeared more frequently in the period preceding a relapse of ocular inflammation. Further, we have reported that the inflammatory response seen in one eye with birdshot retinochoroidopathy seemed directed to the photoreceptor region, the area from which the retinal S-antigen is isolated.[40] One report suggested that the major focus of the inflammatory response is situated in the choroid, with also a lymphocytic infiltrate around the retinal vasculature.[57] The collection of lymphocytes in the choroid could explain the white-cream colored lesions. The striking number of patients with birdshot retinochoroidopathy who demonstrate evidence of retinal autoimmunity suggests that this mechanism is important in this disease. Further, the disease elicited in monkeys immunized with the retinal S-antigen can take on certain characteristics not dissimilar to those seen in the human condition. The strong HLA association would add further support to the notion of an inbred error of immune regula-

tion. In this disease, HLA-A29 positivity can be used as strong corroborative evidence to support the clinical diagnosis. One might expect a strong familial association with this disorder, but this has not been the case in our experience. However, Fich and Rosenberg[58] did report birdshot retinochoroidopathy in monozygotic twins. In this case, in one of the twins the initial diagnosis was a chorioretinal dystrophy.

Why then is HLA-A29 associated with this disorder? The simple answer is that we do not know. It has been suggested that the disorder may be initiated by exogenous factors such as a virus. One could conjecture that a viral antigen may bear sequences similar to an HLA sequence, or that a new epitope consisting of a viral particle and the HLA motif becomes the target of the immune response. However, this does not completely explain the cell-mediated responsiveness against retinal antigens that has been noted in these patients. The report by Boisgérault and associates[59] offers another provocative explanation. They reported that two peptides from the carboxyl terminal sequence of the human retinal antigen bound efficiently to HLA-A29, suggesting a direct role for this HLA phenotype in the autoimmune response. Szpak et al.[60] created a transgenic mouse that expressed HLA-A29. These animals develop uveitis spontaneously, and the disease is similar to that seen in experimentally induced chorioretinitis (**Fig. 25-10**) but was not seen in all animals. The spontaneous disease was noted in 12 of 15 animals (80%) that were more than 12 months old (aged mice).[61] The mechanisms leading to the uveitis still need to be defined.

Long-term studies of patients with retinal vasculitis have yielded interesting observations. In two patients with retinal vasculitis, Soubrane and colleagues[62] reported the appearance of typical lesions of birdshot retinochoroidopathy 7 and 8 years after the first symptoms. They suggest evaluating patients for the presence of HLA-A29 even late in the course of a retinal vasculitis. A similar evolution of clinical findings was reported by Godel and coworkers.[63] An additional provocative observation was that of Bloch-Michel and Frau,[64] who reviewed the records of 20 patients with birdshot retinochoroidopathy and 36 with idiopathic retinal vasculitis. The HLA-A29 phenotype was seen in 95% of the birdshot retinochoroidopathy group, as opposed to 61% of the other group. Long-term follow-up of patients with vasculitis showed that only one developed lesions compatible with birdshot retinochoroidopathy. However, the HLA-A29 phenotype in the idiopathic vasculitis group was associated with more posterior pole involvement, a more severe disease course, and a poorer visual prognosis than in those without this phenotype. The authors suggested that the presence of this gene portends ill for its bearer, with or without lesions typical of birdshot retinochoroidopathy.

Humoral studies have not been particularly useful in further defining any underlying immunologic abnormality. This includes the absence of circulating anticardiolipin antibodies associated with thrombosis and diseases with a significant vascular component.[65] Kuhne and coworkers[66] reported two cases of retinal vasculitis associated with Q fever, induced by *Coxiella burnetii*. One patient showed HLA-A29 positivity; although the authors speculate on the role of this agent in birdshot retinochoroidopathy, they are unable to show a definitive role for this organism.

Table 25-1 A compilation of clinical characteristics

Authors	Shah et al. 2005	Monnet et al. 2006	Kiss et al. 2005	Thorne et al. 2005	Becker et al. 2005	Rothova et al. 2004
Design	Review	Cross-sectional	Retrospective	Retrospective	Retrospective	Retrospective
Period of study	1980–2002	2002/2003	1980–2003	1984–2004	1985–2001	1990–2001
Number of patients	NA	80	28	40	11	55
Female (%)	54	64	50	42.5	54	47
HLA-A29+ (%)	95.7	100	96.4	85.7	100	100
Age diagnosis (years)	NA	52.4	50.6	56	NA	53
Study time (years)	53	55.6	NA	NA	45	NA
Follow-up (months)	NA	NA	81.2	30	72 (treated patients)	NA
Range (months)	NA	NA	12–276	0–246	8–156	12–120
Main outcome measures	NA	Birdshot lesion symptoms, VA	VA, ERG complications	VA, visual field complications	VA, treatment	VA, systemic diseases, visual fields, angiography, treatment
VA						
Baseline	20/40 (LP-20/15)	0.8[a] (CF-1.2)	0.64–0.59[a] (R-L)	20/32	NA	NA
≤20/200-LP (% eyes)	14.4	5	NA	12.8	NA	8
End follow-up	20/30	NA	0.74–0.71[a]	NA	NA	NA
≤20/200-LP (% eyes)	20.6	NA	NA	20 (at 5 years)	NA	30 (at 5 yrs)
Cystoid macular edema						
Baseline	NA	23.8[b]	NA	20.5[c]	NA	NA
At any point (cumulative incidence)	70.4%	NA	35.7%[b]	50%[b] (5 years)	NA	84%[b] (5 years)
Treatment (percentage of patients treated)						
Systemic steroids	NA	35	46	67	100	65
Immunosuppressive agents	NA	41	100	54	45	53
		CI	CI, MM, AZ, others	CI, MM, AZ, MTX	AZ, MTX, MM, CI, IVIG	CI, MTX, AZ, others

NA, not applicable; VA, visual acuity; ERG, electroretinography; LP, light perception; CF, counting fingers; R–L, right to left eye; CI, cyclosporine; MM, mycophenolate mofetil; AZ, azathioprine; MTX, methotrexate; IVIG, intravenous immunoglobulin.
[a]Decimal visual acuity.
[b]Percentage of eyes.
[c]Percentage of patients.

It is worth noting that we have had at least two cases of an HLA laboratory reporting false-negative typing results for HLA-A29. One should consider repeating the HLA typing if the clinical picture strongly suggests a diagnosis of birdshot retinochoroidopathy and the HLA report does not show the presence of HLA-A29.

Therapy

A well-planned therapeutic regimen for the treatment of patients with birdshot retinochoroidopathy still needs to be devised. Three-quarters of those we have seen received either periocular or systemic steroids as part of their therapeutic regimen, and use of steroids still is the mainstay of therapy. Some patients' visual acuities will linger around the 20/30 to 20/40 range, and in the past we elected not to treat these

persons. Also, we did not institute systemic therapy unless there was a significant drop in visual acuity (to <20/40) in both eyes, with the most common reason for decreased visual acuity being cystoid macular edema (**Fig. 25-11**). However, we will now treat patients if they have good visual acuity and evidence of cystoid macular edema. Our recent observations suggest that macular edema is a harbinger of a long-term drop in visual acuity. Further, ancillary testing mentioned above supports the notion that there are physiologic changes even if the visual acuity seems normal. The patient with good vision who is being treated requires a full understanding of why this is being done. Rarely one will see subretinal neovascular nets that need prompt attention, with consideration of the use of laser photocoagulation (**Fig. 25-12**). If steroid therapy is initiated, a slow taper of systemic steroids should be considered followed by low-dose maintenance therapy. A second agent needs to be added if it is

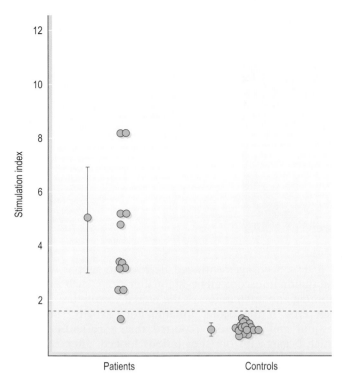

Figure 25-9. Lymphocytes of patient with birdshot retinochoroidopathy demonstrate in vitro proliferative response to retinal S-antigen whereas those of control subjects do not. This in vitro anamnestic response is thought to parallel what occurs in vitro when T cells (and other immune cells) become activated. *(From Nussenblatt RB, Mittal KK, Ryan S et al. Birdshot retinochoroidopathy associated with HLA-A29 antigen and immune responsiveness to retinal S-antigen. Am J Ophthalmol 94: 147–158, 1982. Copyright by The Ophthalmic Publishing Company.)*

Table 25-2 Immunologic parameters in patients with birdshot retinochoroidopathy

	Nussenblatt et al.[44]	Le Hoang et al.[48]
Number of patients	20	21
HLA-A29		
Patients (%)	80	90.5
Control subjects (%)	7.4	7.9
In vitro cellular responses to S-antigen		
Number tested	13	18
Patients positive (%)	12 (92.3%)	11 (61%)
Basophil degranulation to the S-antigen		
Number tested	–	18
Patients positive (%)	–	8 (44%)

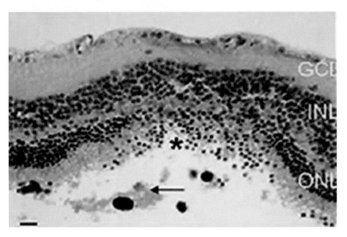

Figure 25-10. Spontaneous uveitis in A29 transgenic mouse with destruction of the photoreceptor region noted. A serous detachment was also noted by the authors. *(From de Kozak Y. Pathological aspects of spontaneous uveitis and retinopathy in HLA-A29 transgenic mice and in animal models of retinal autoimmunity: relevance to human pathologies. Ophthalmic Res 2008; 40: 175–180.)*

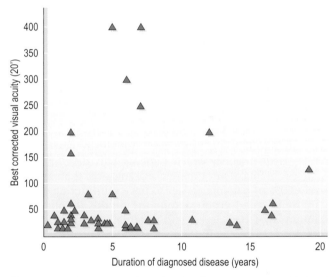

Figure 25-11. Best corrected visual acuity of 55 patients seen at National Eye Institute. Visual acuity in the better-seeing eye is charted to the duration of diagnosed disease. *(From Gasch AT, Smith JA, Whitcup SM. Birdshot retinochoroidopathy. Br J Ophthalmol 83: 241–249, 1999, with permission from the BMJ Publishing Group.)*

clear that steroid therapy is needed for more than 3–4 months. Others[67] have suggested using nonsteroidal antiinflammatory agents, but we have not found them helpful and they are not usually within our armamentarium for the treatment of this entity. Ladas and coworkers[68] reported that they were able to treat patients adequately after an initial prednisone dose of 1 mg/kg/day and then long-term (54–81 months) treatment with 5 mg or less. Zacks and associates[29] reported that abnormalities in the ERG can be associated with recurrence of disease. Changes in the bright scotopic response amplitudes and flicker implicit times were associated with recurrence. A periocular steroid is used for patients in whom disease severity is asymmetric or for treatment of exacerbations occurring while patients are receiving systemic therapy. Martidis and colleagues[69] reported the use of intraocular triamcinolone acetonide for the treatment of cystoid edema. Shah and Branley[70] treated one patient who refused systemic therapy with five intravitreal injections in each eye over a 3-year period; as expected, cataract and increased intraocular pressure were seen. In one of the cases reported, the OCT scan measured macular thickening of 540 μm, and clinically there was evidence of macular cystoid changes. After an injection of 4 mg triamcinolone acetonide (in 0.1 mL; Kenalog 40 mg/mL) using a 27-gauge needle through the pars plana, the vision ultimately improved to 20/25 and macular thickness returned to a normal 190 μm.

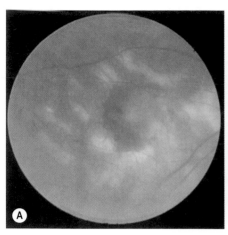 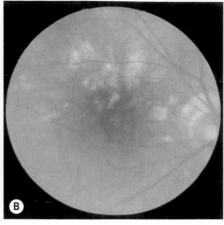

Figure 25-12. Patient with birdshot lesions strewn throughout the posterior pole of both eyes. **A,** The right eye has a subfoveal net that has bled and raised the macula. **B,** The left eye has a lesion in the macula.

The patient did experience visual perturbations in that eye for 2 days after the injection, but there was no increase in pressure. In patients with relatively good visual acuities who need occasional therapy, we really do not know whether these therapeutic approaches have a significant effect on the final visual outcome. De Geronimo and colleagues[21] reported that the retinal thickness analyzer was better than OCT to measure retinal thickness in a patient with birdshot retinochoroidopathy but no macular edema.

As with many uveitic entities, we do not know the natural history of this one. It has been the belief of some that the long-term visual prognosis for these patients is guarded, yet others have thought that the disease has a tendency to stabilize. We have seen both extremes and are unable to distinguish which patients will develop severe visual problems. Our experience[10] suggests that approximately 20% of patients appear to have self-limiting disease, maintaining good vision despite the fundus lesions. Some maintain that few eyes will maintain good vision if untreated.[71] In our published series,[10] 27 patients were followed for 5–13 years: 52% had worsening of visual acuity, 30% had stable vision, and 18% had improved vision. A visual acuity of 20/40 or better was noted in at least one eye in two-thirds of these patients, whereas 22% had a visual acuity of <20/200 in the better eye.

Any patient requiring extended (>3 months) steroid therapy should also receive a second agent. Ciclosporin has been used in some patients, and we have seen good responses.[66] This finding has been corroborated by Le Hoang and associates.[72] Vitale and colleagues[73] corroborated these earlier observations using lower doses of the drug (2.5–5 mg/kg/day) as had been recommended because of the concern for renal toxicity. Some patients needed the addition of azathioprine (1.5–2 mg/kg/day). The investigators found that vitreous inflammation was controlled in 23 eyes (88.5%) treated, and a stabilization or improvement in visual acuity occurred in 20 (83.3%). These results are to be expected because this disorder appears to be mediated by T cells, and therefore an anti-T-cell agent should have a significant effect on the disease course. In Kiss et al.'s[74] study (93%) the vast majority of patients receiving ciclosporin showed an improvement or stabilization of vision of over a median followup of 81 months. A regression model has shown that patients treated with ciclosporin had a better visual acuity than those treated with steroid.[2]

A disconcerting, continued decrease in retinal function and ophthalmoscopically evident alterations, such as retinal thinning and attenuation of the retinal vasculature, may be seen even if the ocular inflammatory activity stabilizes. Rasquin and Pereleux[75] reported that a patient's fundus which began with birdshot lesions looked, after 20 years, like tapedoretinal degeneration. This may be due to the triggering of apoptosis (programmed cell death) of the cells that constitute the retina. Because of these observations, the notion that cytotoxic agents should be given early in the disease has been entertained. We have seen patients who have undergone such therapy, and there seems to be no difference in their clinical course. Further, these patients often require long-term immunosuppressive therapy, which is usually difficult to attain with cytotoxic agents.

Other medications have been used. Becker et al.[76] used a combination of immunosuppressive approaches and achieved control of the inflammatory response. LeHoang and colleagues[77] conducted an interventional nonrandomized study involving 18 patients with birdshot retinochoroidopathy who received intravenous polyclonal immunoglobulin (IVIg). Patients were given 1.6 g/kg of IVIg every 4 weeks for 6 months as sole treatment. Afterwards, they received injections of 1.2–1.6 g/kg at 6–8-week intervals. There was a mean follow-up of 39 months. Of the 26 eyes with vision <20/30, 14 improved by two lines or more, and vision decreased in two. Transient systemic hypertension, headache, eczematous lesions, and hyperthermia were reported to have occurred during the treatment period. Hesse and colleagues[8] described a patient with birdshot retinochoroidopathy with psoriasis in whom treatment with aromatic retinoids led to resolution of both the ocular and dermatologic problems.

The use of biologics has entered into the therapeutic armamentarium as well. Although anti-TNF-α is widely used for other indications, it is less used here. Based on anectdotal information, daclizumab, the anti-IL-2 receptor-blocking agent, seems to have a positive long-term effect. We have also noted this. In eight patients treated by Sobrin et al.[78] a resolution of vasculitis was noted in six, and in seven there was a stabilization of or improvement of vision and control of inflammation. There was, however, a decline in ERG parameters in some despite control of the inflammation. This further supports the concept of an early therapeutic intervention for this disorder, as do the retinal physiologic observations in eyes that see well. To reverse the inflammatory process more rapidly, we have used high doses of daclizumab.[79] This study involved a small number of patients, including one with birdshot. In a report by Rothova and coworkers,[80] the authors put forward the concept that therapy for this disorder is not helpful, as they found a increase in those with poor vision over the years, due mostly to cystoid macular edema and macular atrophy. However, follow-up for all patients was not included at the beginning of the study. It can be argued once again that aggressive early therapy would be the best way to prevent such results long term.

If need be, cataract surgery can be performed on these patients, with adequate perioperative antiinflammatory therapy, which should result in an abatement of ocular inflammatory activity for at least 3 months. The placement of an intraocular lens is always debated. We would usually consider placement if the eye does not have extensive posterior synechiae and, of course, has good control of the intraocular inflammatory process.

Case 25-1

A 54-year-old white man was referred to the National Eye Institute with a complaint of increased floaters and shimmering. He was in good general health. His visual acuity was 20/32 in the right eye and 20/32-1 in the left. The anterior chambers both had an occasional cell, and the tensions were normal. The media had 1+ cells and 1+ haze in both eyes. Scattered yellow white lesions were strewn throughout the fundus, with more concentration in the posterior pole. They appeared deep, probably at the level of the retinal pigment epithelium or photoreceptor region. There were occasional superficial retinal hemorrhages and faint, but not definitive, cystoid edema in the left eye. There was no snowbanking.

A fluorescein angiogram demonstrated rather diffuse retinal vascular leakage, with staining of the disc in both eyes as well, and evidence of mild cystoid edema in the left eye. Goldmann fields were full, but there were patches of nonabsolute scotomas. HLA typing demonstrated the presence of HLA-A29. In vitro cell culturing showed an anamnestic response to the retinal S-antigen.

Our diagnosis was birdshot retinochoroidopathy. We elected not to treat the patient. After a follow-up period of more than 5 years the patient continues to have good central vision. He complains that he has an occasional increase in floaters, that his vision varies from day to day, and that his night vision is not as good as it used to be. We believed that prolonged therapy would carry more risk than no therapy.

Case 25-2

A 47-year-old white man had symptoms for 2 years before coming to the National Eye Institute. Although he had no anterior segment inflammatory disease, vitreitis without snowbanking was noted. He had cream-colored lesions typical of birdshot retinochoroidopathy throughout the fundus, as well as a subretinal neovascular net in the right eye. His vision was 20/400 in the right eye and 20/70 in the left. The left eye had evidence of cystoid macular edema and testing revealed HLA-A29 positivity. A subretinal net had formed despite a trial of oral steroids. It was our belief that the duration of steroid use was not sufficient, and the patient was given prednisone 80 mg/day with a slow taper that brought the maintenance dose to 20 mg/day by 3 months. The patient had a slow improvement of vision to 20/32 in the left eye and continued to receive 20 mg/day of prednisone for 6 months, which was tapered to 15 mg/day. His vision is maintained with this regimen, with minimal systemic secondary effects.

References

1. Cassoux N, Le Hoang P. Birdshot retinochoroidopathy. Ann Med Interne (Paris) 2000; 151(Suppl 1): 1S45–1S47.
2. Shah KH, Levinson RD, Yu F, et al. Birdshot chorioretinopathy. Surv Ophthalmol 2005; 50(6): 519–541.
3. Kiss S, Anzaar F, Stephen Foster C. Birdshot retinochoroidopathy. Int Ophthalmol Clin 2006; 46(2): 39–55.
4. Monnet D, Brezin AP. Birdshot chorioretinopathy. Curr Opin Ophthalmol 2006; 17(6): 545–550.
5. Levinson RD, Monnet D, Yu F, et al. Longitudinal cohort study of patients with birdshot chorioretinopathy. v. quality of life at baseline. Am J Ophthalmol 2008.
6. Ryan SJ, Maumenee AE. Birdshot retinochoroidopathy. Am J Ophthalmol 1980; 89: 31–45.
7. Gass J. Vitiligious chorioretinitis. Arch Ophthalmol 1981; 99: 1778–1787.
8. Hesse S, Berbis P, Chemila JF, et al. Psoriasis and birdshot chorioretinopathy : response to aromatic retinoids. Dermatology 1993; 187: 137–139.
9. Heaton J, Mills R. Sensineural hearing loss associated with birdshot retinochoroidopathy. Arch Otolaryngol Head Neck Surg 1993; 119: 680–681.
10. Gasch AT, Smith JA, Whitcup SM. Birdshot retinochoroidopathy. Br J Ophthalmol 1999; 83: 241–249.
11. Fuerst DJ, Tessler HH, Fishman GA, et al. Birdshot retinochoidopathy. Arch Ophthalmol 1984; 102: 214–219.
12. Rothova A, van Schooneveld MJ. The end stage of birdshot retinochoroidopathy. Br J Ophthalmol 1995; 79(11): 1058–1059.
13. Koizumi H, Pozzoni MC, Spaide RF. Fundus autofluorescence in birdshot chorioretinopathy. Ophthalmology 2008; 115(5): e15–e20.
14. Monnet D, Brézin AP, Holland GN, et al. Longitudinal cohort study of patients with birdshot chorioretinopathy. I. Baseline clinical characteristics. Am J Ophthalmol 2006; 141(1): 135–142.
15. Thorne JE, Jabs DA, Peters GB, et al. Birdshot retinochoroidopathy: ocular complications and visual impairment. Am J Ophthalmol 2005; 140(1): 45–51.
16. Lim L, Harper A, Guymer R. Choroidal lesions preceding symptom onset in birdshot chorioretinopathy. Arch Ophthalmol 2006; 124(7): 1057–1058.
17. Duprat F, Leveque Q, Le Hoang P. Birdshot chorioretinopathy: a case with delayed detection. J Fr Ophtalmol 1998; 21(7): 525–528.
18. Witkin AJ, Duker JS, Ko TH, et al. Ultrahigh resolution optical coherence tomography of birdshot retinochoroidopathy. Br J Ophthalmol 2005; 89(12): 1660–1661.
19. Monnet D, Levinson RD, Holland GN, et al. Longitudinal cohort study of patients with birdshot chorioretinopathy. III. Macular imaging

Behçet's Disease

Robert B. Nussenblatt

Key concepts

- This is a multisystem disease, with the posterior ocular complications potentially being devastating.
- The posterior pole disease should not be treated with corticosteroid alone.
- Newer approaches, such as IFN therapy and biologics such as infliximab, have been suggested as being effective for the ocular manifestations, but randomized studies still need to be done.

Retinal vascular involvement is a common finding in many patients with posterior and intermediate uveitis. Behçet's disease may be the best example of a disorder characterized mainly by its retinal vascular involvement, often with devastating effects on the patient's eyesight.

Behçet's disease is a multisystem disorder named after the Turkish dermatologist, Hulusi Behçet (1889–1948),[1] who in 1937 recognized and reported a triad of symptoms: recurrent intraocular inflammatory episodes with oral and mucosal ulcerations. These observations were based on three patients, two of whom had ocular symptoms atypical of the disorder we recognize today. It should be noted that in the 20th century at least two other clinicians reported cases with similar findings earlier than did Behçet: Adamantiades in 1931 (publishing in the French literature)[2] and Shigeta from Japan in 1924.[3] However, their reports did not stimulate the universal interest that Behçet's did. The disease was known in ancient times, with Hippocrates probably being the first to describe an association between ocular inflammation and oral and genital lesions.[4] Familial occurrence is seen in 8–18% of Turkish patients with the disease, 15% of Koreans, and 13% of Jews, but much less in a Chinese population (2.6%).[5,6] In a more recent study reviewing 761 patients in Turkey, almost 57% of patients with an identifiable diagnosis had Behçet's disease, with 10.4% being juvenile onset.[7] The prevalence has been calculated to be 80–370/100 000.[6] It is interesting to note that the frequency of the disease is 18 times less in Turks living in Germany than in those in Anatolia. In one center in the United States Behçet's disease constituted 2.5% of uveitis referrals.[8] One report from Iran[9] put at 8.6% the number of patients seen in a uveitis clinic in Teheran having Behçet's disease, with more cases of ocular toxoplasmosis being seen. The complete form of Behçet's disease is rare in Northern Italy, with a prevalence calculated at 3.8/100 000 (incidence of 0.24/100 000).[10] The disease has been noted to be especially common in the Far East and in the Mediterranean basin, and is very frequently noted between 30° and 45° north latitude in Asian and European populations.[11] This corresponds to the old Silk Route used for centuries by traders making the dangerous passage from the East to the West (**Fig. 26-1**). It appears that the disease is changing in character, severity and prevalence. About 40 years ago Japan appeared to have the greatest frequency of this disorder,[12] with an overall prevalence of 70–85 cases/1 000 000 population, as calculated in the late 1970s.[13] In the early 1990s it was estimated that the total number of patients with this disease in Japan was 16 570, with a prevalence of 135 cases/1 000 000 population.[14] However, the northern portions of Japan have a higher incidence than do the southern areas. Of the estimated 15 000 patients in Japan with Behçet's disease in 1986, 11 000 were under treatment.[15] This diagnosis was applied to more than 20% of the patients with uveitis seen in the uveitis clinic of the University of Tokyo's Department of Ophthalmology from 1965 through 1977.[13] Other studies have suggested a lower prevalence of 13.5–20/100 000 in Japan and Korea.[6]

This disorder may have devastating consequences for the eyes, and has therefore attracted a great deal of attention. Insight into its mechanisms has led to an improvement in our treatment of this disorder.

Clinical manifestations

The diagnosis of Behçet's disease is based firmly on the presence of a constellation of clinical findings. Therefore, clinical criteria have been established that help the clinician decide whether a patient has the disease. Numerous sets of clinical criteria have been proposed for the diagnosis of Behçet's disease.[16,17] For our service we have adapted the criteria established by the Behçet's Disease Research Committee of Japan (**Box 26-1**). As can be seen, these criteria add an additional major finding to the original three: skin lesions. Further, the presence of ocular inflammatory disease is given greater weight in the diagnosis. It should also be noted that the minor criteria are not considered in this grading system. The Behçet's Disease Research Committee of Japan recognizes three special cases: intestinal Behçet's, vasculo-Behçet's, and neuro-Behçet's (essentially the minor criteria). It has also specifically included three laboratory tests: a pathergy test (a skin-prick test), HLA testing for HLA-B51, and screening for nonspecific factors indicative of immune system activation, such as an elevated erythrocyte sedimentation rate, positive results for C-reactive protein, and an increase in the number of peripheral blood leukocytes.

Box 26-1 Criteria for diagnosis of Behçet's disease

MAJOR CRITERIA

Recurrent aphthous ulcers of oral mucosa

Skin lesions

Erythema nodosum, acne, cutaneous hypersensitivity thrombophlebitis

Genital ulcers

Ocular inflammatory disease

Recurrent anterior and posterior

MINOR CRITERIA

Arthritis

Intestinal ulcers

Epididymitis

Vascular disease

Obliteration, occlusion, aneurysm

Neuropsychiatric symptoms

Complete type

Four major symptoms simultaneously or at different times

Incomplete type

Three major symptoms simultaneously or at different times

or

Typical recurrent ocular disease with one other major criterion

Suspect type

Two major symptoms, excluding ocular

Possible type

One main symptom

Modified from Behçet's Disease Research Committee: Clinical research section recommendations, Jpn J Ophthalmol 1974; 18: 291–294.

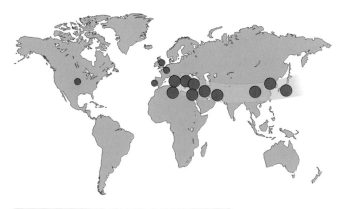

● Country with high incidence of Behçet's disease

Figure 26-1. Map of a broad band through Asia and Europe where Behçet's disease is common. This coincides with the old Silk Route. *(Courtesy of S. Ohno, MD.)*

Another system that the reader should be familiar with is the one suggested by the International Study Group for Behçet's Disease,[18,19] which requires the presence of oral aphthous ulcers for the diagnosis in all patients (**Box 26-2**). These investigators emphasize the importance of oral aphthous ulcers as a sign of this disease on the basis of data collection from a large number of patients and control subjects, in which they found that 97% of patients with Behçet's disease had oral aphthae.[19]

Other systems have used the minor criteria by equating two of those to one major criterion. Others have tried to

Box 26-2 Diagnostic criteria of international study group for Behçet's disease

RECURRENT ORAL ULCERATION

Minor or major aphthous lesions or herpetiform-like lesions need to have been observed by the physician or patient at least three times within a 12-month period.

PRESENCE OF TWO OTHER CRITERIA

Recurrent genital ulceration

Observation by the physician or patient of the aphthous ulceration or scar is required.

Eye lesions

The ocular disease can include anterior and/or posterior uveitis, cells in the vitreous, or the presence of a retinal vasculitis.

Skin lesions

These changes, noted by the physician or patient, include erythema nodosum, pseudofolliculitis, and papulopustular lesions. In addition, lesions would include an acneiform nodule in postadolescent patients not receiving corticosteroid therapy.

Positive pathergy test result

Read by physician at 24–48 hours.

Modified from International Study Group for Behçet's Disease: Criteria for diagnosis of Behçet's disease, Lancet 1990; 335: 1078–1080.

introduce a standardized scoring system for all parts of the disease.[20] There is no question that some degree of uncertainty is built into any system, because the various criteria may manifest at different times during the clinical course. Until we have a better way to diagnose this disease, we have favored a strict adherence to the Japanese criteria, as the patients in whom we have diagnosed Behçet's disease have fairly homogeneous clinical findings.

In a 1991 survey of 3316 patients with Behçet's disease in Japan, oral aphtha was the most frequently seen major criterion, occurring in 97.7%.[21] Other commonly seen problems were skin lesions (90.4%), with genital ulcers and ocular attacks having a similar incidence (79.8% and 78.6%, respectively)[13] (**Table 26-1**). Oral aphthae are by far the most common major criterion at presentation[13] (**Table 26-2**). After the oral aphthae, the order of appearance of the major criteria is skin lesions, ocular symptoms (25.4% in males), genital ulceration in males, and ocular lesions in females (8.6%). Of the minor criteria the most frequently seen in Japan was arthritis (see Table 26-1). The ratio of males to females with this disease in Japan was 1.2 : 1 in 1972, whereas in 1981 it had changed to 0.77 : 1.[15] A study involving 25 eye centers and 14 countries identified 1465 patients with ocular lesions. In those patients 94.5% had oral ulcers, with skin lesions and genital ulcers found in over 60%. Differences over 20 years have been noted in the various aspects of the disease and their presence in men and women (**Table 26-3**). In Israel, Krause and colleagues[22] evaluated 100 patients with Behçet's disease, 66 of whom were Jewish (with origins from Iran, Turkey, and North Africa) and 34 of whom were Arab. The expression of the disease seemed to be the same, but the patients of Arab ethnicity appeared to have more serious eye disease. In Turkey, however, the male-to-female ratio is 3.3 : 1.[15] More males have the complete form of the disease than do females. Although it is a disease with onset during early adulthood, childhood onset

Table 26-1 Percentage of patients manifesting criteria for Behçet's disease*. (Data from Mishima S, Masuda K, Izawa Y et al. Behçet disease in Japan: ophthalmologic aspects. Trans Am Ophthalmol Soc 1979; 76: 225–229.)

Criteria	Men	Women	Total
Major			
Ocular	86.2	67.8	78.6
Aphthae	97.9	98.8	98.3
Skin	89.8	91.3	90.4
Genital	76.8	83.8	79.8
Minor			
Arthritis	56.1	62.6	58.9
Intestinal	27.7	25.9	26.9
Vascular	8.7	6.3	7.7
Psychiatric	10.3	6.4	8.6

*At least 1700 patients were analyzed for each criterion.

Table 26-2 Incidence (%) of major criteria as initial manifestation

	Japan*			Israel[†]
	Men	Women	Total	Total
Criteria	n = 139	n = 70	n = 209	n = 54
Ocular	25.4	8.6	19.7	9
Oral aphthae	59.4	84.3	67.8	80
Genital ulcers	14.5	25.7	18.3	2
Skin lesions	41.7	34.3	39.2	2

*Data from Mishima S, Masuda K, Izawa Y et al.: Behçet disease in Japan: ophthalmologic aspects, Trans Am Ophthalmol Soc 1979; 76: 225–229.
[†]Data from Chajek T, Fairanu M: Behçet's disease: report of 41 cases and a review of the literature, Medicine (Baltimore) 1975; 54: 179–196.

Table 26-3 Epidemiologic changes in Behçet's disease in Japan from 1972 to1991. (Reproduced with permission from Nakae K, Masaki F, Hashimoto T et al. Recent epidemiological features of Behçet's disease in Japan. In Godeau P, Wechster B, Behçet's disease. Copyright 1993 Elsevier.)

Disease Type	No. Male 1972	No. Female 1991	Gender 1972	Ratio 1991
Complete type	594/334	588/551	1.78	1.07
Incomplete type				
With ocular disease	403/230	750/402	1.75	1.87
Without ocular disease	172/298	300/725	0.58	0.41
Incomplete type				
With genital ulcers	260/352	338/806	0.74	0.42
Without genital ulcers	315/176	712/321	1.79	2.22
Incomplete type				
With both ocular and genital	88/54	73/104	1.63	0.7
Ocular without genital	315/176	674/298	1.79	2.26
Genital without ocular	172/298	300/725	0.58	0.41

disease. Being male, presenting initially with poor visual acuity to the eye clinic, and posterior or panuveitis were all associated with a poor visual outcome.[28,29] Being female and having the disease at a young age were associated with non-recurrence of ocular inolvement.[30]

The majority of our patients with Behçet's disease are male. We recently reviewed 120 Behçet's disease patients seen at the National Eye Institute[31] and compared those we have seen over several decades (late 1960s to the early 2000s). Over the three decades the majority (68%) were Caucasian, and the median age at diagnosis was remarkably similar over the three decades (**Table 26-4**); 95% of the patients had bilateral disease. All the patients presented with oral ulcers, with genital and skin lesions being next most common. Over the three decades 8–22% of patients had central nervous system disease (**Table 26-5**). The reader can compare these extraocular findings with the frequency of clinical findings and onset of manifestations reported in 661 Turkish patients (**Table 26-6**).[32] **Table 26-7** compares the therapies used over the three decades. We have seen a marked improvment in the initial visual acuity in those patients treated in the 1990s and 2000s as compared to earlier groups. The mean inflammation score decreased as well.

Barra and colleagues[33] from Brazil reviewed 49 patients with Behçet's disease, representing 2% of the total number of patients with uveitis they saw over a 16-year period. Of their patients 71% were male, and more than three-quarters of all patients were white; in 34.5% the ocular attack was the first symptom of their disease, whereas on the whole it took a little more than 3 years for the ocular symptoms to appear after the first manifestation of disease. In a review of 31

has been reported to occur in rare cases.[23,24] Laghmari and associates[25] studied 13 patients with childhood Behçet's disease and found that familial Behçet's disease as well as articular and digestive manifestations were more commonly seen in younger children, whereas neurologic and vascular involvement, including panuveitis, seemed to occur more frequently in the older children. Ando and colleagues[26] compared patients seen in a Tokyo eye clinic from 1974 to 1983 with those seen from 1984 to 1993. The number of women presenting with the disease increased to about one-quarter of the patients. Initially 70% of patients manifested ocular symptoms (in the third and fourth decades), and by 1993 almost two-thirds of the patients seen had the incomplete form of the disease. What was striking was the observation that the patients seen between 1984 and 1993 had a much better visual course, ascribed by the authors to better therapy (see below). In one study of 520 patients with Behçet's disease in North Africa,[27] 83% were male and patients had a mean age of 20 years, which is very young based on our experience. Eighty percent of the patients had ophthalmic involvement, with one-quarter being blind because of their

Table 26-4 Comparison of demographic characteristics and follow-up duration of patients with ocular Behçet's disease. (Reproduced with permission from Kump et al. Behcet's disease: Comparing 3 decades of treatment response at the National Eye Institute. Can J Opthalmol 2008;43:468.)

Characteristic	1960s	1980s	1990s	Total
Total, n (%)	45 (38)	26 (21)	49 (41)	120 (100)
Sex, n (%)				
Female	19 (42)	10 (38)	24 (49)	53 (44)
Male	26 (58)	16 (62)	25 (51)	67 (56)
Race, n (%)				
Caucasian	35 (78)	19 (73)	28 (57)	82 (68)
African-American	4 (9)	1 (4)	6 (12)	11 (9)
Hispanic	2 (4)	2 (8)	2 (4)	6 (5)
Asian	2 (4)	1 (8)	4 (8)	8 (7)
American-Indian	1 (2)	1 (4)	3 (6)	5 (4)
Other/unknown	1 (2)	1 (4)	6 (12)	8 (7)
Age at diagnosis, median (yrs) (range)	28 (13–50)	28 (15–46)	30.5 (6–59)	28 (6–59)
Missing age at diagnosis, n	4	3	3	10
Follow-up, median (yrs) (range)	0.5 (0–9.3)	2.9 (0–16.8)	1.8 (0–13.1)	1.7 (0–16.8)
Period between ocular onset and first visit (yrs)	3.8	3.4	4.0	3.8

Table 26-5 Comparison of extraocular manifestations of Behçet's disease over three decades*. (Reproduced with permission from Kump et al. Behcet's disease: Comparing 3 decades of treatment response at the National Eye Institute. Can J Opthalmol 2008;43:468.)

Manifestation	1960s, n (%)	1980s, n (%)	1990s, n (%)	Total, n (%)
Total patients	45 (38)	26 (21)	49 (41)	120 (100)
Oral ulcers	45 (100)	26 (100)	49 (100)	120 (100)
Genital ulcers	32 (71)	16 (62)	35 (71)	83 (69)
Skin lesions	26 (58)	17 (65)	27 (55)	70 (58)
Arthritis	13 (29)	12 (46)	20 (41)	45 (38)
Central nervous system	10 (22)	5 (19)	4 (8)	19 (16)
Vascular lesions	3 (7)	–	3 (6)	6 (5)
Epididymitis	2 (4)	1 (4)	2 (4)	5 (4)

*No significant difference among decades, Fisher's exact test.

TABLE 26-6 The frequency of clinical findings and onset manifestations. (Reproduced with permission from Alpsoy et al. Clinical features and natural course of Behçet's disease in 661 cases: a multicentre study. British Journal of Dermatology 2007;157:901.)

Clinical Features	Patients (n = 661)	%
Oral ulcer	661	100.0
Genital ulcer	564	85.3
Papulopustular lesions	366	55.4
Erythema nodosum	292	44.2
Articular involvement	221	33.4
Ocular involvement	193	29.2
Thrombophlebitis	71	10.7
Vascular involvement	29	4.4
Neurological involvement	20	3.0
Gastrointestinal involvement	11	1.6
Skin pathergy reaction	250	37.8
Onset lesions		
Oral ulcer	586	88.7
Genital ulcer	94	14.2
Erythema nodosum	38	5.7
Ocular involvement	28	4.2
Simultaneous occurrence of the symptoms (n = 79)		
Oral and genital ulcer	65	9.8
Oral ulcer and erythema nodosum	21	3.1
Oral ulcer and ocular involvement	15	2.2
Oral ulcer, genital ulcer and erythema nodosum	16	2.4
Oral ulcer, genital ulcer and ocular involvement	11	1.6

the disease seen at Moorfields Hospital in London with 35 patients seen at the Kurume University Eye Clinic in southern Japan over the same period. The Japanese patients were older (43 years) than those seen in London (35 years). No significant differences were noted in extraocular findings. More of the Japanese patients had acute uveitis and posterior pole disease and received treatment with topical steroids. Those in London were more often treated with systemic steroids.

Oral aphthous ulcers

An almost universal finding in Behçet's disease is the amount of discomfort the oral lesions can cause. The number of patients with oral aphthae in the general population is quite high. However, in our experience the lesions in patients with Behçet's disease can occur in clusters and may be found not only on the gums but also on the lips, posterior pharynx, uvula, palate, and tongue. They can be small but painful, and they recur (**Fig. 26-2**). They usually heal in 7–10 days without scarring, but scarring occurs when a particularly large ulcer heals. It has been suggested that in contrast to the regular flat borders of the aphthae seen in this disorder, the lesions in the Stevens–Johnson syndrome tend to be irregular, whereas in

French patients, an ocular manifestation was the first symptom in 29%.[34]

How similar is the presentation of the ocular complications of Behçet's disease in various parts of the world? It would appear that there are more similarities than differences. Muhaya and colleagues[35] compared 19 patients with

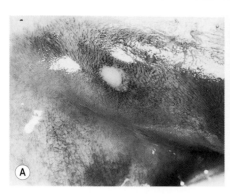

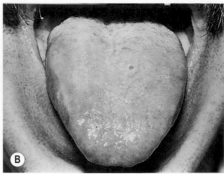

Figure 26-2. Aphthous ulcers are common in Behçet's disease. They usually appear several at a time, sometimes on common surfaces such as the mucosa of the lip (**A**), or on less common regions such as the tonsils and tongue (**B**).

Table 26-7 Comparison of ocular complications in patients with ocular Behçet's disease over three decades. (Reproduced with permission from Kump et al. Behçet's disease: Comparing 3 decades of treatment response at the National Eye Institute. Can J Opthalmol 2008;43:468.)

Complication	1960s, n (%)	1980s, n (%)	1990s, n (%)	Total, n (%)
Total patients	45 (38)	26 (21)	49 (41)	120 (100)
Cataract	19 (42)	11 (42)	15 (31)	45 (38)
Macular edema	13 (29)	9 (35)	16 (32)	38 (32)
Optic atrophy	13 (29)	8 (31)	9 (18)	30 (25)
Epiretinal membrane	8 (18)	5 (19)	8 (16)	21 (18)
Glaucoma	7 (16)	5 (19)	6 (12)	18 (15)
Papillitis	13 (29)	8 (31)	2 (4)	23 (19)
Intra/subretinal hemorrhage	10 (22)	5 (19)	3 (6)	18 (15)
Intravitreal hemorrhage	5 (11)	6 (23)	3 (6)	14 (12)
Branch retinal vein occlusion	9 (20)	3 (12)	3 (6)	15 (13)
Maculopathy	5 (11)	2 (8)	3 (6)	10 (8)
Retinal detachment	2 (4)	2 (8)	3 (6)	7 (6)
Disc/retinal neovascularization	1 (2)	3 (12)	1 (2)	5 (4)
Phthisis bulbi	2 (4)	1 (4)	–	3 (2.5)
Corneal ulcer	2 (4)	–	–	2 (2)
Macular hole	–	1 (4)	1 (2)	2 (2)

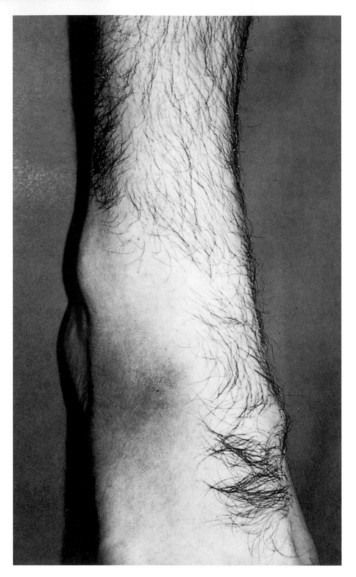

Figure 26-3. Examination of the peripheral extremities is important in evaluating patients with Behçet's disease. Just below this patient's ankle (which was painful) is an area of erythema nodosum.

Reiter's syndrome they can have heaped-up edges.[36] Some patients can provoke the appearance of these lesions by eating certain foods, whereas Wray and colleagues[37] have shown that trauma to the oral mucosa can cause them to appear, strikingly reminiscent of the prick test.

Skin lesions

Erythema nodosum-like lesions are frequently noted on the anterior surface of the legs (**Fig. 26-3**) but can be seen on the face, neck, buttocks, and elsewhere. These lesions involute without ulceration after several weeks.

Acne-like lesions or folliculitis are also common dermatologic lesions. They can appear on the back and face and are histologically identical to those of the 'typical' disorder. Thrombophlebitis is found usually in the extremities. This finding surely denotes a more general vascular disease that

can be life-threatening (discussed later). The thrombophlebitis in the extremities can be migratory and can also follow an injection or the taking of a blood sample.

Cutaneous hypersensitivity is a characteristic feature of Behçet's disease. Dermatographs can be observed in one-third to one-half of patients. Scratching the skin with a needle or taking a blood sample often results in a pustule at that site. This phenomenon – pathergy – has become the basis for the 'prick' test, with some researchers believing that this is an important criterion that can be used in diagnosing the disease (discussed later), as first suggested by Curth.[38] In our experience this phenomenon seems to be less common in patients with Behçet's disease.

Genital ulcers

In males the lesions may appear on the scrotum and penis and are therefore quite evident, sending the patient for professional help early in the disease. Females usually have their lesions on the vulva or on the vaginal mucosae. Other lesions may be perianal. Kobayashi and colleagues[39] reported that lesions on the vulva occur in the premenstrual portion of the month. It has been suggested that the genital lesions in males are more painful, but this has not been our experience. We have seen female patients with particularly painful and distressing genital lesions, frequently diagnosed initially as being herpetic in origin.

The genital lesions can be deep and therefore leave scars. Thus an examination of the genital region in a patient with suspected Behçet's disease can be useful as signs of old disease may be present.

Ocular disease

The ocular manifestations in Behçet's disease have serious implications for the patient. Mamo[40] estimated that vision was lost 3.36 years after the onset of ocular symptoms. The ominous clinical course makes us especially careful in our evaluation of these patients. This has led us to be highly cautious in our use of the diagnosis, and the presence of 'ocular inflammation' associated with other symptoms does not equate in our minds to the diagnosis of Behçet's disease.

The disease can affect both the anterior and posterior portions of the globe, but certain characteristic signs can and should be looked for. Statistically ocular disease manifests some 2–3 years after the initial symptoms are noted.[41] The disease is bilateral, with unilateral cases occurring rarely (see Case 26-1). One important aspect is the recurrent, explosive nature of the ocular disease. Patients do not have 'chronic' ocular inflammatory disease, that is, a lingering inflammatory episode that can be chronically noted. Rather, the disease will appear and be floridly active for a set period (2–4 weeks) and then disappear, with the patient's ocular disease being quiescent for some time, whether one treats or not. Therefore, therapeutic strategies and their evaluation must be undertaken with this in mind (see later discussion).

An anterior uveitis or iridocyclitis is seen frequently, with an associated hypopyon in about one-third of patients[11] (**Fig. 26-4**). Although a typical occurrence, it is not pathognomonic for the disease.[42] The hypopyon may not be visible to the naked eye but seen only with the slit lamp. On occasion a small hypopyon can be seen cradled in the angle when gonioscopic examination is performed. The inflammatory disease has a nongranulomatous appearance. The cells will move easily and slide over the corneal endothelium if the patient's head is tilted in the right direction. Using confocal microscopy, Mocan and colleagues[43] identified that the KPs in Behçet's disease are made up of small round cells, one of five types identified in ocular inflammatory disease.

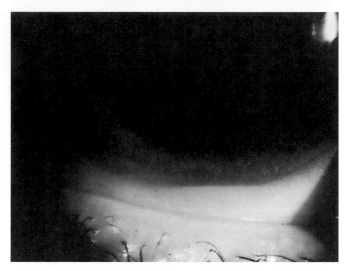

Figure 26-4. Hypopyon is considered a classic symptom in Behçet's disease. However, it is not always present during anterior segment inflammation and sometimes will be seen only on gonioscopic examination.

When the disease is particularly severe and long-standing, cyclitic membranes can form, putting these eyes at risk of developing phacoanaphylaxis.[44] Posterior synechiae can obscure the view of the posterior pole. In our experience an isolated vitreous reaction is not characteristic of this disorder. We have observed this when a patient is receiving therapy that is insufficient to completely prevent the ocular inflammation, and then a smoldering response ensues. Smoldering disease or impending reactivation remain significant problems. Although one does not measure acute activity by the flare in the anterior segment in patients who have had chronic or repeated attacks, Tugal-Tutkan et al.,[45] using the laser cell flare meter and examing a large number of Behçet patients, felt that those eyes with flare measured at >6 photons/s had a higher possibility of recurrence.

Retinal disease

Retinal disease is the most disquieting aspect of Behçet's disease and can ultimately lead to blindness. These recurrent retinal vasoocclusive episodes ultimately cause irreversible alterations. Macular ischemia, even bilateral, has been reported,[46,47] leading to a severe depression in visual acuity with a guarded possibility for a return in vision. Bilateral central retinal vein thrombosis has been described.[48] A funduscopic examination during the acute attack will, in addition, reveal areas of retinal hemorrhage and edema, accompanied by an inflammatory response in the vitreous. The retinitis often has the appearance of a virally induced lesion, and the decision as to what has caused the lesion usually is based on the overall context in which it is being observed (**Fig. 26-5**). Indeed, the disease can readily mimic acute retinal necrosis.[49] The sequelae of the retinal vasoocclusive episodes can be best seen with fluorescein angiography, and we follow disease activity using this tool (**Fig. 26-6**). Some of the changes can be extensive, far more so than imagined on clinical examination alone. Areas of capillary dropout and vascular-tree rearrangement are not uncommon. The loss of a clearly defined capillary-free zone is commonly seen but is not unique to this type of intraocular inflammation. In addition, the angiogram may

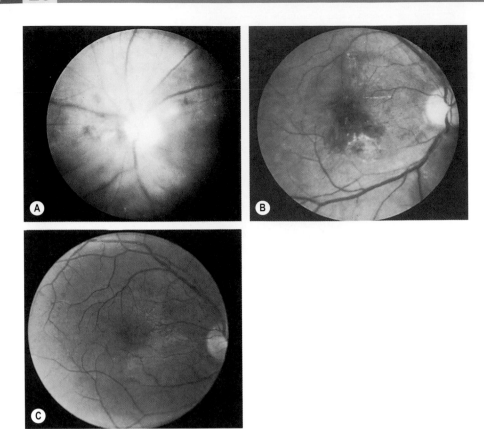

Figure 26-5. Vasoocclusive episodes of the posterior pole resulting from Behçet's disease can cause severe visual impairment (**A and B**). **C,** Fundus (**B**) after an acute episode. Note the preretinal membrane that has begun to form.

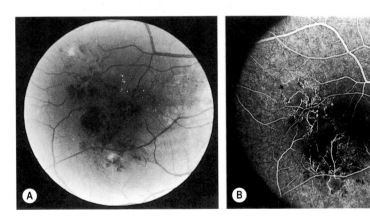

Figure 26-6. Fluorescein angiography can often better show vascular effects that occur with Behçet's disease. This patient has had several vasoocclusive attacks of the posterior pole (**A**), with fluorescein angiography showing capillary dropout and vascular remodeling, particularly temporal to the macula (**B**).

show diffuse retinal vascular leakage, late staining of the vasculature, leakage from the disc, and neovascularization. It is most important when evaluating a Behçet patient to consider performing a fluorescein angiogram, as although the clinical examination may not demonstrate dramatic changes, angiography may show extensive changes (**Fig. 26-7**). It has been thought that the posterior pole disease is essentially retinal disease. However, one can see evidence of choroidal, outer retinal, or retinal pigment epithelial involvement, raising the question that in some patients choroidal involvement is probably of some importance. An example of this is seen in **Figure 26-8**. This patient with Behçet's disease had fluorescein angiographic evidence of a central serous retinopathy associated with retinal edema, further suggesting an occlusion of the choriocapillaris. Indocyanine green (ICG) angiographic evaluation of the disease has been used and reported. In one study, Bozzoni-Pantaleoni and associates[50] noted several patterns of dye

accumulation. In 50% of eyes, poorly defined areas of intermediate and late hyperfluorescence were seen. Atmaca et al.[51] reported choroidal areas of hyper- and hypofluorescence in 53 of 69 (76.8%) of the eyes they studied. Therefore, subretinal alterations are not a rare event. However, it still appears that the retinal alterations are the most damaging. In most studies, the presence on the ICG angiogram of hyperfluorescent areas up to the late phase was related to disease duration.

Other ocular manifestations include episcleritis, filamentary keratitis, conjunctivitis, and subconjunctival hemorrhages.[52] Extraocular muscle paralysis may be a result of neuro-Behçet's disease.[12]

Complications

The complications of repeated inflammatory bouts are of major concern and depend somewhat on where the inflammation is located. Anterior segment inflammation can

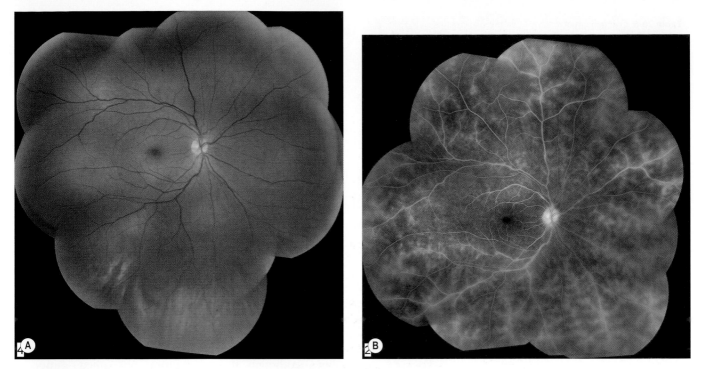

Figure 26-7. This 23-year-old woman with Behçet's disease had bouts of anterior uveitis but recently was complaining of minor visual alterations. **A,** The fundus examination was not particularly alarming. **B,** The fluorecein angiogram demonstrated diffuse retinal vascular alterations with leakage.

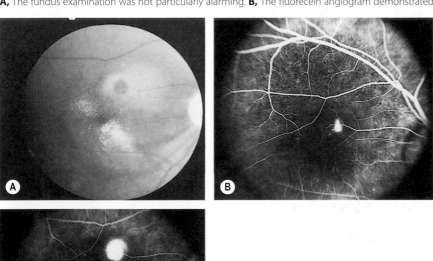

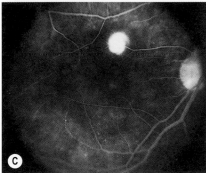

Figure 26-8. A to C, Fluorescein angiographic evidence of eccentrically placed serous retinopathy associated with retinal edema and a large cyst. These findings suggest occlusion of the choriocapillaris rather than retinal disease resulting from this change.

lead to glaucoma, particularly angle-closure glaucoma. Iris atrophy may be seen as well. Cataract formation is not unusual, due to either the inflammation or the medications added to treat the condition. Iris neovascularization and secondary glaucoma are ominous findings and can accompany recurrent posterior globe inflammatory episodes. The visual prognosis for a patient with anterior segment uveitis only in Behçet's disease is thought to be good. More women than men in the Japanese experience have this type of disease, and therefore their visual prognosis is less guarded than that for men. We have not seen this subgroup of patients – that is, those with only anterior segment disease. In our experience the disease most frequently involves both segments of the eye. This was the opinion of the late Dr David Ben Ezra in Israel as well (personal communication, 1987). The reader can see that the ocular complications we have seen over three decades has been relatively similar in percentage distribution (**Table 26-8**).

The posterior segment sequelae of Behçet's disease can lead to serious visual handicap (**Fig. 26-9**). In a recent report,

Table 26-8 Comparison of systemic treatment in patients with ocular Behçet's disease over three decades. (Reproduced with permission from Kump et al. Behçet's disease: Comparing 3 decades of treatment response at the National Eye Institute. Can J Opthalmol 2008;43:468.)

Medication	1960s, n (%)	1980s, n (%)	1990s, n (%)	Total, n (%)
Total patients	45 (38)	26 (21)	49 (41)	120 (100)
Systemic corticosteroids	43 (96)	26 (100)	41 (84)	110 (92)
Systemic corticosteroids alone	31 (69)	2 (8)	8 (16)	41 (34)
Topical/periocular corticosteroids only	2 (4)	–	4 (8)	6 (5)
Ciclosporin	–	23 (89)	27 (55)	50 (42)
Daclizumab	–	–	15 (31)	15 (13)
Chlorambucil	6 (13)	4 (15)	4 (8)	14 (12)
Azathioprine	1 (2)	2 (8)	10 (20)	13 (11)
Methotrexate	2 (4)	–	8 (16)	10 (8)
Mycophenolate mofetil	–	–	8 (16)	8 (7)
Infliximab	–	–	7 (14)	7 (6)
Cyclophosphamide	2 (4)	3 (12)	2 (4)	7 (6)
Sirolimus	–	–	1 (2)	1 (1)
6-Mercaptopurine	1 (2)	–	–	1 (1)

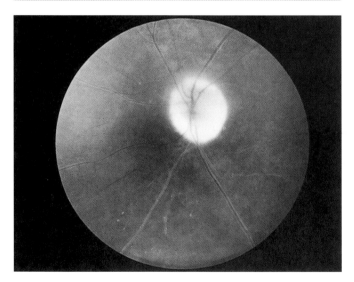

Figure 26-9. End stage of repeated Behçet's disease attacks of the posterior pole. Note optic atrophy and sheathed and markedly attenuated vessels. The retina is atrophic.

Sakamoto and colleagues[53] studied 51 patients with Behçet's disease and found that in addition to posterior pole attacks, skin lesions and arthritis were associated with a loss of vision. In women with the disease, anterior segment attacks and increased intervals between attacks were related to retention of vision. Retinal atrophy is the end result of the multiple ocular inflammatory episodes. With this there will be an associated optic atrophy and often markedly attenuated retinal vessels. In a percentage of patients an associated neovascular component will be seen, leading to recurrent vitreous hemorrhages, subsequent vitreous contraction, and retinal detachment.

In patients with full-blown disease there is little problem in establishing this clinical diagnosis. However, as with all entities, there is overlap in clinical presentation. Further, because parts of the disease spectrum may have occurred some time before presentation and cannot be verified, some uncertainty may arise. The anterior uveitis can mimic almost any severe recurrent process, and particularly the HLA-B27-associated entities, because hypopyon uveitis is seen with these disorders as well. However, these diseases should be unilateral in their presentation, whereas in Behçet's disease unilateral presentation occurs only in a small number of patients. Sarcoidosis can mimic some of the posterior pole lesions. However, the clinical course of sarcoidosis is generally more indolent than the explosive episodes seen in Behçet's disease. The retinitis of Behçet's disease in its most florid form is highly suggestive of a viral retinitis, which should certainly be included in the differential diagnosis.

Minor criteria

As previously mentioned, the symptoms associated with this disorder are legion. As was so aptly emphasized by Geraint James and Spiteri,[54] patients with Behçet's disease can first be seen by practitioners from many different medical disciplines. Although these symptoms are called 'minor,' it should be stressed that the term refers only to their importance in the determination of the diagnosis. Three of these minor criteria deserve comment.

Arthritis

At least half of patients with Behçet's disease manifest a nonmigrating, nondestructive arthritis, with the knee being the most common joint affected. The arthritis is linked often to a general systemically active state of the disease, accompanied at times by other criteria, such as fever, skin lesions, acute-phase reactants, and, on occasion, ocular lesions. One of our patients could predict an ocular attack when his joints became involved, signaling to him a general activation of his disease. Firestein and colleagues[55] reported the coexistence of relapsing polychondritis and Behçet's disease, in which inflamed cartilage was noted.

Vascular alterations

Vessels of all sizes can be involved in this disorder, and angio-Behçet's or cardio-Behçet's disease (aortitis) is associated with a poor prognosis.[56,57] Müftüoglu and coworkers[58] observed vascular involvement in 24% of the 531 patients they reviewed, mostly a deep and superficial thrombophlebitis of the legs. These thromboocclusive episodes can cause an elevation of the erythrocyte sedimentation rate. Aneurysms are not uncommon, and their rupture can be the cause of death. Further, deep vessel thrombosis may occur, often involving the large vessels of the body such as the vena cava.[59] A vasculitis of the small veins may also occur, as in the case of gastrointestinal involvment. The ileocecal region is most commonly involved and can perforate, with rare esophageal and gastric ulcerations. A CT scan will demonstrate initially bowel wall thickening.[60]

Neurologic involvement (neuro-Behçet's disease)

This grave complication may affect about 8% of Japanese patients with Behçet's disease.[13] Of interest was the fact that

Inaba[61] reported that most patients who had neuro-Behçet's did not have ocular disease, with 83.9% of them having the incomplete form of the disease and 90.4% having no ocular disease during their clinical course. In 68 autopsies, Inaba found that the thalamus, basal ganglia, and the brainstem were involved in 85–95%. In addition to neurologic findings, Behçet's disease can also induce frank psychiatric symptoms.

In patients with neuro-Behçet's disease the cerebrospinal fluid (CSF) shows evidence of pleocytosis. During the acute stage neutrophils may predominate, leading to a possible diagnosis of aseptic meningitis, whereas in other patients mononuclear cells may predominate. Inaba[61] reported a predominance of OKT4+ T cells in the CSF, and the α_2-macroglobulin levels were markedly increased. Of interest was the fact that the β_{1A} fraction of C3 was greatly increased during the active stage, suggesting that the alternate pathway of the complement system may be involved. Oligoclonal banding is usually not seen, but Sharief and coworkers[62] have reported the presence of immunoglobulin (Ig) A and IgM oligoclonal bands in the CSF of patients with active neuro-Behçet's disease and documented the disappearance of the bands with remission of neurologic disease. Wang and colleagues[63] found that levels of anticardiolipin antibodies (particularly the IgM isotype) and interleukin (IL)-6 were elevated in the CSF of patients with neuro-Behçet's disease and fell as disease activity abated.

CT examination of the brain shows defects in a large number of patients, as will electroencephalography, but some lesions may not be well seen using these types of studies. The use of gadolinium–diethylenetriamine pentaacetic acid-enhanced magnetic resonance imaging (MRI) studies is another approach that appears to provide good definition of central nervous system (CNS) lesions. Of interest were the reports by Ogawa and Sawada[64] and Edem and coworkers[65] that the unenhanced MRI images continued to show lesions even after therapy initiation and resolution of clinical disease, whereas the enhanced images showed resolution (**Fig. 26-10**). Kobayashi and colleagues,[66] using T_2-weighted MRI scans, were able to detect a hemorrhagic focus located in the right pontine base.

Immunologic and histologic considerations

The histopathologic appearance of the lesions seen in Behçet's disease is that of a perivasculitis associated with tissue destruction (**Fig. 26-11**). In a case from the National Eye Institute, a nongranulomatous uveitis with CD4+ T lymphocytes as well as some B cells and plasma cells infiltrated the eye. There was extensive expression of adhesion molecules on the vascular endothelium.[67] In one report Winter and Yukins[68] believed the underlying lesion was an obliterative vasculitis. Mullaney and Collum[69] noted that in an eye they examined there was a necrotizing arteriolitis and phlebitis with thromboses. Mural IgG, IgA, and C3 deposits were noted in the episclera and some choroidal veins, but not in the retina. The notion has been that the underlying mechanism leading to this histologic alteration was immune complex deposition.[36] Indeed, the deposition of complement components has been reported in some lesions.[70] This notion has been supported by the presence of circulating

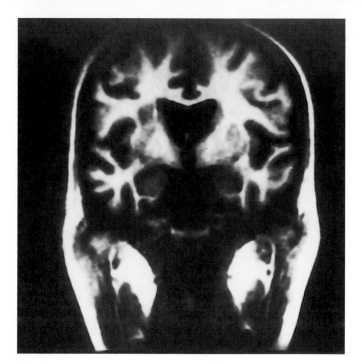

Figure 26-10. MRI brain scan of a patient with neuro-Behçet's disease. Gray-matter lesions are interpreted to be evidence of CNS activity of disease.

immune complexes (CICs) in patients with Behçet's disease,[71] as well as neutrophils in the aqueous of eyes with hypopyon uveitis. Increased chemotactic activity of neutrophils has been observed in Behçet's disease.[72,73] Reports describing histologic findings in Behçet's eyes are listed in **Table 26-9**. The neurologic lesions include perivascular cuffing with mononuclear cells, focal necrosis, demyelinization, and gliosis.[73]

Some observers have suggested that other mechanisms may be at play in this disorder. Kasp and coworkers[74] noted that of 32 patients with Behçet's disease, only one-third had elevated CIC levels. Further, the presence of CICs was associated with quiescent periods, which suggested that the CIC may play a beneficial role in the course of the disease (see Chapter 1).

Role of T cells (but other cells count too!)

The role of T cells in the underlying mechanism of Behçet's disease is stressed by many. Recent immunohistologic studies of the recurrent mouth ulcers seen with this disorder demonstrated that most of the lymphocytes infiltrating into the lesion were DR-negative T cells, whereas the macrophages were DR positive.[75] We have seen a predominance of T cells rather than neutrophils in the recurrent hypopyon uveitis of a patient with Behçet's disease. In 1982 the late David Cogan reviewed 18 eyes for a joint Japanese-American workshop on Behçet's disease. Although a perivasculitis was noted, evidence of typical fibrinoid changes associated with immune complex-mediated disease was not present (personal communication, 1984). Charteris and colleagues[76] carried out a postmortem examination of the eyes from a patient with Behçet's disease who suffered from severe recurrent retinal vasculitis. They found a hyaline thickening of the retinal vessels, with a perivascular infiltrate made up of mostly CD4+ T cells bearing large numbers of IL-2 receptors. In another study of five enucleated eyes from patients with

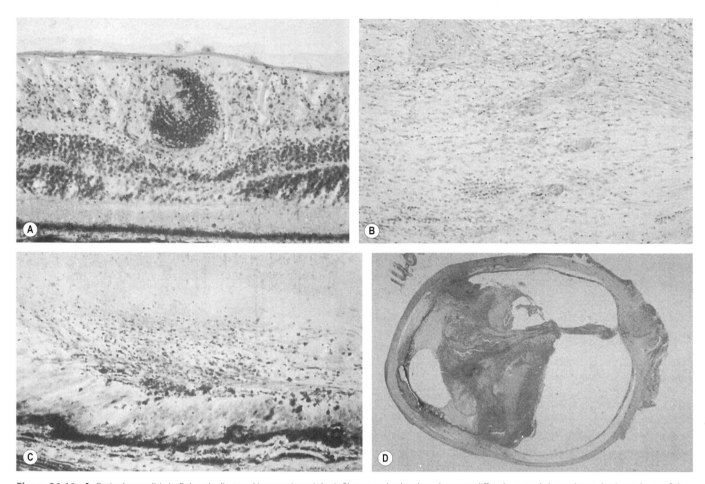

Figure 26-11. A, Retinal vasculitis in Behçet's disease. Note periarteriolar infiltrate and other lymphocytes diffusely spread throughout the inner layer of the retina. **B,** Occlusive retinitis in the retinal vessels of a 37-year-old with long-standing complete Behçet's disease. **C,** Early stage of ocular disease in a patient with neuro-Behçet's disease, with severe pars plana inflammation, macrophages and lymphocytes, and fibrous proliferation. **D,** Enucleated eye of a 37-year-old patient with complete Behçet's disease shows complete detachment of the sensory retina with preretinal and subretinal granulation tissue. *(Courtesy of Professor J. Inomata, Fukuoka, Japan. From Vasculitis and intraocular neovascularization in Behçet's disease: histopathology of the early and advanced late stages. In Dernouchamps JP, Verougstraete C, Caspers-Velu L et al., editors: Recent advance in uveitis [Proceedings of the Third International Symposium on Uveitis, Brussels, Belgium, May 24–27, 1992], Amsterdam, 1993, Kugler.)*

Behçet's disease, Charteris and coworkers[77] again found a predominance of CD4+ T cells, with no complement or immunoglobulin deposits. We have found essentially the same type of T-cell infiltrate in an eye that we have examined. The notion that T cells in the eyes of patients with Behçet's disease are expanded by specific antigen-driven stimulation is supported by the report of Keino and associates,[78] who showed a restricted number of T-cell receptors (BV3, BV5, and BV7) in a patient's eye.

Indeed, perturbations of the systemic T-cell circuitry can be found in patients with Behçet's disease. Valesini and coworkers[79] noted an increase in the number of T4 (CD4) cells in the blood of patients with Behçet's disease who have ocular disease, as well as an elevated T8 (CD8) fraction, thereby lowering the T4 : T8 ratio, a finding we have noted in other ocular inflammatory conditions. Essentially the same observations have been noted in Japan by Kikkawa and Shirotsuki,[80] who studied 11 patients with Behçet's disease and uveitis. Other evidence for an intrinsic T-cell problem includes the work of Sakane and colleagues,[81] in which they noted a defect in a T-cell-mediated suppressor system. Further, interferon-γ, a T-cell product, was detected at a higher level in the sera of patients with Behçet's disease than in sera of control subjects,[82] particularly during the convalescent stage of the disease. Serum IL-2 levels of patients with Behçet's disease with ocular involvement were elevated compared to those of control subjects and patients with intermediate uveitis.[83] Others have reported an increase in tumor necrosis factor (TNF)-α, soluble IL-1 receptor, IL-6, and IL-8 levels.[84] As with other patients whose uveitis involves the posterior segment, patients with Behçet's disease demonstrate evidence of cell-mediated responses to uveitogenic antigens and to their fragments.[85] Other antigens to which Behçet's disease patients have cell-mediated or humoral responses include resistin[86] (adipocyte hormones antagonize insulin action), selenium,[87] and α-tropomyosin.[88] These responses could be blocked by the addition of anti-CD4, anti-HLA, and anti-CD11a antibodies.[89] Yamamoto and associates[90] were able to establish S-antigen-specific CD4+ and CD8+ clones from the blood of a patient with Behçet's disease. Intraocularly, much evidence suggests a strong Th1 profile. Ahn et al.[91] found that TNF-α was higher in the aqueous of Behçet patients than in the aqueous of other uveitis patients, whereas IFN-α was high in the aqueous of Behçet's disease patients as well. No IL-10 was noted. Ahn and colleagues[92] also reported that CD8^bright CD56+ cytotoxic

Table 26-9 Histologic reports describing the ocular complications of Behçet's disease

Authors	No. Reports	Findings
Fenton and Easom*	4	Lymphocytes, PMNs, macrophages
Winter and Yukins[68]	2	Lymphocytes, macrophages
Green and Koo*	1	PMNs, lymphocytes, macrophages
Kaneko and colleagues*	1	Round cells
Okabe and associates[190]	2	Macrophages, lymphocytes
Mullaney and colleagues*	1	Lymphocytes, plasma cells, PMNs, IgG, IgA, C3
Charteris and associates[76]	2	CD4 T cells, HLA-DR+ cells
Charteris and associates[77]	5	T cells, macrophages, PMNs, HLA-DR+ cells
Inomata and colleagues*	25	Lymphocytes, macrophages, PMNs
George and associates[67]	1	T and B cells, plasma cells, macrophages PMNs, HLA-DR+ cells, HLA-DQ+ cells, ICAM-1, LFA-1, VCAM, E-selectin

PNM, polymorphonuclear leukocytes; ICAM-1, intercellular adhesion molecule-1; LFA-1, lymphocyte function antigen-1; VCAM, vascular cell adhesion molecule. *Fenton R, Easom H. Behçet's syndrome, Arch Ophthalmol 72: 71–81, 1964; Green WR, Koo BS. Behçet's disease: a report of ocular histopathology of one case, Surv Ophthalmol 12: 324–332, 1967; Kaneko H, Nakajima H, Okamura A et al.. Histopathology of Behçet's disease. Review of literature with a case report, Acta Pathol Jpn 26: 765–779, 1976; Mullaney J, Collum LM. Ocular vasculitis in Behçet's disease. A pathological and immunohistochemical study, Int Ophthalmol 7: 183–191, 1985; Inomata H, Kohno T, Rao NA et al.. Vasculitis and intraocular neovasuclarization in Behçet's disease. Histopathology of the early and advanced late stages. In Dernouchamps JP, Verougstraete C, Caspers-Verlu L et al.. Recent advances in uveitis, Amsterdam, 1992, Kugler.

effector cells, producing IFN-α and high amounts of preformed perforin, were seen in the aqueous of these patients. Yu et al.[93] reported similar findings, with CD8+ cells predominating in Behçet patients whereas CD4+ cells predominated in other uveitis patients' aqueous; also, NKT CD3+ CD56+ cells were higher in Behçet patients' blood and aqueous.

Our experience and that of others with ciclosporin further support the role of T cells in this disease, as the disease appears to be effectively controlled in many patients with this anti-T-cell medication (see later discussion). Although the evidence overwhelmingly incriminates the T cell in this disease, it is clear that there is a rather general and severe immune alteration. Perhaps under T-cell control in the beginning, the immune system's delicate checks and balances seem to have gone almost universally awry. Indeed, one finds alterations in many parts of the immune system, including circulating immune complexes. It also includes neutrophils. Polymorphonuclear lymphocytes in the peripheral blood of Behçet's disease patients appear to undergo less spontaneous apoptosis in the remission phase of the disease,[94] the reason for which is unclear.

A full elaboration of all the immune system alterations that have been reported in Behçet's disease is beyond the scope of this chapter.

HLA typing and single nucleotide polymorphisms (SNPs)

HLA typing has proved helpful in the diagnosis of Behçet's disease. HLA-B51, a split product of HLA-B5, has been found to be associated with the disease in Japanese patients,[11] with a calculated relative risk of 9.4. The frequency of this antigen in control subjects was 12%, whereas in patients it was 57% (58% in patients with the complete form of the disease versus. 54% in those with the incomplete form). A more recent study using polymerase chain reaction–restriction fragment length polymorphism methodology to evaluate 90 Japanese patients yielded a relative risk for HLA-B51 of 7.9.[95] Some disagreement has arisen as to the strength of these observations when applied to non-Japanese patients. Most of these studies were performed before the 'B5' antigen was split. Godeau and colleagues[96] found an incidence of 54% of HLA-B5 in patients with Behçet's disease (most of Mediterranean origin) versus 13% in the control population. Several other studies, from Israel,[59] Turkey,[97] and Greece[98] have supported the HLA-B5 association. Further support for the association of HLA-B51 and this disorder came with a publication by Villanueva and colleagues.[99] These investigators reported on three siblings, all females, with Behçet's disease, including the ocular manifestations. They all had the same HLA phenotype, which included HLA-B51. Gül and associates[100] found no association between HLA-B51 positivity and severity of disease. However, in a German study, those with HLA-B51 were more likely to have ocular involvement (63% vs 43%), and in addition those of German descent (as opposed to Turkish) with the disease were less likely to bear B51 on their cells.[101] In familial Behçet's disease[102] parent–child involvement was more common in patients without ocular lesions than in those with them. An interesting case that emphasizes how little we know was reported by Horie et al.[103] They reported a 54-year-old woman who developed blurry vision and was diagnosed with Behçet's disease. Two years later her sister developed an ocular inflammation which was diagnosed as Vogt–Koyanagi–Harada's (VKH) disease. Both of the sisters had the same HLA typing – positive for B5101 and both negative for DR4 (associated with VKH).

However, O'Duffy and coworkers[104] found no such association in the 26 patients they typed in the United States, nor did Ohno and colleagues[105] when they typed six white patients. The reason for this may be lack of association, but on the other hand it may reflect the different criteria for diagnosis used in these American studies as opposed to the Japanese studies. In the very small group of Ohno and coworkers 'atypical' cases were studied, so that the diagnosis was not presumptive in only two of them. In an effort to explain this lack of association with B51 in some ethnic groups, it has been suggested that the HLA B exon sequence that encodes B51 is the real pathogenic factor.[106]

In addition to HLA typing and polymorphisms, there has been much interest in evaluating single-nucleotide polymorphisms (SNPs) of various mediators of the immune response. Recently 102 patients of middle Eastern descent with Behçet's disease were tested for a possible link between a specific tumor necrosis factor SNP and the disease. Although HLA-B51 was again found to be strongly linked with the disease, no TNF gene polymorphisms were found to be associated.[107] TNF-α SNP −1031C was found associated with the disease in a study performed in the United Kingdom.[108] In Turks, an association with the disease has been reported with the IL-1A −889 allele and the IL-1B +5887 haplotype.[109] Another portion of the genome that has been investigated has been a novel family of the major histocompatibility complex (MHC) class I genes, located near the HLA B gene and termed MIC (MHC class I chain-related genes). Yabuki and associates[110] reported an association between one MICA (one of the transmembrane regions) microsatellite polymorphism A6 in patients with Behçet's disease compared with control subjects (86.8% vs 50%). However, Salvarani and coworkers[111] did not find such a linkage. No association was seen in CTLA (cytotoxic T-lymphocyte associated antigen 4, an adhesion molecule important in cell trafficking) SNPs distributions between controls and Behçet's patients.[112]

Various investigators have attempted to identify an exogenous cause for this disease, particularly a viral one. The incidence of the disease is greater in the northern portions of Japan, although there is no known genetic difference, such as a higher incidence of HLA-B51, between the people in the north of Japan as opposed to those in the south. A somewhat dated report emphasized that there had been no documented cases of the disease in Nisei living in Hawaii,[113] suggesting that an exogenous source may indeed act at least as a triggering mechanism. As mentioned above, Turks living in Germany have a much smaller chance of developing the disease than those living in Anatolia.[6]

The search for the presence of live virus in the retina has not been successful, and therapeutic approaches with this concept as its underlying logic have not been rewarding (see later discussion). Denman and colleagues[114] offered a more provocative theory on the role of virus in this disorder. They noted that mononuclear cells from these patients have a high concentration of the interferon-induced enzyme 2′,5′-oligoadenylate synthetase, which is suggestive, but not confirmatory, of a viral infection.[115] They speculate that the virus may act as a 'promoter' by stimulating the expansion of clones of abnormal lymphocytes that will induce disease. Bonass and coworkers,[116] using DNA dot-blotting techniques, found evidence of the presence of herpes simplex virus type 1 DNA in a high percentage of patients with Behçet's disease. More recent work has centered on the possible role of streptococcal-related antigens as an etiologic agent of this disease. Hirohata and colleagues[117] showed that when *Streptococcus sanguis*-related antigens (RRE KTH-1 antigens) were added to T cells of patients with Behçet's disease in in vitro cultures, the amount of IL-6, an 'inflammatory' cytokine, is higher than that produced by T cells from control subjects stimulated in a similar fashion. This suggests that a hypersensitivity response to these bacterial antigens could be a triggering mechanism for this disease. Tanaka and coworkers[118] reported finding titers of the 65-kDa heat shock protein of *Streptococcus* in patients with Behçet's disease. Pervin and colleagues[119] demonstrated a responsiveness of T-cell clones from patients with Behçet's disease to four peptide determinants within the 65-kDa heat shock proteins derived from *Mycobacterium tuberculosis*. The inflammatory response seen in these patients could in part be due to a heightened response to bacterial antigens.[120] The potential role of these findings still needs to be elucidated. Recently, Kurhan-Yavuz and coworkers[121] have shown a relationship to an endogenous antigen, a common sequence found in various HLA-B molecules that is shared by HLA-B7 and HLA-B51 (B27PD). Increased amounts of IL-2 and TNF-2 were seen in the supernatants from lymphocytes of patients with Behçet's disease after stimulation with this molecule.

No truly specific tests for the diagnosis of Behçet's disease exist. The skin-prick test looking for evidence of pathergy has been suggested to be highly diagnostic for Behçet's disease by some, particularly the Turkish. Skin hyperreactivity has not been a markedly striking feature in the patients we have seen in the United States. Wechsler and colleagues[122] have applied immunofluorescence techniques to skin from which biopsy specimens were obtained after an intradermal injection of distilled water. About 60% of those thought to have Behçet's disease had complement and/or IgM deposition, compared to 14% of control subjects. There was no concordance with HLA-B5. Dogan and colleagues[123] found that total serum sialic acid levels, as well as the proportion of total serum sialic acid to total protein levels, can help to distinguish Behçet's disease from other uveitic entities. Michaelson and coworkers[124] investigated the presence of anticytoplasmic antibodies in this disease by means of an indirect immunofluorescence technique, using guinea pig lip as the tissue substrate. Although eight of eight American patients with Behçet's disease had positive test reactions, only 10 of 16 Turkish patients showed positivity. Anticardiolipin antibodies, which have been observed in several patients with lupus erythematosus accompanied by retinal vascular disease, were reported to be present in high serum titers in one patient with neuro-Behçet's disease.[125] These antibodies were looked for in patients with Behçet's with uveitis, and no correlation could be made by Efthimiou and coworkers,[126] but Bergman and colleagues[127] claimed that IgM isotypes were increased in these patients. However, Aydintug and coworkers[128] found no evidence of anticardiolipin or antineutrophil cytoplasmic antibodies in 72 Turkish patients they screened. Rather, they found that 18% had evidence of antiendothelial cell antibodies (AECAs), which did not induce complement-mediated cytotoxicity; nor was the binding due to immune complexes. However, they did find that those with evidence of AECAs were more apt to develop acute thrombotic events and retinal vasculitis.

Therapy

The responsibility of the ophthalmologist in the treatment of Behçet's disease is a heavy one. The visual course of the patient is often a major factor in the evaluation of whether therapy is successful, or should be altered or stopped. Because of the difficulty in treating the posterior pole aspects of this disorder, a litany of therapies has been proposed. Despite these sometimes intensive attempts, loss of useful visual acuity may occur in about three-quarters of the eyes 6–10 years after the initiation of ocular symptoms.[129]

The most commonly used agents in the past have been systemic corticosteroids, cytotoxic agents (alkylating agents), colchicine, and ciclosporin and tacrolimus (FK506). More recently, IFN-a and anti-TNF therapy have begun to be used. So far, most of these latter medications have been used in a noncontrolled fashion in relatively small numbers of patients, and in case reports with relatively short follow-up. It is important to remember that few medications have been evaluated in randomized studies, and even fewer in the ocular realm. An evaluation of evidenced-based studies shows 21 randomized controlled studies (**Table 26-10**). To date, only azathioprine and ciclosporin have been shown to be effective for the ocular complications of Behçet's disease. At the time of writing IFN-a has been shown in a controlled trial to be effective against mucocutaneous lesions, whereas none have been reported for anti-TNF-α agents.[130] This may change in the near future.

Systemic corticosteroids

Although Behçet's disease may initially respond to systemic corticosteroids, it will invariably become 'resistant,' with a further drop in vision and the need for additional therapeutic modes.[129] Reed[131] has given high-dose intravenous methylprednisolone followed by oral immunosuppressive therapy to rapidly reverse retinal disease. Some Japanese observers never give corticosteroids for this disease because they believe that in the long term the addition of these agents will result in an even worse visual prognosis.

Cytotoxic and antimetabolic agents

In several reports from the Mediterranean basin the efficacy of cytotoxic agents (particularly alkylating agents) in the treatment of the ocular component of Behçet's disease has been demonstrated.[132-134] Mamo[132] noted no ocular recurrences in most patients treated. In a retrospective clinical study Pivetti-Pezzi and coworkers[135] found that the visual prognosis for patients treated with chlorambucil early in their disease course was considerably better than that for those treated early with steroid. A reappraisal by Tabbara[136] of the role of chlorambucil in the treatment of this disorder was considerably less favorable. He underlined the significant side effects seen with the drug, and noted that three-quarters of the eyes studied had a visual acuity of 20/200 or less when chlorambucil was used as the sole therapeutic agent. Kazokoglu and coworkers[137] evaluated the long-term effects of cyclophosphamide and colchicine and concluded that in their 64 patients there was no statistically significant positive change in visual acuity or the attack rate compared with the posttreatment period. These observations essentially corroborate those of BenEzra and Cohen[129] as well as ours. A disturbing report by Takeuchi and Takeuchi[138] found an increased frequency of chromosomal aberrations (dicentrics) in patients with Behçet's disease treated with cytotoxic agents as well as colchicine. Another approach has been to use intravenous pulse cyclophosphamide therapy (which may have fewer side effects) to treat Behçet's disease, an approach similar to that used for severe renal disease. Our experience with this method has not been especially promising, whereas Hamza and colleagues[139] reported some advantage with this method over pulse steroid therapy. Yazici and colleagues[140] reported that azathioprine was superior to placebo in the treatment of this disease. Although any controlled trial deserves attention, it has been noted that maintenance of visual acuity was a goal that was met with only modest success.[141,142] However, long-term results demonstrated that maintenance of visual acuity was better achieved in the azathioprine-treated group than in the control group.[143] Greenwood and coworkers[144] reported their experience with the use of azathioprine in treating the ocular manifestations of Behçet's disease and found that it was only partially effective in allowing a reduction of steroid dosage, and overall was not overwhelmingly effective.

Colchicine

Because the results of leukocyte migration studies showed abnormalities, the use of colchicine was thought ideal because it would inhibit such migration.[145] Most practitioners use it to prevent recurrences, not to treat active disease. Hijikata and colleagues[134] found that the visual prognosis for patients receiving colchicine was better than that for those receiving steroid. A masked, randomized study in Turkey, in which patients received colchicine or placebo, demonstrated no differences between the groups.[146]

A randomized (colchicine versus placebo) study[147] treating active mucocutaneous disease demonstrated that the colchicine-treated group had a reduced incidence of genital ulcers, erythema nodosum, and arthritis. This effect was seen particularly in women. This medication is being used less and less, as other medications for ocular disease, at least, seem to give better control.

Interferon-α

The use of interferon-α in the treatment of the ocular complications of Behçet's disease has been reported. Kötter and colleagues[148] used an initial dose of 6×10^6 IU subcutaneously daily and then 3×10^6 IU every day for 1 month, followed by 3×10^6 IU subcutaneously every other day. This group saw an improvement in all seven patients treated. Pivetti-Pezzi and associates[149] and Wechsler and coworkers[150] used a dose of 3×10^6 IU three times a week. Pivetti-Pezzi and associates saw a 50% reduction of ocular relapses. In two patients the medication was stopped, and there was a recurrence of disease. All patients had a flu-like illness during therapy. Sakane and Takeno[151,152] stressed the potential secondary effects of this therapy, such as immune reactivity, thyroiditis, and a Behçet's disease-like retinopathy, all having been associated with IFN-a therapy.

Ciclosporin and tacrolimus (FK506)

Our observation early on in using ciclosporin suggested clearly that patients with Behçet's disease appeared to have a particularly positive therapeutic response to this agent.[153] These observations were confirmed in a randomized, double-masked multicenter study in Japan, in which ciclosporin was found to be superior to the original standard therapy.[154] In their study, Ando and associates[26] wrote: 'The introduction of ciclosporin in 1985 is probably responsible for the improvement of the visual prognosis in Behçet's disease patients.' Observations have been made in Israel, where the drug was compared with cytotoxic agents in a masked study,[155] as well as in Turkey.[156] Özyazgan and colleagues,[157] in a single masked study, compared 5 mg/kg/day of ciclosporin with intravenous administration of 1 g

Table 26-10 A review of several randomized controlled studies in Behçet's disease

Trial	Agent	Duration	Patient Selection	Comments
Buggage RR et al.[179] (2007)	Daclizumab (1 mg/kg) infusions monthly vs. placebo added to immunosuppressive therapy	15 month median	17 (8M, 9F) with recurrent ocular attacks	No suggestion that daclizumab was beneficial. However, low attack rate for both arms limited ability to make a definitive comparison.
Mat CM et al.[191] (2006)	Methylprednisolone acetate 40 mg IM/3 times weekly vs placebo	27 weeks	86 (43M, 43F) patients with mainly genital ulcers	Effective for erythema nodosum in females but not in males. The drug is more effective among females, similar to colchicine trial.
Melikoglu M et al.[192] (2005)	Etanercept 25 mg SC 2 times weekly vs placebo	4 weeks	40 males with positive pathergy, monosodium urate tests and mucocutaneous lesions	No effect on pathergy and monosodium urate tests, but effective for oral ulcers, nodular lesions, and papulopustular lesions.
Alpsoy E et al.[193] (2002)	IFN-á2a 6 MU 3 times weekly vs placebo	3 months	50 (31M, 19F) with mucocutaneous lesions	Favorable effects on oral and genital ulcers and papulopustular lesions. Adverse effects and high cost limit its use.
Sharquie KE et al.[194] (2002)	Dapsone 100 mg daily vs placebo	3 months	20 patients with mucocutaneous lesions	Favorable effect on mucocutaneous lesions.
Yurdakul S et al.[147] (2001)	Colchicine 1–2 mg daily vs placebo	2 years	116 (60M, 56F) with active mucocutaneous lesions	Effective for genital ulcers, erythema nodosum and arthritis in females, but only for arthritis in males.
Hamuryu-dan V et al.[195] (1998)	Thalidomide 100 mg or 300 mg daily vs placebo	24 weeks	96 male patients with active mucocutaneous lesions	Both dosages are effective for oral and genital ulcers and follicular lesions. Polyneuropathy and teratogenesis limit its use.
Moral F et al.[196] (1995)	Azapropazone 300 mg daily vs placebo	3 weeks	63 with acute arthritis	No difference from placebo on arthritis.
Yazici H et al.[140] (1990)	Azathioprine 2.5 mg/kg body weight daily vs placebo	2 years	73 males (48 with and 25 without eye disease)	Effective for the preservation of visual acuity and the prevention of the emergence of new eye disease, as well as mucocutaneous lesions and arthritis.
Masuda K et al.[154] (1989)	Ciclosporin 10 mg/kg body weight daily vs colchicine 1 mg daily	16 weeks	96 patients with active eye disease	Ciclosporin is more effective for eye and mucocutaneous lesions than colchicine.
Davies UM et al.[171] (1988)	Acyclovir 4 g, then 800 mg daily vs placebo	12 week	22 (7M, 15F) patients with mainly mucocutaneous lesions	No difference in the frequency of orogenital lesions between groups.
Aktulga E et al.[146] (1980)	Colchicine 0.5 mg daily vs placebo	6 months	35 patients with mainly mucocutaneous lesions	Beneficial for erythema nodosum and arthralgia.
Denman AM et al.[197] (1979)	Transfer factor vs placebo	6 months	20 (11M, 9F) patients with mainly mucocutaneous lesions	No difference between the groups.

cyclophosphamide (Cytoxan) per month. In this small study of 23 patients, they found that the ciclosporin group had a significantly marked improvement of their vision compared to the other group, but at 24 months it was not clear whether this improvement was sustained, leaving the observers with the call for further long-term studies. Kotake and colleagues[158] treated 20 Japanese patients with Behçet's disease with low doses of ciclosporin (5 mg/kg/day), and found it to be effective in 70%. Chavis and coworkers[159] in Saudi Arabia reported a salutary effect of ciclosporin on loss of vision due to papillitis, optic neuritis, macular neuro-retinitis, and retinal phlebitis, but not with retinal arteritis. Their approach to therapy is different from the one we have outlined here, with a taper of ciclosporin therapy once clinical improvement is seen; this is therefore intermittent low-dose therapy, as opposed to continuous low-dose ciclosporin therapy as described by us. We have reported our long-term results with ciclosporin in 19 patients with Behçet's disease.[160] We found that combined ciclosporin and prednisone therapy appeared to be an effective means to treat this disorder. The combination permits the use of lower doses of both medications, thereby helping to reduce the possibility of untoward secondary effects. Also of interest was the positive therapeutic effect of ciclosporin therapy reported by Elidan and colleagues[161] on the hearing loss that occurred during Behçet's disease.

With a mechanism that is essentially the same as that of ciclosporin, it is logical to assume that tacrolimus would be a useful therapy for this disorder. It has been used in the treatment of presumed pulmonary vasculitis due to Behçet's disease, with resolution of the pulmonary lesion, as well as amelioration of the uveitis.[162]

Anti-TNF therapy (infliximab)

Infliximab, a chimeric monoclonal antibody directed against TNF-α was reported effective in treating five patients with Behçet's disease. When one dose was given at the last relapse, remission was evident within 24 hours. However, remission is the natural history of this disease even without therapy, but several reports have appeared suggesting its usefulness. Abu El-Asrar et al.[163] reported the response over a relatively long period (16–36 months). When given at 5 mg/kg at time 0, week 2 and then week 6, followed by every 8 weeks, they found that three of six patients were attack free, but that two developed positive ANAs. This reflects our general experience. One patient has been infused for 4 years,[164] and another's optic disc neovascularization regressed with this therapy[165] (no real surprise if the neovascularization is inflammatorily driven). It appears useful, but just to what degree remains to be determined. Sakellariou et al.[166] described a Behçet's patient who developed scleromalacia perforans while receiving infliximab. The implication is that the disease was not necessarily caused by the medication, but rather that it was not effective in controlling the full span of the disease; we see this in all medications as they are more widely used. It is important to remember that it is a chimeric antibody (see Chapter 7) and therefore more prone to the devleopment of antibody reactions; it is often given in conjunction with methotrexate in order to minimize these responses. Further, it is contraindicated in patients with suspected multiple sclerosis,[167] and there have been several

alerts calling attention to the risk of systemic infection (tuberculosis and fungal disease). Like many of the biologics, it is not cheap, with the annual cost for rheumatoid arthritis treatment estimated at £11,000 sterling.[168] Finally, others have begun to examine the role of humanized antibodies directed against the same cytokine, using adalimumab (Humira). Mushtaq et al.[169] transferred three patients from infliximab to adalimumab and achieved control of their disease. The same caveats apply here, in that it is a small series and we need to see whether this antibody is generally as effective as the one it might replace.

Other approaches

Brief comments should be made about some of the other therapeutic approaches suggested for Behçet's disease. The use of agents that augment the immune response appears not to be based on any recent information dealing with potential mechanisms for this disease. Plasmapheresis may be a helpful adjunct in an emergency, but in our mind is not practical for long-term use and must usually be accompanied by immunosuppressive therapy. Bonnet and colleagues[170] treated seven patients with plasma exchange to remove circulating immune complexes and simultaneously gave high doses of aciclovir, with most discouraging results. The use of antiviral agents cannot currently be supported by information in the literature. However, a randomized study using aciclovir for the treatment of Behçet's disease showed no value, at least for the orogenital ulcers.[171] Some centers both inside and outside the United States have used thalidomide to treat various components of Behçet's disease. Although some aspects of the disease may respond positively to this approach,[172] the ocular lesions do not seem particularly amenable.[173] An interesting observation has been the use of thalidomide in the treatment of a patient with neuro-Behçet's disease, in whom no relapses were seen when this agent was added to chlorambucil and prednisone.[174] Stuebiger and associates[175] reported regression of neovascularization with IFN-α therapy. Oral prostaglandin E_1, a potent vasodilator, has been used to treat the leg ulcers sometimes seen with the peripheral vascular complications of Behçet's disease.[176] Rituximab, an antibody directed against CD20, a marker for B cells, induced a 24-month remission in one patient.[177] Additionally, a clinical trial using CAMPATH-1H directed to the CD52 marker, a marker for T cells, induced tolerance in the majority of 18 Behçet's disease patients treated.[178] A randomized study looking at the usefulness of daclizumab in treating the ocular manifestations of the disease did not show it effective as a sole agent. However, the relatively few recurrences in randomized groups prevented an in-depth evaluation.[179]

Our approach to the patient with Behçet's disease who has severe ocular involvement is as follows (**Fig. 26-12**). For patients with bilateral disease having their first attack, we usually use systemically administered prednisone and then slowly taper the medication. We know that long-term therapy of this nature will not protect the patient, but our diagnosis may still be wrong or the patient may indeed have only one attack, although this happens rarely. In some cases it might be useful to observe the patient, particularly if one has not witnessed the attack at its peak and sees only

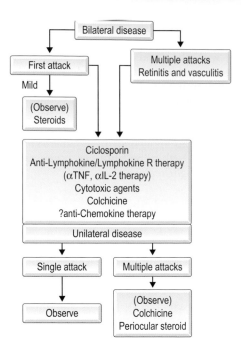

Figure 26-12. General outline for treatment of ocular complications of Behçet's disease.

minimal residua. If the attacks become repetitive, or if the initial attack is particularly severe, then alternative therapeutic agents should be considered. Based on our experience and that of several groups worldwide, we believe that ciclosporin is the initial drug to consider for this disorder, but only after an evaluation determining the feasibility of its use. The goal of therapy is to prevent the recurrent explosive episodes affecting the posterior portion of the globe, and if this is not met we might then consider additional immunosuppressive agents, and then finally add infliximab. Others may turn to IFN-α first, but we have not done so over recent years.

It must be stressed that many agents we use are not approved for the treatment of this disorder in the United States, but certainly some have become standard of care. The patient must be fully aware of the side effects, which one hopes can be minimized. If good control is achieved, it may be that the patient needs to be treated for an extended period, that is, 1–4 years, during which time there can certainly be an attempt to slowly taper the medication. An additional secondary effect of ciclosporin therapy needs to be mentioned here – so far one that has been noted only in patients with Behçet's disease in Japan. In those patients, CNS symptoms, including pleocytosis in the spinal fluid, have been noted. Because uveitis and neuro-Behçet's disease are not commonly seen together, these findings are thought to be due to the ciclosporin. Indeed, Kotter and colleagues[180] carried out a retrospective review of their patients treated with a variety of agents and found that all of those who developed CNS involvement were receiving ciclosporin. Retrospective studies are difficult to evaluate without randomization. Were the most difficult to control cases receiving ciclosporin? Is ciclosporin adequate for ocular disease but simply not effective in treating CNS involvement? We have not so far recognized this in the patients we have treated, nor was this seen in the randomized study comparing ciclosporin to colchicine.[154]

If an alternative therapeutic approach is needed, the practitioner might consider the use of colchicine. The usefulness of colchicine for this disorder is still in doubt, and strict criteria for its continuation or stoppage must be established. We have not used it for bilateral sight-threatening disease. Alternatively, cytotoxic agents should be considered as well. The vast bulk of the literature supports the use of alkylating agents (chlorambucil or cyclophosphamide) for both the uveitis and the CNS findings in this disease.[181] Once again, patients need to know about the potential side effects of these drugs, and the appropriate authorities, if necessary, need to be apprised of the situation. The place of monoclonal antibody therapy still needs to be defined.

In instances of unilateral disease, we usually observe this rare patient with just one attack. If the disease becomes unilaterally recurrent, we might continue to observe the patient if the vision is already markedly diminished because of previous attacks. However, if intervention appears indicated, we would consider using either a periocular steroid or colchicine. Some practitioners have reported the use of intravitreal traimacinolone injections, often giving them repeatedly.[182,183] This should not be considered for long-term treatment, but can be used to deal with acute problems needing immediate action. Constant local steroid therapy is not necessarily benign. Ufret-Vincently et al.[184] reported the development of cytomegalovirus retinitis in an eye from a Behçet's disease patient who received a fluorocinolone implant. For these patients we generally do not use ciclosporin. The alternative argument is that most will develop bilateral disease, and the eye initially involved may ultimately be the better one. These are difficult questions that both practitioner and patient must consider on an individual basis.

Surgery is usually not part of the initial therapeutic approach for these patients. In one report of 26 eyes from patients with Behçet's disease needing vitreoretinal surgery, 15 (58%) had an improvement in vision after surgery, whereas 11 eyes (41%) had no change over a mean follow-up of 23 months. Ahn et al.[185] also suggest that vitrectomy resulted in an improvement in visual acuity and inflammation in the Behçet's patients they operated on. Evaluating nonrandomized data, and in particular vitrectomy studies, is exceptionally difficult, as medical therapy is usually part of the treatment strategy. The important measure is that Behçet patients need surgery but that it should be performed with under-aggressive immunosuppressive coverage; just what the ideal coverage is not defined. For our group it is any combination that renders the patient's ocular activity quiescent and that recurrences have not occurred over the past 3 months or longer. There are numerous reports in the literature regarding the need for adequate immunosuppressive coverage, including the use of IFN-α.[186] Park and colleagues report the large number of postoperative complications in Behçet's patients.[187] Kawaguchi and co-workers[188] reported that such patients had significantly worse outcomes after phacoemulsification and IOL placement than did other uveitis patients, and 35% of the Behçet's patients suffered relapses. Retinal tears, some at the periphery of an active lesion, may occur and membrane removal may be necessary.[181,189] Laser surgery can be performed if the patient is adequately immunosuppressed.

Case 26-1

A 38-year-old Korean man had a 2-year history of symptoms supporting the diagnosis of Behçet's disease. He had had biopsy-proved erythema nodosum, as well as several episodes of painful and tender joints, including the knee, ankle, and foot. He had several mouth ulcers present simultaneously, as well as a penile ulcer. He showed HLA-B51 positivity. For the past year he had noticed that the vision in his left eye was blurry. Attempts were made to treat the condition with eyedrops, but the problem appeared to wax and wane despite therapy. The patient seemed to have on average an attack only in the left eye once a month. When we first saw him, visual acuity was 20/12.5 in the right eye and 5/125 in the left. The right eye showed no evidence of current or prior uveitic episodes. The left eye had trace evidence of flare and cells in the anterior segment. There were 3% cells and 2% haze in the vitreous. The retina had areas of gliosis, with diffuse sheathing and markedly attenuated retinal vessels. Because the patient had unilateral disease and a recent recurrence was resolving, he was given a regimen of 0.6 mg colchicine three times daily. He was able to tolerate this dose schedule, and repeated complete blood cell counts showed no alterations. The number of ocular attacks in the left eye decreased from once a month to one every 7–9 months. He has continued this treatment regimen.

Case 26-2

A 39-year-old man of Scottish-Irish ancestry had a 6-year history of arthritis, mouth ulcers, acne-like lesions on his back and penile ulcers. In addition, recurrent anterior and posterior uveitis developed 2 years before he was seen by us. These episodes were treated initially with systemic steroids, but because of the increasing frequency of ocular attacks he was given chlorambucil. This regimen was maintained for 6 months, with some reduction in the number of ocular attacks. However, his white blood cell count began to decrease to < 3000/mm³. This medication was discontinued because a dose reduction of chlorambucil did not increase the number of circulating white blood cells, and he began to have increased bouts of uveitis. At this point he was seen by us. His visual acuity was 20/30 OD and 20/60 OS, with mild retinal vascular alterations noted. An electroretinogram showed slightly reduced rod- and dark-adapted cone responses in both eyes. The patient was given ciclosporin after the cytotoxic agent had been stopped for more than 1 month. His condition has been maintained with ciclosporin for 5 years at ever-decreasing doses to 3 mg/kg for an extended period of time. His vision is 20/15 OD and 20/30 OS. There have been no recurrences of his ocular disease. On occasion he will develop a mouth ulcer.

Case 26-3

A 35-year-old man of Greek extraction developed all four major criteria for Behçet's disease within the span of 1.5 years. Initial therapy with chlorambucil and then cyclophosphamide (Cytoxan) resulted in some reduction in his retinal vasoocclusive attacks. The best-corrected vision decreased to 20/80 OD and 20/30 OS. Fluorescein angiographic examination showed marked areas of capillary dropout, and there was some retinal atrophy, with the optic nerve in the right eye beginning to look pale. The patient was given ciclosporin therapy and a marked resolution of his nonocular symptoms was seen; his ocular attacks dissipated. Over a period of 3 years his vision dropped markedly in both eyes despite the absence of inflammatory disease. When he returned several years later, his vision was reduced to hand movements OD and 20/400 OS. His therapy was stopped.

Comment 26-3. This patient presents a most frustrating scenario. It would seem that once retinal alterations due to the uveitis have progressed extensively, the degenerative changes become autonomous of the inflammatory disease that initiated them. We assume that apoptosis – programmed cell death – has been initiated. Once this has occurred, vision will irreversibly decrease, even if the uveitis has been controlled.

References

1. Behçet H. Ueber rezideivierende, aphthöse, durch ein Virus verursachte Geschwüre am Mund, am Auge und an den Genitalien. Dermatol Wochenschr 1937; 46: 414–419.
2. Adamantiadis B. Sur un cas d'iritis a hypopyon recidevante. Ann Ocul 1931; 168: 271–274.
3. Shigeta T. Recurrent iritis with hypopyon and its pathological findings. Acta Soc Ophthalmol Jpn 1924; 28: 516–521.
4. Feigenbaum A. Description of Behçet's syndrome in the Hippocratic third book of endemic diseases. Br J Ophthalmol 1956; 40: 355–357.
5. Onal S, Tugal-Tutkun I, Urgancioglu M, et al. Clinical course of ocular Behçet's disease in siblings. Ocular Immunology and Inflammation 2001; 9: 111–124.
6. Fietta P. Behçet's disease: familial clustering and immunogenetics. Clin Exp Rheumatol 2005; 23(4 Suppl 38): S96–105.
7. Kazokoglu H, Onal S, Tugal-Tutkun I, et al. Demographic and clinical features of uveitis in tertiary centers in Turkey. Ophthalmic Epidemiol 2008; 15(5): 285–293.
8. Rodriguez A, Calonge M, Pedroza-Seres M, et al. Referral patterns of uveitis in a tertiary eye care center. Arch Ophthalmol 1996; 114: 593–599.
9. Soheilian M, Heidari K, Yazdani S, et al. Patterns of uveitis in a tertiary eye care center in Iran. Ocul Immunol Inflamm 2004; 12(4): 297–310.
10. Salvarani C, Pipitone N, Catanoso MG, et al. Epidemiology and clinical course of Behçet's disease in the Reggio Emilia area of Northern Italy: a seventeen-year population-based study. Arthritis Rheum 2007; 57(1): 171–178.
11. Ohno S, Matsuda H. Studies of HLA antigens in Behçet's disease in Japan. In: Lehner T, Barnes C, eds. Recent Advances in Behçet's Disease, 1986, Royal Society of Medicine Services: London. pp. 11–16.
12. Bietti G, Bruna F. An ophthalmic report on Behçet's disease. In: Monacelli M, Nazzaro P, eds. Behçet's Disease, 1966, Karger: Basel. p. 79.

13. Mishima S, Masuda K, Izawa Y, et al. Behçet's disease in Japan: Ophthalmologic aspects. Tr Am Ophth Soc 1979; 76: 225–279.

14. Nakae K, Masaki F, Hashimoto T, et al. Recent epidemiological features of Behçet's disease in Japan. In: Godeau P, Wechsler B, eds. Behcceet's Disease, 1993, Elsevier Science Publishers B.V. pp. 145–151.

15. Ohno S. Behçet's disease in the world. In: Lehner T, Barnes C, eds. Recent Advances in Behçet's, 1986, Royal Society of Medicine Services: London. pp. 181–186.

16. Dilsen N, Konice M, Aral O. Our diagnostic criteria of Behçet's disease – an overview. In: Lehner T, Barnes C, eds. Recent Advances in Behçet's Disease, 1986, Royal Society of Medicine Services: London. pp. 177–180.

17. Barnes CG. Behçet's syndrome – classification criteria. Ann Med Interne 1999; 150(6): 477–482.

18. ISGBD, International Study Group for Behçet's disease. Criteria for diagnosis of Behçet's disease. Lancet 1990; 335: 1078–1080.

19. ISGBD, The International Study Group for Behçet's disease. Evaluation of diagnostic ('classification') criteria in Behçet's disease – towards internationally agreed criteria. Br J Rheumatol 1992; 31: 299–308.

20. Bhakta BB, Brennan P, James TE, et al. Behçet's disease: evaluation of a new instrument to measure clinical activity. Rheumatology 1999; 38: 728–733.

21. Nakae K, Masaki F, Inaba G, et al. A nation-wide epidemiological survey on Behçet's disesae, report 2: association of HLA-B51 with clinico-epidemiological features. Report of Behçet's disease research committee. 1993, Ministry of Health and Welfare: Japan.

22. Krause I, Mader R, Sulkes J, et al. Behçet's disease in Israel: the influence of ethnic origin on disease expression and severity. J Rheumatol 2001; 28: 1033–1036.

23. Hafner R, Truckenbrodt H. Behçet's syndrome with childhood onset. Acta Univ Carol [Med] (Praha) 1991; 37: 25–30.

24. Losieau-Corvez M, de Kerdanet MM, Chevrant-Breton J, et al. Phlebothrombosis revealing Behçet's disease in a 13-year-old adolescent. Arch Fr Pediatr 1992; 49: 815–817.

25. Laghmari M, Karim A, Allali F, et al. La maladie de Behçet chez l'enfant, aspects cliniques et evolutifs. A propos de 13 cas. J Fr Ophthalmol 2002; 25: 904–908.

26. Ando K, Fujino Y, Hijikata K, et al. Epidemiological features and visual prognosis of Behçet's disease. Jpn J Ophthalmol 1999; 43: 312–317.

27. El Belhadji M, Hamdani M. L'attente ophtalmologique dans la maladie de Behçet. A propos de 520 cas. Journal francais d'ophtalmologie 1997; 20: 592–598.

28. Cho YJ, Kim WK, Lee JH, et al. Visual prognosis and risk factors for Korean patients with Behçet uveitis. Ophthalmologica 2008; 222(5): 344–350.

29. Kitaichi N, Miyazaki A, Iwata D, et al. Ocular features of Behçet's disease: an international collaborative study. Br J Ophthalmol 2007; 91(12): 1579–1582.

30. Matsuo T, Itami M. Recurrent versus non-recurrent or no eye involvement in Behçet's disease. Ocul Immunol Inflamm 2005; 13(1): 73–77.

31. Kump LI, Moeller KL, Reed GF, et al. Behçet's disease: comparing 3 decades of treatment response at the National Eye Institute. Can J Ophthalmol 2008; 43(4): 468–472.

32. Alpsoy E, Donmez L, Onder M, et al. Clinical features and natural course of Behçet's disease in 661 cases: a multicentre study. Br J Dermatol 2007; 157(5): 901–906.

33. Barra C, Belfort Jr R, Abreu MT, et al. Behçet's disease in Brazil – a review of 49 cases with emphasis on ophthalmic manifestations. Jpn J Ophthalmol 1991; 35: 339–346.

34. Cochereau-Massin I, Wechsler B, Le Hoang P, et al. Ocular prognosis in Behçet's disease. J Fr Ophthalmol 1992; 15: 343–347.

35. Muhaya M, Lightman S, Ikeda E, et al. Behçet's disease in Japan and in Great Britain: a comparative study. Ocul Immunol Inflamm 2000; 8: 141–148.

36. Michaelson J, Chisari F. Behçet's disease. Surv Ophthalmol 1982; 26: 190–203.

37. Wray D, Graykowski E, Notkins A. Role of mucosal injury in initiating recurrent aphthous stomatitis. Br Med J [Clin Res] 1981; 283: 1569–1570.

38. Curth H. Behçet's syndrome, abortive form (?): recurrent aphthous oral lesions and recurrrent genital ulcerations. Arch Dermatol Syphilol 1946; 54: 179–196.

39. Kobayashi T, Matsumaya E, Sugimoto T. Gynecological aspect of mucocutaneous–ocular syndromes. World Obstet Gynecol 1959; 11: 995–999.

40. Mamo J. The rate of visual loss in Behçet's disease. Arch Ophthalmol 1970; 84: 451–452.

41. Imai Y. Studies on prognosis and symptoms of Behçet's disease in long-term observation. Jpn J Clin Ophthalmol 1971; 25: 665–694.

42. Ramsay A, Lightman S. Hypopyon uveitis. Surv Ophthalmol 2001; 46: 1–18.

43. Mocan MC, Kadayifcilar S, Irkec M. Keratic precipitate morphology in uveitic syndromes including Behçet's disease as evaluated with in vivo confocal microscopy. Eye 2008; 23: 1221–1227.

44. Inomata H, Yoshikawa H, Rao NA. Phacoanaphylaxis in Behçet's disease: a clinicopathologic and immunohistochemical study. Ophthalmology 2003; 110(10): 1942–1945.

45. Tugal-Tutkun I, Cingü K, Kir N, et al. Use of laser flare-cell photometry to quantify intraocular inflammation in patients with Behçet uveitis. Graefes Arch Clin Exp Ophthalmol 2008; 246(8): 1169–1177.

46. Yilmaz G, Akova Y, Aydin P. Macular ischaemia in Behçet's disease. Eye 2000; 14(Pt 5): 717–720.

47. Garcher C, Bielefeld P, Desvaux C, et al. Bilateral loss of vision and macular ischemia related to Behçet's disease. Am J Ophthalmol 1997; 124: 115–117.

48. Abu El-Asrar AM, al-Momen AK, Alamro SA, et al. Bilateral central retinal vein thrombosis in Behçet's disease. Clin Rheumatol 1996; 15: 511–513.

49. Balansard B, Bodaghi B, Cassoux N, et al. Necrotising retinopathies simulating acute retinal necrosis syndrome. Br J Ophthalmol 2005; 89(1): 96–101.

50. Bozzoni-Pantaleoni F, Gharbiya M, Pirraglia MP, et al. Indocyanine green angiographic findings in Behçet's disease. Retina 2001; 21: 230–236.

51. Atmaca LS, Sonmez PA. Fluorescein and indocyanine green angiography findings in Behçet's disease. Br J Ophthalmol 2003; 87(12): 1466–1468.

52. Furusawa T. A clinical study on mucocutaneous ocular syndrome. Gank Rinsho Iho 1958; 52: 1143–1146.

53. Sakamoto M, Akazawa K, Nishioka Y, et al. Prognostic factors of vision in patients with Behçet's disease. Ophthalmology 1995; 102: 317–321.

54. Geraint James D, Spiteri M. Behçet's disease. Ophthalmology 1982; 89: 1279–1284.

55. Firestein G, Gruber H, Weisman MH, et al. MAGIC syndrome: mouth and genital ulcers with inflamed cartilage. In: Lehner T, Barnes C, eds. Recent Advances in Behçet's Disease, 1986, Royal Society of Medicine Services: London. pp. 275–280.

56. Shimizu T, Ehrlich GE, Inaba G, et al. Behçet's disease (Behçet's syndrome). Semin Arthritis Rheum 1979; 8: 223–260.

57. Tai Y, Fong PC, Ng WF, et al. Diffuse aortitis complicating Behçet's disease leading to severe aortic regurgitation. Cardiology 1991; 79: 156–160.

58. Muftuoglu U, Yurdakul S, Yurdakul S, et al. Vascular involvement in Behçet's disease – a review of 129 cases. In: Lehner T, Barnes C, eds. Recent Advances in Behçet's Disease, 1986, Royal Society of Medicine Services: London. pp. 255–260.

59. Chajek T, Fairnau M. Behçet's disease. Report of 41 cases and a review of

the literature. Medicine 1975; 54: 179–196.

60. Ebert EC. Gastrointestinal Manifestations of Behçet's Disease. Dig Dis Sci 2008.

61. Inaba G. Clinical features of neuro-Behçet's syndrome. In: Lehner T, Barnes C, eds. Recent Advacnes in Behçet's disease, 1986, Royal Society of Medicine Services: London. pp. 235–246.

62. Sharief M, Hentges R, Thomas E. Significance of CSF immunoglobulins in monitoring neurologic disease activity in Behçet's disease. Neurology 1991; 41: 1398–1401.

63. Wang C, Chuang C, Chen C. Anticardiolipin antibodies and interleukin-6 in cerebrospinal fluid and blood of Chinese patients with neuro-Behçet's syndrome. Clin Exp Rheumatol 1992; 10: 599–602.

64. Ogawa M, Sawada T. Sequential gadolinium-DTPA enhanced MRI studies in neuro-Behçet's disease. Neuroradiology 1991; 33: 136–139.

65. Edem E, Carlier R, Idir AB, et al. Gadolinium-enhanced MRI in central nervous system Behçet's disease. Neuroradiology 1993; 35: 142–144.

66. Kobayashi H, Saito Y, Kaneko Y, et al. A case of neuro-Behçet's disease with hemorrhagic brain stem lesion detected by MRI. Rinsho Shinkeigaku 1992; 32: 763–766.

67. George RK, Chan CC, Whitcup SM, et al. Ocular immunopathology of Behçet's disease. Surv Ophthalomol 1997; 42: 157–162.

68. Winter F, Yukins R. The ocular pathology of Behçet's disease. Am J Ophthalmol 1966; 62: 257–262.

69. Mullaney J, Collum L. Ocular vasculitis in Behçet's disease. A pathological and immunohistochemical study. Int Ophthalmol 1985; 7: 183–191.

70. Gamble C, Wiesner KB, Shapiro RF, et al. The immune complex pathogenesis of glomerulonephritis and pulmonary vasculitis in Behçet's disease. Am J Med 1979; 66: 1031–1039.

71. Levinsky R, Lehner T. Circulating soluble immune complexes in recurrent oral ulceration and Behçet's syndrome. Clin Exp Immunol 1978; 32: 193–198.

72. Matsumura N, Mizushima Y. Leucocyte movement and colchicine treatment in Behçet's disease. Lancet 1975; 2: 813.

73. Fukuda Y, Hayashi H. Pathologic studies on neuro-Behçet's disease. 1980, Annual Report of Behçet's disease research committee: Japan.

74. Kasp E, Graham EM, Stanford MR, et al. Retinal autoimmunity and circulating immune complexes in ocular Behçet's disease. In: Lehner T, Barnes C, eds. Recent Advances in Behçet's Disease, 1986, Royal Society of Medicine Services: London. pp. 67–72.

75. Poulter L, Lehner T, Duke O. Immunohistological investigation of recurrent oral ulcers ad Behçet's disease. In: Lehner T, Barnes C, eds. Recent Advances in Behçet's Disease, 1986, Royal Society of Medicine Services: London. pp. 123–128.

76. Charteris D, Barton K, McCartney AC, et al. CD4+ lymphocyte involvement in ocular Behçet's disease. Autoimmunity 1992; 12: 201–206.

77. Charteris D, Champ C, Rosenthal AR, et al. Behçet's disease: activated T lymphocytes in retinal perivasculitis. Br J Ophthalmol 1992; 76: 499–501.

78. Keino H, Sakai J, Nishioka K, et al. Clonally accumulating T cells in the anterior chamber of Behçet's disease. Am J Ophthalmol 2000; 130: 243–245.

79. Valesini G, Pivetti-Pezzi P, Mastrandrea F, et al. Evaluation of T cell subsets in Behçet's syndrome using anti-T cell monoclonal antibodies. Clin Exp Immunol 1985; 60: 55–60.

80. Kikkawa T, Shirotsuki H. Imbalance in T lymphocyte subsets in panuveitis type of Behçet's disease. J Eye 1984; 1: 1007–1010.

81. Sakane T, Kotani H, Takada S, et al. Functional aberration of T cell subsets in patients with Behçet's disease. Arthritis Rheum 1982; 25: 1343–1351.

82. Ohno S, Kato F, Matsuda H, et al. Studies on spontaneous production of gamma-interferon in Behçet's disease. Ophthalmologica 1982; 185: 187–192.

83. BenEzra D, Maftzir G, Kalichman I, et al. Serum levels of interleukin-2 receptor in ocular Behçet's disease. Am J Opthalmol 1993; 115: 26–30.

84. Evereklioglu C, Er H, Türköz Y, et al. Serum levels of TNF-alpha, sIL-2R, IL-6, and IL-8 are increased and associated with elevated lipid peroxidation in patients with Behçet's disease. Mediators Inflamm 2002; 11(2): 87–93.

85. Yamamoto J, Minami M, Inaba G, et al. Cellular Autoimmunity to retinal specific antigens in patients with Behçet's disease. Br J Ophthalmol 1993; 77: 584–589.

86. Yalcindag FN, Yalçindag A, Batioglu F, et al. Evaluation of serum resistin levels in patients with ocular and non-ocular Behçet's disease. Can J Ophthalmol 2008; 43(4): 473–475.

87. Okunuki Y, Usui Y, Takeuchi M, et al. Proteomic surveillance of autoimmunity in Behçet's disease with uveitis: selenium binding protein is a novel autoantigen in Behçet's disease. Exp Eye Res 2007; 84(5): 823–831.

88. Mahesh SP, Li Z, Buggage R, et al. Alpha tropomyosin as a self-antigen in patients with Behçet's disease. Clin Exp Immunol 2005; 140(2): 368–375.

89. Hamzaoui K, Mili Boussen E, Hamzaoui A, et al. Cellular autoimmunity to retinal specific antigens in Behçet's disease. Soc Tunisienne Sci Med Tunis 1998; 76: 66–70.

90. Yamamoto JH, Fujino Y, Lin C, et al. S-antigen specific T cell clones from a patient with Behçet's disease. Br J Ophthalmol 1994; 78: 927–932.

91. Ahn JK, Yu HG, Chung H, et al. Intraocular cytokine environment in active Behçet's uveitis. Am J Ophthalmol 2006; 142(3): 429–434.

92. Ahn JK, Chung H, Lee DS, et al. CD8brightCD56+ T cells are cytotoxic effectors in patients with active Behçet's uveitis. J Immunol 2005; 175(9): 6133–6142.

93. Yu HG, Lee DS, Seo JM, et al. The number of CD8+ T cells and NKT cells increases in the aqueous humor of patients with Behçet's uveitis. Clin Exp Immunol 2004; 137(2): 437–443.

94. Fujimori K, Oh-i K, Takeuchi M, et al. Circulating neutrophils in Behçet's disease is resistant for apoptotic cell death in the remission phase of uveitis. Graefes Arch Clin Exp Ophthalmol 2008; 246(2): 285–290.

95. Mizuki N, Inoko H, Mizuki N, et al. Human leukocyte antigen serologic and DNA typing of Behçet's disease and its primary association with B51. Invest Ophthalmol Vis Sci 1992; 33: 3332–3340.

96. Godeau P, Torre D, Campanchi R, et al. HLA-B5 and Behçet's disease. In: Dausset J, Svejgaard A, eds. HLA and disease, 1976, PUB: Paris. p. 101.

97. Ersoy F, Berkel I, Firat T, et al. HLA antigens associated with Behçet's disease. In: Dausset J, Svejgaard A, eds. HLA and disease, 1976, PUB: Paris. p. 100.

98. Palimeris G, Papakonstantinov P, Mantas M. The Adamantiadis–Behçet syndrome in Greece In: Saari K, ed. Uveitis update, 1984, Excerpta Medica: Amsterdam. p. 321.

99. VIllaneuva J, Gonzalez-Dominguez J, Gonzalez-Fernandez R, et al. HLA antigen familial study in complete Behçet's syndrome affecting three sisters. Ann Rheum Dis 1993; 52: 155–157.

100. Gul A, Uyar FA, Inanc M, et al. Lack of association of HLA-B*51 with a severe disease course in Behçet's disease. Rheumatology 2001; 40: 668–672.

101. Krause L, Köhler AK, Altenburg A, et al. Ocular involvement is associated with HLA-B51 in Adamantiades–Behçet's disease. Eye 2008.

102. Nishiyama M, Nakae K, Umehara T. A study of familial occurrence of Behçet's disease with and without ocular lesions. Jpn J Ophthalmol 2001; 45: 313–316.

103. Horie Y, Namba K, Kitaichi N, et al. Sister cases of Behçet's disease and

Vogt–Koyanagi–Harada disease. Br J Ophthalmol 2008; 92(3): 433–434.

104. O'Duffy J, Taswell H, Elveback L. HL-A antigens in Behçet's disease. J Rheumatol 1976; 3: 1–3.

105. Ohno S, Char DH, Kimura SJ, et al. Studies on HLA antigens in American patients with Behçet's disease. Jpn J Ophthalmol 1978; 22: 58–61.

106. Sano K, Yabuki K, Imagawa Y, et al. The absence of disease-specific polymorphisms within the HLA-B51 gene that is the susceptible locus for Behçet's disease. Tissue Antigens 2001; 58(2): 77–82.

107. Verity DH, Wallace GR, Vaughan RW, et al. HLA and tumour necrosis factor (TNF) polymorphisms in ocular Behçet's disease. Tissue Antigens 1999; 54: 264–272.

108. Ahmad T, Wallace GR, James T, et al. Mapping the HLA association in Behçet's disease: a role for tumor necrosis factor polymorphisms? Arthritis Rheum 2003; 48(3): 807–813.

109. Karasneh J, Hajeer AH, Barrett J, et al. Association of specific interleukin 1 gene cluster polymorphisms with increased susceptibility for Behçet's disease. Rheumatology (Oxford) 2003; 42(7): 860–864.

110. Yabuki K, Mizuki N, Ota M, et al. Association of MICA gene and HLA-B*5101 with Behçet's disease in Greece. Invest Ophthalmol Vis Sci 1999; 40: 1921–1926.

111. Salvarani C, Boiardi L, Mantovani V, et al. Association of MICA alleles and HLA-B51 in Italian patients with Behçet's disease. J Rheumatol 2001; 28: 1867–1870.

112. Bye L, Modi N, Stanford MR, et al. CTLA-4 polymorphisms are not associated with ocular inflammatory disease. Tissue Antigens 2008; 72(1): 49–53.

113. Hirohata T, Kuratsume M, Nomura A. Prevalence of Behçet's syndrome in Hawaii. Hawaii Med J 1975; 34: 244–246.

114. Denman A, Hylton W, Pelton BK, et al. The viral aetiology of Behçet's disease. In: Lehner T, Barnes C, eds. Recent Advances in Behçet's Disease, 1986, Royal Society of Medicine Services: London. pp. 23–30.

115. Hylton W, Cayley J, Dore C, et al. 2´5´-oligoadenylate synthetase induction in lymphocytes of patients with connective tissue diseases. Ann Rheum Dis 1986; 45: 220–224.

116. Bonass W, Bird-Stewart JA, Chamberlain MA, et al. Molecular studies in Behçet's syndrome. In: Lehner T, Barnes C, eds. recent Advances in Behçet's Disease, 1986, Royal Society of Medicine Services: London. pp. 37–42.

117. Hirohata S, Oka H, Mizushima Y. Streptococcal-related antigens stimulate production of IL6 and interferon gamma by T cells from patients with Behçet's disease. Cell Immunol 1992; 140: 410–419.

118. Tanaka T, Yamakawa N, Koike N, et al. Behçet's disease and antibody titers to various heat-shock protein 60s. Ocul Immunol Inflamm 1999; 7: 69–74.

119. Pervin K, Childerstone A, Shinnick T, et al. T cell epitope expression of mycobacterial and homologous human 65-kilodalton heat shock protein peptides in short term cell lines from patients with Behçet's disease. J Immunol 1993; 151: 2273–2282.

120. Evereklioglu C. Current concepts in the etiology and treatment of Behçet's disease. Surv Ophthalmol 2005; 50(4): 297–350.

121. Kurhan-Yavuz S, Direskeneli H, Bozkurt N, et al. Anti-MHC autoimmunity in Behçet's disease: T cell responses to an HLA-B-derived cross-reactive with retinal-S antigen in patients with uveitis. Clin Exp Immunol 2000; 120: 162–166.

122. Wechsler J, Wechsler B. Behçet's disease: an immunofluorescent study of intradermal distilled water injection by studying 48 patients – value for diagnosis. In: International Academy of Pathology. 1980. Paris, France.

123. Dogan H, Pasaoglu H, Ekinciler OF, et al. A comparative study of total protein, total and lipid associated serum sialic acid levels in patients with Behçet's disease and control groups. Acta Ophthalmol (Copenh) 1992; 70: 790–794.

124. Michaelson J, Chisari F, Kansu T. Antibodies to oral mucosa in patients with ocular Behçet's disease. Ophthalmology 1985; 92: 1277–1281.

125. Salvarani C, Massai G, Macchioni P, et al. Anticardiolipin antibodies in a case of neuro- Behçet's with superior vena caval obstruction. Clin Rheumatol 1987; 6: 88–91.

126. Efthimiou J, Cambridge G, Harris E N, et al. Anticardiolipin antibodies and vascular complications in Behçet's syndrome. In: Lehner T, Barnes C, eds. Recent Advances in Behçet's Disease, 1986, Royal Society of Medicine Services: London. pp. 151–154.

127. Bergman R, Lorber M, Lerner M, et al. Anticardiolipin antibodies in Behçet's disease. J Dermatol 1990; 17: 164–167.

128. Aydintug A, Tokgöz G, D'Cruz DP, et al. Antibodies to endothelial cells in patients with Behçet's disease. Clin Immunol Immunopathol 1993; 67: 157–162.

129. BenEzra D, Cohen E. Treatment and visual prognosis in Behçet's disease. Br J Ophthalmol 1986; 70: 589–592.

130. Hatemi G, Silman A, Bang D, et al. EULAR recommendations for the management of Behçet's disease. Ann Rheum Dis 2008; 67(12): 1656–1662.

131. Reed JB, Morse LS, Schwab IR. High-dose intravenous pulse methylprednisolone hemisuccinate in acute Behçet's retinitis. Am J Ophthalmology 1998; 125: 410–411.

132. Mamo J. Treatment of Behçet's disease with chlorambucil. Arch Ophthalmol 1976; 94: 580–583.

133. Tricoulis D. Treatment of Behçet's disease with chlorambucil. Br J Ophthalmol 1976; 60: 55–57.

134. Hijikata K, Masuda K. Visual prognosis in Behçet's disease: Effects of cyclophosphamide and colchicine. Jpn J Ophthalmol 1978; 22: 506–519.

135. Pivetti-Pezzi P, Gasparri V, De Liso P, et al. Prognosis in Behçet's disease. Ann Ophthalmol 1985; 17: 20–25.

136. Tabbara K. Chlorambucil in Behçet's disease. A reappraisal. Ophthalmology 1983; 90: 906–908.

137. Kazokoglu H, Saatçi O, Cuhadaroglu H, et al. Long-term effects of cyclophosphamide and colchicine treatment in Behçet's disease. Ann Ophthalmol 1991; 23: 148–151.

138. Takeuchi F, Takeuci A. Chromosome aberration in lymphocytes from Behçet's disease. J Rheumatol 1991; 18: 1207–1210.

139. Hamza M, Meddeb S, Mili I, et al. Bolus of cyclophosphamide and methylprednisolone in uveitis in Behçet's disease. Preliminary results with the use of new criteria of evaluation. Ann Med Interne (Paris) 1992; 143: 438–441.

140. Yazici H, Pazarli H, Barnes CG, et al. A controlled trial of azathioprine in Behçet's syndrome. N Engl J Med 1990; 322: 281–285.

141. O'Duffy JD. Behçet's syndrome. N Engl J Med 1990; 326–328.

142. Tabbara K. Azathioprine in Behçet's syndrome. N Engl J Med 1990; 322: 326–328.

143. Hamuryudan V, Ozyazgan Y, Hizli N, et al. Azathioprine in Behçet's Syndrome. Effects on long-term prognosis. Arthritis Rheum 1997; 40: 769–774.

144. Greenwood AJ, Stanford MR, Graham EM. The role of azathioprine in the management of retinal vasculitis. Eye 1998; 12(Pt 5): 783–788.

145. Lange U, Schumann C, Schmidt KL. Current aspects of colchicine therapy classical indications and new therapeutic uses. Eur J Med Res 2001; 6: 150–160.

146. Aktulga E, Altaç M, Müftüoglu A, et al. A double blind study of colchicine in Behçet's disease. Haematologica 1980; 65: 399–402.

147. Yurdakul S, Mat C, Tüzün Y, et al. A double-blind trial of colchicine in Behçet's syndrome. Arthritis Rheum 2001; 44: 2686–2692.

148. Kotter I, Eckstein AK, Stübiger N, et al. Treatment of ocular symptoms of Behçet's disease with interferon alfa

2a: a pilot study. Br J Ophthalmol 1998; 82: 488–494.

149. Pivetti-Pezzi P, Accorinti M, Pirraglia MP, et al. Interferon alpha for ocular Behçet's disease. Acta Ophthalmol Scand 1997; 75: 720–722.

150. Wechsler B, Bodaghi B, Huong DL, et al. Efficacy of interferon alfa-2a in severe and refractory uveitis associated with Behçet's disease. Ocul Immunol Inflamm 2000; 4: 293–301.

151. Sakane T, Takeno M. Interferon therapy in Behçet's disease. Intern Med (Tokyo) 2000; 39: 604–605.

152. Sakane T, Takeno M. Novel approaches to Behçet's disease. Exp Opin Invest Drugs 2000; 9: 1993–2005.

153. Nussenblatt R, Palestine AG, Chan CC, et al. Effectiveness of cyclosporin therapy for Behçet's disease. Arthritis Rheum 1985; 28: 671–679.

154. Masuda K, Nakajima A, Urayama A, et al. Double-masked trial of cyclosporin versus colchicine and long-term open study of cyclosporin in Behçet's disease. Lancet 1989; 1(8647): 1093–1096.

155. BenEzra D, Brodsky M, Pe'er J, et al. Ciclosporin (CyA) versus conventional therapy in Behçet's disease. Preliminary observations of a masked study. In: Schindler R, ed. Ciclosporin in Autoimmune Diseases, 1985, Springer-Verlag: Berlin. pp. 158–161.

156. Assuman U, Müftüoglu H. Treatment of ocular involvement in Behçet's disease with ciclosporin A (preliminary report). In: Schindler R, ed. Ciclosporin in Autoimmune Diseases, 1985, Springer-Verlag: Berlin. pp. 147–151.

157. Ozyazgan Y, Yurdakul S, Yazici H, et al. Low dose cyclosporin A versus pulsed cyclophosphamide in Behçet's syndrome: a single masked trial. Br J Ophthalmol 1992; 76: 241–243.

158. Kotake S, Ichiishi A, Kosaka S, et al. Low dose cyclosporin treatment for ocular lesions of Behçet's disease. Nippon Ganka Gakkai Zasshi 1992; 96: 1290–1294.

159. Chavis P, Antonio S, Tabbara K. Cyclosporine effects on optic nerve and retinal vasculitis in Behçet's disease. Doc Ophthalmol 1992; 80: 133–142.

160. Whitcup S, Salvo EJ, Nussenblatt R. Combined cyclosporine and corticosteroid therapy for sight threatening uveitis in Behçet's disease. Am J Ophthalmol 1994; 118: 39–45.

161. Elidan J, Levi H, Cohen E, et al. Effect of cyclosporine A on the hearing loss in Behçet's disease. Ann Otol Rhinol Laryngol 1991; 100: 464–468.

162. Koga T, Yano T, Ichikawa Y, et al. Pulmonary infiltrates recovered by FK506 in a patient with Behçet's disease. Chest 1993; 104: 309–311.

163. Abu El-Asrar AM, Abboud EB, Aldibhi H, et al. Long-term safety and efficacy of infliximab therapy in refractory uveitis due to Behçet's disease. Int Ophthalmol 2005; 26(3): 83–92.

164. Takamoto M, Kaburaki T, Numaga J, et al. Long-term infliximab treatment for Behçet's disease. Jpn J Ophthalmol 2007; 51(3): 239–240.

165. Giansanti F, Barbera ML, Virgili G, et al. Infliximab for the treatment of posterior uveitis with retinal neovascularization in Behçet's disease. Eur J Ophthalmol 2004; 14(5): 445–448.

166. Sakellariou G, Berberidis C, Vounotrypidis P. A case of Behçet's disease with scleromalacia perforans. Rheumatology (Oxford) 2005; 44(2): 258–260.

167. van Oosten BW, Barkhof F, Truyen L, et al. Increased MRI activity and immune activation in two multiple sclerosis patients treated with the monoclonal anti-tumor necrosis factor antibody cA2. Neurology 1996; 47: 1531–1534.

168. Murray PI, Sivaraj RR. Anti-TNF-alpha therapy for uveitis: Behçet and beyond. Eye 2005; 19(8): 831–833.

169. Mushtaq B, Saeed T, Situnayake RD, et al. Adalimumab for sight-threatening uveitis in Behçet's disease. Eye 2007; 21(6): 824–825.

170. Bonnet M, Ouzan D, Trepo C. Plasma exchange and acyclovir in Behçet's disease. J Fr Ophthalmol 1986; 9: 15–22.

171. Davies UM, Palmer RG, Denman AM. Treatment with acyclovir does not affect orogenital ulcers in Behçet's syndrome: a randomized double-blind trial. Br J Rheumatol 1988; 27(4): 300–302.

172. Allen B. The use of thalidomide in orogenital ulceration: an overview. In: Lehner T, Barnes C, eds. Recent Advances in Behçet's Disease, 1986, Royal Society of Medicine Services: London. pp. 355–358.

173. Hamza M. Treatment of Behçet's disease with thalidomide. Clin Rheumatol 1986; 5: 365–371.

174. Ranselaar C, Boone RM, Kluin-Nelemans HC. Thalidomide in the treatment of neuro-Behçet's syndrome. Br J Dermatol 1986; 115: 367-370.

175. Stuebiger N, Koetter I, Zierhut M. Complete regression of retinal neovascularization after therapy with interferon alfa in Behçet's disease. Br J Ophthalmol 2000; 84: 1437–1438.

176. O'Duffy J, Robertson D, Goldstein N. Chlorambucil in the treatment of uveitis and meningoencephalitis of Behçet's disease. Am J Med 1984; 76: 75–84.

177. Sadreddini S, Noshad H, Molaeefard M, et al. Treatment of retinal vasculitis in Behçet's disease with rituximab. Mod Rheumatol 2008; 18(3): 306–308.

178. Lockwood CM, Hale G, Waldman H, et al. Remission induction in Behçet's disease following lymphocyte depletion by the anti-CD52 antibody CAMPATH 1-H. Rheumatology (Oxford) 2003; 42(12): 1539–1544.

179. Buggage RR, Levy-Clarke G, Sen HN, et al. A double-masked, randomized study to investigate the safety and efficacy of daclizumab to treat the ocular complications related to Behçet's disease. Ocul Immunol Inflamm 2007; 15(2): 63–70.

180. Kotter I, Günaydin I, Batra M, et al. CNS involvement occurs more frequently in patients with Behçet's disease under cyclosporin A (CSA) than under other medications–results of a retrospective analysis of 117 cases. Clin Rheumatol 2006; 25(4): 482–486.

181. Akova YA, Yilmaz G, Aydin P. Retinal tears associated with panuveitis and Behçet's disease. Ophthalmic Surg Lasers 1999; 30: 762–765.

182. Ohguro N, Yamanaka E, Otori Y, et al. Repeated intravitreal triamcinolone injections in Behçet disease that is resistant to conventional therapy: one-year results. Am J Ophthalmol 2006; 141(1): 218–220.

183. Atmaca LS, Yalcindag FN, Ozdemir O. Intravitreal triamcinolone acetonide in the management of cystoid macular edema in Behçet's disease. Graefes Arch Clin Exp Ophthalmol 2007; 245(3): 451–456.

184. Ufret-Vincenty RL, Singh RP, Lowder CY, et al. Cytomegalovirus retinitis after fluocinolone acetonide (Retisert) implant. Am J Ophthalmol 2007; 143(2): 334–335.

185. Ahn JK, Chung H, Yu HG. Vitrectomy for persistent panuveitis in Behçet's disease. Ocul Immunol Inflamm 2005; 13(6): 447–453.

186. Krause L, Altenburg A, Bechrakis NE, et al. Intraocular surgery under systemic interferon-alpha therapy in ocular Adamantiades–Behçet's disease. Graefes Arch Clin Exp Ophthalmol 2007; 245(11): 1617–1621.

187. Park MC, Hong BK, Kwon HM, et al. Surgical outcomes and risk factors for postoperative complications in patients with Behçet's disease. Clin Rheumatol 2007; 26(9): 1475–1480.

188. Kawaguchi T, Mochizuki M, Miyata K, et al. Phacoemulsification cataract extraction and intraocular lens implantation in patients with uveitis. J Cataract Refract Surg 2007; 33(2): 305–309.

189. Wu TT, Hong MC. Pars plana vitrectomy with internal limiting membrane removal for a macular hole associated with Behçet's disease. Eye 2009; 23: 1606–1607.

190. Okabe S, Matsuo N, Okamoto S, et al. Electron microscopic studies on retinochoroidal atrophy in the human eye. Acta Med Okayama 1982; 36: 11–21.

191. Mat C, Yurdakul S, Uysal S, et al. A double-blind trial of depot corticosteroids in Behçet's syndrome.

Rheumatology (Oxford) 2006; 45(3): 348–352.

192. Melikoglu M, Fresko I, Mat C, et al. Short-term trial of etanercept in Behçet's disease: a double blind, placebo controlled study. J Rheumatol 2005; 32(1): 98–105.

193. Alpsoy E, Durusoy C, Yilmaz E, et al. Interferon alfa-2a in the treatment of Behçet's disease: a randomized placebo-controlled and double-blind study. Arch Dermatol 2002; 138(4): 467–471.

194. Sharquie KE, Najim RA, Abu-Raghif AR. Dapsone in Behçet's disease: a double-blind, placebo-controlled, cross-over study. J Dermatol 2002; 29(5): 267–279.

195. Hamuryudan V, Mat C, Saip S, et al. Thalidomide in the treatment of the mucocutaneous lesions of the Behçet syndrome. A randomized, double-blind, placebo-controlled trial. Ann Intern Med 1998; 128(6): 443–450.

196. Moral F, Hamuryudan V, Yurdakul S, et al. Inefficacy of azapropazone in the acute arthritis of Behçet's syndrome: a randomized, double blind, placebo controlled study. Clin Exp Rheumatol 1995; 13(4): 493–495.

197. Denman AM, Hollingworth P, Webster ADB, et al. Failure of transfer factor in the treatment of Behçet's syndrome: a double-blind trial. In: Lehner T, Barnes CG, eds. Behçet's Syndrome, 1979 Academic Press: London.

Retinal Vasculitis

Robert B. Nussenblatt

Key concepts

- Retinal vascular changes can be seen in many ocular inflammatory entities, some associated with systemic disease and others not.
- Fluorescein angiography is very important to evaluate the full extent of the vascular disease.
- Therapy for the ocular disease needs to be coordinated with those treating the systemic illness.

Retinal vascular involvement is a common occurrence in many cases of posterior and intermediate uveitis. The use of the term vasculitis is somewhat of a misnomer, because it suggests that the underlying mechanism leading to these alterations is a type III hypersensitivity reaction – that is, one of immune complexes. We simply do not know whether this is true. Indeed, the evidence available in experimental models, as well as from eyes that have been evaluated, suggests that this is not the case. The meager pathologic data available indicate that the most accurate term for these entities probably is perivasculitis and, in most cases, phlebitis. Although there are conditions in which the retinal vascular component is the predominant feature of the ocular disease, the ubiquitous nature of these retinal vascular alterations indicates that 'retinal vasculitis' can also be a clinical sign. Behçet's disease is perhaps the sine qua non of retinal vasculitis (see Chapter 26); however, myriad disorders can have a similar presentation. It has been suggested that the retinal veins are involved in Behçet's disease, tuberculosis, sarcoidosis, multiple sclerosis, pars planitis, Eales' disease, and the ocular manifestations of human immunodeficiency virus (HIV). Arteriolar involvement is more common in systemic disorders with predominantly arterial involvement, such as polyarteritis nodosa and systemic lupus erythematosus (SLE).[1] Lymphoma, albeit rare, should always be considered as a possible underlying cause of retinal vasculitis.[2]

Clinical characteristics

Although this chapter deals with multiple mechanisms, patients with retinal vasculitis most often report a painless decrease in or marked loss of vision, which may at times be accompanied by floaters. There can also be large areas of scotomata relating to the areas of ischemia. If the retinal vascular changes are in the periphery of the fundus, then patients may report minimal symptoms or none at all, even in light of marked changes noted on ocular examination.

An examination of the retina shows striking vascular alterations, sometimes best seen with fluorescein angiography. Active vascular disease is characterized by sheathing of the vessels or, in some conditions, such as sarcoidosis, an immense inflammatory response around the vessels that has been described as 'candle-wax drippings.' Sheathing can skip along the length of a vessel. Although we can only presume what is occurring histologically, it is thought that a perivasculitis is underlying what we describe clinically as sheathing: large numbers of cells either leaving or entering the vessels. What is drawing them there? We do not know, and speculation abounds. It could be due to the expression of vascular endothelial antigens, to the presence of adhesion molecules, to simple passage of immune cells through the vessel wall to reach the retina and its uveitogenic antigens, or to a mixture of all of these.

Another characteristic of retinal vasculitis is the occlusive retinopathy that can be prominent in some patients. Large areas of capillary dropout are commonly seen. In many inflammatory conditions of the retina the capillary-free zone takes on a markedly jagged and enlarged appearance. Often, in addition to capillary dropout one sees vascular architectural alterations just temporal to the macula, sometimes manifesting as arteriolar/venular anastomoses and crossing of vessels over the horizontal raphe.

The involvement of primarily the retinal vasculature in an inflammatory disorder is rather commonly seen, the best example being Behçet's disease, discussed in Chapter 26. However, other well-recognized entities, such as birdshot retinochoroidopathy (see Chapter 25) and sarcoidosis (see Chapter 22), as well as infectious processes, have or can have marked involvement of the retinal vasculature, although we frequently do not think of these diseases in that sense. Indeed, the entities with a significant retinal vasculature component are listed in **Box 27-1**. It is important to note that noninflammatory conditions can also lead to what appears to be a retinal vasculitis. Venous obstruction, Coats' disease, and diabetes mellitus can mimic the changes seen in an inflammation-driven process.

Although a systemic evaluation for the patient with ocular vasculitis being seen for the first time makes sense, the reader should be aware of our experience. We reviewed our evaluation of 25 patients with 'primary' ocular vasculitis. Only one had a history suggestive of systemic disease (lupus erythematosus). False-positive diagnostic test results were obtained in five of 24 (20.8%) of these patients. No underlying disease was found in any of these patients at review some 4 years later.[3]

Box 27-1 Disorders with retinal vasculitis as a common finding

SYSTEMIC DISORDERS

Behçet's disease
Sarcoidosis
Systemic lupus erythematosus
Postvaccination
Multiple sclerosis
Wegener's granulomatosis
Takayasu's disease
Buerger's disease
Polyarteritis nodosa
Polymyositis
Dermatomyositis
Whipple's disease
Crohn's disease
Sjögren's A antigen
Kikuchi–Fujimoto disease
Susac's syndrome

INFECTIOUS DISORDERS

Syphilis
Cat scratch fever
Hepatitis C[2]
Chickenpox[3]
Toxoplasmosis
Toxocariasis
Coccidiomycosis
Tuberculosis
Cytomegalovirus infection
Herpes simplex
Herpes zoster
Rift Valley fever virus
West Nile virus
Acute retinal necrosis
Candidiasis
Leptospirosis
Rickettsia
Mediterranean spotted fever
Brucellosis
Amebiasis
Mononucleosis
Lyme disease
Hepatitis B

OCULAR DISORDERS

Birdshot retinochoroidopathy
Pars planitis
Eales' disease
Choroiditis
Retinal arteritis and aneurysms
Behçet's retina sine systemic disease
Vein occlusion

NEOPLASMS

Paraneoplastic syndromes
Ocular and systemic lymphoma
Acute leukemia

Reproduced with permission from Samuel, M.A., et al. Idiopathic retinitis, vasculitis, aneurysms, and neuroretinitis (IRVAN): new observations and a proposed staging system. Ophthalmology 2007;114(8): pp. 1526–1529.

Ocular vasculitic disorders without systemic disease

We have seen patients with ocular findings that are indistinguishable from those in patients with Behçet's disease. These patients have none of the typical systemic findings but yet will have recurrent episodes of retinal vasculitis. In addition, some of these persons show HLA-B51 positivity. The possibility that they may develop Behçet's disease certainly exists. However, on a statistical basis one would expect other features of the disorder to develop within 3 years of the appearance of the first criteria, and this has not been the case. The recurrent episodes of retinal vasculitis (and retinitis) are frequently difficult to control and may require the use of other immunosuppressive agents in addition to prednisone. Lueck and coworkers[4] reported the case of a patient with recurrent steroid-sensitive uveitis and central nervous system (CNS) disease thought to be due to sarcoidosis. Postmortem examination revealed a histologic picture compatible with that for Behçet's disease, despite the patient's lack of any of the systemic stigmata associated with this diagnosis. The authors have called this entity the Behçet's MINUS syndrome (multifocal intermittent neurologic and uveitic syndrome).

We have seen other patients with severe retinal vasculitis that appears to be unassociated with systemic disease; often attempts to identify an underlying abnormality (e.g., immune complexes or sedimentation rate) prove fruitless. The disorder frequently may continue despite aggressive immunotherapy (**Fig. 27-1**).

Eales' disease

Although Eales' disease had been discussed by others, the disorder carries the name of Henry Eales who, in 1880,[5] described five young men with recurring vitreal and retinal hemorrhages associated with constipation and epistaxis. The definition of the condition has varied considerably over the years. Our group defines Eales' disease as an idiopathic condition that manifests as an obliterative perivasculitis (particularly involving the venule side) affecting the retina in multiple quadrants, starting at or anterior to the equator and progressing posteriorly. The disease sometimes is accompanied by neovascularization, without vitritis, obvious uveal inflammation, or obvious systemic disease. It is in essence a diagnosis of exclusion and probably includes a heterogeneous patient population. There is a strong association with purified protein derivative skin test positivity,[6] and Moura and colleagues[7] reported that strongly positive Mantoux test results were found in 87% of 141 patients. Biswas and colleagues[8] published two papers further evaluating the relationship between tuberculosis and Eales' disease in India. In one study, polymerase chain reaction (PCR) was performed on 12 vitrectomy specimens from patients with Eales' disease and on 45 specimens from patients without Eales' disease. This methodology had the sensitivity to detect 2.5 pg of *Mycobacterium tuberculosis*. Five of the 12 specimens (41.6%) from the patients with Eales' disease versus one of 45 specimens (2.2%) from the patients without Eales disease were positive for *M. tuberculosis*. In their second study[9] 11 of 23 epiretinal membranes (47.8%) versus three of 27 control epiretinal membranes (11.1%) (p = 0.001) were positive for the *M. tuberculosis* genome. In another study from India,

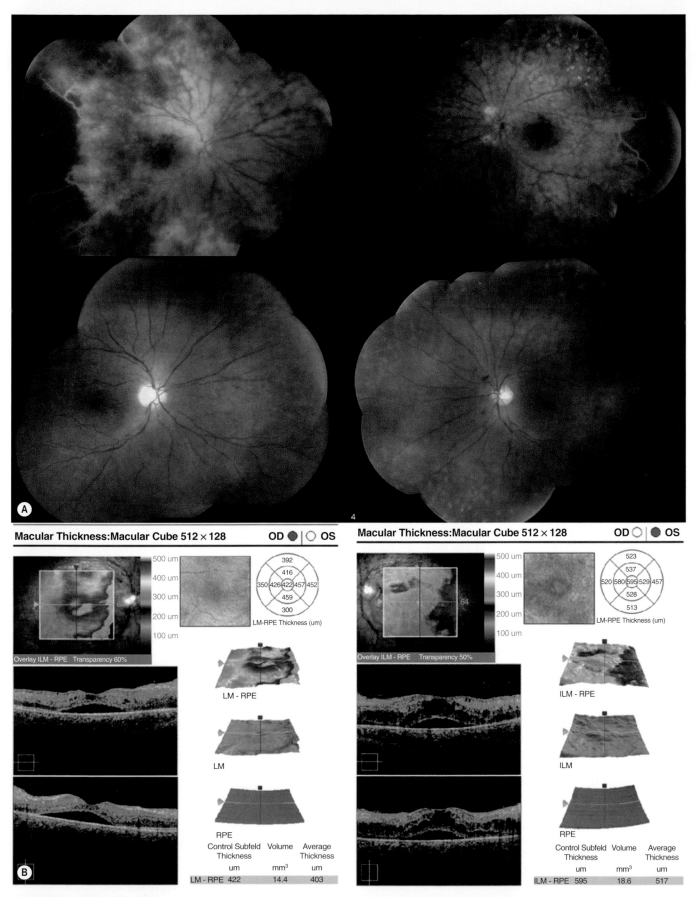

Figure 27-1. This 17-year-old Hispanic woman complained of decreased vision. She was found to have a retinal vasculitis in both eyes. **A,** Montage and fundus findings. Note the peripheral retinal capillary loss. Laser photocoagulation had been started in the periphery of the OS before referral to the NEI. **B,** OCT of both eyes showing macular edema and subretinal fluid. An extensive evaluation revealed no systemic abnormality. She was stabilized on prednisone and ciclosporin in the short term.

Therese and coworkers,[10] using PCR, reported finding *M. fortuitum* and *M. chelonae* in vitrectomy specimens, thereby suggesting that other mycobacteria could initiate similar immune responses. The disease has been estimated to affect 1% of adult males in India and usually occurs in patients under 40 years of age. The process has minimal inflammation associated with it.

The disorder may start with retinal edema, followed by a progressive cuffing of the venules (periphlebitis), and then by peripheral retinal vascular nonperfusion and retinal neovascularization.[11] The condition affects the retinal periphery, but on occasion it can begin at the optic nerve head, mimicking a vein occlusion. Only with the more characteristic peripheral retinal signs will the diagnosis become clear. The arteries are not involved. Unlike occlusions that result from arteriosclerotic plaques, this occlusion does not usually occur at an arteriovenous crossing. The periphlebitis may occlude substantial portions of a vein, but in an irregular fashion. Unlike vein occlusions in the posterior pole, those in the periphery will not cause cottonwool spots.[12] The development of neovascularization may be rapid. Fluorescein angiographic examination of the retinal vasculature may show nonperfusion, arteriovenous shunting, and neovascularization (**Fig. 27-2**). Recurrent vitreous hemorrhage, with ensuing vitreous contraction and retinal detachment, is a serious risk in this disorder. Although the disease is thought to be an ocular disorder, Biswas and associates[13] reported three patients with seizures and/or migraine. An MRI scan in two patients showed a putaminal infarct with white matter edema.

Although the disease may proceed with its full-blown clinical picture as described, in some patients the process may spontaneously reverse itself. The visual prognosis in these patients is not totally hopeless. Elliot[14] reported that 25 of 46 eyes he followed for an average of 6 years had a visual acuity of 20/50 or better, whereas 26% had a vision of 20/200 or worse. The exact role of the immune system remains unclear. However, Murugeswari et al.[15] have shown a correlation between VEGF and IL-6 levels in the vitreous specimens of Eales' disease patients, with IL-8 and MCP-1 also being elevated compared to controls. This would suggest that at least locally active inflammatory factors are being produced. Part of the definition calls for minimal or no evidence of inflammatory disease. Muthukkaruppan and associates[16] found circulating immune complexes in these patients. Rennie and associates[17] have also noted vestibulo-auditory problems associated with the ocular condition, suggesting that this is indeed a systemic ailment. The notion that the disease is due to tuberculosis hypersensitivity is difficult to support because it does not seem to be found in greater numbers of patients in countries in which the population is actively immunized with bacille Calmette–Guérin vaccine. It may be that mycobacterial antigens are particularly good initiators of a still-undefined disease mechanism, but that other antigens are probably capable of producing the same effect. Alternatively a specific genetically determined immune background may put some patients at higher risk for development of the disease.

For patients with capillary dropout and neovascularization, laser ablation could be contemplated. Vitrectomy certainly plays a role in the management of patients who have recurrent vitreous hemorrhages. Dehghan et al.[18] observed

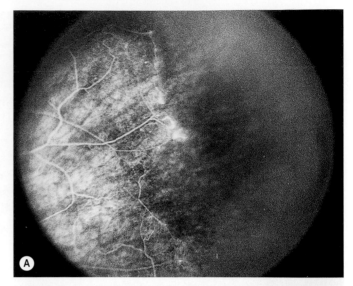

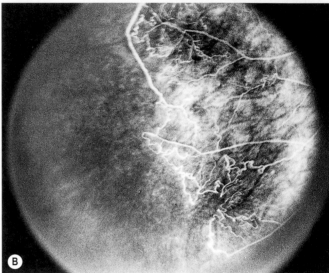

Figure 27-2. A and B, Peripheral retinal vasoocclusive disease with neovascularization due to Eales' disease. *(Courtesy of R. Murphy, MD.)*

that in their study of 67 eyes, vitrectomy and laser photocoagulation resulted in improved visual acuity and regression of neovascularization. Most other observers will consider other therapy. Some have resorted to systemic immunosuppression, including methotrexate,[19] observing an improvement in visual acuity. Others have used intravitreal injections of steroid. Ishaq et al.[20] saw reduction of leakage, but their follow-up was short, whereas Agrawal et al.[21] saw a reduction in inflammatory activity in the eye in two cases, one of which recurred (**Fig. 27-3**). Others have reported the use of anti-VEGF thearpies. Akova et al.[22] reported regression and no recurrence of disease after 12 months in a patient whose disorder was not responsive to panretinal photocoagulation and who received 1.25 mg of bevacizumab intravitreally. Kumar and Sinha[23] reported a similarly positive result in a patient they treated. The evaluation of these therapies is made very difficult by the natural history of the disease, which suggests that it may regress by itself. Moreover, it appears that many approaches may be valuable, but the difficulty is choosing the best one for your patient.

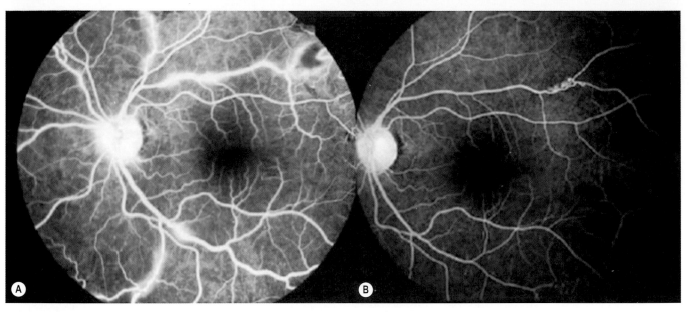

Figure 27-3. Fundus photographs of eye with Eales' disease. **A,** Before intravitreal steroid therapy and **B,** 8 weeks after the injection. *(Reproduced with permission from Ishaq, M, et al. Intravitreal steroids may facilitate treatment of Eales' disease (idiopathic retinal vasculitis): an interventional case series. Eye. 2007;21(11): 1403–1405.)*

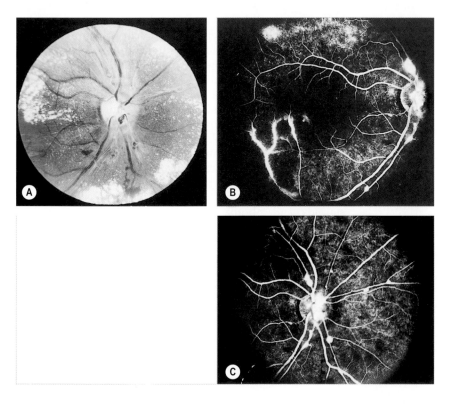

Figure 27-4. A to C, A patient with retinal aneurysms and arteritis. Note extensive exudate and hemorrhage, sheathing of vessels, and macroaneurysms. Extensive capillary dropout was seen just beyond these areas of exudate.

Idiopathic retinal vasculitis, aneurysms, and neuroretinitis (IRVAN syndrome)

A rare condition with multiple saccular and fusiform aneurysms involving the larger arterioles, combined with peripheral vascular nonperfusion and uveitis, has been reported.[24,25] The degree of nonperfusion can be quite profound (**Fig. 27-4**). A neuroretinitis, as well as retinal neovascularization, optic nerve head swelling, and anterior uveitis, can be associated with this disorder, which occurs in younger persons. The underlying nature of the disorder remains in doubt. It is interesting that the disease appears quite dynamic, with

the aneurysms reported to regress and appear elsewhere sometimes quite rapidly.[26,27] It is not clear whether immunosuppressive agents are beneficial for this condition. Some suggest it may be a matter of dose, as Ishikawa and colleagues[28] reported the case of a 15-year-old whose ocular disease did not respond to oral steroid, but did respond with 500 mg of intravenously administered prednisolone. This may reflect that the disease is at the level of the retinal vasculature rather than the immune system. Jampol and colleagues[29] reported a patient with occlusive retinal arteriolitis with neovascularization. Although the disease course in the 34-year-old white woman had some similarities to the entity

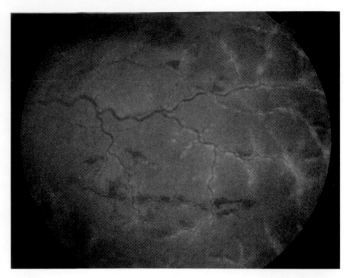

Figure 27-5. Fundus of a young boy with idiopathic frosted branch angiitis. Yannuzzi has suggested that angiitis is seen in children, whereas periphlebitis generally is noted in young adults. *(Courtesy of L. A. Yannuzzi, MD.)*

just described, no aneurysms were noted. The disease has been seen in a pregant woman in a hypercoaguable state,[30] and peripheral venule and arteriolar occlusions have been noted,[31] again suggesting the local, vascular element to the disorder. Laser photocoagulation has been shown to have a benefit in only a relatively small number of patients. Abu El-Asrar and colleagues[32] reported regression of IRVAN aneurysms in a patient with allergic fundal sinusitis, and Tomita and coworkers[33] reported that the regression remained long after photocoagulation of the nonperfused areas of retina. Samuel et al.[34] reviewed 44 eyes with this condition and offer a scoring system for the disease (**Box 27-2**). They conclude that retinal laser photocoagulation should be performed as early as possible if there are areas of widespread retinal nonperfusion.

Frosted branch angiitis

Frosted branch angiitis has been described by Walker et al.[35] as 'florid translucent retinal perivascular sheathing.' It was first reported in a 6-year-old boy with vessels resembling frosted branches,[36] and is generally found in younger individuals. The disorder usually results in a severe drop in visual acuity, at least during the acute period. Although both arteries and veins may be involved, the venules tend to be more commonly affected (**Fig. 27-5**). About three-quarters of reported cases have been bilateral; it has no gender preference, and more than 65–70% of patients have been reported to have retinal edema and an intermediate uveitis. One case reported macular choroidal neovascularization associated with the disorder.[37] This is an ocular sign and can have many causes, some of which are infectious. It has been reported to occur before and after the appearance of ocular toxoplasmosis,[38,39] and after influenza A exposure,[40] but it can be idiopathic with no obvious systemic cause.[41] One can speculate that it is an extreme example of a diffuse perivasculitis. The 'frosting' around the vessels could be in fact thousands (millions?) of cells that are moving through the vascular wall into the retina.

The condition will disappear with proper and aggressive therapy, but of course the key is choosing the 'proper' therapy. Frosted branch angiitis has been associated with ocular cytomegalovirus in patients with AIDS. Resolution of the findings in adults is seen with aggressive anticytomegalovirus (CMV) therapy. In an HIV-positive child we saw, the angiitis persisted even after therapy with intravenous ganciclovir and foscarnet and resolution of the antigenemia.[42] This suggested that even in the context of HIV infection, CMV is not the sole cause of this ocular finding. Other infectious conditions in which this sign has developed include tuberculosis, syphilis, and herpes simplex type 2 virus infection.[43] Others have found it to be associated with aseptic meningitis,[44] lymphoma, leukemia, sarcoidosis, multiple sclerosis, pars planitis, and SLE. Masuda and coworkers[45] reported a patient with frosted branch angiitis with yellow-white placoid lesions, with an evaluation suggesting an occlusion of the choriocapillaris. Borkowski and Jampol[46] reported retinal and disk neovascularization in a patient with bilateral frosted branch angiitis who also had peripheral retinal ischemia. Retinal neovascularization was noted by Kleiner and colleagues[47] after multiple branch vein occlusions. Borkowski and Jampol's patient was treated with steroids and photocoagulation, with a good outcome. Responsiveness of this disorder to steroid therapy was also reported by Sykes and Horton[48] in a patient who also had Crohn's disease.

Scleritis

Although scleritis certainly is not a disease of the retinal vasculature, it seems important to discuss it and how it may relate to intraocular inflammatory disease. The vasculature near the scleritis appears to be integrally involved in the inflammatory/pathologic process, with medial necrosis, perivasculitis, or thrombosis often seen.[49,50] The inflammatory reaction associated with anterior scleritis can spill over into the eye, leading to anterior or even intermediate uveitis. Posterior scleritis is an entity that is frequently not included in the differential diagnosis of posterior pole lesions[51] (**Fig. 27-6**). This disorder may not be associated with anterior segment changes. Patients frequently report ocular pain, although the eye does not appear inflamed. At times the conjunctiva may be slightly boggy. There may be a mild vitreous inflammatory response associated with a drop in visual acuity. Careful examination of the posterior segment may reveal choroidal folds or even a thickening of the retina, although these processes are often subtle and difficult to determine. Ultrasound examination of the

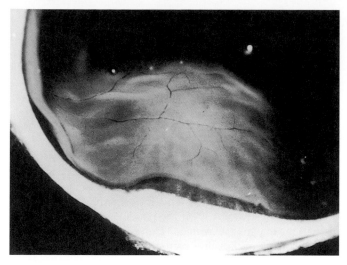

Figure 27-6. Although not retinal vasculitis, posterior scleritis should be considered in patients with poor vision, pain, uveitis, and striae of choroid. *(Courtesy of David Cogan, MD.)*

globe is a very useful tool to help in the diagnosis. In many patients the disease responds to corticosteroid therapy, although relapse may occur once the dosage is reduced.

A note of caution is warranted. Although most cases of posterior scleritis are not associated with a systemic disorder, it is fitting to consider this caveat. The ophthalmologist always needs to be aware of the fact that this entity can manifest as a systemic disorder, and a careful rheumatologic evaluation seems warranted for most patients (see Chapter 20).

Ocular vasculitic disorders with systemic disease

Perhaps the most common systemic entities that we see with a marked vascular component are sarcoidosis (**Fig. 27-7**), Behçet's disease, and multiple sclerosis. Although sarcoidosis is usually not thought of as the basis for a retinal vasculitis, it can cause myriad ocular manifestations, including severe involvement of the retinal vasculature (see Chapter 22). Multiple sclerosis was first associated with

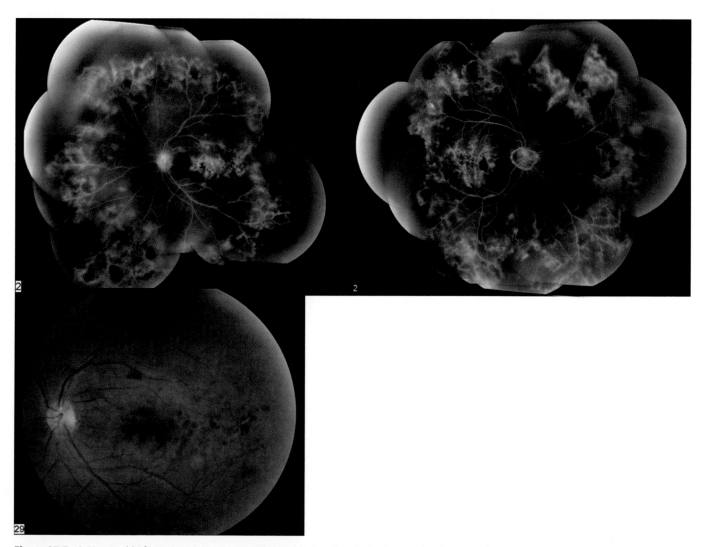

Figure 27-7. A 50-year-old African-American woman with sarcoidosis and marked pulmonary involvement who presented with a bilateral retinal vasculitis. The fundus picture of the left eye shows multiple retinal hemorrhages.

ocular inflammatory disease at the turn of the 20th century. In an early article, Rucker[52] suggested that perhaps 20% of patients with multiple sclerosis may have retinal sheathing (i.e., vasculitis); others, such as Breger and Leopold,[53] have reported this finding in an even higher percentage of patients (14 of 52, 27%). In our experience, it would seem that generally less than 5–8% of these patients have this complication.

Apart from the more common ocular entities, retinal vasculitis can be associated with several systemic entities, many of which are among the collagen-vascular group of disorders. A key point to consider in making these diagnoses is that usually the patient's complaints are associated with a subacute chronic disorder. The findings include malaise, weight loss, arthritis, fever, and rash. An important finding is mononeuritis multiplex. This is an acute neuropathy that begins at one named nerve root and then progresses to one or more other nerve roots, one at a time. It more commonly affects the nerve roots of the lower extremities and can have an abrupt painful onset, with the patient reporting deep muscle pain. It is a common presenting sign in polyarteritis nodosa and occurs in a significant number of patients with SLE and rheumatoid arthritis later in the course of their disease. The ophthalmologist should be aware that other disorders can cause mononeuritis multiplex, including diabetes, paraneoplastic syndromes, and even jellyfish stings.[54,55]

Some of the diseases that need to be considered in the search for a systemic cause for retinal vasculitis include those discussed in the following sections.

Systemic lupus erythematosus

SLE is a common systemic disorder that is diagnosed by use of a combination of clinical and laboratory criteria. A more mild form of the ocular disease may have a microangiopathy in which vasoocclusion and vasculitis are less common. Retinal vasculitis can rarely be the presenting finding.[56] Histology of such eyes has shown capillary lumen obliteration and the deposition of IgG.[57] Thought to be the classic immune complex disorder,[58] it affects the eye with severe intraocular complications in a relatively small number of patients. However, when it does, it can be extremely problematic because it is sometimes difficult to provide adequate therapy. Jabs and coworkers[59] reported on 11 patients with severe retinal vasoocclusive disease and poor visual outcome often associated with CNS involvement in SLE (**Figs 27-8, 27-9, 27-10**). Antiphospholipid antibodies are associated with the vasoocculusive ocular disease, leading, it is thought, to microthrombi.[60] Therefore, anticoagulation must be considered in preventing further thrombosis. Proliferative retinopathy can be a serious problem as well.[61] It should be mentioned that antiphospholipid antibodies may cross-react with cardiolipin, which is used in some syphilis testing.[62] This condition raises the intellectually interesting but also practically important question as to whether therapy should consist of laser photocoagulation or systemic immunotherapy to stop the underlying inflammatory process that presumably induces the retinal vascular alterations. Although aggressive systemic immunosuppression therapy is often needed, plasmapharesis[63] has been used acutely in conjunction with immunosuppression to reverse the ocular pathology.

Polyarteritis nodosa

Polyarteritis nodosa was first described by Kussmaul and Maier in 1866. It is a necrotizing vasculitis that involves the medium-sized muscular arteries and smaller arterioles. It can present as a bilateral iritis, vitreitis, and retinal vasculitis involving both the veins and arteries, which can very aggressive in nature,[64,65] with one case reported manifesting a central retinal artery occlusion as well.[66] It has been estimated that up to 20% of these patients may have ocular involvement.[67] Mononeuritis multiplex, an acute neuropathy described earlier, has been estimated to develop in two-thirds of patients with polyarteritis nodosa. The most common sites are in the lower extremities. This is a potentially fatal disorder: 5-year survival is 13% if the patient is untreated, versus 80% in those who are treated.[68] Current therapy usually consists of corticosteroids and cyclophosphamide.[22]

Wegener's granulomatosis

Wegener's granulomatosis is characterized by a necrotizing granulomatous vasculitis of the upper and lower respiratory tract, systemic small vessel vasculitis that can involve multiple organs, and a focal necrotizing glomerulonephritis. Ocular complications, including uveitis, scleritis, and retinal vasculitis, can occur in 16% of patients.[69,70] One must remember that, except for mild anterior segment disease, the eye disease does not respond to topical medications, and that the systemic therapy usually indicated for the disease needs to be employed.[71] It is also important to remember that the cytoplasmic antineutrophil antibody (ANCA) test is highly specific for this disease. Soukasian and coworkers[72] reported that the ANCA test result was positive in seven patients with scleritis due to Wegener's granulomatosis but negative in 54 patients with ocular inflammatory disease due to other causes. Others have reported the usefulness of this test, not only for diagnosis but also for following the course of the disease.[73,74] Antinuclear cytoplasmic antibodies are a marker not only for Wegener's granulomatosis, but also for necrotizing vasculitis, Churg–Strauss syndrome, microscopic polyangiitis, and idiopathic crescentic glomerulonephritis. Indeed, Gallagher[75] found ANCA-positive patients with retinal vasculitis having microscopic polyangiitis.

Two caveats should be kept in mind by the eyecare physician. Two patterns of ANCA are reported – a cytoplasmic pattern (cANCA), which is believed to be more specific for Wegener's granulomatosis, and a peripheral pattern (pANCA), which is less useful in making the diagnosis. Young,[76] in testing patients with uveitis, used the ANCA test and found positive results in those with chronic uveitis of various underlying causes. Because this test is interpreted manually, so that there can be great variation in results, an enzyme-linked immunosorbent assay, directed towards proteinase 3, is now being used. The second caveat is that if a high suspicion remains in the physician's mind it is useful to repeat the cANCA test, because results may initially be negative in patients with Wegener's granulomatosis localized to the orbit or eye, but will become positive with time.

Whipple's disease

Whipple's disease is a multisystem disorder, usually manifested by malabsorption, diarrhea, and polyarthritis, that

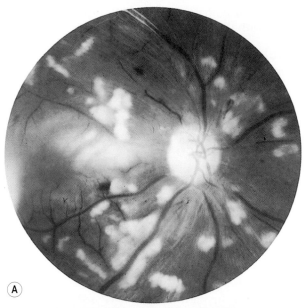

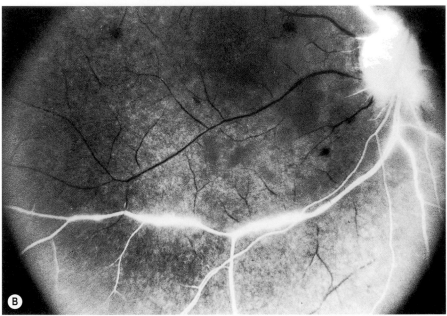

was described by George Hoyt Whipple at the beginning of the last century.[77] The first case report with eye findings was ascribed to Jones and Paulley in 1949;[78] it has been estimated that <5% of patients will have uveitis. The disease is believed to be caused by the Whipple's disease bacillus *Tropheryma whippleii*, which can be found in vitreous specimens using electron microscopy and PCR, along with foamy macrophages.[79] In some patients, fluorescein angiographic results show diffuse vasculitis with hemorrhages, exudates, retinal capillary occlusion, and choroidal folds.[80] Although the gastrointestinal complaints are typically present, others have reported patients with minimal symptoms related to that organ system,[81] and Bodaghi and colleagues[82] reported a similar constellation of problems due to *Arthrobacter* infection. Lo Monaco and colleagues[83] have stressed the neurologic signs found in one patient who had a retinal vasculitis, and who was treated with high-dose steroid and cyclosphosphamide. Chan and associates[84] emphasized the need for early diagnosis, because early antibiotic therapy leads to a greater chance of resolution.

Inflammatory bowel disease

Crohn's disease commonly affects the eye in several ways, including uveitis (pars planitis), retinitis, scleritis, and keratitis. However, Duker and colleagues[85] reported the case of a patient with a severe bilateral, obliterative, retinal arteritis, and phlebitis. There are case reports of both bilateral and unilateral retinal vasculitis with Crohn's disease.[86,87] The disorder appeared to respond to systemic corticosteroid and cyclophosphamide therapy. Ruby and Jampol[88] reported two patients with retinal vascular disease, one of whom had disease involving both the retinal arteries and veins, with an apparent branch retinal artery occlusion. In one report, Felekis and coworkers[89] evaluated 60 patients with inflammatory bowel disease of whom 23 had Crohn's disease.

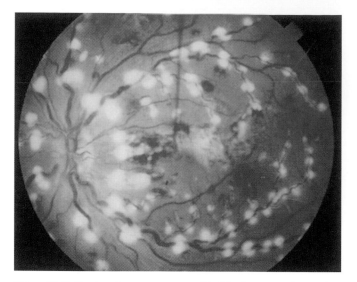

Figure 27-9. Fundus of a young woman with difficult-to-control systemic lupus erythematosus. Extensive nerve fiber infarcts and hemorrhage create a dramatic picture, with maintenance of good visual acuity. Retinopathy resolved after disease was controlled.

Only one case of retinal vasculitis was noted, and this was in a patient with ulcerative colitis.[89]

Autoantibodies to Sjögren's syndrome A antigen

This systemic lupus-like illness may be systemically mild, but retinal arteriolitis that leads to retinal ischemia, optic disk, and retinal neovascularization may occur.[90]

Retinal vein occlusion

It is important to note that putative nonimmune mechanisms may lead to ophthalmoscopic findings that mimic an immune-driven pathologic condition[91] such as retinal vein occlusion. After thrombosis, the vein occlusion can develop a secondary perivasculitis.

Relapsing polychondritis

Relapsing polychondritis is a systemic inflammatory disease of connective tissue that may have associated ocular manifestations. The diagnosis is characteristically made by

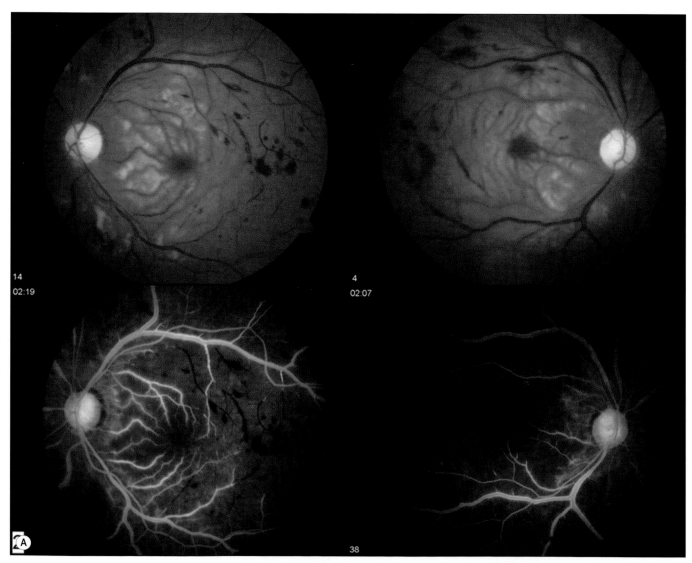

Figure 27-10. This 15-year-old African-American girl presented with a decrease in vision and systemic symptoms compatible with SLE. **A,** The fundus as it appeared at the initial examination at the NEI. Note the retinal hemorrhages and remarkable degree of loss of vasculature seen on the angiogram.

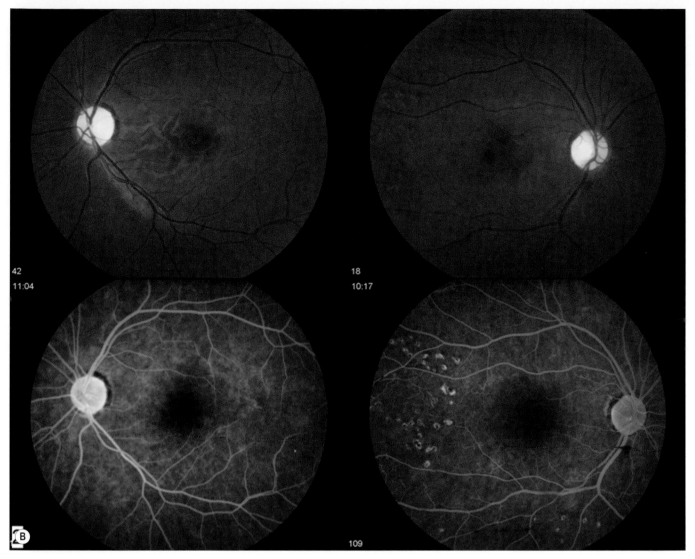

Figure 27-10, Cont'd B, One year later, after systemic immunosuppressive therapy and laser. The patient has retained good central vision but the optic nerve changes remain disquieting.

observation of inflammation of the cartilage of the nose, earlobes, or trachea. Inflammation at two of these sites suffices for the diagnosis. Alternately, inflammation of one such site combined with two of the following associated signs is consistent with a diagnosis: hearing loss, vestibular imbalance, ocular inflammation, or rheumatoid factor-negative arthritis. In a review of 112 patients, Isaak and colleagues[92] found ocular signs or symptoms in 21 at the time of diagnosis. Ocular involvement occurred in 57 of these patients at some time during the course of their disease. The most common ocular findings were episcleritis (39%) and scleritis (14%). Iridocyclitis has been observed in as many as 30% of patients with this disease,[93] but was found in only 9% of patients in the series of Isaak and coworkers. Retinopathy, primarily exudates, and hemorrhages were seen in 9% as well. Occasionally retinal vascular occlusions, serous retinal detachments, and optic neuropathy develop. A systemic vasculitis was reported in 9% of patients,[92] demonstrating the systemic inflammatory nature of this syndrome. Vessels of any caliber may be involved. It is possible that although the episcleral and scleral involvement in this disease is immunologically similar to the mechanisms

that lead to inflammation of the cartilage, the other ocular manifestations that are seen are not tissue specific but part of the varied accompanying systemic vascular involvement.

Viral diseases

The exact role of viruses in the development of a vasculitis of the retinal vasculature with no overt destruction of the retina itself remains to be defined. It is clear that viruses can cause vascular endothelial cells to express receptors that might make them more susceptible to involvement in an immune event. Iwase and coworkers[94] reported on a 6-year-old child who first developed a dendritic corneal ulcer and iritis due to herpes simplex virus type 1, followed by a drop in vision due to a retinal periphlebitis and vitreal inflammatory reaction that responded to aciclovir therapy. Herpes zoster has been implicated in several cases. Retinal vasculitis has been reported in association with chickenpox.[95,96] Yet another patient had a unilateral retinal varicella zoster retinitis with no systemic symptomology, proven by PCR performed on the aqueous. The patient was treated with antiviral

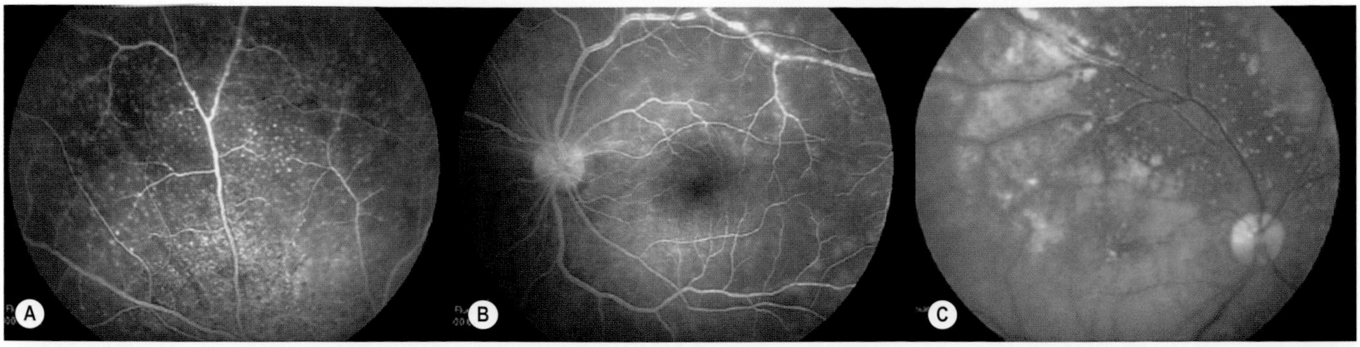

Figure 27-11. A very rare instance of retinal vasculitis and retinal infiltrates associated with HTLV-1 systemic disease. **A,** Punctate hyperfluorescent subretinal infiltrates along with a retinal periphlebitis. **B,** Subretinal infiltrates and superior temporal periphlebitis. **C,** Fundus photograph showing subretinal infiltrates with periphlebitis and macular edema. *(Reproduced with permission from Merle, H, et al. Retinal vasculitis caused by adult T-cell leukemia/lymphoma. Jpn J Ophthalmol 2005;49(1): 41–45.)*

therapy.[97] Retinal vasculitis has been noted in a patient with chronic hepatitis C infection.[98]

Other viral entities that can present with a retinal vasculitis include Rift Valley fever, dengue, West Nile disease and HTVL-1[2] (**Fig. 27-11**). Dengue has been reported by observers in Southeast Asia. In a report by Chan et al.[99] from Singapore, 12 of 13 patients with dengue had central visual impairment, which seemed to coincide with the nadir of the patients' thrombocytopenia. All recovered vision to 20/30 or better. In a case report, a patient who suffered from a C4 deficiency that predisposes to autoimmune disorders presented with a retinal vasculitis and a macular detachment.[100] In addition, West Nile virus can present with an ischemic and hemorrhagic retinal vasculitis.[101,102] In a review of the disease in North America, Chan[103] described that of 14 eyes, 86% had multifocal chorioretinal changes, 43% a vitritis, and 29% sheathing and vasculitis.

Multiple sclerosis

It has been suggested that 9–23% of multiple sclerosis patients will have a perpheral uveitis and retinitis.[104] Although these numbers seem high it is clear that it does happen. Friedman[105] reported a case where the retinal vasculitis was the initial finding in a case of multiple scleritis.

Tuberculosis

Central retinal artery vasculitis leading to occlusion[106] (see Chapter 9) has been noted. A recent study from India of 360 uveitis patients with a positive PPD were found to have fewer recurrences (16% vs 47%) when their steroid treatment was combined with four-drug antitubercular therapy.[107]

Rheumatoid arthritis

In a report by Giordano and colleagues,[108] 11 of 60 patients (18.3%) with rheumatoid arthritis had fluorescein angiographic evidence of retinal vasculitis. Matsuo and coworkers[109] reported the case of a 37-year-old woman who developed choroiditis and retinal vasculitis while receiving low-dose steroid therapy for her rheumatoid arthritis.

Kikuchi–Fujimoto disease

This necrotizing lymphadenitis is usually self-limiting. Zou and colleagues[110] reported a case with bilateral occlusive retinal vasculitis which developed neovascularization. The patient was treated with methotrexate and prednisone.

Susac syndrome

This syndrome is characterized by a microangiopathy of the brain, retina and cochlea. It affects mostly young women. In one recently reported case[111] there were focal nonperfused retinal arterioles with staining of the vessel walls, but no intraocular inflammation was reported. The patient was treated with cyclosphosphamide and improved retinal perfusion was seen.

Sweet syndrome

Acute febrile neutrophilic dermatosis, or Sweet syndrome, is a skin disorder characterized by reddish papules and nodules along with fever, circulating neutrophilia, and neutrophils infiltrating into the dermis.[112] Systemic corticosteroids are used to treat the disorder. Anterior segment problems, such as scleritis, glaucoma, and keratitis, have been reported, as has been choroiditis. It has been associated with Crohn's disease and malignancies. It has been estimated that about a quarter of these patients will have ocular complications.[113] In addition, a bilateral retinal vasculitis has been described with this syndrome which was treated with prednisone, colchicine, and diaphenylsulfone.[114]

Tattoo- and drug-induced vasculitis

Moschos et al.[115] reported the case of a 21-year-old man who, after having mulitple tattoos placed, developed retinal vasculitis and macular edema. He was aggressively treated with immunosuppressive therapy. Another patient was reported to develop retinal vasculitis after trimethoprin sulfamethoxazole-induced urticaria.[116] The disease, however, manifested 2 years after the cutaneous problem began. It is possible to theorize that both tattooing and a severe enough cutaneous inflammatory reacton released skin antigens (perhaps melanin like) that are shared with the eye.

In summary, this group of disorders that primarily affect the retinal vasculature frequently presents great challenges to treating physicians. It is remarkable how many disorders can manifest as a retinal vasculitis.[117,118] We are learning more about the underlying immune mechanisms of this group of diseases. Whereas immune complexes have traditionally been hailed as the underlying cause, we are now seeing alternative hypotheses. One example is the possible role of effector T cells and their ability to activate endothelial cells leading to effector cell homing, whereas Müller cells may be attempting to modulate this response.[119] Wallace and coworkers[120] have reported a CX3CR1 genotype association (particularly the I249/M280 haplotype) in retinal vasculitis patients in the United Kingdom. These variants may be implicated in leukocyte migration and neuronal protection. We are beginning to learn more of the kinds of inflammatory cell product that are elevated in retinal vasculitis.

Wallace et al. reported that macrophage inflammatory protein (MIP) 1α and 1β were elevated in the sera of retinal vasculitis patients. Lee et al.[121] reported that IFN-β was elevated in the sera of 47% of retinal vasculitis patients tested and stayed elevated for 6–12 months; E-Selectin (an adhesion molecule) was also elevated.

The potential workup for these patients can be very long[122,123] (**Boxes 27-3–27-5**). For well-defined disorders such as Behçet's disease aggressive therapy is imperative, with various options for immunosuppression available. There

---

Box 27-3 Laboratory tests (From Abu El-Asrar AM, Herbort CP, Tabbara KF. Retinal vasculitis. Ocul Immunol Inflamm 2005; 13(6): 415–33.)

- Complete blood count with differential
- Erythrocyte sedimentation rate
- C-reactive protein
- Serum chemistry panel with tests for renal and liver functions
- Blood sugar
- Urinalysis
- Venereal Disease Research Laboratory (VDRL) test, fluorescent treponemal antibody absorption (FTA-ABS) test
- Tuberculin skin testing
- Toxoplasmosis serology
- Lyme disease serology
- Cat-scratch disease serology
- Human immunodeficiency virus, human T-cell lymphoma virus type 1, cytomegalovirus, herpes simplex virus, varicella zoster virus, hepatitis virus, and West Nile virus serology
- Polymerase chain reaction to identify pathogens in ocular specimens
- Serum angiotensin-converting enzyme
- Rheumatoid factor
- Antinuclear antibody

- Anti-DNA
- Antineutrophil cytoplasmic antibody
- Antiphospholipid antibodies (lupus anticoagulants and anticardiolipin antibodies)
- Serum complement, CH50, AH50
- Extractable nuclear antigen
- Serum protein electrophoresis
- Serum cryoglobulins
- Human leukocyte antigen testing
- Vitreous biopsy
- Cerebrospinal fluid cytology and cell count Imaging
- Fluorescein angiography
- Optical coherence tomography
- Ultrasonography
- Chest X-ray
- CT scanning
- Magnetic resonance imaging
- Gallium scan
- Sacroiliac X-ray

Box 27-4 Disorders associated with retinal vasculitis

Infectious disorders

- Bacterial disorders (tuberculosis, syphilis, Lyme disease, Whipple's disease, brucellosis, cat-scratch disease, endophthalmitis)
- Viral disorders (human T-cell lymphoma virus type 1, cytomegalovirus, herpes simplex virus, varicella zoster virus, Rift Valley fever virus, hepatitis, acquired immunodeficiency syndrome, West Nile virus infection)

Parasitic disorders (toxoplasmosis)

- Rickettsial disorders (Mediterranean spotted fever)

Neurologic disorders

- Multiple sclerosis
- Microangiopathy of the brain, retina, and cochlea (Susac syndrome)

Malignancy

- Paraneoplastic syndromes
- Ocular lymphoma
- Acute leukemia

Systemic inflammatory disease

- Behçet's disease
- Sarcoidosis

- Systemic lupus erythematosus
- Wegener's granulomatosis
- Polyarteritis nodosa
- Churg–Strauss syndrome
- Relapsing polychondritis
- Sjögren's A antigen
- Rheumatoid arthritis
- HLA-B27-associated uveitis
- Crohn's disease
- Post vaccination
- Dermatomyositis
- Takayasu's disease
- Buerger's disease
- Polymyositis

Ocular disorders

- Frosted branch angiitis
- Idiopathic retinal vasculitis, aneurysms, and neuroretinitis
- Acute multifocal hemorrhagic retinal vasculitis
- Idiopathic recurrent branch retinal arterial occlusion
- Pars planitis
- Birdshot retinochoroidopathy

Box 27-5 Diagnostic studies performed on patients with retinal vasculitis

Laboratory tests

- Complete blood count with differential
- Erythrocyte sedimentation rate
- C-reactive protein
- Serum chemistry panel with tests for renal and liver functions
- Blood sugar
- Urinalysis
- Venereal Disease Research Laboratory (VDRL) test, fluorescent treponemal antibody absorption (FTA-ABS) test
- Tuberculin skin testing
- Toxoplasmosis serology
- Lyme disease serology
- Cat-scratch disease serology
- Human immunodeficiency virus, human T- cell lymphoma virus type 1, cytomegalovirus, herpes simplex virus, varicella zoster virus, hepatitis virus, and West Nile virus serology
- Polymerase chain reaction to identify pathogens in ocular specimens
- Serum angiotensin-converting enzyme
- Rheumatoid factor
- Antinuclear antibody
- Anti-DNA

- Antineutrophil cytoplasmic antibody
- Antiphospholipid antibodies (lupus anticoagulants and anticardiolipin antibodies)
- Serum complement, CH50, AH50
- Extractable nuclear antigen
- Serum protein electrophoresis
- Serum cryoglobulins
- Human leukocyte antigen testing
- Vitreous biopsy
- Cerebrospinal fluid cytology and cell count

Imaging

- Fluorescein angiography
- Optical coherence tomography
- Ultrasonography
- Chest X-ray
- CT scanning
- Magnetic resonance imaging
- Gallium scan
- Sacroiliac X-ray

The diagnostic workup should be tailored according to the patient's medical history, review of systems, and physical examination.

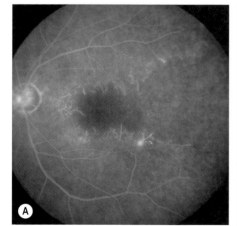 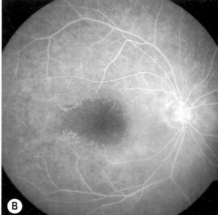 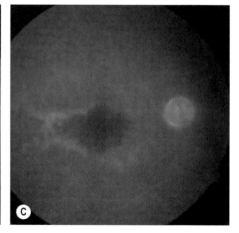

Figure 27-12. **A and B,** Fluorescein angiogram of the eyes of a middle-aged patient of Scandinavian background who had moderate intermediate uveitis associated early on with macular edema. The fundus examination was never striking and one needed to look carefully to perceive retinal vascular changes. However, the fluorescein angiogram shows striking symmetric loss of retinal vasculature which extended into the periphery. **C,** The edges of the areas of loss hyperfluoresced and then would appear to be pruned by the next time angiography was performed. No systemic disease was ever found over the course of many years.

have been several references to the use of steroids in this chapter. Howe and colleagues[124] reported on the effectiveness of steroid therapy for retinal vasculitis. Of their patients, 29 were given ≥1 mg/kg of prednisolone, and therapy was maintained at a dose of ≥40 mg for at least 5 weeks. Of these 29 patients, 60% had an increase in visual acuity with therapy, and this number increased to 77% when other agents were added to the regimen in eight additional patients. Stanford and Verity[125] also spoke of patients with ischemic retinal vasculitis who did not do well with steroid therapy.

However, some cases of retinal vascular disease may be quite severe but are neither associated with a systemic disorder nor well-characterized in the literature. Such an example is seen in **Figure 27-12**, a patient with intermediate uveitis and severe retinal vascular disease. Not only is the

natural history of severe retinal vascular disease unknown, but frequently it is also not associated with impressive inflammatory disease (**Figs 27-13 and 27-14**). The therapeutic approach to these patients is problematic and often compounded by the presence of neovascularization. Panretinal photocoagulation (PRP) may have a beneficial effect on the course of retinal vascular disease such as IRVAN. Indeed, this therapy has seemed to be the only modality that has stabilized some severe occurrences of retinal vasculitis. The use of anti-VEGF therapies opens up a new avenue for treatment of these patients. It should be added that we have seen severe inflammatory episodes apparently provoked by PRP. However, even with that risk, it may still be the indicated approach – clearly if there is evidence of capillary dropout on the angiogram, but perhaps even if there is not.

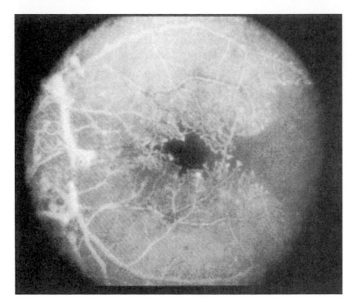

Figure 27-13. Fluorescein angiogram of the left eye in a 16-year-old girl with decreased vision who suffered from recurrent vitreous hemorrhages. Extensive work-up failed to demonstrate any systemic disorder. High-dose oral prednisone was not successful in preventing progression of the disorder.

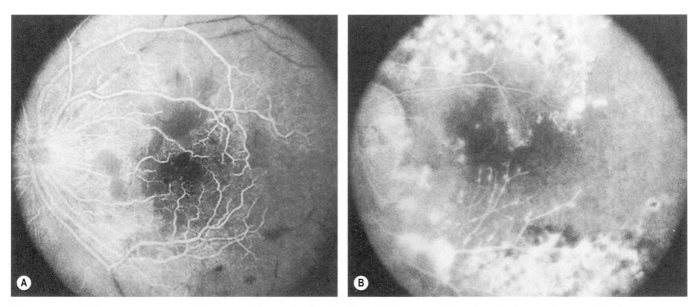

Figure 27-14. A, Fluorescein angiogram of a 46-year-old man who developed poor vision associated initially with a low-grade intraocular inflammatory response. Extensive systemic evaluation revealed no abnormalities. Note the extensive capillary loss involving a significant portion of the posterior pole, as well as nonperfusion of larger vessels. Aggressive immunosuppression to the point of toxicity was initiated with no therapeutic effect. **B,** Angiogram obtained 9 months later shows further loss of retinal vasculature. Areas of circular hyperfluorescence are from panretinal photocoagulation, which had been recently initiated, resulting in some stabilization of the disorder. However, with such extensive loss already, long-term visual prospects are most guarded.

References

1. Abu el-Asrar AM, Tabbara KF. Retinal vasculitis. Curr Opin Ophthalmol 1997; 8(3): 68–79.
2. Merle H, Donnio A, Gonin C, et al. Retinal vasculitis caused by adult T-cell leukemia/lymphoma. Jpn J Ophthalmol 2005; 49(1): 41–45.
3. George RK, Walton RC, Whitcup SM, et al. Primary retinal vasculitis. Systemic associations and diagnostic evaluation. Ophthalmology 1996; 103: 384–389.
4. Lueck C, Pires M, McCartney AC, et al. Ocular and neurological Behçet's disease without orogenital ulceration? J Neurol Neurosurg Psychiatry 1993; 56: 505–508.
5. Eales H. Cases of retinal hemorrhage associated with epistaxis and constipation. Birmingham Med Rev 1880; 9: 262–273.
6. Ashton N. Pathogenesis and aetiology of Eales's disease. In: 19th Internatinal Congress of Ophthalmology. 1962. Bombay: Times of India Press.
7. Moura R, Orefice F. Retinal vasculitis. In: Orefice F, Belfort RJ, eds. Uveites, 1987; Roca: São Paulo. 315–319.
8. Biswas J, Therese L, Madhavan HN. Use of polymerase chain reaction in detection of *Mycobacterium tuberculosis* complex DNA from vitreous sample of Eales' disease. Br J Ophthalmol 1999; 83: 994–997.
9. Madhavan HN, Therese KL, Gunisha P, et al. Polymerase chain reaction for detection of *Mycobacterium tuberculosis* in epiretinal membrane in Eales'

disease. Invest Ophthalmol Vis Sci 2000; 41: 822–825.

10. Therese KL, Deepa P, Therese J, et al. Association of mycobacteria with Eales' disease. Indian J Med Res 2007; 126(1): 56–62.

11. Das T, Biswas J, Kumar A, et al. Eales' Disease. Indian J Ophthalmol 1994; 42: 3–18.

12. Wise G, Dollery C, Henkind P. The Retinal Circulation. 1971, New York: Harper and Row.

13. Biswas J, Raghavendran R, Pinakin G, et al. Presumed Eales' disease with neurologic involvement. Report of three cases. Retina 2001; 21: 141–145.

14. Elliot A. Recurrent intraocular hemorrhage in young adults (Eales' disease). Trans Amer Ophthalmol Soc 1954; 52: 811.

15. Murugeswari P, Shukla D, Rajendran A, et al. Proinflammatory cytokines and angiogenic and anti-angiogenic factors in vitreous of patients with proliferative diabetic retinopathy and Eales' disease. Retina 2008; 28(6): 817–824.

16. Muthukkaruppan V, Rengarajan K, Chakkalath HR, et al. Immunological status of patients of Eales' disease. Indian J Med Res 1989; 90: 351–359.

17. Rennie W, Murphy RP, Anderson KC, et al. The evaluation of patients with Eales' disease. Retina 1983; 3: 243–247.

18. Dehghan MH, Ahmadieh H, Soheilian M, et al. Therapeutic effects of laser photocoagulation and/or vitrectomy in Eales' disease. Eur J Ophthalmol 2005; 15(3): 379–383.

19. Bali T, Saxena S, Kumar D, et al. Response time and safety profile of pulsed oral methotrexate therapy in idiopathic retinal periphlebitis. Eur J Ophthalmol 2005; 15(3): 374–378.

20. Ishaq M, Feroze AH, Shahid M, et al. Intravitreal steroids may facilitate treatment of Eales' disease (idiopathic retinal vasculitis): an interventional case series. Eye 2007; 21(11): 1403–1405.

21. Agrawal S, Agrawal J, Agrawal TP. Intravitreal triamcinolone acetonide in Eales' disease. Retina 2006; 26(2): 227–229.

22. Akova YA, Jabbur NS, Foster CS. Ocular presentation of polyarteritis nodosa. Clinical course and management with steroid and cytotoxic therapy. Ophthalmology 1993; 100(12): 1775–1781.

23. Kumar A, Sinha S. Intravitreal bevacizumab (Avastin) treatment of diffuse diabetic macular edema in an Indian population. Indian J Ophthalmol 2007; 55(6): 451–455.

24. Karel I, Peleska M, Divisova G. Fluorescence angiography in retinal vasculitis in children's uveitis. Ophthalmologica 1973; 166: 251–264.

25. Kincaid J, Schatz H. Bilateral retinal arteritis with multiple aneurysmal dilations. Retina 1983; 3: 171–178.

26. Yeshurun I, Recillas-Gispert C, Navarro-Lopez P, et al. Extensive dynamics in location, shape, and size of aneurysms in a patient with idiopathic retinal vasculitis, aneurysms, and neuroretinitis (IRVAN) syndrome. Idiopathic retinal vasculitis, aneurysms, and neuroretinitis. Am J Ophthalmol 2003; 135(1): 118–120.

27. Sashihara H, Hayashi H, Oshima K. Regression of retinal arterial aneurysms in a case of idiopathic retinal vasculitis, aneurysms, and neuroretinitis (IRVAN). Retina 1999; 19(3): 250–251.

28. Ishikawa F, Ohguro H, Sato S, et al. A case of idiopathic retinal vasculitis, aneurysm, and neuroretinitis effectively treated by steroid pulse therapy. Jpn J Ophthalmol 2006; 50(2): 181–185.

29. Jampol L, Isenberg S, Goldberg M. Occlusive retinal arteriolitis with neovascularization. Am J Ophthalmol 1978; 81: 583–589.

30. McDonald HR. Diagnostics and therapeutic challenges. IRVAN syndrome. Retina 2003; 23(3): 392–399.

31. Venkatesh P, Verghese M, Davde M, et al. Primary vascular occlusion in IRVAN (idiopathic retinal vasculitis, aneurysms, neuroretinitis) syndrome. Ocul Immunol Inflamm 2006; 14(3): 195–196.

32. Abu El-Asrar AM, Jestaneiah S, Al-Serhani AM. Regression of aneurysmal dilatations in a case of idiopathic retinal vasculitis, aneurysms and neuroretinitis (IRVAN) associated with allergic fungal sinusitis. Eye 2004; 18(2): 197–199; discussion 199–201.

33. Tomita M, Matsubara T, Yamada H, et al. Long term follow up in a case of successfully treated idiopathic retinal vasculitis, aneurysms, and neuroretinitis (IRVAN). Br J Ophthalmol 2004; 88(2): 302–303.

34. Samuel MA, Equi RA, Chang TS, et al. Idiopathic retinitis, vasculitis, aneurysms, and neuroretinitis (IRVAN): new observations and a proposed staging system. Ophthalmology 2007; 114(8): 1526–1529 e1.

35. Walker S, Iguchi A, Jones NP. Frosted branch angiitis: a review. Eye 2004; 18(5): 527–533.

36. Ito Y, Nakano M, Kyu N et al. Frosted branch angiitis in a child. Jpn J clin Ophthalmol 1976; 30: 797–803.

37. Liu Y, Ma Z, Tso MO, et al. Frosted branch angiitis secondary to macular choroidal neovascularization in a Chinese woman. Jpn J Ophthalmol 2005; 49(3): 228–230.

38. Oh J, Huh K, Kim SW. Recurrent secondary frosted branch angiitis after toxoplasmosis vasculitis. Acta Ophthalmol Scand 2005; 83(1): 115–117.

39. Díaz-Valle D, Díaz-Rodríguez E, Díaz-Valle T, et al. Frosted branch angiitis and late peripheral retinochoroidal scar in a patient with acquired toxoplasmosis. Eur J Ophthalmol 2003; 13(8): 726–728.

40. Jo T, Mizota A, Hatano N, et al. Frosted branch angiitis-like fundus following presumed influenza virus type A infection. Jpn J Ophthalmol 2006; 50(6): 563–564.

41. Taban M, Sears JE, Crouch E, et al. Acute idiopathic frosted branch angiitis. J AAPOS 2007; 11(3): 286–287.

42. Fine HF, Smith JA, Murante BL, et al. Frosted branch angiitis in a child with HIV infection. Am J Ophthalmol 2001; 131: 394–396.

43. Markomichelakis NN, Barampouti F, Zafirakis P, et al. Retinal vasculitis with a frosted branch angiitis-like response due to herpes simplex virus type 2. Retina 1999; 19(5): 455–457.

44. Johkura K, Hara A, Hattori T, et al. Frosted branch angiitis associated with aseptic meningitis. Eur J Neurol 2000; 7: 241.

45. Masuda K, Ueno M, Watanabe I. A case of frosted branch angiitis with yellowish-white placoid lesions: fluorescein and indocyanine green angiography findings. Jpn J Ophthalmol 1998; 42: 484–489.

46. Borkowski LM, Jampol LM. Frosted branch angiitis complicated by retinal neovascularization. Retina 1999; 19(5): 454–455.

47. Kleiner RC, Kaplan HJ, Shakin JL, et al. Acute frosted retinal periphlebitis. Am J Ophthalmol 1988; 106: 27–33.

48. Sykes SO, Horton JC. Steroid-responsive retinal vasculitis with a frosted branch appearance in Crohn's disease. Retina 1997; 17(5): 451–454.

49. Watson P. The nature and treatment of scleral inflammation. Trans Ophthalmol Soc UK 1982; 102: 257–281.

50. Watson P. Chapter 23: Diseases of the sclera and episclera. In: Duane T, Jaeger E, eds. Clinical Ophthalmology, 1987, Harper and Row: Philadelphia.

51. Benson W. Posterior scleritis. Surv Ophthalmol 1988; 32: 297–316.

52. Rucker C. Sheathing of the retinal veins in multiple sclerosis. JAMA 1945; 127: 970–973.

53. Breger B, Leopold I. The incidence of uveitis in multiple sclerosis. Am J Ophthalmol 1966; 62: 540–545.

54. Hellman D, Laing TJ, Petri M, et al. Mononeuritis multiplex: The yield of evaluations for occult rheumatic diseases. Medicine 1988; 67: 145–153.

55. Hellmann D. Mononeuritis Multiplex. In: Klippel J, Dieppe P, eds. Rheumatology, 1991, Mosby-Yearbook-Europe Limited: London. p. 6.26.2–6.26.5.

56. Bandyopadhyay SK, Moulick A, Dutta A. Retinal vasculitis – an initial presentation of systemic lupus erythematosus. J Indian Med Assoc 2006; 104(9): 526–527.

57. Nag TC, Wadhwa S. Histopathological changes in the eyes in systemic lupus erythematosus: an electron microscope and immunohistochemical study. Histol Histopathol 2005; 20(2): 373–382.

58. Nag TC, Wadhwa S. Vascular changes of the retina and choroid in systemic lupus erythematosus: pathology and pathogenesis. Curr Neurovasc Res 2006; 3(2): 159–168.

59. Jabs D, Fine SL, Hochberg MC, et al. Severe retinal vaso-occlusive disease in systemic lupus erythematosus. Arch Ophthalmol 1986; 104: 558–563.

60. Au A, O'Day J. Review of severe vaso-occlusive retinopathy in systemic lupus erythematosus and the antiphospholipid syndrome: associations, visual outcomes, complications and treatment. Clin Exp Ophthalmol 2004; 32(1): 87–100.

61. Vine A, Barr C. Proliferative lupus retinopathy. Arch Ophthalmol 1984; 102: 852–854.

62. Read RW. Clinical mini-review: systemic lupus erythematosus and the eye. Ocul Immunol Inflamm 2004; 12(2): 87–99.

63. Papadaki TG, Zacharopoulos IP, Papaliodis G, et al. Plasmapheresis for lupus retinal vasculitis. Arch Ophthalmol 2006; 124(11): 1654–1656.

64. Curi AL, Freeman G, Pavesio C. Aggressive retinal vasculitis in polyarteritis nodosa. Eye 2001; 15(Pt 2): 229–231.

65. Morgan D, Foster C, Gragoudas E. Retinal vasculitis in polyarteritis nodosa. Retina 1986; 6: 205–209.

66. Emad Y, Basaffar S, Ragab Y, et al. A case of polyarteritis nodosa complicated by left central retinal artery occlusion, ischemic optic neuropathy, and retinal vasculitis. Clin Rheumatol 2007; 26(5): 814–816.

67. Stillermen M. Ocular manifestations of diffuse collagen disease. Arch Ophthalmol 1951; 45: 239–250.

68. Leib ES, Restivo C, Paulus HE. Immunosuppressive and corticosteroid therapy of polyarteritis nodosa. Am J Med 1979; 67(6): 941–947.

69. Fauci A, Haynes BF, Katz P, et al. Wegener's granulomatosis: Prospective clinical and therapeutic experience with 85 patients for 21 years. Ann Intern Med 1983; 98: 76–85.

70. Mangouritsas G, Ulbig M. Cotton-wool spots as the initial ocular manifestation in Wegener's granulomatosis. German J Ophthalmol 1994; 3: 68–70.

71. Pakrou N, Selva D, Leibovitch I. Wegener's granulomatosis: ophthalmic manifestations and management. Semin Arthritis Rheum 2006; 35(5): 284–292.

72. Soukasian S, Foster CS, Niles JL, et al. Diagnostic value of anti-neutrophil cytoplasmic antibodies in scleritis associated with Wegener's granulomatosis. Ophthalmology 1992; 99: 125–132.

73. Nolle B, Specks U, Ludemann J, et al. Ann Intern Med 1989; 111: 28–40.

74. Cohen Tervaert J, van der Woude FJ, Fauci AS, et al. Association between active Wegener's granulomatosis and anticytoplasmic antibodies. Arch Intern Med 1989; 149: 2461–2465.

75. Gallagher MJ, Ooi KG, Thomas M, et al. ANCA associated pauci-immune retinal vasculitis. Br J Ophthalmol 2005; 89(5): 608–611.

76. Young D. The antineutrophil antibody in uveitis. Br J Ophthalmol 1991; 75: 208–211.

77. Whipple GH. A hitherto undescribed disease characterized anatomically by deposits of fat and fatty acids in the intestinal and mesenteric lymphatic tissues. Johns Hopkins Hosp Bull 1907; 18: 382–391.

78. Jones FA, Paulley JW. Intestinal lipodystrophy. Lancet 1949; 1: 214–216.

79. Rickman LS, Freeman WR, Green WR, et al. Brief report: uveitis caused by *Tropheryma whipplei* (Whipple's bacillus). N Engl J Med 1995; 332: 363–366.

80. Avila M, Jalkh AE, Feldman E, et al. Manifestations of Whipple's disease in the posterior segment of the eye. Arch Ophthalmol 1984; 102: 384–390.

81. Nishimura JK, Cook BE, Pach JM. Whipple disease presenting as posterior uveitis without prominent gastrointestinal symptoms. Am J Ophthalmol 1998; 126: 130–132.

82. Bodaghi B, Dauga C, Cassoux N, et al. Whipple's syndrome (uveitis, B27-negative spondylarthropathy, meningitis, and lymphadenopathy) associated with *Arthrobacter* sp. infection. Ophthalmology 1998; 105: 1891–1896.

83. Lo Monaco A, Govoni M, Zelante A, et al. Whipple disease: unusual presentation of a protean and sometimes confusing disease. Semin Arthritis Rheum 2008; 38: 403–406.

84. Chan RY, Yannuzzi LA, Foster CS. Ocular Whipple's disease. Ophthalmology 2001; 108: 2225–2231.

85. Duker J, Brown G, Brooks L, Retinal vasculitis in Crohn's disease. Am J Ophthalmol 1987; 103: 664–668.

86. Garcia-Diaz M, Mira M, Nevado L, et al. Retinal vasculitis associated with Crohn's disease. Postgrad Med J 1995; 71(833): 170–172.

87. Saatci OA, Koçak N, Durak I, et al. Unilateral retinal vasculitis, branch retinal artery occlusion and subsequent retinal neovascularization in Crohn's disease. Int Ophthalmol 2001; 24(2): 89–92.

88. Ruby A, Jampol L. Crohn's disease and retinal vascular disease. Am J Ophthalmol 1990; 110: 349–353.

89. Felekis T, Katsanos K, Kitsanou M, et al. Spectrum and frequency of ophthalmologic manifestations in patients with inflammatory bowel disease: A prospective single-center study. Inflamm Bowel Dis 2008.

90. Farmer S, Kinyoun JL, Nelson JL, et al. Retinal vasculitis associated with autoantibodies to Sjögren's syndrome A antigen. Am J Ophthalmol 1985; 100: 814–821.

91. Green W, Chan CC, Hutchins GM, et al. Central retinal vein occlusion: a prospective histopathologic study of 29 eyes in 28 cases. Trans Am Soc Ophthalmol 1981; 79: 371–422.

92. Issak B, Liesegang T, Michet C. Ocular and systemic findings in relapsing polychondritis. Ophthalmology 1986; 93: 681–689.

93. Matas B. Iridocyclitis associated with relapsing polychondritis. Arch Ophthalmol 1970; 84: 474–476.

94. Iwase K, Murao M, et al. A case of dendritic corneal ulcer associated with retinal periphlebitis and uveitis. A new diagnostic method and treatment. Rinsho Ganka 1986; 40: 403–407.

95. Kuo Y-H, Yip Y, Chen S-N. Retinal vasculitis associated with chickenpox. Am J Ophthalmol 2001; 132: 584–585.

96. Wolf AH, Thurau SR, Kook D, et al. Ocular manifestation of primary VZV infection in a splenectomized patient. Ocul Immunol Inflamm 2008; 16(4): 199–201.

97. Wimmersberger Y, Gervaix A, Baglivo E. VZV retinal vasculitis without systemic infection: diagnosis and monitoring with quantitative polymerase chain reaction. Int Ophthalmol 2008.

98. Perez-Alvarez AF, Jiménez-Alonso J, Reche-Molina I, et al. Retinal vasculitis and vitritis in a patient with chronic hepatitis C virus. Arch Intern Med 2001.

99. Chan DP, Teoh SC, Tan CS, et al. Ophthalmic complications of dengue. Emerg Infect Dis 2006; 12(2): 285–289.

100. Chang PE, Cheng CL, Asok K, et al. Visual disturbances in dengue fever: an answer at last? Singapore Med J 2007; 48(3): e71–73.

101. Garg S, Jampol LM, Wilson JF, et al. Ischemic and hemorrhagic retinal vasculitis associated with West Nile virus infection. Retina 2006; 26(3): 365–367.

102. Garg S, Jampol LM. Systemic and intraocular manifestations of West Nile virus infection. Surv Ophthalmol 2005; 50(1): 3–13.

103. Chan CK, Limstrom SA, Tarasewicz DG, et al. Ocular features of West Nile virus infection in North America: a study of 14 eyes. Ophthalmology 2006; 113(9): 1539–1546.

104. Engell T, Anderson PK. The frequency of periphlebitis in multiple sclerosis. Acta Neurol Scand 1982; 65: 601–608.

105. Friedman SM. Retinal vasculitis as the initial presentation of multiple sclerosis. Retina 2005; 25(2): 218–219.

106. Fountain J, Werner R. Tuberculous retinal vasculitis. Retina 1984; 4: 48–50.

107. Bansal R, Gupta A, Gupta V, et al. Role of anti-tubercular therapy in uveitis with latent/manifest tuberculosis. Am J Ophthalmol 2008; 146: 772–792

108. Giordano N, D'Ettorre M, Biasi G, et al. Retinal vasculitis in rheumatoid arthritis: an angiographic study. Clin Exp Rheumatol 1990; 8: 121–125.

109. Matsuo T, Masuda I, Matsuo N. Geographic choroiditis and retinal vasculitis in rheumatoid arthritis. Jpn J Ophthalmol 1998; 42(1): 51–55.

110. Zou W, Wen F. Bilateral occlusive retinal vasculitis in Kikuchi–Fujimoto disease. Clin Exp Ophthalmol 2007; 35(9): 875–877.

111. Martinet N, Fardeau C, Adam R, et al. Fluorescein and indocyanine green angiographies in Susac syndrome. Retina 2007; 27(9): 1238–1242.

112. Gottlieb CC, Mishra A, Belliveau D, et al. Ocular involvement in acute febrile neutrophilic dermatosis (Sweet syndrome): new cases and review of the literature. Surv Ophthalmol 2008; 53(3): 219–226.

113. Fett DL, Gibson LE, Su WP. Sweet's syndrome: systemic signs and symptoms and associated disorders. Mayo Clin Proc 1995; 70(3): 234–240.

114. Sato M, Kawamura T, Hase S, et al. A case of bilateral retinal vasculitis associated with Sweet syndrome. Retina 2005; 25(6): 800–802.

115. Moschos MM, Guex-Crosier Y. Retinal vasculitis and cystoid macular edema after body tattooing: a case report. Klin Monatsbl Augenheilkd 2004; 221(5): 424–426.

116. Batioglu F, Taner P, Aydintuǧ OT, et al. Recurrent optic disc and retinal vasculitis in a patient with drug-induced urticarial vasculitis. Cutan Ocul Toxicol 2006; 25(4): 281–285.

117. Abu El-Asrar AM, Herbort CP, Tabbara KF. Retinal vasculitis. Ocul Immunol Inflamm 2005; 13(6): 415–433.

118. Herbort CP, Cimino L, Abu El Asrar AM. Ocular vasculitis: a multidisciplinary approach. Curr Opin Rheumatol 2005; 17(1): 25–33.

119. Hughes EH, Dick AD. The pathology and pathogenesis of retinal vasculitis. Neuropathol Appl Neurobiol 2003; 29(4): 325–340.

120. Wallace GR, Vaughan RW, Kondeatis E, et al. A CX3CR1 genotype associated with retinal vasculitis in patients in the United Kingdom. Invest Ophthalmol Vis Sci 2006; 47(7): 2966–2970.

121. Lee MT, Hooper LC, Kump L, et al. Interferon-beta and adhesion molecules (E-selectin and s-intracellular adhesion molecule-1) are detected in sera from patients with retinal vasculitis and are induced in retinal vascular endothelial cells by Toll-like receptor 3 signalling. Clin Exp Immunol 2007; 147(1): 71–80.

122. Levy-Clarke GA, Nussenblatt R. Retinal vasculitis. Int Ophthalmol Clin 2005; 45(2): 99–113.

123. Walton RC, Ashmore ED. Retinal vasculitis. Curr Opin Ophthalmol 2003; 14(6): 413–419.

124. Howe LJ, Stanford MR, Edelsten C, et al. The efficacy of systemic corticosteroids in sight-threatening retinal vasculitis. Eye 1994; 8(Pt 4): 443–447.

125. Stanford MR, Verity DH. Diagnostic and therapeutic approach to patients with retinal vasculitis. Int Ophthalmol Clin 2000; 40(2): 69–83.

Serpiginous Choroidopathy

Robert B. Nussenblatt

Key concepts

- Although the typical serpiginoid lesion, when present, is distinctive, one needs to be aware that other conditions can simulate the clinical appearance, including tuberculosis.
- Reactivation is typically at the borders of older lesions and will show blockage in the early phase of the angiogram.
- High-dose prednisone or other forms of aggressive therapy can be used to stop the reactivation.

Serpiginous choroidopathy is a clinically defined disorder characterized by destruction of the inner choroid and the retinal pigment epithelium (RPE) as well as secondary involvement of the retina. This entity has been known by a multitude of names, including serpiginous choroiditis, geographic choroiditis, geographic choroidopathy, geographic helicoid peripapillary choroidopathy, and macular geographic helicoid choroidopathy.[1–5] Although by the early part of the last century it had been recognized as a distinct but poorly defined entity,[6] our understanding of this disease remains limited. We still are not sure whether the retinal destruction seen in serpiginous choroidopathy is mediated predominantly by an inflammatory process or by an abiotrophy. In fact, the clinical spectrum of serpiginous choroidopathy may represent several different diseases. One notion is that it is an extreme form of the white-dot syndromes. Until we know more about these entities, the author prefers not to lump them together. In most uveitis clinics it is a fairly rare entity, comprising no more than 5% of posterior uveitis.[7]

Clinical features

The typical patient with serpiginous choroidopathy is middle-aged and has no major underlying medical problems. Although the disease has been reported in patients of varying ethnic backgrounds, it may be seen more commonly in white persons. In some series there is a slight male preponderance.[8]

Patients usually report blurred vision or a central or pericentral scotoma in one eye, although examination usually reveals bilateral disease. Serpiginous choroidopathy primarily affects the choroid, choriocapillaris, and RPE. The terms serpiginous, helicoid, and geographic describe the appearance of the chorioretinal disease, which progresses in a serpentine fashion, usually starting at the optic disc and winding through the posterior pole (**Fig. 28-1**). Acute lesions appear gray-white or yellow and involve the choriocapillaris and RPE. On careful examination these new lesions appear to have 'substance,' and they subtly elevate the overlying retina. Acute lesions last up to several months, but over time they become atrophic, with disappearance of the choriocapillaris and involvement of the underlying large choroidal vessels.[9] Thinning of the overlying neurosensory retina usually follows disease of the choroid and RPE, and scarring with clumps of RPE are common late in the course of the disease.

Patients rarely have a solitary active lesion involving the posterior pole. Much more commonly, active lesions occur adjacent to an area of choroidal and RPE atrophy. An area of chorioretinal atrophy often can be found next to the optic disc in a symptom-free contralateral eye.

Reports in the literature concerning the inflammatory component associated with the choroidal and RPE lesions of serpiginous choroidopathy vary greatly. Hamilton and Bird,[10] for example, observed no inflammatory disease in the patients they studied. In our experience, however, cellular reaction in the posterior vitreous can occur, especially in patients with acute lesions, and mild vitritis has been reported in about one-third of patients.[11,12] Anterior uveitis has also been described in patients with serpiginous choroidopathy, but is more rare.[13] It is important to look for evidence of inflammatory disease, because this finding may help in deciding whether a therapeutic intervention with antiinflammatory agents has a reasonable chance for success (see Chapter 7).

Choroidal neovascularization can also occur in serpiginous choroidopathy. Gass[11] stated that choroidal neovascularization occurs in as many as 25% of patients, although we have observed it in fewer than 10% of our patients at the National Eye Institute. Blumenkranz and coworkers[8] reported active choroidal neovascularization in seven of 53 patients with the disease. Choroidal neovascularization may be seen at the time the disease is diagnosed, and when located in the macula may cause a visual disturbance (**Fig. 28-2**). Although the choroidal neovascularization may regress spontaneously in some patients,[14] we have treated membranes threatening the fovea with laser photocoagulation. Serous detachments of the neurosensory retina, as well as RPE detachments, have been reported in patients with serpiginous choroidopathy.[13,15] Retinal vasculitis may also occur, and branch vein occlusions have been reported.[11,13]

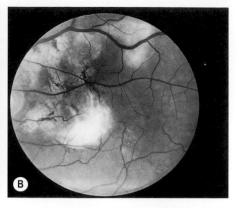

Figure 28-1. A, A large serpiginous lesion surrounding the optic disc. An active lesion is seen inferior to the disc. Older, atrophic regions can be seen both to right and left of the active lesion. Some choroidal vessels can be noted through the lesion. **B,** White active lesion, seen at the edge of an old atrophic area.

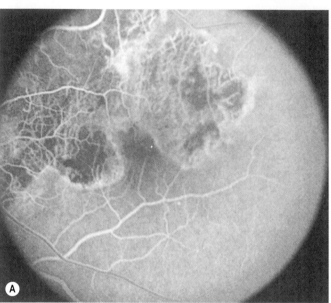

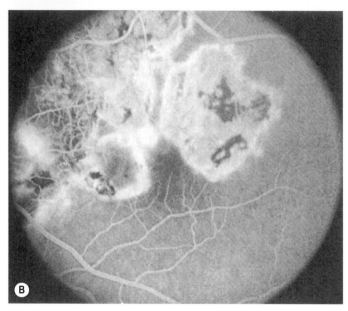

Figure 28-2. Fluorescein angiogram showing choroidal neovascular membrane in a patient with serpiginous choroidopathy. **A,** Early frame showing lacy hyperfluorescence. **B,** Late frame showing late leakage in the area of the choroidal neovascular membrane.

The disorder usually begins near the disc, with new areas of activity being evident at the margin of old lesions. This centripetal or helicoid extension can continue for years. Laatikainen and Erkkilä[16] followed 15 patients for a mean of 4.9 years and noted new lesions in eight. These acute lesions can cause a decrease in visual acuity that may return after a long recovery period. Weiss and coworkers[12] observed that visual acuity decreased in nine of 17 eyes after an acute episode, and that the visual acuity returned to the preattack level once the acute lesions resolved, although this could take a number of months. They further noted that 15 of 17 eyes ultimately developed lesions involving the fovea, although Laatikainen and Erkkilä[16] noted a loss of central vision in only six of 28 eyes.

The diagnosis of serpiginous choroidopathy is made purely on clinical grounds, with the major criteria listed in **Box 28-1**. Fluorescein angiography and serial fundus photographs are also helpful in following the disease. Fluorescein angiographic examination of an active lesion will show early blockage with late hyperfluorescent borders that spread toward the center of the lesion (**Fig. 28-3**). The early hypofluorescence of active lesions may be due to blockage of the underlying choroidal fluorescence by swollen RPE cells, but more likely represents the impaired choroidal vasculature.

Box 28-1 Findings supporting the diagnosis of serpiginous choroiditis

Patient

White
Both genders
Late teens to 60s

Ocular examination

Inflammatory response in the anterior chamber or vitreous sometimes occurs
Lesion begins in the peripapillary region; centripetal or helicoid progression, giving 'geographic' distribution
New white-yellow lesions begin at edge of old ones
Bilateral involvement

Additional tests

Fluorescein angiography
Serial fundus photographs

Old atrophic lesions will show diffuse staining, and hyperfluorescence is noted in areas of RPE clumping. Late staining of the retinal vessels is seen in patients with a vasculitis or perivasculitis. There have been several reports describing the

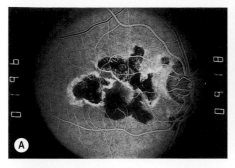 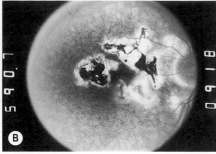

Figure 28-3. Fluorescein angiogram of serpiginous lesion showing (**A**) early phase of angiogram with central blockage and (**B**) late phase with more diffuse hyperfluorescence. Areas that continue to block fluorescence had overlying RPE clumping.

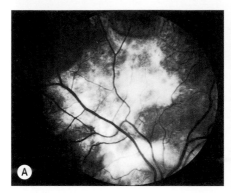 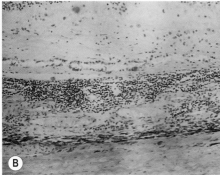

Figure 28-4. Clinical (**A**) and histologic (**B**) photographs of the eye of a young man with serpiginous choroiditis. Note marked lymphocytic infiltrate into choroid. *(Courtesy of JDM Gass, MD.)*

use of indocyanine green (ICG) angiography to evaluate this disorder. What seems to be a recurring theme is that although fluorescein angiography appears to be more effective for showing active and inactive lesions, ICG methodology usually demonstrates many more lesions than are seen with fluorescein. Therefore, the use of ICG methodology may help to better describe the extent of the disease, even before it is seen with fluorescein angiography. It can help the observer to determine the ultimate clinical progression of the disease.[17-21] Fundus autofluorescence can be used in addition to OCT[22] and ICG observations. In one study reported by Cardillo-Piccolino and colleagues,[23] autofluorescence, OCT and ICG were used to follow the course of disease in two patients with serpiginous choroiditis. They found that the fundus hyperautofluorescence was noted 2–5 days after the appearance of the clinical lesion, delineating what could be the area of real RPE damage, as this area was smaller than the defects seen on ICG. As the disorder became quiescent, these same areas showed hypoautofluorescence, whereas the OCT still demonstrated lesions in the photoreceptor region.

It is probably fair to say that the appearance of the lesions we recognize as serpignous choroiditis is not a single disease but also can be a manifestation of infectious processes. Although most patients with serpiginous choroidopathy have no associated medical illnesses and therefore are treated with immunosuppressive agents, it has become clear through several reports that a careful medical evaluation is critical to rule out an underlying infectious process.

Pathology

Unfortunately, few eyes with serpiginous choroidopathy have been studied in the pathology laboratory. Histologic examination shows an extensive loss of the RPE and destruc-

tion of the overlying retina. Portions of the choriocapillaris and part of the choroid are filled with a lymphocytic infiltrate, suggesting that the disease has an inflammatory component (**Fig. 28-4**).[11,24] Areas of RPE hypertrophy and subretinal scarring have also been described. An eye evaluated for the presence of virus (see below) showed a lymphocytic infiltration as in the previous case.[24] On the basis of these few observations it would seem reasonable to consider this lesion a choroiditis.

Etiology

The cause of serpiginous choroidopathy is unknown. It had been suggested that the disorder is the result of a vascular abiotrophy and should therefore be considered degenerative. Laatikainen and Erkkilä[16] indicated that an immune-mediated vasculitis might induce occlusion of the choroidal vessels. The finding of a lymphocytic infiltrate in the choroid and an accompanying vitritis suggests an inflammatory etiology. In one study the incidence of HLA-B7 was higher in 15 Finnish patients with serpiginous choroiditis than in the control group (54.5% versus 24.3%, $p < 0.05$).[25] In addition, increased levels of antibacterial antibodies, such as antistreptolysin O, were found in eight of the patients with serpiginous choroiditis. The clinical course of the disease, characterized by multiple recurrent inflammatory episodes, is compatible with an infectious disease process such as herpes virus infection. Serpiginous choroidopathy has been reported after viral meningitis, and some clinicians give anecdotal reports of improvement after treatment with aciclovir. Nevertheless, firm evidence to suggest an infectious cause is lacking. Indeed, in a report by Akpek and colleagues,[24] using the polymerase chain reaction (PCR), no evidence of herpes simplex virus (HSV) P1/P2 (for HSV-1, HSV-2, Epstein–Barr virus [EBV], cytomegalovirus [CMV] and human herpes virus [HHV]-8), and varicella-zoster virus (VZV) P1/P2 (for VZV, HHV-6, HHV-7) can be demonstrated in the infiltrating lymphocytes or the choroidal tissue. Theoretically it is possible that the the inflammatory disease may be a secondary phenomenon unrelated to previous infection that may have originally been directed against a viral antigen. Retinal degeneration after the impairment of the choroidal vasculature could release potentially antigenic moieties, which in genetically prone persons leads to an inflammatory response.

Differential diagnosis

A number of disorders should be considered in the differential diagnosis of serpiginous choroidopathy. Several authors have reported the association of serpiginous-like lesions associated with tuberculosis. Gupta and Gupta[26] reported seven patients in India with choroidal tuberculosis that presented as what clinically appeared to be serpiginous chorodi-tis. The clincial presentation included multifocal lesions that progressed to a wavelike confluence; others were plaque-like with an ameboid presentation. Teyssot and coworkers[27] emphasized the need to evaluate their French patients with all types of disorder at the level of the retinal pigment epithelium/choroid/choriocapillaris. In 14 patients with disorders at that level of the eye, six (including those with serpiginous choroidopathy) had a family history of tuberculosis or active infection. Recently Mackensen et al.[28] performed a retrospective evaluation of German patients with a serpiginous-like choroiditis. Eleven of the 21 patients tested for tuberculous exposure using the QuantiFERON test were positive. Many of these were known to have had positive Mantoux skin tests; 13% of other uveitis patients tested positive. All of this emphasizes how important a thorough evaluation is. Tuberculosis may also explain the relatively high percentage (19%) of serpiginous patients seen in a large uveitis center in India.[29] Other infectious processes have been reported to present with a serpiginous-like lesion as well. Such an example is a 32-year-old woman who presented with blurred vision in her left eye. The ocular examination revealed extensive serpiginoid lesions. Blood serology and PCR performed on aqueous from her eye were both positive for toxoplasmosis[30] (**Fig. 28-5**).

Noninfectious disorders may present with similar clinical findings to serpiginous choroiditis. Posterior scleritis may mimic a macular serpiginous lesion, though this is associated with pain[31] (**Fig. 28-6**). The bilateral lesions of acute posterior multifocal placoid pigment epitheliopathy (APMPPE) may appear similar to those of serpiginous choroidopathy. Acute lesions in both diseases may be yellowish and involve the choroid and retina at the level of the RPE, and RPE clumping can be seen late in the course of both diseases (**Fig. 28-7**). Acute lesions of both APMPPE and serpiginous choroidopathy show early blockage of fluorescence and late hyperfluorescence. However, the acute lesions of APMPPE resolve within 2 weeks, and recurrence is uncommon. In addition, choroidal atrophy and choroidal neovascularization are atypical in APMPPE but common in serpiginous choroidopathy, and the prognosis for good visual outcome is far better for patients with APMPPE. Nevertheless, we have seen a number of patients with a

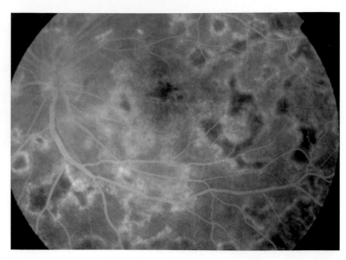

Figure 28-5. A case of toxoplasmosis that resembles serpiginous choroiditis. *(Reproduced with permission from Mahendradas, P., et al. Serpiginous choroiditis-like picture due to ocular toxoplasmosis. Ocul Immunol Inflamm. 2007;15(2): 127–130.)*

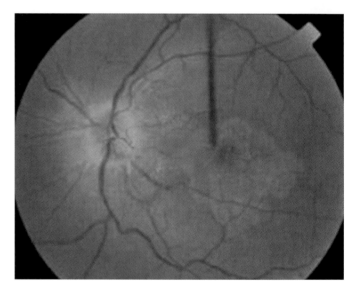

Figure 28-6 Posterior scleritis resembling macular serpiginous choroiditis. *(Reproduced with permission from Sonika, et al. Posterior scleritis mimicking macular serpiginous choroiditis. Indian J Ophthalmol 2003;51(4): 351–353.)*

disease that falls between the classic findings of serpiginous choroidopathy and those of APMPPE. We have informally termed this condition ampiginous choroidopathy because these patients have fundus lesions typical of those seen in APMPPE but develop recurrent disease more typical for the patient with serpiginous choroidopathy (Fig. 28-7).[32] They do, however, maintain relatively good central vision and do not have the relentless, helical progression characteristic of serpiginous choroidopathy. However, large portions of the retina may be involved. Jones and colleagues[33] described a condition similar to the one we have described with a prolonged progressive clinical course and widespread lesions. Perhaps a variant of ampiginous is what has been termed persistent placoid maculopathy,[34] which presents as a macular choroiditis (**Fig. 28-8**) and with many eyes developing choroidal neovascularization (this is described in the chapter on white-dot syndromes).

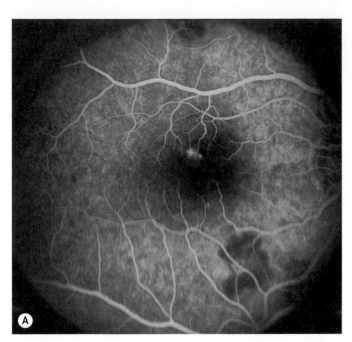 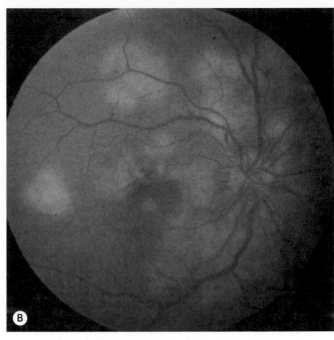

Figure 28-7. Case of ampiginous choroidopathy. This 32-year-old man began having vague visual complaints. **A,** Angiogram on presentation showed areas of blockage from the macula, but one small area of hyperfluorescence was seen in the posterior pole. He was thought to have AMPPE (see Chapter 29). About 2 weeks later he presented with new lesions and a drop in visual acuity (**B**). Lesions were numerous but still were thought to represent severe APMPPE. Because of poor vision he was given immunotherapy. Six months later (and after medication was stopped) he was seen again because of disease recurrence in his other eye (the appearance was very unlike that of APMPPE). An angiogram demonstrated very extensive changes in the choroid. Seven years later his vision was 20/40 + 2 in this eye.

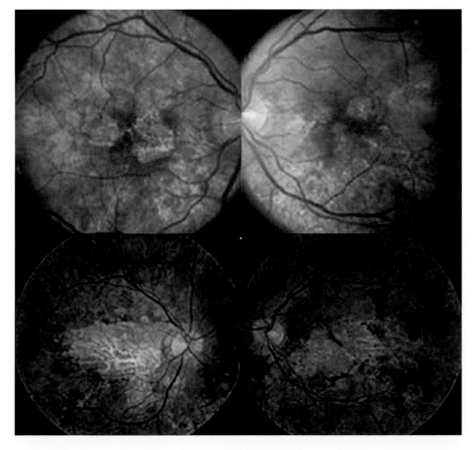

Figure 28-8. A case of posterior placoid chorioretinitis. The top photos were taken as the new lesions developed. Those below are the lesions after therapy and stabilization. Compare with ampiginous choroiditis fundus photo (Fig. 28-7). *(Reproduced with permission from Yeh, S., et al. Retentless placoid chorioretinitis associated with central nervous system lesions treated with mycophenolate mofetil. Arch Ophthalmol 2009;127(3): 941–943.)*

Diseases that cause peripapillary chorioretinal scarring can be confused with serpiginous choroidopathy. Age-related macular degeneration, angioid streaks, idiopathic choroidal neovascularization, toxoplasmosis as mentioned above, the presumed ocular histoplasmosis syndrome, and previous retinal laser photocoagulation are other entities to be considered in the evaluation of patients suspected of having serpiginous choroidopathy. Edelstein and associates[35] described an unusual case of ocular sarcoidosis with manifestations similar to those of serpiginous choroidopathy. An occurrence of systemic non-Hodgkin's lymphoma was reported to present with lesions suggestive of this entity as well.[36]

Therapy

In our experience, patients with a significant inflammatory response, manifested by vitritis and acute yellowish lesions, appear to have a beneficial response to corticosteroid therapy. We have observed improvement in visual acuity in patients treated with oral prednisone, but again these data are anecdotal. Nevertheless, it appears logical to treat eyes with serpiginous choroidopathy that have evidence of inflammatory disease with a trial of corticosteroids, as long as one predetermines the definition of a therapeutic response and the amount of time that therapy will be continued before this response is reached. We have also used ciclosporin in combination with corticosteroids to treat some patients with serpiginous choroidopathy,[37] whereas others did not find this combination useful.[38] However, Araujo and colleagues[39] found that ciclosporin, given at 3–5 mg/kg/day, seemed to be safe and effective for serpiginous choroidopathy, with remissions being seen in all but one of seven patients in their series. In addition, we have treated one patient – in whom an active lesion was threatening the fovea – with pulse intravenous methylprednisolone at a dose of 1 g/day for 3 days. Recently, Markomichelakis et al.[40] described their experience using pulse methyprednisolone in five patients, seeing a recognizable response within 10 days. We have not often seen cystoid macular edema in our patients with serpiginous choroidopathy, but periocular steroid injections can be considered. Intravitreal injections have been reported to have been used to treat this condition,[41] with one report suggesting that one injection was sufficient to control the active lesion.[42] Single injections seem a problematic solution for a chronic problem. Taking into account the long-term nature of the disease process, Seth and Gaudio[43] placed a fluorocinolone acetonide implant intravitreally, with reported control over 14 months. Other antiinflammatory drug regimens, including corticosteroids and cytotoxic agents, have been used but have never been evaluated in controlled clinical trials.[9] Hooper and Kaplan[44] used the combination of azathioprine (1.5 mg/kg of body weight/day), ciclosporin (5 mg/kg/day), and prednisone (1 mg/kg/day) to treat patients with serpiginous choroidopathy and observed a rapid remission of active disease in five of them. In two patients disease recurred immediately after discontinuation of low-dose therapy, but was arrested when therapy was resumed. Vonmoos and associates[45] reported a good result using triple therapy in one patient. Vianna and colleagues reported that azathioprine (1.5–2.0 mg/kg/day) and steroid

(1 mg/kg) alone could control the disease.[46] Akpek and coauthors[47] reported the use of an alkylating agent (either chlorambucil or cyclophosphamide) to treat this entity: seven of nine patients experienced long-term drug-free remissions. Side effects included bone marrow suppression (transient), nausea, and fatigue, with one patient developing a carcinoma of the bladder. However, because the clinical course of serpiginous choroidopathy is often characterized by sporadic remissions and recurrences, it is impossible to determine the therapeutic efficacy of any regimen reported to date. Sometimes a serous detachment of the retina may occur adjacent to an area of inflammatory activity, and these detachments tend to resolve with corticosteroid therapy. Hoyng and colleagues[48] used oral prednisone to treat a patient with serpiginous choroidopathy with an RPE detachment and serous detachment, similar to what we have also seen. Steinmetz and coworkers[49] reported that acetazolamide was useful in treating cystoid macular edema in one patient with serpiginous choroidopathy. Sobaci and coworkers[50] have suggested that interferon (IFN) therapy could be used effectively to treat this disorder. In their study they used IFN-α_{2a}, 4 500 000 IU, three times a week for the first 3 months, followed by once a week for the next 3 months. Corticosteroids were used simultaneously and then tapered. Argon laser therapy was also used. They reported that half of the eyes (four of eight) had no recurrence or maintained good vision. This type of report, like many others, is very difficult to interpret without randomization and the use of other concurrent medication. Also, the natural course of this disease is variable. An example of this is a report of a serpiginous choroiditis patient maintaining good vision for 18 years with only occasional corticosteroid therapy.[51] As in the case reported above, laser photocoagulation could be considered in patients with choroidal neovascularization that may threaten central vision. Photodynamic therapy has been reported[52] to have been employed as well, with stabilization of vision but no improvement. In both cases, antineovascular therapy alone would not be treating the underlying problem that may very well be at the basis of the neovascularization, the ongoing inflammatory response.

In earlier studies, antituberculous medications had been tried for patients with this disease but with little definitive proof of efficacy.[9] However, recent studies have suggested that tuberculosis can present ocularly as a serpiginous-like lesion (mentioned above), and therefore antituberculous therapy needs to be considered in some cases. A small number of uveitis specialists consider using aciclovir to treat this disorder, but its use is based on anecdotal reports of a possible therapeutic effect in a very small number of patients.

What is clear is that the ideal therapeutic approach to this disease remains to be discovered, but with so few patients affected, a randomized clinical trial with appropriate statistical power will be difficult to conduct. We have usually treated those patients with periocular steroid injections. However, it must be admitted that some instances of this disease force one to think very hard about the efficacy of therapy. Such an example is seen in **Figure 28-9**. This patient was being treated with triple therapy and her disease seemed to be stable (Fig. 28-6A). She returned 1 month later with a large newer lesion, now with the disorder completely surrounding the fovea. Figure 28-6B shows the early blockage of the superior lesion, and Figure

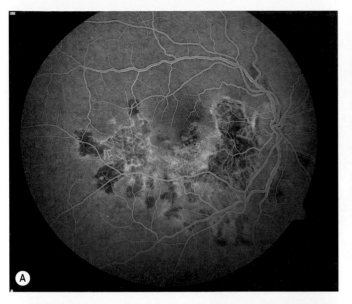

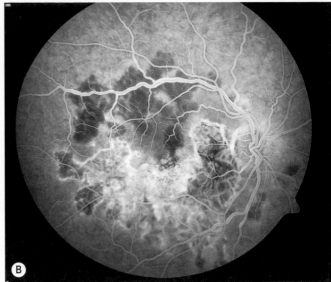

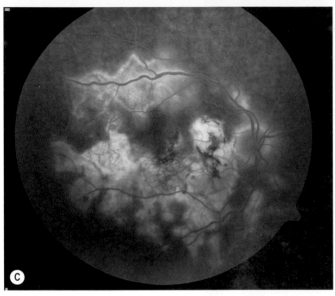

Figure 28-9. A and B, Angiogram from a patient with serpiginous choroidopathy treated with immunosuppressive drugs, whose disease was thought to be clinically quiescent. The patient returned 1 month after therapy was started with a large recurrence involving the superior part of the posterior pole **(B and C)**.

28-6C shows the late hyperfluorescence typical of the disorder.

We need to always be mindful of the potential harm that can result from our interventions. Cordero-Coma and coworkers[53] describe the case of a 48-year-old woman who was treated with the anti-TNF biologic remicade. In spite of a negative evaluation for tuberculosis before beginning therapy, the patient ultimately expired of disseminated tuberculosis.

Case 28-1

A 64-year-old white man was referred to the National Eye Institute because of a gradual loss of vision in the right eye over the previous 6 months. The left eye was amblyopic. The visual acuity was 20/100 in the right eye and 20/200 in the left. There were 1+ cells and flare in both eyes, and the vitreous of each eye had 1+ cells, with some strands. There were choroidal lesions in both eyes compatible with the diagnosis of

serpiginous choroiditis, and these were perifoveal in both eyes. The patient was given a regimen of 50 mg prednisone for 1 week, with a slow taper to 20 mg/day over several months. His vision improved to 20/25 in the right eye after 3 weeks. We elected to keep treating the patient with low-dose prednisone (10–15 mg/day) for 1 year. A repeat fluorescein angiogram showed no further progression of the lesion in that eye. Good vision in that eye has been maintained for 3 years after prednisone was discontinued.

Case 28-2

A 49-year-old white man had first noted blurring of vision in his right eye 5 years before being seen by us. He was noted to have a peripapillary lesion extending into the macular region, giving him poor vision in that eye. An inactive 'scar' had been noted inferonasally in the left eye. The patient had a past history of possible tuberculosis. Two years before being seen at the

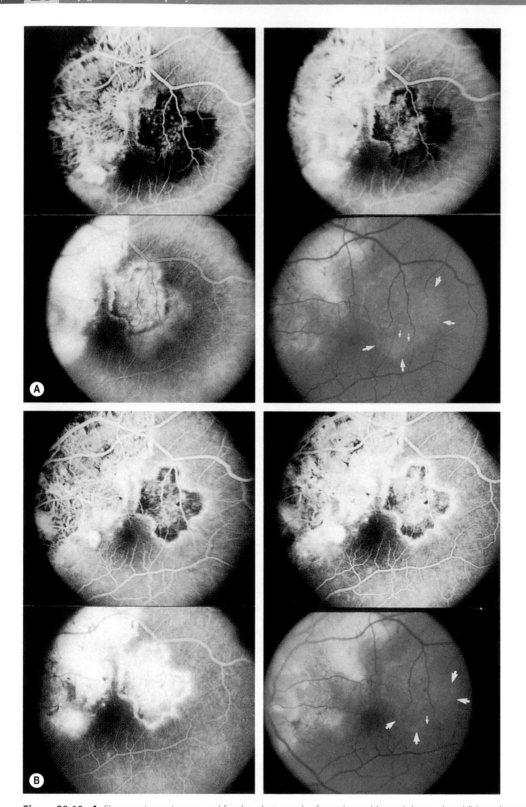

Figure 28-10. A, Fluorescein angiogram and fundus photograph of a patient with serpiginous choroiditis and complaints of slightly decreased visual acuity and metamorphopsia in the left eye. Early blocked fluorescence and late leakage are seen at the borders of active lesions. Late frame also shows late leakage compatible with serous detachment of adjacent retina (arrows). **B,** Fluorescein angiogram and fundus photograph of same patient 9 days after pulse intravenous methylprednisolone therapy. The patient had noted decreased metamorphopsia. Early blocked fluorescence is no longer seen at the border of the lesion, and serous retinal detachment has resolved (arrows). *(Reproduced with permission from Ophthalmology 98:952, Copyright Elsevier 1991.)*

National Eye Institute he noted changes in the vision in his left eye, and was subsequently given prednisone therapy (80 mg/day), as well as antituberculous medication. His vision in both eyes varied dramatically, sometimes being as good as 20/25–20/40. However, with continued prednisone therapy his vision began to fail in both eyes, with extension of the lesions toward the fovea. When seen at the National Eye Institute, his fluorescein angiogram showed central involvement in both eyes and a vision of 20/200. There was no inflammatory response. The patient was given ciclosporin therapy, and no improvement of his vision was seen after 3 months. At this point the ciclosporin was discontinued.

Case 28-3

A 43-year-old man, in whom bilateral serpiginous choroiditis had been diagnosed 11 years before being seen at the National Eye Institute, had decreased vision that was worse in the right eye. He lost good central vision in the right eye despite medical and laser therapy. He had exacerbations of inflammatory disease in his left eye 8 and 10 years after the initial flare-up, each resolving after periocular injections of betamethasone (Celestone). One year after the last flare-up he was first seen at the National Eye Institute with no active disease. He returned with a flare-up of his disease about 5 months later, with complaints of metamorphopsia and changes on Amsler grid testing. Although his visual acuity remained 20/20, he was treated with periocular and systemic corticosteroids and his vision returned to baseline. Ten months later, he returned with similar complaints of metamorphopsia. An active lesion with a cream-colored and slightly elevated border was noted on fundus examination. A fluorescein angiogram showed blocked fluorescence in the early frames with late hyperfluorescence. Hyperfluorescence suggestive of a serious detachment of the retina adjacent to the lesion was also noted in the late frames (**Fig. 28-10A and B**).

The patient was treated with pulse intravenous methylprednisolone at a dose of 1 g/day for 3 days. He was then given a regimen of oral prednisone (20 mg/day) and ciclosporin (7 mg/kg body weight/day). Within the first 3–4 days the patient noted diminished metamorphopsia, and the angiogram showed resolution of the area of blocked fluorescence (Fig. 28-10B). His subsequent course has been marked by development of a choroidal neovascular membrane (see Fig. 28-2), which was treated with laser photocoagulation. Recently the patient has developed inflammatory activity despite therapy with oral prednisone (60 mg/day) and ciclosporin (6 mg/kg of body weight/day). We have therefore added azathioprine to his therapeutic regimen.

References

1. Schatz H, Maumenee AE, Patz A. Geographic helicoid peripapillary choroidopathy: clinical presentation and fluorescein angiographic findings. Trans Am Acad Ophthalmol Otolaryngol 1974; 78: 747–761.
2. Orth D, Daily MJ, Babb MF. Subretinal neovascularization with geographic (serpiginous) choroiditis. Am J Ophthalmol 1979; 88: 683–689.
3. Bock CJ, Jampol LM. Serpiginous choroiditis, In: Principles and practice of ophthalmology, Albert DM, Jacobiec FA, eds. 1974, Mosby: Philadelphia. p. 517–523.
4. Schatz H, McDonald HR. Geographic helicoid peripapillary choroidopathy (serpiginous choroiditis), In: Retina, Ryan SJ, et al. eds. 1989, Mosby: St. Louis.
5. Hardy RA, Schatz H. Macular geographic helicoid choroidopathy. Arch Ophthalmol 1987; 105: 1237–1242.
6. Junius P. Seltene augenspielgelbilder zum klinischen phanomen des retinitis exsudativa Coats und der retinochoroiditis 'parapapillaris'. Arch AugenheilkD 1932; 106: 475.
7. Chang JH, Wakefield D. Uveitis: a global perspective. Ocul Immunol Inflamm 2002; 10(4): 263–279.
8. Blumenkranz MS, Gass JDM, Clarkson JG. Atypical serpiginous choroiditis. Arch Ophthalmol 1982; 100: 1773–1775.
9. Laatikainen I, Erkkilä H. Serpiginous choroiditis. Br J Ophthalmol 1974; 58: 777–783.
10. Hamilton AM, Bird AC. Geographical choroidopathy. Br J Ophthalmol 1974; 58: 784–797.
11. Gass JDM, Stereoscopic atlas of macular diseases: diagnosis and treatment. 1987, Mosby: St. Louis. p. 136.
12. Weiss H, Annesley WH Jr, Shields JA, et al. The clinical course of serpiginous choroidopathy. American Journal of Ophthalmology 1979; 87: 133–142.
13. Masi RJ, O'Connor R, Kimura SJ. Anterior uveitis in geographic or serpiginous choroiditis. Am J Ophthalmol 1978; 86: 228–232.
14. Laatikainen I, Erkkilä H. Subretinal and disc neovascularization in serpiginous choroiditis. Br J Ophthalmol 1982; 66: 326–331.
15. Wojno T, Meredith TA. Unusual findings in serpiginous choroiditis. Am J Ophthalmol 1982; 94: 650–655.
16. Laatikainen I, Erkkilä H. A follow-up study on serpiginous choroiditis. Acta Ophthalmol (Copenh) 1981; 59: 707–718.
17. Salati C, Pantelis V, Lafaut BA, et al. A 8 months indocyanine angiographic follow-up of a patient with serpiginous choroidopathy. Bull Soc belge Ophtalmol 1997; 265: 29–33.
18. Squirrell DM, Bhola RM, Talbot JF. Indocyanine green angiographic findings in serpiginous choroidopathy: evidence of a widespread choriocapillaris defect of the peripapillary area and posterior pole. Eye 2001; 15(Pt 3): 336–338.
19. Giovannini A, Ripa E, Scassellati-Sforzolini B, et al. Indocyanine green angiography in serpiginous choroidopathy. European Journal of Ophthalmology 1996; 6: 299–306.
20. Giovannini A, Mariotti C, Ripa E, et al. Indocyanine green angiographic findings in serpiginous choroidopathy. British Journal of Ophthalmology 1996; 80: 536–540.
21. van Liefferinge T, Sallet G, De Laey JJ. Indocyanine green angiography in cases of inflammatory chorioretinopathy. Bull Soc Belge Ophtalmol 1995; 257: 73–81.
22. Punjabi OS, Rich R, Davis JL, et al. Imaging serpiginous choroidopathy with spectral domain optical coherence tomography. Ophthalmic Surg Lasers Imaging 2008; 39(4 Suppl): S95–S98.
23. Cardillo Piccolino F, Grosso A, Savini E. Fundus autofluorescence in serpiginous choroiditis. Graefes Arch Clin Exp Ophthalmol 2008.
24. Akpek EK, Chan CC, Shen D, et al. Lack of herpes virus DNA in choroidal tissues of a patient with serpiginous choroiditis. Ophthalmology 2004; 111(11): 2071–2075.
25. Erkkilä H, Laatikainen I, Jokinen E. Immunological studies on serpiginous chorodits. Graefes Arch Clin Exp Ophthalmol 1982; 219: 131–134.
26. Gupta V, Gupta A, Arora S, et al. Presumed tubercular serpiginous-like choroiditis: clinical presentations and management. Ophthalmology 2003; 110(9): 1744–1749.

27. Teyssot N, Bodaghi B, Cassoux N, et al. Acute posterior multifocal placoid pigment epitheliopathy, serpiginous and multifocal choroiditis: etiological and therapeutic management. J Fr Ophtalmol 2006; 29(5): 510–518.

28. Mackensen F, Becker MD, Wiehler U, Max R, et al. QuantiFERON TB-Gold – a new test strengthening long-suspected tuberculous involvement in serpiginous-like choroiditis. Am J Ophthalmol 2008; 146:761–767.

29. Biswas J, Narain S, Das D, et al. Pattern of uveitis in a referral uveitis clinic in India. Int Ophthalmol 1996; 20(4): 223–228.

30. Mahendradas P, Kamath G, Mahalakshmi B, et al. Serpiginous choroiditis-like picture due to ocular toxoplasmosis. Ocul Immunol Inflamm 2007; 15(2): 127–130.

31. Sonika, Narang S, Kochhar S, et al. Posterior scleritis mimicking macular serpiginous choroiditis. Indian J Ophthalmol 2003; 51(4): 351–353.

32. Lim WK, Buggage RR, Nussenblatt RB. Serpiginous choroiditis. Surv Ophthalmol 2005; 50(3): 231–244.

33. Jones BE, Jampol LM, Yannuzzi LA, et al. Relentless placoid chorioretinitis. A new entity or an unusual variant of serpiginous chorioretinitis. Archives of Ophthalmology 2000; 118: 931–938.

34. Golchet PR, Jampol LM, Wilson D, et al. Persistent placoid maculopathy: a new clinical entity. Ophthalmology 2007; 114(8): 1530–1540.

35. Edelstein C, Stanford MR, Graham EM. Serpiginous choroiditis: an unusual presentation of ocular sarcoidosis. Br J Ophthalmol 1994; 78: 70–71.

36. Rattray KM, Cole MD, Smith SR. Systemic non-Hodgkin's lymphoma presenting as a serpiginous choroidopathy: report of a case and review of the literature. Eye 2000; 14: 706–710.

37. Nussenblatt RB, Palestine AG, Chan CC. Cyclosporine A therapy in the treatment of intraocular inflammatory disease resistant to systemic corticosteroids and cytotoxic agents. Am J Ophthalmol 1983; 96: 275–282.

38. Laatikainen I, Tarkkanen A. Failure of cyclosporin A in serpiginous choroditis. J Ocul Ther Surg 1984; 3: 280–283.

39. Araujo AAQ, Wells AP, Dick AD, et al. Early treatment with cyclosporin in serpiginous choroidopathy maintains remission and good visual outcome. British Journal of Ophthalmology 2000; 84: 979–982.

40. Markomichelakis NN, Halkiadakis I, Papaeythymiou-Orchan S, et al. Intravenous pulse methylprednisolone therapy for acute treatment of serpiginous choroiditis. Ocul Immunol Inflamm 2006; 14(1): 29–33.

41. Pathengay AO. Intravitreal triamcinolone acetonide in serpiginous choroidopathy. Indian J Ophthalmol 2005; 53(1): 77–79.

42. Adiguzel U, Sari A, Ozmen C, et al. Intravitreal triamcinolone acetonide treatment for serpiginous choroiditis. Ocul Immunol Inflamm 2006; 14(6): 375–378.

43. Seth RK, Gaudio PA. Treatment of serpiginous choroiditis with intravitreous fluocinolone acetonide implant. Ocul Immunol Inflamm 2008; 16(3): 103–105.

44. Hooper PL, Kaplan HJ. Triple agent immunosuppression in serpiginous choroiditis. Ophthalmology 1991; 98: 948–952.

45. Vonmoos F, Messerli J, Moser HR, et al. Immunosuppressive therapy in serpiginous choroiditis – case report and brief review of literature. Klin Monatsbl Augenheilkd 2001; 218: 394–397.

46. Vianna RN, Ozdal PC, Deschênes J, et al. Combination of azathioprine and corticosteroids in the treatment of serpiginous choroiditis. Can J Ophthalmol 2006; 41(2): 183–189.

47. Akpek EK, Jabs DA, Tessler HH, et al. Successful treatment of serpiginous choroiditis with alkylating agents. Ophthalmology 2002; 109: 1506–1513.

48. Hoyng C, Tilanus M, Deutman A. Atypical central lesions in serpiginous choroiditis treated with oral prednisone. Graefes Arch Clin Exp Ophthalmol 1998; 236: 154–156.

49. Steinmetz RL, Fitzke FW, Bird AC. Treatment of cystoid macular edema with acetazolamide in a patient wih serpiginous choroidopathy. Retina 1991; 11: 412–415.

50. Sobaci G, Bayraktar Z, Bayer A. Interferon alpha-2a treatment for serpiginous choroiditis. Ocul Immunol Inflamm 2005; 13(1): 59–66.

51. Karagiannis DA, Sampat V, Dowler J. Serpiginous choroidopathy with bilateral foveal sparing and good visual acuity after 18 years of disease. Retina 2007; 27(7): 989–990.

52. Lim JI, Flaxel CJ, LaBree L. Photodynamic therapy for choroidal neovascularisation secondary to inflammatory chorioretinal disease. Ann Acad Med Singapore 2006; 35(3): 198–202.

53. Cordero-Coma M, Benito MF, Hernández AM, et al. Serpiginous choroiditis. Ophthalmology 2008; 115(9): 1633, 1633 e1–2.

White-Dot Syndromes

Robert B. Nussenblatt

Key concepts

- These entities comprise disorders that are usually transient compared to those that cause long-term visual handicap.
- Nuances of these disorders, such as 'ampiginous', can take on the characteristics of two entities.
- It is not yet clear whether these clinical entities are manifestations of the same disease process.

Localized, well-circumscribed areas of inflammatory disease in the fundus are a common manifestation of many intraocular inflammatory disorders (see Chapters 13, 22, 23, and 25). In addition, several entities have been noted to occur with multiple white dots in the fundus, usually in the deeper layers of the posterior segment. They are grouped here because of their sometimes overlapping features and the belief by some that these disorders may represent the broad spectrum of one underlying entity[1] and that the underlying histopathologic lesion is a microgranuloma.[2] Recently, we are seeing that many investigators appear to be 'lumpers,' suggesting that all these are really the expression of one disease, as suggested many years ago by Gass.[3] Most occur acutely, sometimes leaving minimal or no permanent long-term visual loss. An infectious cause has been suggested for some,[3] although more recent evidence does not support this theory, and other disorders due to presumed infectious causes may not easily fit into the better-defined entities.[4]

Multiple evanescent white-dot syndrome

Clinical findings

Jampol and colleagues[5] reported on 11 patients in whom similar funduscopic changes were noted. The alterations are unilateral and are predominantly seen in young women. Numerous small (100–200 μm), discrete white lesions are noted deep in the retina or at the level of the retinal pigment epithelium (RPE) (**Fig. 29-1**) – hence the term multiple evanescent white-dot syndrome (MEWDS). The lesions appear in the posterior pole and extend to the midperiphery. They tend to be concentrated in the perifoveal region, but seem usually to spare the fovea itself. In addition, there is often a granular appearance to the macula. The granularity may take the appearance of tiny white or orange specks, which do not approach the size of the deeper circular lesions.

The macular changes cause an irregularity to the internal limiting membrane reflex. Other ocular findings include vitreous cells and occasional sheathing of the retinal venules (**Box 29-1**). There is usually no significant anterior chamber reaction. Although the lesions appear to fade with time, they can evolve into chorioretinal scars.[6]

Patients with MEWDS usually do not report a preceding flu-like episode. The mean age at onset of symptoms is about 28 years,[5,7] but Lim and coworkers[8] reported two patients in their seventh decade. The decrease in visual acuity is usually quite sudden. The disease may cause a marked drop in visual acuity even to the level of 20/200, and an afferent pupillary defect may be noted. The disease runs its course over an average of 7 weeks, after which a return to a visual acuity of between 20/20 and 20/40 usually ensues. The white lesions and macular granularity will fade with time, but subtle RPE alterations can be noted. Recurrences of the disorder are seen rarely.[9,10] Aaberg and colleagues[9] reported a recurrence in a previously affected eye 3 years after the initial visual loss, as well as recurrences in the contralateral eye. Although most reports have come from North America, this disorder has been seen in Europe.[11] Asano and colleagues[12] found that the degree of myopia was statistically higher in Japanese patients than that seen in controls. It is usually not associated with systemic disease. Lu and associates[13] reported fundus lesions as seen in MEWDS after murine typhus, and Stangos et al.[14] reported similar fundus changes in a 50-year-old after hepatitis A and yellow fever vaccination. An interesting observation was made by Landolfi and coworkers[15] in reporting that sympathetic ophthalmia appeared to mimic MEWDS. A patient whose eye was promptly repaired after a ruptured globe developed in the other eye a decrease in vision and 100–500 mm grey-white lesions.

Laboratory findings

Although no formal evaluation of these patients has been undertaken, there appear to be neither systemic manifestations of this disorder nor characteristic blood test results. Jampol and colleagues[5] reported collecting acute and convalescent sera for viral titers from one patient, but no antibody to a specific virus was identified.

Findings on the electroretinogram (ERG), early receptor potential (ERP), and visual pigment regeneration tests have been noted to be abnormal in these patients during the acute phase of the disease, with a return to normal during the recovery phase.[16] Indeed, during the acute phase a wave of the ERG and the ERP amplitudes were markedly affected. Feigl and colleagues[17] performed multifocal ERGs on four

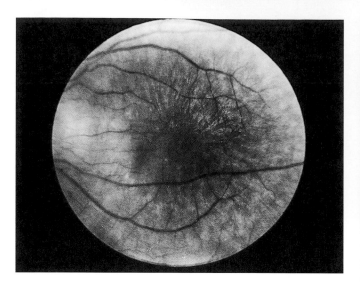

Figure 29-1. Fundus photograph showing alterations noted in MEWDS.

Box 29-1 Clinical findings in multiple evanescent white-dot syndrome

Sudden drop in visual acuity
Patients are mostly young females
Small discrete white dots at RPE level
'Grainy' macula
ERG changes that reverse after episode
Minimal RPE pertubation after episode
Condition rarely recurs
Vision returns without medication

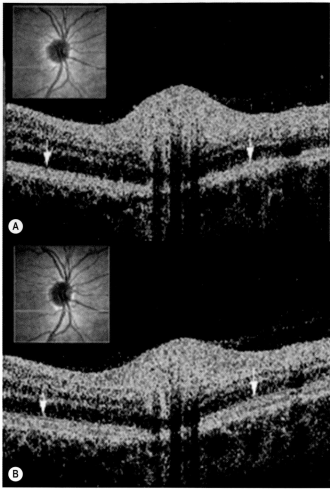

Figure 29-2 A, Case of MEWDS with initial loss of inner segment/outer segment boundary. **B,** Spontaneous resolution with segment boundary restored. *(From Spaide RF, Koizumi H, Bailey Freund K. Photoreceptor outer segment abnormalities as a cause of blind spot enlargement in acute zonal occult outer retinopathy-complex diseases. Am J Ophthalmol 2008; 146: 111–120. © 2008, Elsevier Inc.)*

patients with MEWDS. Although results were varied, first-order kernel amplitudes seemed to reflect early disturbances of the photoreceptors. van Meel and colleagues[18] performed scanning laser densitometry on a patient with MEWDS and noted small areas of absent visual pigment that did not correspond to the white fundic spots. Even with recovery, these abnormal areas of pigment loss were still faintly seen. The authors believed that their study supported the notion that this disorder is the result of a metabolic disturbance at the level of the RPE. MP1 mapping areas of retinal sensitivity can show enlarged blind spots in these patients.[19] Fundus autofluorescence (FAF) will show areas of hyperfluorescence. Yeneral et al.[20] reported that FAF showed lesions before the clinical exam became apparent.

Fluorescein angiography frequently shows early hyperfluorescence with late staining. This is unlike the angiographic findings associated with acute posterior multifocal placoid pigment epitheliopathy (APMPPE) (see later discussion). There is staining also of the macula and late staining of the disc. Gross and colleagues[21] reported recognizing new angiographic features in a subgroup of patients with MEWDS – dots and spots. Small dots noted on fluorescein angiography were interpreted to be at the level of the inner retina or the RPE, whereas larger spots were more external, in the subpigment epithelial level. These findings would suggest varying degrees of choroidal and retinal involvment in this disorder. Indocyanine green (ICG) angiography shows hypofluorescent lesions throughout the posterior pole, which are more visible on the ICG angiogram than is apparent on clinical examination[22] and appear to be seen longer on the ICG angiogram than with clinical examination.[23]

High-resolution optical coherence tomography (OCT) repeatedly show changes in the outer retina.[24–26] What appears to be most often reported is the loss of the retinal photoreceptor inner and outer segments, which can return to a more normal apppearance after the acute episode (**Fig 29-2**). It should be noted that Spaide and colleagues[26] found these changes in patients with various acute zonal occult outer retinopathy-complex diseases. Sikorski and colleagues[24] suggest that the spectral mapping they performed suggests that the alterations noted are better explained by alterations in the RPE/photoreceptor juncture rather than sites of active inflammatory disease.

Several entities have ocular manifestations similar to those seen in MEWDS. APMPPE is usually a bilateral disease with considerably larger lesions. With resolution there is often considerable RPE perturbation in this disorder, whereas in MEWDS the changes are more subtle. In APMPPE, the fluorescein angiographic picture is one of initial blockage with late staining, unlike that seen in MEWDS. Multifocal choroiditis, as first reported by Nozik and Dorsch,[27] can be distinguished from MEWDS by the more severe inflammatory response in the vitreous, long-standing lesions, and cystoid edema in the former, as well as the different evolution of the spots and probable normal electrophysiologic results in the latter. Birdshot retinochoroidopathy causes ERG and electrooculogram (EOG) changes that do not improve with time, and the involvement of the retinal vasculature with cystoid edema is quite striking (see Chapter 25). Sarcoidosis should be ruled out in patients with MEWDS, because lesions similar to those in this disorder can be seen. Usually, however, the lesions of sarcoidosis are bilateral, have more vitreous involvement, and can cause far more RPE alterations than are seen in MEWDS. As mentioned above, some researchers, including Callanan and Gass,[1] have stressed the notion that there may be an overlap of symptoms in the white-dot syndromes. To confuse matters, Bryan and colleagues[28] reported MEWDS to have occurred in the eyes of four patients with multifocal choroiditis. Gass and Hamed[29] reported MEWDS in an eye that 5 years previously had acute macular neuroretinopathy; with lesions in this entity being red-orange and some appearing in the central macula. **Table 29-1** describes three white dot syndromes. Please see comments below.

Therapy

To date, patients with MEWDS who have been reported have rarely needed to be treated. Sequelae to the acute episode seem to be minimal, with an expected return to near-preattack vision in about 7 weeks on average.[5] However, some patients may have recurrences. Figueroa and colleagues[30] used ciclosporin to treat one such patient who had multiple recurrences. The recurrences stopped while the patient was taking a therapeutic dose of the medication.

Multifocal choroiditis and panuveitis

Several investigators reported a fundic condition with the characteristics of presumed ocular histoplasmosis syndrome. This began with the report of Nozik and Dorsch[27] of two patients with bilateral uveitis associated with a distinctive chorioretinopathy. The identification of these patients is relevant because of the associated sequelae that may lead to irreversible visual handicap.

Clinical findings

Patients have a multifocal choroiditis that strongly suggests the ocular histoplasmosis syndrome (**Fig. 29-3**). However, they also have a significant vitreitis and often an anterior uveitis. The lesions, 50–200 mm in diameter, can be strewn throughout the fundus, but in our experience are posterior to the equator. They have a punched-out appearance and appear to be at the level of the RPE or inner choroid. At times pigment is heaped around the edge of the lesion. The

Table 29-1 Comparison of three white-dot syndromes (From Golchet PR, et al. Persistent placoid maculopathy: a new clinical entity. Ophthalmology 2007; 114(8): 1530–40)

	Persistent Placoid Maculopathy	**Macular Serpiginous choroiditis**[4, 6–9, 11–13, 23]	**Acute Posterior Multifocal Placoid Pigment Epitheliopathy**[8, 18–21]
Lesion characteristics	Long-standing geographic central whitish plaques involving the fovea	Variable sizes and shapes, heal to scars and atrophy in weeks	Multiple postequatorial cream-colored placoid lesions of varying sizes, fade in 1–2 wks
Visual acuity	Normal to mildly affected (20/20–20/60) with good prognosis for recovery unless complicated by CNV	Rapid decrease in central vision to counting fingers with poor prognosis for recovery	Sudden onset of moderate vision loss, photopsia, and scotomas with excellent prognosis for recovery
Gender	Only 6 patients	Male = female	Male = female
Laterality	Bilateral, symmetric (6/6 patients)	Eventually all bilateral, usually asymmetric	Usually bilateral and symmetric
FA characteristics	Early hypofluorescence followed by partial filling-in in the late phase	Early hypofluorescence of the central portion of the lesion surrounded by progressive hyperfluorescence at the margins with eventual late staining	Early hypofluorescence followed by late hyperfluorescence and staining; window defects appear in the quiescent stage
ICG angiography characteristics	Persistent hypofluorescence throughout the angiogram	Early hypofluorescence with some resolution in the late phase; no staining of lesion borders	Hypofluorescence of the active and healed lesions
Complications	CNV in 11/12 eyes, with 9 resulting in disciform mascular scars so far, RPE mottling in 1/12 eyes	CNV and disciform macular scars in up to 35%; RPE mottling and subretinal scar formation common; RPE detachments, vein and artery occlusions described	Most patients spontaneously recover; rare cases of permanent loss of vision secondary to RPE alterations or CNV; also, reports of CME, papillitis, bilateral central vein occlusions, and associated CNS vasculitis
Clinical course	Persistent lesions with mild decrease in VA unless complicated by CNV or RPE damage	Multiple discrete recurrences usually adjacent to old lesions, variably spaced over many years	Acute transient decrease in VA associated with a viral prodrome and rare recurrences

CME, cystoid macular edema; CNV, choroidal neovascularization; FA, fluorescein angiography; ICG, indocyanine green; RPE, retinal pigment epithelium; VA, visual acuity.

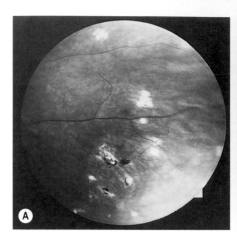
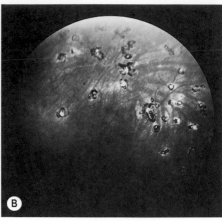

Figure 29-3. A and B, Multiple histoplasmosis-like lesions in periphery of patients with focal choroiditis and uveitis. These eyes, unlike those with ocular histoplasmosis syndrome, have a profound vitreous inflammatory response and cystoid macular edema. Both conditions carry the risk of subretinal neovascularization of the fovea.

pigmentary changes around the disc that are associated with the histoplasmosis syndrome can be seen here as well. The disorder is bilateral and occurs more frequently in women. In the review of Dreyer and Gass[31] the median age of onset was 33 years, and in the group reported by Morgan and Schatz[32] 28 years. Most of our group of 24 patients (19 females and five males) came to us after having had a long, chronic course of inflammation and averaged 52 years of age. Morgan and Schatz found that all but one of the patients they examined had myopia. Patients with this disorder do not necessary come from an area that is endemic for histoplasmosis, and a relatively low percentage show a response to the histoplasmin skin test.[31]

The inflammatory activity in the vitreous is marked, and retinal involvement can be noted on close examination. Cystoid macular edema has been found in 14% of the eyes studied by Dreyer and Gass,[31] whereas 41% of our patients had sequelae of this disorder. At least one-third of the eyes will ultimately have a subretinal neovascular net in the macula.[31] Nets from these patients are similar to others removed from eyes with other entities; many have the extra-domain B-containing fibronectin.[33] Mild disc edema can also be seen. However, acute and symptomatic blind-spot enlargements with no signs of optic nerve abnormalities have been reported by Khorram and coworkers,[34] who conjectured that this is a manifestation of peripapillary retinal dysfunction. Callanan and Gass[1] also reported an acutely enlarged blind spot in seven of their patients. Also, in four of these, white dots similar to those of MEWDS were transiently noted, suggesting a similar cause for these two disorders. Peripheral chorioretinal streaks, once thought to be seen only in the ocular histoplasmosis syndrome, were noted in three of 47 eyes with multifocal choroiditis.[35]

Punctate inner choroidopathy

Watzke and colleagues[36] described a group of patients with a condition they termed punctate inner choroidopathy (PIC), which we consider to be a variant of multifocal choroiditis until proved otherwise. In their report of 10 moderately myopic women the ocular changes noted were essentially the same as those already described, except that there were no signs of ocular inflammation. The women had blurred vision associated with light flashes and paracentral scotomas. The lesions were 100–300 mm in diameter and initially appeared yellow. Reddy and Folk[37] believe that PIC

and multifocal choroiditis, although quite similar, can be distinguished. In multifocal choroiditis there is vitreous inflammation and the retinal lesions are less discrete and shallower, whereas PIC lesions are deep, punched out, and cylindric. Also, new lesions can appear with multifocal choroiditis, which is unusual in PIC. In our mind these distinctions are blurred, and thus we generally consider PIC as a subgroup of multifocal choroiditis. Although macular edema may be somewhat less common with PIC, both PIC and multifocal choroiditis are associated with the real risk of subretinal membranes. A recent comparison of 66 patients with multifocal choroiditis and 13 with PIC does suggest some differences clinically.[38] Those with PIC presented earlier with symptoms (29 years versus 45 years). At presentation, in the comparison reported, PIC patients presented more frequently with CNV (76.9% versus 27.7%); however they appeared to have fewer structural complications due to the intraocular inflammation, such as cataract, CME, and epiretinal membranes. Those with PIC also tended not to have as great a decrease in visual acutiy. A questionnaire sent to members of the PIC society essentially corroborated those clinical findings.[39] Those who responded confirmed the impression that the typical patient was a young, myopic Caucasian woman. Self-reporting, they said that most had the development of CNV and subretinal fibrosis within the first year of diagnosis. Often observers are intoning a dual diagnosis, i.e. an initial diagnosis of PIC but then with time and findings of unexplained visual field changes, sometimes eleectrophysiologic alterations, a diagnosis of AZOOR is then made.[40,41] This blurring of diagnoses can sometimes be a bit confusing unless one is convinced these clinical disorders are really the same, which yet needs to be proved.

Laboratory findings

Patients with multifocal choroiditis do not appear to originate from areas that are endemic for histoplasmosis. However, some give a history of an antecedent febrile illness.

Fluorescein angiographic evaluation of the punched-out lesions shows early hyperfluorescence, typical of a RPE window defect. Morgan and Schatz[32] noted a fuzzy hyperfluorescent leakage late in the angiogram in some lesions. ICG angiography[41,42] tends to show more presumptive lesions than are noted on a clinical examination or on fluorescein angiography. Electrophysiologic testing does not demonstrate typical findings in multifocal choroiditis.

Indeed, the results of the ERG will tend to be normal or borderline in most patients.[13]

The disorders that need to be excluded when diagnosing this condition include many of those mentioned for MEWDS. One to note in particular is birdshot retinochoroidopathy (see Chapter 25). HLA typing has not been performed on many of these patients, and no information to date suggests any linkage, whereas HLA-A29 is strongly associated with birdshot retinochoroidoopathy (see Chapter 25). In addition, the lesions in this entity tend to be smaller and more punched-out or discrete in appearance than those in birdshot retinochoroidopathy. Birdshot retinochoroidopathy tends to occur in older persons who have less anterior segment inflammatory disease, more optic nerve involvement, and problems with night vision and color discrimination. The presence of cystoid macular edema appears to be as common in both entities in our experience, but the incidence of subretinal foveal nets is higher in this condition. In ocular histoplasmosis vitreous cells should not be present, and the lesions are generally larger. The incidence of subfoveal neovascular nets is higher in ocular histoplasmosis. Deutsch and Tessler[43] reported their observations in 28 patients with a pseudohistoplasmosis syndrome; 43% were African-American and 32% had disciform scars. Further, 32% of the patients were presumed to have sarcoidosis, 29% tuberculosis, and 11% syphilis. Multifocal, creamy choroidal infiltrates in older patients can be due to a masquerade syndrome (see Chapter 30).[44] Patients with familial juvenile systemic granulomatosis (Blau syndrome) have been shown to have multifocal choroiditis lesions[45] **(Fig. 29-4)**. MEWDS patients will more often have unlateral disease, with yellow lesions at the level of outer retina, and often with spontaneous resolution.

Visual field changes need to be documented. Holz et al.,[46] in an early description of these patients, noted the presence of an enlarged blind spot and that the visual field alterations could not be explained on the basis of the fundus changes, i.e. the field defects were larger than the spots. This could be used as evidence that both multifocal choroiditis and PIC are just one manifestion of AZOOR, as has been suggested by some. However, one could argue that the spots are simply the tip of the iceberg, reflective of changes surrounding these funduscopically apparent lesions that disrupt the neighboring photoreceptors and RPE.

A provocative hypothesis is that this disorder is virally induced. Grutzmacher and coworkers[47] ascribed RPE punched-out lesions to herpes retinitis in an otherwise healthy patient. Tiedeman[48] evaluated 10 patients with the multifocal choroiditis and panuveitis syndrome for evidence of Epstein–Barr virus-specific antibodies. These patients were noted to have antibodies directed against the viral capsid antigen (immunoglobulin [Ig] M) or the Epstein–Barr early antigen. None of the control subjects tested was found to have these antibodies, but most did have viral capsid antigen IgG or Epstein–Barr nuclear antigen antibodies, indicating previous exposure to this virus. Although none of the patients had overt systemic disease, it was hypothesized that these responses suggested an active or persistent state of viral infection and that the patients might be immunologically unable to clear the virus. Because we know that the ocular disease can continue for years, this hypothesis suggests that such persons would in theory have a higher risk of developing the systemic complications of Epstein–Barr virus, an association not so far made. Further, chronic Epstein–Barr infection has been reported by Wong and coworkers[49] to manifest a different intraocular inflammatory disease picture that responds to treatment with aciclovir. More recent studies have not borne out these observations. Spaide and colleagues[50] evaluated 11 patients with multifocal choroiditis whom they compared with 11 gender- and age-matched control subjects for the presence of anti-Epstein–Barr virus antibodies. They found that neither the antiviral capsid antigen IgG nor the antinuclear antigen antibody titers were significantly different between the two groups. None of the patients in either group had IgM antibodies to the antiviral capsid antigen. One patient with multifocal choroiditis and three control subjects had positive anti-early antigen antibody titers.

For patients with the PIC subgroup of disease, a novel mechanistic explanation was offered by Scheider.[51] He hypothesized that young myopic women are more prone to develop this syndrome because of their tendency to have bacteremia, which, coupled with the attenuated choroidal vessels of myopia, would increase their risk of infectious thromboses.

Chorioretinal biopsies of the lesions in multifocal choroiditis have shown the presence not of virus (see Case 29-2) but of a large number of B cells in the choroid.[52] Shimada et al.[53] reported the histopathology of choroidal neovascular lesions removed from 14 eyes with multifocal choroiditis and PIC. VEGF was seen in all the specimens (no surprise), and in three of the eight multifocal choroiditis specimens CD20+ B cells were noted. Overall there apeared to no be no real histopathologic differences between the specimens from the multifocal choroiditis and the PIC eyes. These are in contrast to the report of Nölle and Eckardt[54] that in nine vitrectomy specimens from patients with this disorder there were a large number of T cells – about one-third of the cell population being macrophages – and only rare B cells. Charteris and Lee[55] reported the necropsy results of eyes from a 59-year-old woman with this disorder. They noted that 70–80% of the lymphocytes were identified as T cells; less than 20% were B cells. In situ hybridization for identification of herpes simplex virus showed negative

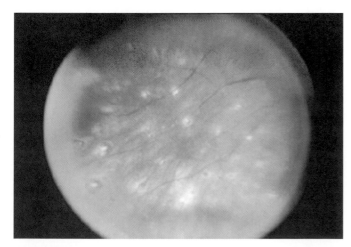

Figure 29-4. Multifocal choroiditis in patient from family with familial juvenile systemic granulomatosis (Blau syndrome). *(From Latkany PA, Jabs DA, Smith JR et al. Multifocal choroiditis in patients with familial juvenile systemic granulomatosis. Am J Ophthalmol 2002; 134: 897–904.)*

results. The finding of a large number of T cells, presumably in the choroid, in this study reflects the fact that different underlying mechanisms will result in similar clinical entities, which we had also seen with this entity[52] (see Case 29-2). An eye that was evaluated showed B cells as well as substantial numbers of CD3+ lymphocytes. No microgranulomas were noted.[56]

Therapy for multifocal choroiditis has centered on the use of immunosuppressive agents (see following discussion), with varying success. An interesting hypothesis is that an initial viral disorder may have triggered an immune response that no longer requires the presence of the virus but rather needs immunosuppressive therapy to be controlled.

Therapy

Periocular or systemic corticosteroids have been used to treat multifocal choroiditis. In the report by Dreyer and Gass,[31] six of 18 patients had improvement of vision with steroid therapy, whereas nine had no change and in two it was thought that this form of therapy halted a rapid decline in vision. Morgan and Schatz[32] reported that in their patients the inflammatory disease responded very well to steroid therapy, and that most patients were left with good vision, as did Levy et al.[57] Of our 24 patients to date, 10 of the 17 who needed steroid therapy had cystoid macula edema. We have seen a moderately good response to steroid therapy, but the disorder can be stubbornly chronic, requiring at least consideration of the addition of other immunosuppressive agents. In our experience the visual prognosis is guardedly optimistic. Of great interest was the observation of Morgan and Schatz[32] that subretinal neovascular lesions regressed with steroid therapy. This was not seen by Dreyer and Gass[31] in one patient. We have not observed regression in our patients. Foster's group[58] reported their experience in treating 19 patients with multifocal choroiditis. In their series, no patient had visual loss after they were given immunosuppressive therapy. Laser ablation of the subretinal net appears to be indicated; however, several caveats apply. The first is that there is the potential for an increase in the inflammatory response after such an intervention, something to avoid if we theorize that the inflammatory response is the underlying 'initiator' of the neovascular net. Second, the experience of Dreyer and Gass suggests that laser ablation has not been particularly successful in preventing a further deterioration of vision. The combination of PDT and an intravitreal injection of triamcinolone has been reported to yield a positive therapeutic result.[59] Cirino and colleagues[60] reported the resolution of a CNV lesion secondary to PIC when a multiple sclerosis patient began receiving regular therapy with interferon (IFN)-β_{1A}. It would seem reasonable to suppose that the CNV is inflammatorily driven, and therefore treating the inflammation as well as giving some agent directed against the neovascular component, would be a good approach.

Nölle and Eckardt[54] saw no impressive therapeutic effect of vitrectomy in nine patients with this disease. We have limited experience with the removal of submacular neovascular nets in such patients, who often, unlike those with histoplasmosis syndrome, have a great deal of fibrosis associated with the net, making removal difficult, if at all possible. Spaide and colleagues[61] used photodynamic therapy to treat seven patients with multifocal choroiditis with subretinal neovascular membranes. All were myopic, and in four of the seven corticosteroid therapy was unsuccessful. The mean improvement in visual acuity was 0.86 line.

Acute retinal pigment epitheliitis

Clinical findings

Acute retinal pigment epitheliitis was first reported by Krill and Deutman,[62] who described a group of relatively young patients with fairly subtle alterations at the level of the RPE. The condition resulted in an acute drop in visual acuity or metamorphopsia. This appears to be an acute inflammation of the retinal pigment epithelium, with a usually benign course. Some of the changes may be so mild that patients do not see a physician. Clusters of lesions, usually in the posterior pole, are noted. The lesions themselves are deep, fine, dark-gray, or black spots which in their acute stage are surrounded by a yellow halo. With resolution the halo may disappear and the lesions may appear darker in color. Fine subfoveal pigmentary clumping may be present, and could be due to an inflammation of the neurosensory retina.[63,64]

Central serous retinopathy has been noted in this entity, presumably due to the perturbation of the RPE. Retinopathy may be either bilateral or unilateral and can affect both men and women. A gradual resolution with complete or near-complete return to good vision occurs within 6–12 weeks.

This 'disorder' seems to be a sign and not a real disease. So many things can affect the RPE, as this chapter suggests. We may see more and more of these RPE alterations as we become better as seeing RPE changes that were not obvious to the naked eye; an example today would be fundus autofluorescence. It may help to better understand the mechanisms. One example is the report by Hsu and Fineman[65] using OCT. They showed outerneurosensory retinal involvement rather than RPE changes, suggesting that RPE alterations may be secondary. One can argue that recognizing the phenomenon is valuable in having some idea about its natural history.

Laboratory findings

The fluorescein angiogram will demonstrate an area of hypofluorescence surrounded by an area of hyperfluorescence. As the disorder progresses it leaves a somewhat depigmented background, and a 'lacy' hyperfluorescence may be noted. Central serous retinopathy may also be documented on angiographic examination.

Electrophysiologic testing may show an abnormal EOG during the acute phase of the disease, which will return toward normal as the disorder wanes. The finding does, however, strongly suggest that the disorder affects the RPE in a far more widespread manner than is recognized on the basis of ophthalmoscopic observations. ERG results and visually evoked cortical responses have been reported as being normal.[66]

Because of the acute nature of the illness, it has been assumed that it is viral in origin. To date, however, no studies have corroborated this hypothesis. It appears to be an adverse event secondary to drug therapy. Zoledronate, a bisophonate used to treat tumor-induced hypercalcemia, was reported to induce acute retinal pigment epitheliitis in a patient (it has also been reported to induce uveitis).[67] Loh et al.[68] reported similar changes in a patients with Dengue fever.

Therapy

No therapy is generally called for because the disease should resolve spontaneously, although one patient was treated with nonsteroidal antiinflammatory drugs and vision returned to normal.[69]

Acute posterior multifocal placoid pigment epitheliopathy

APMPPE is a term first used by Gass in 1968[70] to describe a syndrome of multiple large plaque-like lesions at the level of the RPE associated with temporary visual loss. Although there is no histologic confirmation that this is an inflammatory disease, the transient nature of the lesions and a possible association with a viral prodrome have led most authors to consider APMPPE as a manifestation of inflammation or infection at the level of the RPE or superficial choroid. It is probable that the clinical entity of benign diffuse external exudative retinitis first described by Scuderi and colleagues[71] in 1948 represents part of the clinical spectrum that we now include in the diagnosis of APMPPE.

Clinical findings

The disease usually manifests with a sudden onset of visual blurring or flashing lights in a patient younger than 30 years of age.[72–74] There is no gender predilection. Older patients have occasionally been reported. In some patients flashing lights precede the visual loss by several weeks. Most cases are bilateral and appear simultaneously in both eyes. However, unilateral cases and a delay in the appearance of the disease in the second eye by several weeks have also been noted. The anterior segments may have no significant inflammation, or there may be a 1+ to 2+ nongranulomatous inflammation. The vitreous may also have a mild to moderate inflammatory response. The characteristic clinical finding is multiple flat yellow-white (cream-colored) plaques at the level of the RPE (**Fig. 29-5**). These vary in size and are clearly defined. The placoid lesions typically begin in the macula or posterior pole, with later-developing lesions noted more peripherally. The lesions do not extend beyond the equator. Cystoid macular edema is not a prominent part of this syndrome and is rarely seen, if ever. In the acute phase the vision is often moderately decreased but rarely falls below 20/400. Some patients may have only a mild decrease, with vision in the 20/25 to 20/40 range. Visual field testing will demonstrate a central or pericentral scotoma.[75]

Papillitis is occasionally seen in association with this disease.[76,77] Characteristically the vision begins to improve spontaneously within a few weeks after the onset of symptoms, but may be somewhat slower in resolving.[72–75] Usually preceding the visual improvement by a few weeks is the initial resolution of the cream-colored placoid lesions. As the fundus lesions resolve, they lose their cream-colored appearance. Older lesions may resolve while new lesions are still appearing. There is often a residual RPE stippling, mottling, and depigmentation (**Fig. 29-6**). Vision usually returns

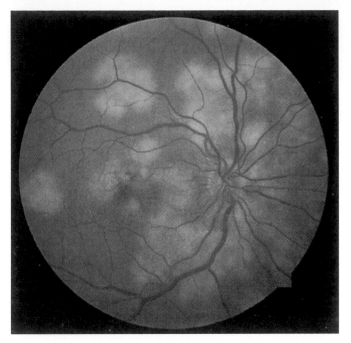

Figure 29-5. Acute lesions of APMPPE.

to near normal, but some patients may have mild residual visual deficits. Snellen acuity returns rapidly in most patients, but residual defects in visual fields, color vision, and the Stiles–Crawford effect may persist for up to a year.[49] A few patients will have significant residual visual loss.[78]

Although APMPPE is thought to be a nonrecurrent disorder and the prognosis has been considered favorable, there are reports of recurrences. Of 13 patients in one study, five had late recurrences in previously unaffected eyes.[78] We observed one patient who had recurrent episodes of APMPPE leading to significant visual loss. We have seen disease begin as what appears as a severe form of APMPPE and take on more of a serpiginous character (see Chapter 28). We have called this condition ampiginous choroiditis (see Comment 29-2 and **Fig. 29-7**), an entity that seems very similar to that described in the literature as relentless placoid chorioretinitis.[79]

APMPPE typically occurs in otherwise healthy persons. There have been occasional reports associating it with systemic disorders, suggesting as with many of these white dot syndromes that they are not really one 'disorder' but a sign of RPE/photoreceptor disfunction induced by a number of factors. Fine and co-workers[80] reported it presenting after varicella vaccination. It has been reported to occur after swine flu, hepatititis B, and meningicoccal C conjugate vaccination. Many authors have noted a viral prodrome in some patients,[72–74] and there is a report of its occurring after mumps.[81] Occasional reports of erythema nodosum,[66] episcleritis,[74] neurosensory hearing loss,[82] and cerebral vasculitis[83] associated with APMPPE have reinforced the concept that this is an immune-driven vascular alteration. Hsu and coworkers[65] reported APMPPE associated with a systemic necrotizing vasculitis (there is another case associated with more typical Wegener's granulomatosis, mentioned below), and there is a report of the fundus changes arising in a patient with clear cell renal cell carcinoma.[84] Bilateral central retinal vein occlusions have been associated with APMPPE as well, perhaps reflecting a vasculitis of the ciliary vessels.[85]

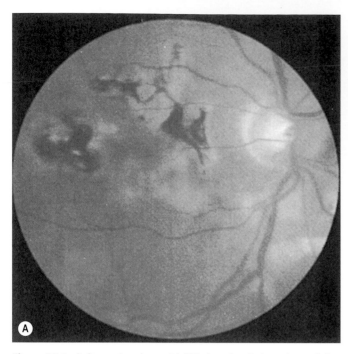 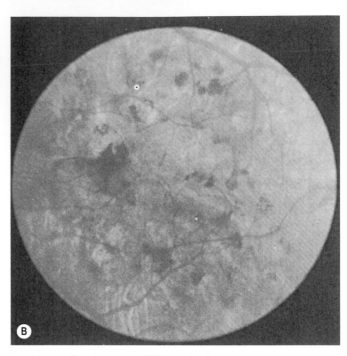

Figure 29-6. A, Reparative phase with RPE clumping. **B,** Late phase of disease, showing a profound amount of RPE perturbation.

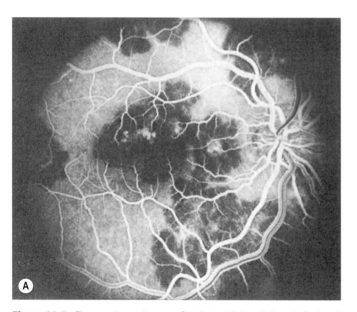 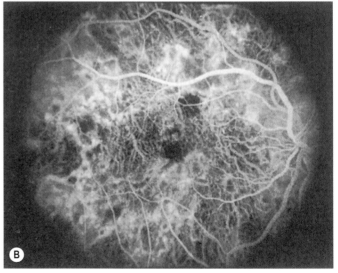

Figure 29-7. Fluorescein angiogram of patient with 'ampiginous' chorioretinopathy. **A,** Clinical picture of APMPPE confirmed by angiogram. **B,** Angiogram (taken about 1.5 years later) shows findings more typical of serpiginous choroiditis.

Others have reported a neurosensory detachment, retinal vasculitis, and papillitis.[86] There is no coherent explanation for the development of this disease.

In addition to the striking clinical appearance of the fundus, the fluorescein angiography findings are characteristic in APMPPE[72–74,87] (**Fig. 29-8**). In the acute stage of the disease, during which there are active cream-colored lesions, the choroidal fluorescence is blocked in the early phases of the angiogram. In the late stages there is staining of the lesions that had previously blocked fluorescence. Hypofluorescence followed by hyperfluorescence in combination with appropriately sized and colored fundic lesions is diagnostic of APMPPE. Fluorescein angiographic findings in the late or resolved stage of the disease are less characteristic and

demonstrate transmission defects in the RPE without leakage. There are hypofluorescent dots during the active stage which later become hyperfluorescent. Autofluorescence shows areas of hypofluorescence that do not always correlate with the fundus lesions that are visible (**Fig. 29-9**).

Usually the disorder is limited to the eye. However, in several patients APMPPE has been associated with cerebral vasculitis.[88] This can occur at the time of the ocular disease or months later. A pleocytosis may be seen in the cerebrospinal fluid. In one report,[89] multifocal white-matter lesions were seen on an MRI scan, and the neurologic symptoms disappeared with steroid therapy. It has been associated with diseases that may have a significant vasculitis component, such as Wegener's granulomatosis[90] and scleritis.[91] APMPPE

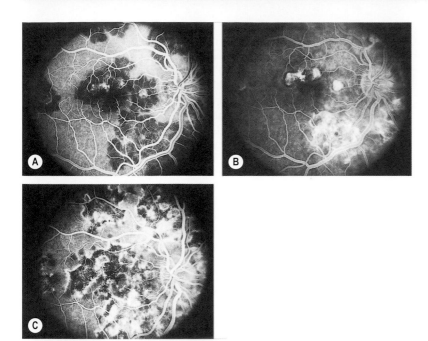

Figure 29-8. A, Early blockage of lesions seen on fluorescein angiography. **B,** Late hyperfluorescence seen in the inferior portion of the same lesion. **C,** Extensive hyperfluorescence seen in the angiogram of an eye with old APMMPE.

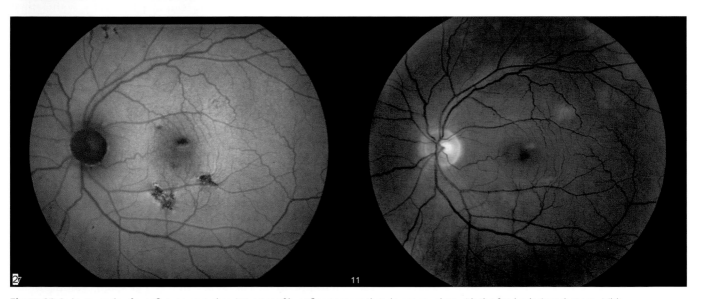

Figure 29-9 An example of autofluorescence showing areas of hypofluorescence that do not correlate with the fundus lesions that are visible.

has been diagnosed in a patient with juvenile rheumatoid arthritis and was treated with ciclosporin and prednisone.[92] APMPPE may not be a specific disease but rather a response of the RPE or choroid to various disease processes (**Fig. 29-10**).

Etiology

In his initial description Gass[70] believed that the site of the lesion in APMPPE was at the level of the RPE or was due to an abnormality in choroidal perfusion with secondary involvement of the RPE. The EOG is markedly impaired during the acute phase of the disease, supporting the concept of RPE involvement.[75] Isolated areas of choroidal nonperfusion inside placoid lesions suggest that the primary lesion is impaired filling of the choroid,[87] perhaps due to a choroidal vasculitis.[93] It is now thought that the choroidal vasculature is obstructed at the level of the precapillary arterioles.

It is interesting to note that a true vasculitis such as Wegener's granulomatosis can produce ocular lesions that resemble those of APMPPE.[94] The varying size of the APMPPE lesions could support a choroidal hypoperfusion hypothesis. It is possible that APMPPE is part of a spectrum of choroidal perfusion abnormalities, and, as Young and colleagues[87] suggest, patients with more confluent lesions may have a less favorable clinical course than those with APMPPE; yet the lesions appear to have the same root cause: choroidal ischemia with secondary involvement of the RPE. The photoreceptors are most likely involved in this ischemic process, accounting for the visual loss and the slow recovery of sensitive measures of photoreceptor function such as the Stiles–Crawford effect.[75] Patients with unilateral lesions but bilateral perfusion abnormalities have been described, further supporting the choroidal location of the disease process. The variability in the degree of choroidal ischemia may explain some of the unusual sequelae of APMPPE, such

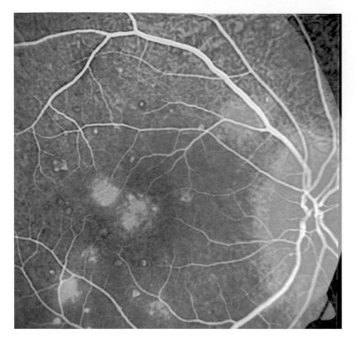

Figure 29-10. ICG angiogram superimposed on the fluorescein angiogram of a patient in the early stages of 'ampiginous' choroiditis. 'White' lesions are those seen on fluorescein angiography, and dark lesions are those seen on ICG angiography. Here, curiously, there is a good correlation between the two tests. This is unlike other observations, which found more lesions on ICG than on fluorescein angiography. *(Courtesy of Ronald Buggage, MD and Sunil Srivastava, MD.)*

as subretinal neovascular membranes. Preceding viral illnesses are certainly often reported and raise the possibility of a localized viral infection. Bodine and colleagues[95] reported one case they believed was associated with Lyme disease.

Therapy

Most patients with APMPPE have a good visual prognosis and do not require therapy. Some authors have used systemic corticosteroid therapy, but it is difficult to assess its value in view of the overall favorable prognosis (see Case 29-2). In one study[96] in which patients with APMPPE were followed for an extended period, the lack of steroid responsiveness was corroborated and more than one-quarter of the eyes had a vision of 6/24 or less. However, in one patient with CME secondary to APMPPE an intravitreal injection of steroid was reported to improve vision and cause regression of the CME.[97] In severe cases with papillitis and retinal vasculitis, we would wait some time to see a resolution, but then we would certainly be tempted to intervene therapeutically as was done in one report.[86] The various responses reported may reflect the fact that we are seeing a manifestation of many different inflammatory mechanisms, some that are short lived and clear without intervention, and others that are chronic and need therapy.

Subretinal fibrosis and uveitis syndrome

Clinical findings

We reported on the first three patients with this disorder.[98] This rare entity[99,100] is characterized by chronic inflammation

in the vitreous with whitish-yellow subretinal lesions that appear to be gliotic or fibrotic (**Fig. 29-11A** and **B**). These lesions can coalesce to form a large sheet of this fibrotic-appearing material and progress to encompass the whole posterior pole, with loss of vision. However, in some patients the progression may not continue and a steady state may be reached, or the lesion may encircle but not encroach on the macula (Fig. 29-11, C). Sometimes, although the macula is not directly involved, cystoid macular edema may result, with a subsequent drop in visual acuity. The vitreal inflammatory response may be quite marked, and there may be a low-to-moderate anterior chamber response. In our experience the patients have all been young women, mostly African-American, and in all but one the disease has been bilateral. Others have reported this entity in males (Rubens Belfort Jr, personal communication). The number of cases followed is still too small to define the ultimate visual outcome in these patients. A similar clinical finding of progressive subretinal fibrosis has been seen after ocular surgery and has been conjectured to be a variant of sympathetic ophthalmia.[101] Our patients had no such history. Subretinal fibrosis can be a sequela to almost any inflammatory condition stimulating the RPE region, particularly with retinal elevation. It has been noted in conjunction with multifocal choroiditis,[102] and associated with long-standing ulcerative colitis.[103]

It is interesting to note that the entity may have been reported by Fuchs in his 1949 *Atlas of the Ocular Fundus*.[104] In it, Fuchs described an 'extremely rare' bilateral condition in which there were large areas of connective tissue formation under the retina that led to a severe drop in visual acuity.

Laboratory findings

In patients with more advanced disease the ERG and EOG show markedly diminished results. The ERG may show changes of both rod and cone function.[98] The fluorescein angiogram shows predominantly subretinal alterations. In the early phase of the angiogram one may see multiple areas of blockage of choroidal fluorescence as well as hyperfluorescence. In the later phase of the angiogram, staining of the lesions without leakage can be noted.

Laboratory testing does not appear to be contributory. Culturing of peripheral lymphocytes has not demonstrated an in vitro anamnestic response to retinal antigens, such as the S-antigen.

We performed an immunohistochemical evaluation of two eyes with this entity[105,106] (**Fig. 29-12**) which revealed a markedly inflamed choroid with a predominance of B cells and plasma cells. Complement and IgG were deposited above Bruch's membrane. In one eye a granulomatous lymphocytic infiltrate was present in the choroid. Of the T-cell subpopulations, there was a predominance of the helper/inducer subset. Müller cells expressed class II antigens. There were no circulating antiretinal antibodies, and virus could not be cultured from the specimen. The subretinal fibrosis contained islands of cells that were interpreted as originating from the RPE. The impression was that a dysregulation leading to a B-cell disorder with antibody and complement deposition occurs. This leads to retinal and RPE damage, as well as to the development of fibrosis. Without any

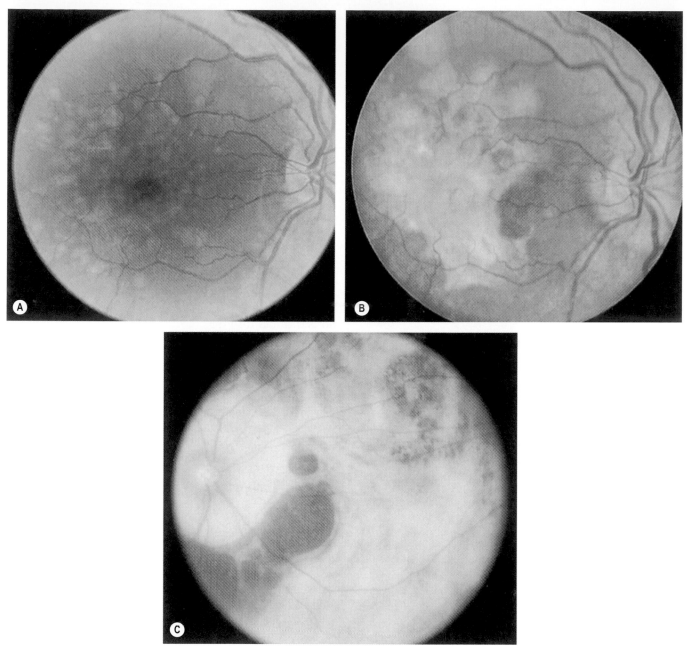

Figure 29-11. A, Early changes of subretinal fibrosis syndrome and uveitis. With time these changes coalesced to form the picture seen in **B. C,** Extensive subretinal fibrosis involving the disc and then extending into the macular region.

definitive data to date, one can speculate what is at the basis of this B-cell dysregulation and whether the B cells are the cause of the fibrosis. One possible explanation is that the two are not related but rather cause a shift in T-cell subsets, from a Th1 response to a Th2 profile. Whereas Th1 cells would produce IFN and IL-2, the Th2 inducer cells would produce a lymphokine cascade rich in IL-4, which could stimulate B cells, and transforming growth factor-b, a lymphokine associated with scarring and fibrosis.

Although we believe that this entity is a distinct condition, as do Cantrill and Folk,[107] several other conditions could mimic its clinical features. A long-standing retinal detachment can lead to subretinal fibrosis. Ocular inflammatory conditions to consider include sarcoidosis, ocular histoplasmosis syndrome, APMPPE, syphilis, tuberculosis, birdshot retinochoroidopathy, pathologic myopia, acute macular neuroretinopathy,[108] syphilis, sympathetic ophthalmia, and toxoplasmosis.

Therapy

Therapeutic interventions to date have not been universally successful in stopping the disorder. One exception is that if cystoid macular edema is present the edema seems to respond to corticosteroid therapy, resulting in an increase in visual acuity. However, we have not found that our therapeutic intervention has slowed or in any way altered the fibrotic changes, at least in the most advanced or fulminant cases. Fortunately for some persons, the disease can progress very slowly or stop altogether, for reasons that are not

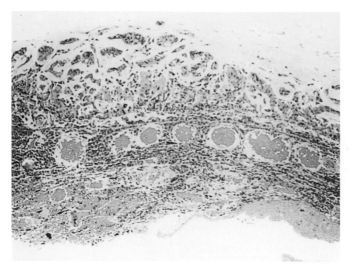

Figure 29-12. Chorioretinal biopsy specimen from a patient with subretinal fibrosis and uveitis syndrome. There is marked choroidal infiltration by lymphocytes, as well as replacement of normal retinal structures by islands of irregular cells and amorphous connective tissue. Electron microscopic examination revealed that the connective tissue consisted of collagen fibrils and these islands of cells had characteristics suggestive of RPE. Both T and B lymphocytes were seen, but there was a differential increase in the number of B cells compared to that in peripheral blood. No virus or other organisms were found either by culture or by electron microscopy. *(From Palestine AG, Nussenblatt RB, Chan CC et al. Histopathology of the subretinal fibrosis and uveitis syndrome. Ophthalmology 1985; 92: 838–844.)*

known. Corticosteroid therapy would seem appropriate in light of the B-cell nature of the disease. However, it is known that the factors stimulating fibroblast proliferation may not be affected by this kind of therapy. One patient has been treated with aggressive cytotoxic therapy[107] (cyclophosphamide), and the course of the disease was not altered. The disease of one of our patients seems to have been controlled with methotrexate. One recent report[109] suggested that infliximab was successful in treating one case. Although subretinal changes were seen in that case, it lacked the overwhelming fibrotic appearance that we noted. However, it is possible that spectra of the disease exist.

Acute zonal occult outer retinopathy (AZOOR) and the azoor complex diseases

Gass[110] reported on 13 patients, predominantly young women (77%), with a group of findings that he named acute zonal occult outer retinopathy (AZOOR). These changes include a rapid loss of one or more large zones of outer retinal function, manifested by progressive scotomata as well as photopsia (an important complaint), with minimal funduscopic changes, at least initially. There is little or no clinical evidence of inflammatory disease, but later there may be RPE atrophy. Thus the disorder is characterized by the development of one or more scotomas (readily documented with visual field testing), usually associated with photopsia, in one or both eyes. In spite of the initially minimal funduscopic changes, the ERG findings will be abnormal.[111] Francis et al.[112] suggested that in addition to the clinical findings, the diagnostic criteria should include electrophysiologic changes that show a consistent pattern of

dysfunction both at the photoreceptor/RPE complex and at the inner retinal levels. In addition, they found a delayed 30 Hz flicker ERG as well as a reduction in the EOG light rise. Full-field ERGs performed by Zibrandtsen et al.[113] also revealed an alteration in the 30 Hz flicker responses and subnormal photopic responses and a subnormal scotopic responses in one case. They felt that the findings suggested photoreceptor atrophy. Multifocal electroretinography (mERG) revealed localized outer retinal dysfunction. Several groups have reported OCT abnormalities at the level of the inner and outer retinal segments, abnormalities seen in many of these white dot syndromes.[26,114, 115] With time there are striking RPE changes (**Fig. 29-13**). Spaide[116] has reported extensive autofluorescence, and atrophy of the choriocapillaris was seen on ICG. During the early phase of the disease a large number of disorders need to be excluded, including retrobulbar neuritis, a pituitary or intracranial tumor, and cancer-associated retinopathy. Results of the medical and neurologic investigation are usually unrewarding.[110] No autoantibodies to the photoreceptor region have been reported.[111] In the later disease phases the differential diagnosis includes disorders that cause retinal vascular narrowing and RPE alterations, including syphilis, retinal vasculitis, and diffuse unilateral subacute neuroretinitis. In a long-term follow-up of 51 patients[117] (37 female and 14 male, average age 33 years) AZOOR was present in one eye of 31 patients (61%) and in both eyes of 20 patients (39%). Eighty-eight percent of patients presented with photopsias, and the fundus was deemed to be normal in 82 eyes. The ERG was depressed in all eyes, and this finding has been seen by others as well.[118] In the long-term study by Gass (**Table 29-2**), visual field changes stabilized within 6 months in 37% of patients, progressed in 4%, and partially improved in 24%. A final visual acuity of 20/40 was seen in 68% of eyes, and 18% were legally blind. Changes at the level of the RPE were seen in 43 eyes (48%). Of the patients reviewed, 28% had an autoimmune disease. Immunosuppressive therapy has been given, as has antiviral medication. The results are difficult to assess, but it would appear that dramatic results have not been seen with these therapies (see Table 29-2). Perhaps a variant of AZOOR is the acute idiopathic blind-spot enlargement syndrome.[119] Findings are similar to those in AZOOR, including photopsias, but findings on the ERG are usually normal and findings on the focal ERG are abnormal.

Gass described a group of entities identified as 'AZOOR complex,' which has been referred to recently as AZOOR complex of diseases. These include MEWDS, multifocal choroiditis and PIC, acute idiopathic blind spot enlargement, acute macular neuroretinopathy[108] (**Fig. 29-14**), acute anular outer retinopathy, and AZOOR. It has been Gass' belief that they have an infectious cause.[3] There have been several reports describing patients with one of the these entities, such as multifocal choroiditis, who then develop what the authors feel is AZOOR.[40,41] An interesting exchange between Gass on one side and Jampol and Becker on the other is found in the literature. Jampol and Becker[120] take the view that these entities are probably discrete, but that patients with these diseases share common nondisease-specific genes and that the environment or other factors triggers the expression of disease seen clinically. I would agree with the latter view. We are beginning to see this

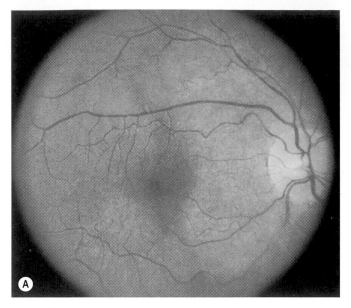
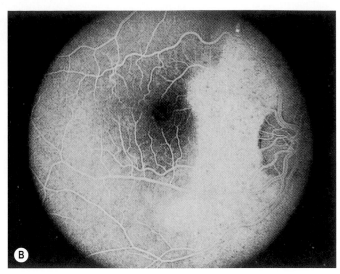

Figure 29-13. A, Fundus photograph. **B,** Fluorescein angiogram of a patient with AZOOR.

appellation applied to many disorders where the visual field alterations may not fit the clinical fundus appearance, moving away from Gass' original group of disorders.[121] One example is AZOOR described as being associated with pars planitis.[122]

So are they one disease or several?

The entities discussed here have been nicely described in the past.[123-125] They are believed by some to be essentially one entity that expresses itself clinically in multiple ways, but it is our belief that they can be clinically differentiated. Further, until we learn more about the underlying mechanisms, we cannot really speculate as to whether these are all separate entities or simply variations on a theme. However, there are strong reasons to distinguish them on the basis of their clinical findings, because doing so is helpful in predicting the ultimate visual outcome in an individual patient. Because we are dealing with a range of disorders – from those that are not sight-threatening and which resolve without therapy, to others for which we have no effective therapy and which have the potential for severe visual handicap – it would seem that their recognition on clinical grounds and their very different natural histories would justify our noting them as separate conditions. It is, however, important to remember that many believe that these disorders represent a spectrum of basically the same underlying disorder. Gass,[110] for instance, would place disorders such as MEWDS, multifocal choroiditis, and geographic atrophy of the RPE under the rubric of AZOOR with focal fundus lesions. To date, no direct viral etiology has been substantiated. It is also true that several reports seem to indicate various white dot syndrome entitities in the same eye at different points in time.[40,41,46] Even the presence of CNV may be the first manifestation of many of these white dot syndromes, MEWDS, multifocal choroiditis, and PIC.[126] However, it may be that the eye can react at the level of the RPE in only a limited number of ways, despite the fact that the initiating event may be quite different. AZOOR has been described after a car accident.[127] Hence the reason for similar or overlapping clincal syndromes. Time will tell.

Case 29-1

A 24-year-old Hispanic woman came to the eye clinic because of poor vision in her right eye for 3 months. Testing revealed hand motion vision in the right eye and 20/20 in the left.

Examination of the right eye showed extensive subretinal fibrosis, extending from around the disc and encompassing essentially all of the posterior pole. The left eye was normal. A work-up was performed to rule out several disorders, including syphilis, tuberculosis, and sarcoid, and testing results supported none of these diagnoses. Results of the patient's toxoplasmosis titer were positive. She was thought to have subretinal fibrosis with uveitis syndrome. Because the right eye had such poor vision, it was decided not to treat her. She returned 3 months later with a complaint of decreased vision in the left eye. The visual acuity was hand motions in the right eye, 20/200 in the left eye. Patches of white subretinal fibrosis associated with a vitreal response were noted. The patient was given a regimen of 80 mg prednisone daily, but her vision continued to decrease and new lesions were noted. An alkylating agent was begun along with the prednisone. Despite this therapy vision in the left eye continued to decrease until it reached that of the right eye.

Comment 29-1. Many cases of subretinal fibrosis will not proceed inexorably to poor vision. We have noted patients whose vision will stabilize, and a few of these had unilateral disease. However, the ideal therapy for this potentially sight-threatening, predominantly B-cell disease, is lacking.

Case 29-2

A 27-year-old white man was treated with laser therapy 2 years before being seen for a small retinal hole in the periphery of the right eye. He came for an ophthalmologic evaluation because of a 1-month history of scotomas and flashing lights in the left eye, with the same findings now in the right eye. He was given prednisone (60 mg/day) but no change in the symptoms was

Table 29-2 Minimum 3-year follow-up study of 51 patients (90 eyes with 113 eye episodes of visual loss) with AZOOR (Reproduced with permission from Golchet, P.R., et al. Persistent placoid maculopathy: a new clinical entity. Ophthalmology 2007;14(8):1530–1540)

	Number of Patients	Number of Recurrences	Number of Eye Episodes
Duration of follow-up	51 (100)		
Median, 96 months			
Mean, 100 months			
Range, 36–420 months			
Gender			
Female	37 (73%)		
Male	14 (27%)		
Age at onset of AZOOR	51 (100%)		
Median, 33 years			
Mean, 36 years			
Range, 13–63 years			
Race (recorded in 43 patients)			
Caucasian	39 (91%)		
Hispanic	3 (7%)		
Asian	1 (2%)		
Unilateral involvement at onset*	31 (61%)		
Bilateral involvement at onset[†]	20 (39%)		
Unilateral at final examination	12 (24%)		
Bilateral at final examination	39 (76%)		
Delayed involvement in fellow eye			
Median, 31 months			
Mean, 50 months			
Range, 2–192 months			
Recurrence of AZOOR	16 (31%)	23	
Median time from onset of AZOOR			
39 months; mean 52 months			
Range, 12–156 months			
Course of visual field loss			
Improvement[‡]	13 (20%)		21 (19%)
Stable within 6 months after onset	40 (78%)		87 (77%)
Stepwise progression of visual loss[§]	2 (4%)		4 (4%)
Follow-up <6 months	1 (2%)		1 (1%)
Totals	56[‖]	23	113

AZOOR, acute zonal occult outer retinopathy.
*One patient monocular.
[†]Occult in one eye of five (25%) cases.
[‡]One patient with improvement worsened after a recurrence and was stable thereafter. Improvement in the visual field in 12 patients persisted for duration of follow-up.
[§]Two patients with 3- and 10-year intervals between onset in the first and second eye had stepwise loss of vision in both eyes.
[‖]Five patients had a different course in the two affected eyes.

seen. He was in good health, was taking no medication, and had no significant past medical history. When seen, his visual acuity was 20/20 in the right eye and 20/200 in the left. No anterior segment inflammation was present, but there were 1+ cells in the vitreous of both eyes. White-yellow subretinal infiltrates were seen in both the posterior pole and the retinal periphery that became more yellowish in appearance with time.

Some areas had subretinal scarring and RPE clumping. The fluorescein angiogram revealed that some lesions showed initial blockage with late staining, typical of APMPPE. There was no macular edema. The EOG findings were 188% in the right eye and 142% in the left. The ERG showed diminished oscillatory potentials. Hardy–Rand–Rittler plates showed that color vision testing results were highly abnormal in the left eye. As the

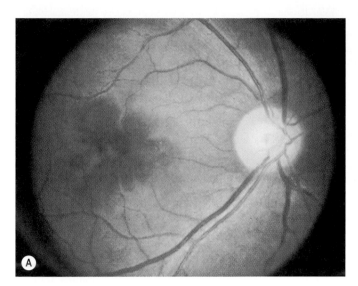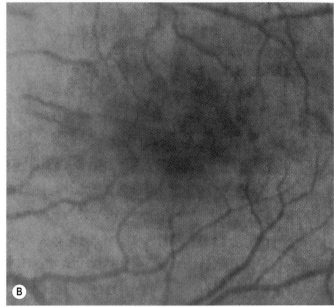

Figure 29-14. A and B, Two example of acute macular neuroretinopathy. Note the reddish-orange color of the lesions. *(Reproduced with permission from Turbeville SD, Cowan LD, Gass JD et al. Acute macular neuroretinopathy, a review of the literature. Surv Ophthamol 48:1, 2003.)*

disease progressed, new lesions appeared in the right eye, and the central vision seemed to be threatened. Ciclosporin was added to the therapeutic regimen for 3 months. Although there appeared to be resolution of the lesions, the disease now resembled serpiginous choroiditis (see Fig. 29-6). The patient has been followed for 10 years and his vision has been maintained at 20/32 in the right eye and 20/63 in the left eye. He has had no recurrences. The fundus in both eyes shows marked RPE clumping extending out to the retinal periphery.

Comment 29-2. Those who have followed this patient coined the term 'ampiginous' chorioretinopathy to describe his retinopathy. Did our therapy play any role in maintaining his vision? We do not know. He did not suffer a recurrence, typical of APMPPE. The retinal appearance was not typical of this disease, however; the extensive changes and scarring were more typical of serpiginous chorioretinopathy.

Case 29-3

A 53-year-old myopic Japanese-American woman had a small symptomatic retinal hole noted on a routine ocular examination. This was treated with laser therapy. Some months later, she noticed floaters and decreased visual acuity. She was found to have in the right eye 1+ vitreal cells and multiple creamy-white lesions strewn throughout the posterior pole and extending toward the equator. Despite prednisone therapy her vision continued to decline in that eye. After a macular hemorrhage her vision dropped to 20/400 and fibrosis ensued. Some months later the same problem developed in her left eye. Her vision decreased somewhat to 20/30, with multiple creamy-white lesions being seen in the fundus. She underwent an extensive evaluation to uncover an underlying problem for what was diagnosed as a multifocal choroiditis. Results of a lumbar puncture were normal, as were a gallium scan and conjunctival biopsy. Of interest was the finding of elevated

serum titers for herpes simplex 1 (1 : 2560), herpes simplex 2 (1 : 320), and herpes zoster (1 : 640). Because of this finding, the patient was given a short course of aciclovir, but the lesions continued to evolve and new ones were seen. The progression in the left eye continued along the same course as that seen in the right, and neither antiviral nor immunosuppressive therapy was effective in altering the course of the disease.

Thus the ophthalmologist was presented with a diagnostic dilemma, and because the macula in the left eye was threatened it was decided to perform a chorioretinal biopsy. There was mild atrophy of the inner retinal layers. The choroid was filled with B cells and plasma cells. There were nodules at the level of the RPE that resembled Dalen–Fuchs nodules but were made up predominantly of B cells. Virus could not be detected using immunofluorescence, electron microscopy or culture. It was decided to treat the patient with cyclophosphamide. The reasons for this decision were that (1) there was no evidence of active infection and (2) with a predominantly B-cell infiltrate, ciclosporin – with its effect being essentially on the T-cell arm of the immune response – would not be indicated. The patient's ocular disease responded rapidly to cyclophosphamide (initial dose 2 mg/kg, then lowered) combined with 17.5 mg of prednisone. The lesions involuted, and cytotoxic medication was stopped after about 1 year. Her eyes have shown no inflammatory activity for more than 3 years after therapy was stopped. The patient required a cataract extraction in the right eye, from which a biopsy specimen was obtained, but visual acuity of 20/400 in the right eye and 20/30 in the left eye has been maintained.

Comment 29-3. The white-dot syndromes still remain problematic. The chorioretinal biopsy helped enormously in determining a therapeutic approach. In addition, the finding of B cells in this disease was quite unexpected. We have seen a similar finding in a biopsy specimen of another patient with this disorder. It is interesting to note that T-cell infiltrates at this level of the eye can look clinically essentially the same.[31]

References

1. Callanan D, Gass J. Multifocal choroiditis and choroidal neovascularization associated with the multiple evanescent white dot and acute idiopathic blind spot enlargement syndrome. Ophthalmology 1992; 99(11): 1678–1685.

2. Ben Ezra D, Forrester JV. Fundal white dots: the spectrum of a similar pathological process. Br J Ophthalmol 1995; 79: 856–860.

3. Gass JD, Editorial: Are acute zonal occult outer retinopathy and the white spot syndromes (AZOOR complex) specific autoimmune diseases. Am J Ophthalmol 2003; 135: 380–381.

4. Grand MG, Storch GA. Presumed parvovirus B19-associated retinal pigment epitheliopathy. Retina 2000; 20: 199–202.

5. Jampol L, Sieving PA, Pugh D, et al. Multiple evanescent white dot syndrome. I. clinical findings. Arch Ophthalmol 1984; (102): 671–674.

6. Kozielec GF, Wyhinny GJ, Jampol LM. Evolution of distinct chorioretinal scars in recurrent MEWDS. Retina 2001; 21: 180–182.

7. Mamalis N, Daily M. Multiple evanescent white-dot syndrome. A report of eight cases. Ophthalmology 1987; 94: 1209–1212.

8. Lim JI, Kokame GT, Douglas JP. Multiple evanescent white dot syndrome in older patients. Am J Ophthalmol 1999; 127: 725–728.

9. Aaberg T, Campo R, Joffe L. Recurrences and bilaterality in the multiple evanescent white-dot syndrome. Am J Ophthalmol 1985; 100: 29–37.

10. Meyer R, Jampol L. Recurrences and bilaterality in the multiple evanescent white-dot syndrome. Am J Ophthalmol 1986; 101: 388–389.

11. Borruat F, Othenin-Girard P, Safran A. Multiple evanescent white dot syndrome. Klin Monatsbl Augenheilkd 1991; 198: 453–456.

12. Asano T, Kondo M, Kondo N, et al. High prevalence of myopia in Japanese patients with multiple evanescent white dot syndrome. Jpn J Ophthalmol 2004; 48(5): 486–489.

13. Lu TM, Kuo BI, Chung YM, et al. Murine typhus presenting with multiple white dots in the retina. Scan J Infect Dis 1997; 29: 632–633.

14. Stangos A, Zaninetti M, Petropoulos I, et al. Multiple evanescent white dot syndrome following simultaneous hepatitis-A and yellow fever vaccination. Ocul Immunol Inflamm 2006; 14(5): 301–304.

15. Landolfi M, Bhagat N, Langer P, et al. Penetrating trauma associated with findings of multiple evanescent white dot syndrome in the second eye: coincidence or an atypical case of sympathetic ophthalmia? Retina 2004; 24(4): 637–645.

16. Sieving P, Fishman GA, Jampol LM, et al. Multiple evanescent white dot syndrome. II. Electrophysiology of the photoreceptors during retinal pigment epithelial disease. Arch Ophthalmol 1984; (102): 675–679.

17. Feigl B, Haas A, El-Shabrawi Y. Multifocal ERG in multiple evanescent white dot syndrome. Graefe's Arch Clin Exp Ophthalmol 2002; 240: 615–621.

18. van Meel G, Keunen JE, van Norren D, et al. Scanning laser densitometry in multiple evanescent white dot syndrome. Retina 1993: (13): 29–35.

19. Boscarino MA, Johnson TM. Microperimetry in multiple evanescent white dot syndrome. Can J Ophthalmol 2007; 42(5): 743–745.

20. Yenerel NM, Kucumen B, Gorgun E, et al. Atypical presentation of multiple evanescent white dot syndrome (MEWDS). Ocul Immunol Inflamm 2008; 16(3): 113–115.

21. Gross NE, Yannuzzi LA, Freund KB, et al. Multiple evanescent white dot syndrome. Arch Ophthalmol 2006; 124(4): 493–500.

22. Ie D, Glaser BM, Murphy RP, et al. Indocyanine Green Angiography in Multiple Evanescent White-Dot Syndrome. Am J Ophthalmol 1994; (117): 7–12.

23. Tsukamoto E, Yamada T, Kadoi C, et al. Hypofluorescent spots on indocyanine green angiography at the recovery stage in multiple evanescent white dot syndrome. Ophthalmologica 1999; 213: 336–338.

24. Sikorski BL, Wojtkowski M, Kaluzny JJ, et al. Correlation of spectral optical coherence tomography with fluorescein and indocyanine green angiography in multiple evanescent white dot syndrome. Br J Ophthalmol 2008; 92(11): 1552–1557.

25. Nguyen MH, Witkin AJ, Reichel E, et al. Microstructural abnormalities in MEWDS demonstrated by ultrahigh resolution optical coherence tomography. Retina 2007; 27(4): 414–418.

26. Spaide RF, Koizumi H, Freund KB. Photoreceptor outer segment abnormalities as a cause of blind spot enlargement in acute zonal occult outer retinopathy-complex diseases. Am J Ophthalmol 2008; 146(1): 111–120.

27. Nozik R, Dorsch W. A new chorioretinopathy associated with anterior uveitis. Am J Ophthalmol 1973; 76: 758–762.

28. Bryan RG, Freund KB, Yannuzzi LA, et al. Multiple evanescent white dot syndrome in patients with multifocal choroiditis. Retina 2002; 22: 317–322.

29. Gass JD, Hamed LM. Acute macular neuroretinopathy and multiple evanescent white dot syndrome occurring in the same patients. Arch Ophthalmol 1989; 107: 189–193.

30. Figueroa MS, Ciancas E, Mompean B, et al. Treatment of multiple evanescent white dot syndrome with cyclosporine. Eur J Ophthalmol 2001; 11: 86–88.

31. Dreyer R, Gass J. Multifocal choroiditis and panuveitis. A syndrome that mimics ocular histoplasmosis. Arch Ophthalmol 1984; 102: 1776–1784.

32. Morgan C, Schatz H. Recurrent multifocal choroiditis. Ophthalmol 1986; 93: 1138–1147.

33. Nicolo M, Birò A, Cardillo-Piccolino F, et al. Expression of extradomain-B-containing fibronectin in subretinal choroidal neovascular membranes. American Journal of Ophthalmology 2003; 135: 7–13.

34. Khorran K, Jampol L, Rosenberg M. Blind spot enlargement as a manifestation of multifocal choroiditis. Arch Ophthalmol 1991; 109: 1403–1407.

35. Spaide R, Yannuzzi L, Freund K. Linear streaks in multifocal choroiditis and panuveitis. Retina 1991; 11: 229–231.

36. Watzke R, Packer AJ, Folk JC, et al. Punctate inner choroidopathy. Am J Ophthalmol 1984; (98): 572–584.

37. Reddy CV, Brown J Jr, Folk JC, et al. Enlarged blind spots in chorioretinal inflammatory disorders. Ophthalmology 1996; 103: 606–617.

38. Kedhar SR, Thorne JE, Wittenberg S, et al. Multifocal choroiditis with panuveitis and punctate inner choroidopathy: comparison of clinical characteristics at presentation. Retina 2007; 27(9): 1174–1179.

39. Gerstenblith AT, Thorne JE, Sobrin L, et al. Punctate inner choroidopathy: a survey analysis of 77 persons. Ophthalmology 2007; 114(6): 1201–1204.

40. Taira K, Nakazawa M, Takano Y, et al. Acute zonal occult outer retinopathy in the fellow eye 5 years after presentation of punctate inner choroidopathy. Graefes Arch Clin Exp Ophthalmol 2006; 244(7): 880–882.

41. Saito A, Saito W, Furudate N, et al. Indocyanine green angiography in a case of punctate inner choroidopathy associated with acute zonal occult outer retinopathy. Jpn J Ophthalmol 2007; 51(4): 295–300.

42. Vadala M, Lodato G, Cillino S. Multifocal choroiditis: Indocyanine green angiographic features. Ophthalmologica 2001; 215: 16–21.

43. Deutsch T, Tessler H. Inflammatory pseudohistoplasmosis. Ann Ophthalmol 1985; 17: 461–465.

44. Jakobiec F, Sacks E, Kronish JW, et al. Multifocal static creamy choroidal

infiltrates. An early sign of lymphoid neoplasia. Ophthalmology 1987; (94): 397–406.

45. Latkany PA, Jabs DA, Smith JR, et al. Multifocal choroiditis in patients with familial juvenile systemic granulomatosis. American Journal of Ophthalmology 2002; 134: 897–904.

46. Holz FG, Kim RY, Schwartz SD, et al. Acute zonal occult outer retinopathy (AZOOR) associated with multifocal choroidopathy. Eye 1994; 8(Pt 1): 77–83.

47. Grutzmacher R, Henderson D, McDonald PJ, et al. Herpes simplex chorioretinitis in a healthy adult. Am J Ophthalmol 1983; (96): 788–794.

48. Tiedeman J. Epstein–Barr viral antibodies in multifocal choroiditis and panuveitis. Am J Ophthalmol 1987; 103: 659–663.

49. Wong K, D'Amico DJ, Hedges TR 3rd, et al. Ocular involvement associated wlith chronic Epstein-Barr virus disease. Arch Ophthalmol 1987; (105): 788–792.

50. Spaide R, Sugin S, Yannuzzi LA, et al. Epstein-Barr virus antibodies in multifocal choroiditis and panuveitis. Am J Opthalmol 1991; 112(4): 410–413.

51. Scheider A. Multifocal inner choroiditis. Ger J Opthalmol 1993; 2: 1–9.

52. Martin D, Chan CC, de Smet MD, et al. The role of chorioretinal biopsy in the managment of posterior uveitis. Opthalmology 1993; (100): 5.

53. Shimada H, Yuzawa M, Hirose T, et al. Pathological findings of multifocal choroiditis with panuveitis and punctate inner choroidopathy. Jpn J Ophthalmol 2008; 52(4): 282–288.

54. Nolle B, Eckardt C. Vitrectomy in multifocal choroiditis. Ger J Ophthalmol 1993; 2: 14–19.

55. Charteris D, Lee W. Multifocal posterior uveitis: clinical and pathological findings. Br J Ophthalmol 1990; 74: 688–693.

56. Dunlop AAS, Cree IA, Hague S, et al. Multifocal choroiditis. clinicopathologic correlation. Arch Ophthalmol 1998; 116: 801–803.

57. Levy J, Shneck M, Klemperer I, et al. Punctate inner choroidopathy: resolution after oral steroid treatment and review of the literature. Can J Ophthalmol 2005; 40(5): 605–608.

58. Michel SS, Ekong A, Baltatzis S, et al. Multifocal choroiditis and panuveitis. Ophthalmology 2002; 109: 378–383.

59. Chan WM, Shneck M, Klemperer I, et al. Combined photodynamic therapy and intravitreal triamcinolone for choroidal neovascularization secondary to punctate inner choroidopathy or of idiopathic origin: one-year results of a prospective series. Retina 2008; 28(1): 71–80.

60. Cirino AC, Mathura JR Jr., Jampol LM. Resolution of activity (choroiditis and choroidal neovascularization) of chronic recurrent punctate inner choroidopathy after treatment with interferon B-1A. Retina 2006; 26(9): 1091–1092.

61. Spaide RF, Freund KB, Slakter J, et al. Treatment of subfoveal choroidal neovascularization associated with multifocal choroiditis and panuveitis with photodynamic therapy. Retina 2002; 22: 545–549.

62. Krill A, Deutman A. Acute retinal pigment epitheliitis. Am J Ophthalmol 1972; 74: 193–205.

63. Luttrull JK, Chittum ME. Acute retinal pigment epitheliitis. Am J Ophthalmol 1995; 120: 389–391.

64. Lutrull JR, Chittum ME. Acute retinal pigment epitheliitis. Am J Ophthalmol 1997; 123: 127–129.

65. Hsu CT, Harlan JB, Goldberg MF, et al. Acute posterior multifocal placoid pigment epitheliopathy associated with a systemic necrotizing vasculitis. Retina 2003; 23(1): 64–68.

66. Deutman A, Oosterhuis JA, Boen-Tan TN, et al. Acute posterior multifocal placoid pigment epitheliopathy. Br J Ophthalmol 1972; (56): 863–874.

67. Gilhotra JS, Gilhotra AK, Holdaway IM, et al. Acute retinal pigment epitheliitis associated with intravenous bisphosphonate. Br J Ophthalmol 2006; 90(6): 798–799.

68. Loh BK, Chee SP. Optical coherence tomography findings in acute retinal pigment epitheliitis. Am J Ophthalmol 2007; 143(6): 1071; author reply 1071.

69. Poyato P, et al. Acute retinal pigment epitheliitis: uncommon symptoms in a case report. Arch Soc Esp Oftalmol 2000; 1: 51–54.

70. Gass J. Acute posterior multifocal placoid pigment epitheliopathy. Arch Ophthalmol 1968; 80: 177–185.

71. Scuderi G, Recupero S, Valvo A. Acute posterior multifocal placoid pigment epitheliopathy. Ann Ophthalmol 1977; 9: 189–194.

72. Ryan S, Maumenee A. Acute posterior multifocal placoid pigment epitheliopathy. Am J Ophthalmol 1972; 81: 403–412.

73. Holt W, Regan A, Trempe C. Acute posterior multifocal placoid pigment epitheliopathy. Am J Ophthalmol 1976; 81: 403–412.

74. Savino P, Weinberg RJ, Yassin JG, et al. Diverse manifestations of acute posterior multifocal placoid pigment epitheliopathy. Am J Ophthalmol 1974; (77): 659–662.

75. Smith V, Pokorny J, Ernest JT, et al. Visual function in acute posterior multifocal placoid pigment epitheliopathy. Am J Ophthalmol 1978; (85): 192–199.

76. Abu El-Asrar AM, Alijazairy AH. Acute posterior multifocal placoid pigment epitheliopathy with retinal vasculitis and papillitis. Eye 2002; 16: 642–644.

77. Kirkham T, Ffytche T, Sanders M. Placoid pigment epitheliopahty with retinal vasculitis and papillitis. Br J Ophthalmol 1972; 56: 875–880.

78. Damato B, Nanjiani M, Foulds W. Acute posterior multifocal placoid pigment epitheliopathy. A followup study. Trans Ophthalmol Soc UK 1983; 103: 517–522.

79. Jones BE, Jampol LM, Yannuzzi LA, et al. Relentless placoid chorioretinitis. A new entity or an unusual variant of serpiginous chorioretinitis. Arch Ophthalmol 2000; 118: 931–938.

80. Fine HF, Kim E, Flynn TE, et al. Acute posterior multifocal placoid pigment epitheliopathy following varicella vaccine. Br J Ophthalmol 2008 DOI: 10.1136. 144501.

81. Borruat FX, Piguet B, Herbort CP. Acute posterior multifocal placoid pigment epitheliopathy following mumps. Ocul Immunol Inflamm 1998; 6: 189–193.

82. Clearkin L, Hung S. Acute posterior multifocal placoid pigment epitheliopathy associated with transient hearing loss. Trans Ophthalmol Soc UK 1983; 103: 562–564.

83. Kersten D, Lessell S, Carlow T. Acute posterior multifocal placoid pigment epitheliopathy and late-onset meningo-encephalitis. Ophthalmology 1987; 94: 393–396.

84. Parmeggiani F, Costagliola C, D'Angelo S, et al. Clear cell renal cell carcinoma associated with bilateral atypical acute posterior multifocal placoid pigment epitheliopathy. Oncology 2004; 66(6): 502–509.

85. Allee SD, Marks SJ. Acute posterior multifocal placoid pigment epitheliopathy with bilateral central retinal vein occlusion. Am J Ophthalmol 1998; 126: 309–312.

86. Vedantham V, Ramasamy K. Atypical manifestations of acute posterior multifocal placoid pigment epitheliopathy. Indian J Ophthalmol 2006; 54(1): 49–52.

87. Young N, Bird A, Sehmi K. Pigment epithelial diseases with abnormal choroidal perfusion. Am J Ophthalmol 1980; 90: 607–618.

88. Althaus C, Unsöld R, Figge C, et al. Cerebral complications in acute posterior multifocal placoid pigment epitheliopathy. Ger J Ophthalmol 1993; (2): 150–154.

89. Stoll G, Reiners K, Schwartz A, et al. Acute posterior multifocal placoid pigment epitheliopathy with cerebral involvement. J Neurol Neurosurg Psychiatry 1991; (54): 77–79.

90. Chiquet C, Lumbroso L, Denis P, et al. Acute posterior multifocal placoid pigment epitheliopathy associated with Wegener's granulomatosis. Retina 1999; 19: 309–313.

91. Matsuo T, Horikoshi T, Nagai C. Acute posterior multifocal placoid pigment epitheliopathy and scleritis in a patient with pANCA-positive

systemic vasculitis. Am J Ophthalmol 2002; 133: 566–568.

92. Bridges WJ, Saadeh C, Gerald R. Acute posterior multifocal placoid pigment epitheliopathy in a patient with systemic-onset juvenile rheumatoid arthritis: treatment with cyclosporin A and prednisone. Arthritis Rheum 1995; 38: 446–447.

93. Spaide R, Yannuzzi L, Slakter J. Choroidal vasculitis in acute posterior multifocal placoid epitheliopathy. Br J Ophthalmol 1991; 75: 685–687.

94. Kinyoun J, Kalina R, Klein M. Choroidal involvement in systemic necrotizing vasculitis. Arch Ophthalmol 1987; 105: 939–942.

95. Bodine S, Marino J, Camisa TJ, et al. Mutlifocal choroiditis with evidence of Lyme disease. Am J Ophthalmol 1992; 24: 169–173.

96. Roberts TV, Acute posterior multifocal placoid pigment epitheliopathy: A long-term study. Aust NZ J Ophthalmol 1997; 25: 277–281.

97. Yenerel NM, Gorgun E, Dinc UA, et al. Treatment of cystoid macular edema due to acute posterior multifocal placoid pigment epitheliopathy. Ocul Immunol Inflamm 2008; 16(1): 67–71.

98. Palestine A, Nussenblatt RB, Parver LM, et al. Progressive subretinal fibrosis and uveitis. Br J Ophthalmol 1984; (68): 667–673.

99. Gandorfer A, Ulbig MW, Kampik A. Diffuse subretinal fibrosis syndrome. Retina 2000; 20: 561–563.

100. Kaiser PK, Gragoudas ES. The Subretinal fibrosis and uveitis syndrome. Int Ophthalmol Clin 1996; 36: 145–152.

101. Wang RC, Zamir E, Dugel PU, et al. Progressive subretinal fibrosis and blindness associated with multifocal granulomatous chorioretinitis. A variant of sympathetic ophthalmia. Ophthalmology 2002; 109: 1527–1531.

102. Amaro MH, Muccioli C, Motta MM. Progressive subretinal fibrosis and multifocal granulomatous chorioretinitis. Arq Bras Oftalmol 2006; 69(3): 413–415.

103. Fuentes-Paez G, Martínez-Osorio H, Herreras JM, et al. Subretinal fibrosis and uveitis syndrome associated with

ulcerative colitis. Int J Colorectal Dis 2007; 22(3): 333–334.

104. Fuchs A, Diseases of the fundus oculi with atlas. 1949, Philadelphia: The Blakiston Co.

105. Palestine A, Nussenblatt RB, Chan CC, et al. Histopathlogy of the subretinal fibrosis and uveitis syndrome. Ophthalmology 1985; (92): 838–844.

106. Kim M, Chan CC, Belfort R Jr, et al. Histopathologic and immunohistopathologic features of subretinal fibrosis and uveitis syndrome. Am J Ophthalmol 1987; (104): 15–23.

107. Cantrill H, Folk J. Multifocal choroiditis associated with progressive subretinal fibrosis. Am J Ophthalmol 1986; 101: 170–180.

108. Turbeville SD, Cowan LD, Gass JD. Acute macular neuroretinopathy: A review of the literature. Surv Ophthalmol 2003; 48: 1–11.

109. Adan A, Sanmartí R, Burés A, et al. Successful treatment with infliximab in a patient with Diffuse Subretinal Fibrosis syndrome. Am J Ophthalmol 2007; 143(3): 533–534.

110. Gass J. Acute zonal occult outer retinopathy. Donders lecture: the Netherlands Ophthalmological Society. Maastricht Holland. June 19 1992; J Clin Neuroophthalmol 1993; 13: 79–97.

111. Jacobson SG, Morales DS, Sun XK, et al. Pattern of retinal dysfunction in acute zonal occult outer retinopathy. Ophthalmology 1995; 102: 1187–1198.

112. Francis PJ, Marinescu A, Fitzke FW, et al. Acute zonal occult outer retinopathy: towards a set of diagnostic criteria. Br J Ophthalmol 2005; 89(1): 70–73.

113. Zibrandtsen N, Munch IC, Klemp K, et al. Photoreceptor atrophy in acute zonal occult outer retinopathy. Acta Ophthalmol 2008; 86(8): 913–916.

114. Takai Y, Ishiko S, Kagokawa H, et al. Morphological study of acute zonal occult outer retinopathy (AZOOR) by multiplanar optical coherence tomography. Acta Ophthalmol 2008.

115. Li D, Kishi S. Loss of photoreceptor outer segment in acute zonal occult outer retinopathy. Arch Ophthalmol 2007; 125(9): 1194–1200.

116. Spaide RF. Collateral damage in acute zonal occult outer retinopathy. Am J Ophthalmol 2004; 138(5): 887–889.

117. Gass JD, Agarwal A, Scott IU. Acute zonal occult outer retinopathy: A long-term follow-up study. Am J Ophthalmol 2002; 134: 329–339.

118. Jacobson DM, Acute zonal occult outer retinopathy and central nervous system inflammation. J Neuro-ophthalmol 1996; 16: 172–177.

119. Volpe NJ, Rizzo JFI, Lessell S. Acute idiopathic blind spot enlargement syndrome. A review of 27 new cases. Arch Ophthalmol 2001; 119: 59–63.

120. Jampol LM, Becker KG. Perspective: White spot syndromes of the retina: A hypothesis based on the common genetic hypothesis of autoimmune/inflammatory disease. Am J Ophthalmol 2003; 135: 376–379.

121. Song ZM, Sheng YJ, Chen QS, et al. Clinical characteristics of acute zonal occult outer retinopathy in Chinese patients. Ophthalmologica 2008; 222(3): 149–156.

122. Sharma SM, Watzke RC, Weleber RG, et al. Acute zonal occult outer retinopathy (AZOOR) and pars planitis: a new association? Br J Ophthalmol 2008; 92(4): 583–584.

123. Jampol LM, Wiredu A. MEWDS, MFC, PIC, AMN, AIBSE, and AZOOR: one disease or many? Retina 1995; 15(5): 373–378.

124. Teyssot N, Bodaghi B, Cassoux N, et al. Acute posterior multifocal placoid pigment epitheliopathy, serpiginous and multifocal choroiditis: etiological and therapeutic management. J Fr Ophthalmol 2006; 29(5): 510–518.

125. Matsumoto Y, Haen SP, Spaide RF. The white dot syndromes. Compr Ophthalmol Update 2007; 8(4): 179–200; discussion 203–204.

126. Machida S, Fujiwara T, Murai K, et al. Idiopathic choroidal neovascularization as an early manifestation of inflammatory chorioretinal diseases. Retina 2008; 28(5): 703–710.

127. Sadaba LM, Moreno J, Sáinz C, et al. AZOOR. After whiplash injury. Rev Med Univ Navarra 2001; 45(4): 35–38.

Masquerade Syndromes

Scott M. Whitcup

Key concepts

- The masquerade syndromes comprise a group of disorders that occur with intraocular inflammation and are often misdiagnosed as a chronic idiopathic uveitis.
- Because many of the masquerade syndromes are malignancies or infectious processes, early diagnosis and prompt treatment are critical.
- Intraocular lymphomas are frequently non-Hodgkin's lymphomas involving the central nervous system.
- Diagnosis can be made by identifying malignant cells in the vitreous or cerebral spinal fluid; however, prompt and correct handling of specimens and review by an experienced cytopathologist are critical to the correct diagnosis.
- Nonmalignant masquerade syndromes are often treated with unnecessary antiinflammatory therapy.
- Response to antiinflammatory therapy does not rule out a masquerade syndrome; however, lack of a response to therapy should suggest the possibility of a masquerade syndrome.
- The diagnosis of masquerade syndrome should be considered in all cases of idiopathic uveitis.

The masquerade syndromes comprise a group of disorders that occur with intraocular inflammation and are often misdiagnosed as a chronic idiopathic uveitis. The term masquerade syndrome was first used in the ophthalmic literature in 1967 to describe a conjunctival carcinoma manifesting as a case of chronic conjunctivitis;[1] today, however, it is used most commonly to describe disorders simulating chronic uveitis. Because many of the masquerade syndromes are malignant processes, early diagnosis and prompt treatment are critical (**Box 30-1**). Other disorders such as retinal degenerations and intraocular foreign body can also masquerade as a uveitis, and, again, misdiagnosis frequently leads to inappropriate therapy. The focus of this chapter is on the malignant conditions that can masquerade as uveitis, but nonmalignant disorders often misdiagnosed as chronic idiopathic ocular inflammatory disease are also discussed.

Intraocular lymphoma

Although intraocular lymphoma is a lethal disease, early diagnosis and treatment can improve the prognosis. This disease was previously misnamed reticulum-cell sarcoma because the large malignant cells resembled sarcoma cells. However, these tumors are more appropriately classified as intraocular large-cell lymphomas.

Several types of lymphoma can involve the eye and mimic uveitis. Hodgkin's disease, which is characterized by painless lymphadenopathy, fever, night sweats, weight loss, and the presence of Reed–Sternberg cells on histologic examination, can involve the eye. Ocular involvement in Hodgkin's lymphoma is relatively rare and usually occurs late in the course of the disease.[2] There is one case in the ophthalmic literature in which a patient with Hodgkin's disease had retinal periphlebitis as the initial clinical finding.[3] Other ocular manifestations include iritis or chorioretinitis with associated vitritis. In addition, a paraneoplastic retinopathy associated with Hodgkin's lymphoma has been reported.[4]

Two clinically distinct forms of non-Hodgkin's lymphoma more frequently involve the eye: non-Hodgkin's lymphoma of the central nervous system (NHL-CNS), and systemic non-Hodgkin's lymphoma that metastasizes to the eye. Patients with systemic non-Hodgkin's lymphoma metastatic to the eye are usually quite sick, with fever, lymphadenopathy, and weight loss. Diagnosis in these patients is rarely puzzling. In contrast, the patient with NHL-CNS that first manifests ocular findings often poses a diagnostic dilemma.

Non-Hodgkin's lymphoma of central nervous system

NHL-CNS, also known as primary CNS lymphoma, arises from the brain, spinal cord, leptomeninges, or the eye, and may then spread throughout the CNS.[5–7] Systemic spread outside the CNS occurs more rarely and has been reported in fewer than 10% of autopsies.[8,9] Although NHL-CNS is a rare tumor, its incidence has trebled over the last 10 years, an increase that cannot be fully explained by AIDS or other causes of immunosuppression.[10] The median age for patients with NHL-CNS is between 50 and 60 years; there is a slight male preponderance.[5,10] Cases in children have been reported, however,[11,12] and the two youngest patients with reported cases of intraocular lymphoma were 15 and 27 years old.[13,14] As for NHL-CNS, immunosuppression appears to be a risk factor for the development of ocular lymphoma. Ocular lymphoma has now been associated with AIDS.[15] In addition, ocular lymphoma has been reported in a number of patients undergoing immunosuppression after organ transplantation.[16]

In a large case series of Hochberg and Miller,[10] patients with NHL-CNS showed four distinct clinical profiles: (1)

Box 30-1 Ophthalmic conditions masquerading as idiopathic uveitis

MALIGNANT DISORDERS

Intraocular lymphomas
> Non-Hodgkin's lymphoma of central nervous system
> Systemic non-Hodgkin's lymphomas metastatic to eye
> Hodgkin's lymphoma

Leukemia

Carcinoma metastatic to eye
> Lung
> Renal
> Breast

Uveal melanoma

Childhood malignancies
> Retinoblastoma
> Leukemia
> Medulloepithelioma
> Juvenile xanthogranuloma

Paraneoplastic syndromes
> Cancer-associated retinopathy
> Melanoma-associated retinopathy
> Bilateral diffuse uveal melanocytic proliferation

NONMALIGNANT DISORDERS

Intraocular foreign body

Retinal detachment

Myopic degeneration

Pigment dispersion syndrome

Retinal degenerations

Postoperative infections
> Fungal
> *Propionibacterium acnes*

Postvaccination disorders and drug reactions
> Rifabutin
> Didanosine (ddl)

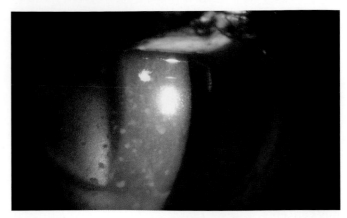

Figure 30-1. Anterior segment of the eye of a patient with biopsy-proven intraocular large-cell lymphoma demonstrating corneal keratitic precipitates.

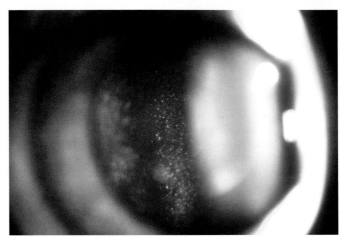

Figure 30-2. Slit-lamp biomicroscopy examination revealing sheets of vitreous cells characteristic of intraocular lymphoma.

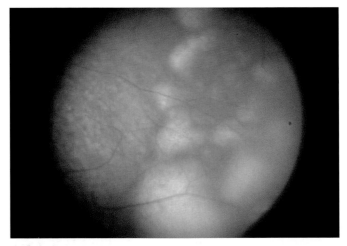

Figure 30-3. Retinal photograph of a patient with biopsy-proven intraocular lymphoma demonstrating multiple yellow lesions deep to retina.

solitary or multiple discrete intracranial nodules, (2) diffuse meningeal or periventricular lesions, (3) subretinal infiltrates or vitritis, and (4) localized intradural spinal masses. Ocular involvement may precede detectable disease in other parts of the CNS, although the percentage of patients in whom this occurs may be overestimated in the ophthalmic literature, in which there is a selection bias for patients who have ocular disease. In a study performed at the National Eye Institute, two-thirds of the patients with ocular disease had undiagnosed CNS disease at the time of their diagnosis.[17] The mean time between the onset of ocular symptoms and the onset of CNS symptoms in one study was 29 months (range, 7–108 months).[18] In this study, systemic spread outside the CNS was noted in 6% of patients and disease was limited to the eye in 22%.

The most common ocular symptoms associated with intraocular lymphoma are blurred vision and floaters; redness and pain are rare. Patients have reduced visual acuity, although the vision is usually better than one would expect from the clinical examination. Slit-lamp biomicroscopic examination often reveals mild anterior segment inflammation, with aqueous cells and flare and keratic precipitates on the corneal endothelium (**Fig. 30-1**).[7,13,17–19]

Vitreous cells, occurring in sheets, are typical of the disease (**Fig. 30-2**), and examination of the fundus usually shows subretinal yellow infiltrates through a hazy vitreous (**Fig. 30-3**). Atypical presentations have been reported, including a hemorrhagic retinal vasculitis that resembled a viral retinitis (**Fig. 30-4**).[20] In some patients the fundus may appear

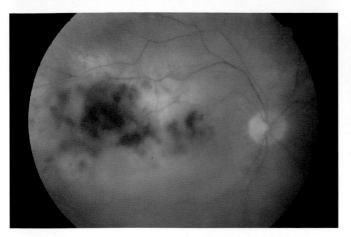

Figure 30-4. Fundus photograph of patient with intraocular lymphoma showing retinal infiltrates and hemorrhage mimicking cytomegalovirus retinitis. Findings resolved with therapy for lymphoma.

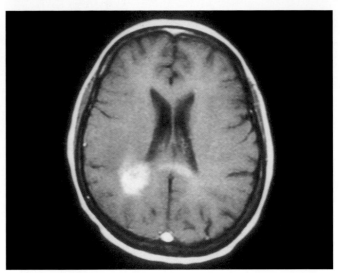

Figure 30-6. MRI scan showing a mass lesion in the temporal lobe of a patient with intraocular lymphoma.

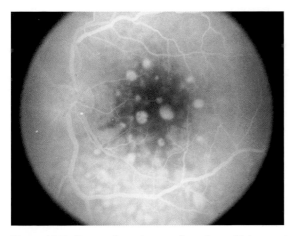

Figure 30-5. Fluorescein angiogram of a patient with intraocular lymphoma showing multiple circular areas of hyperfluorescence corresponding to tumor infiltration.

normal, and subretinal lesions may be noted only with fluorescein angiography (**Fig. 30-5**). Although the disease may start in one eye, bilateral disease is common after several months.[13,17]

Diagnosis

Many patients with intraocular lymphoma have CNS disease at the time of presentation, and a thorough history and neurologic examination are warranted. CNS findings such as headaches, focal weakness, sensory deficits, confusion, and difficulty with gait are common. A history of recent seizure is also a strong indication of CNS involvement. Magnetic resonance imaging (MRI) and a lumbar puncture should be performed on all patients suspected of having an intraocular lymphoma, even if neurologic symptoms are absent (**Fig. 30-6**). Because lymphoma cells can be fragile, samples should be immediately hand-carried to the cytology laboratory for processing, and at least 5–10 mL of cerebrospinal fluid (CSF) should also be sent for cytologic examination. A repeat lumbar puncture may be necessary for the diagnosis.

If the CSF shows no malignant cells, we perform a standard three-port pars plana vitrectomy in an attempt to make

the diagnosis of lymphoma. Tissue culture medium (RPMI-1640, Roswell Park Memorial Institute, Mediatech, Inc., Herndon, VA.) enriched with 10% fetal calf serum is added to the collection chamber of the vitrectomy machine to improve cell viability. An initial sample of core vitreous is also obtained at the start of the vitrectomy and taken immediately to the cytology laboratory for processing.

The methods used to process vitreous specimens have been delineated previously.[21,22] Briefly, the vitreous specimen is centrifuged at 1000 rpm for 8 minutes at 4°C. The cell pellet is resuspended in 4 mL of fresh tissue culture medium and cytocentrifuged for 10 minutes. The machine places centrifuged specimens directly onto gelatinized slides. Giemsa-, Gram-, or Diff Quick-stained slides are prepared, and additional slides are prepared for immunohistochemical staining for B- and T-cell markers and for κ and λ light chains. We prefer a more complete surgical vitrectomy to obtain as much vitreous as possible for analysis, but some investigators have used a vitreous aspiration needle tap in patients with possible intraocular lymphoma.[23]

Even when vitreous specimens are properly processed, diagnosis of an intraocular lymphoma can be difficult. Multiple vitreous specimens may be needed to make the diagnosis. Char and colleagues[24] reported that in three of 14 patients in whom ocular lymphoma was later diagnosed more than one vitreous specimen was required, and we found that multiple samples were needed to make the correct diagnosis in three of 10 patients.[17] In another series of 84 vitrectomy specimens, 14% were diagnosed as definite 'malignant lymphoma', 6% as 'suspicious of neoplastic disease', 74% as 'reactive cellular infiltrate', and 5% 'insufficient for diagnosis'.[25] Although mishandling of vitreous samples partially accounts for some of the difficulty in making the correct diagnosis, treatment with corticosteroids may obscure the diagnosis of intraocular lymphoma. Corticosteroids can be cytolytic in CNS lymphoma, and this exquisite sensitivity of tumor cells appears to be unique to NHL-CNS. In a number of patients corticosteroid therapy caused CNS lymphoma lesions to reduce in size or disappear, hindering the ability to make the correct diagnosis. Because many patients with intraocular lymphoma are treated with corticosteroids at the time of vitrectomy, the viability of tumor cells in the samples may be diminished, which may contribute to the difficulty in diagnosing this disease. Finally, because the number of malignant cells in a vitreous specimen may be few, it is critical that the cytologist be experienced in the diagnosis of lymphoma.

Recent data suggest that intravitreal cytokine levels can be useful in the diagnosis of intraocular lymphoma. Interleukin (IL)-10 can be produced by lymphoma cells and levels of IL-10 are elevated in both the serum and vitreous of patients with intraocular lymphoma. In contrast, levels of IL-6 are elevated in the vitreous of patients with intraocular inflammation unrelated to a malignant neoplasm. We reported that levels of IL-10 exceeded those of IL-6 in all five patients with intraocular lymphoma examined, but in none of the 13 patients with uveitis.[26] This test, however, is neither 100% sensitive nor 100% specific. We have seen patients with intraocular lymphoma with higher levels of IL-6 than IL-10.[27] However, when IL-10 is elevated in vitreous specimens, the clinician should remain suspicious about an underlying malignancy, and these patients should be closely followed. A study of 51 patients with proven intraocular lymphoma and 108 patients with uveitis of other causes showed that measurement of IL-10 in the aqueous humor can be a good screening test for NHL-CNS.[28] A cutoff of 50 pg/mL in the aqueous humor was associated with a sensitivity of 0.89 and a specificity of 0.93, and the area under the respective ROC curves was only slightly higher for vitreous levels (0.989) than for aqueous levels (0.962).

Typical lymphoma cells are large and pleomorphic with scanty cytoplasm, and hypersegmented nuclei with prominent nucleoli are often diagnostic (**Fig. 30-7**). However, only a few of these characteristic cells are present in any single specimen, and most vitreous samples contain mainly reactive lymphocytes, histiocytes, necrotic debris, and fibrinous material. The diagnosis of NHL-CNS is usually confirmed by the finding of malignant cells showing B-cell markers with either a κ or a λ light chain monoclonal response. Gross examination of eyes with NHL-CNS shows large gray patches of subretinal and retinal infiltration above a thickened choroid (**Fig. 30-8**). Collections of lymphoma cells are characteristically found between Bruch's membrane and the retinal pigment epithelium (RPE) (**Fig. 30-9**). Reactive T lymphocytes can be seen in the retina and choroid in areas surrounding the tumor cells.

The differential diagnosis for patients suspected of having an intraocular lymphoma often includes sarcoidosis. Therefore, evaluation of these patients should include a chest X-ray, angiotensin-converting enzyme (ACE) measurement, serum and urine calcium levels, and pulmonary function testing to rule out this diagnosis. A limited gallium scan of the chest and lacrimal glands may also be useful. If patients have a diminished diffusing capacity on pulmonary function testing, we often obtain a pulmonary consultation

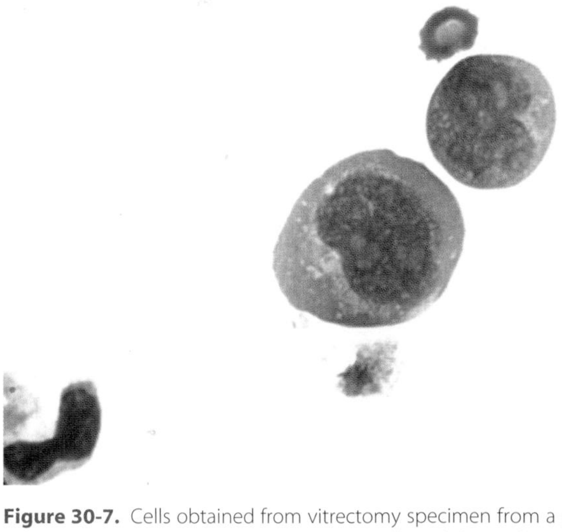

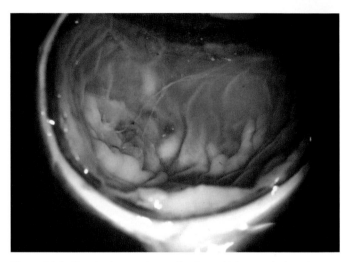

Figure 30-8. Enucleation specimen of patient with intraocular lymphoma shows multiple white areas of retinal and subretinal tumor infiltration with adjacent areas of retinal hemorrhage.

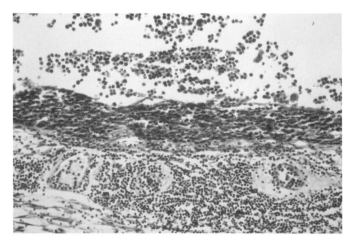

Figure 30-9. Photomicrograph of enucleated globe shown in Figure 30-8 reveals tumor infiltration between Bruch's membrane and the retinal pigment epithelium. Reactive lymphocytes and some tumor cells are seen in the overlying vitreous. (Hematoxylin & eosin stain; original magnification ×200.)

Figure 30-7. Cells obtained from vitrectomy specimen from a patient with large-cell lymphoma demonstrating large cells with hyperchromatic, pleomorphic nuclei. (Diff Quick stain; Original magnification ×1000.)
(Reproduced with permission from Whitcup et al: Intraocular lymphoma: clinical and histopathologic diagnosis. Ophthalmology 100:1399–1406, 1993.)

and consider a CT scan of the chest and bronchoscopic examination to make the diagnosis of sarcoidosis. Other diseases to consider include syphilis, tuberculosis, acute retinal necrosis, and cytomegalovirus retinitis.

Treatment

The treatment of NHL-CNS is controversial and the ideal therapy is as yet unproven. Radiation therapy was first proposed for the treatment of a chronic uveitis in 1911,[29] and historically, radiotherapy has been recommended as the initial therapy for NHL-CNS.[30] In patients with detectable lymphoma limited to the eyes, controversy centers on whether to limit therapy to the eye or to treat the CNS prophylactically. Char and colleagues[24] reported on two patients with isolated ocular involvement treated with only ocular radiation who had no recurrent disease 24 and 109 months after treatment. NHL-CNS tends to be quite radiosensitive and responds well to 15–45 Gy. However, many researchers recommend cranial irradiation (45 Gy to the whole brain) in addition to orbital radiation in patients with isolated ocular involvement, as many patients have subclinical CNS involvement by the time intraocular lymphoma manifests.[24,31] In the series of Peterson and colleagues,[14] 10 of 11 patients with lymphoma limited to the eyes at initial presentation later developed CNS disease. In fact, Rouwen and colleagues[31] advise using a combination of chemotherapy and radiotherapy for intraocular lymphoma even if CNS disease cannot be documented on MRI or lumbar puncture. Chemotherapy is recommended to treat possible CNS disease, and radiotherapy is given because penetration of the blood–retinal barrier by chemotherapeutic agents is uncertain. If CNS disease is documented, there is less controversy surrounding the treatment of intraocular lymphoma. In these patients, the combination of radiotherapy and chemotherapy is more frequently recommended, although this therapeutic approach may not be ideal because of its induced CNS toxicity.

A number of chemotherapy regimens have been used for the treatment of intraocular lymphoma. The use of high-dose cytarabine (Ara-C) can lead to therapeutic drug levels in the CSF, and there have been reports of successful treatment of intraocular lymphomas with this therapy alone.[32] However, some studies indicate that CSF levels of systemically administered chemotherapeutic agents may be variable and short-lived.[33] We therefore recommend placement of an Ommaya reservoir for delivery of intrathecal methotrexate to ensure adequate drug levels in the CSF. A number of researchers have used intrathecal methotrexate for the treatment of intraocular lymphoma, but always in combination with radiotherapy.[24] DeAngelis and colleagues[5] showed that the addition of chemotherapy to cranial radiotherapy significantly improved disease-free survival and contributed to overall survival in patients with primary CNS lymphoma.

However, combined radiotherapy and chemotherapy can cause significant toxicity. Cranial radiotherapy produces significant CNS toxicity in long-term survivors. Furthermore, Bleyer[34] and DeAngelis and colleagues[5] emphasize that chemotherapy can exacerbate the toxicity produced by radiotherapy, especially with methotrexate. In contrast to the usual sequence of therapy for intraocular lymphoma, in which radiotherapy is administered before chemotherapy,

the use of chemotherapy before radiotherapy may reduce the risk of leukoencephalopathy and protect against late toxicity.[34,35]

The National Cancer Institute and the National Eye Institute investigated a treatment protocol using systemic and intrathecal chemotherapy for the treatment of NHL-CNS.[36] In this trial, 14 nonimmunocompromised patients received a chemotherapy regimen that incorporated a 24-hour infusion of high-dose methotrexate with leucovorin rescue, thiotepa, vincristine, dexamethasone, and intrathecal Ara-C and methotrexate. The chemotherapy was administered in 21-day cycles and the response rate was 100%. Eleven patients (79%) had a complete response and three (21%) had a partial response. At more than 4.5 years of follow-up the cumulative survival rate was 68.8%, and the progression-free survival rate was 34.3%. The median survival had not been reached at the time of publication, and the progression-free survival was 16.5 months. Toxicity of the treatment regimen included severe drug-related leukoencephalopathy in two patients, grade 3 or 4 neutropenia in 50% of the cycles, ileus in one patient, and seizures in two. Although this was a small trial, we believe that the use of chemotherapy alone as initial therapy should be investigated further. Finally, high-dose thiotepa, busulfan and cyclophosphamide followed by autologous bone marrow transplantation appeared to be effective in some patients with refractory intraocular lymphoma.[37]

Local recurrence of NHL-CNS in the eye can be difficult to diagnose and treat. Definitive diagnosis requires obtaining a vitreous specimen for cytologic examination. One therapeutic option for ocular recurrence is radiation. However, we have seen a number of patients with ocular recurrence who had already received maximal radiation to the eyes. Intravitreal injections of chemotherapeutic agents may be a useful therapeutic approach for these patients. Combinations of intravitreal methotrexate, fluorouracil, and dexamethasone have been studied.[38–41] The safety of intravitreal injections of retuximab is being assessed.[42]

The presence of intraocular lymphoma is usually associated with concomitant brain disease, and survival is similar to that for other presentations of primary CNS lymphoma.[43] Some data suggest that patients whose ocular disease was identified and treated before CNS progression had a significantly improved survival,[44] thereby emphasizing the importance of early diagnosis and therapy. Although many patients with NHL-CNS have a good initial response to therapy, recurrence is common, and in some studies the 5-year survival is <5%. Hochberg and Miller[10] reported an overall median survival time from diagnosis of 13.5 months in patients with primary CNS lymphoma, and Freeman and colleagues[18] reported a mean survival time of 26 months for patients with intraocular lymphoma. However, some reports suggested that intrathecal chemotherapy combined with radiotherapy of the orbits and whole brain may improve survival.[24] Hopefully, additional research into new therapeutic approaches will lead to improved survival in this disease.

Systemic Non-Hodgkin's lymphoma metastatic to eye

Systemic NHL can metastasize to the eye and cause an anterior or a posterior uveitis. Unlike the location of NHL-CNS cells between the RPE and Bruch's membrane, lymphoma cells in patients with systemic NHL characteristically infiltrate the choroid and may be mistaken for an ocular melanoma.[45] Metastatic lymphoma may also cause a hypopyon or hyphema in an otherwise uninflamed eye.[46] Although most patients with NHL have symptoms of lymphadenopathy, fever, and weight loss, ocular involvement may be the initial presentation of the disease.[45]

Lymphoid hyperplasia of uvea

Lymphoid hyperplasia of the uvea is a disorder characterized by infiltration of the uveal tract by well-differentiated small lymphocytes. The disease was initially referred to as inflammatory pseudotumors of the uveal tract or intraocular pseudotumor.[47,48] Although the disease is usually unilateral, bilateral cases have been reported. Clinical features include anterior uveitis, vitritis, choroidal infiltrates (**Fig. 30-10**), and iris heterochromia.[48,49] Open angle glaucoma is common, owing to infiltration of the anterior chamber angle. Extraocular extension may occur, leading to conjunctival salmon-colored lesions, as well as orbital masses that cause proptosis and diplopia.[48,50] The disease is usually painless unless severe glaucoma develops.

Diagnosis has been based on histologic findings in enucleation specimens or biopsy specimens obtained from extraocular extensions of the tumor. We recently were able to make the diagnosis on the basis of a chorioretinal biopsy specimen in a 39-year-old man with painless choroidal thickening.[51] A number of pathologists believe that lymphoid hyperplasia of the uvea is probably a low-grade lymphoid neoplasia. Ten cases of reactive lymphoid hyperplasia of the uvea were reevaluated using immunohistochemical and molecular analyses at the Armed Forces Institute of Pathology.[52] Eight of the 10 were low-grade lymphomas histologically and by immunohistochemistry. The tumor often responds to therapy with corticosteroids, although some tumors warrant the use of moderate doses of radiotherapy; unlike patients with NHL-CNS, the long-term prognosis for these patients is quite favorable.[49,50]

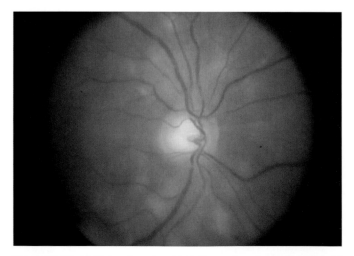

Figure 30-10. Multiple yellow choroidal infiltrates in patient with lymphoid hyperplasia of uvea.

Other malignant processes manifesting as uveitis

A uveal melanoma can manifest as a unilateral uveitis.[53] Melanomas involving the ciliary body can produce dilated episcleral vessels called sentinel vessels, which may be misdiagnosed as an episcleritis. Melanomas of the iris can produce anterior chamber cells and flare,[54] and choroidal melanomas are often associated with cataract and a focal choroidal mass that may be mistaken for a sarcoid or tuberculous granuloma or a posterior scleritis.[55] Leukemia can masquerade as uveitis in adults. Chronic myeloid leukemia in blast crisis and relapsing acute myeloid leukemia have been reported as masquerade syndromes.[56,57] These patients often develop a severe anterior segment cellular infiltration with hypopyon. Diagnosis can often be made on cytologic findings from an anterior chamber paracentesis. A panuveitis has been described more rarely in patients with leukemia.[58]

Choroidal metastases can produce signs and symptoms of uveitis. In some case series, up to half of the ocular metastases are recognized before the diagnosis of an underlying malignant process.[59] Renal and lung carcinomas are the malignant conditions most likely to manifest with ocular metastases. Although breast carcinomas frequently metastasize to the eye, in more than 90% of patients the primary lesion is known at the time the ocular lesion is noted. Patients with possible metastatic disease to the eye should undergo a thorough medical evaluation to determine the underlying primary cancer. In some patients, needle aspiration of the ocular tumor may be helpful in the diagnosis.[60]

In children, retinoblastoma may manifest with tumor cells floating in the anterior chamber and be mistaken for iritis.[61] Because retinoblastoma is the most common intraocular malignant process in childhood, the possibility of retinoblastoma should be excluded in any young child with leukokoria, strabismus, or an undiagnosed uveitis. Acute myelogenous leukemia can also manifest as uveitis in children, and in some cases, an anterior chamber paracentesis can be diagnostic.[62,63] Other tumors, such as medulloepitheliomas, and benign lesions such as juvenile xanthogranuloma can masquerade as idiopathic uveitis.[64]

Paraneoplastic syndromes

Paraneoplastic syndromes may cause intraocular inflammation with an autoimmune retinopathy and masquerade as a uveitis. Cancer-associated retinopathy (CAR) is a paraneoplastic syndrome that was initially described in three patients with oat cell carcinoma of the lung,[65] but has now been reported with a number of malignant conditions. Patients usually have loss of vision, and although the fundus can appear normal early in the course of the disease, vascular sheathing, disturbances of the RPE, and optic disc pallor may ensue. Histologic studies show destruction of the photoreceptors.[66] Thirkill and coworkers[67] identified retinal autoantibodies in patients with CAR, and some have responded favorably to corticosteroid therapy. These findings suggest that the retinal destruction may be partly immune mediated.

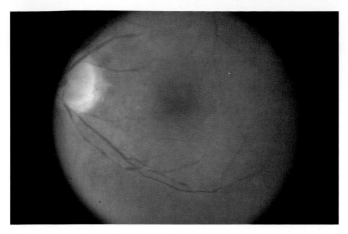

Figure 30-11. Retina photograph of a patient with recoverin-associated retinopathy. Optic disc pallor, attenuated retinal vessels, and areas of retinal pigment epithelial atrophy are seen.

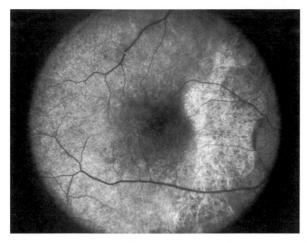

Figure 30-12. Late-phase fluorescein angiogram from a patient with acute zonal occult outer retinopathy showing a large patch of hyperfluorescence extended from the optic disc to the macula. *(Courtesy Muriel Kaiser-Kupfer, MD.)*

We have seen a patient with a clinical picture similar to that of CAR but with no underlying malignancy (**Fig. 30-11**).[68] This patient had elevated levels of antibody against recoverin, and we termed this immunologically and clinically distinctive condition recoverin-associated retinopathy. These cases of nonparaneoplastic autoimmune retinopathy may also include disorders such as acute zonal occult outer retinopathy (AZOOR) (**Fig. 30-12**); however, more research is needed to determine the pathogenesis of these diseases.[69]

Another paraneoplastic disorder that can masquerade as an idiopathic uveitis has recently been named bilateral diffuse uveal melanocytic proliferation (BDUMP). Machemer[70] first reported bilateral diffuse uveal melanocytic tumors in a patient with a large retroperitoneal mass thought to be pancreatic carcinoma, and Barr and colleagues[71] reported on four similar bilateral diffuse melanocytic uveal tumors in patients with an associated systemic malignant process diagnosed by biopsy or at autopsy. Although the condition occurs in patients with carcinomas, the underlying malignant processes are often occult.[72] Gass and Glatzer[73] characterize the ocular findings by the presence of multiple subtle round and oval subretinal red patches that demonstrate early hyperfluo-

rescence on angiographic examination; multiple, slightly elevated, pigmented and nonpigmented uveal melanocytic tumors with evidence of diffuse thickening of the uveal tract; exudative retinal detachment; and the rapid development of cataracts. Episcleral injection, vitreous cells, and other signs of mild ocular inflammation can be seen.

Histopathologic findings in the ocular lesions are diffuse uveal tract infiltrates with apparently benign, spindle-shaped melanocytic cells. Some of these cells have vesiculated nuclei with prominent nucleoli, and many have foamy cytoplasm, but mitotic figures are not characteristic.[71] BDUMP should be suspected in patients with bilateral diffuse melanocytic uveal tumors, serous retinal detachments, and cataract. It is important to recognize this condition so that patients can be evaluated for underlying malignant conditions that may warrant immediate therapy to improve prognosis.

Multiple sclerosis

Ocular inflammatory disease classified as intermediate uveitis may occur in patients with multiple sclerosis. Although some authors classify multiple sclerosis in a list of masquerade syndromes, we prefer to consider multiple sclerosis as a cause of uveitis – like other uveitides with both CNS and ocular manifestations, such as Vogt–Koyanagi–Harada syndrome. Multiple sclerosis as a cause of uveitis is discussed in the chapter on intermediate uveitis (Chapter 21).

Other nonmalignant conditions

A number of nonmalignant conditions can masquerade as idiopathic uveitis. An intraocular foreign body may elicit an anterior or a posterior uveitis. Patients with uniocular uveitis should be questioned about possible antecedent trauma. Gonioscopic examination should be performed to rule out a foreign body in the angle, and patients at high risk for an intraocular foreign body, such as construction workers, may require an ultrasound or CT scan to make the diagnosis. Metastatic squamous epithelial downgrowth after cataract surgery has masqueraded as chronic inflammation.[74] Retinal detachment in atopic dermatitis can masquerade as a panuveitis.[75]

A number of retinal diseases can masquerade as ocular inflammatory disease. Retinal detachment can sometimes produce enough intraocular inflammation to be misdiagnosed as a uveitis, and myopic degeneration can produce cream-colored atrophic lesions that may be confused with a focal choroiditis. We have also seen patients with advanced atrophic age-related macular degeneration misdiagnosed as an idiopathic white-dot syndrome.

Mydriatic agents can cause pigmented cells in the aqueous humor and may lead to improper grading of anterior chamber inflammation. Pigment dispersion syndrome is characterized by accumulation of pigment on the posterior surface of the central cornea in a vertical, spindle-shaped pattern (Krukenberg's spindle) (**Fig. 30-13**). Pigment granules may also be deposited on the anterior surface of the lens and on the iris, leading to heterochromia. Pigment dispersion may be associated with glaucoma, and in some patients may be mistaken for a uveitis.[76] Patients with retinal

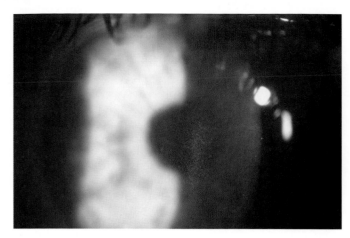

Figure 30-13. Kruckenberg's spindle in a patient with pigment dispersion syndrome that masqueraded as anterior uveitis. *(Courtesy of Muriel Kaiser-Kupfer, MD.)*

Table 30-1 Uveitis associated with medications

Medication	Uveitis
Anticholinesterases and direct-acting agonists	Anterior uveitis
Hydralazine	Lupus-like syndrome with episcleritis and retinal vasculitis
Nitrogen mustard	Necrotizing uveitis with retinal vasculitis
Rifabutin	Hypopyon uveitis
Procainamide	Lupus-like syndrome with episcleritis
Intraocular gases	
Air	Anterior uveitis
Perfluorocarbons	Fibrinous anterior uveitis
Silicone oil	Anterior uveitis
α-Chymotrypsin	Severe vitritis
Topical prostaglandin analogues	Anterior uveitis, cystoid macular edema

degenerations, such as retinitis pigmentosa (RP), may have a number of signs consistent with underlying inflammatory disease. Vitreous cells, posterior subcapsular cataract, and cystoid macular edema may occur,[77-79] and in patients in whom the characteristic bone spicule pigment is minimal the underlying diagnosis of RP may be missed. It is of interest that some have suggested that the ocular inflammation in these patients may be due to a secondary immunologic reaction against retinal antigens released into the vitreous as the retina degenerates. Thirkill and colleagues[80] showed that sera from 11 of 52 patients with RP (21%) exhibited a minimum of twice the clinically normal reactivity with retinal antigens when assayed by enzyme-linked immunosorbent assay, and of these 11 patients eight possessed antibodies to the retinal S-antigen. The authors concluded that patients with RP who have indications of immunologic hypersensitivity to known uveitopathogenic retinal antigens are at higher risk for autoimmune retinopathies. Williams and coworkers[81] demonstrated that activated RP peripheral lymphocytes adhered to and altered cultured human RPE cells, suggesting that immune-mediated cytopathologic effects may contribute to the retinal degeneration in RP. If this secondary immunologic response contributes to the deterioration of visual function in patients with RP, immunosuppressive therapy may have a role in the treatment of some patients with retinal degeneration, although this hypothesis needs to be tested in controlled studies.

Indolent ocular infections may mimic a chronic idiopathic uveitis, and these are discussed in detail in Chapters 9 and 10. Fungal infections of the choroid, retina, and vitreous may occur in immunosuppressed patients, in patients with systemic fungal infections, or in patients who have recently had surgery. *Propionibacterium acnes*, a pathogen that has recently been recognized as a cause of uveitis, may not appear clinically for months after cataract surgery. *P. acnes* endophthalmitis is discussed in detail in Chapter 18.

Finally, uveitis may occur after vaccination and has also been associated with a vast number of medications, some which are listed in **Table 30-1**. Even topical administration of corticosteroids has been associated with the development of an anterior uveitis.[82] Many of the associations between uveitis and medications may not represent a direct causal effect, but patients with an anterior uveitis should still be asked whether they have recently started taking any new medications.

It is clear that a number of entities can masquerade as idiopathic uveitis, and in the absence of a correct diagnosis inappropriate therapy may be prescribed. The diagnosis of a masquerade syndrome should therefore be considered in the evaluation of all patients with undiagnosed inflammatory eye disease.

References

1. Theodore FH. Conjunctival carcinoma masquerading as chronic conjunctivitis. Eye Ear Nose Throat Mon 1967; 46: 1419–1420.
2. Kamellin S. Uveitis associated with Hodgkin's disease: report of a case. Arch Ophthalmol 1944; 31: 517–519.
3. Barr CC, Joondeph HC. Retinal periphlebitis as the initial clinical finding in a patient with Hodgkin's disease. Retina 1983; 3: 253–257.
4. To KW, Thirkill CE, Jakobiec FA, et al. Lymphoma-associated retinopathy. Ophthalmology 2002; 109: 2149–2153.
5. DeAngelis LM, Yahalom J, Thaler H, et al. Combined modality therapy for primary CNS lymphoma. J Clin Oncol 1992; 10: 635–643.
6. Appen RE. Posterior uveitis and primary cerebral reticulum cell sarcoma. Arch Ophthalmol 1975; 93: 123–124.
7. Rockwood EJ, Zakov ZN, Bay JW. Combined malignant lymphoma of the eye and CNS (reticulum-cell sarcoma). J Neurosurg 1984; 61: 369–374.
8. Henry JM, Heffner RR Jr, Dillard SH, et al. Primary malignant lymphomas of the central nervous system. Cancer 1974; 34: 1293–1302.
9. Murray K, Kun L, Cox J. Primary malignant lymphoma of the central nervous system: results of treatment of

11 cases and review of the literature. J Neurosurg 1986; 65: 600–607.

10. Hochberg FH, Miller DC. Primary central nervous system lymphoma. J Neurosurg 1988; 68: 835–853.

11. Helle TL, Britt RH, Colby TV. Primary lymphoma of the central nervous system: clinicopathological study of experience at Stanford. J Neurosurg 1984; 60: 94–103.

12. Cohen IJ, Vogel R, Matz S, et al. Successful non-neurotoxic therapy (without radiation) of a multifocal primary brain lymphoma with methotrexate, vincristine, and BCNY protocol (DEMOB). Cancer 1986; 57: 6–11.

13. Qualman SJ, Mendelsohn G, Mann RB, et al. Intraocular lymphomas: natural history based on a clinicopathologic study of eight cases and review of the literature. Cancer 1983; 52: 878–886.

14. Peterson K, Gordon KB, Heinemann M-H, et al. The clinical spectrum of ocular lymphoma. Cancer 1993; 72: 843–849.

15. Schanzer CM, Font RL, O'Malley RE. Primary ocular malignant lymphoma associated with the acquired immune deficiency syndrome. Ophthalmology 1991; 98: 88–91.

16. Johnson BL. Intraocular and central nervous system lymphoma in a cardiac transplant recipient. Ophthalmology 1992; 99: 987–992.

17. Whitcup SM, de Smet MD, Rubin BI, et al. Intraocular lymphoma: clinical and histopathologic diagnosis. Ophthalmology 1993; 100: 1399–1406.

18. Freeman LN, Schachat AP, Knox DL, et al. Clinical features, laboratory investigations, and survival in ocular reticulum cell sarcoma. Ophthalmology 1987; 94: 1631–1639.

19. Barr CC, Green WR, Payne JW, et al. Intraocular reticulum-cell sarcoma: clinicopathologic study of four cases and review of the literature. Surv Ophthalmol 1975; 19: 224–239.

20. de Smet MD, Nussenblatt RB, Davis JL, et al. Large cell lymphoma masquerading as a viral retinitis. Int Ophthalmol 1990; 14: 413–417.

21. Davis JL, Solomon D, Nussenblatt RB, et al. Immunocytochemical staining of vitreous cells: indications, techniques, and results. Ophthalmology 1992; 99: 250–256.

22. Ljung BM, Char D, Miller TR, et al. Intraocular lymphoma: cytologic diagnosis and the role of immunologic markers. Acta Cytol 1988; 32: 840–847.

23. Lobo A, Lightman S. Vitreous aspiration needle tap in the diagnosis of intraocular inflammation. Ophthalmology 2003; 110: 595–599.

24. Char DH, Ljung B-M, Miller T, et al. Primary intraocular lymphoma (ocular reticulum cell sarcoma): diagnosis and management. Ophthalmology 1988; 95: 625–630.

25. Coupland SE, Bechrakis NE, Anastassiou G, et al. Evaluation of vitrectomy specimens and chorioretinal biopsies in the diagnosis of primary intraocular lymphoma in patients with Masquerade syndrome. Graefes Arch Clin Exp Ophthalmol 2003; 241: 860–870.

26. Whitcup SM, Stark-Vancs V, Wittes RE, et al. Association of interleukin 10 in the vitreous and cerebrospinal fluid and primary central nervous system lymphoma. Arch Ophthalmol 1997; 115: 1157–1160.

27. Buggage RR, Velez G, Myers-Powell B, et al. Primary intraocular lymphoma with a low interleukin 10 to interleukin 6 ratio and heterogeneous IgH gene rearrangement. Arch Ophthalmol 2000; 118: 731–732.

28. Cassoux N, Giron A, Bodaghi B, et al. IL-10 measurement in aqueous humor for screening patients with suspicion of primary intraocular lymphoma. Invest Ophthalmol Vis Sci 2007; 48: 3253–3259.

29. Koster W. Über die Direkte Behandlung von Augenerkrankungen mit Radium und Metothorium. Strahlentherapie 1913; 3.

30. Margolis L, Fraser R, Lichter A, et al. The role of radiation therapy in the management of ocular reticulum cell sarcoma. Cancer 1980; 45: 688–692.

31. Rouwen AJP, Wijermans PW, Boen-Tan TN, et al. Intraocular non-Hodgkin's lymphoma treated with systemic and intrathecal chemotherapy and radiotherapy: a case report and review of the literature. Graefes Arch Clin Exp Ophthalmol 1989; 227: 355–359.

32. Baumann MA, Ritch PS, Hande KR, et al. Treatment of intraocular lymphoma with high-dose Ara-C. Cancer 1986; 57: 1273–1275.

33. Shapiro WR, Young DF, Tehta BM. Methotrexate: distribution in cerebrospinal fluid after intravenous, intraventricular and lumbar injections. N Engl J Med 1975; 293: 161–166.

34. Bleyer WA. Neurologic sequelae of methotrexate and ionizing radiation: a new classification. Cancer Treat Rep 1981; 65(suppl 1): 89–98.

35. Geyer JR, Taylor EM, Milstein JM. Radiation, methotrexate, and white matter necrosis: laboratory evidence for neural radioprotection with pre-irradiation methotrexate. Int J Radiat Oncol Biol Phys 1988; 15: 373–375.

36. Sandor V, Stark-Vancs V, Pearson D, et al. Phase II trial of chemotherapy alone for primary CNS and intraocular lymphoma. J Clin Oncol 1998; 16: 3000–3006.

37. Soussain C, Merle-Beral H, Reux I, et al. A single-center study of 11 patients with intraocular lymphoma treated with conventional chemotherapy followed by high-dose chemotherapy and autologous bone marrow transplantation in 5 cases. Leuk Lymphoma 1996; 23: 339–345.

38. Fishburne BC, Wilson DJ, Rosenbaum JT, et al. Intravitreal methotrexate as an adjunctive treatment of intraocular lymphoma. Arch Ophthalmol 1997; 115: 1152–1156.

39. de Smet MD. Management of non-Hodgkin's intraocular lymphoma with intravitreal methotrexate. Bull Soc Belge Ophtalmol 2001; 279: 91–95.

40. Velez G, Yuan P, Sung C, et al. Pharmacokinetics and toxicity of intravitreal chemotherapy for primary intraocular lymphoma. Arch Ophthalmol 2001; 119: 1518–1524.

41. Sou R, Ohguro N, Maeda T, et al. Treatment of primary intraocular lymphoma with intravitreal methotrexate. Jpn J Ophthalmol 2008; 52: 167–174.

42. Kitzmann AS, Pulido JS, Mohney BG, et al. Intraocular use of retuximab. Eye 2007; 21: 1524–1527.

43. Ferreri AJ, Blay JY, Reni M, et al. International Extranodal Lymphoma Study Group (IELSG). Relevance of intraocular involvement in the management of primary central nervous system lymphomas. Ann Oncol 2002; 13: 531–538.

44. Hormigo A, Abrey L, Heinemann MH, et al. Ocular presentation of primary central nervous system lymphoma: diagnosis and treatment. Br J Haematol 2004; 126: 202–208

45. Fredrick DR, Char DH, Ljung BM, et al. Solitary intraocular lymphoma as an initial presentation of widespread disease. Arch Ophthalmol 1989; 107: 395–397.

46. Guzak SV. Lymphoma as a cause of hyphema. Arch Ophthalmol 1970; 84: 229–231.

47. Ryan SJ, Frank RN, Green WR. Bilateral inflammatory pseudotumors of the ciliary body. Am J Ophthalmol 1971; 72: 586–591.

48. Ryan SJ, Zimmerman LE, King FM. Reactive lymphoid hyperplasia: an unusual form of intraocular pseudotumor. Trans Am Acad Ophthalmol Otolaryngol 1972; 76: 652–671.

49. Jakobiec FA, Sacks E, Kronish JW, et al. Multifocal static creamy choroidal infiltrates: an early sign of lymphoid neoplasia. Ophthalmology 1987; 94: 397–406.

50. Desroches G, Abrams GW, Gass JDM. Reactive lymphoid hyperplasia of the uvea: a case with ultrasonographic and computed tomographic studies. Arch Ophthalmol 1983; 101: 725–728.

51. Cheung MK, Martin DF, Chan CC, et al. Diagnosis of reactive lymphoid hyperplasia by chorioretinal biopsy. Am J Ophthalmol 1994; 118: 457–462.

52. Cockerham GC, Hidayat AA, Bijwaard KE, et al. Re-evaluation of 'reactive lymphoid hyperplasia of the uvea': an immunohistochemical and molecular analysis of 10 cases. Ophthalmology 2000; 107: 151–158.

53. Read RW, Zamir E, Rao NA. Neoplastic masquerade syndromes. Surv Ophthalmol 2002; 47: 81–124.

54. Litricin O. Diffuse malignant ring melanoma of the iris and ciliary body. Ophthalmologica 1979; 178: 235–238.

55. Char DH, Schwartz A, Miller TR, et al. Ocular metastases from systemic malignant melanoma. Am J Ophthalmol 1980; 90: 702–707.

56. Lipton JH, McGowan HD, Payne DG. Ocular masquerade syndrome in lymphoid blast crisis of chronic myeloid leukemia. Leuk Lymphoma 1995; 20: 161–163.

57. Ayliffe W, Foster CS, Marcoux P, et al. Relapsing acute myeloid leukemia manifesting as hypopyon uveitis. Am J Ophthalmol 1995; 119: 361–364.

58. Dhar-Munshi S, Alton P, Ayliffe WH. Masquerade syndrome: T-cell prolymphocytic leukemia presenting as panuveitis. Am J Ophthalmol 2001; 132: 275–277.

59. Ferry AP, Font RL. Carcinoma metastatic to the eye and orbit. I. A clinicopathologic study of 227 cases, Arch Ophthalmol 1974; 92: 276–286.

60. Shields JA, Shields CL, Ehya H, et al. Fine-needle aspiration biopsy of suspected intraocular tumors (the 1992 Urwick lecture). Ophthalmology 1993; 100: 1677–1684.

61. Croxatto JO, Fernandez MR, Malbran ES. Retinoblastoma masquerading as ocular inflammation. Ophthalmologica 1983; 186: 48–53.

62. Kincaid MC, Green WR. Ocular and orbital involvement in leukemia. Surv Ophthalmol 1983; 27: 211–232.

63. Rosenthal AR. Ocular manifestations of leukemia: a review. Ophthalmology 1983; 90: 899–905.

64. DeBarge LR, Chan CC, Greenberg S, et al. Chorioretinal, iris, and ciliary body infiltration by juvenile xanthogranuloma masquerading as uveitis. Am J Ophthalmol 1994; 39: 65–71.

65. Sawyer RA, Selhorst JB, Zimmerman LE, et al. Blindness caused by photoreceptor degeneration as a remote effect of cancer. Am J Ophthalmol 1976; 81: 606–613.

66. Buchanan TAS, Gardiner TA, Archer DB. An ultrastructural study of retinal photoreceptor degeneration associated with bronchial carcinoma. Am J Ophthalmol 1984; 97: 277–287.

67. Thirkill CE, Roth AM, Keltner JL. Cancer-associated retinopathy. Arch Ophthalmol 1987; 105: 372–375.

68. Whitcup SM, Vistica BA, Milam AH, et al. Recoverin-associated retinopathy: a clinically and immunologically distinctive disease. Am J Ophthalmol 1998; 126: 230–237.

69. Heckenlively JR, Ferreyra HA. Autoimmune retinopathy: A review and summary. Semin Immunopathol 2008; 30: 127–134.

70. Machemer R. Zur Pathogenese des flachenhaften malignen Melanoms. Klin Monatsbl Augenheilkd 1966; 148: 641–652.

71. Barr CC, Zimmerman LE, Curtin VT, et al. Bilateral diffuse melanocytic uveal tumors associated with systemic malignant neoplasms: a recently recognized syndrome. Arch Ophthalmol 1982; 100: 249–255.

72. Ryll DL, Campbell RJ, Robertson DM, et al. Pseudometastatic lesions of the choroid. Ophthalmology 1980; 87: 1181–1186.

73. Gass JDM, Glatzer RJ. Acquired pigmentation simulating Peutz–Jeghers syndrome: initial manifestation of diffuse uveal melanocytic proliferation. Br J Ophthalmol 1991; 75: 693–695.

74. Stone DU, Char DH, Crawford JB, et al. Metaplastic squamous epithelial downgrowth after clear corneal cataract surgery. Am J Ophthalmol 2006; 142: 695–697.

75. Lim WK, Chee SP. Retinal detachment in atopic dermatitis can masquerade as acute panuveitis with rapidly progressive cataract. Retina 2004; 24: 953–956.

76. Char DH. Intraocular masquerade syndromes. In Tasman W, Jaeger EA, editors: Duane's clinical ophthalmology. Philadelphia, 1989, Lippincott.

77. Heckenlively JR. The frequency of posterior subcapsular cataract in the hereditary retinal degenerations. Am J Ophthalmol 1982; 93: 733–738.

78. Fetkenhour CL, Choromokos E, Weinstein J, et al. Cystoid macular edema in retinitis pigmentosa. Trans Am Acad Ophthalmol Otolaryngol 1977; 83: 515–521.

79. Fishman GA, Maggiero JM, Fishman M. Foveal lesions seen in retinitis. Arch Ophthalmol 1977; 95: 1993–1996.

80. Thirkill CE, Roth AM, Takemoto DJ, et al. Antibody indications of secondary and superimposed retinal hypersensitivity in retinitis pigmentosa. Am J Ophthalmol 1991; 112: 132–137.

81. Williams LL, Lew HM, Shannon BT, et al. Activated retinitis pigmentosa peripheral lymphocytes adhere to and alter cultured human retinal pigment epithelial cells. Invest Ophthalmol Vis Sci 1992; 33: 2848–2860.

82. Krupin T, LeBlanc RP, Becker B, et al. Uveitis in association with topically administered corticosteroid. Am J Ophthalmol 1970; 70: 883–885.

Other Ocular Disorders and the Immune Response: Who Would Have Thought?

Robert B. Nussenblatt

Key concepts

- Evidence is rapidly accruing to support the notion that these entities, particularly AMD, have a significant immune component.
- Immunosuppressive therapy has been shown in a few patients to have a positive therapeutic effect in AMD.
- Understanding these disorders furthers our knowledge of the multiple mechanisms that make up the downregulatory immune environment of the eye.

Introduction

It seems fitting to include this chapter in a book on uveitis. Diseases that have not traditionally (at least by most eyecare specialists) been thought of as immune mediated are being considered to be within the immune sphere. We will deal with three very common ocular disorders: age-related macular degeneration (AMD), diabetic retinopathy, and glaucoma. It is clear that as we gather more information about glaucoma and AMD we are seeing striking parallels with other 'degenerative' disorders, such as atherosclerosis and Alzheimer's disease. Diabetes has been long thought of an immune-mediated disease, but these concepts have not percolated to the eye particularly. It is clear that we will be able to support immune involvement in all three of the diseases. It is not whether the immune system is involved: rather, the more important question is just how central the immune mechanism is to the clinical manifestations we observe, and whether, with this knowledge, it can be manipulated in such a way as to arrive at a positive therapeutic response.

Age-related macular degeneration

Age related macular degeneration is the most common cause of irreversible blindness in the United States and the United Kingdom. It is estimated that 1.75 million people in the United States are affected with the more advanced form of the disease.[1] Indeed, it is now considered the most common cause of irreversible blindness in the world.[1] If there is no change in lifestyle or treatment strategies, it has been estimated that by 2020 this number will increase to 3 million Americans with the severe form of the disease. The disorder probably begins years before the patient is aware of visual alterations. It is characterized by the presence of large drusen, which can coalesce, disappear, and appear elsewhere. More about drusen later. Suffice to say that large drusen and the small drusen seen in many patients do not seem to be related. The risk increases with each risk factor in the eye. The two significant ones are large drusen and pigment changes. If you have four risk factors, that is, the two in each eye, the 5-year risk of developing advanced AMD in either eye is 50%.[2]

In addition to the presence of large drusen, the disease will show loss of RPE (geographic atrophy) as well as hyperplasia of the RPE, and in a minority of patients in the United States, choroidal neovascularization (CNV).

Much work has centered on this condition. There have been several reviews, and the interested reader should consult them.[3,4] This chapter will be a short synopsis of what has become a large corpus of information.

Animal work

Animal laser model

Punching a hole through Bruch's membrane in a mouse or rat will result in a choroidal neovascular lesion which will appear 2–3 weeks after the insult (**Fig. 31-1**). Using this model for CNV, several investigators have evaluated inflammatory responses as well as potential therapeutic approaches. Work using this model would suggest that macrophages limit the size of a CNV lesion, at least produced in this injury model.[5] In addition, dendritic cells were found next to the induced CNV site, and immature dendritic cells appeared to enhance the CNV size.[6] The same group identified genes in the mouse that appear to control the size of the angiogenic lesion after laser injury.[6] Semkova et al.[7] reported that overexpression of FasL in the RPE resulted in less CNV. Of interest was that the three most commonly used anti-VEGF agents in humans showed no effect in diminishing leakage from laser-induced CNV lesions in rats.[8] The data from this model are sometimes contradictory, perhaps suggesting the complex interactions of subtypes of cells that may be involved.

Ccl2 and Ccr2 knockout model

Ccr2, a chemokine receptor, is present on macrophages. Its ligand is MCP1 (Ccl2) and it aids in the adhesion of macrophages to vasculature and helps them move into the tissues. Ambati et al.[9] showed that by 9 months, these mice develop drusen and a thickening of Bruch's membrane. By 16–18 months, they can demonstrate RPE atrophy and in some cases neovascularization. Impaired

PART 5 · Uveitic Conditions not Caused by Active Infection

Chapter **31** Other Ocular Disorders and the Immune Response: Who Would Have Thought?

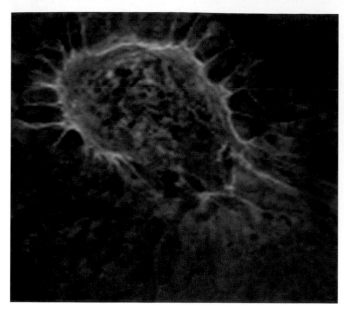

Figure 31-1. Confocal microscopic photo of laser lesion in a mouse retina. This computer-enhanced photo shows the hole in red/pink with the surrounding retinal pigment epithelium outlined in green. The CNV will grow from the lesion. *(Courtesy of Zhuqing Li and Robert Fariss, NEI, NIH.)*

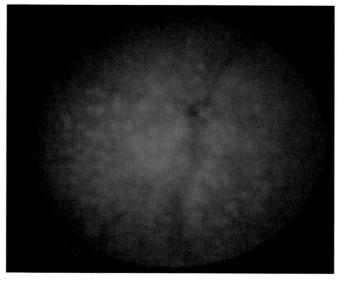

Figure 31-2. The fundus lesions in the Ccl2 and Cx3cr1 double knockout model. Multiple retinal lesions suggestive of drusen. *(Courtesy of Chi Chao Chan, MD, NEI, NIH.)*

macrophage function leads to an accumulation of immune components such as C5 in the areas of AMD-like change. Bear in mind that Tsutsumi et al.[10] showed that a reduced number of macrophages at a laser-induced lesion yielded less CNV.

Ccl2 and Cx3cr1 double knockout model

This model, developed at the Laboratory of Immunology of the NEI,[11,12] develops drusen-like lesions after 4–6 weeks (**Fig. 31-2**).

There is increased complement activity with deposition at the drusen-like lesions, Bruch's membrane, the RPE and the choroidal capillaries. These mice also demonstrated anti-retinal antibodies as seen in AMD patients.

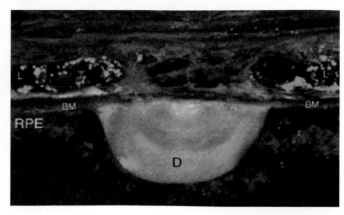

Figure 31-3. Druse from a human retina (D). The druse has been stained from the presence of CFH (green) and co-staining of CFH with C5b-9 (yellow). *(From Bok D. Evidence for an inflammatory process in age-related macular degeneration gains new support. Proc Natl Acad Sci USA 2005; 102: 7053.)*

CEP induced AMD-like disease

Carboxyethylpyrrole (CEP), a unique oxidation fragment of docosahexaenoic acid, is found within the large drusen of patients with AMD. Hollyfield et al.[13] immunized mice with this material, and over a period ranging from 3 to 9 months the animals developed posterior segment lesions that were AMD-like. Macrophages were noted near the RPE and there were areas of RPE loss (**Fig. 31-3**). The significance of this model is that it was induced by immunization, and so a T-helper response, and that it was induced with material found in human eyes with this disease.

There are other knockout models showing fundus changes that are reminiscent of AMD. These include knockouts of CFH, ABCR, and Cx3Cr1.[3]

Human data

There is an increasing amount of information about AMD and the possible role of the immune system. Some of it dates back to the 1990s.

Autoimmunity

Penfold and colleagues[14] reported the presence of retinal autoantibodies in patients with AMD. More recently, Patel and coworkers[15] reported that patients with choroidal neovascularization and large drusen had autoantibodies to retinal elements far more often than did controls (82.2%, 93.75% and 8.69%, respectively).

Gene associations

Recently there has been a flurry of interest in evaluating gene variants (single nucleotide polymorphisms) with AMD. This has led to many different associations. Perhaps the finding that received that most interest was the association of the complement factor H variant Y402H with AMD.[16–19] Although other variants have been associated with AMD, such as complement factor B (BF), complement component 2 (C2), C3, C7, and complement factor I (FI) and CX3CR1,[3] the association of Y402H was seen to be particularly strong ($\chi^2 = 54.4$ and $P = 1.6 \times 10^{-13}$), and much speculation has centered around the implications of the association. CFH is encoded on chromosome 1. It is a major regulator of complement activity, blocking activation of the complement cascade. Complement is traditionally associated with the innate immune system, the oldest part of our immune system which reacts rapidly to invading organisms. It has been speculated that the Y402H variant does not inhibit complement activity as efficiently as the wildtype molecule, thus leading to the immune activation and AMD.[20] However, to date no functional studies have definitively shown alterations in activity with the variant rather than the wild type of CFH.

Another variant that has been studied and associated with AMD is that of high temperature requirement serine protease (HTRA-1) (rs11200638). This variant, which is located on chromosome 10q26, is a major genetic risk factor for wet AMD. As with CFH HTRA-1, in initial studies in a population with a very low presence of the Y402H variant, i.e., a group of Eastern Asians in Hong Kong, the P value was as essentially as robust as that with CFH[10,11,21] Of interest was the strong association of the same variant found in a Caucasian population of 581 patients and 309 normal controls in Utah.[22] It was estimated that this variant conferred an attributable risk of 49.3%. In addition, Yang and coworkers,[22] using anti-HTRA1 antibody to label drusen, demonstrated the presence of this variant in the centerpoint of AMD. In addition, Yoshida et al.[23] found the same variant in a Japanese population.

What is special about HTRA-1? It appears to have several functions that may be important in the pathogenesis of AMD. It is part of the heat shock proteases that are induced with stress. In addition, it is a regulator of TGF-β activity.[24] TGF-β is considered a downregulatory immune molecule,[25,26] one of the major molecules in maintaining a downregulatory immune environment in the eye.[27] Further, a substrate of HTRA-1 is fibronectin. Fibronectin fragments stimulate proinflammatory and catabolic elements from murine RPE, including IL-6, MMP-3, MMP-9, and MCP-1.[28] All of these products could contribute to inflammation, catabolism, and attraction of monocytes, which are all elements of AMD.

Are there others associations? Indeed, several others have been made, mostly with molecules that are somehow involved with the immune response. These include the CXCR1 variant V294I,[29] complement factor B, complement components including C2, C3, and C7,[3] the PLEKHA1 gene,[30] IL-8,[31] ARMS2,[32,33] and the toll-like receptor 3 variant L412F,[34] which has been associated with protection from the atrophic form of AMD.

How do we then have so many molecules already considered as such dominant players in AMD? One possibility is that they are players in a larger downregulatory environment, as discussed below.

Macrophages and other cells

As mentioned both above and below, macrophages/monocytes appear to be a major player in the pathogenesis of this disease. The real question is, exactly what is it? Is it that they are not functionally efficient enough, or are they being overactive? The animal work has provided us with mixed information. Cousins et al.[35] evaluated circulating macrophages from patients with AMD and from controls (**Table 31-1**). In this study, 'activated' macrophages were defined as those making large quantities of the proinflammatory lymphokine TNF-α. This is a lymphokine discussed in several other chapters. Cousins et al. found that the macrophages of patients

with the wet form of AMD produced statistically significantly greater amounts of TNF-α than did those from controls and the dry type of AMD.

It is important to bear in mind that macrophage subtypes may be very significant factors in this the induction of this disease. As discussed in the Fundamentals chapters, the M_1 subtype of macrophage can conceivably present antigen and produce proinflammatory substances. This is in contrast to the M_2 subtype, which may scavenge but may not present antigen, maintaining a downregulatory atmosphere.

Bear in mind also the possible role of microglia, resident immune cells, as well as dendritic cells. All of these cells have been shown to potentially interact with immune cells when they enter the eye.

Histopathology

The attempt here is not to discuss the pathologic changes classically described as associated with AMD, but whether there are implications of an immune response. Penfold et al.,[36] in 1985, reported the presence of macrophage, fibroblasts, lymphocytes and mast cells not only at the level of the neovascular lesion, but also in the atrophy of the RPE and the breakdown of Bruch's membrane. It is quite possible that the inflammatory process occurs early on in the disease, at a time when there are minimal or no visual alterations. What we see as the disease is the consequence of something that occurred quite some time earlier. Large drusen, the most reliable harbinger of AMD, have been extensively evaluated. Using liquid chromatography tandem mass spectrometry analyses of drusen, Crabbe et al.[37] identified 129 different proteins in both small and hard and large and soft drusen. Crystallins, heat shock proteins, and products of oxidative reactions were noted. Anderson et al.[38] evaluated the drusen and surrounding tissue in more than 400 AMD eyes. They noted RPE cells undergoing cell death with the accumulation of C5 in their cytoplasm. Drusen in AMD were also noted to harbor C3 and C5 activation fragments, in addition to HTRA1 noted above.[22]

The downregulatory immune environment

Can this be the underlying link? We have noted evidence of autoantibodies implicating T- and B-cell activation. Macrophages seem somehow central to the underlying disease. We know that ocular resident cells, particularly the RPE, can interact readily with the immune system. We have seen that drusen contain fragments of molecules involved with the immune response, both innate and acquired. Finally, the genetic associations constantly increase, and almost always involve genes associated with immune regulation. All these genetic associations are suggested as the underlying cause of the disease. How is that possible? Another possible explanation is that all of these associations are really affecting a major characteristic of the ocular environment, which we have termed the downregulatory immune environment (DIE).[1] With this concept it really does not matter what the genetic alterations are, and we are sure to find others. It is the disruption of DIE that leads to the disorder, and it can occur through multiple mechanisms. We know that the multiple molecules in the eye create an environment that suppresses immune responses. It would not be in the organism's best interest to have inflammatory responses in the eye except when absolutely necessary. ACAID is one of the

Table 31-1 Prevalence of neovascular AMD and high TNF-α mRNA levels in freshly isolated monocytes. (Reproduced with permission from Cousins, S.W., D.G. Espinosa-Heidmann, and K.G. Csaky, Monocyte activation in patients with age-related macular degeneration: a biomarker of risk for choroidal neovascularization? Arch Ophthalmol 2004;122(7):1013–1018)

| TNF-α mRNA Levels in Fresh Monocytes | Prevalence of Test Result, No. (%) | | | |
	Dry AMD (n = 22)	Neovascular AMD (n = 25)	OR (95% CI)	P Value
Low	11 (50)	5 (20)	NA	NA
Medium	4 (18)	4 (16)	2.20 (1.99–2.38)	0.32
High	7 (32)	16 (64)	5.03 (4.99–5.06)	0.02

AMD, age-related macular degeneration; CI, confidence interval; mRNA, messenger RNA; NA, not applicable; OR, odds ratio; TNF-α, tumor necrosis factor-α.

Table 31-2 Factors that affect the downregulatory intraocular environment

Cellular	Cell Surface and Soluble Factors	Physical
NKT cells	Transforming growth factor-β	Light
Müller cells	IL-11	
RPE	IL-10	
Microglia	GITR/GITR ligand	
F4/80 macrophages	CD95 ligand	
	IL-1 receptor antagonist	
	Cortisol	
	Antigens	
	Crystallins, arrestin	
	Complement factors	
	CD55, CD59, CD46	
	Soluble inhibitors of C1q and C3 convertase	
	Somatostatin	
	α-Melanocyte-stimulating hormone	
	Vasoactive intestinal peptide	
	Thrombospondin	
	Calcitonin gene-related peptide	

better-described ways that this occurs. Table 31-2 lists many of the ways in which this downregulatory environment is maintained, involving many of the cells found in the back of the eye as well. One could explain the possible scenario leading to AMD as follows:

- The RPE produces debris which is excreted into the environment. This includes immunogenic antigens such as β crystallins and retinal antigens such as arrestin. The multiple mechanisms associated with DIE are in play. This would include the presence of TGF-β and CFH.
- Macrophages: we could hypothesize that the M₂ type – those that clear debris but do not necessarily induce an inflammatory response – come in small numbers to

help clean up the debris. However, if there is a defect in macrophage recruitment then the debris will collect in larger amounts. Perhaps this explains some of the animal models. This clearing of debris is a lifelong process.

- With aging, DIE is not as an effective immune downregulatory mechanism. More macrophages and a small number of inflammatory cells now gather. There are also Th cells present, and macrophages are producing the proinflammatory cytokine IL-17. Activation with proinflammatory cytokine production and autoantibodies occurs.
- Over a long a period of time the proinflammatory cytokines and autoantibodies are toxic to the RPE and could cause apoptosis of these cells. TLR3 variants may protect this from happening.
- For those with either the CFH or HTRA1 SNPs (and others) that put individuals at higher risk for AMD, DIE's control is further diminished. The presence of drusen is the body's attempt to wall off the active components of the immune system to prevent a heightened immune response. The drusen are thus a sign of a chronic inflammatory response that has overcome DIE's control.
- A more rigorous inflammatory response will lead to further loss of RPE (because of toxic lymphokines) and the development of CNV with the recruitment of bone marrow cells (**Fig. 31-4**).

Should we consider immunotherapy?

The use of anti-VEGF agents has changed the clinical picture for the minority of patients with the wet form of AMD. However, no good therapy yet exists for the dry form. There seems little doubt the immune system is involved in the pathologic process that leads to AMD, but that is not the real question: from a clinical perspective this is: just how central is the immune mechanism(s) and can it be manipulated in such a way as to have a positive effect on patients' vision?

There are initial indications that perhaps the immune system's involvement is significant enough in AMD or CNV production so that treatment will have a positive clinical effect. It has been suggested that steroids may be useful in treating AMD, with mixed results. However, in the more recent past we have reported the effective treatment of a CNV secondary to inner punctate choroidopathy with rapamycin.[39] If AMD CNV is secondary to an immune

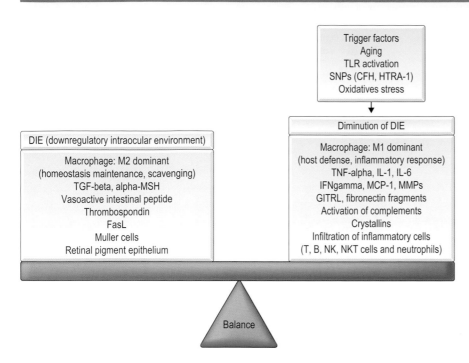

Figure 31-4. The maintenance of DIE is a balance. The many contributing factors leading to this downregulatory environment can be counteracted by proinflammatory events. *(From Nussenblatt RB, Liu B, Li Z. Age-related macular degeneration: an immunologically driven disease. Curr Opin Invest Drugs. 2009; 10(5): 434–42.)*

response, this medication could be useful. So far there have been only anecdotal oral reports, but these have been suggestive. An anti-TNF-α monoclonal antibody, remicade, has been used both systemically and intravitreally in the treatment of wet AMD, with diminishing retinal fluid and a possible effect on the CNV.[40,41] Intravitreal methotrexate has also been shown to have a positive effect on AMD (Shree Kurup, MD, personal communication). Finally the NEI, in a joint study with the retinal and immunology groups, are evaluating three agents, daclizumab, rapamycin, and remicade, in a randomized pilot study. Initial results should be available shortly.

The immunotherapy has emphasized the treatment of the wet type of disease, though the NEI has its own study evaluating rapamycin in the treatment of the dry form. However, one can very readily argue that therapy should begin much earlier than when the clinical signs of the disease become evident. This would mean treating years before, perhaps when the large drusen first appear. Treating with immunosuppressive agents, whether intravitreal or systemic, for 20 years is simply not feasible, for many reasons. One must begin to consider other therapeutic modalities that will be easily adhered to and not have signficant side effects: clearly a challenge for the future.

Diabetic retinopathy

Diabetes is becoming epidemic in the United States. It has been estimated that almost 13% of adults over the age of 20 have diabetes, and that 40% of these have not been diagnosed. Nearly one-third of those 65 and older have the disorder. The diagnosis has been estimated to be 60–70% higher in the African-American and Hispanic communities. Further, perhaps 30% of adults have prediabetic status, with blood sugars elevated albeit not in the diabetic range.[42] The United States is also seeing an epidemic of obesity in children, with a marked increase in diabetes in that population as well. As we will see, the underlying mechanisms have implicated the immune response. Diabetic retinopathy is one of the most commonly seen problems in medical ophthalmology. Some the most important early clinical studies performed under the auspices of the National Eye Institute, NIH, dealt with this entity, and in particular the value of laser photocoagulation.

Diabetes and the immune process

Diabetes is generally divided clinically into types I and II. Type I is usually seen in the young, requires insulin replacement, and is often associated with more severe complications. Type II until recently was seen in older individuals, was associated with obesity, and could often be controlled with diet, exercise or agents that stimulate the body's own insulin production. Certainly retinopathy is seen in both types. But what of the underlying disease? Is there a suggestion of an immune-mediated cause? The information is very strong to suggest that there is.

The concept of autoantibodies being associated with diabetes has been offered for some time. In the late 1970s Bottazzo et al.[43] reported that within 3 months of their diagnosis 74% of juvenile diabetics had antibodies directed towards islet cells of the pancreas. This dropped to 20% 3 years after the diagnosis, presumably because the antigenic stimulus, the islet cells, was largely destroyed. Those with antibodies had a higher probability of thyrogastric autoimmunity. Indeed, others have shown that in type I diabetics thyroid and endomysial antibodies were seen at diagnosis.[44] This finding put them at greater risk of developing both thyroid and celiac disease. Therefore, type I diabetes falls into a group of disorders thought to be autoimmune. Immune complexes have been reported to be found in patients with diabetes. Serum fibrillin–antifibrillin autoantibodies may be associated with the microangiopathy seen in the disorder.[45] With regard to cellular responses, Zykova et al.[46] noted that macrophages from diabetics were stimulated with lipopolysaccharide to produce TNF-α as well as in normal controls. These find-

PART 5 · Uveitic Conditions not Caused by Active Infection

Chapter **31** Other Ocular Disorders and the Immune Response: Who Would Have Thought?

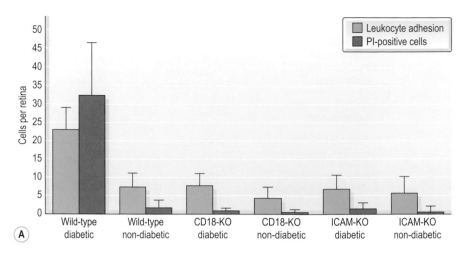

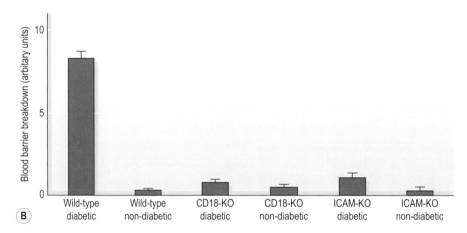

Figure 31-5. Inducing diabetes in CD18 and ICAM-1 (intercellular adhesion molecule-1) knockout mice results in a marked decrease in cellular adherence of vessels and a breakdown of the blood–ocular barrier. CD18 and ICAM-1 are important immune markers for immune cells. *(From Adamis AP, Berman AJ. Immunological mechanisms in the pathogenesis of diabetic retinopathy. Semin Immunopathol, 2008; 30(2): p. 65–84.)*

ings correlated with levels of apolipoprotein and the presence of retinopathy.

Animal work

Cellular stasis and vascular leakage appear to be seen in both animal models and humans with diabetes. Increased cellular numbers and capillary damage have been seen in rats with induced diabetes,[47] and also in monkeys with spontaneously occurring disease.[48] These cellular accumulations are associated with an increase in the expression of ICAM-1 levels in the retina; ICAM-1 is part of the adhesion cell family, with its ligand present on infiltrating cells.[49] Indeed, the use of antiadhesion molecule therapy will markedly diminish the induction of diabetic retinopathy in animals. Further, mice genetically altered so as not to express either ICAM or CD18 (the ligand) on their cell surface showed a dramatic reduction in cellular adherence as well as retinal damage (**Fig. 31-5**).[50]

Treating animals with antibody to block FasL–Fas interactions (inducing apoptosis) will inhibit endothelial cell apoptosis in the retina and reduce blood–retinal barrier breakdown.[51]

Human observations

The information to date concerning diabetic retinopathy and the immune response is highly suggestive, but a full understanding of the mechanisms awaits discovery. It has been seen that an asymmetric rapid progression of diabetic retinopathy was noted in a patient whose posterior uveitis exacerbated only in one eye.[52] Diabetes has been known to become worse during pregnancy, when there is an upregulation of adhesion molecules and increases in IL-6 and 8, all proinflammatory mediators.[53] Other factors have been noted to appear to be protective of diabetic retinopathy. Such an example is glutamic acid decarboxylase (GAD). Antibodies against GAD have been shown to be inversely related to the presence of retinopathy,[54,55] whereas HLA-DQ4 and DR4/ -DQ4 haplotypes were indeed associated.[54] An interesting association between a polymorphism in toll-like receptor 4, a receptor important in innate immune responses, was noted by Buraczynska et al.[56] with early-onset diabetic retinopathy in patients with type 2 diabetes.

Perhaps the most provocative findings are in the vitreous. Adamiec-Mroczek et al.[57] have shown that IL-6 and TNF-α levels were high in the vitreous of patients with diabetic retinopathy compared to vitreous samples from patients with other disorders. Others have not only found elevated IL-6 levels in the vitreous, but also IL-8,[58] and s-IL-2 was also elevated in the sera of diabetics.[59] In addition, activated fragments of complement, T and B cells as well as monocytes can be found in the preretinal membranes of diabetics.[60] In addition, McLeod et al.[30] showed increased cellular infiltrations in both the choroid and retina, with an increase in ICAM-1 expression. All of these findings have led some to suggest that diabetic retinopathy is an autoimmune disease.[61]

Can we begin to think about immune therapy for diabetes and diabetic retinopathy?

Antiinflammatory therapy is already being evaluated in the treatment of systemic type II diabetes. The evidence suggests that a low-grade inflammatory response in patients with a sedentary lifestyle and a western diet contributes to the development of type II diabetes. Investigators have begun evaluating the use of Salsalate, an NSAID used in the treatment of arthritic pain, in treating difficult-to-control type II diabetes. In a proof of principle study involving 20 patients, Fleischman et al.[62] evaluated the effects of Salsalate in a double-masked randomized study. They found that fasting glucose was reduced, as was the glucose level after a glucose challenge. In a randomized study of 54 patients (40 were analyzed), patients receiving Salsalate, 3 g/day for 7 days, once again showed lowered glucose levels. However, the conclusion of these investigators was that the effect was not greater effective insulin activity but rather was due to increased insulin concentrations, which salicylates are known to induce.[63] These findings have resulted in a large randomized study supported by the National Institute of Diabetes and Digestive and Kidney Diseases (NIDDK) to evaluate this therapy, which is currently in its active recruitment phase.[64]

Others have suggested using antidendritic cell therapy for the treatment of systemic diabetes. It is known that mature dendritic cells will serve as antigen-presenting cells to T cells; such antigen transfer would induce an inflammatory response. Such a concept would have potential value in the eye as well.

Another approach for the eye is to use the information gained from both animal and some human studies concerning the upregulation of adhesion molecules in the eye. Anti-CD11a antibodies (Raptiva, see Chapter 7), directed against part of the adhesion molecule complex, are being used in uveitis and do appear to have a positive clinical effect. All the information would suggest that interfering with the upregulated response in the eye would be beneficial. However, Raptiva appears to have long-term potential problems that would limit its use at present. Intravitreal application remains to be investigated.

One final word about gene therapy. This area has received much attention, both good and bad. Gene therapy in the eye has certainly attracted interest, with some success. Investigators treating diabetes have thought about this as well, and although it does not directly affect the eye it is possible that altering the systemic course could have a significant effect on the ocular complications.[65] These concepts include reducing inflammatory cytokine production, reducing the interaction of antigen-presenting cells with activating T cells, and blocking the interactions that lead to apoptosis of islet cells. We can conceive of similar scenarios in the eye.

Glaucoma

Glaucoma is one of the most common ocular disorders encountered by the eyecare specialist. It has been estimated that by the age of 70, 7% of the population will have glaucoma.[66] Glaucoma is clinically thought of a problem of increased intraocular pressure, whereas really it is a progressive loss of retinal ganglion cells and their associated axons. Certain ethnic groups appear to have not only a high incidence of the disease but also the most severe disease (for example African-Americans).[67-69] Albeit easy to describe when in its full-blown clinical presentation, it has been particularly difficult to develop adequate screening techniques for its detection. The Baltimore Eye Study concluded that there was no cutoff for which reasonable sensitivity and specificity could be obtained.[70] It has been reported that 16% of patients will have clinically diagnosed glaucoma without a pressure reading > 21 mmHg.[71] The goal of a better understanding of the underlying mechanisms of this disorder so as to develop better ways to screen for the disease and treat it has yet to be reached. One approach is to consider screening the sera of glaucoma suspects for possible immune mediators.

Autoantibodies and glaucoma

Autoantibodies in glaucoma were first reported by Wax et al.[72] in patients with normal tension glaucoma. Initial reports centered on antibodies directed against a heat shock protein (HSP 60). Subsequent to these initial observations, antibodies directed against several other proteins have been reported. These include α A and B crystallins and HSP27. HSP 27 antibodies have been reported to induce apoptosis in neuronal cells. Grus and coworkers have also reported antibodies directed against α foldrin, which is a neuronal cytoskeletal protein.[73,74] What is particularly interesting about foldrin is that it can be the target of caspase-3, destructive enzymes in the retina that could destroy retinal infrastructural integrity. Further, α foldrin has been implicated in the CNS process leading to Alzheimer's disease.[73,75]

Grus and coworkers have evaluated autoantibodies from the sera of patients with normal tension glaucoma (NTG), primary open angle glaucoma (OAG), and controls (**Fig. 31-6**). The group evaluated the presence of these natural

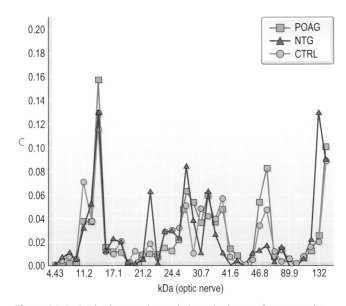

Figure 31-6. Antibody screening techniques in the sera from controls; the antibodies appear to be directed against different antigens compared to sera from patients with normal tension glaucoma and primary open angle glaucoma. *(From Grus F, Sun D. Immunological mechanisms in glaucoma. Semin Immunopathol 2008; 30: 121–126.)*

PART 5 · Uveitic Conditions not Caused by Active Infection

Chapter **31** Other Ocular Disorders and the Immune Response: Who Would Have Thought?

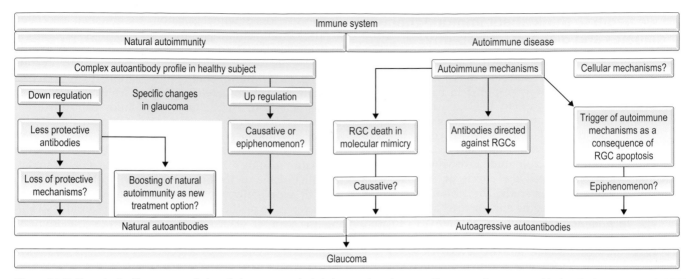

Figure 31-7. Hypothesis of immune mediation of glaucoma, particularly low-tension glaucoma. The suggestion presented is that the innate system in NTG patients has lost several of it protective antibodies, leading to disease, and at the same time has developed autoaggressive antibodies that could be causative as well. Other antibody changes that occur later might be epiphenomena. *(From Grus FH, Joachim SC, Wuenschig D, et al. Autoimmunity and glaucoma. J Glaucoma 2008; 17: 79–84.)*

autoantibodies based on their molecular weight and reactivity. They noted that NTG patients had the greatest difference compared to POAG and controls, but POAG patients' profiles were also different from that seen in healthy controls.

It was thus felt that what is being observed is a dysregulation of the immune system in its normal mechanisms to protect retinal ganglion cells. This concept is illustrated in **Figure 31-7**.

The complex natural autoantibody profile found in healthy subjects protects cells from apoptosis or direct attack by antibodies. In patients with autoimmune disease, noxious antibodies are formed and are not counteracted by the protective antibodies. These noxious antibodies may be a result of molecular mimicry – that is, antibodies originally directed against invading organisms whose molecular sequence is similar to the proteins found in retinal ganglion cells. Therefore, the antibodies meant to kill invading cells now kill cells in the retina. It should be emphasized that this is currently a hypothesis.

Cellular immunity and glaucoma

A growing collection of literature is looking at glaucoma no longer as a simple elevation of intraocular pressure but rather as a neuropathy that can be manipulated with neuroprotective measures. Of course, this then requires an understanding of the basic mechanisms that lead to the degenerative changes. One important concept has been particularly championed by Michal Schwartz and coworkers,[76] i.e., that low-grade autoimmune responses are necessary for the continued repair and protection of retinal ganglion cells, and presumably for other cells in the retina as well. **Figure 31-8** shows the various factors that could be considered with regard to cellular and cell product mechanisms. Some of the factors that lead to neural degeneration include: oxidative stress and the development of free radicals, which cause damage to the retinal ganglion cell; in addition, although glutamic acid is an important mediator in the neural circuitry, excessive levels are toxic; there may be a lack of neurotropins and

other growth factors in patients with glaucoma; and there is an abnormal accumulation of proteins in the retina of glaucoma patients. Tezel et al.[77] showed that oxidatively modified proteins are present during glaucomatous neurodegeneration, proteins similar to what is found in Alzheimer's disease. Indeed, many of the factors outlined as underlying the pathology leading to glaucoma are seen in neurodegenerative diseases in general.[78]

These factors lead to the concept that low-grade autoimmunity may result in the protection of these cells. Experiments have supported this. Using a crush injury of the optic nerve, Schwartz and coworkers,[76] in a series of papers, showed that the immune system – indeed, T cells – played a key role in protecting the optic nerve. When T cells specific to myelin basic protein are present then the loss of ganglion cells is less after a traumatic nerve injury. Activated T cells provide cytokines and growth factors, and may help stimulate microglia and monocytes. It has been found that myelin-associated antigens only protect white matter (myelinated fibers). In an experiment using the R-16 fragment of IRBP, Bakalash et al.[79] showed that this antigen, which normally resides in the retina, could protect retinal ganglion cells. In the case of the IRBP fragment it also induced a uveitis, so the results are both good and bad. However, as a proof of principle it was an important observation. Interestingly, the use of steroids resulted in a further loss of retinal ganglion cells. These observations naturally lead to the question of whether immune intervention would help.

Can immune intervention help alter the course of glaucoma?

At present we have only case reports to support the notion that altering the immune system pharmacologically could be beneficial to glaucoma patients. Fellman et al.[80] report the case of a patient with glaucoma who was treated with methotrexate for rheumatoid arthritis. During this period her visual fields improved. In addition, the patient's serum,

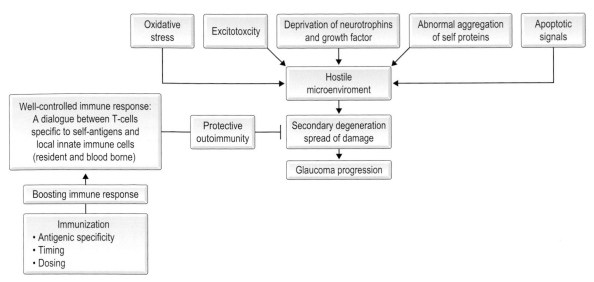

Figure 31-8. The concept of cellular immune protection in glaucoma as suggested by Schwartz and colleagues. Degenerating neurons will create a very toxic environment for the surrounding retinal cells, with increased oxidative stress, production of glutamate, apoptosis, and lack of growth factors. The immune system, both innate and acquired, creates a protective barrier against further progression of the disorder. It is further suggested that the immune response may not be adequate and needs to be augmented by immunization techniques. *(From Schwartz M, London A. Glaucoma as a neuropathy amenable to neuroprotection and immune manipulation. In: Nucci C et al., eds. Progress in Brain Research, Vol. 173 © 2008 Elsevier.)*

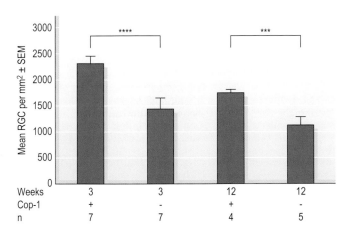

Figure 31-9. Retinal ganglion cell counts after copolymer-1 vaccination. In this elevated pressure model in rats, protection was noted even after 12 weeks. Rats lacking T cells were not protected. *(From Bakalash S, Ben Shlomo G, Aloni E, et al. T-cell-based vaccination for morphological and functional neuroprotection in a rat model of chronically elevated intraocular pressure. J Mol Med 2005; 83: 904–916.)*

which was reactive to several retinal proteins, including heat shock protein 60-kDa (hsp60) and rhodopsin, showed reduced reactivity as measured by Western blotting.

From experimental work on cellular immunity, a concept of 'protective immunity' has evolved and the idea that a T-cell vaccination for glaucoma might be considered.[81,82] Bakalash and coworkers[82] reported on the use of copolymer-1, a weak agonist of self-antigens, which has been used in multiple sclerosis. It was conjectured that the T-cell-mediated response seen after vaccination with copolymer-1 could cross-react with self-antigens, thereby boosting the protective immunity proposed. Copolymer-1 vaccination was capable of protecting retinal ganglion cells in a model of chronic elevation of intraocular pressure (**Fig. 31-9**). Protection occurred early on and appeared sustained, at least till 12 weeks into the experiment. Interestingly, when this approach was tried in rats lacking T cells, no such protection could be elicited.

References

1. Nussenblatt RB, Ferris F, III. Age-related macular degeneration and the immune response: implications for therapy. Am J Ophthalmol 2007; 144(4): 618–626.
2. Ferris FL, Davis MD, Clemons TE, et al. A simplified severity scale for age-related macular degeneration: AREDS Report No. 18. Arch Ophthalmol 2005; 123(11): 1570–1574.
3. Ding X, Patel M, Chan CC. Molecular pathology of age-related macular degeneration. Prog Retin Eye Res, 2008.
4. Patel M, Chan CC. Immunopathological aspects of age-related macular degeneration. Semin Immunopathol 2008; 30(2): 97–110.

5. Apte RS, Richter J, Herndon J, et al. Macrophages inhibit neovascularization in a murine model of age-related macular degeneration. PLoS Med 2006; 3(8): e310.
6. Nakai K, Fainaru O, Bazinet L, et al. Dendritic cells augment choroidal neovascularization. Invest Ophthalmol Vis Sci 2008; 49(8): 3666–3670.
7. Semkova I, Fauser S, Lappas A, et al. Overexpression of FasL in retinal pigment epithelial cells reduces choroidal neovascularization. FASEB J 2006; 20(10): 1689–1691.
8. Lu F, Adelman RA. Are intravitreal bevacizumab and ranibizumab effective in a rat model of choroidal

neovascularization? Graefes Arch Clin Exp Ophthalmol 2009; 247(2): 171–177.
9. Ambati J, Anand A, Fernandez S, et al. An animal model of age-related macular degeneration in senescent Ccl-2- or Ccr-2-deficient mice. Nat Med 2003; 9(11): 1390–1397.
10. Tsutsumi C, Sonoda KH, Egashira K, et al. The critical role of ocular-infiltrating macrophages in the development of choroidal neovascularization. J Leukoc Biol 2003; 74(1): 25–32.
11. Tuo J, Bojanowski CM, Zhou M, et al. Murine ccl2/cx3cr1 deficiency results in retinal lesions mimicking human

PART 5 · Uveitic Conditions not Caused by Active Infection

Chapter **31** Other Ocular Disorders and the Immune Response: Who Would Have Thought?

age-related macular degeneration. Invest Ophthalmol Vis Sci 2007; 48(8): 3827–3836.

12. Chan CC, Ross RJ, Shen D, et al. Ccl2/Cx3cr1-deficient mice: an animal model for age-related macular degeneration. Ophthalmic Res 2008; 40(3–4): 124–128.

13. Hollyfield JG, Bonilha VL, Rayborn ME, et al. Oxidative damage-induced inflammation initiates age-related macular degeneration. Nat Med 2008; 14(2): 194–198.

14. Penfold PL, Provis JM, Furby JH, et al. Autoantibodies to retinal astrocytes associated with age-related macular degeneration. Graefes Arch Clin Exp Ophthalmol 1990; 228(3): 270–274.

15. Patel N, Ohbayashi M, Nugent AK, et al. Circulating anti-retinal antibodies as immune markers in age-related macular degeneration. Immunology 2005; 115(3): 422–430.

16. Hageman GS, Anderson DH, Johnson LV, et al. A common haplotype in the complement regulatory gene factor H (HF1/CFH) predisposes individuals to age-related macular degeneration. Proc Natl Acad Sci U S A 2005; 102(20): 7227–7232.

17. Edwards AO, Ritter R 3rd, Abel KJ, et al. Complement factor H polymorphism and age-related macular degeneration. Science 2005; 308(5720): 421–424.

18. Haines JL, Hauser MA, Schmidt S, et al. Complement factor H variant increases the risk of age-related macular degeneration. Science 2005; 308(5720): 419–421.

19. Klein RJ, Zeiss C, Chew EY, et al. Complement factor H polymorphism in age-related macular degeneration. Science 2005; 308(5720): 385–389.

20. Johnson PT, Betts KE, Radeke MJ, et al. Individuals homozygous for the age-related macular degeneration risk-conferring variant of complement factor H have elevated levels of CRP in the choroid. Proc Natl Acad Sci U S A 2006; 103(46): 17456–17461.

21. Dewan A, Liu M, Hartman S, et al. HTRA1 promoter polymorphism in wet age-related macular degeneration. Science 2006; 314(5801): 989–992.

22. Yang Z, Camp NJ, Sun H, et al. A variant of the HTRA1 gene increases susceptibility to age-related macular degeneration. Science 2006; 314(5801): 992–993.

23. Yoshida T, DeWan A, Zhang H, et al. HTRA1 promoter polymorphism predisposes Japanese to age-related macular degeneration. Mol Vis 2007; 13: 545–548.

24. Launay S, Maubert E, Lebeurrier N, et al. HtrA1-dependent proteolysis of TGF-beta controls both neuronal maturation and developmental survival. Cell Death Differ 2008; 15(9): 1408–1416.

25. Wahl SM. Transforming growth factor-beta: innately bipolar. Curr Opin Immunol 2007; 19(1): 55–62.

26. Lehner T. Special regulatory T cell review: The resurgence of the concept of contrasuppression in immunoregulation. Immunology 2008; 123(1): 40–44.

27. Stein-Streilein J, Streilein JW. Anterior chamber associated immune deviation (ACAID): regulation, biological relevance, and implications for therapy. Int Rev Immunol 2002; 21(2–3): 123–152.

28. Austin BA, Liu B, Li Z, et al. Biologically Active Fibronectin Fragments Stimulate Release of MCP-1 and Catabolic Cytokines from Murine Retinal Pigment Epithelium. Invest Ophthalmol Vis Sci 2009.

29. Tuo J, Smith BC, Bojanowski CM, et al. The involvement of sequence variation and expression of CX3CR1 in the pathogenesis of age-related macular degeneration. FASEB J 2004; 18(11): 1297–1299.

30. Leveziel N, Souied EH, Richard F, et al. PLEKHA1-LOC387715-HTRA1 polymorphisms and exudative age-related macular degeneration in the French population. Mol Vis 2007; 13: 2153–2159.

31. Goverdhan SV, Ennis S, Hannan SR, et al. Interleukin-8 promoter polymorphism -251A/T is a risk factor for age-related macular degeneration. Br J Ophthalmol 2008; 92(4): 537–540.

32. Kanda A, et al. A variant of mitochondrial protein LOC387715/ARMS2, not HTRA1, is strongly associated with age-related macular degeneration. Proc Natl Acad Sci U S A 2007; 104(41): 16227–16232.

33. Conley YP, Jakobsdottir J, Mah T, et al. CFH, ELOVL4, PLEKHA1 and LOC387715 genes and susceptibility to age-related maculopathy: AREDS and CHS cohorts and meta-analyses. Hum Mol Genet 2006; 15(21): 3206–3218.

34. Yang Z, Stratton C, Francis PJ, et al. Toll-like receptor 3 and geographic atrophy in age-related macular degeneration. N Engl J Med 2008; 359(14): 1456–1463.

35. Cousins SW, Espinosa-Heidmann DG, Csaky KG. Monocyte activation in patients with age-related macular degeneration: a biomarker of risk for choroidal neovascularization? Arch Ophthalmol 2004; 122(7): 1013–1018.

36. Penfold PL, Madigan MC, Gillies MC, et al. Immunological and aetiological aspects of macular degeneration. Prog Retin Eye Res 2001; 20(3): 385–414.

37. Crabb JW, Miyagi M, Gu X, et al. Drusen proteome analysis: an approach to the etiology of age-related macular degeneration. Proc Natl Acad Sci U S A 2002; 99(23): 14682–14687.

38. Anderson DH, Mullins RF, Hageman GS, et al. A role for local inflammation in the formation of drusen in the aging eye. Am J Ophthalmol 2002; 134(3): 411–431.

39. Nussenblatt RB, Coleman H, Jirawuthiworavong G, et al. The treatment of multifocal choroiditis-associated choroidal neovascularization with sirolimus (rapamycin). Acta Ophthalmol Scand 2007; 85(2): 230–231.

40. Markomichelakis NN, Theodossiadis PG, Sfikakis PP. Regression of neovascular age-related macular degeneration following infliximab therapy. Am J Ophthalmol 2005; 139(3): 537–540.

41. Theodossiadis PG, Liarakos VS, Sfikakis PP, et al. Intravitreal Administration of the Anti-Tumor Necrosis Factor Agent Infliximab for Neovascular Age-related Macular Degeneration. Am J Ophthalmol 2009.

42. National Institute of Diabetes and Digestive and Kidney Diseases (NIDDK). N. New survey results show huge burden of diabetes. 2009 [cited January 26, 2009 February 22, 2009]; Available from: http://www.nih.gov/news/health/jan2009/niddk-26.htm.

43. Bottazzo GF, Mann JI, Thorogood M, et al. Autoimmunity in juvenile diabetics and their families. Br Med J 1978; 2(6131): 165–168.

44. Glastras SJ, Craig ME, Verge CF, et al. The role of autoimmunity at diagnosis of type 1 diabetes in the development of thyroid and celiac disease and microvascular complications. Diabetes Care 2005; 28(9): 2170–2175.

45. Nicoloff G, Angelova M, Nikolov A. Serum fibrillin-antifibrillin immune complexes among diabetic children. Vasc Pharmacol 2005; 43(3): 171–175.

46. Zykova SN, Svartberg J, Seljelid R, et al. Release of TNF-alpha from in vitro-stimulated monocytes is negatively associated with serum levels of apolipoprotein B in patients with type 2 diabetes. Scand J Immunol 2004; 60(5): 535–542.

47. Schroder S, Palinski W, Schmid-Schonbein GW. Activated monocytes and granulocytes, capillary nonperfusion, and neovascularization in diabetic retinopathy. Am J Pathol 1991; 139(1): 81–100.

48. Kim SY, Johnson MA, McLeod DS, et al. Neutrophils are associated with capillary closure in spontaneously diabetic monkey retinas. Diabetes 2005; 54(5): 1534–1542.

49. Miyamoto K, Khosrof S, Bursell SE, et al. Prevention of leukostasis and vascular leakage in streptozotocin-induced diabetic retinopathy via intercellular adhesion molecule-1 inhibition. Proc Natl Acad Sci U S A 1999; 96(19): 10836–10841.

50. Adamis AP, Berman AJ. Immunological mechanisms in the pathogenesis of diabetic retinopathy. Semin Immunopathol 2008; 30(2): 65–84.

51. Joussen AM, Poulaki V, Mitsiades N, et al. Suppression of Fas-FasL-induced endothelial cell apoptosis prevents diabetic blood-retinal barrier

breakdown in a model of streptozotocin-induced diabetes. FASEB J 2003; 17(1): 76–78.

52. Knol JA, van Kooij B, de Valk HW, et al. Rapid progression of diabetic retinopathy in eyes with posterior uveitis. Am J Ophthalmol 2006; 141(2): 409–412.

53. Kastelan S, Tomić M, Mrazovac V, et al. Does maternal immune system alternation during pregnancy influence the progression of retinopathy in diabetic women? Med Hypotheses 2008; 71(3): 464–465.

54. Mimura T, Funatsu H, Uchigata Y, et al. Glutamic acid decarboxylase autoantibody prevalence and association with HLA genotype in patients with younger-onset type 1 diabetes and proliferative diabetic retinopathy. Ophthalmology 2005; 112(11): 1904–1909.

55. Mimura T, Funatsu H, Uchigata Y, et al. Development and progression of diabetic retinopathy in patients with Type 1 diabetes who are positive for GAD autoantibody. Diabet Med 2004; 21(6): 559–562.

56. Buraczynska M, Baranowicz-Gaszczyk I, Tarach J, et al. Toll-like receptor 4 gene polymorphism and early onset of diabetic retinopathy in patients with type 2 diabetes. Hum Immunol 2009; 70(2): 121–124.

57. Adamiec-Mroczek J, Oficjalska-Mlynczak J. Assessment of selected adhesion molecule and proinflammatory cytokine levels in the vitreous body of patients with type 2 diabetes – role of the inflammatory-immune process in the pathogenesis of proliferative diabetic retinopathy. Graefes Arch Clin Exp Ophthalmol 2008; 246(12): 1665–1670.

58. Canataroglu H, Varinli I, Ozcan AA, et al. Interleukin (IL)-6, interleukin (IL)-8 levels and cellular composition of the vitreous humor in proliferative diabetic retinopathy, proliferative vitreoretinopathy, and traumatic proliferative vitreoretinopathy. Ocul Immunol Inflamm 2005; 13(5): 375–381.

59. Yuuki T, Kanda T, Kimura Y, et al. Inflammatory cytokines in vitreous fluid and serum of patients with diabetic vitreoretinopathy. J Diabetes Complications 2001; 15(5): 257–259.

60. Baudouin C, Fredj-Reygrobellet D, Brignole F, et al. MHC class II antigen expression by ocular cells in proliferative diabetic retinopathy. Fundam Clin Pharmacol 1993; 7(9): 523–530.

61. Kastelan S, Zjacic-Rotkvic V, Kastelan Z. Could diabetic retinopathy be an autoimmune disease? Med Hypotheses 2007; 68(5): 1016–1018.

62. Fleischman A, Shoelson SE, Bernier R, et al. Salsalate improves glycemia and inflammatory parameters in obese young adults. Diabetes Care 2008; 31(2): 289–294.

63. Koska J, Ortega E, Bunt JC, et al. The effect of salsalate on insulin action and glucose tolerance in obese non-diabetic patients: results of a randomised double-blind placebo-controlled study. Diabetologia 2009; 52(3): 385–393.

64. National Institute of Diabetes and Digestive and Kidney Diseases (NIDDK). N. Study tests anti-inflammatory drug for poorly controlled type 2 diabetes. 2009 [cited February 3, 2009 Available from: http://www.nih.gov/news/health/feb2009/niddk-03.htm.

65. Giannoukakis N, Rudert WA, Robbins PD, et al. Targeting autoimmune diabetes with gene therapy. Diabetes 1999; 48(11): 2107–2121.

66. Quigley HA, Broman AT. The number of people with glaucoma worldwide in 2010 and 2020. Br J Ophthalmol 2006; 90(3): 262–267.

67. Girkin CA. Primary open-angle glaucoma in African Americans. Int Ophthalmol Clin 2004; 44(2): 43–60.

68. Girkin CA, McGwin G Jr, McNeal SF, et al. Racial differences in the association between optic disc topography and early glaucoma. Invest Ophthalmol Vis Sci 2003; 44(8): 3382–3387.

69. Merritt JC. Glaucoma blindness in African Americans: have 55 years of therapies, technologies, and talent altered blindness rates? J Natl Med Assoc 1996; 88(12): 809–819.

70. Tielsch J, Katz J, Singh K, et al. A Population-based Evaluation of Glaucoma Screening: The Baltimore Eye Survey. American Journal of Epidemiology 1991; 134(10): 1102–1110.

71. Sommer A, Tielsch JM, Katz J, et al. Relationship between intraocular pressure and primary open angle glaucoma among white and black Americans. The Baltimore Eye Survey. Arch Ophthalmol 1991; 109(8): 1090–1095.

72. Wax MB, Barrett DA, Pestronk A. Increased incidence of paraproteinemia and autoantibodies in patients with normal-pressure glaucoma. Am J Ophthalmol 1994; 117(5): 561–568.

73. Grus F, Sun D. Immunological mechanisms in glaucoma. Semin Immunopathol 2008; 30(2): 121–126.

74. Grus FH, Joachim SC, Wuenschig D, et al. Autoimmunity and glaucoma. J Glaucoma 2008; 17(1): 79–84.

75. Fernandez-Shaw C, Marina A, Cazorla P, et al. Anti-brain spectrin immunoreactivity in Alzheimer's disease: degradation of spectrin in an animal model of cholinergic degeneration. J Neuroimmunol 1997; 77(1): 91–98.

76. Schwartz M, London A. Glaucoma as a neuropathy amenable to neuroprotection and immune manipulation. Prog Brain Res 2008; 173: 375–384.

77. Tezel G, Yang X, Cai J. Proteomic identification of oxidatively modified retinal proteins in a chronic pressure-induced rat model of glaucoma. Invest Ophthalmol Vis Sci 2005; 46(9): 3177–3187.

78. Schwartz M. Lessons for glaucoma from other neurodegenerative diseases: can one treatment suit them all? J Glaucoma 2005; 14(4): 321–323.

79. Bakalash S, Kessler A, Mizrahi T, et al. Antigenic specificity of immunoprotective therapeutic vaccination for glaucoma. Invest Ophthalmol Vis Sci 2003; 44(8): 3374–3381.

80. Fellman RL, Tezel G, Wax MB. Effects of methotrexate treatment on serum immunoreactivity of a patient with normal-pressure glaucoma. Am J Ophthalmol 1999; 127(6): 724–725.

81. Schori H, Kipnis J, Yoles E, et al. Vaccination for protection of retinal ganglion cells against death from glutamate cytotoxicity and ocular hypertension: implications for glaucoma. Proc Natl Acad Sci U S A 2001; 98(6): 3398–3403.

82. Bakalash S, Shlomo GB, Aloni E, et al. T-cell-based vaccination for morphological and functional neuroprotection in a rat model of chronically elevated intraocular pressure. J Mol Med 2005; 83(11): 904–916.

Index